Atlas of Psychiatry

Waguih William IsHak
Editor

Atlas of Psychiatry

Springer

Editor
Waguih William IsHak
Cedars-Sinai Health System
Department of Psychiatry and Behavioral Neurosciences
University of California Los Angeles
David Geffen School of Medicine
Los Angeles, CA, USA

ISBN 978-3-031-15400-3 ISBN 978-3-031-15401-0 (eBook)
https://doi.org/10.1007/978-3-031-15401-0

This Springer imprint is published by the registered company Springer Nature Switzerland AG
The registered company address is: Gewerbestrasse 11, 6330 Cham, Switzerland

To my love Asbasia (Hanan) Mikhail-IsHak, MD, FACEP, our sons William and Michael, our parents William Makram IsHak, MD, Nawara Yacoub Dawoud-IsHak, MD, Mrs. Aziza Mikhail and Mr. Aboelkhair Mikhail, and our siblings Rafik William IsHak, MD, FRCS, Albert Mikhail, MD, and Mrs. Lamia Maalouf, for their inspiration, encouragement, and love.

Foreword

The *Atlas of Psychiatry* is the first of its kind in psychiatry, currently the only discipline that does not have a comprehensive atlas for visual learning about the whole field. The Atlas has been developed for clinicians, trainees, and students who need a visual guide describing basic, clinical, and scholarly information. It is a large full-color hardback with extensive drawings and clinical images, printed on glossy paper and also available in various electronic formats. The audience is a wide-scope readership adopting a user-friendly method to familiarize with psychiatry and psychiatric disorders, in contrast to the traditional text-only-based volumes.

The *Atlas of Psychiatry* chapters have been written by world-class experts in the field, in addition to a number of chapters that Dr. IsHak has written with his team on a variety of topics. Each chapter includes figures, illustrations, and tables covering each psychiatric disorder, with images and tables potentially describing epidemiology, etiology, pathophysiology, phenomenology, and treatment. The psychiatric disorders are classified using the latest diagnostic classification systems, with images created or curated and described by authors in each scientific area and diagnosis. Experts in each aspect of psychiatry and psychiatric disorders have synchronized the text and imagery content with the mission of delivering a clear and lucid explanation of each topic. The *Atlas of Psychiatry* is an innovative and important contribution to the field.

Maurizio Fava, MD
Harvard Medical School, Psychiatrist-In-Chief, Department of Psychiatry Director, Division of Clinical Research, Mass General Research Institute; Executive Director, Clinical Trials Network & Institute Associate Dean for Clinical & Translational Research, Slater Family Professor of Psychiatry, Boston, MA, USA

Preface

The *Atlas of Psychiatry* is a visual guide intended for a diverse readership looking for a visual method to learn cutting-edge, and scholarly information about psychiatry and psychiatric disorders. The goal is to inform the reader by describing basic science and theory, as well as clinical and therapeutic information using imagery and text to show and tell about the field.

We hope that the Atlas will be useful for physicians of all specialties especially internal medicine, primary care, family medicine, psychiatry, and neurology, health care professionals especially nurses, nurse practitioners, physician assistants, and medical assistants, mental health care professionals especially psychologists, social workers, psychotherapists, substance use counselors, and spiritual counselors, trainees especially medical students, residents, fellows, and graduate students, researchers, as well as hospital, clinic, and treatment programs staff especially leaders, middle management, and program personnel.

Chapters 1–11 cover the landmark theories and concepts, key contributors, illustrations, must-see images, and detailed tables to describe the aspects of topic in each chapter. Chapters 12–24 describe the psychiatric disorders including epidemiology, etiology, pathophysiology, phenomenology, and treatment, using illustrations, must-see images, and detailed tables as well. Chapter 25 ends the book with a futuristic collection of directions where the field could be following in the next decade.

This Atlas was only made possible because of so many supportive and nurturing individuals for whom this editor is eternally grateful. I truly hope that the *Atlas of Psychiatry* will be a helpful and useful contribution.

Los Angeles, CA — Waguih William IsHak

Acknowledgments

I am deeply grateful for supportive and nurturing figures throughout my career, and it gives utmost pleasure to acknowledge them in the *Atlas of Psychiatry*. I begin with William Makram IsHak, MD (may he rest in peace) who instilled psychological mindedness and reading the master pieces in psychological sciences, then Cairo University amazing Professors Yehia El Rakhaway, Emad Hamdy Ghoz, Tarek S. Gawad, Abdelhamid Hashem, Samir Aboelmagd, Nahed Khairy, Zeinab Nasser, Zakaria Halim, Salwa Erfan, and Soad Moussa, followed by the Milieu Therapy psychiatry masters: Professors Refaat Mahfouz, Ahmed Abdallah, Yehia Jaffer, and Hassib El-Defrawi, to NYU's incredible Professors Robert Delgado, Brian Ladds, Zebulon Taintor, Eric Peselow, Adam Wolkin, Leonard Adler, Martin Kahn, Richard Hanson, Kim Hopper, David Nardacci, Martin Geller, Asher Aladjem, Samuel Slipp, Richard Oberfield, Howard Silbert, Henry Weinstein, Howard Welsh, Murray Alpert, George Nicklin, Bertina Baer, and Bruce Rubenstein.

I am very thankful for the phenomenal care of Samy Rizk, MD, and Mrs. Mary-Terez Rizk, the life-changing fortunes by Norman Sussman, MD, and Nancy Hanna, MD as well as the priceless mentorship of Professors Carol Bernstein, Manuel Trujillo, Virginia Sadock, and Benjamin Sadock. I continue to cherish the invaluable advice and career opportunities from Professor Shlomo Melmed Cedars-Sinai's Dean of the Medical Faculty, Peter Panzarino, MD, Thomas Trott, MD, PhD, Saul Brown, MD, PhD, and Mark Rappaport, MD, and continue to value the precious guidance from Professors Lloyd Sederer, Sherwyn Woods, Laura Roberts, Robert Cohen, Robert Pechnick, Daniel Berman, Russell Poland, Fawzy I. Fawzy, Thomas Strouse, George Awad, Edward Feldman, Rebecca Hedrick, and especially Bruce Gewertz, MD —Cedars-Sinai's Surgeon-in-Chief, as well as Professor and STAR*D PI A. John Rush, Nobel Laureate Louis Ignarro, and Harvard Mass General's Psychiatrist-in-Chief Maurizio Fava, for having the most profound impact on my career involvements. I remain appreciative of Itai Danovitch, MD unwavering and genuine support of all my professional endeavors at Cedars-Sinai.

I was inspired and given growth opportunities and learned a great deal from leaders, teachers, colleagues, collaborators, and dear friends over the years, who appear on page xi and xii of The Textbook of Clinical Sexual Medicine. I gratefully acknowledge my debt to them, as they have contributed in a fundamental way (albeit indirectly) to the creation of the *Atlas of Psychiatry*.

I also would like to especially thank Nadina Persaud, Lee Klein, and Melanie Zerah the staff at Springer for their outstanding professional work and patience throughout the duration of this project.

This book is dedicated to the medical students, residents, and faculty at Cairo University School of Medicine, Dar El-Mokattum Milieu Therapy Hospital, New York University School of Medicine (NYU), Cedars-Sinai Medical Center, and the David Geffen School of Medicine at the University of California at Los Angeles (UCLA).

Waguih William IsHak

Contents

Contributors

Scott T. Aaronson, MD Sheppard Pratt Health System, Baltimore, MD, USA

Rasha Abdelsalam, MD Department of Psychiatry and Behavioral Neurosciences, Cedars-Sinai Medical Center, Los Angeles, CA, USA

Leslie Aguilar-Hernandez, BA Department of Psychiatry and Behavioral Neurosciences, Cedars-Sinai Medical Center, Los Angeles, CA, USA

Samoon Ahmad, MD Department of Psychiatry, NYU Grossman School of Medicine, New York, NY, USA

Luma Bashmi, MA Department of Health Psychology, School of Medicine, Royal College of Surgeons in Ireland-Bahrain, Busaiteen, Kingdom of Bahrain

Neeltje M. Batelaan, MD, PhD Department of Psychiatry, Amsterdam UMC, Vrije Universiteit Amsterdam, Amsterdam Public Health, Amsterdam, Netherlands

Dinesh Bhugra, CBE, PhD, MPhil, MSc, MA Institute of Psychiatry, Psychology & Neuroscience, King's College London, London, UK

Philippe-Edouard Boursiquot, MD Department of Psychiatry and Behavioural Neurosciences, McMaster University, Dundas, ON, Canada

Adam Brenner, MD Department of Psychiatry, The University of Texas Southwestern Medical Center, Dallas, TX, USA

Alaina V. Burns, MD, MPH Department of Psychiatry and Biobehavioral Sciences, Adult Division, UCLA-Semel Institute for Neuroscience and Human Behavior, Los Angeles, CA, USA

Shane S. Bush, PhD, ABPP Long Island Neuropsychology, PC, Lake Ronkonkoma, NY, USA

Francesca Casoni, MD, PhD Department of Clinical Neurosciences, Neurology, Sleep Disorders Center, IRCCS San Raffaele Scientific Institute, Milan, Italy

Shawna T. Chan, MD Department of Psychiatry and Biobehavioral Sciences, David Geffen School of Medicine at UCLA, Los Angeles, CA, USA

Taolin Chen, PhD Huaxi MR Research Center (HMRRC), Department of Radiology, West China Hospital of Sichuan University, Chengdu, China

Functional and Molecular Imaging Key Laboratory of Sichuan Province, West China Hospital of Sichuan University, Chengdu, China

Ying Chen, PhD Huaxi MR Research Center (HMRRC), Department of Radiology, West China Hospital of Sichuan University, Chengdu, China

Research Unit of Psychoradiology, Chinese Academy of Medical Sciences, Chengdu, China

Samantha Cohen, MA Department of Psychiatry and Behavioral Neurosciences, Cedars-Sinai Medical Center, Los Angeles, CA, USA

Alexander Cohn, MD Department of Psychiatry and Biobehavioral Sciences, David Geffen School of Medicine at UCLA, Los Angeles, CA, USA

Itai Danovitch, MD, MBA Department of Psychiatry and Behavioral Neurosciences, Cedars-Sinai Medical Center, Los Angeles, CA, USA

Katrina DeBonis, MD Department of Psychiatry and Biobehavioral Sciences, David Geffen School of Medicine at UCLA, Los Angeles, CA, USA

Elizabeth Dohrmann, MD Los Angeles County Department of Mental Health, Los Angeles, CA, USA

William W. Eaton, PhD Department of Mental Health, Johns Hopkins Bloomberg School of Public Health, Baltimore, MD, USA

Lidia Younan, MD Cedars-Sinai Medical Center, Los Angeles, CA, USA

Maurizio Fava, MD Harvard Medical School, Boston, MA, USA

Luigi Ferini-Strambi, MD Università Vita-Salute San Raffaele, Milan, Italy

Department of Clinical Neurosciences, Neurology, Sleep Disorders Center, IRCCS San Raffaele Scientific Institute, Vita-Salute San Raffaele University, Milan, Italy

Sophie M. D. D. Fitzsimmons, MBBCh, MSc Department of Psychiatry and Department of Anatomy and Neurosciences, Amsterdam UMC, Vrije Universiteit Amsterdam, Amsterdam Neuroscience, Amsterdam, Netherlands

Andrea Galbiati, PhD Università Vita-Salute San Raffaele, Milan, Italy

Department of Clinical Neurosciences, Neurology, Sleep Disorders Center, IRCCS San Raffaele Scientific Institute, Vita-Salute San Raffaele University, Milan, Italy

Paloma Garcia, BA Brown University, Providence, RI, USA

Lucas E. Gelfond, BA Brown University, Providence, RI, USA

Sam Nishanth Gnanapragasam, BSc, MBBS, MRCPsych South London and Maudsley NHS Foundation Trust, London, UK

Yasmine Gohar, MA, PhD, AMFT, APCC Psychiatry Department, The Behman Hospital, Cairo, Egypt

Eric L. Goldwaser, DO, PhD Department of Psychiatry, Weill Cornell Medicine, New York, NY, USA

Qiyong Gong, MD, PhD Huaxi MR Research Center (HMRRC), Department of Radiology, West China Hospital of Sichuan University, Chengdu, China

Department of Radiology, West China Xiamen Hospital of Sichuan University, Xiamen, China

Nathalie Herrera, MD Cedars-Sinai Medical Center, Los Angeles, CA, USA

Odile A. van den Heuvel, MD, PhD Department of Psychiatry and Department of Anatomy and Neurosciences, Amsterdam UMC, Vrije Universiteit Amsterdam, Amsterdam Neuroscience, Amsterdam, Netherlands

Robert Higgo, MB ChB, MSc, FRCPsych Centre for Mental Health and Society, Prifysgol Bangor University,, Wrexham, Wales, UK

Michael W. Ishak, BA Candidate Princeton University, Princeton, NJ, USA

Waguih William IsHak, MD, FAPA Cedars-Sinai Health System, Department of Psychiatry and Behavioral Neurosciences, University of California Los Angeles, David Geffen School of Medicine, Los Angeles, CA, USA

William W. Ishak, BA Brown University, Providence, RI, USA

Zhiyun Jia, PhD Department of Nuclear Medicine, West China Hospital of Sichuan University, Chengdu, China

Noah K. Kaufman, PhD, ABN, ABPdN, ABPP Center for Neuropsychological Studies, Las Cruces, NM, USA

Darlene Rae King, MD Department of Psychiatry, The University of Texas Southwestern Medical Center, Dallas, TX, USA

Maria Kleinstäuber, PhD Department of Psychology, Utah State University, Logan, UT, USA

Fei Li, PhD Huaxi MR Research Center (HMRRC), Department of Radiology, West China Hospital of Sichuan University, Chengdu, China

Functional and Molecular Imaging Key Laboratory of Sichuan Province, West China Hospital of Sichuan University, Chengdu, China

Russell Lim, MD Department of Psychiatry, University of California, Davis, Davis, CA, USA

Paul S. Links, MD, FRCPC Department of Psychiatry and Behavioural Neurosciences, McMaster University, Dundas, ON, Canada

Nian Liu, PhD Huaxi MR Research Center (HMRRC), Department of Radiology, West China Hospital of Sichuan University, Chengdu, China

Department of Radiology, Affiliated Hospital of North Sichuan Medical College, Nanchong, China

Tom Lorenz, MB, ChB, BSc, MRCPsych Department of Child and Adolescent Psychiatry, Betsi Cadwaladr University Health Board, Flintshire, Wales, UK

Su Lui, PhD Huaxi MR Research Center (HMRRC), Department of Radiology, West China Hospital of Sichuan University, Chengdu, China

Department of Radiology, West China Xiamen Hospital of Sichuan University, Xiamen, China

Matthew Macaluso, DO Department of Psychiatry and Behavioral Neurobiology, UAB Depression and Suicide Center, Heersink School of Medicine, The University of Alabama at Birmingham, Birmingham, AL, USA

Naira Magakian, MD Cedars-Sinai Medical Center, Los Angeles, CA, USA

Stephen Marder, MD Semel Institute for Neuroscience at UCLA, VA Desert Pacific Mental Illness Research, Education, and Clinical Center (VISN 22 MIRECC), Los Angeles, CA, USA

Christopher Martin, MD David Geffen School of Medicine at UCLA, Charles R. Drew University of Medicine and Science, Los Angeles, CA, USA

Krista Q. Mercado, BS Department of Ecology and Evolutionary Biology, University of California, Los Angeles, Los Angeles, CA, USA

Asbasia A. Mikhail, MD, FACEP Department of Emergency Medicine, Huntington Hospital, Pasadena, CA, USA

Adith Mohan, MRCPsych Department of Psychiatry, Northern Beaches Hospital, Frenchs Forest, NSW, Australia

Ashley Ngor University of California, Los Angeles, Los Angeles, CA, USA

David Okikawa, MD David Geffen School of Medicine, University of California, Los Angeles, Los Angeles, CA, USA

Sarin Pakhdikian, DO Kirk Kerkorian School of Medicine, University of Nevada, Las Vegas, Las Vegas, NV, USA

Demetria Pizano, MA University of Alabama at Birmingham, Birmingham, AL, USA

Netasha Pizano, MA University of California, Santa Barbara, Santa Barbara, CA, USA

Rob Poole, MBBS, FRCPsych Centre for Mental Health and Society, Prifysgol Bangor University, Wrexham, Wales, UK

Basant K. Puri, PhD, MB, MSc, FRMS, FRSB University of Winchester, Winchester, UK

Jothi Ramalingam, MBBS Department of Psychiatry, Northern Beaches Hospital, Frenchs Forest, NSW, Australia

James Ross, MD, MHPE, FRCPC Department of Psychiatry, Schulich School of Medicine and Dentistry, University of Western Ontario, Parkwood Mental Health Institute, London, ON, Canada

Perminder S. Sachdev, MD, PhD Department of Psychiatry, Northern Beaches Hospital, Frenchs Forest, NSW, Australia

Maria Salsone, MD, PhD Department of Clinical Neurosciences, Neurology, Institute of Molecular Bioimaging and Physiology, National Research Council, Sleep Disorders Center, IRCCS San Raffaele Scientific Institute, Milan, Italy

Benjamin Schneider, MD David Geffen School of Medicine, University of California at Los Angeles, Los Angeles, CA, USA

Tiffany E. Schwasinger-Schmidt, MD, PhD Department of Internal Medicine, University of Kansas School of Medicine-Wichita, Wichita, KS, USA

Fraser Scott, BA, BMBCh, MRCPsych South London and Maudsley NHS Foundation Trust, London, UK

Marco Sforza, MSc Università Vita-Salute San Raffaele, Milan, Italy

Department of Clinical Neurosciences, Neurology, Sleep Disorders Center, IRCCS San Raffaele Scientific Institute, Vita-Salute San Raffaele University, Milan, Italy

Alexander J. Steiner, PsyD Executive Mental Health, Inc., Los Angeles, CA, USA

Alexandra M. Taran, BS Department of Integrative Biology, Oregon State University, Corvallis, OR, USA

Gabriel Tobia, MD Department of Psychiatry, Brigham and Women's Faulkner Hospital, Boston, MA, USA

Manuel Trujillo, MD Department of Psychiatry, New York University School of Medicine, New York, NY, USA

Raymond Y. Wen, BS, PharmD-c San Diego Health, Skaggs School of Pharmacy and Pharmaceutical Sciences, University of California, San Diego, CA, USA

Haoyang Xing, PhD Huaxi MR Research Center (HMRRC), Department of Radiology, West China Hospital of Sichuan University, Chengdu, China

Research Unit of Psychoradiology, Chinese Academy of Medical Sciences, Chengdu, China

Mira Zein, MD, MPH Department of Psychiatry and Behavioral Sciences, Department of Primary Care and Population Health, Stanford University School of Medicine, Stanford, CA, USA

About the Editor

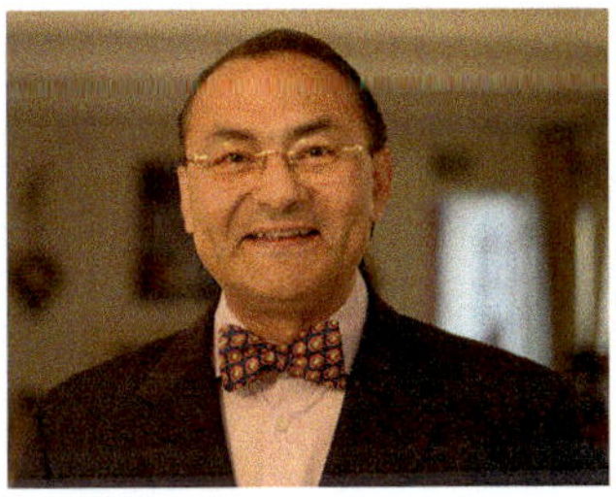

Waguih William IsHak, MD, FAPA is Professor and Clinical Chief of Psychiatry at Cedars-Sinai and Clinical Professor of Psychiatry at the David Geffen School of Medicine at the University of California Los Angeles (UCLA). Dr. IsHak has nearly 35 years of experience in psychiatry, psychotherapy, and psychopharmacology, with specific training and expertise in sexual medicine and outcome measurement in psychiatric disorders particularly depressive symptom severity, functioning, and quality of life. He is researching innovative ways to measure and improve the detection and treatment of depression in people seeking medical care, in order to remove behavioral barriers to wellness. Dr. IsHak has lectured and published on quality of life as a critical outcome measure of healthcare interventions, mood disorders especially depression, sexual medicine, and outcome measurement in psychiatry as well as computer applications in psychiatry. He was also the author and designer of Health Education Programs for the Public, including the Online Depression Screening Test (ODST), Online Screening for Anxiety (OSA), and Online Screening Tests for Sexual Disorders. He has edited and authored six books: this volume, *The Handbook of Wellness Medicine* (Cambridge University Press, 2020), the *Textbook of Clinical Sexual Medicine* (Springer Nature, 2017), *Guidebook of Sexual Medicine* (A&W Publishing, 2008), *Outcome Measurement in Psychiatry: A Critical Review* (APPI, 2002), and *On Call Psychiatry* (WB Saunders, 2001). Dr. IsHak's research has been funded by NARSAD, National Institute of Health, and the Patient Centered Outcomes Research Institute (PCORI) especially on depression in heart disease. The Personalized Wellness Program is the latest program aiming at enhancing patient-centered care to promote health and wellness. His articles have appeared in many prestigious journals, such as *JAMA Psychiatry, Journal of Clinical Psychiatry, Harvard Review of Psychiatry, Journal of Affective Disorders, Journal of Sexual Medicine, Journal of Graduate Medical Education, and Quality of Life Research.* He is a member of several professional societies, including the American Psychiatric Association, the American Association of Directors of Psychiatry Residency Training, and the International Society of Sexual Medicine. Dr. IsHak was awarded the 2002 and 2010 *Golden Apple Teaching Award*, Department of Psychiatry, Cedars-Sinai Medical Center; 2007 *Outstanding Medical Student Teaching Award*,

Department of Psychiatry and Biobehavioral Science at UCLA; 2011 *Excellence in Education Award*, David Geffen School of Medicine at UCLA; 2012 *Parker J. Palmer Courage to Teach Award*, Accreditation Council for Graduate Medical Education; and 2012 *Nancy Roeske Award for Excellence in Medical Student Education*, American Psychiatric Association, was elected to the *Gold Humanism Honor Society* in 2012, and has been on Super Doctors list from 2012 to 2023. Dr. IsHak served as a Chief proctor and examiner for the American Board of Psychiatry and Distinguished fellow of the American Psychiatric Association.

1 Introduction to Psychiatry

Darlene Rae King and Adam Brenner

What's going through your mind? How do billions of cells orchestrate life, generate the experience of the soul, and create who we are as a person? What then are mental disorders, and how do we treat them? These are questions psychiatrists ponder. Modern science has led to marvelous breakthroughs in medicine for diseases that can be physically described and modeled, but diseases of the mind remain perplexing. The mind is the final frontier, and much remains to be understood and discovered. For those that are afflicted by mental illness, discoveries cannot come fast enough, and as psychiatrists, it is our privilege to work at the intersection of medicine, neuroscience, culture, and technology to help alleviate patient suffering and incorporate new knowledge as it becomes available. We set out to treat mental illness and understand the inner workings of the mind: things that are in some ways still mysterious but are clearly highly complex. Those who enter psychiatry understand the lifelong learning involved and feel comfortable operating within a gray space. Patients must be considered from multiple viewpoints to construct an accurate formulation and help treat their mental illness. If the state of the specialty is still appealing after hearing all the above, then know that Psychiatry is one of the up-and-coming fields of medicine (Fig. 1.1).

D. R. King (✉) · A. Brenner
Department of Psychiatry, The University of Texas Southwestern Medical Center, Dallas, TX, USA
e-mail: darlene.king@utsouthwestern.edu; adam.brenner@UTSouthwestern.edu

W. W. IsHak (ed.), *Atlas of Psychiatry*, https://doi.org/10.1007/978-3-031-15401-0_1

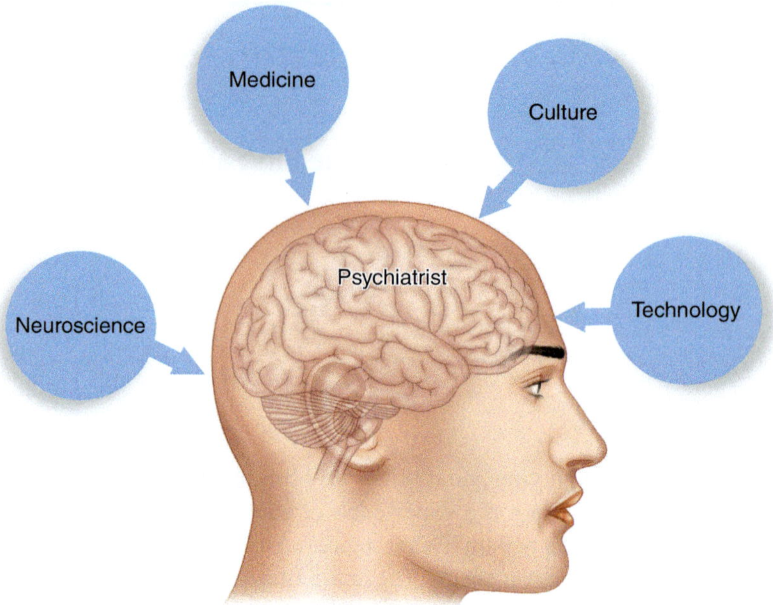

Fig. 1.1 Aspects of psychiatry

Brief History

The history of psychiatry is filled with fascinating narratives, breakthroughs, and cautionary tales. It is easy to look upon earlier attempts to ease psychological suffering and see them as outlandish or even horrifying. But, as you look through the following timeline, consider that we are still operating with very little understanding of how the mind works and that even today, it is possible we are making our own mistakes. If history has anything to offer up, it is that the pathophysiology of psychosis, depression, or other mental pathologies are extraordinarily complex, and as we work to uncover their mysteries, we must remain humble and thoroughly consider hypotheses and their evidence to prevent harming future patients (Fig. 1.2) [1].

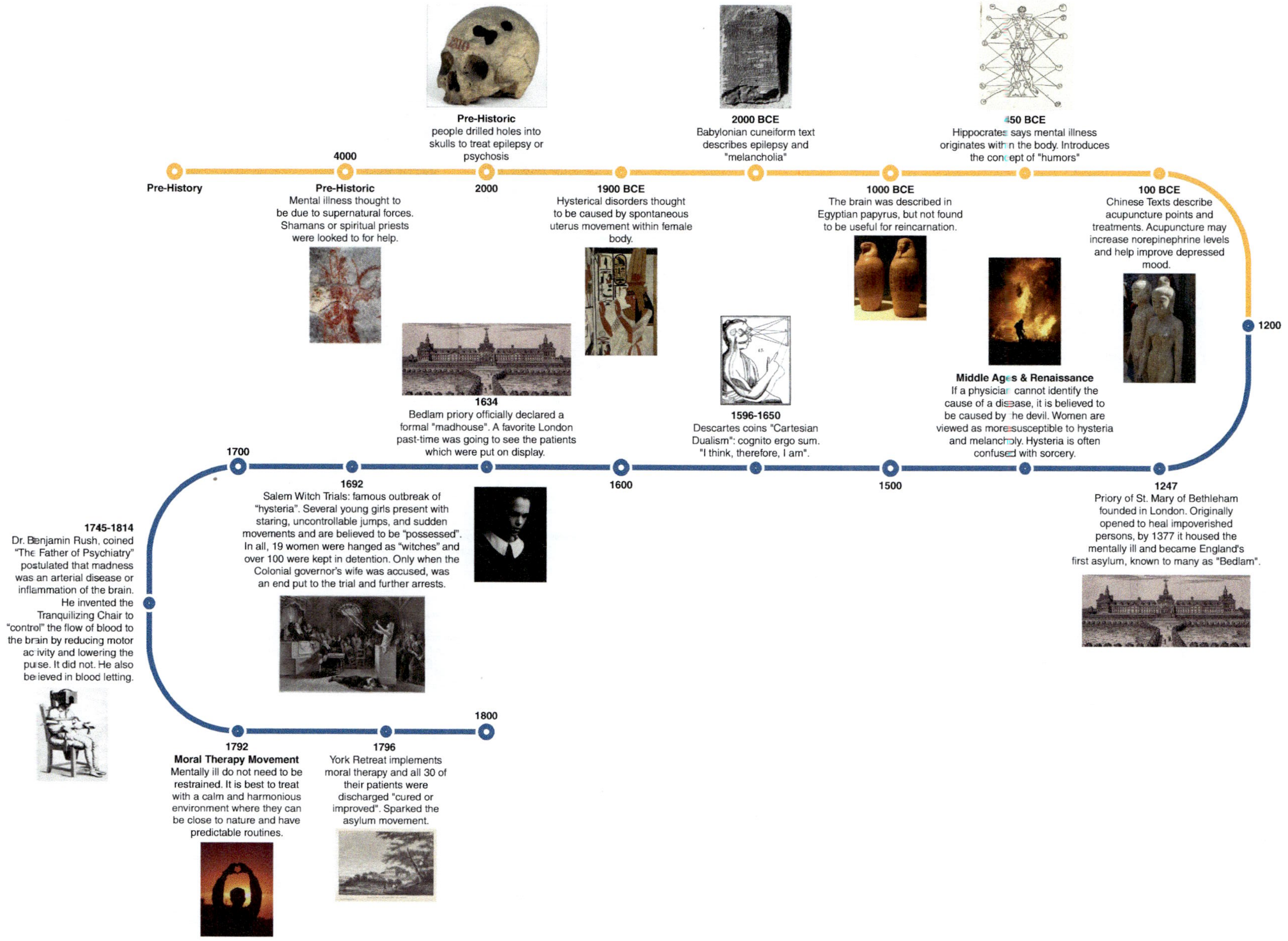

Fig. 1.2 History of psychiatry timeline. *Top Images from left to right*: Trepanned cranium; Cuneiform text; Humors; Bedlam; Moral Therapy; York Retreat; Alzheimer Neurons; Freud Sofa; Kraepelin; Camphor Seizure; ECT Machine; Thorazine; Lithium; Deinstitutionalization. *Bottom Images from left to right*: Shaman; Egyptian; Canopic jars; Acupuncture; middle ages fire; Descartes; Salem witch trials; Tranquility Chair; Thirteen Founders; Bleuler; Brain atrophy; Tooth; AA recovery symbol; Lobotomy MRI; Community; Anti-Psychiatrists; DSM; fMRI [2–9]

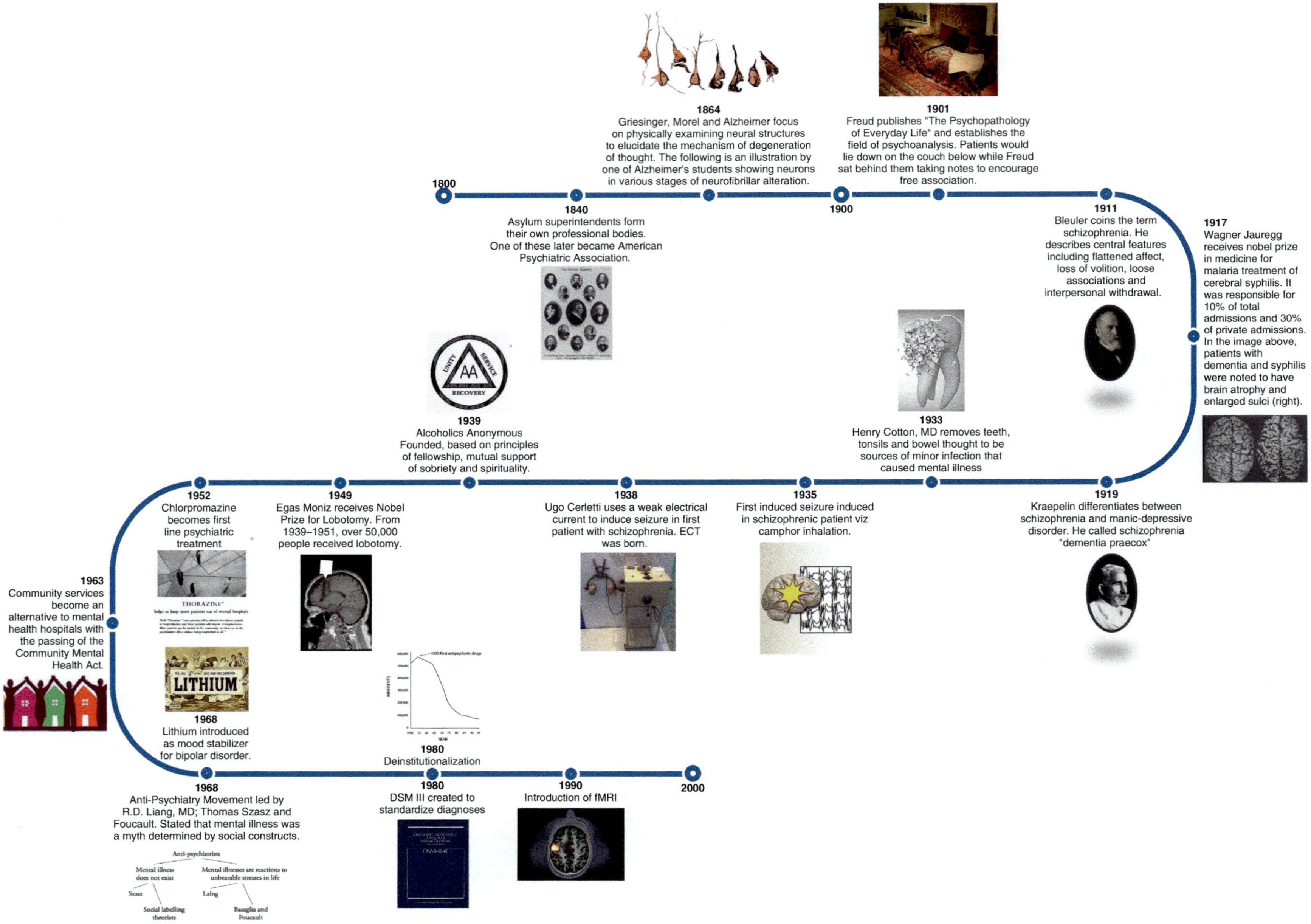

Fig 1.2 (continued)

Medicine

What is the difference between a psychologist, psychiatrist, and neurologist (Fig. 1.3)?

A psychologist is someone with an academic degree, usually a masters or PhD, who specializes in the study of thought and behavior. They conduct experiments to test theories of human behavior. The graduate degree can be more research-focused (PhD) or clinically focused (PsyD). Clinical psychologists can do additional training in a clinical setting to provide talk therapy to patients, such as cognitive behavioral therapy, or perform neuropsychological assessments better to describe a person's deficits or personality pathology. Clinical psychologists do at least 1 year of clinical training as an intern prior to graduation [10].

Psychiatry is a branch of medicine. It is not based on theory but on practice. When someone has symptoms of mental illness, treatments that have been shown to decrease those symptoms are used, even if the mechanism behind that treatment is not fully known. Mental health and the treatments for mental illness determine the scope of psychiatry. Psychiatrists are medical doctors and as such have experience in prescribing medication. Psychiatrists are also educated in and perform a variety of psychotherapy modalities.

Neurology is another branch of medicine. Neurologists focus on treating illnesses that originate from lesions in the brain or nervous system. While there is a lot of overlap between neurology and psychiatry in that many neurological illnesses are complicated by abnormalities in cognition or behavior, psychiatry remains the field of medicine that focuses on illnesses that affect the mind. It is crucial to have a specialty that is an expert in illnesses whose manifestation is in subjective experience and changes in behavior. An often-used analogy is that the brain is the hardware, and the mind is the software. The difference between neurology and psychiatry falls along these lines.

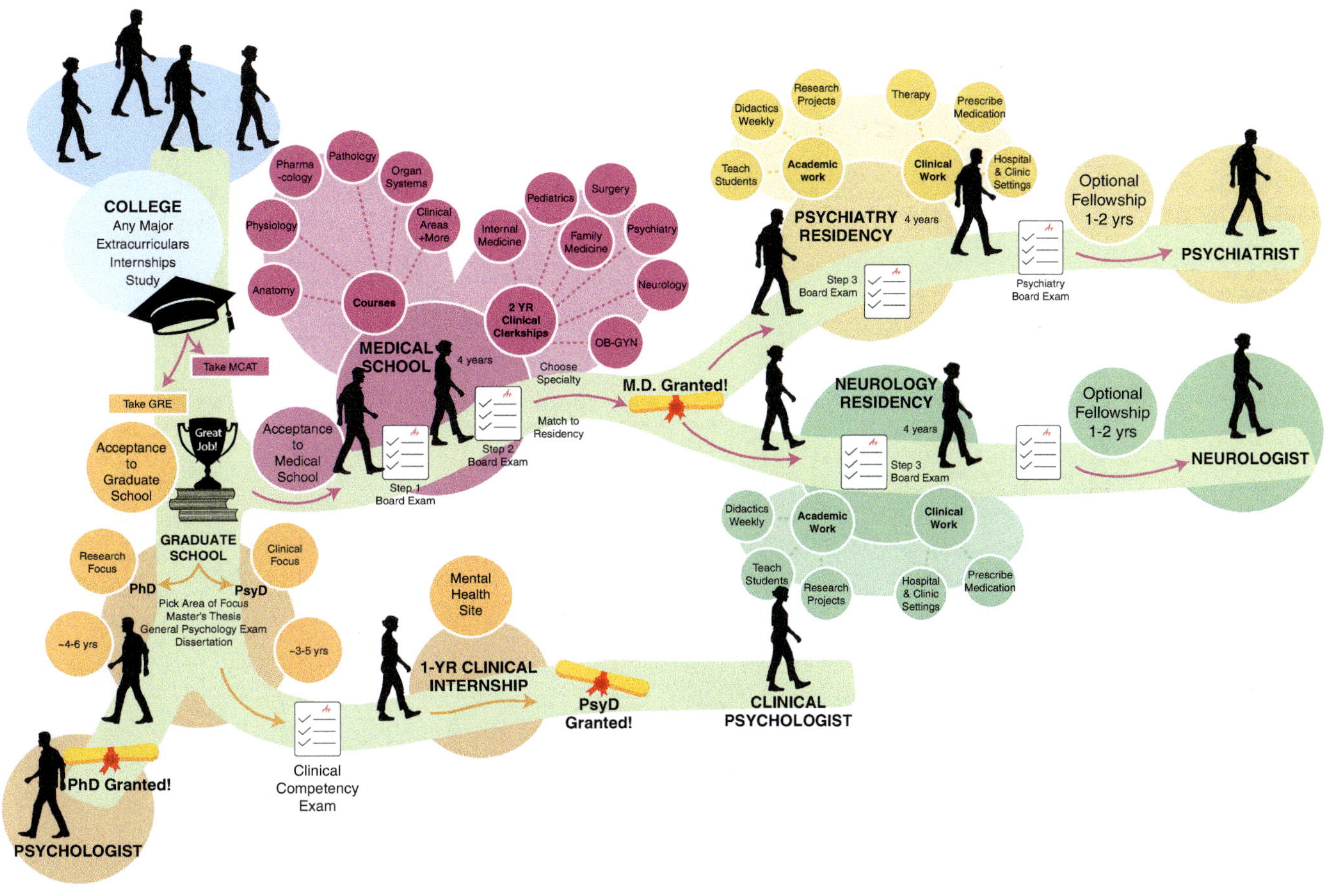

Fig. 1.3 Career paths for psychiatry, psychology, and neurology

Psychopharmacology

Psychopharmacology is a valuable part of psychiatry. For patients suffering from mental illness, medications can make all the difference. Psychiatry relies most heavily on three major classes of medications: antidepressants, antipsychotics, and mood stabilizers. It is important to understand the mechanism of action of these drugs, what they are useful in treating and how to manage their side effects. It is so rewarding to see a patient who is afflicted by symptoms take medication, experience relief, and return to baseline functioning.

The administration of psychiatric medications has challenges though. While prejudice against mental illness has been declining, stigma remains a major barrier for patients and is most obvious during discussions about medication. Unlike drugs for diabetes or bacterial infection, patients are much more hesitant to start an antidepressant or mood stabilizer. It is important to explore all the concerns a patient has and continue the discussion over time. It is vital to teach patients about the indication for medication, why it will be helpful to them, and common side effects [11].

In addition to overcoming stigma, another challenge faced in the realm of psychopharmacology is that patients may lack insight into their mental illness. In these cases, adherence is a major problem that, if not addressed, results in a repetitive cycle of hospitalization improvement on medication discharge nonadherence to medication decline in readmission. Fortunately, effective interventions are possible to break this cycle, such as access to regular community care, working closely with family, and/or recommending a long-acting injectable. Lastly, it is also important to be aware of the cost of medications because the best medication is one that a patient can and will take. If a medication is too expensive, the added financial stress or the inability to access the medication will negate its clinical benefit. Overall, psychopharmacology is a crucial piece of psychiatry requiring medical knowledge of the medications and when to use them, but also how to overcome challenges such as stigma, nonadherence, and cost to deliver the best care to the patient (Figs. 1.4 and 1.5) [11].

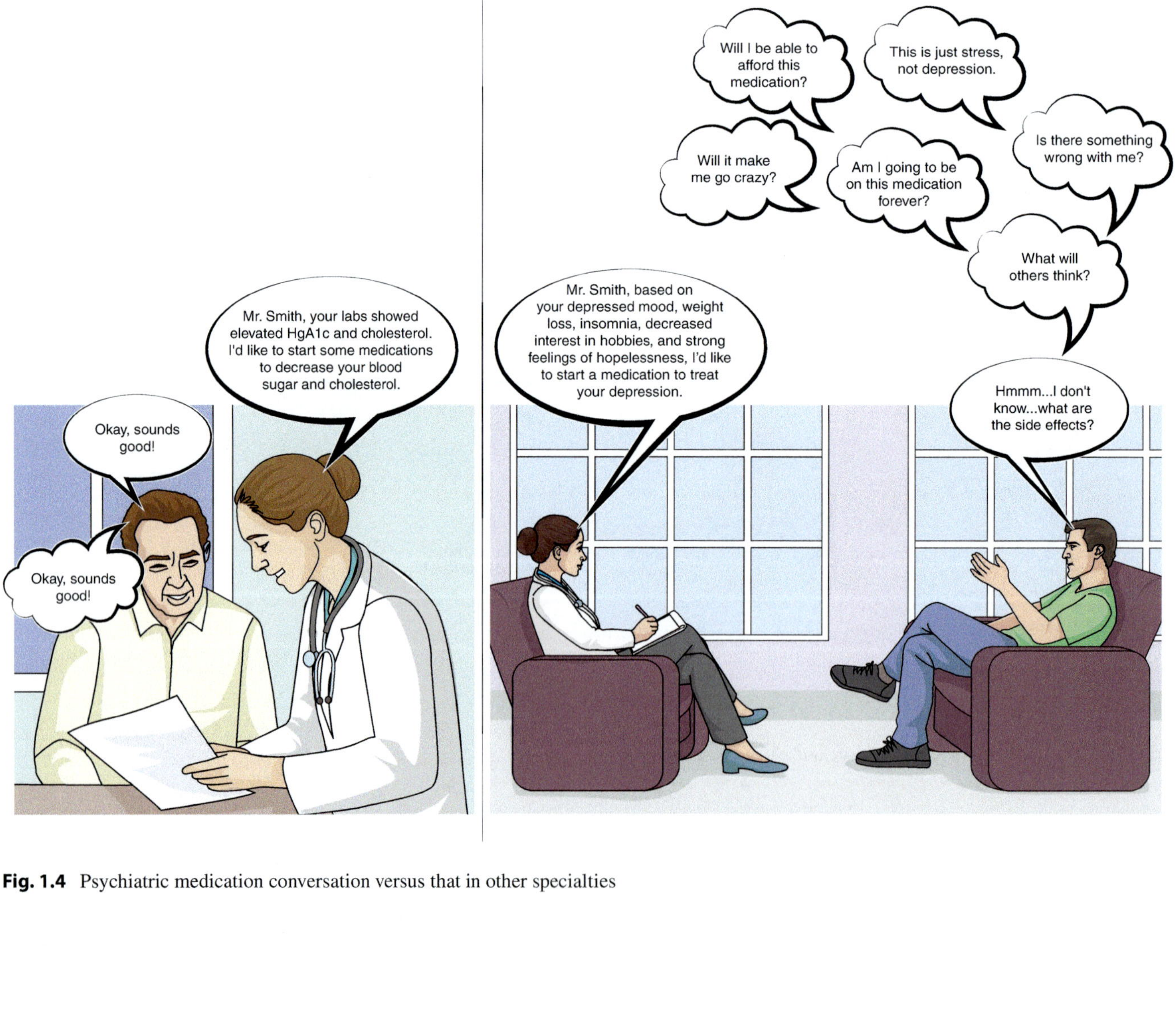

Fig. 1.4 Psychiatric medication conversation versus that in other specialties

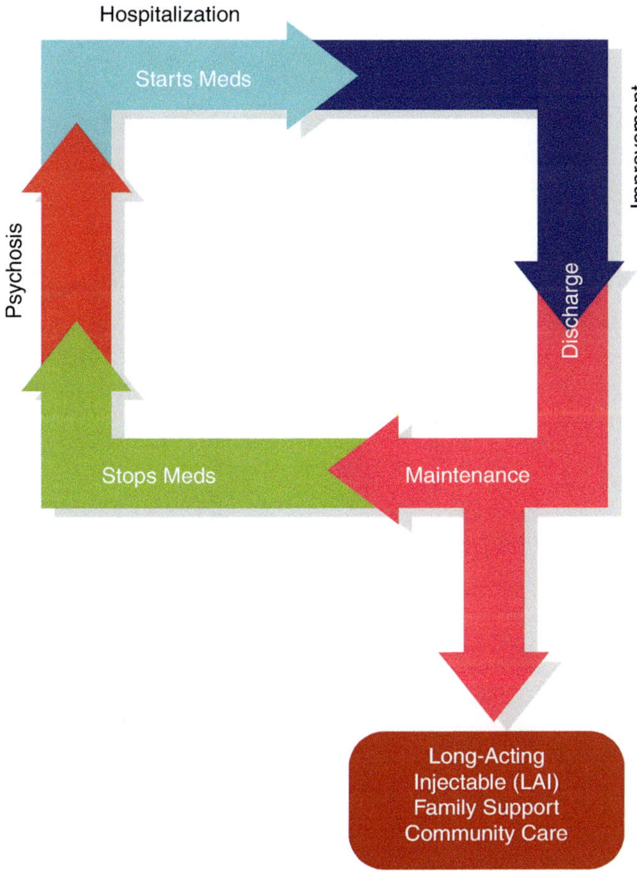

Fig. 1.5 Pharmacology and psychosis cycle

Interventional Psychiatry

Interventional psychiatry utilizes modalities such as electroconvulsive therapy, magnetic seizure therapy, transcranial magnetic stimulation, or ketamine/esketamine to treat psychiatric conditions, especially treatment resistant-depression. Some interventions are aimed at the induction of seizures, while others intervene through more focused stimulation of areas of the brain. Growing an understanding of circuit dysfunction (how different focal areas of the brain interact) is central to the development work in neurostimulation. This is an exciting area of psychiatric practice, offering novel ways to ameliorate and treat psychiatric illness.

We are still in the early days of interventional psychiatry, with new modalities continuing to appear and optimal use of older modalities still being defined. It has long been appreciated that ECT is one of the most effective treatments for depression, but it is not risk-free. Some patients have significant cognitive side effects. However, MST has been shown to be just as effective as ECT, with fewer memory effects [12]. There is still much work to be done in studying the frequency of treatments and the intensity of treatments for optimum recovery in the areas of interventional psychiatry (Fig. 1.6).

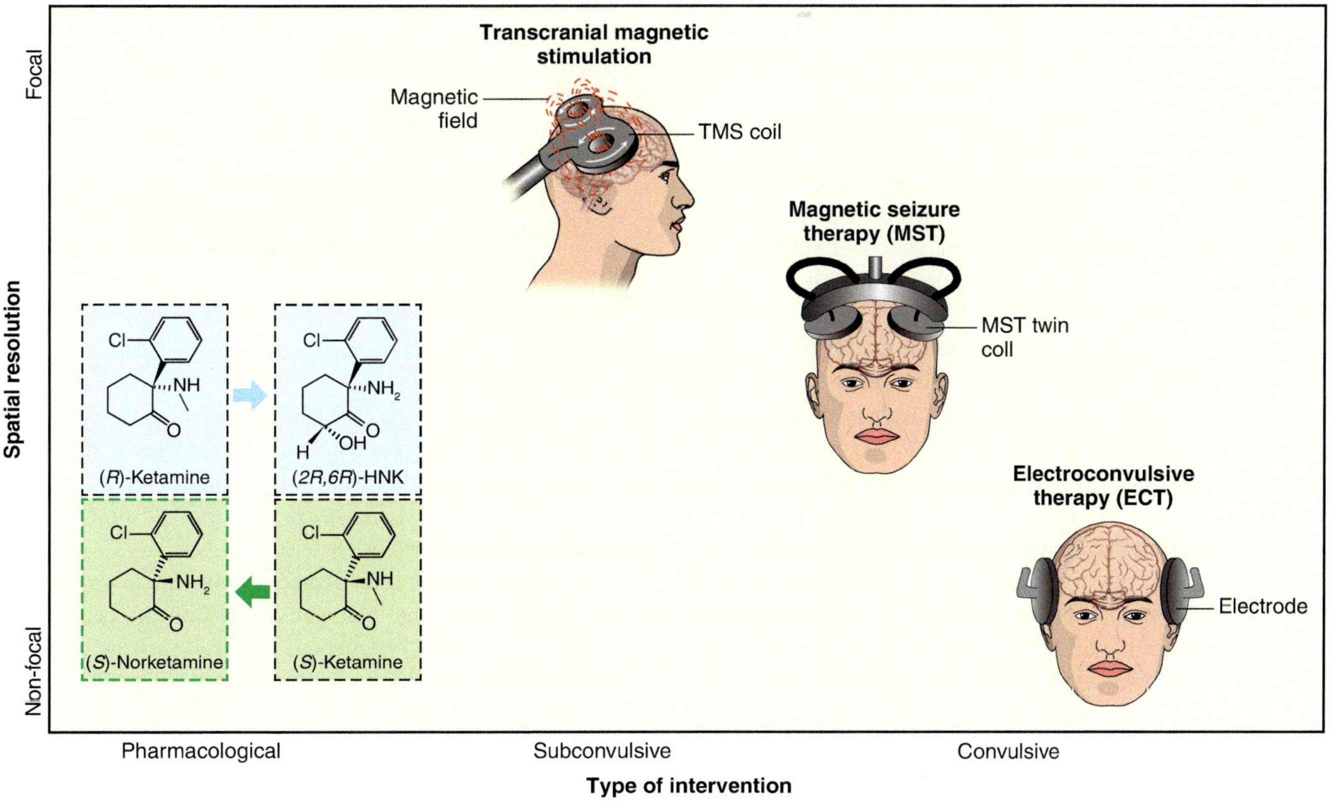

Fig. 1.6 Interventional Psychiatry treatments. (*From* Hashimoto et al. [13]; *with permission*)

Neuroscience

The Diagnostic and Statistical Manual of Mental Disorders (DSM) was written to standardize diagnoses across the country and minimize subjectivity. This yielded reliability in diagnosis, but did these diagnostic criteria accurately reflect underlying pathology in the brain or specific genetic abnormalities? Psychiatric illnesses are often called syndromes in that they usually present with common clinical symptoms, but the exact cause of the constellation of symptoms may be different or unknown [14]. Schizophrenia, for example, can present in a variety of ways with high interindividual variability. Such variability often calls into question whether it is one illness or several different illnesses that have not yet been differentiated. Genetics research into DSM disorders has repeatedly found that a given disorder might be associated—though weakly—with genetic polymorphisms at many sites resulting in numerous potential disease mechanisms. In addition, a particular mechanism might be found to be implicated in several different DSM disorders (Fig. 1.7) [15].

Several decades of research had accordingly produced relatively little to show in terms of defining the etiologies of psychiatric disorders. The NIMH developed a new strategy to 'deconstruct' the current disorders into intermediate areas of neurobiological function and aim research efforts at these 'domains.' This new Research Domain Criteria (RDoC) is aimed at relating core psychological processes to biological processes, with the hope that this will provide a new framework for defining the boundaries of psychiatric disorders and their subtypes based on empirical data from genetics and neuroscience. The emphasis will be on neural circuits but will extend 'downwards' to the genetic and molecular elements and 'upwards' to the level of individuals, families, and social contexts. This approach may yield progress. RDoC was applied in subjects with psychosis who would typically be diagnosed with schizophrenia. Based on a large biomarker panel, subjects were able to be classified into three categories which have become known as "biotypes" (Fig. 1.8; Table 1.1) [16, 17].

In addition to biotypes, neuroscience research is also elucidating more models to help describe behaviors and link behavior to anatomy and neural pathways within the brain. Nervous tissue varies depending on its location inside the brain. Cortical neurons and the global organization of such neurons can be seen in Fig. 1.9.

When thinking about neurons and brain connectivity, it is helpful to know what a synapse is, and what neurotransmitters are most common at these synapses. An understanding of synapses and neurotransmitters is very useful for understanding how medication and other chemical substances interfere with these biological components (Fig. 1.10; Table 1.2).

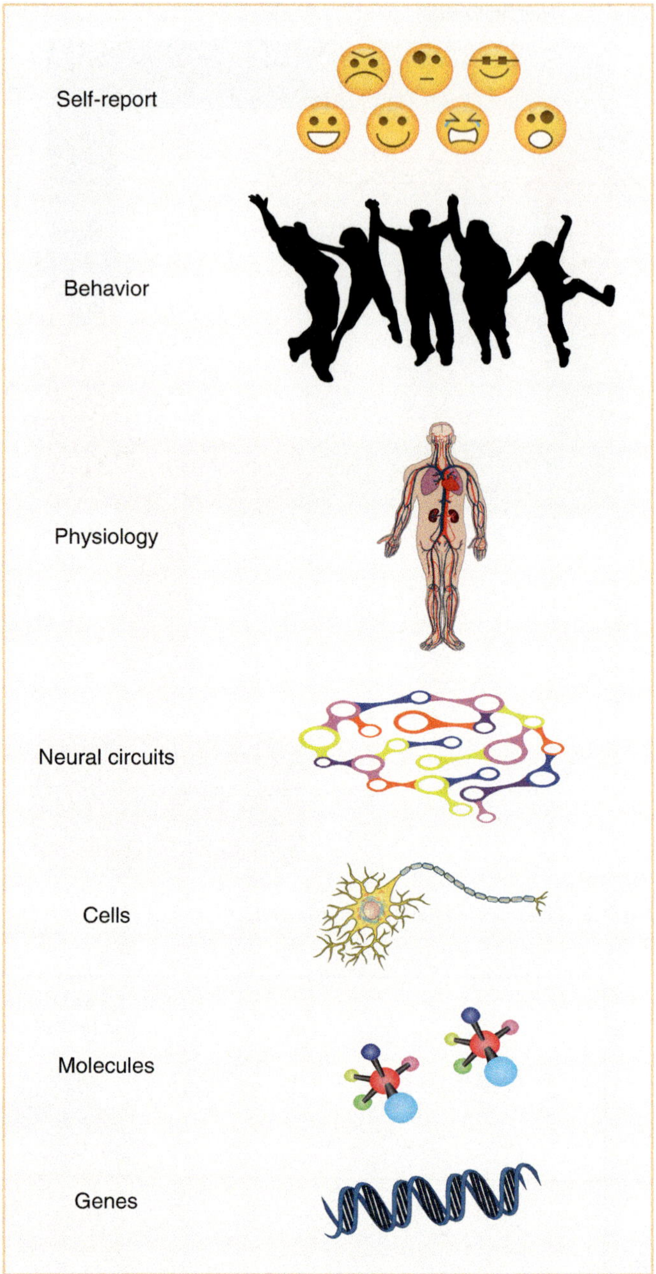

Fig. 1.7 Psychiatric factors that influence the mental illness

Another way to think about brain connectivity is to map functional areas in the cortex. Functional cortex maps today have usually been made by stimulating small areas and noting the effect. Figure 1.11 shows approximate functions of different regions of the cortex.

The human connectome project is also underway which seeks to map functional connectivity within the brain [18]. Connectomes use MRI sequences to build a wiring diagram based on water molecules diffusing across white matter tracts where spontaneous fluctuations contribute to positive and negative correlates that are then used to form a lesion

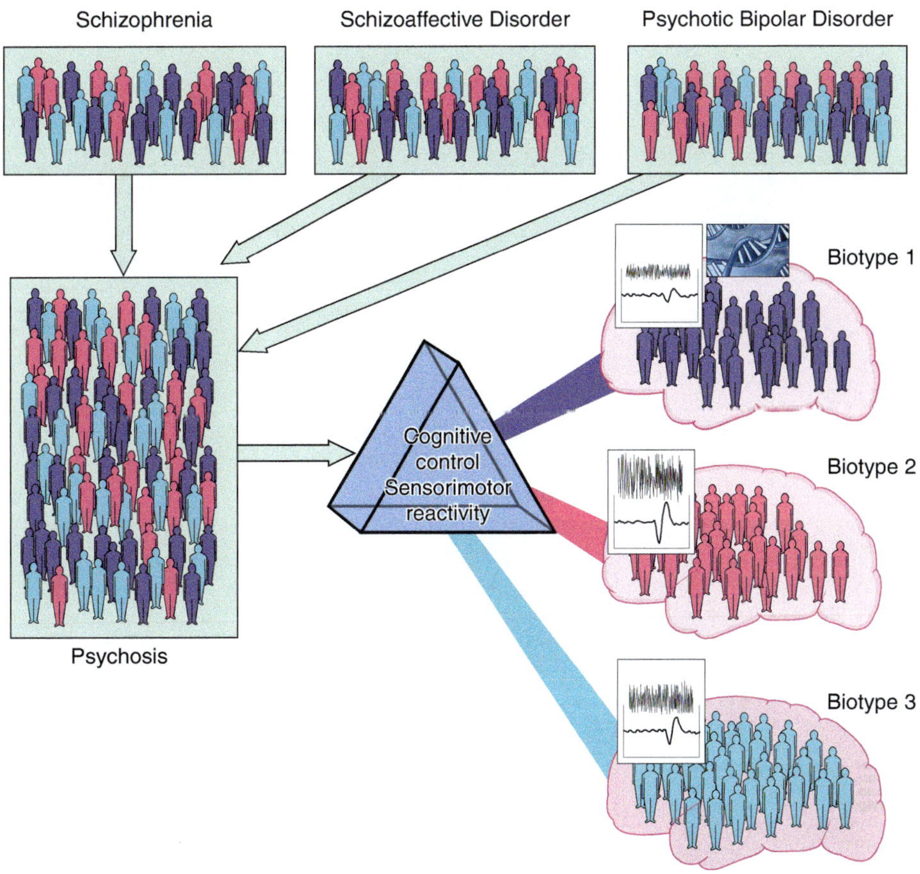

Fig. 1.8 Schema of the bipolar and schizophrenia network

Table 1.1 Summary of research domains and biologic correlates

Negative affect	**Positive affect**	**Cognition**
Fear	Reward seeking	Attention
Distress	Gratification	Perception
Aggression	Habit formation	Memory
		Executive function
Basolateral amygdala	Mesolimbic dopamine system	Parietal areas (attention)
Hippocampus	Orbital frontal cortex	Thalamic and occipital (perception)
Ventral medial prefrontal cortex	Ventral and dorsal striatum	Dorsolateral prefrontal cortex
		Hippocampus
		Anterior cingulate
Social processes	**Regulatory systems**	**Sensorimotor systems**
Attachment	Arousal	Motor actions
Parenting	Sleep	Agency
Separation anxiety	Circadian rhythms	Habit
Facial recognition		Innate motor patterns
Oxytocin	Reticular activating systems	Inferior parietal cortex
Vasopressin	Ventral tegmental area	Posterior parietal cortex
	Locus ceruleus	Premotor cortex
		Thalamus
		Cerebellum
		Somatosensory cortex
		Sensorimotor basal ganglia
		Hypothalamus
		Motor cortex
		Brainstem
		Occulomotor system

From Tamminga et al. [16]; with permission

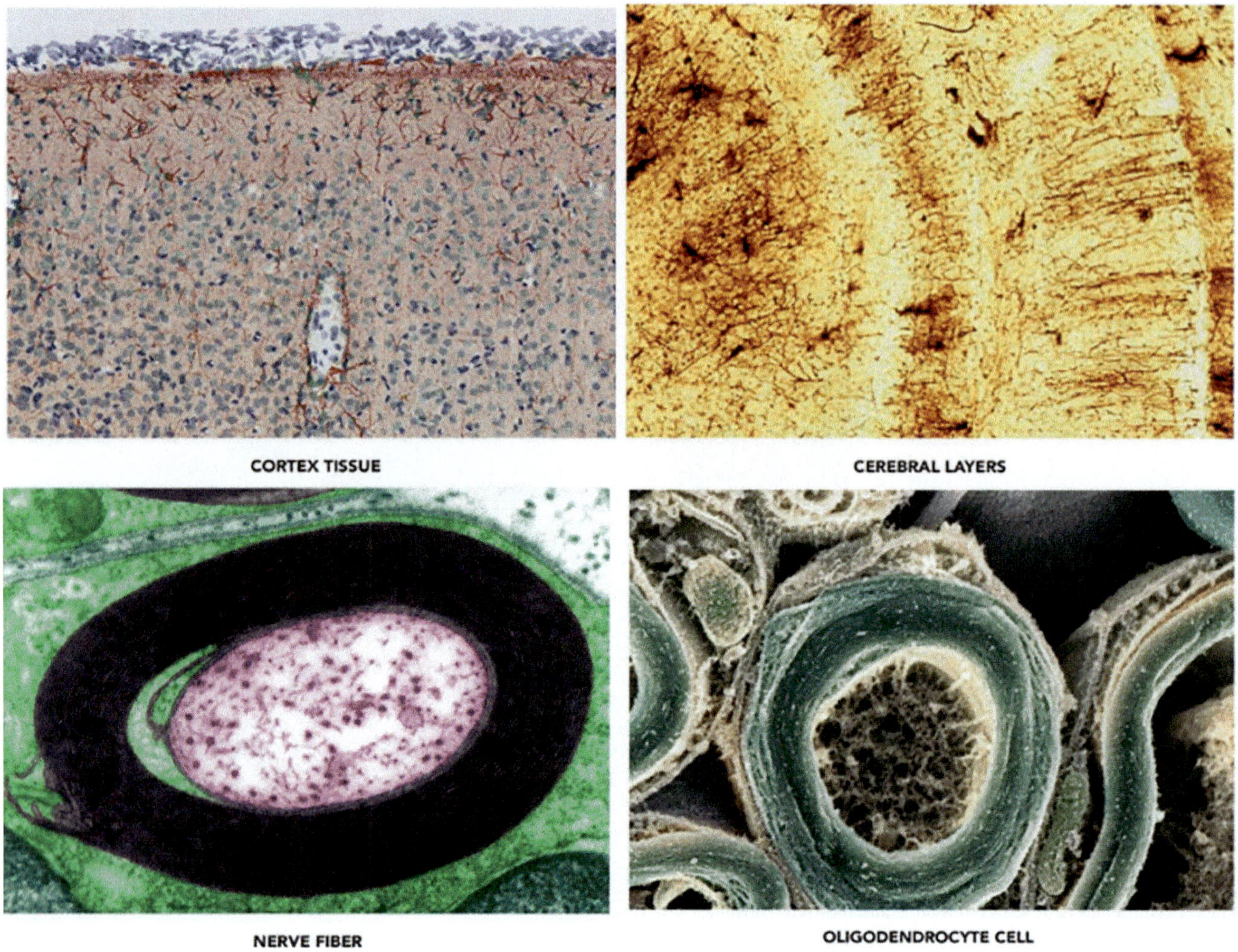

Fig. 1.9 Cortical and cerebral tissue

network with the goal of localizing neuropsychiatric symptoms (Fig. 1.12). Figure 1.13 shows the process by which connectomes are created. Data is obtained from MRI images. Images are labeled with five tissue types which are used to create a fiber orientation distribution (FOD) that is then used to create tractograms using anatomical constraints. A connectivity matrix is generated from the tractogram and network-based statistics test for the white matter connectivity effects [19].

One of the major systems that concern psychiatry is the limbic system shown in Fig. 1.14.

The limbic system is associated with basic emotional and motivational processes such as anger, pleasure, sex, and general survival. It consists of the limbic lobe (cingulate gyrus, cingulate sulcus, and parahippocampal gyrus), hippocampus, amygdala, hypothalamus, mammillary bodies, thalamus, and fornix. Neurons in the limbic system also extend down into the brainstem and into other areas of the brain such as the frontal cortex. Sensory neurons of the olfactory system are also linked to the limbic system and influence memory formation and bring olfactory sensation into consciousness. These structures are explained in more detail in Fig. 1.15.

Emotions are thought to arise in the amygdala, brainstem, and hypothalamus. An anatomic correlation with how emotions may be initiated, expressed, and become conscious is illustrated in Fig. 1.16. The frontal lobe is one area involved in maintaining consciousness.

The amygdala can be considered the emotional "sensor" of the brain. It receives emotional inputs from the rest of the body, cortex, sensory cells, and hypothalamus. When the amygdala fires, it sends information through the emotional circuit shown in Fig. 1.17 and causes physical changes in the body. Input from the frontal lobe evokes conscious awareness of emotions. Positive emotions follow a slightly separate circuit to include an area of the brainstem to produce dopamine and a sense of positive reinforcement [20]. The amygdala's role in whether sensory information becomes conscious or not is depicted in Fig. 1.18. The figure shows two routes, a slow and accurate route, and a quick route. The

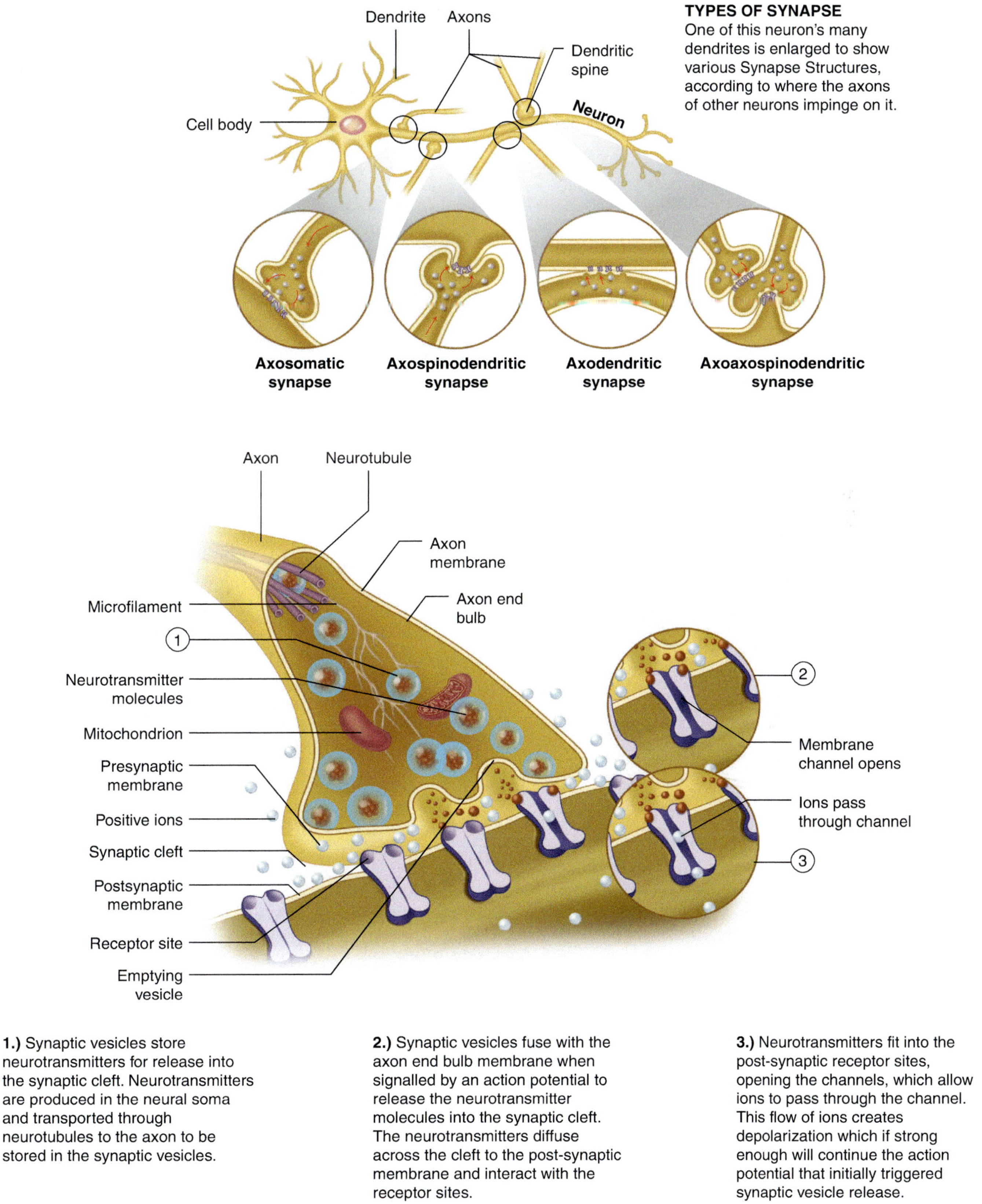

Fig. 1.10 Structure of a synapse. (1) Synaptic vesicles store neurotransmitters for release into the synaptic cleft. Neurotransmitters are produced in the neural soma and transported through neurotubules to the axon to be stored in the synaptic vesicles. (2) Synaptic vesicles fuse with the axon end bulb membrane when signaled by an action potential to release the neurotransmitter molecules into the synaptic cleft. The neurotransmitters diffuse across the cleft to the post-synaptic membrane and interact with the receptor sites. (3) Neurotransmitters fit into the post-synaptic receptor sites, opening the channels, which allow ions to pass through the channel. This flow of ions creates depolarization which if strong enough, will continue the action potential that initially triggered synaptic vesicle release

Table 1.2 Common neurotransmitters and their post-synaptic effects [20]

Inhibitory	Excitatory and inhibitory	Mostly excitatory	Excitatory
Serotonin	Dopamine	Acetylcholine	Glutamate
Glycine		Noradrenaline	Aspartate
Gamma aminobutyric acid (GABA)			Histamine

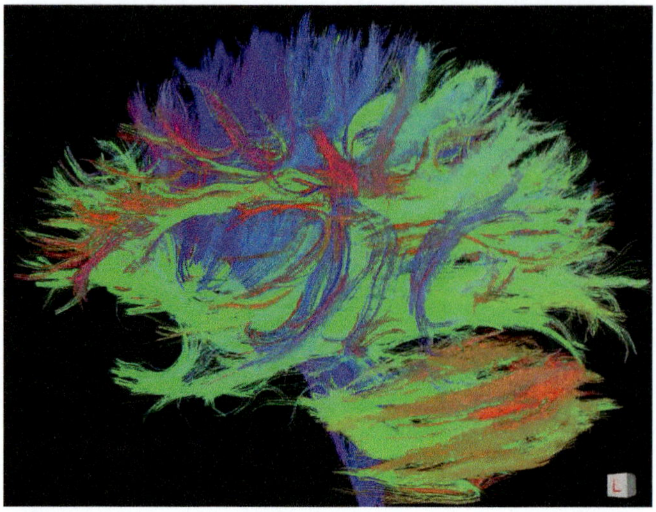

Fig. 1.12 Sagittal view of human connectome or tractogram (*From* Wikicommons. Author jgmarcelino from Newcastle upon Tyne, UK. 22 April 2010. https://creativecommons.org/licenses/by/2.0/deed.en. No changes)

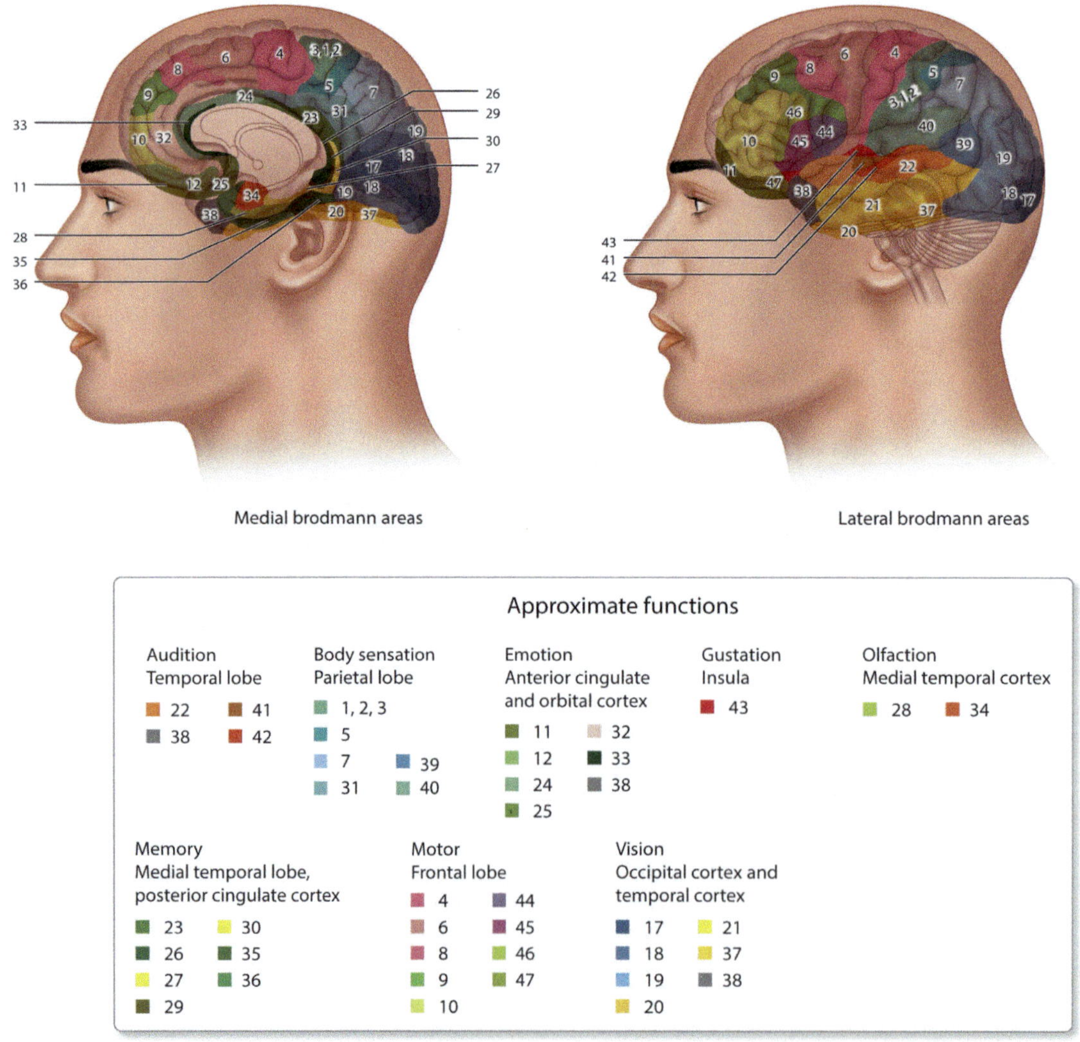

Fig. 1.11 Functional areas of the brain. The medial brodmann areas link areas that are associated with hearing, vision, memory, emotional insight, and emotional reactions. The lateral brodmann areas include Broca's area and are based on nerve-cell body arrangements

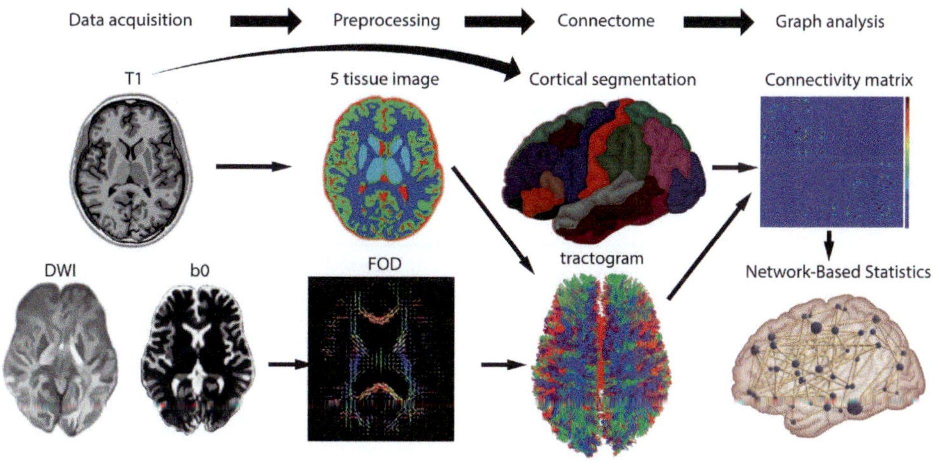

Fig. 1.13 Process of creating a connectome

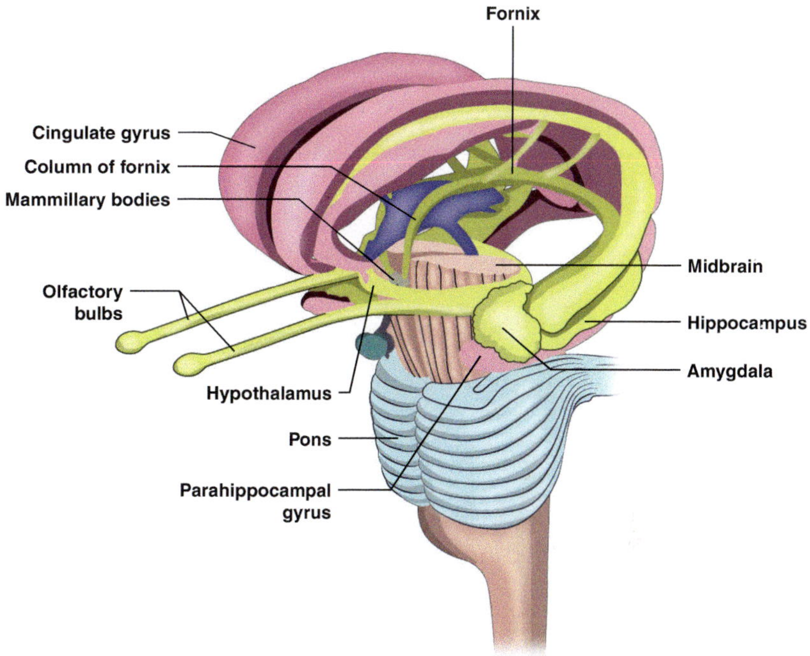

Fig. 1.14 Anatomy of the limbic system

Fig. 1.15 A focus on structures of the limbic system. **Cingulate Cortex:** The cingulate cortex shares extensive neural pathways with other brain regions. It is involved in motivational processing as it connects to the reward centers of the brain (orbitofrontal cortex, basal ganglia, and insula). It also contributes to orienting attention, consolidation of long-term memory, and processing of emotionally relevant stimuli [21]. **Stria Terminalis:** Pathways from the stria terminalis link the amygdala to the rest of the brain and play a role in anxiety and stress responses [21]. **Frontal Cortex:** The frontal cortex works in conjunction with the limbic system to produce conscious feelings. It then modifies these emotions to fit socially acceptable norms. It is also considered the "action cortex" as it contributes to skeletal and ocular movement as well as speech control. The prefrontal cortex is the largest part of the frontal cortex and is responsible for reasoning [22]. **Olfactory Complex:** Olfactory bulbs carry information directly to the amygdala and hypothalamus to mediate behavioral, emotional, motivational, and physiological effects of odors and smell. Information is also projected through the thalamus to the orbitofrontal cortex to help with the perception and discrimination of odors [23]. **Thalamus:** The thalamus is a structure located near the center of the brain, which allows for nerve fiber connections to the cerebral cortex in all directions. It is a major relay station filtering information between the brain and body. Its connection to the limbic system allows the thalamus to be involved in learning and episodic memory. It is also involved in sleep regulation and wakefulness. The thalamus is divided into five major functional components: reticular and intralaminar nuclei (arousal, pain), sensory nuclei (medial geniculate nucleus for auditory, lateral geniculate nucleus for visual, and ventrobasal complex for somatosensory and vestibular), effector nuclei (motor language), associative nuclei (cognitive functions), and limbic nuclei (mood and motivation) [24]. **Hippocampus:** The hippocampus plays a crucial role in the storage and retrieval of episodic memories. Episodic memory is recollections about a specific event occurring at a certain time and place. Patients with hippocampal damage struggle to create new episodic memories [25]. **Amygdala:** The amygdala receives afferent input from many sites within the brain, including the olfactory bulb, olfactory nucleus, medial frontal cortex, dorsomedial thalamic nucleus, hypothalamus, and dorsal raphe nuclei. These sites provide internal and external information that contribute to threat analysis and emotional responses. The amygdala plays a role in acquired and innate emotional reactions, particularly fear, anxiety, and rewarding properties of stimuli [23]. **Corpus Callosum:** The corpus callosum facilitates communication between the left and right hemispheres. Hypothalamus and mammillary body: The hypothalamus integrates autonomic response and endocrine function with behavior concerned with controlling blood pressure, body temperature, drive for water or salt, emergency responses to stress, energy metabolism, and hormonal control. The mammillary bodies assist with recollective memory, emotion, and goal-directed behaviors [26]

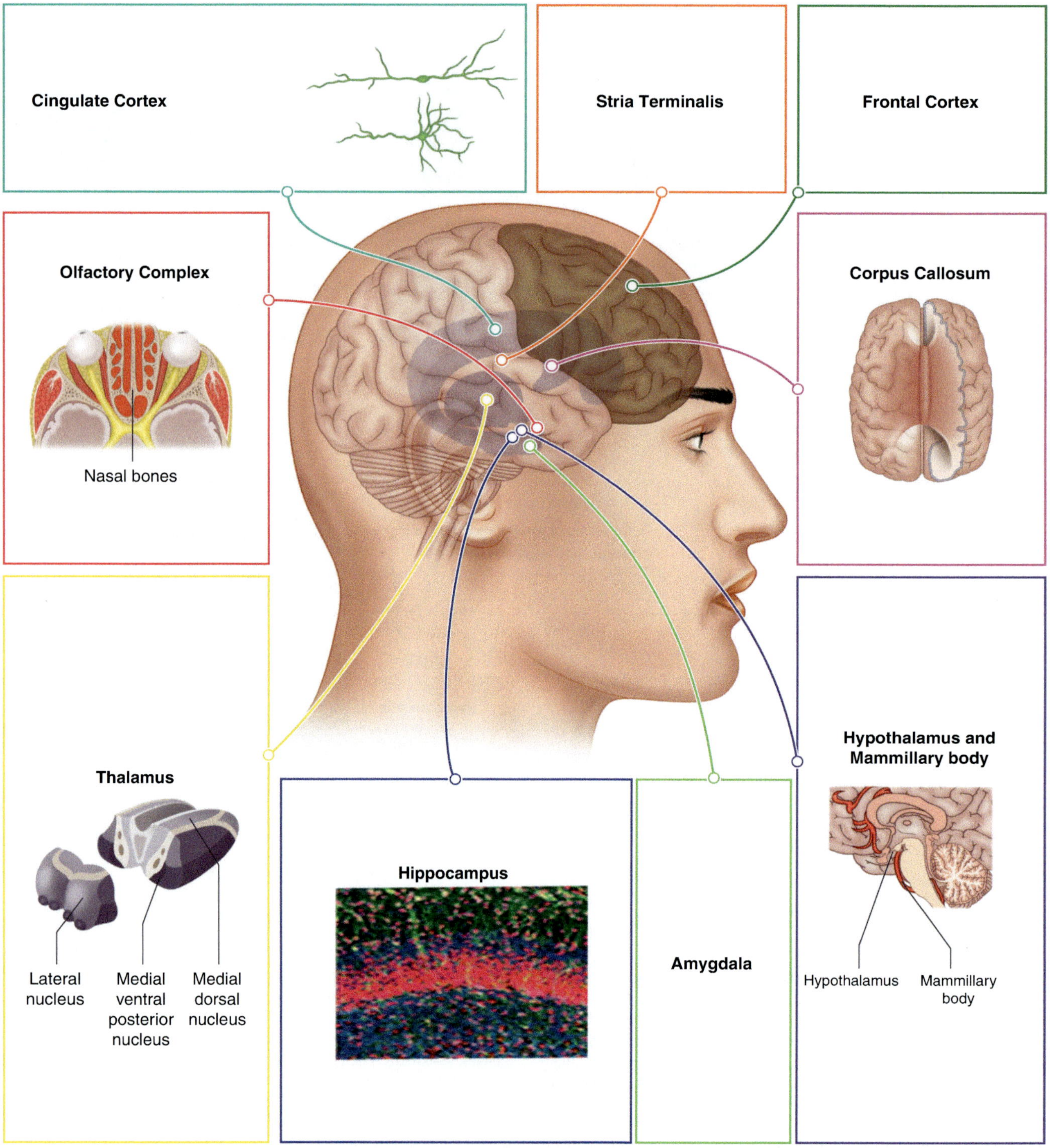
Cingulate Cortex
Stria Terminalis
Frontal Cortex
Olfactory Complex
Nasal bones
Corpus Callosum
Thalamus
Lateral nucleus
Medial ventral posterior nucleus
Medial dorsal nucleus
Hippocampus
Amygdala
Hypothalamus and Mammillary body
Hypothalamus
Mammillary body

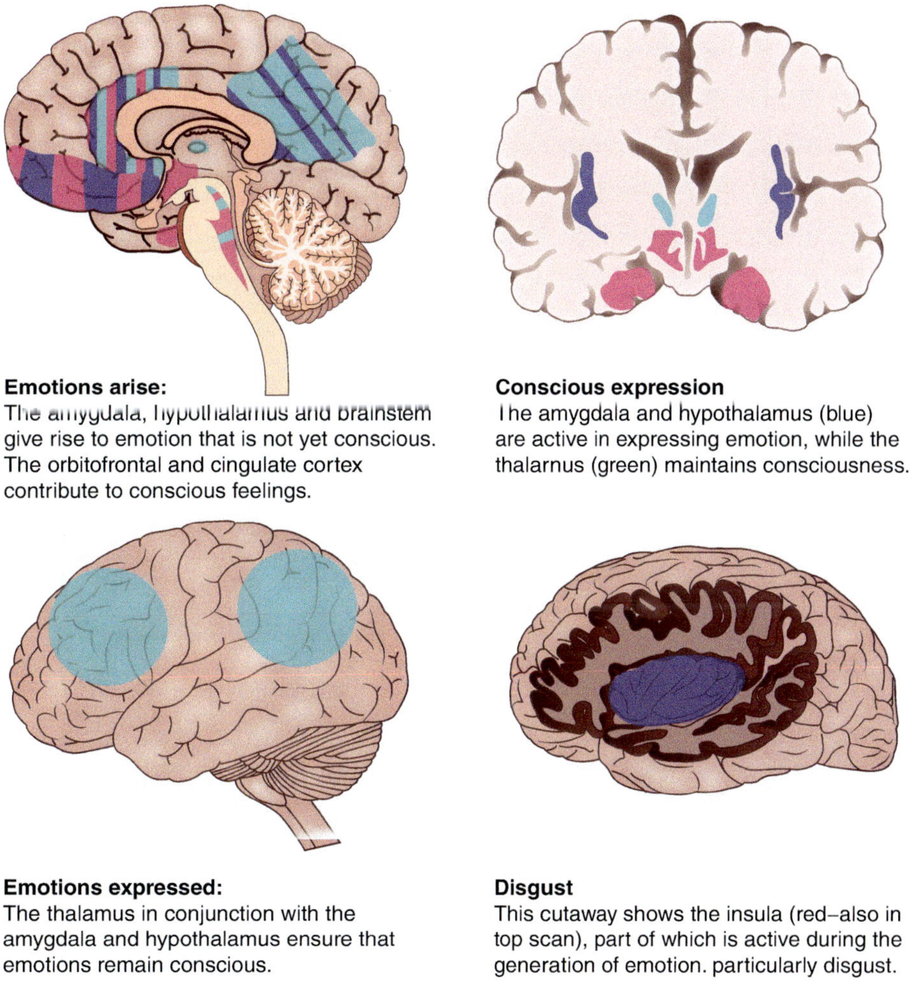

Fig. 1.16 Anatomical representation of the expression of emotions

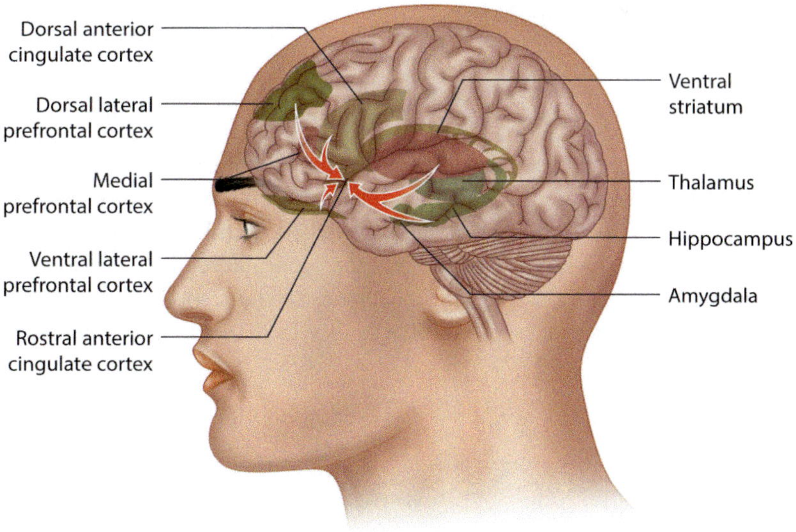

Fig. 1.17 Processing emotions through an emotion circuit in the brain

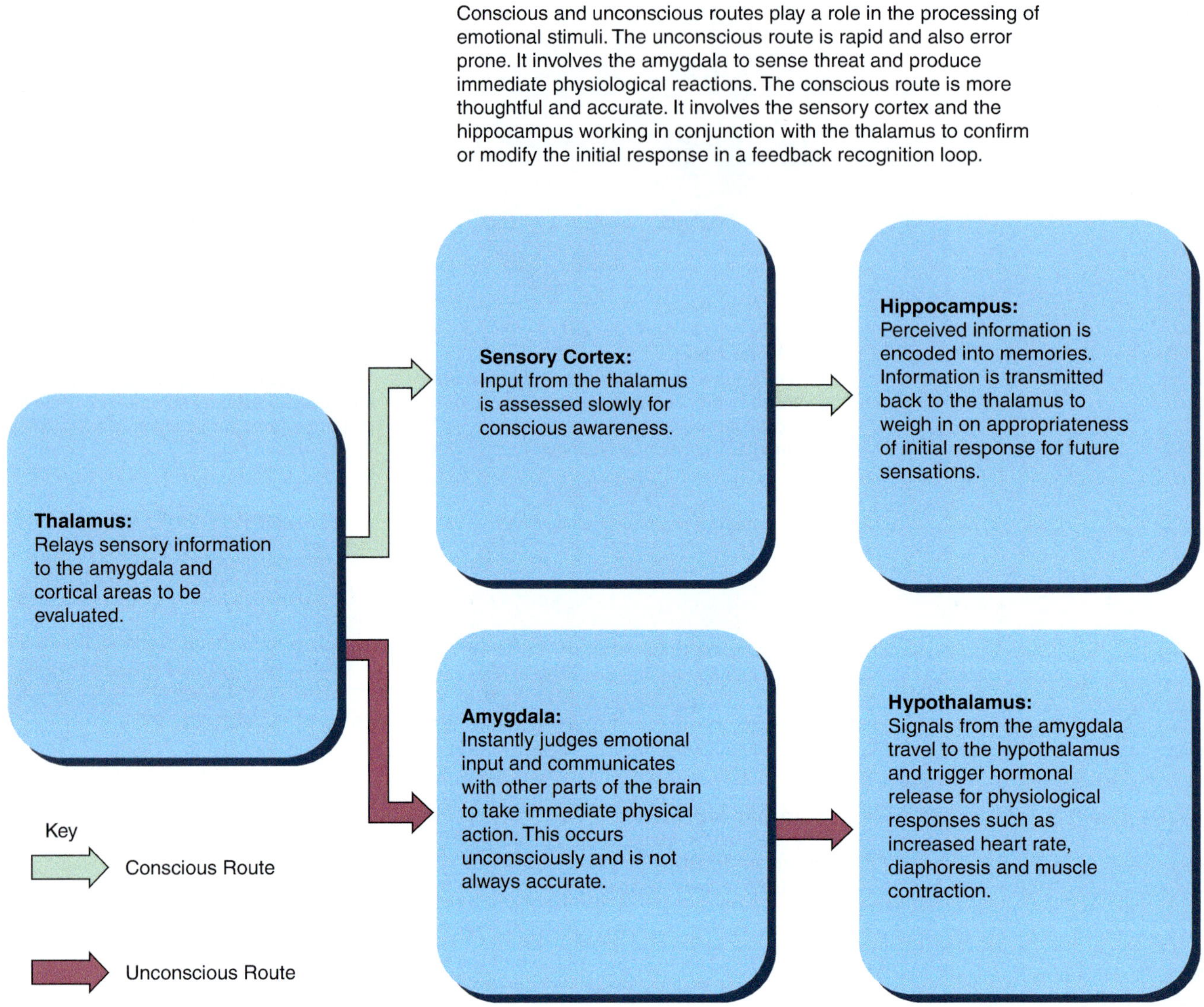

Fig. 1.18 Conscious and unconscious routes

quick route is in place to react very quickly to threats or rewards which involves the amygdala. The slow route is processed through the frontal lobes and is more thoughtful.

In addition to the limbic system, another important region of the brain is the insula. The insula is thought to be responsible for the feeling of "self" and the ability to distinguish ourselves from others. In being aware of others, the insula also plays a role in triggering empathic feelings. fMRI scans had shown insula activity when participants watched another person in pain. This phenomenon is shown in Fig. 1.19. The insula also works as part of the process of bringing our emotional state into consciousness.

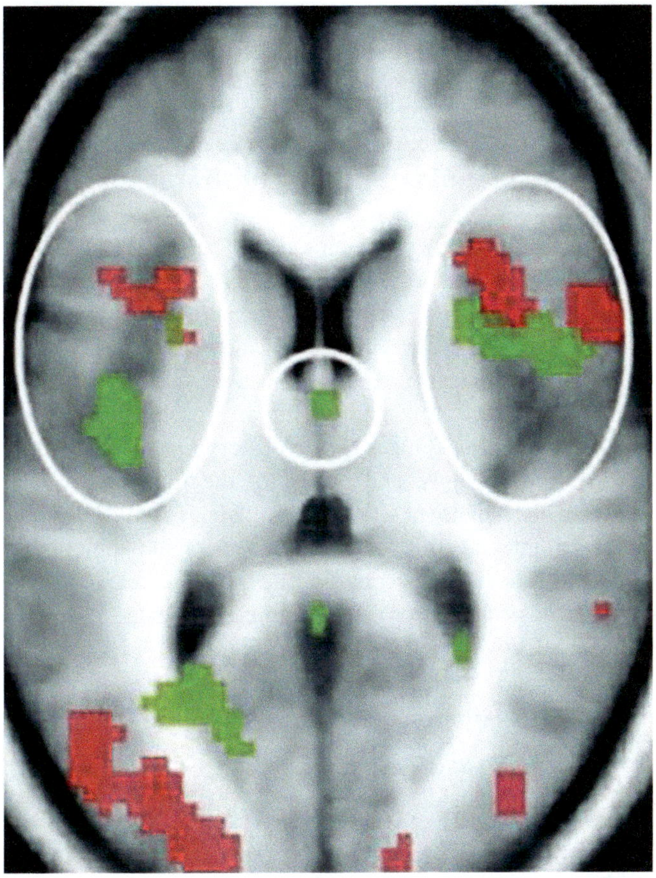

Fig. 1.19 fMRI showing insula activity when participants witnessed another individual in pain

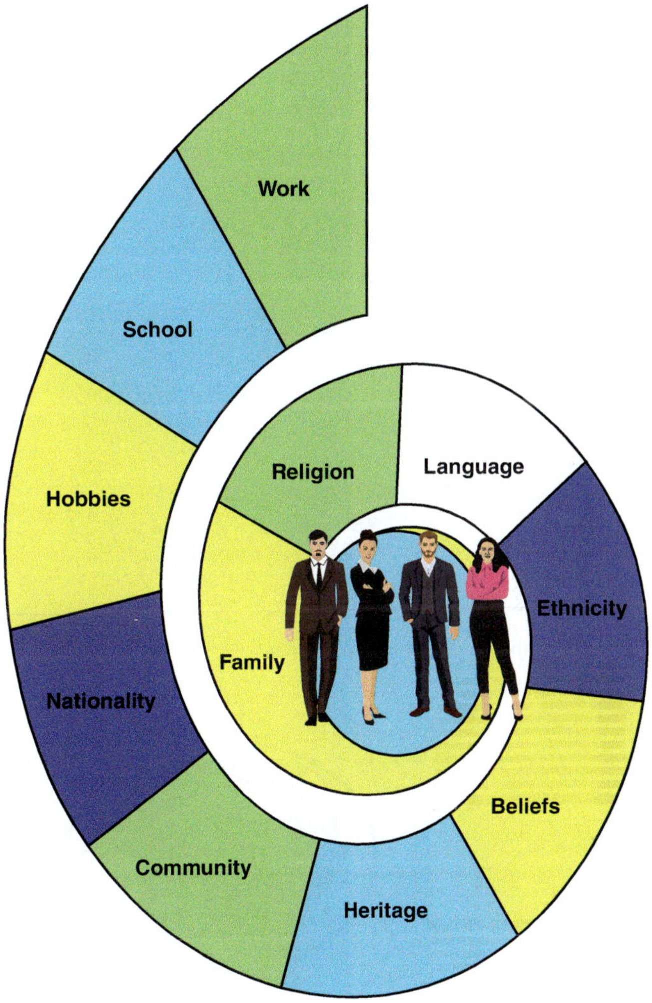

Fig. 1.20 Cultural factors

Culture and Society

Treating mental illness requires more than knowing the psychopathology, psychopharmacology, or presentation of an illness. The missing piece is knowledge about the context within which the illness arose. We have a growing evidence base demonstrating that childhood trauma and deprivation lead to adult psychiatric illnesses and that the social environment has an enormous impact on whether and how adults recover from serious mental illness. Different racial and ethnic communities are subject to very different exposure to these 'social determinants of mental health,' leading to significant disparities and inequities in mental health and treatments [27]. In addition, humans are interpersonal creatures, and our close attachments shape our development and impact our health throughout our lives. Friendship has been shown to decrease inflammation and extend longevity [28]. While we see an individual patient in our office, it is important to realize that each patient is a member of a complex network of relationships that further exist within a larger societal structure ruled by various cultural dynamics (Fig. 1.20) [29].

Pathology often arises out of isolation or when an individual begins to struggle to function within the cultural and societal framework. This should not be surprising—the human brain and human culture co-evolved over millennia, creating a new kind of primate that was both gifted at and dependent on accumulated social learning. Different social structures and cultures have a profound impact on the prevalence and presentation of many psychiatric illnesses. As psychiatrists, we often see patients afflicted by environments so harsh or isolation so intense that medication will do very little to improve their psyche (Fig. 1.21).

It is only when their environment improves or they gain more support in their life that change occurs. In this way, we see that relationships can help or hinder a person's growth and well-being. When treating patients from a culture different from your own—and even your own, it is also important to be both humble and curious and know that false assumptions can be made that might lead to the wrong diagnosis and ineffective treatment. The DSM encourages the use of the

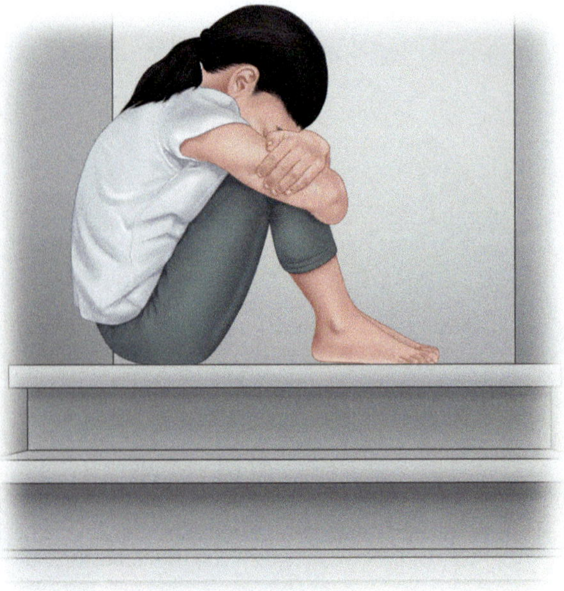

Fig. 1.21 Child trauma has a lasting effect

cultural formulation to thoroughly explore cultural factors with patients to ensure that patients are well understood so that an individualized treatment plan can be established [30].

Narrative Meaning and Psychotherapy

A unique aspect of human beings, compared to all other social animals, is our use of language to create narrative meaning from our experiences. Each patient's experience of childhood adversities or social determinants of mental health is unique because what it meant to them subjectively cannot be understood without careful listening. Similarly, each patient with a serious mental illness has a powerful story to tell of how their identity, relationships, and hopes for the future have been impacted. Psychiatrists learn how to listen carefully to their patients to integrate this subjective dimension into their understanding of the patient's condition. At the same time, connecting with the patient's story is one of the most powerful ways to build an effective treatment alliance (Fig. 1.22) [31].

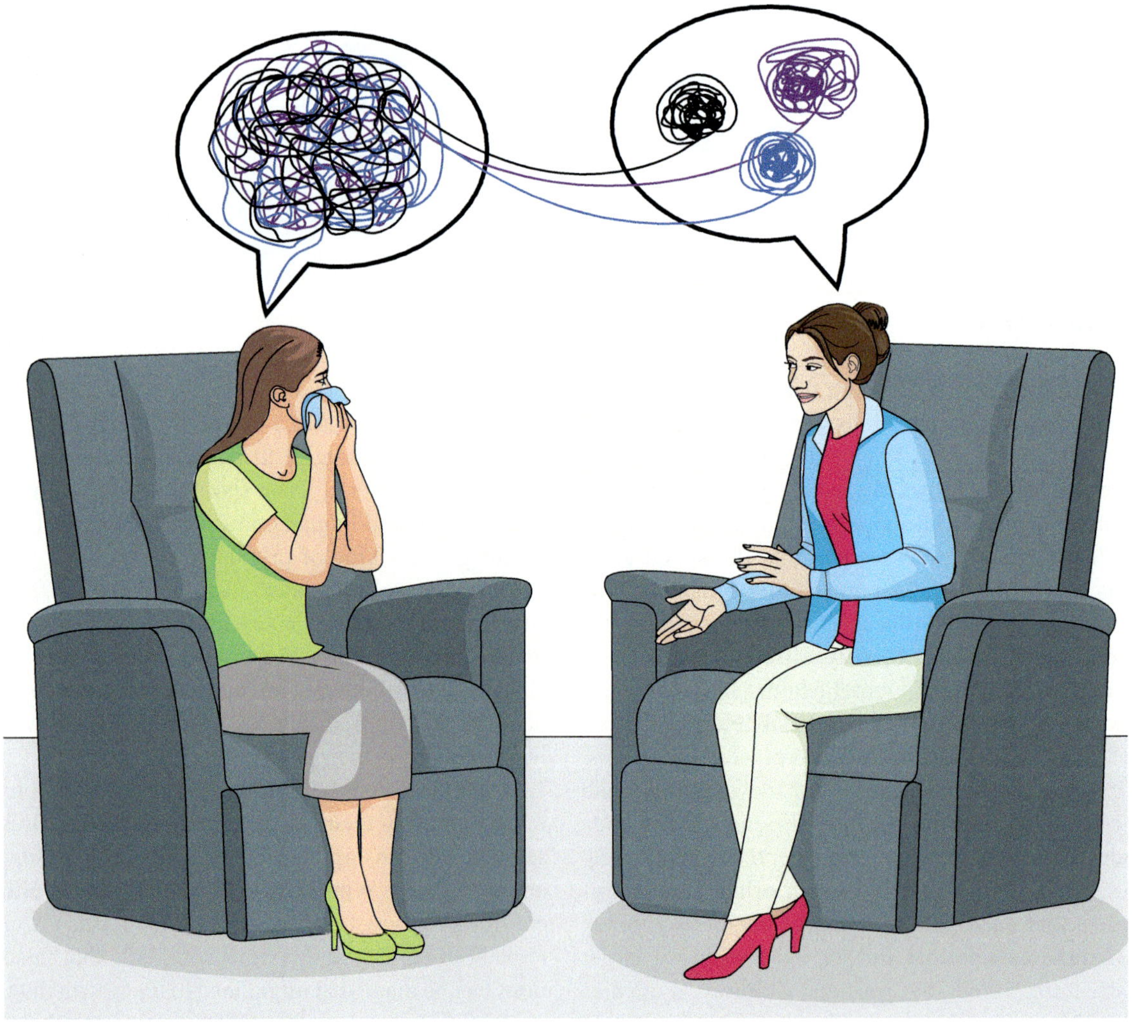

Fig. 1.22 Psychiatrist listening to a patient

Technology

Technology can be both a blessing and a curse. As new technologies are created, new opportunities to study how they influence our mental health also arise as well as new ethical dilemmas. While computers have made information more convenient and accessible than ever before, online gaming and social media introduce new challenges, as many users are finding some of these sites highly addictive. What implications will this have on the future and on the mental health of children and adolescents? Social media and mobile phone apps not only provide information with one swipe but also collect information just as easily. What do your online use patterns tell us about your mental health? How ethical is it to collect this anonymously and utilize it for research, marketing, or health care? With the creation of more technology, we must also think about how it may be influencing our community and us.

Another area of innovation and development is in the arena of mobile phone applications. There are already many apps in the marketplace that say they promote mental wellness by offering meditation, CBT, journaling, mood tracking, and even smoking cessation. The effectiveness of these apps and whether they are beneficial or not remains to be seen and is an area of active research. For any app, it is important to evaluate it, considering your overall goal, privacy settings, evidence, and usability of the app. This method is described in more detail on the APA website and is known as the app evaluation model (Fig. 1.23) [32, 33].

Technology is expanding to offer new mental health treatments, but as always, ethics and evidence must take priority to avoid repeating the mistakes of the past.

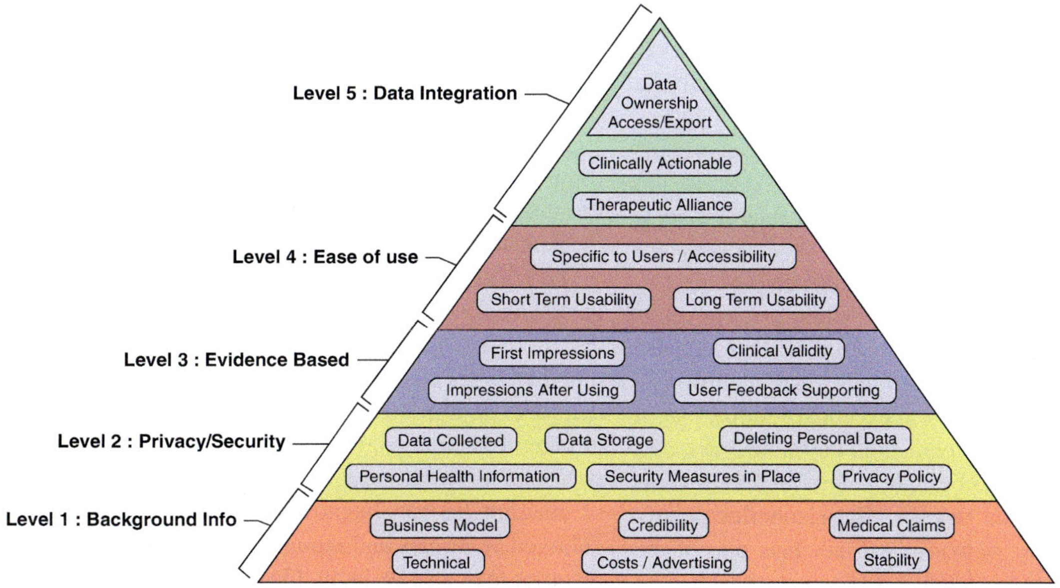

Level 1 : Background Info

- Does the app identify funding sources and conflicts of interest?
- Does the app identify ownership?
- Does the app come from a legitimate source?
- Where does app info originate?
- Are there additonal or hidden costs?
- Does the app need an active internet connection?
- On what plaforms does the app operate?
- Has the app been updated in the last 180 days?

Level 2 : Privacy/Security

- Is there a privacy policy?
- Does the app declare data use and purpose?
- Does the app describe use of PHI?
- Can you opt out of data collection or delete data?
- Are data maintained on the device or the web?
- Does the app explain security systems used?

Level 3 : Evidence Based

- Does the app do what it claims to do?
- Is app content correct, well-written and relevant?
- Are references included with the app?
- Is there evidence of benefit from end user feedback?

Level 4 : Ease of use

- Are there potential barriers to access?
- Can the user easily understand how to use the app?
- Is the app easy to use on a long-term basis?
- Does the app clearly define its functional scope?

Level 5 : Data Integration

- Do you own your data?
- Can you easily access your data?
- Can you easily share your data?
- Does the app lead to any postive behavior change?
- Does the app improve therapeutic alliance between patient and provider?

Fig. 1.23 App Evaluation model (*From* Lagan et al. [32]; Creative Commons Attribution 4.0 International License, http://creativecommons.org/licenses/by/4.0/)

Subspecialties of Psychiatry

Entering a career in psychiatry means choosing to work in a field that is still forming, growing, and constantly reassessing its identity. Psychiatrists often report greater career satisfaction and lower levels of burnout compared to other specialties. It is highly customizable with options to further specialize by doing a fellowship after completing residency.

Addiction Psychiatry

In 2014, it was estimated that 20.1 million adults in the United States have a substance use disorder, and of those, about 7.9 million adults have both a substance use disorder and mental illness [34]. The COVID-19 pandemic has also greatly affected those with substance use disorders. According to the CDC, over 81,000 drug overdose deaths have occurred in the United States from June 2019 to May 2020. This is the highest number of overdose deaths ever recorded in a 12-month period and is thought to be due to the covid-19 pandemic (Fig. 1.24) [35].

Addiction psychiatry focuses on helping individuals compelled to use addictive chemical substances despite the adverse consequences that severely limit their function, relationships, and mental health. Addiction psychiatrists are trained in understanding the psychosocial, environmental, and genetic factors that all play a role in addiction. They prescribe medications such as naltrexone or opioid replacement therapies, which have shown to be effective in reducing cravings and compulsive use. Addiction psychiatry fellows learn how to effectively combine medication, psychotherapy, and motivational interviewing to be optimally effective in helping patients with addiction recover. The alcoholics anonymous model is free and welcoming to all. It is one of the most effective paths to abstinence and lowers health care costs. There are over two million members in AA worldwide (Fig. 1.25) [35].

Child and Adolescent Psychiatry

The CDC reports that 1 in 6 children aged 2–8 has a mental, behavioral, or developmental disorder. The percentage of children diagnosed with depression or anxiety between the ages of 2–17 increases each year. As children age, it becomes more common to receive a diagnosis of depression or anxiety (Fig. 1.26).

Child and adolescent psychiatrists work with children and their families to effectively manage and treat mental, behavioral, and developmental disorders. Early diagnosis and treatment of children with these conditions can make all the difference in their quality of life going forward. Childhood symptoms can differ from those that appear in adult mental illness. It is important to recognize moderate to severe symptoms that persist over time that may indicate either progression towards a mental illness or neurobiological disorder. Symptoms in children can change, overlap, and appear very different from those found in adults. Figure 1.27 shows how the brain continues developing throughout childhood to adulthood, a likely contributor to these differences.

The National Institute of Mental Health (NIMH) recommends that children with depression plus severe attention deficit hyperactivity disorder (ADHD) symptoms such as mood changes and temper outbursts be evaluated for bipolar disorder [36]. Figure 1.28 shows a SPECT scan of a 7-year-old boy with enlarged ventricles and symptoms of irritability, paranoia, and auditory and visual hallucinations. At the time of imaging, he was diagnosed with Bipolar I, but due to the enlarged ventricles and thought disorder, the schizoaffective disorder may also be likely [36].

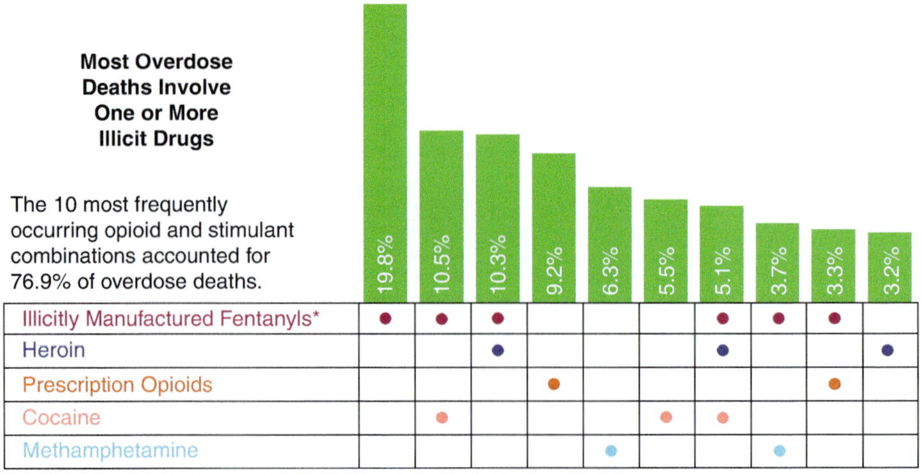

Fig. 1.24 Percentage of overdose deaths involving opioid and stimulant combinations (Data from CDC [37])

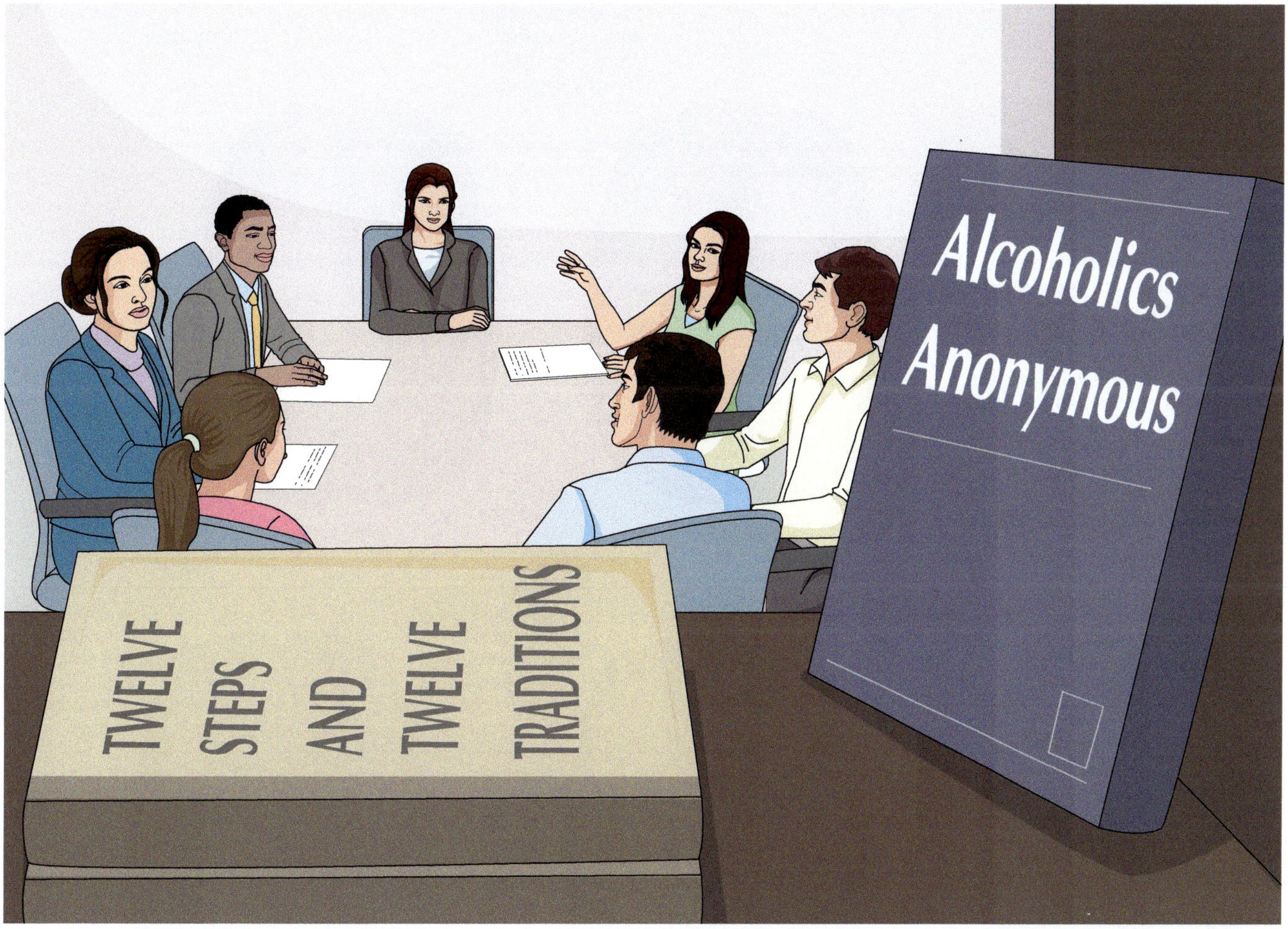

Fig. 1.25 Alcoholics Anonymous Group

Fig. 1.26 Prevalence of mental disorders in children varies by age

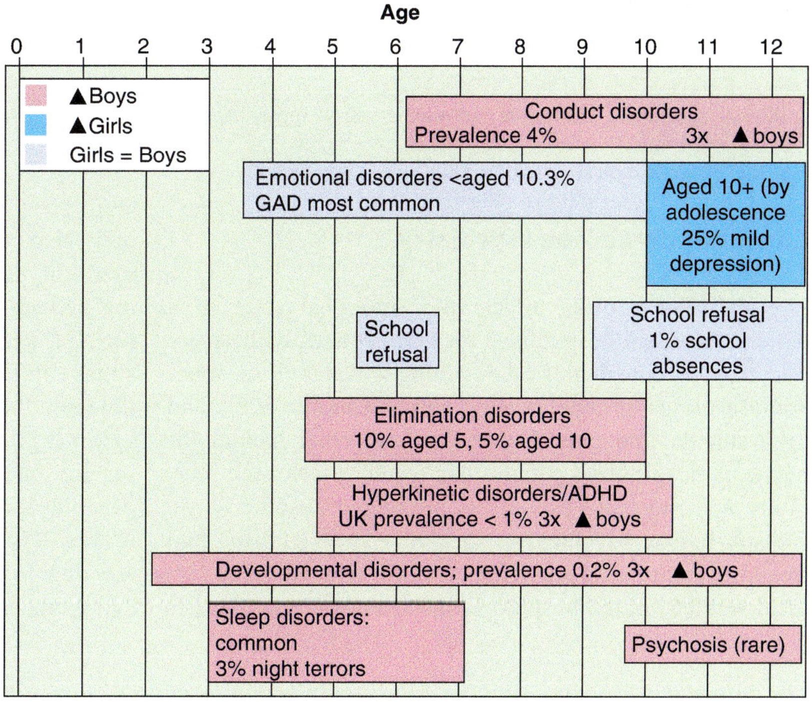

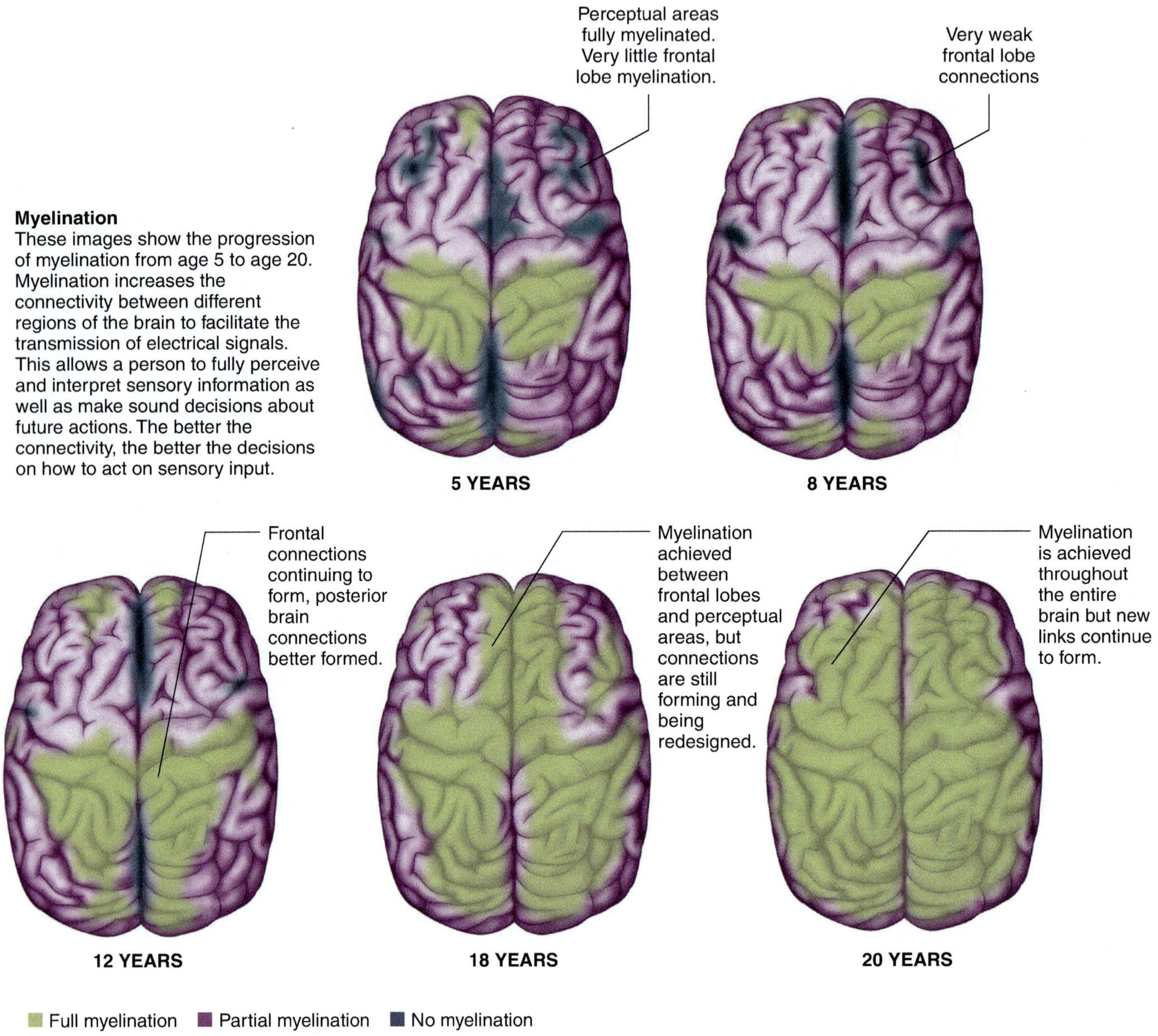

Fig. 1.27 Myelination process from childhood to adulthood

Consultation-Liaison Psychiatry

Physical illness often affects the emotional state of a patient. A patient hospitalized for burn wounds with severe pain may become depressed, resulting in weight loss, anhedonia, feelings of hopelessness, decreased motivation, and even suicidal thoughts. Depression and other mental illnesses in hospitalized patients can result in increased morbidity and mortality as well as prolonged hospital stays. Consult-liaison psychiatrists specialize in diagnosing and treating patients who are being cared for on medical or surgical services in the hospital. Consult-liaison psychiatrists may also work closely with services where psychiatric morbidity is the highest and has the greatest effect on treating patient's medical condition as oncology, pain, pediatrics, or geriatric services [38]. Figure 1.29 shows how stress can lead to mental or physical illness. There are few illnesses that only affect the body and not the mind, and vice versa. Many patients referred to the consult-liaison service have medical comorbidities in conjunction with psychiatric illness or behavioral disturbances. Psychiatrists in this field work diligently to determine which symptoms are due to an underlying medical condition and which symptoms are primarily psychiatric in nature.

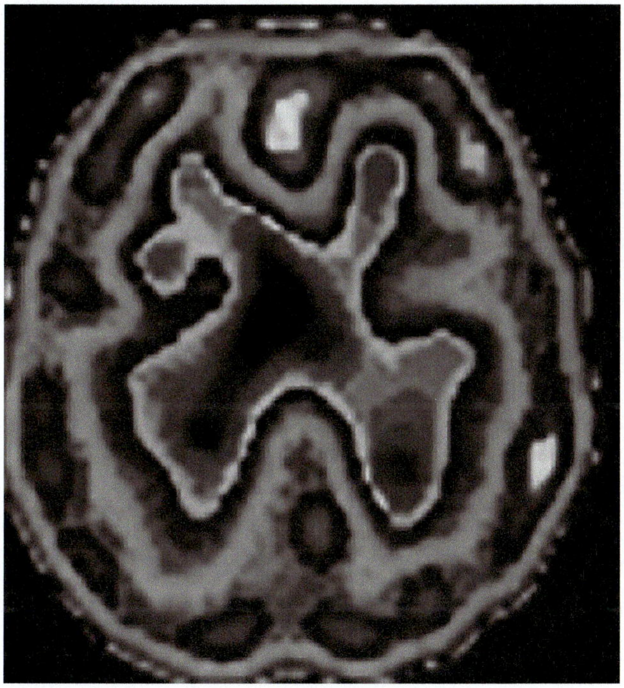

Fig. 1.28 SPECT scan of a 7-year-old boy experiencing paranoia and hallucinations (*Reprinted from* Taylor [36]; *with permission*)

Consult-liaison training provides expertise in the management of delirium and agitation, assessment of capacity to make medical decisions, and conflict resolution between the patient and the primary medical team. Capacity is an important topic to be familiar with and means that a patient can understand their illness, what is recommended for treatment of the illness, and the consequences of accepting or rejecting the treatment. Figure 1.30 describes the key features of capacity.

Forensic Psychiatry

Forensic psychiatry works at the intersection of psychiatry and the law. Forensic psychiatrists perform evaluations for criminal and civil matters. Forensic psychiatrists are experts at analyzing the complex questions of causation and accountability around mental illness and criminal behavior. Forensic psychiatry fellows learn to evaluate referred inmates and civilians. Some of their work includes writing a professional opinion concerning an inmate's consideration for a "Not Guilty By Reason of Insanity (NGRI)" plea. When an individual is unable to work with an attorney for behavioral or

Fig. 1.29 Relationship between stress, mental illness, and physical illness

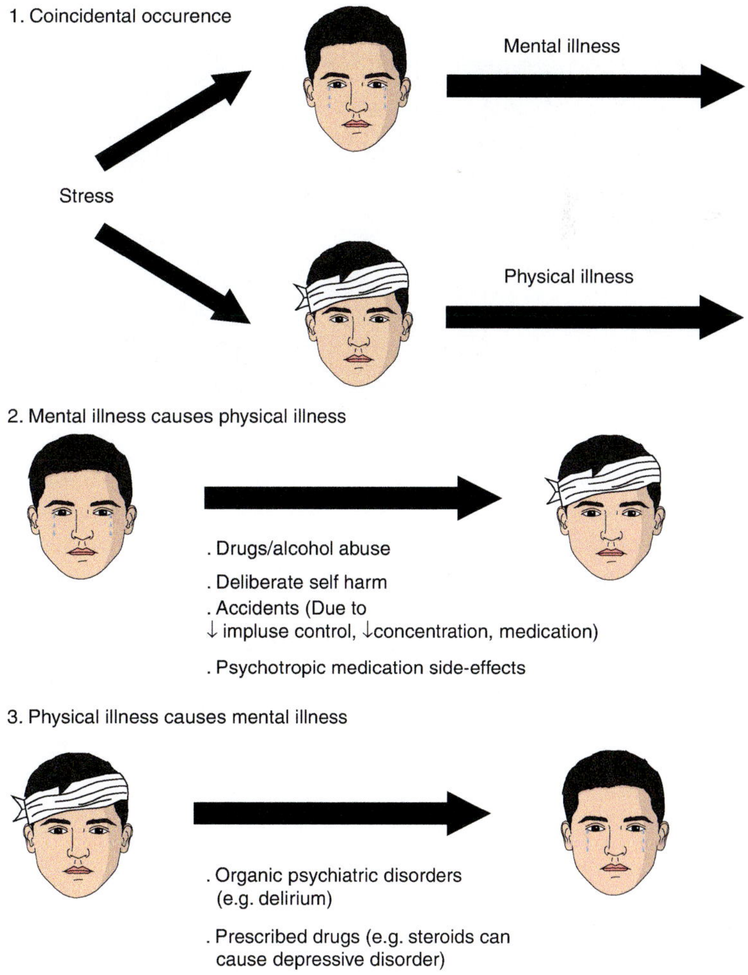

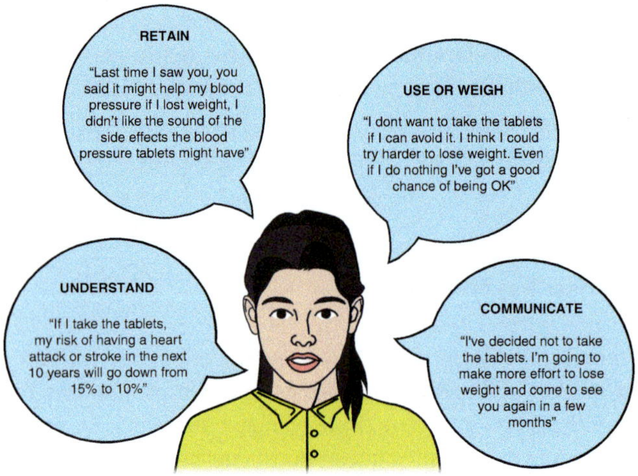

DO	PRINCIPLE	DON'T
Formally assess capacity	ASSUME PEOPLE HAVE CAPACITY UNLESS PROVED OTHERWISE	Assume someone lacks capacity on the basis of factors such as their age or diagnosis
Take the time to help people understand and make decisions. If they may regain capacity and it is possible to wait, then do so	HELP PEOPLE MAKE THEIR OWN DECISIONS	View capacity as a static phenomenon–it will change over time and will be affected by the way in which you communicate information
Base your assessment of capacity on how the person arrives at their decision, not on what they decide	PEOPLE HAVE THE RIGHT TO MAKE WHAT YOU THINK ARE UNWISE DECISIONS	Conclude that someone doesn't have capacity because you disagree with their decision
Use whatever means available to decide what the person would have wanted for themselves if they had capacity	WHEN SOMEONE LACKS CAPACITY, ACT IN THEIR BEST INTERESTS	Assume you know what is best for other people
Think about the least intrusive and restrictive means of achieving what is in the person's best interests	WHEN SOMEONE LACKS CAPACITY DO NOT RESTRICT THEIR LIBERTY MORE THAN IS NECESSARY	Do more than is necessary

Fig. 1.30 Elements of mental capacity

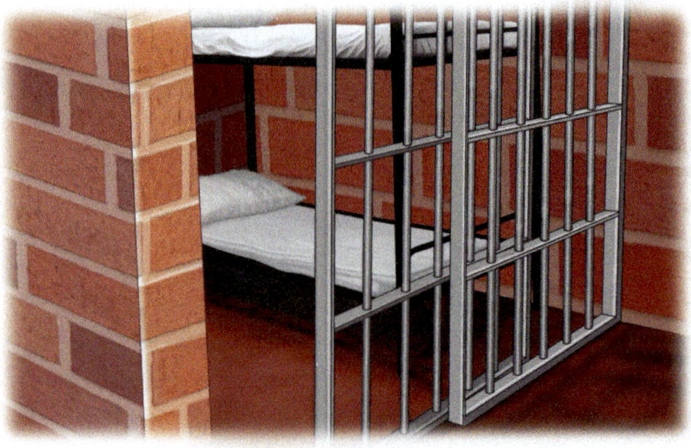

Fig. 1.31 Jail cell

developmental reasons, a forensic psychiatrist will evaluate for competency to stand trial. If a person is deemed incompetent to stand trial because of mental illness, they receive treatment and are periodically reevaluated by a forensic psychiatrist until competency is achieved. On the civil side, some of the things forensic psychiatrists do include disability, return to work, and testamentary capacity evaluations (Fig. 1.31).

Geriatric Psychiatry

It is estimated that about 20% of individuals age 55 and older have a mental health condition, including depression, bipolar disorder, anxiety disorders, or severe cognitive impairment [39]. Depression is not a normal part of aging and can increase the risk of suicide. When treating depression in geriatric patients, it is important to reduce sensory isolation, help with isolation and provide geriatric doses for medications. Figure 1.32 summarizes the management of depression in geriatric adults.

Men age 85 and older have a suicide rate of 45.23 per 100,000, approximately four times as high as the general population [39]. Geriatric psychiatry fellows are trained in the diagnosis and treatment of psychiatric and neurocognitive disorders of the elder. A strong emphasis is placed on learning to help families, patients, and caregivers manage mental illness and neurocognitive impairment in the aging population. Brain changes are normal as a person progresses in age; however, some changes, such as Parkinson's and other dementias, produce pathological changes. The following figures compare a typical adult brain to a normal geriatric brain and finally, compare all three to that of a person with Parkinson's disease (Figs. 1.33 and 1.34).

Fig. 1.32 Treating depression in older people

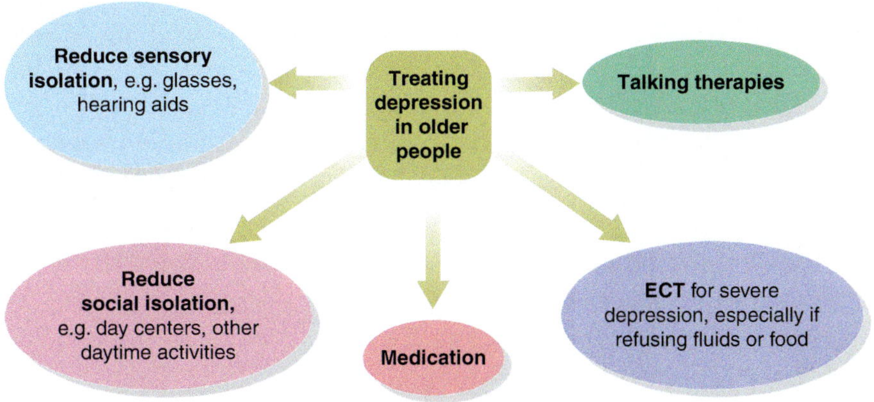

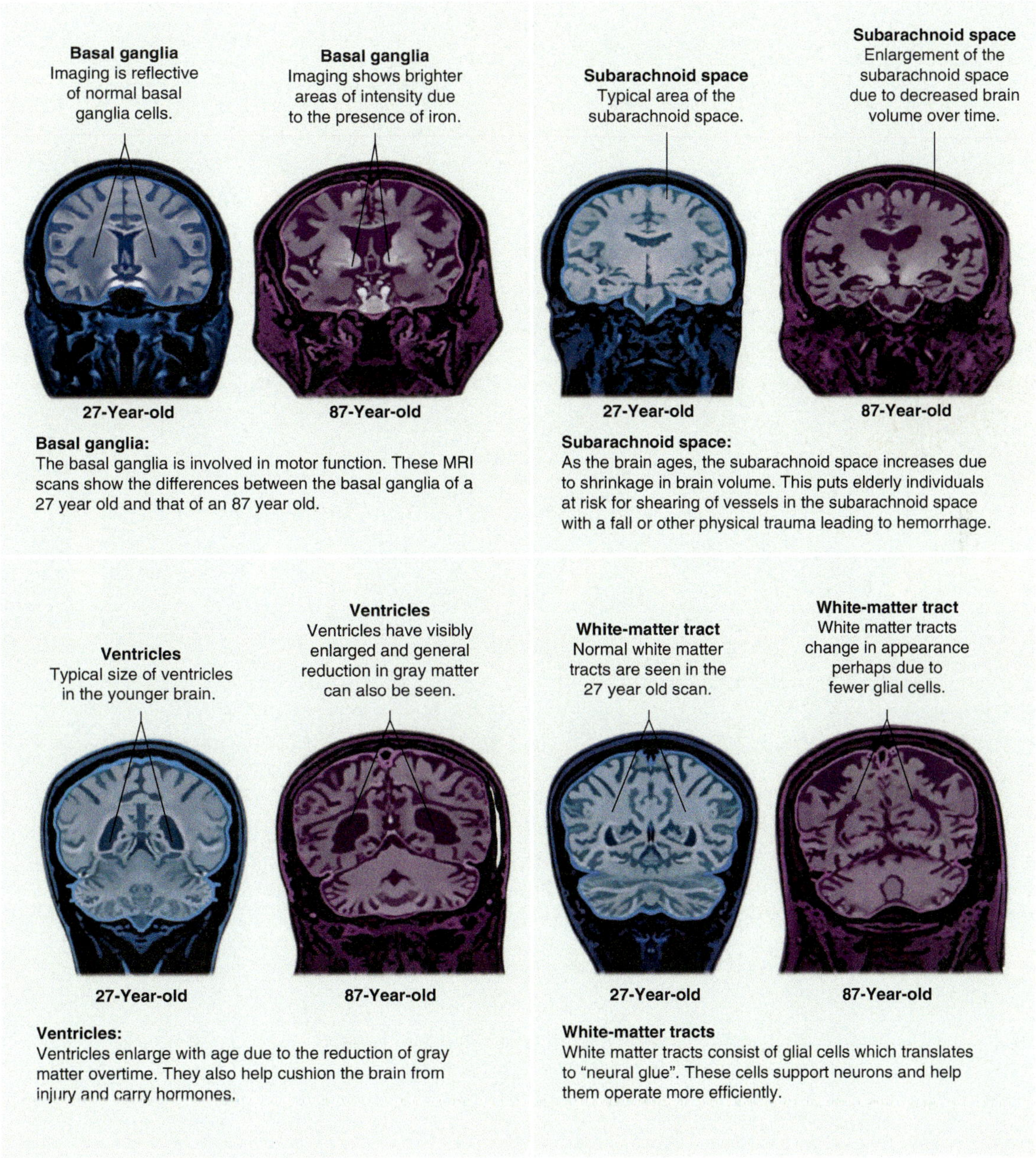

Fig. 1.33 Changes in brain structures with age

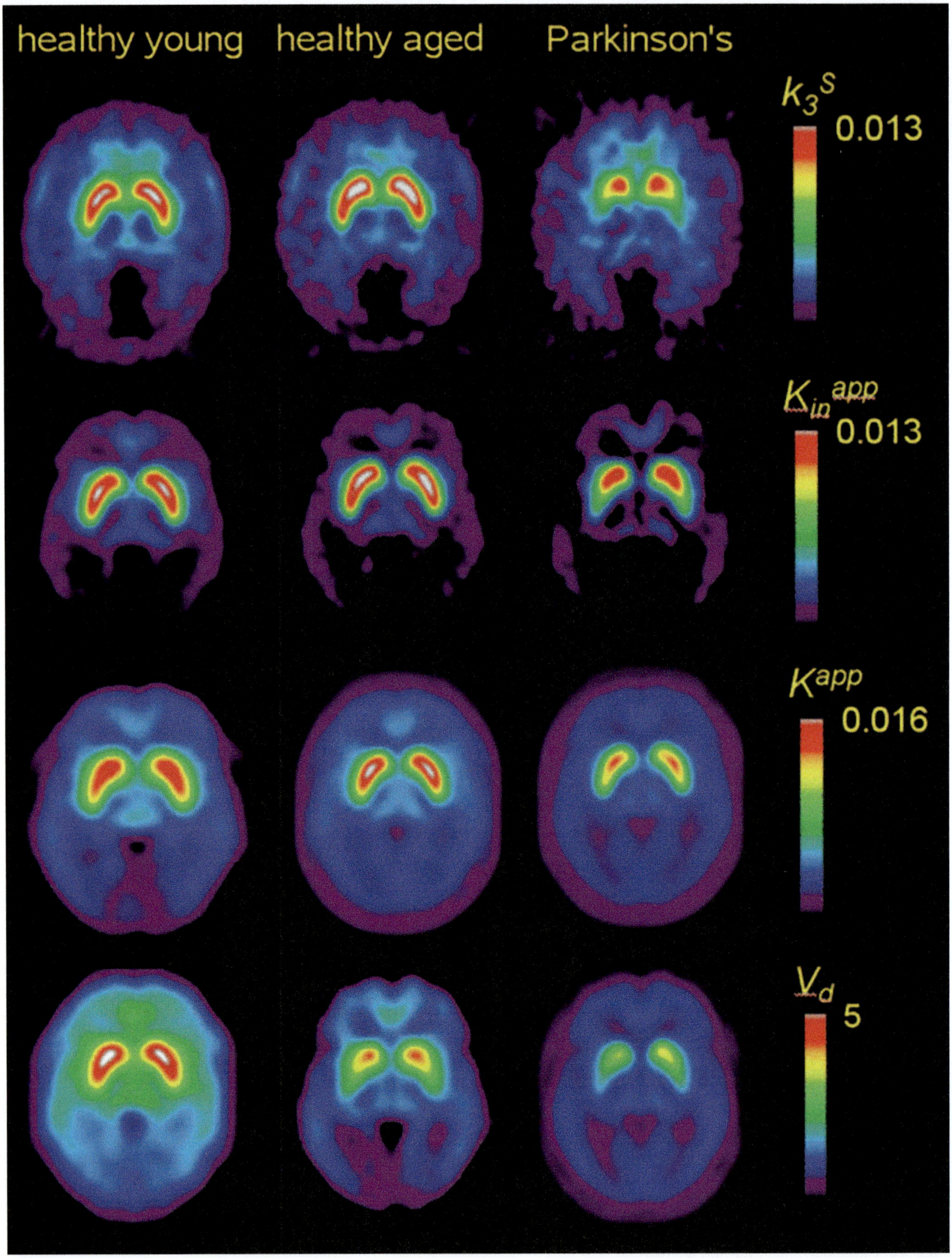

Fig. 1.34 Mean parametric maps of functional dopamine utilization differences between healthy young, healthy aged, and Parkinson's brain [40]

Future of Psychiatry

In addition to providing medication, psychiatrists also provide hope, guidance, and encouragement to patients. To enjoy a career in psychiatry, it helps to be empathic and enjoy talking to patients about their struggles. Overall, psychiatry is a very rewarding field where the treatment of one patient can provide direct relief to them, have a positive impact on their families and communities, and benefit generations to come (Fig. 1.35). For more about the future of psychiatry, see Chap. 25.

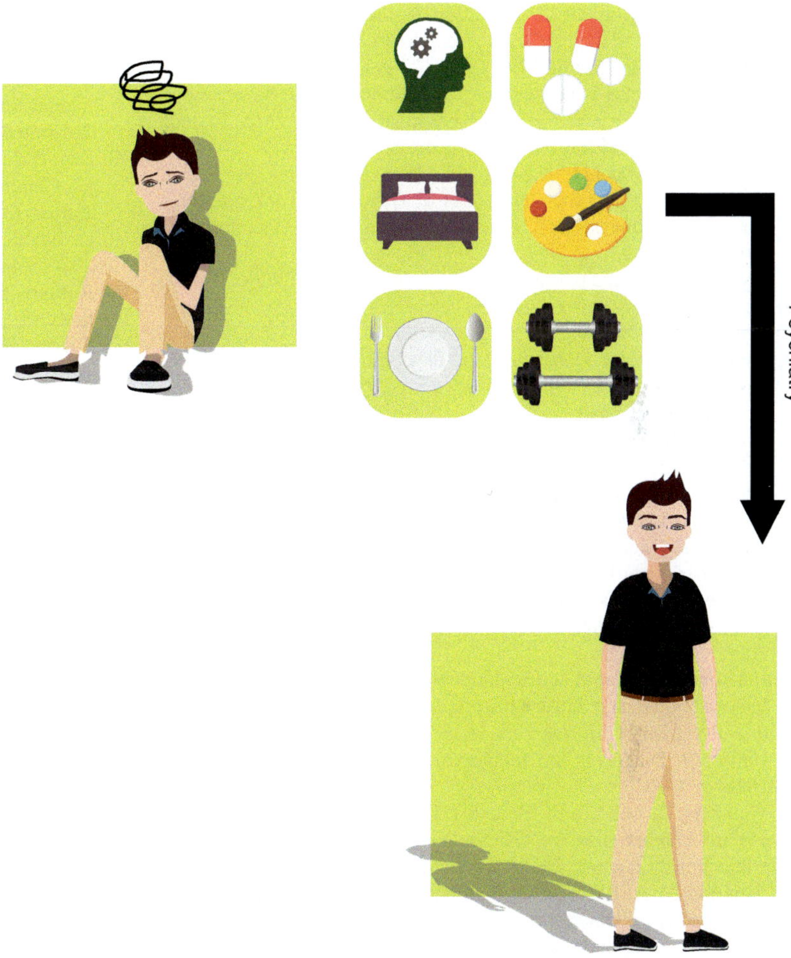

Fig. 1.35 Psychiatry as a tool to improve lives

References

1. Porter R. Madness a brief history. New York: Oxford University Press; 2002.
2. Bynum B, Bynum H. Trepanned cranium. Lancet. 2018;392(10142):112.
3. Wilson J, Reynolds E. Texts and documents. Translation and analysis of a cuneiform text forming part of a babylonian treatise on epilepsy. Med Hist. 1990;34(2):185–98.
4. G. d. Champeaux, I Simboli del medio evo, Milan; 1981.
5. Berchtold N, Cotman C. Evolution in the conceptualization of dementia and Alzheimer's disease: Greco-Roman period to the 1960s. Neurobiol Aging. 1998;19(3):173–89.
6. Rahimi M, Shokri F, Hassanian-Moghaddam H, et al. Severe camphor poisoning, a seven-year observational study. Environ Toxicol Pharmacol. 2017;52:8–13.
7. Dambricourt-Malassé A, Cao B, You Q, Zhang P. Agro-pastoral rituals and shaman dances of Dahongyan rock painting, Guizhou, southwestern China, new investigations. Quanter Int. 2019;507:43–52.
8. Myers D. Klinische psychologie: therapie, In: Psychologie; 2014.
9. Baxter W. American psychiatry celebrates 150 years of caring. Psychiatr Clin N Am. 1994;17(3):683–93.
10. Loyola University Department of Psychology. Clinical psychology program; 2020. https://www.luc.edu/psychology/graduate/. Accessed 5 Oct 2020.
11. Goldberg JF, Ernst CL. The psychiatrist as physician. In: Managing the side effects of psychotropic medications. Washington, DC: American Psychiatric Association; 2019. p. 3–45.
12. National Institute of Mental Health. Brain Stimulation Therapies; June 2016. https://www.nimh.nih.gov/health/topics/brain-stimulation-therapies/brain-stimulation-therapies.shtml#:~:text=Magnetic%20seizure%20therapy%20(MST)%20borrows,than%20that%20used%20in%20rTMS. Accessed 5 Oct 2020.
13. Hashimoto K. Rapid-acting antidepressant ketamine, its metabolites and other candidates: a historical overview and future perspective. Psychiatry Clin Neurosci. 2019;73(10):613–27.
14. Heldt MJ. Diagnosis. In: Memorable psychiatry. Jonathan Heldt; 2018. p. 3–15.
15. Weinberg D, Lenroot R, Jacomb I. Cognitive subtypes of schizophrenia characterized by differential brain volumetric reductions and cognitive decline. JAMA Psychiatry. 2016;73(12):1251–9.
16. Tamminga CA, Pearlson G, Stan A, Gibbons R, Padmanabhan J, Keshavan M, Clementz B. Strategies for advancing disease definition using biomarkers and genetics: the bipolar and schizophrenia network for intermediate phenotypes. Biol Psychiatry Cogn Neurosci Neuroimaging. 2017;2(1):20–7.
17. Clementz B, Sweeney J, Hamm J, Ivleva E, Ethridge L, Pearlson G, et al. Identification of distinct psychosis biotypes using brain-based biomarkers. Am J Psychiatry. 2016;173:373–84.
18. The Human Connectome Project. Neuroimaging and Martinos Center for Biomedical Imaging, Consortium of the Human Connectome Project; 2020. http://www.humanconnectomeproject.org/. Accessed 2 Oct 2020.
19. Osetreich L, Randeniya R, Garrido M. White matter connectivity reductions in pre-clinical continuum of psychosis: a connectome study, vol. 40. Wiley Periodicals; 2019. p. 529–37.
20. Carter R, Aldridge S, Page M, Parker S. The human brain book. New York: DK Publishing; 2019.
21. Jumah F, Dossani R. Neuroanatomy, cingulate cortex. Treasure Island, FL: StatPearls Publishing; 2021.
22. El-Baba R, Schury M. Neuroanatomy, frontal cortex. Treasure Island, FL: StatPearls Publishing; 2021.
23. Kandel E, Schwartz J, Jessell T. Principles of neural science. 4th ed. New York: McGraw-Hill; 2000.
24. Torrico T, Munakomi S. Neuroanatomy, thalamus. Treasure Island, FL: StatPearls Publishing; 2021.
25. Knierim J. The hippocampus. Curr Biol. 2015;25(23):R1116–21.
26. Peterson D, Reddy V, Mayes D. Neuroanatomy, mammillary bodies. Treasure Island, FL: StatPearls Publishing; 2021.
27. Shim R, Compton M. Addressing the social determinants of mental health: if not now, when? If not US, who? Psychiatr Serv. 2018;69:844–6.
28. Snyder-Mackler N, Burger J, Gaydosh L, Belsky D, Noppert G, Campos F, Bartolomucci A, Yang Y, Aiello A, O'Rand A, Harris K, Shively C, Alberts S, Tung J. Social determinants of health and survival in humans and other animals. Science. 2020;368(6493):eaax9553.
29. Robbins M, Howe-Martin L. Beyond the therapy dyad: the importance of systems and culture. In: Psychotherapy: a practical introduction. Philadelphia, PA: Wolters Kluwer; 2021. p. 211–36.
30. American Psychiatric Association. DSM-5® handbook on the cultural formulation interview. Washington, DC: American Psychiatric Association Publishing; 2020.
31. Brenner A, Howe-Martin L. Psychotherapy: a practical introduction. Philadelphia, PA: Wolter-Kluwer; 2020.
32. Lagan S, Aquino P, Emerson MR. Actionable health app evaluation: translating expert frameworks into objective metrics. NPJ Digit Med. 2020;100(3):1–8.
33. American Psychiatric Association. App Advisor; 2020. https://www.psychiatry.org/psychiatrists/practice/mental-health-apps. Accessed 5 Oct 2020.
34. SAMHSA. Substance Use & Mental Illness in U.S. Adults,; 2014. https://www.samhsa.gov/sites/default/files/infographics/nsduh-infographic.jpg. Accessed 3 March 2021.
35. Stanford Medicine News Center. Alcoholics anonymous most effective path to alcohol abstinence. 11 Mar 2020. https://med.stanford.edu/news/all-news/2020/03/alcoholics-anonymous-most-effective-path-to-alcohol-abstinence.html. Accessed 2021.
36. Taylor EH. Atlas of bipolar disorders. Boca Raton, FL: CRC Press; 2006.
37. Center for Disease Control. Overdose Deaths Accelerating During COVID-19 Press Release; 17 December 2020. https://www.cdc.gov/media/releases/2020/p1218-overdose-deaths-covid-19.html. Accessed 3 March 2021.
38. Stevens L, Rodin I. Psychiatry: an illustrated colour text. London: Churchill Livingstone; 2010. p. 16.
39. Centers for Disease Control and Prevention and National Association of Chronic Disease Directors. The State of Mental Health and Aging in America Issue Brief I: What do the data tell us? 2008. https://www.cdc.gov/aging/pdf/mental_health.pdf. Accessed March 2021.
40. Cumming P. Imaging dopamine. New York: Cambridge University Press; 2009.

Epidemiology of Psychiatric Disorders

2

William W. Eaton

Introduction: What Is a Case?

Epidemiology is the study of diseases in populations [1]. Some have simplified the definition to be the study of rates—i.e., the study of a fraction with a numerator including cases of disease and a denominator including the entire population [2]. The purpose of epidemiologic research is to estimate the burden of the disease on the population, to suggest clues to the etiology of the disease, and to help design strategies to prevent or treat the disease in the population [3].

Many diseases have a simple cause (e.g. a germ) and a straightforward and valid test as to the presence of the disease (viewing the presence of the germ in a blood sample), as well as a simple treatment (e.g., an antibiotic). If a disease is viewed as a distinct change in the function of the neurology and physiology of the organism, then it is clear that this strict definition of disease is not appropriate in psychiatry, where the more general term *disorder* is used for describing the illnesses. The complex nature of the target illnesses produces important problems for psychiatric epidemiology. There are five textbooks in psychiatric epidemiology [4–8].

One important problem is deciding which behaviors observed by the therapist or complaints reported by the subject should be treated as symptoms and signs of medical illness. Similar to blood pressure, there is a wide range of thresholds in psychiatric signs and symptoms, which require decisions as to when the disorder is actually present and when treatment is merited. There is added complexity for psychiatry because the co-occurrence of a range of different signs and symptoms at different thresholds will contribute to the decision as to the presence of a disorder. These complexities are an area where psychiatric epidemiology produces useful information facilitating a decision about criteria for the presence or absence of a disorder. In some cases, such as schizophrenia, the presentation of the disorder is relatively similar from country to country, as in Fig. 2.1 from the International Pilot Study of Schizophrenia (IPSS) [9]. The IPSS was one of the earliest international collaborative studies in the field of psychiatric epidemiology based on hospital admissions. The syndrome profiles for persons diagnosed with schizophrenia are similar in high-income countries such as Denmark and London to low-income situations such as Cali, Colombia, and Agra, India. For example, the psychomotor disorder is reported in less than 20% of patients in all five countries, but distorted self-perception is reported in more than 80% of patients in all five countries. For many other psychiatric disorders, the symptom profile is more complex and varies around the world, making it a statistical and clinical challenge to decide precisely how to define a case of disorder [10, 11].

W. W. Eaton (✉)
Department of Mental Health, Johns Hopkins Bloomberg School of Public Health, Baltimore, MD, USA
e-mail: weaton1@jhu.edu

W. W. IsHak (ed.), *Atlas of Psychiatry*, https://doi.org/10.1007/978-3-031-15401-0_2

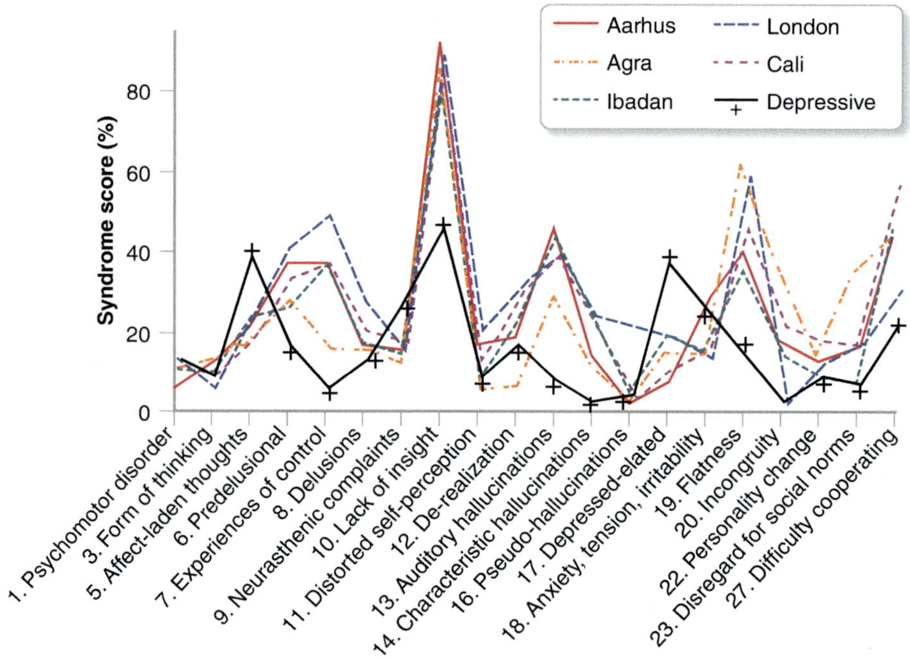

Fig. 2.1 International pilot study of schizophrenia. Syndrome profiles of schizophrenia for five countries

Prevalence and Burden

A central aspect of epidemiology is to estimate the burden of disease using prevalence data. Prevalence is the proportion of the population with the disorder at a given point or period of time. Table 2.1 shows a review of the prevalence of disorders over a single year [12]. The median prevalence ranges from 0.3% for anorexia nervosa to 9.1% for personality disorders, but it may be wise to be cautious about these two disorders where the median is constructed based on only six studies each. There are 42 studies on the one-year prevalence of depressive disorder and 25 studies of simple phobic disorder, with medians of 5.3 and 4.8, respectively. The range of prevalence is not small, with 50% of the studies (i.e., the interquartile range) of simple phobia falling in the range of 3.5–7.3, and the interquartile range for the depressive disorder being 3.6–6.5. The table illustrates several important principles of psychiatric epidemiology. First, there are large numbers of prevalence studies. Second, there is a wide range of results. Third, the prevalences are higher than for many medical illnesses, which helps to explain the large burden that mental disorders embody.

The mental disorders in Table 2.1 display considerable variability in prevalence estimates. Schizophrenia is unusual in having a relatively limited range of prevalence estimates, as well as a relatively unvarying symptom presentation, as shown in Fig. 2.1 [13]. Depressive disorder has much more variation in its prevalence, as shown in Table 2.2 [14], in which the 18 studies are all from the World Mental Health Surveys [15], using standard methods including the same survey diagnostic instrument (Composite International Diagnostic Instrument, or CIDI) across different populations [16]. There is a fivefold variation in prevalence from 2.2% in Japan to 10.4% in Sao Paulo, Brazil. There is little evidence of variation by national income level, but some evidence for regional variation in that the two lowest rates are both in East Asia (Japan and Shenzen, China), possibly due to cultural variation in the presentation of symptoms [17]. It could also be that etiologic factors differ around the world, producing differences in rates of disorder. Despite the variation in prevalence, there is remarkable consistency in the age of onset, with a median between 20 and 30 years in nearly all countries.

Table 2.1 Review of the prevalence in percent of 12 mental disorders

Disorder	Median one year prevalence	Interquartile range	Number of studies
Disorders in children			
Attention deficit hyperactivity	0.5	0.2–0.9	19
Conduct disorder	2.3	1.9–3.3	22
Anorexia nervosa	0.3	0.2-0.3	6
Disorders in adults			
Panic	0.9	0.6–1.9	33
Social phobic	2.8	1.1–5.8	30
Simple phobic	4.8	3.5–7.3	25
Obsessive compulsive	1.0	0.6–2.0	19
Post-traumatic stress	2.2	1.2–5.0	4
Major depressive	5.3	3.6–6.5	42
Personality disorders	9.1	9.0–14.4	6
Schizophrenia	0.5	0.3–0.6	23
Bipolar	0.6	0.3–1.1	16

From Eaton et al. [12]; with permission

Table 2.2 Prevalence and age of onset of depressive disorder in world mental health surveys

	One year prevalence (%)	Age of onset median (IQR)
High-Income Countries		
Japan	2.2	30.1 (20.8–45.3
Italy	3.0	27.7 (19.1–39.1)
Germany	3.0	27.6 (18.6–39.6)
Spain	4.0	30.0 (19.7–44.3)
Netherlands	4.9	27.2 (19.3–39.5)
Belgium	5.0	29.4 (20.9–41.3)
France	5.9	28.4 (19.3–38.9)
Israel	6.1	25.5 (18.1–38.5
New Zealand	6.6	24.2 (16.1–34.5)
United States	8.3	22.7 (15.1–34.6)
Low-Middle Income Countries		
Shenzen, China	3.8	18.8 (14.9–23.4)
Mexico	4.0	23.5 (16.7–34.0)
Pondicherry, India	4.5	31.9 (24.5–42.7)
South Africa	4.9	22.3 (15.8–33.8)
Lebanon	5.5	23.8 (17.5–32.8)
Colombia	6.2	23.5 (15.6–33.6)
Ukraine	8.4	27.8 (18.7–39.6)
Sao Paulo, Brazil	10.4	24.3 (17.2–35.8)

From Bromet et al. [14]; Creative Commons Attribution License (http://creativecommons.org/licenses/by/2.0)

The Global Burden of Disease (GBD) study uses epidemiologic data to estimate disease burden quantitatively, combining data on the mortality associated with illnesses, as well as the disability associated with them [18]. Epidemiologic data on the age of onset and life expectancy by age allows the calculation of the index of Years of Life Lost (YLL). Similar data on the age of onset, chronicity of the disorder, and disability associated with the illness allows calculation of the Years Lost to Disability (YLD). There is considerable variation around the globe in Years Lost to Disability from Depressive Disorder (Fig. 2.2), which results from its relatively early onset and enduring chronicity [19]. When the two measures (YLL and YLD) are combined the result is a general measure of the burden of the illness called the Disability Adjusted Life Years (DALYs). The estimate of disability is made by asking raters to compare the value of a year of life for a healthy person to the value of a year of life for a person with an illness. The result allows comparison of the burden of diseases with high mortality to diseases with low mortality but high associated disability.

An important effect of the GBD study was to reveal the importance of the burden of mental disorders. The study estimated that there were about 2.5 billion DALYs in the world population in the year 2015 (Fig. 2.3) and that about 7% of

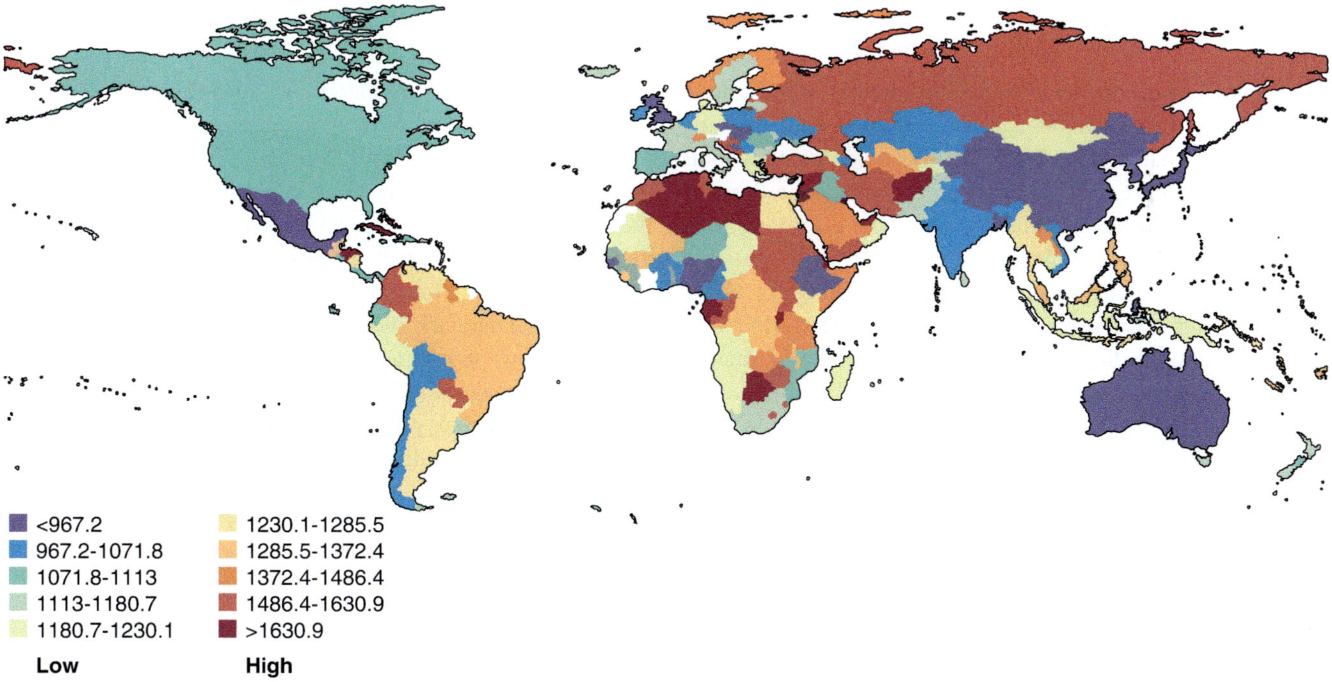

Fig. 2.2 Years lost to disability from depressive disorder by country

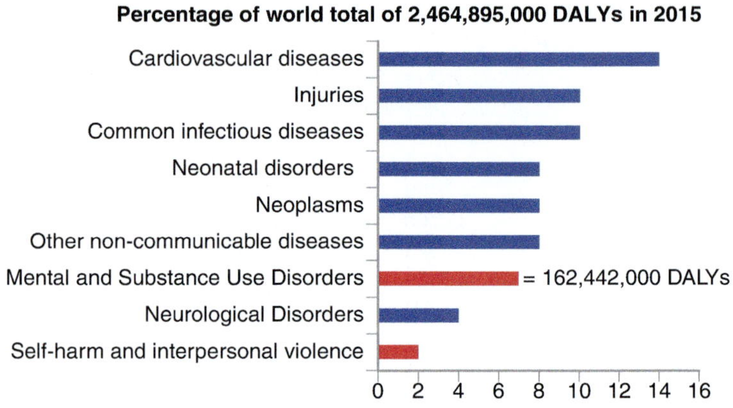

Fig. 2.3 World total of disability adjusted life years in 2015. Percentages due to disease categories

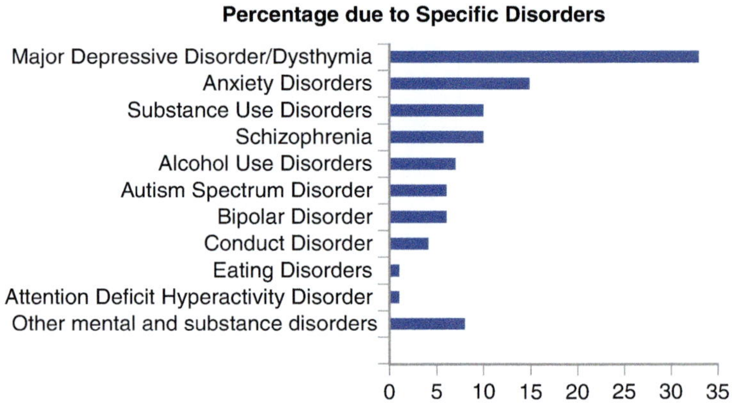

Fig. 2.4 World total of 162,442,000 DALYs in 2015 because of mental and substance use disorders. Percentages due to specific disorders

these, or 162 million, were caused by mental or substance use disorders [20]. Another 2% were accounted for by suicide and self-harm (Fig. 2.3). The most important mental disorder was depression, accounting for about one-third of the 162 million DALYs connected to mental disorders, with anxiety disorders accounting for about 15%, and substance use disorders and schizophrenia each accounting for about 10% of the total of the 162 million DALYs (Fig. 2.4).

Epidemiologic data on incidence and course of mental disorders provided crucial information for the GBD studies, and, with a few exceptions, these data were only available in the second half of the twentieth century, after longitudinal population-based studies were conducted. These studies have taken two basic forms of data collection: surveillance operations, supplying linked data on the use of facilities for the treatment of mental disorders in a defined population; and population-based surveys, supplying data from interviews with household-residing persons in the general population.

Surveillance operations are best for severe disorders such as schizophrenia, which almost always leads to referral to a medical professional or hospital. The best surveillance operations are in countries in which the entire population is able to get medical care without charge and where the nation is sufficiently populated with medical facilities. The prototypes are psychiatric case registers in Scandinavian countries which link the system of medical records across all types of facilities, such as is done in Denmark. Figure 2.5 shows the organization of record systems in Denmark [21], including the Danish Psychiatric Case Register (lower right). The validity of the clinical diagnoses in the Danish psychiatric facilities has been evaluated and is acceptable [22]. There are no areas in Denmark more than 30 miles from a medical clinic, so few people are missed. The population is large enough so that there are sufficient numbers of cases even for rare illnesses. The psychiatric register system has been operating since 1969, facilitating longitudinal studies. The superiority of the Scandinavian register systems is widely recognized.

Population-based surveys are best for disorders that do not always involve medical treatment or hospitalization, such as depression and anxiety disorders, where it is estimated that less than half of those who meet the criteria for disorder actually receive treatment [23]. Population-based surveys involve probabilistic selection of individuals in a defined population, such as people residing in households in a county or state or another area defined by the national census. The probabilistic selection allows generalization to the entire population of interest, with estimable degrees of error. In North America, surveys of the general population began

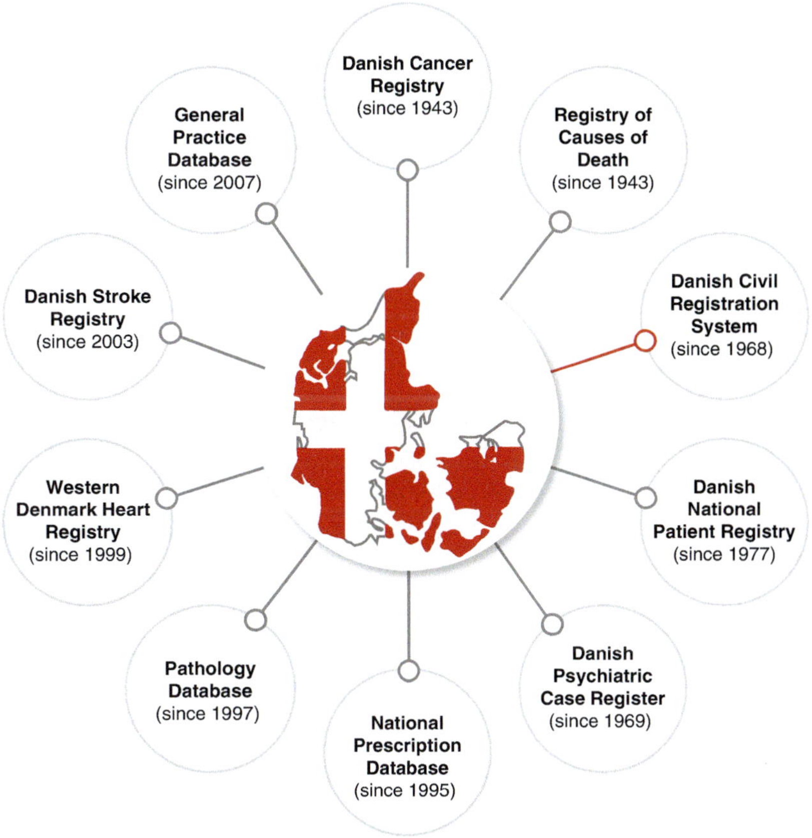

Fig. 2.5 Danish civil registration system

after World War II with surveys such as the Midtown Manhattan Study [24] and the Stirling County Study in Atlantic Canada [25]. The specific diagnostic criteria made available in the third edition of the Diagnostic and Statistical Manual in 1980 were implemented in population-based surveys, using interviews that could generate diagnoses, starting with the use of the Diagnostic Interview Schedule in the NIMH Epidemiologic Catchment Area (ECA) study [26]. This new generation of surveys provided the range of prevalence estimates shown in Tables 2.1 and 2.2.

Incidence and Life Course

Incidence is the rate at which new cases of the disorder occur in a known population during a defined period of time. It is used to study the risk of disorders and is a measure of the force of morbidity in the population. Unlike many physical illnesses, psychiatric disorders occur during many years of the life course and are strongly influenced by social factors whose importance varies during the life course (Fig. 2.6) [27]. The importance of the life course was recognized at about the same time as the population-based surveys were implemented. As the figure shows, different social fields are connected to major life changes at different stages of the life course. The major life changes can influence the onset of the disorders. For example, middle childhood may be a period when emotional or sexual abuse occurs in the context of the family of orientation, raising the risk for the entire range of later disorders. Early adulthood is associated with vocational choice and marriage, during which stresses occur. Epidemiologists have recognized the difficulty in studying slow-acting causal factors for mental disorders with the concept of the "induction period" or the "etiologically relevant period" as shown in Fig. 2.7 [28, 29]. The time between the first action of a cause is divided into the induction period when the future occurrence of the disorder is not predicted with perfect accuracy and the period of latency when the outcome is certain, but the clinical presentation is not complete. Precursors are signs and symptoms that may or may not be visible but predict the future occurrence, whereas prodromal signs and symptoms indicate the disorder will eventually appear in full. Fig. 2.8 represents this process empirically with data on schizophrenia from the Heidelberg psychiatric register [30]. These data show that the prodrome begins with the presentation of negative symptoms and then, about 5 years later, positive symptoms, which precipitate hospital admission. Many psychiatric disorders have induction periods of years or even decades in length, maximizing the importance of long-term studies which follow cohorts of the population over time. Maintaining contact with a population-based cohort over decades is expensive and difficult for disorders in

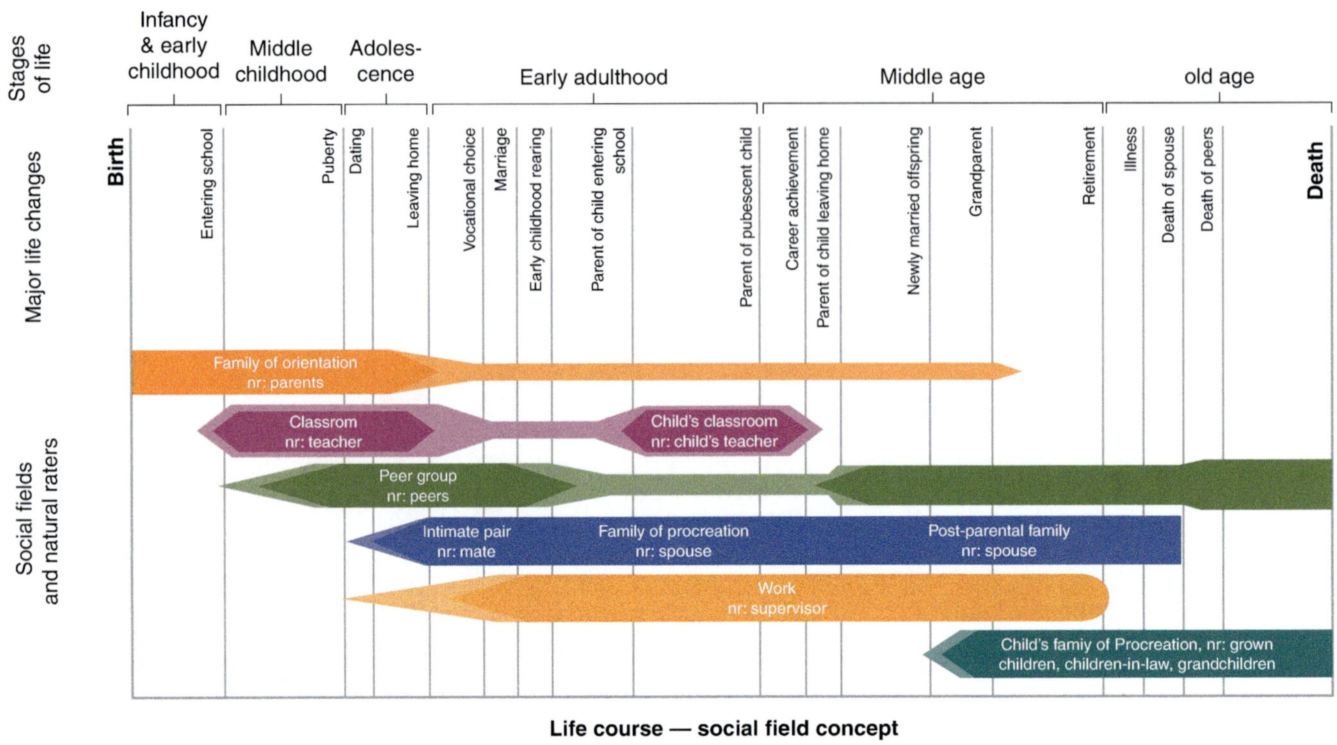

Fig. 2.6 Lifecourse framework for the study of mental disorders (From Kellam [27]; with permission)

Fig. 2.7 Etiologically relevant period

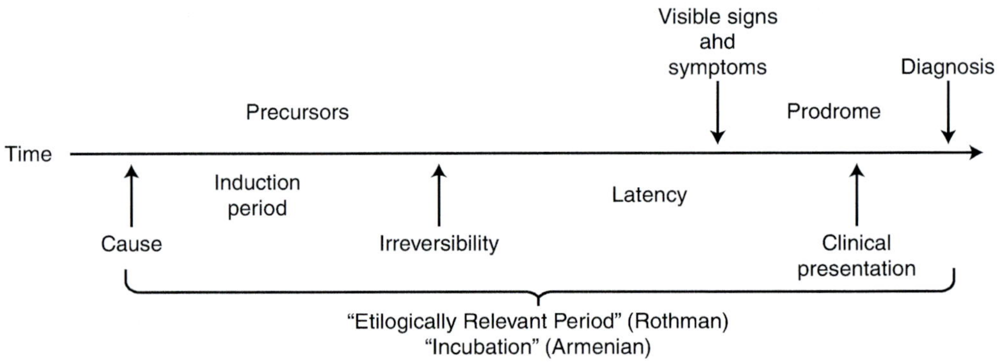

Fig. 2.8 Prodrome of schizophrenia

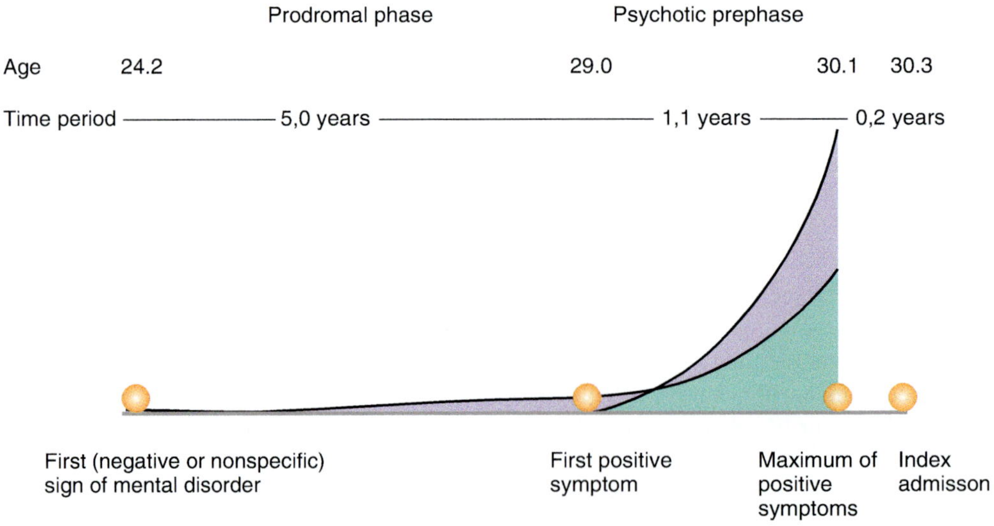

which treatment is often not sought. Three exemplary cohort studies are the Avon Longitudinal Study of Parents and Children (ALSPAC) in England [31], the Baltimore ECA [32], and the Dunedin study in New Zealand [33].

The beginning signs and symptoms of many mental disorders occurs in young adulthood (Fig. 2.9) [34]. There is an early peak for males (solid blue line) at about age 10 (mostly childhood behavioral disorders) with a second peak at about age 20 (dominated by mood and anxiety disorders but including schizophrenia), and the third peak in incidence in old age, dominated by disorders of cognitive decline. The early peaks amount to about 1% annual incidence (i.e., ordinate on the left, about 80 with new onset during each year per 10,000 person-years of exposure. The cumulation of new onsets adds to the cumulative incidence proportion (dotted line, with ordinate on the right), which totals more than 30% by the end of life. The curves for females (orange lines) have a similar shape but slightly higher first lifetime and cumulative incidence.

Epidemiologists use incidence data to discern etiologic patterns which may help in developing possibilities for prevention or treatment. Psychiatric disorders are presumed to include a range of etiologic pathways, including genetics, biology, immune system, and social and physical environment, which interact and combine in complex ways (Fig. 2.10) [35]. Even just the pattern of the age of onset can suggest varying etiologic systems. For example, the pattern

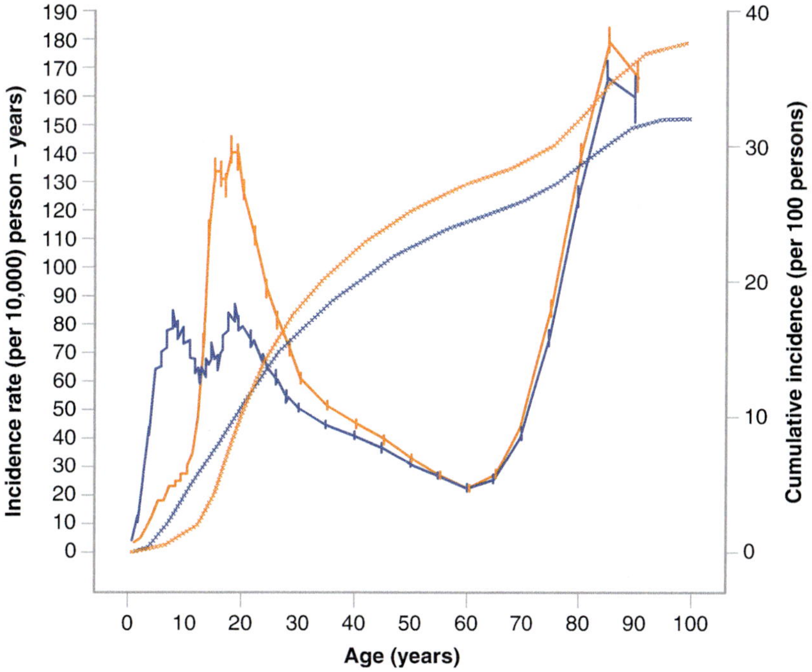

Fig. 2.9 First lifetime and cumulative incidence of any mental disorder

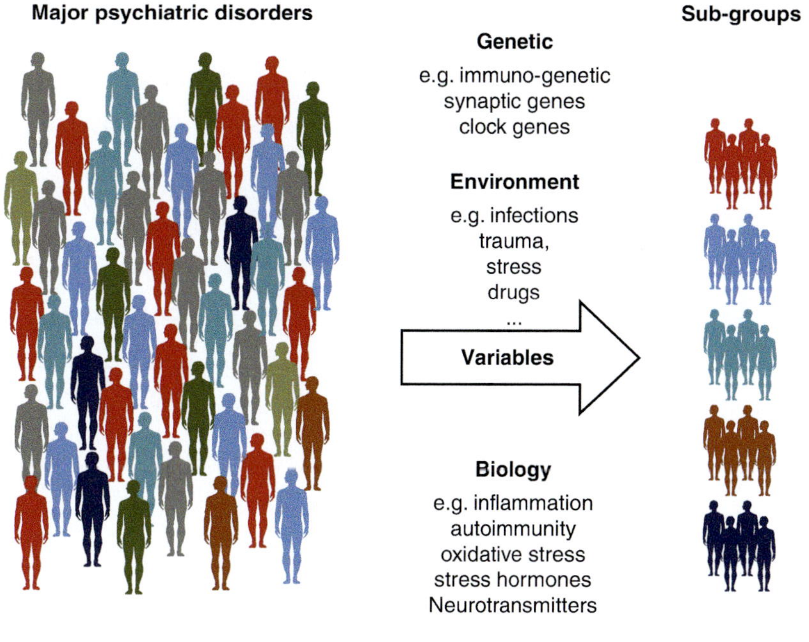

Fig. 2.10 Heterogeneity of psychiatric diagnoses

of the age of onset for depressive disorder appears to have two peaks—one in early adulthood, and one in later life. This pattern has been observed in data originating from surveillance operations like the Danish register [34] (Fig. 2.11a) as well as data from population-based surveys such as the Baltimore ECA [36] (Fig. 2.11b). There is rough consistency in the estimates of incidence for the two sources of data (about 3/1000 per year), as well as for the shapes of the curves, even though the curve from the surveillance method is based on about 59 million person-years of observation, compared to the curve from the survey method based on about 23,000 person-years of observation. The bimodality suggests two forms of depressive disorder, possibly with separate etiologies (discussed below in the section on comorbidity). Depressive disorder with an incidence in early life may be influenced by the stresses occurring during young adulthood, whereas depressive disorder with an incidence in later life has been termed "vascular" depression, possibly associated with inflammation and immune system disturbances occurring later [37].

Risk factors are evaluated by the Relative Risk, that is, a fraction comparing the incidence rate in a group exposed to

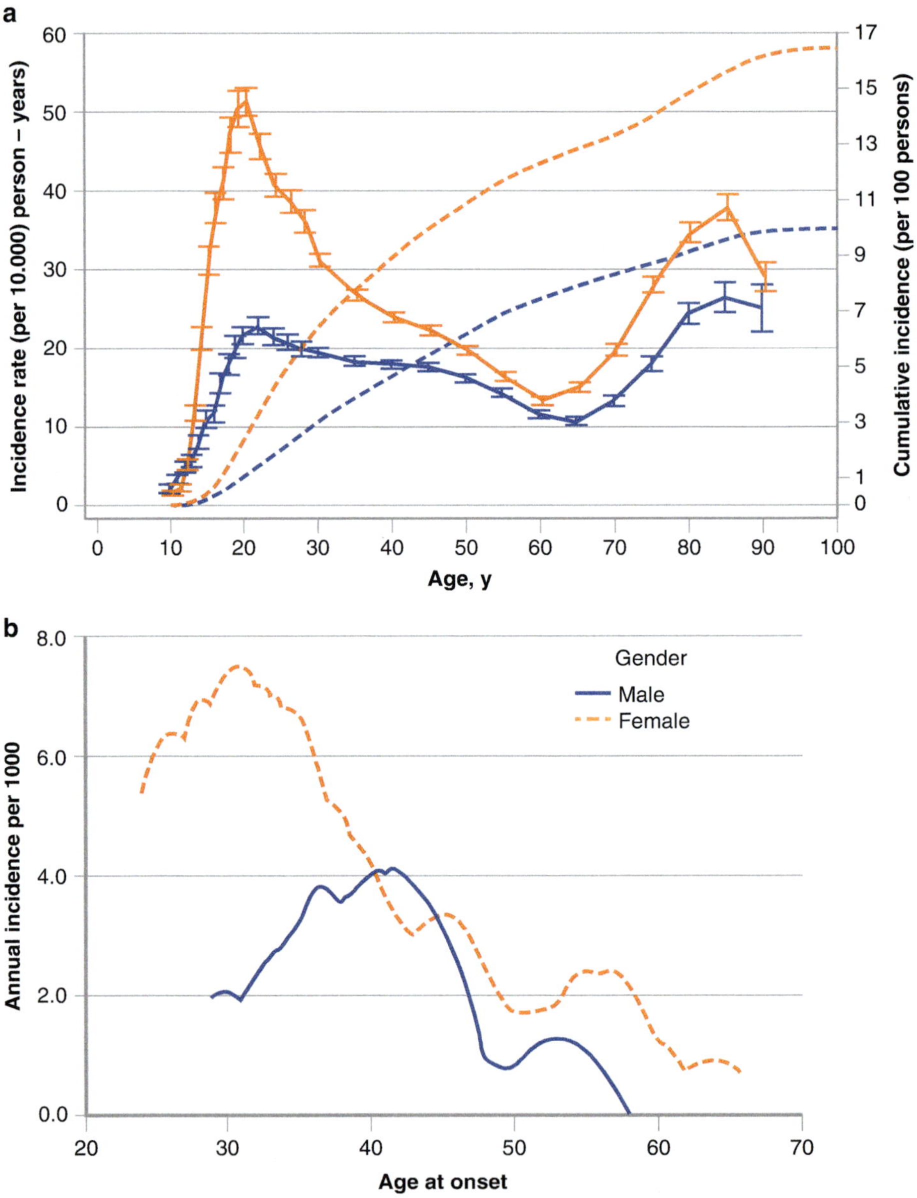

Fig. 2.11 Life course pattern of incidence for depressive disorder. (**a**) Denmark, 2000–2012. 59.5 person-years of exposure. (**b**) Baltimore, 1981–1995. 23,698 person-years of exposure. (*From* Pederson [11]; *with permission*)

a risk factor to those not exposed. The connection of incidence data to risk factors facilitates the calculation of the population-attributable fraction, which is the proportion of the new cases that would not occur if the risk factor is causal and were eliminated. The formula for the PAF is:

$$\frac{P(e)(RR-1)}{1+P(e)(RR-1))}$$

where P(e) is the prevalence of those exposed to the risk factor and RR is the relative risk. The PAF is useful for evaluating the potential benefits of reducing or eliminating risk factors.

The PAF can be applied to signs and symptoms of disorders that occur before the disorder has reached full diagnostic criteria—that is, the prodrome. Table 2.3 gives examples for the diagnosis of depressive disorder, taking advantage of longitudinal data on incidence and relative risk from the Baltimore ECA cohort. The prevalence of the nine symptom groups is shown in the left column; for example, problems with sleeping were present in 13.6% of the cohort in 1981. The relative risk for incidence of depressive disorder, over the time period 1981–1993, in those with sleeping problems versus no sleeping problems, was 7.6. When these numbers are entered into the formula for PAF, the result is 47%—that is if the sleeping problems could be identified and successfully treated, nearly half of the onset of depressive disorder would be prevented.

Table 2.3 Population attributable fraction for depressive disorder

Symptom	Prevalence %	Relative risk	PAF %
Sadness	6.6	7.0	28
Loss of interest	2.2	3.5	5
Weight or appetite problem	10.4	3.0	17
Problems with sleeping	13.6	7.6	47
Fatigue	7.9	4.0	19
Psychomotor problems	4.4	5.3	16
Concentration	5.5	6.1	22
Guilt	3.2	10.4	23
Suicidal ideation	12.1	6.8	41

Genetics as a Primal Risk Factor

Reviewing the range of risk factors for mental disorders gives the opportunity to view the history of psychiatric epidemiology because several risk factors have been studied for more than half a century. Family background was one of the earliest risk factors to be studied (Table 2.4) [38]. The table includes 21 family studies of depressive disorder, showing that about 18% of "cases," that is, persons with first-degree relatives (parents, sibs, or children) with depressive disorder, also had the disorder, compared to 7.7% of the control group in which there was no depression in the first-degree relatives. The 25th–75th percentile (interquartile range) shows a relatively limited range for the results. For schizophrenia, the morbid risk in cases is only about 5%, but this is almost 10 times as high as the risk in the control population of 0.6%. The possible biological causes (DNA) of these results were discounted for many years with the argument that the family culture and socialization of the children were the sources of the higher morbid risk in families. However, several adoption studies were published in the second half of the twentieth century in which the families were completely independent, solidifying the argument that the cause was a biological transmission. Twin studies allow estimation of the percentage of the total variance in the occurrence of the disorder in the population, which is explained by genes, and these show that the additive genetic variance for mental disorders ranges from about 30% for depressive disorder up to more than 80% for schizophrenia.

The focus of genetics can be on single candidate genes, but this has usually proven fruitless because a single gene typically explains very little of the variance in the occurrence of the disorder. In the past decade, the availability of large numbers of cases and controls has enabled the study of the effects of the entire genome on psychiatric disorders in Genome-Wide-Association studies (GWAs). Figure 2.12 is a GWAs study of depressive disorder (so-called "Manhattan plot"), showing that 102 gene loci have statistically credible

Table 2.4 The table includes 21 family studies of depressive disorder, showing that about 18% of "cases," that is, persons with first-degree relatives (parents, sibs or children) with depressive disorder, also had the disorder, compared to 7.7% of the control group in which there was no depression in the first-degree relatives

Disorder	Morbid risk % in first degree relatives median (25th–75th percentile)		
	# Studies	Cases	Controls
Obsessive compulsive	17	7.5 (4.6–7.3)	2.5 (1.2–2.9)
Panic disorder	11	11.6 (10.3–14.8)	1.8 (1.4–2.5)
Major depression	21	17.9 (14.9–22.0)	7.7 (5.9–12.2)
Bipolar disorder	22	5.9 (3.5–8.6)	0.5 (0.4–1.71)
Schizophrenia	25	5.1 (3.6–9.0	0.6 (0.3–0.8)
Attention deficit/HD	13	24.1 (15.8–52.8)	3.5 (2.0–5.8)
Conduct disorder	2	28.0 (23.0–33.0)	4.5 (4.3–4.8)

From Zandi et al. [38]; *with permission*

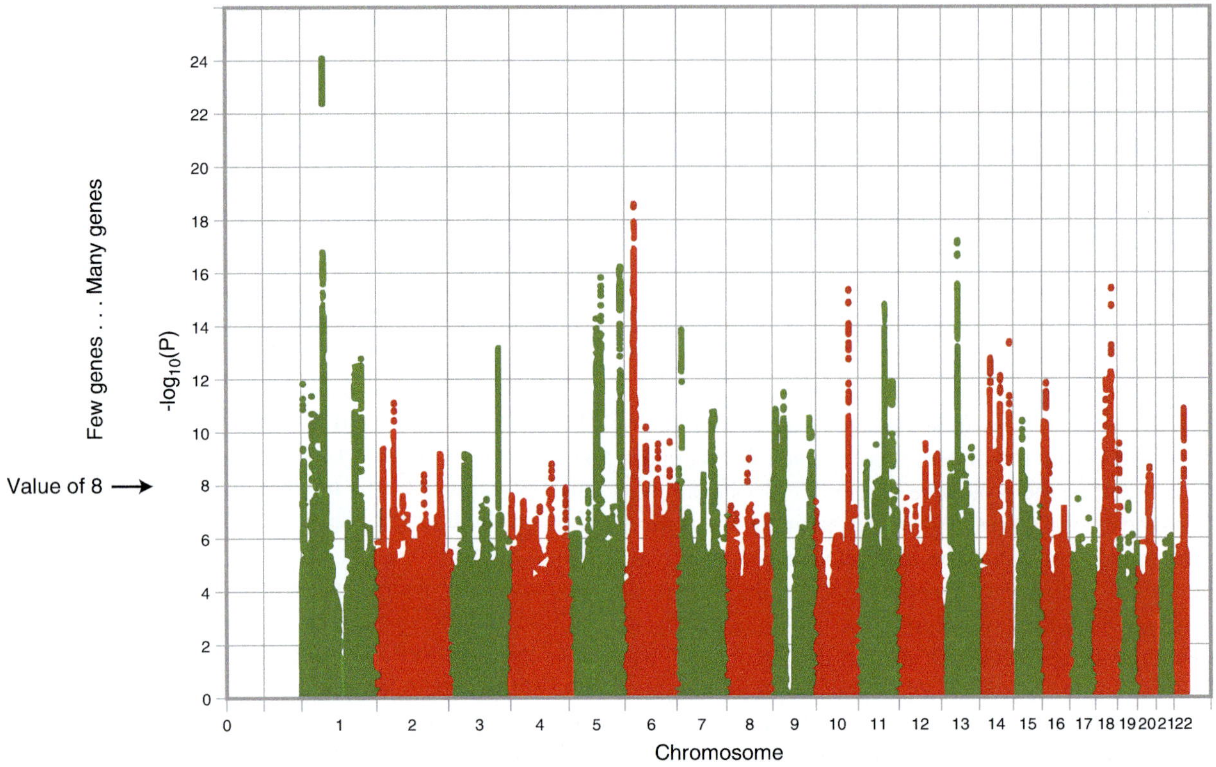

Fig. 2.12 Manhattan plot of depression GWAs. 246,363 cases and 561,190 controls. 102 loci identified

evidence of influence on the occurrence of depressive disorder [39]. The sample size is so large (246,343 cases and 561,190 controls, drawn from extensive cross-national collaborations) that even a tiny effect can be statistically above the typical value of $p < 0.05$, leading to the requirement of much stronger statistical evidence, as shown in a horizontal line with a statistical level of $p < 10^{-8}$ power. The analysis shows that 102 gene loci have an effect this strong (vertical lines passing through the line of 10^{-8} level). Even though these genes have only a tiny effect on risk, their location in the chromosome is interesting—for example, the strongest effect is in the area of the short arm of chromosome 6 where many of the genes are linked to the immune system. When all 102 genes are compiled into a score representing risk, the result explains about 20–30% of the variance—that is, much less than the predicted heritability from twin studies. This has been called the riddle of "missing heritability."

It is important to study the ways in which genetic background interacts with other risk factors. Perhaps the most common environmental risk factor is social stress. Figure 2.13 shows a simplistic version of this potential interaction called the diathesis-stress model [40]. As the genetic load (diathesis) on the individual increases, the risk for disorder is raised, as is the severity of the disorder for those who are above the diagnostic threshold. Some persons are in highly protective (stress-free) environments, and the disorder does not occur, even for those with high genetic loading. Likewise, there are persons with such low genetic load that even under high stress, the disorder does not occur (resistant individuals). The figure shows a simplistic additive model, but the concept of genetic diathesis interacting with the range of risk factors is applied to many situations.

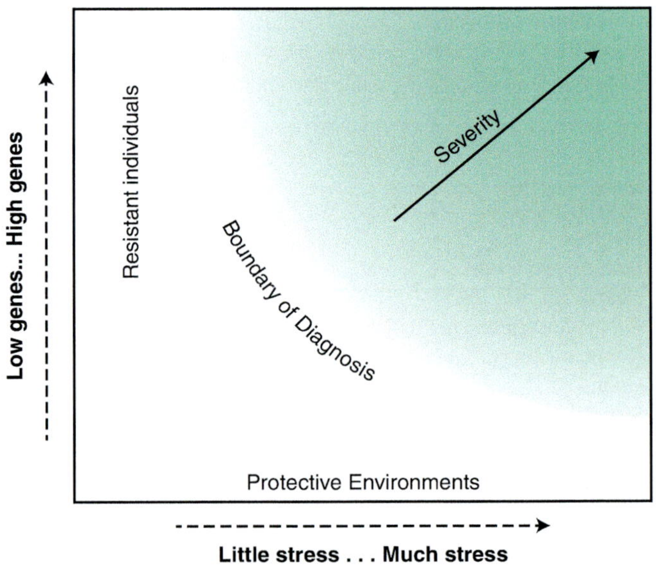

Fig. 2.13 Diathesis stress model

Risk Factors for Schizophrenia

It was noticed as early as 1929 that persons with schizophrenia had a slight tendency to be born in the winter (Fig. 2.14) [41]. Some researchers suspected that the effect was due to persons with weak memories choosing to answer the question about their birth near the passing of the new year, but this was contradicted by three studies in the southern hemisphere, where the winter occurs during June, July, and August. There are more than 30 studies, possibly because the data are so easy to collect (i.e., diagnosis and birth month, easily obtained from hospital statistics). The effect is small, amounting to an increase of about 5%, but was viewed as important, in part, because the cause was presumably due to

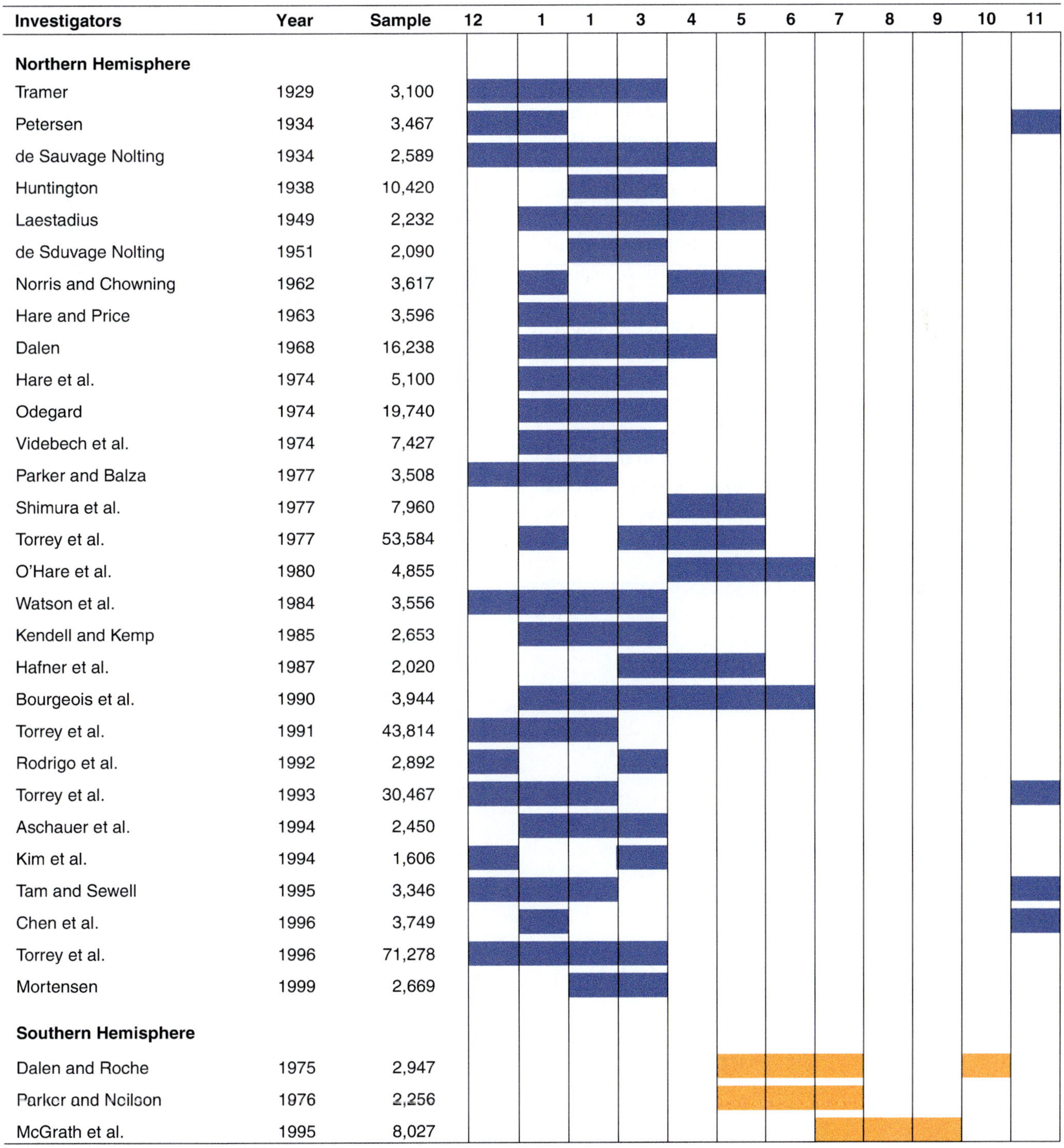

Fig. 2.14 Season of birth of persons with schizophrenia. Dark bars indicate months with increased risk

perinatal influences and was distinct from the genetic etiology. The explanation linking the season of birth to the occurrence of flu in the mother during the second trimester reinforced interest in perinatal origins of schizophrenia [42–44], which have been extensively studied in the years following many of the studies on the season of birth. Table 2.5 reviews many of these studies, revealing a range of pre and perinatal effects on raised risk for psychosis [45]. The research literature is strong: the meta-analytic review included 152 separate studies with 98 risk or protective factors. Table 2.5 focuses on risk factors, and some of the effects shown are strong (e.g., diabetes with relative risk greater than 5), but all of the effects shown are statistically significant at level $p < 0.10$ (selected from a much longer list of perinatal effects including many that were not significant in the review). These effects feed into a range of etiologic possibilities connected to neurodevelopmental hypotheses for schizophrenia [46]. In contrast, there is little evidence of perinatal complications associated with the risk of bipolar disorder [47].

The study of perinatal complications illustrates an important tendency in the study of risk factors: they often interact with genetic risk. Figure 2.15 shows that obstetric complications have a much stronger predictive power for measures of the brain associated with schizophrenia (e.g., ventricular size as measured by the ratio of cerebrospinal fluid to the whole brain) in those with high genetic loading for schizophrenia (e.g., two parents with the disorder) than those with low genetic background for schizophrenia (neither parent with schizophrenia) [48].

Another early risk factor for schizophrenia was urban residence, as noted in the classic Chicago study of 1939

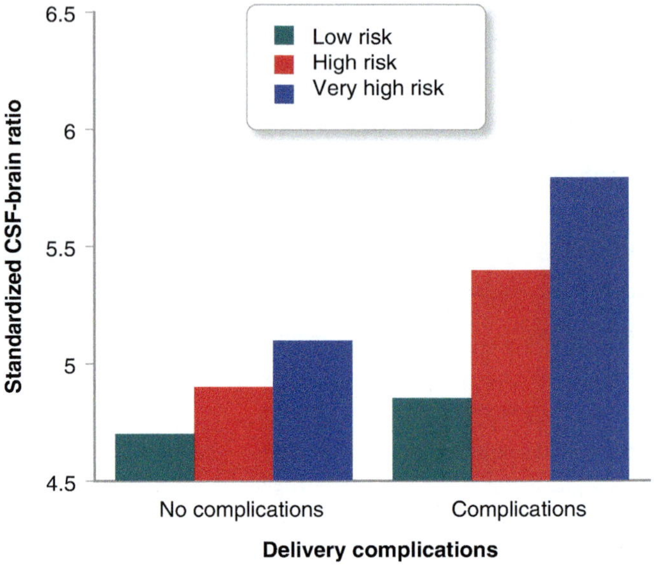

Fig. 2.15 Mean (+SEM) ventricular cerebrospinal fluid (CSF)-brain volume ratios, as affected by the interaction of genetic risk and occurrence of obstetric complications. Danish High-Risk sample: the very high-risk group had two parents with schizophrenia; the high-risk group had one parent with schizophrenia; the low-risk group had no parents with schizophrenia

Table 2.5 Perinatal risk factors for psychosis

Complication	Number of studies	Pooled odds ratio	Significance
Maternal age < 20	22	1.17	0.0004
Maternal age > 35	24	1.44	0.06
Paternal age < 20	11	1.31	<0.0001
Paternal age > 35	13	1.28	0.012
Previous births ≥ 3	10	1.30	<0.0001
Maternal diabetes	3	5.13	0.078
Fever in pregnancy	3	2.18	0.10
Suboptimum antenatal visits	4	1.83	<0.0001
Toxoplasma	4	1.30	0.022
Herpes Simplex 2	5	1.35	0.0002
Famine	3	1.61	<0.0001
Maternal hypertension	5	1.40	0.0058
Preeclampsia	14	1.32	0.059
Premature rupture	4	2.29	0.0013
Polyhydramnios	3	3.05	0.025
Blood loss during pregnancy	11	1.54	0.023
Rhesus incompatibility	9	1.42	0.051
Apgar score < 7 at 5 min	5	1.57	0.084
Aspyhxic state	8	1.93	0.0012
Premature birth	21	1.35	0.0016
Birthweight <2500 g	23	1.53	<0.0001
Small for gestational age	10	1.40	<0.0001
Head circumference < 32 cm	10	1.37	0.057

The risk factors are all those with significance levels $p \leq 0.10$. (*From* Davies et al. [45]; *with permission*)

(Fig. 2.16), showing higher rates of admission for those residing in central city areas [49]. A similar figure was created for Manic Depression (not shown), but the lack of a residential clustering led the authors to conclude that the residential pattern for that disorder was "random." There are many replications of this finding of urban residence for schizophrenia continuing to the present time [50]. The urban risk may be the start of an etiologic chain involving the brain, with epidemiologic data showing that persons brought up in areas of greater urban density have less gray matter volume in the dorsolateral prefrontal cortex (Fig. 2.17).

Fig. 2.16 Rates of first hospital admission for schizophrenia per 100,000 population in Chicago census tracts in 1927. (*From* Faris and Dunham [49]; *with permission*)

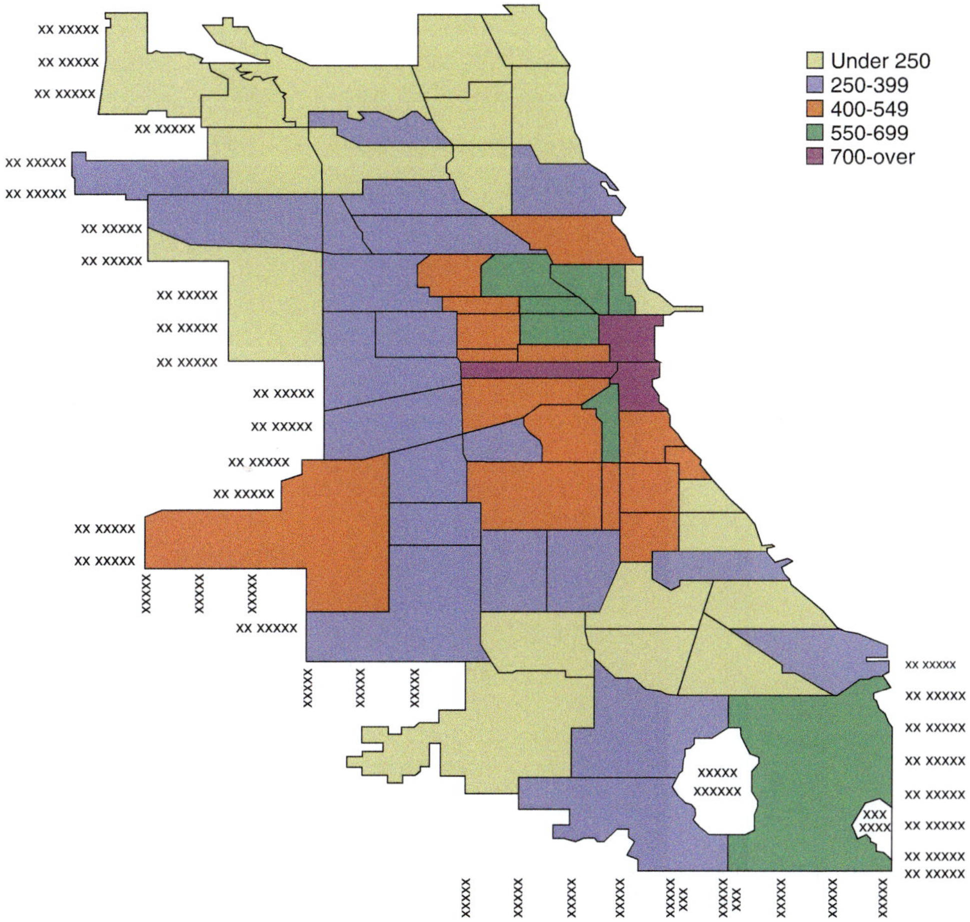

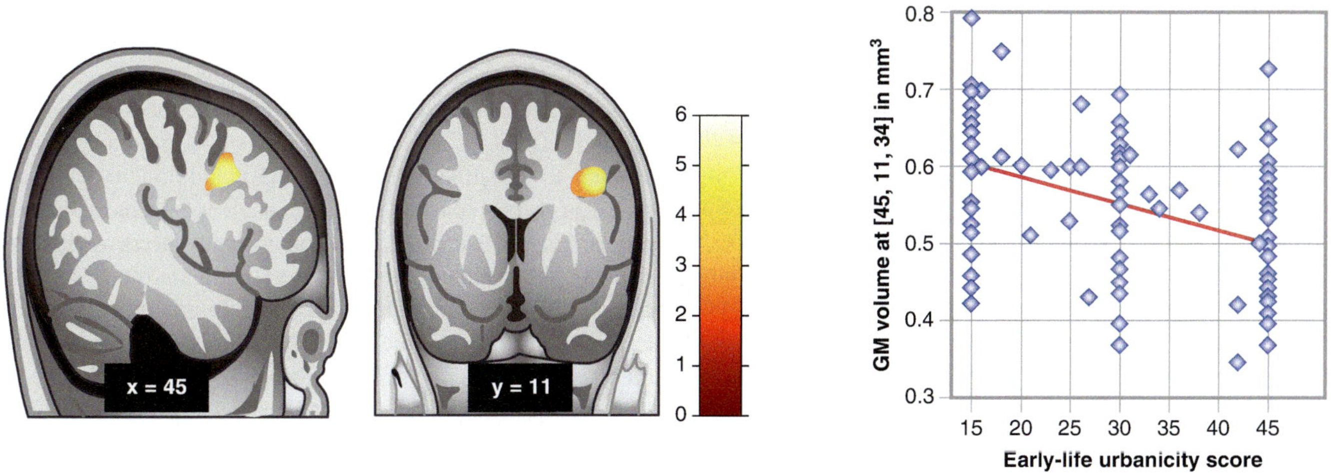

Fig. 2.17 Association of urban density during upbringing with diminished grey matter in the right posterior dorsolateral prefrontal cortex. Colors reflect the strength of negative correlation in brain areas, with significant correlations mapping to the right posterior DLPFC (yellow area). The scatterplot shows the relationships between grey matter volumes of the most significantly correlated voxel ($x = 45$, $y = 11$, $z = 34$) and early-life urbanicity scores. (*Adapted from* Haddad et al. [18]; *with permission*)

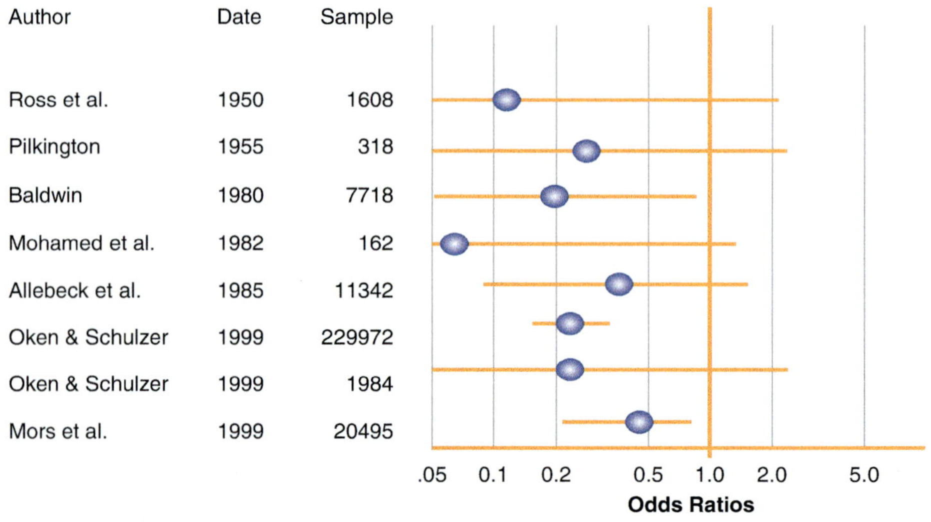

Fig. 2.18 Forest plot of risk for rheumatoid arthritis for persons with schizophrenia. Odds ratios (circles) and 95% confidence intervals (bars)

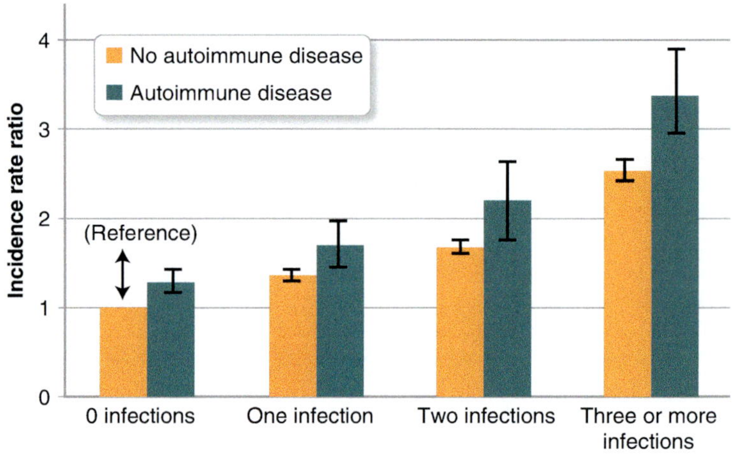

Fig. 2.19 Incidence rate ratios, with confidence intervals, of schizophrenia spectrum disorders in persons with a history of autoimmune disease, and infections, in Denmark, 1977–2006

For many years it has been well-documented that there is a lower risk for Rheumatoid Arthritis among persons with schizophrenia, shown in virtually every study. Figure 2.18 is a Forest Plot reviewing the highest quality studies, showing the risk for rheumatoid arthritis to be as low as one-fifth compared to the general population. Each line of the Forest Plot represents a single study, with the estimated odds ratio shown by the circle and the 95% confidence interval by the horizontal line [51]. Since rheumatoid arthritis is an autoimmune disease, interest has grown in the possibility of an etiologic chain for schizophrenia linked to the immune system. Figure 2.19 shows that persons with a history of autoimmune disease are at higher risk for schizophrenia and also that persons with a history of infections are at higher risk [52]. The predictive relationship of prior autoimmune disease to the incidence of schizophrenia is not affected by statistical control of other risk factors, such as the parental history of schizophrenia, urban birth, or parental wealth [53].

Risk Factors for Stress and Mood Disorders

As with the connection of season of birth, studied since 1929, to perinatal factors, studied in the past two decades, the connection of historical risk factors from epidemiologic studies in the prior century to new etiologic pathways in the prior decade is a current trend. Stress is the most commonly studied risk factor for mood and anxiety disorders. Stress is defined as the situation when the demands of the environment are perceived to exceed the capacity of the individual to respond [54]. The most common form of stress related to depressive disorder is the loss of a significant other, such as occurs in widowhood. One of the early epidemiologic studies showing the relationship of stress to the occurrence of mental disorders was the Midtown Manhattan Study (Fig. 2.20), a population-based survey in New York City [24]. This study included a generic measure of mental disorder, a quantitative measure of stress combined from several

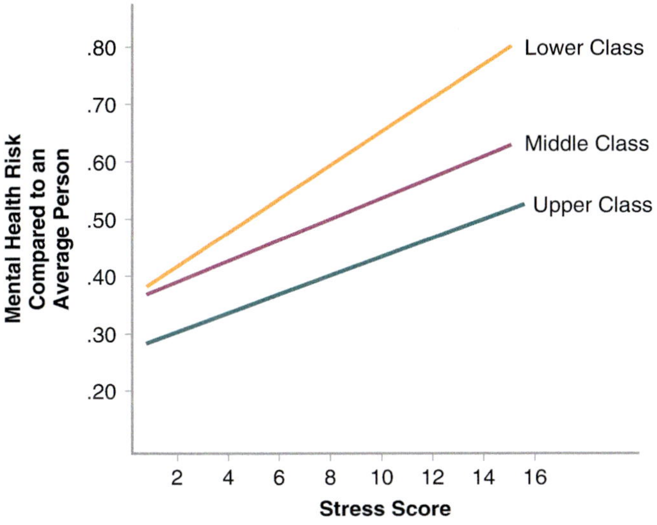

Fig. 2.20 Stress and social class in Manhattan

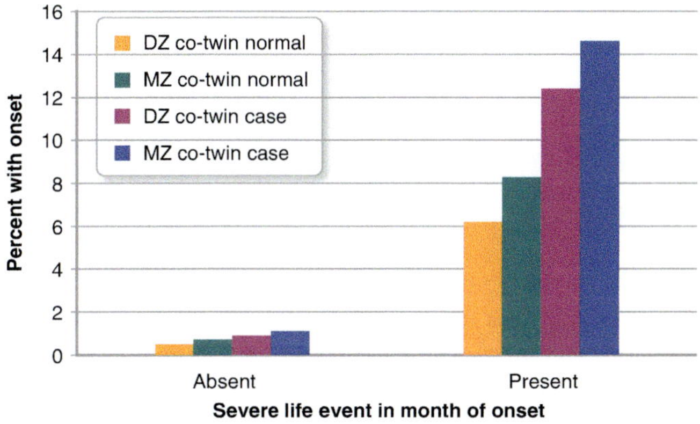

Fig. 2.21 Stress potentiates effects of heredity. Risk of onset of major depression per person-month as a function of genetic liability and the presence or absence of a severe stressful life event in that month among 2060 female twins

items in the questionnaire (on the abscissa), and a statistical technique called a RIDIT, which measures the risk of the disorder compared to the average person. There are three pieces of information in Fig. 2.20. First, the upward slant of the three lines makes it clear that an increase in stress is associated with an increased probability of mental disorder. Second, it is also clear that the risk for the disorder was higher among the lower class (yellow line for the lower class above red and green lines for the middle and upper class). The third piece of information is shown by the higher slope of the stress-to-disorder relationship for the yellow line representing the lower class. The implication of the different slope is that the lower class is somehow less equipped to deal with stress—possibly due to lesser material resources (e.g., money to pay a parking ticket) or to lower psychological coping ability (e.g., mental flexibility or self-confidence).

Stress interacts with genetic background in its influence on risk for major depressive disorder, as noted earlier with respect to the diathesis-stress model in Fig. 2.13. A simple example of this interaction is shown in Fig. 2.21, in which the effect of a genetic background predisposing to depression has only a minimal effect on risk for onset for those with little or no stress; contrasting with a strong effect of genetic background, and much higher risk for onset, if there is a severe life event in the preceding month [55]. A precise version of this interaction has been revealed in studies of the gene responsible for the serotonin transport in the nerve system. The short allele of the serotonin transport (5HTT) gene was identified as expressing this interaction (Fig. 2.22) in one of the most widely cited research articles in the field of psychiatric epidemiology [56]. The study was replicated many times, and the results were challenged in a meta-analysis of 14 studies [57], but then reaffirmed in a later meta-analysis of 56 studies [58], and yet again in a later meta-analysis of 81 studies [59]. The later meta-analyses were consistent with the original study, with a stronger interaction effect for the 5HTT allele and the occurrence of adverse childhood experiences than for adult stresses, as shown on the right side of Fig. 2.22. Table 2.6 shows the results of the Adverse Childhood Experiences (ACE) study, in which a score was formed expressing the degree of stress during childhood, including severe stressors like childhood sexual abuse, to less severe stressors such as marital separation of the parents [60]. The degree of stress experienced during childhood is highly predictive of depressive disorder, with about 15% experiencing a depressive episode among those with low childhood stress, compared to more than 60% among females and 35% among males for those with high scores of childhood stress. The importance of the effects of childhood stress is consistent with the second and third meta-analyses of the interaction of stress and the 5HTT polymorphism, in which the interaction is strongest for those with childhood stress and weak or possibly not existent for those with stress concentrated only in adulthood. This reaffirms the importance of the life course model in psychiatric epidemiology.

The association of lower class status with higher risk for mental disorder, including mood and anxiety disorders as well as schizophrenia, is one of the most consistent findings in the field of psychiatric epidemiology [61]. Social class can be measured by educational level, income, unemployment, or prestige associated with the occupation, among other measures. The social class level can change during the course of life, yielding two interpretations. The *causation* interpretation is that the stresses of lower social class increase the risk for the disorder, as shown in Fig. 2.20. The *selection* interpretation is that persons who will eventually have an

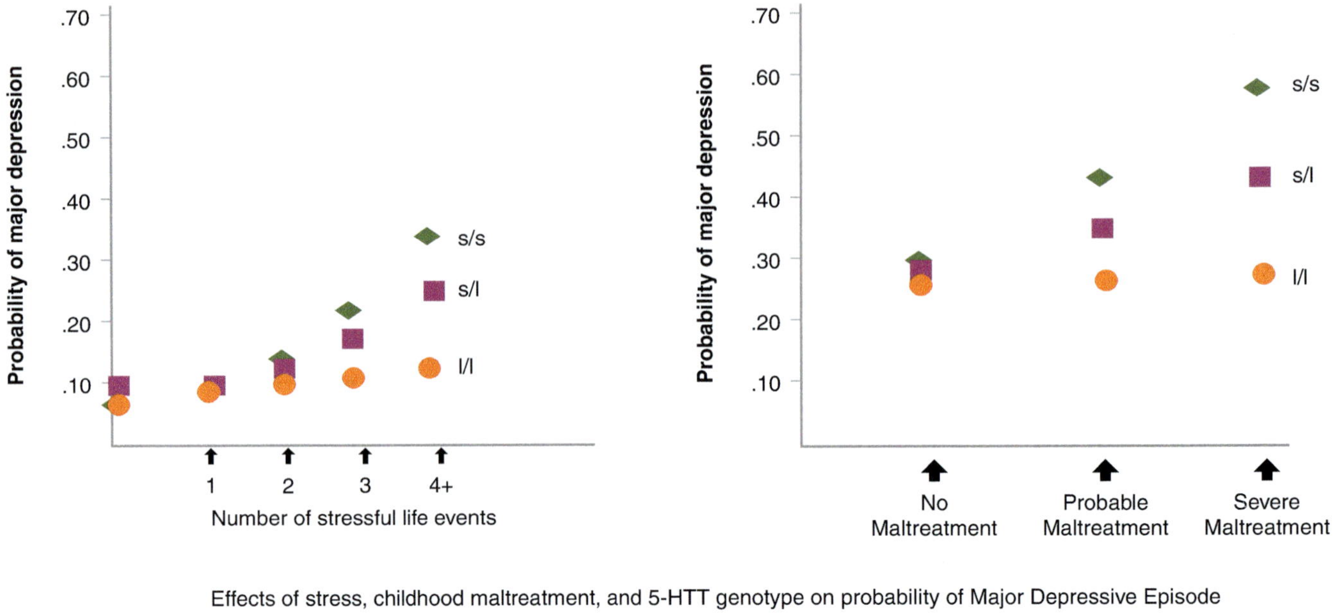

Fig. 2.22 Interaction of child maltreatment and short allele of 5HTT polymorphism. At risk for a major depressive episode as assessed by a diagnostic interview schedule. 1037 subjects in Dunedin, New Zealand

Table 2.6 Lifetime prevalence of depressive disorders

ACE	Males			Females		
Score	*N*	%	OR	*N*	%	OR
0	1823	13.8	1.0	1984	18.5	1.0
1	1256	19.0	1.4	1289	25.8	1.4
2	693	24.4	1.8	742	32.7	1.8
3	340	26.5	1.9	503	44.7	3.0
4	176	36.9	2.9	322	47.5	3.0
5+	96	35.4	2.4	236	61.0	5.0

ACE score includes emotional abuse, physical abuse, sexual abuse, battered mother, household substance abuse, parental separation or divorce, criminal household member, occurring prior to age 18 in 9460 members of the Kaiser Health Plan in San Diego

From Chapman et al. [60]; *with permission*

onset of mental disorder are disadvantaged in the competitive workplace and end up in lower-class occupations. The causation interpretation is more likely to be correct for mood and anxiety disorders which are more reactive to the occurrence of stress, whereas the selection interpretation is more likely to be correct for schizophrenia, in which prodromal symptoms may hinder upward social mobility. The causation interpretation has been applied to schizophrenia by the contention that the stress of formulating a *life plan*, involving complex and unavoidable decisions about future occupations and marital life, occurs during the prodromal period, raises the risk for schizophrenia, and is exacerbated for those in lower socioeconomic status during childhood and adolescence [62]. Data from Sweden in Fig. 2.23 show a higher risk for schizophrenia for those with a lower grade point average in school, which is consistent with the selection interpretation [63]. The results are different for bipolar disorder, in which there is a trend for a higher risk associated with a better grade point average. These results are supported by longitudinal data on employment status and the onset of schizophrenia, as shown in Fig. 2.24, where the rate of unemployment is higher for people with schizophrenia even as far as 15 years before their first admission [64]. The results on social class have been studied in relation to brain structure. Figure 2.25 shows variation in areas of brain volume and surfaces related to a neighborhood level of socioeconomic status (A), parental income (B), and educational level of the parents (C) [65].

A risk factor for schizophrenia that seems to defy explanation is that immigrants to England from Africa or the Caribbean have much higher rates than the general population in England, as shown in Fig. 2.26. The figure shows results from 19 separate studies, all consistently showing higher relative risk for afro-Caribbean immigrants, with a range of relative risk as high as 19. While it might be due to the lower class status of these immigrants, the finding is not

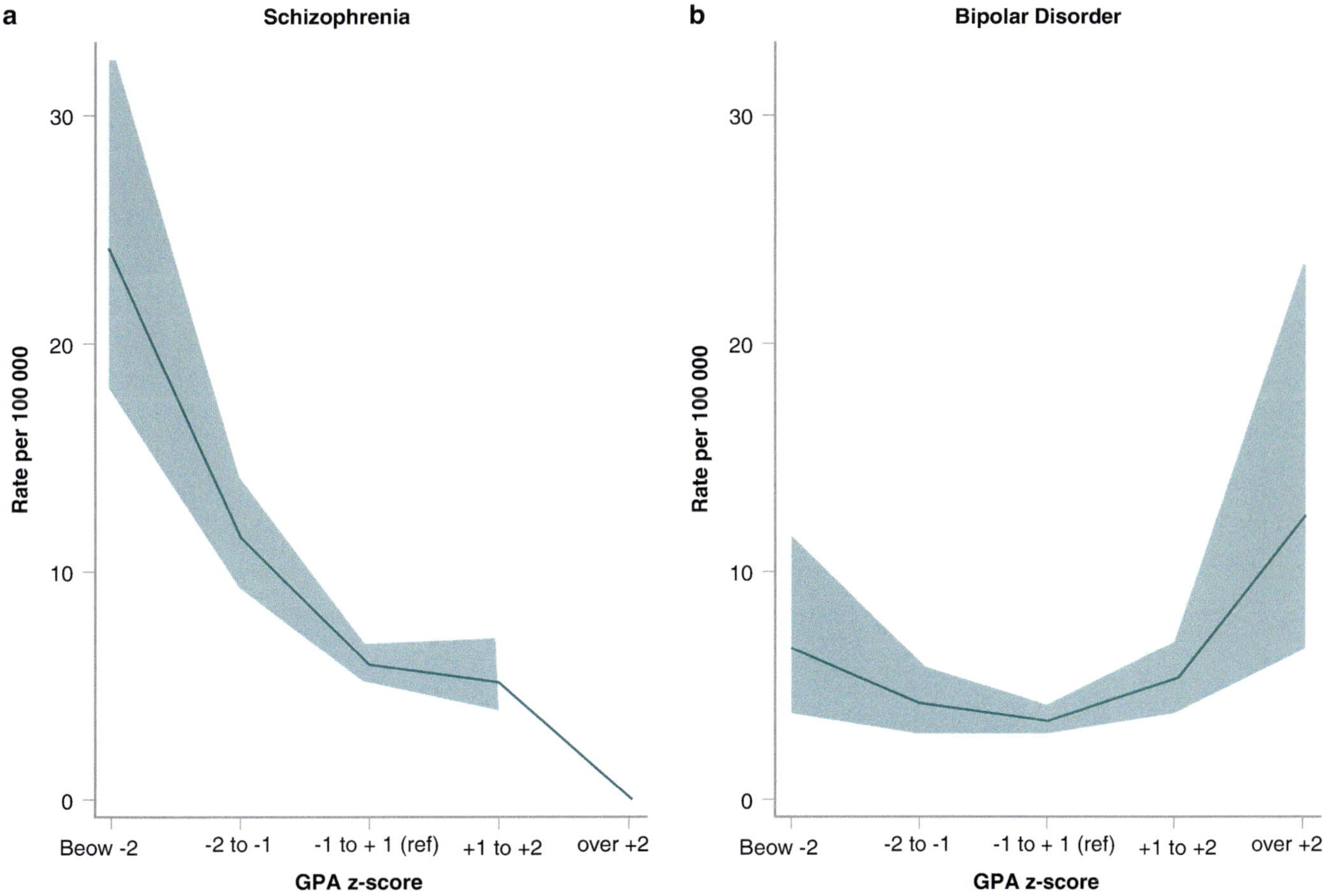

Fig. 2.23 School achievement (grade point average) and risk for schizophrenia (**a**) and bipolar disorder (**b**) students age 15–16 in Sweden; hospital admission age 17–31. (Shaded areas indicate 95% confidence intervals)

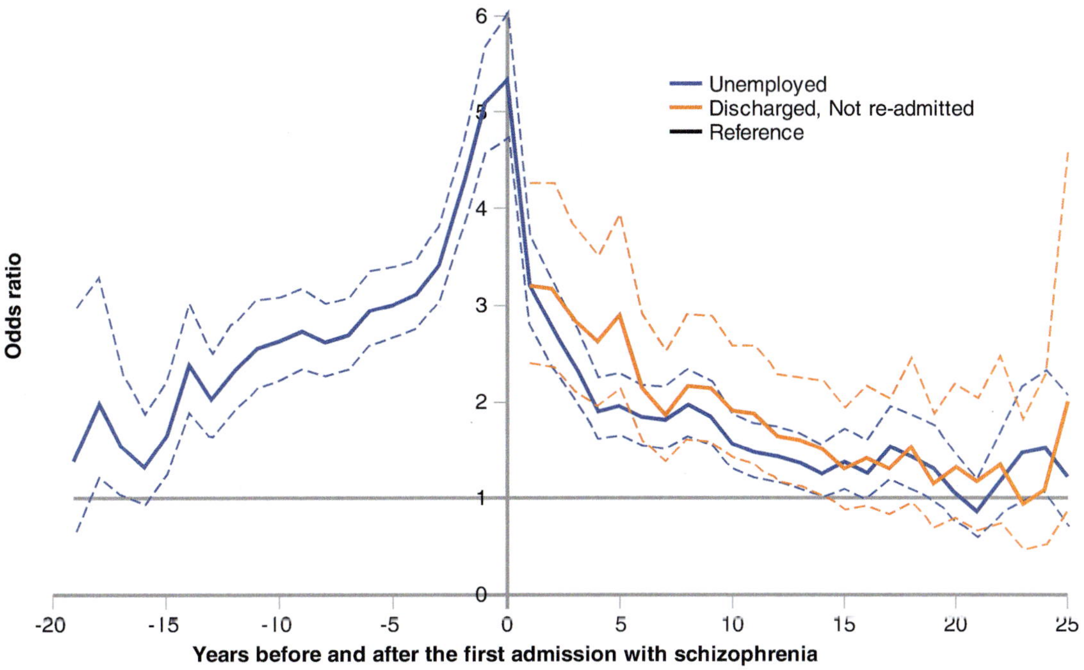

Fig. 2.24 Relative risk of being unemployed for those with schizophrenia as compared to control population: 20 years prior to onset to 25 years post-onset

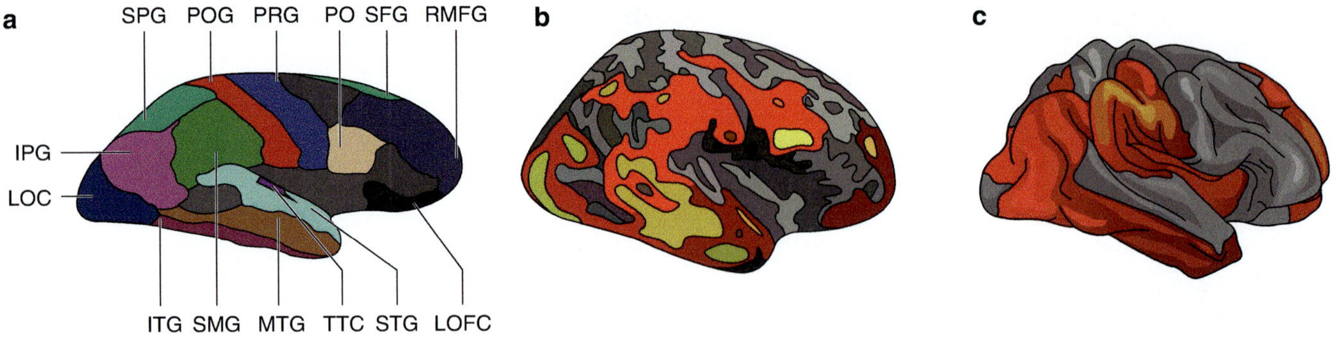

LOC = Lateral Occipital Lobe
IPG = Inferior Parietal Gyrus
POG = Post Central Gyrus
PRG = Precentral Gyrus
PO = Parietal Orbital Frontal Cortex
SFG = Superior Frontal Gyrus
RMFG = Right Medial Frontal Gyrus
ITG = Inferior Temporal Gyrus
SMG = Superior Medial Gyrus
MTG = Medial Temporal Gyrus
TTC = Temporal Cortex
STG = Superior Temporal Gyrus
LOFC = Lateral Orbital Frontal Cortex

Fig. 2.25 Socioeconomic status and brain structure. (**a**) Brain area volumes by neighborhood SES. (**b**) Cortical thickness varies with family income. (**c**), Surface areas vary with parental education

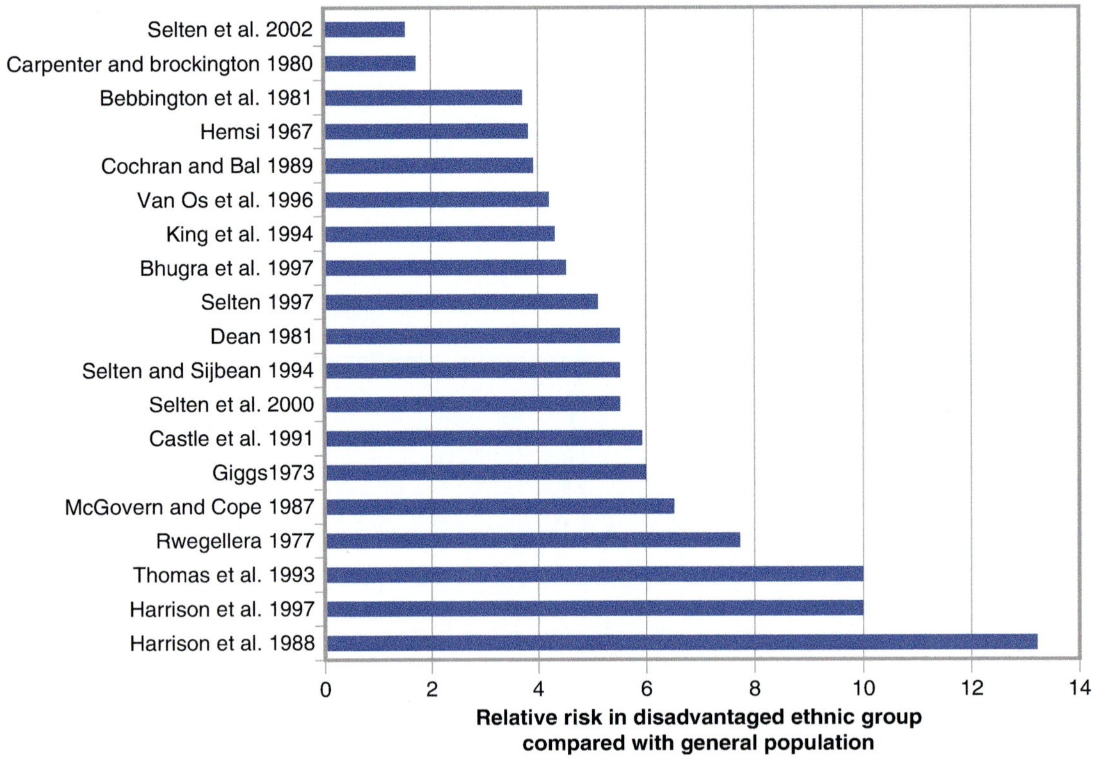

Fig. 2.26 Relative risk of schizophrenia in London for Afro-Caribbean immigrants compared to British citizens

replicated in other ethnic groups. It could also be that these ethnic groups have a higher genetic risk for schizophrenia, but studies in the countries of origin do not reveal the high rates found in London [66]. It has been hypothesized that persons living in Afro-Caribbean countries are more likely to immigrate to Britain due to aspects of their prodromal symptomatology, but the difference survives into the second and third generations of the immigrants, weakening this logic. It is possible that the stress of immigration produces the effect, but this logic is also weakened by the existence of the effect in later generations who have not suffered the stress of immigration. Another possible explanation is that the immigrants suffer from being born in Britain, where better prenatal nutrition produces a larger fetus than the mother can tolerate ("cephalopelvic disproportion"), generating perinatal complications. This logic is inconsistent with the data that the effect of Afro-Caribbean ethnicity is found also in second- and third-generation immigrants [67]. Another explanation is that the formation of vitamin D, which is stimulated by the bright sun passing through dark skin in tropical climates, is hampered by the cloudy atmosphere in Britain, with stronger effects for those with dark skin than for native English [68].

The presence of social support is an important element in the risk structure for depressive and anxiety disorders. The interaction of life stage, social supports, and social class are shown in Fig. 2.27, originating from the classic work of George Brown and Tirril Harris in a survey of women in London, entitled *The Social Origins of Depression* [69]. The figure combines two graphs. The ordinate on the left shows that the prevalence of depression is higher for those in the lower class (red bar) as compared to the middle class (light green bar). The two bars reflecting depressive disorder also show that the effect of social class is concentrated among women raising young children. The ordinate on the right shows that women in the middle class are more likely to have an intimate confidante as social support (dark green bar) than those in the lower class (dark blue bar) and that this effect is strongest for those raising young children. The lack of an intimate confidante, or another form of social support, has been shown both to be an individual risk factor for depressive disorder and to interact with stress (such as may occur in bringing up young children) in raising the risk for depression. Social supports are a stronger risk factor for depression in females than in males (Fig. 2.28) [70]. The data in Fig. 2.28 are drawn from twins, which has the effect of controlling for the possible confounding of genetic effects on social supports.

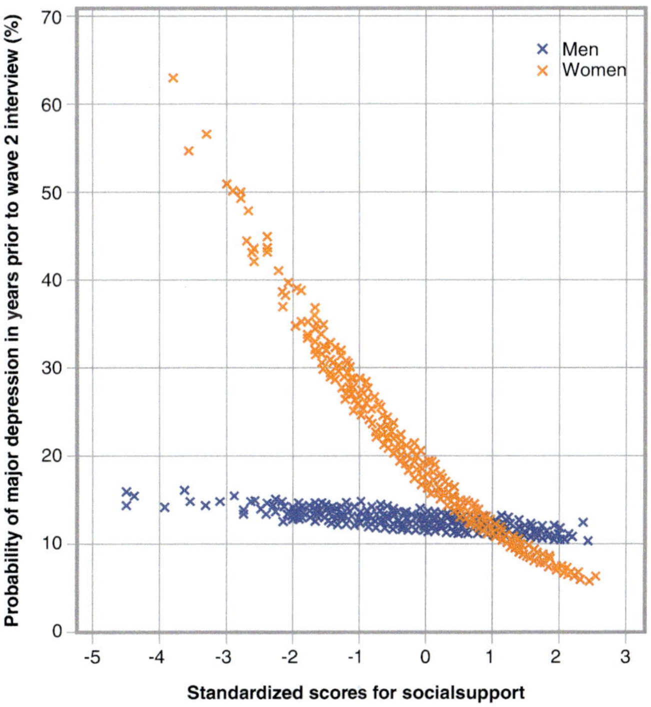

Fig. 2.28 Social support and incidence of depressive disorder between two waves for 1057 opposite-sex twin pairs in the Virginia Study of Twins

Fig. 2.27 Life stage, social support, and social class as influences on depression among women in London. Left ordinate is percent with depressive disorder onset; Right ordinate is percent with a confidante

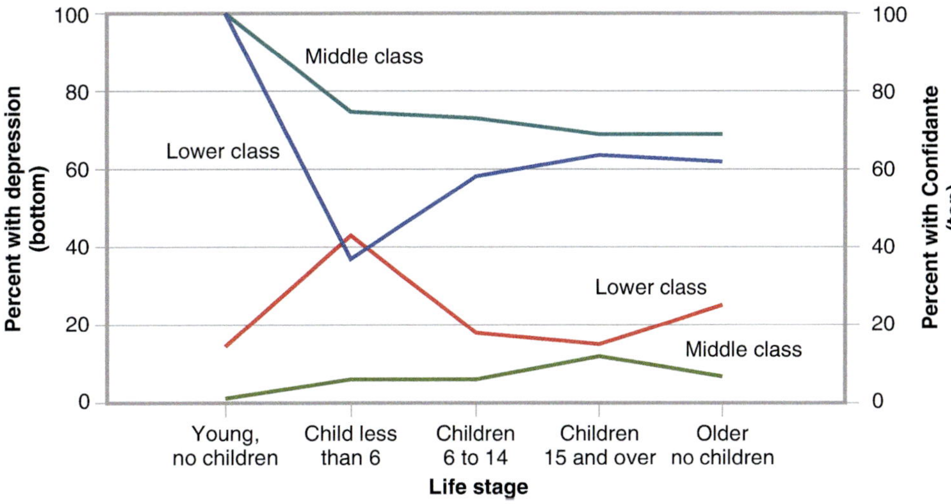

Comorbidity

An important aspect of mental disorders which shows up in epidemiologic research is the high degree of comorbidity with other disorders. Psychiatric disorders are highly comorbid with each other, as well as with a range of physical illnesses. The overlap in disorders is shown in Table 2.7, in which only bipolar disorder never occurs by itself, and in 77% of the cases, three or more disorders occur in the individual with that disorder [71]. Mood and anxiety disorders occur without accompanying disorders in less than 25% of the cases. The overlap in disorders, and the difficulty in deciding upon a threshold of symptoms for the diagnosis, have led researchers to propose dimensional schemas for outcomes in psychiatric symptomatology [72].

Mental disorders occur together with physical disorders, both as consequences of the stress associated with the physical disorder, and also as a potential cause for the physical disorder. Many studies have shown that depressive disorder is associated with elevated risk for diabetes [73], heart attack [74], and dementia [75]. Figure 2.29 reveals the strength of evidence about this relationship in the many replicating studies and also the fact that it takes two forms, with early depression predicting the later onset of diabetes, and early diabetes predicting the later onset of depression. The bimodal pattern of onset for depressive disorder, shown in data from both psychiatric registers (Fig. 2.11a) and population-based surveys (Fig. 2.11b), suggests that depression takes two forms. As noted earlier, it could be that the earlier-occurring form is caused by life stresses occurring at that stage of life, such as obtaining a job and beginning a family, as suggested by the life course framework (Fig. 2.6). The later-occurring form, dubbed "vascular depression" [76], may have physiological causes, such as changes in the immune system and inflammation associated with aging, which is connected to diabetes, heart disease, and dementia. Almost all medical conditions have raised risk associated with the prior occurrence of schizophrenia (part a) and depressive disorder (part b) in both males and females, as shown in Fig. 2.30 [77]. The exception appears to be cancer, which is associated with only an incremental change in risk. The other exception is the lower risk for those with schizophrenia to have musculoskeletal conditions, consistent with the findings on rheumatoid arthritis presented in Fig. 2.18.

Comorbidity with physical illnesses is one likely explanation for the higher rate of mortality for those with mental disorders. Figure 2.30a and b [78] show the much higher risk for mortality in England among persons with schizophrenia (Fig. 2.30a) and bipolar disorder (Fig. 2.31b). These disorders are exceptions in that the data indicate only moderate elevation of mortality for most other mental disorders, with the exception of dementia and drug use disorders [79].

An important consideration when studying comorbidity is the potential effect of the bias identified by Berkson in 1946 [80]. The bias is the tendency for data based on hospital admissions or other treatment to reflect an unmeasured confounder—that is, the occurrence of a comorbid condition that affected the probability that the individual ended up in the treatment setting. This bias must certainly apply to the data in Fig. 2.31, as well as to many other situations in psychiatric epidemiology, such as the genetic data presented in GWAS studies as in Fig. 2.12. This bias is part of the logic for conducting studies of household-residing populations, such as the ECA program and World Mental Health Surveys discussed earlier. However, it is difficult to conduct population-based surveys when the disorder is rare, as it is for schizophrenia, and also, the bias is likely to be less powerful when the disorder is bizarre or severe, so as to almost inevitably involve medical or psychiatric treatment.

Table 2.7 Lifetime comorbidity of mental disorders

	Percent with:				
Primary disorder	No other disorder	One other disorder	Two other disorders	Three or more other disorders	Total no. of respondents
Conduct disorder	28.5	32.3	20.0	19.2	415
Major depressive disorder	25.0	29.8	20.9	24.3	6410
Panic disorder	15.0	19.3	18.4	47.3	2116
Social phobia	11.7	19.1	19.8	49.4	1983
Simple phobia	23.4	25.7	17.9	33.0	4030
Bipolar I disorder	0	5.4	16.9	77.7	935
Alcohol abuse/ dependence	47.7	25.2	12.7	14.4	11,843
Drug abuse/ dependence	5.9	30.1	24.6	39.4	2063
Personality disorder	19.5	28.7	19.9	31.9	6295

National Survey of Alcohol and Related Conditions, wave 1
Disorders in columns include those listed in rows, as well as dysthymia and generalized anxiety disorder

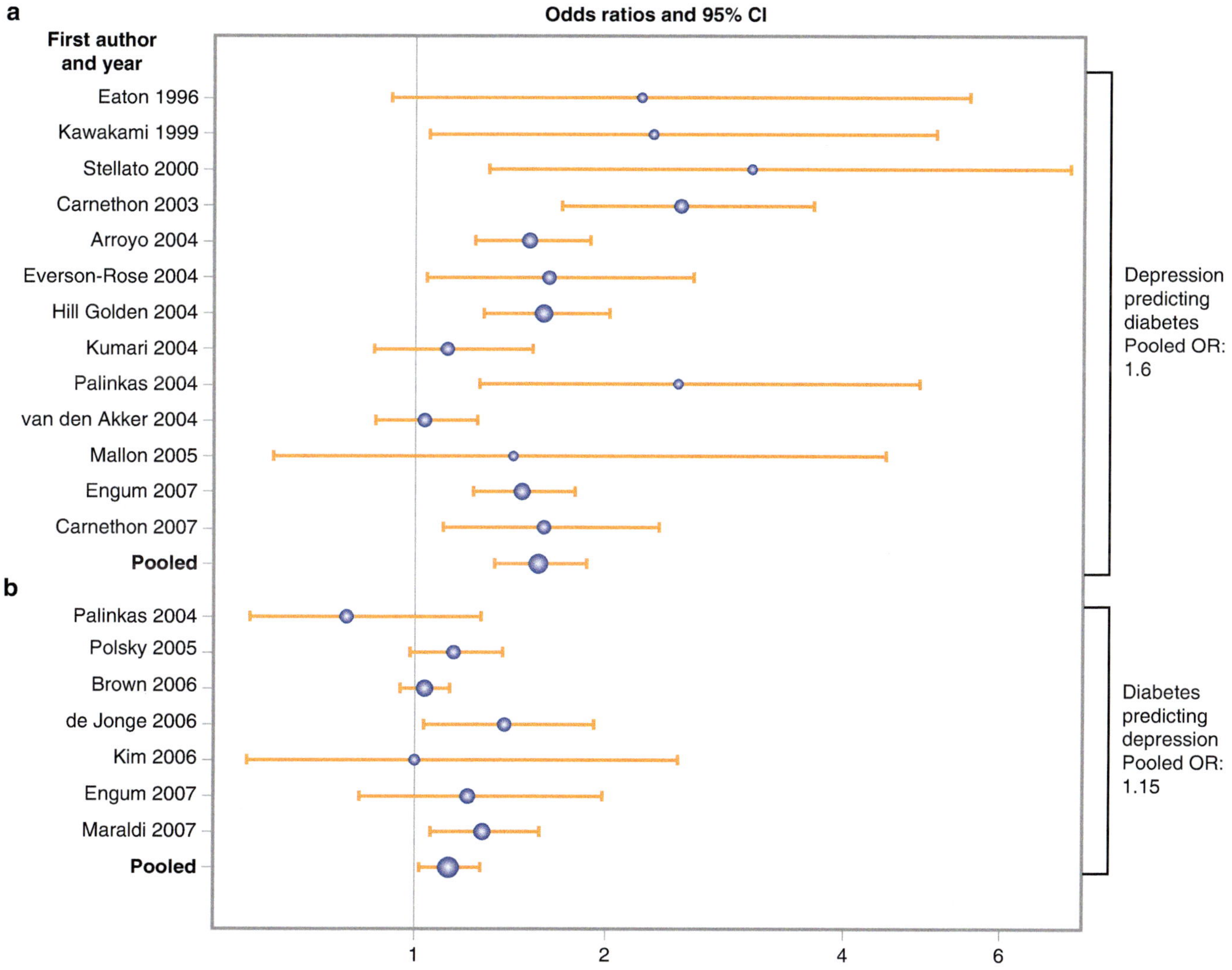

Fig. 2.29 Forest plot of the bidirectional longitudinal relationship between depression and diabetes

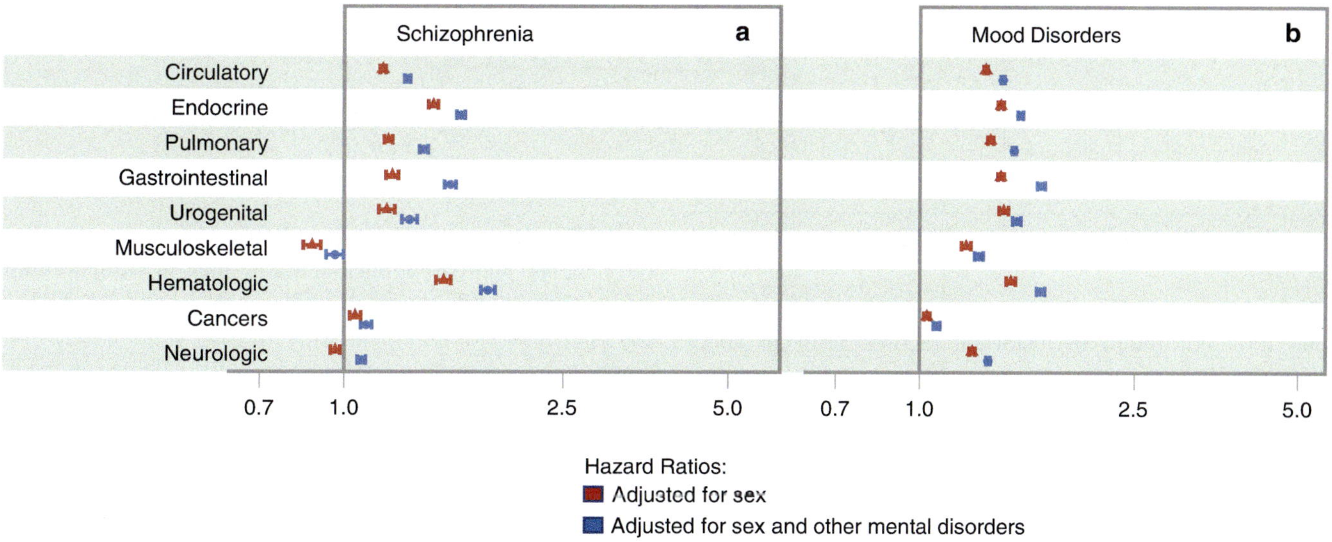

Fig. 2.30 Almost all medical conditions have raised the risk associated with the prior occurrence of depressive disorder and schizophrenia, in both males and females

Fig. 2.31 (**a**) Risk for mortality among persons with schizophrenia compared with the general population, years 1999–2006. (**b**) Risk for mortality among persons with bipolar disorder compared with the general population, years 1999–2006

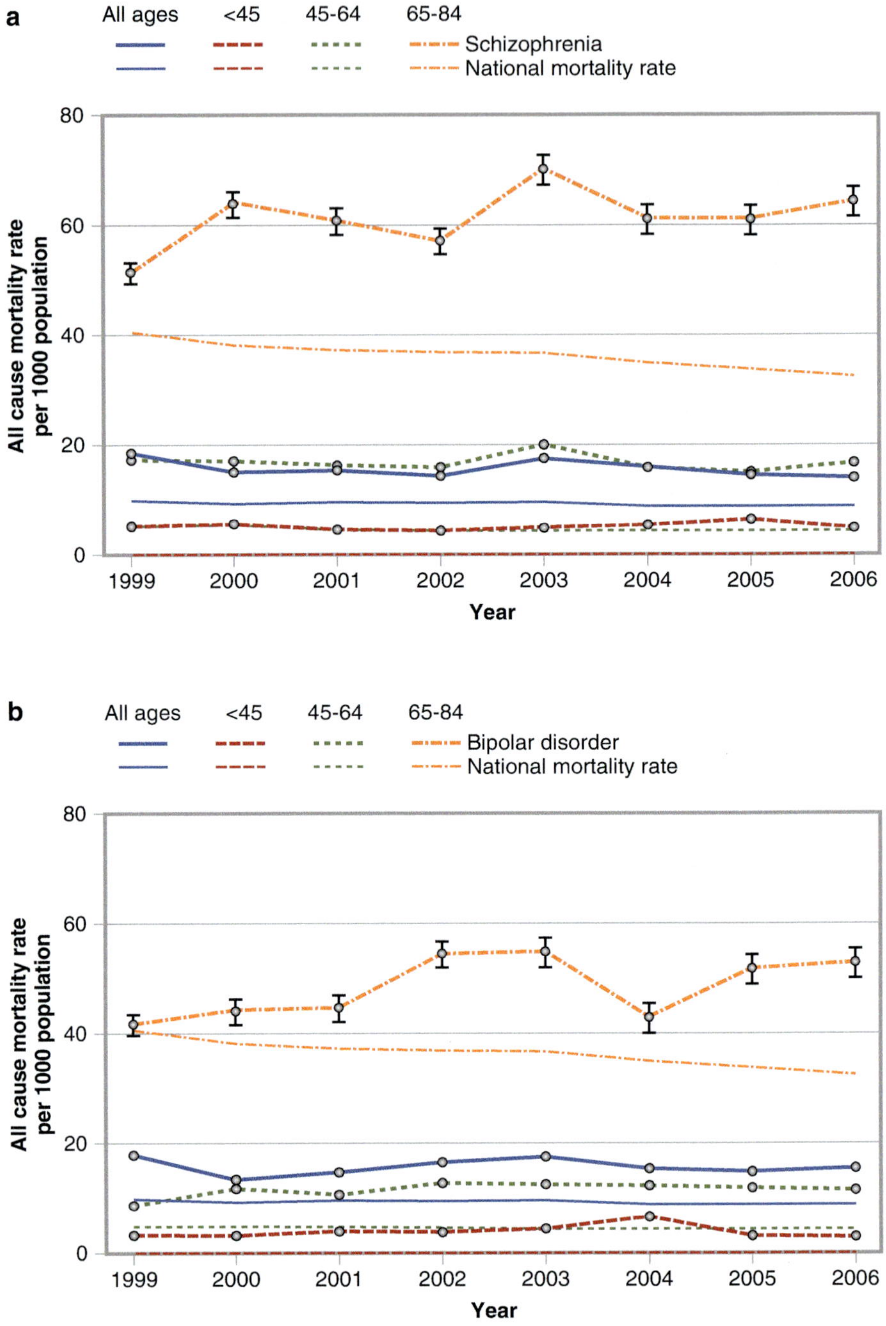

Historical Trends in Mental Disorders

A puzzle in the epidemiology of schizophrenia is the fact that it is not found in historical records prior to about 1500 CE [81]. This contrasts with the repeated descriptions of depressive disorder in ancient texts such as the old testament and the Bhagavad Gita and with the careful description of manic depressive disorder in the Galenic period by Aretaus of Cappadocia. An early appearance relevant to schizophrenia may be the painting of *Dulle Griet* ("Mad Meg") by Pieter Breughel in the sixteenth century. It has been hypothesized that Breughel, who typically carefully painted realistic persons and situations, actually met a woman with schizophrenia and attempted to represent her, including her physical and psychological aspects [82] (Fig. 2.32). The painting has clear allusions to the work of Hieronymous Bosch from an earlier generation, with the *Ship of Fools* (above her head) that he painted, as well as the upturned funnel from Bosch's *Cure of Folly* (lower right corner). Reading a description of Ophelia from Shakespeare's Hamlet, written in about the same time period, gives a sense of schizophrenia symptoms as well. These cultural occurrences fit in with data

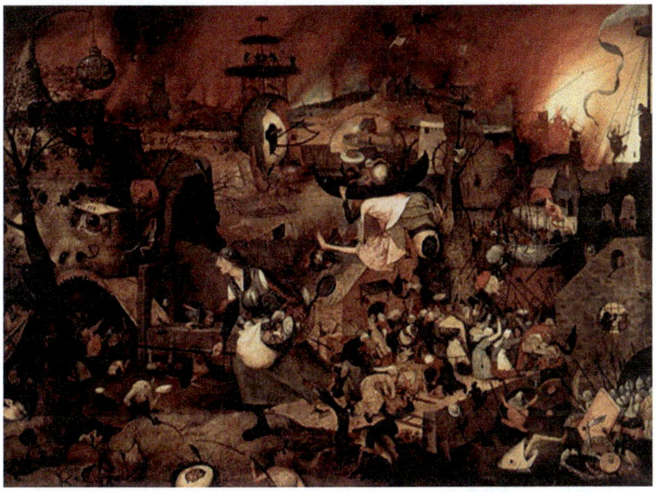

Fig. 2.32 Dulle Griet, by Pieter Breughel, 1564. Public domain

on the epidemiology of mental illness as recorded starting in about 1800 and moving to the present time (Fig. 2.33) [83]. Some researchers have concluded this is the result of the occurrence of a new virus [84], while others suggest it is the result of opening the household to pets that carry infectious agents such as Toxoplasmosis Gondii [85]. Others have suggested that the growth in insanity in this period is due to the emerging psychological difficulties of formulating a life plan in an increasingly complex and challenging social environment [62].

The lack of historical evidence for the existence of schizophrenia contrasts not just with the repeated descriptions of depressive disorder in ancient texts, but with evidence for a rising trend in the prevalence of depression in the second half of the twentieth century. Figure 2.34 shows the lifetime prevalence of depressive disorder for six cohorts, with the more recent cohorts having a higher prevalence [86]. The data

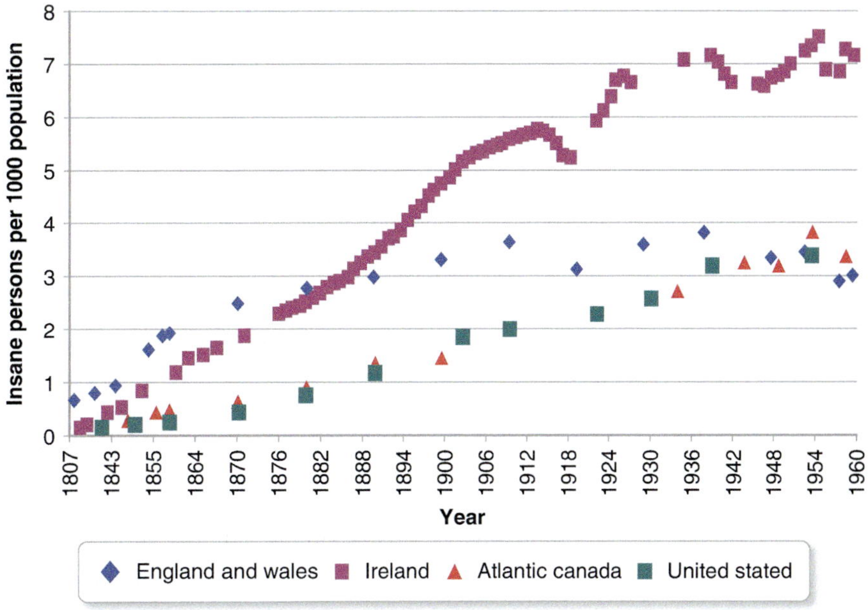

Fig. 2.33 Historical trends in severe mental illness in four countries

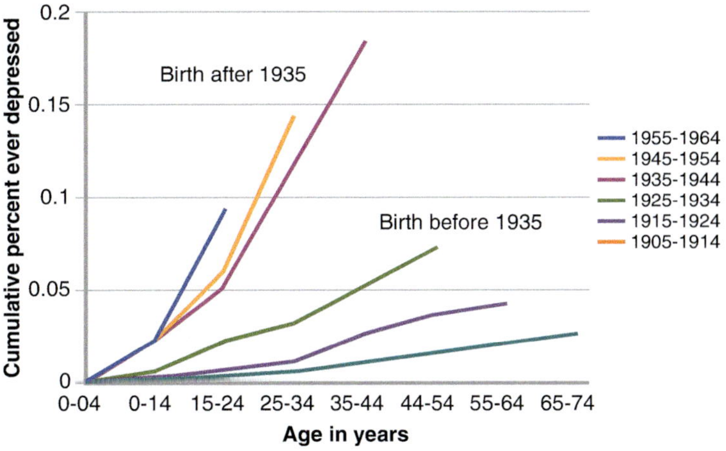

Fig. 2.34 Lifetime prevalence of the depressive disorder in six birth cohorts. Females in five ECA sites

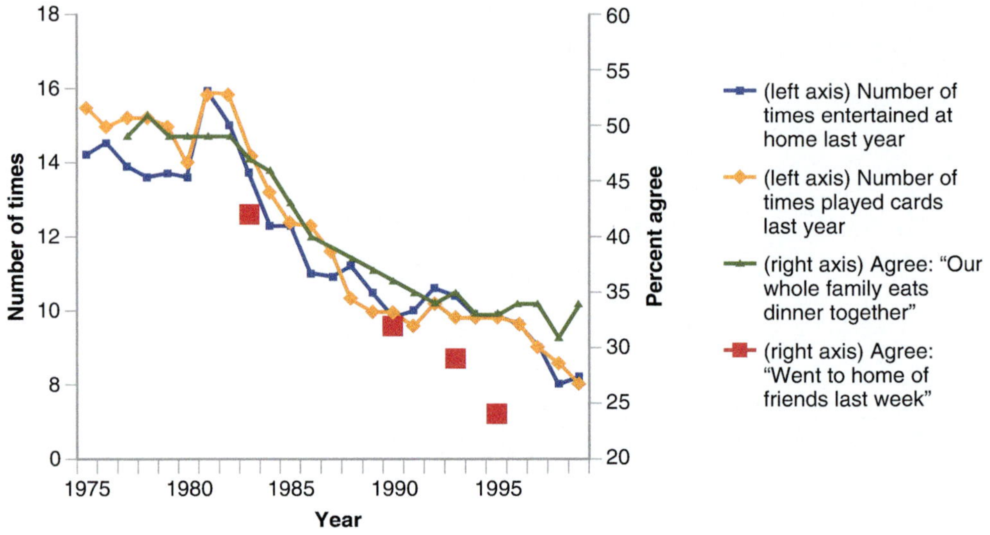

Fig. 2.35 Decline in social connections in America, 1976–2000

were collected in 1981 so that the later births (e.g., the two blue and yellow lines representing the so-called "baby-boom" cohort born between 1945 and 1964) have a cumulative prevalence of depression of about 10–15%, by age 15–35; this compares to the earlier birth cohorts (purple and green lines) whose prevalence of depression by that age was less than 5%. These findings have been replicated many times on sites around the world. Possible explanations are that people with depression die at younger ages and so are not counted in the later years of cohorts born earlier, that the older cohort is culturally different in being less introspective, or that easier access to more available treatment for depression in later periods leads to better recall, or that older subjects forget episodes that occurred a long time prior to the interview than young persons. However, the dominant explanation for this finding connects to the study of social supports (discussed above), which have weakened over the same period of time. The work by Robert Putnam shows the trend in decline in meetings of informal social groups, as in Fig. 2.35, as well as many other social functions such as PTA meetings and church attendance [87]. The effects of the promulgation of social media on social support networks in the last decade is likely to have an as-yet-unknown effect on these relationships.

Conclusion

The origins of psychiatric epidemiology occurred in the nineteenth century, in parallel with other forms of epidemiology. But the progress in developing techniques of prevention and treatment through epidemiologic research has been much slower and less dramatic than in epidemiology devoted to infectious diseases, such as smallpox and TB, and chronic illnesses, such as diabetes and coronary heart disease. Studies conducted over many decades have demonstrated the importance of the mental disorders and have located many risk factors but have barely contributed to their prevention or cure, as has happened for other diseases. This situation may be about to change with a better understanding of biological, immunological, and neurological systems, as well as social systems, now known to be related to the occurrence of mental disorders. These developments will lead to a more precise definition and assessment of mental disorders, moving from the model in Fig. 2.10 to something more like Fig. 2.36 (on the right side). There will be an increasingly strong and wide-ranging measurement of genetic, social, and psychological risk factors, which can be collectively termed the *exposome*. [88] Newly developed risk factors such as the microbiome, as well as the vast array of physiological variables, are summarized in Fig. 2.36 as the "interactome." Understanding the complex relationships intertwining these systems requires large samples, available in electronic data systems such as EPIC and also produced by new developments in assessment via the web and cell phones. The complex etiologic pathways can now be investigated in large datasets with new mathematical techniques such as those involved in computational psychiatry and other new forms of mathematical investigation [89]. These developments will produce much finer and more specific definitions of disorders than currently used (as in Fig. 2.10). More precise definitions of disorders generated by this new form of psychiatric epidemiology will lead to improvement in the prevention and treatment of mental disorders. The future of psychiatric epidemiology is likely to be productive in the coming decades.

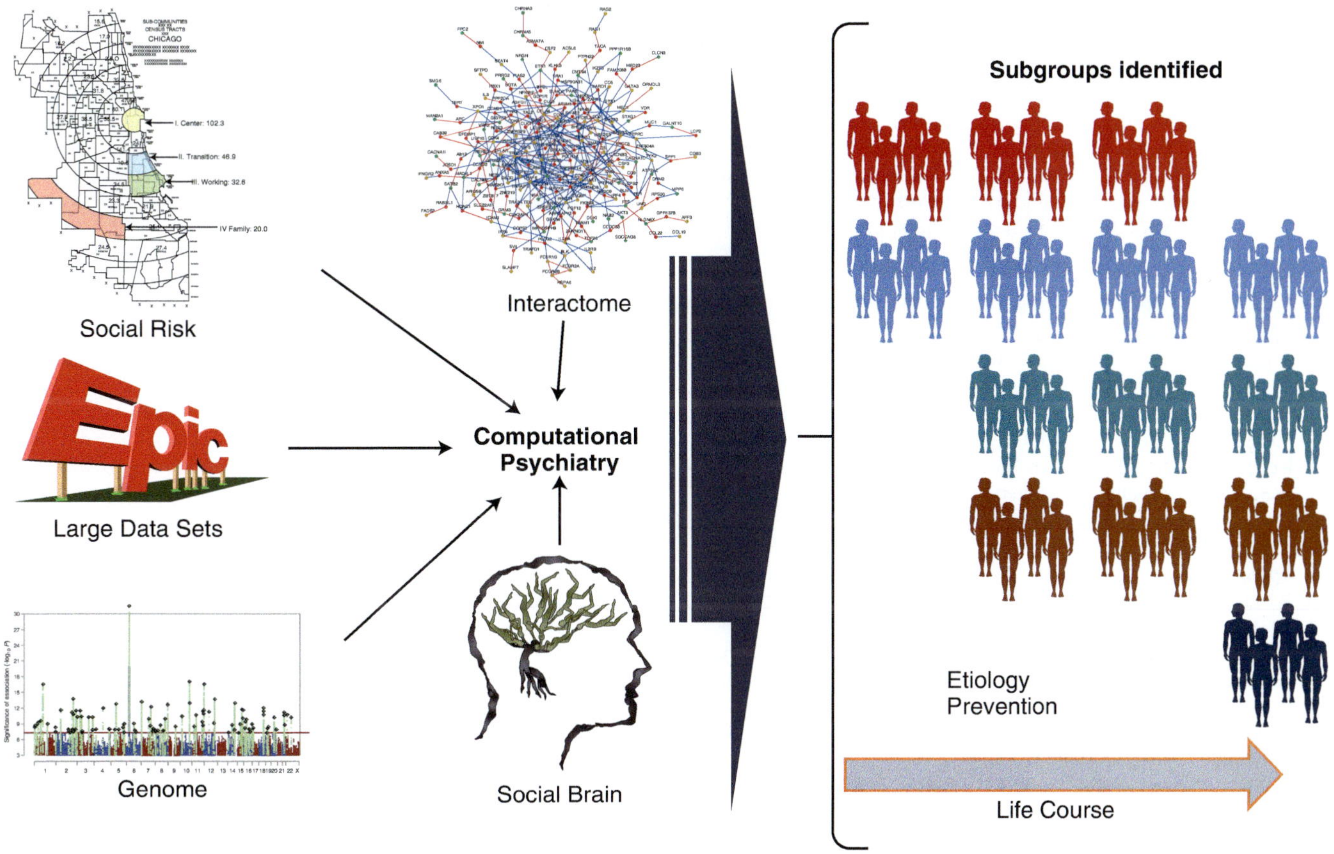

Fig. 2.36 The future of psychiatric epidemiology. Large samples combined with a large array of risk factors across many disciplines were analyzed via new mathematical methods

References

1. Gordis L. Epidemiology. Third ed. Philadelphia, PA: Elsevier; 2004.
2. Foege WH, Alexander D. Langmuir—his impact on public health. Am J Epidemiol. 1996;144(8 Suppl):S11–S5.
3. Morris JN. Uses of epidemiology. 3rd ed. Edinburgh: Churchill Livingstone; 1975.
4. Cooper B, Morgan HG. Epidemiological psychiatry. Springfield, IL: Charles C. Thomas; 1973.
5. Prince M, Stewart R, Ford T, Hotopf M. Practical psychiatric epidemiology. New York: Oxford University Press; 2003.
6. Cooper B. The epidemiology of psychiatric disorders. Baltimore, MD: The Johns Hopkins University Press; 1987.
7. Susser E, Schwartz S, Morabia A, Bromet EJ. Psychiatric epidemiology: searching for the causes of mental disorders. New York: Oxford University Press; 2006.
8. Tsuang M, Tohen M, Jones P. Textbook in psychiatric epidemiology. 3rd ed. New York: John Wiley & Sons, Ltd.; 2011.
9. Carpenter WT. Flexible system for the diagnosis of schizophrenia: report from the WHO international pilot study of schizophrenia. Science. 1973;182:1275–8.
10. Eaton WW, Bohrnstedt G. Latent variable models for dichotomous outcomes: analysis of data from the NIMH epidemiologic catchment area program. Newbury Park: Sage Publications, Inc.; 1989.
11. Krueger RF. The structure of common mental disorders. Arch Gen Psychiatry. 1999;56:921–6.
12. Eaton WW, Bienvenu OJ, Nestadt G, Volk HE, Anthony JC. The burden of mental disorders. In: Eaton WW, Fallin MD, editors. Public mental health. 2nd ed. New York: Oxford University Press; 2019.
13. World Health Organization. Schizophrenia: a multinational study. Geneva: World Health Organization; 1975.
14. Bromet E, Andrade LH, Hwang I, Sampson NA, Alonso J, de Girolamo G, et al. Cross-national epidemiology of DSM-IV major depressive episode. BMC Med. 2011;9:90.
15. Kessler RC, Haro JM, Heeringa SG, Pennell BE, Ustun TB. The world health organization world mental health survey initiative. Epidemiol Psichiatr Soc. 2006;15(3):161–6.
16. Essau CA, Wittchen H-U. An overview of the composite international diagnostic interview (CIDI). Int J Methods Psychiatr Res. 1993;3:79–85.
17. Kleinman A. Neurasthenia and depression: a study of somatization and culture in China. Cult Med Psychiatry. 1982;6:117–90.
18. Haddad, Leila, Schäfer A, Streit F, Lederbogen F, Grimm O, Wüst S, Deuschle M, Kirsch P, Tost H, Meyer-Lindenberg A. Brain Structure Correlates of Urban Upbringing, an Environmental Risk Factor for Schizophrenia Schizophrenia Bulletin. 2015;41(1):115–122.
19. Global Burden of Disease [Internet]. IHME. [cited 2020]. https://ourworldindata.org/mental-health.
20. Collaborators GDaH. Global, regional, and national disability-adjusted life-years (DALYs) for 315 diseases and injuries and healthy life expectancy (HALE), 1990-2015: a systematic

analysis for the Global Burden of Disease Study 2015. Lancet. 2016;388:1603–58.
21. Pedersen CB. The Danish civil registration system. Scand J Public Health. 2011;39(7 Suppl):22–5.
22. Kessing LV. Validity of diagnoses and other clinical register data in patients with affective disorder. Eur Psychiatry. 1998;13:392–8.
23. Mojtabai R, Muray S, Eaton WW. Pathways to care: need, attitudes, barriers. In: Eaton WW, Fallin MD, editors. Public mental health. 2nd ed. New York: Oxford University Press; 2019. p. 439–65.
24. Langner TS, Michael ST. Life Stress and mental health. New York: Free Press; 1963. p. 1963.
25. Leighton DC, Harding JS, Macklin DB, Macmillan AM, Leighton AH. The character of danger: psychiatric symptoms in selected communities. New York: Basic Books; 1963. p. 1963.
26. Eaton WW, Regier DA, Locke BZ, Taube CA. The epidemiologic catchment area program of the national institute of mental health. Public Health Rep. 1981;96(4):319–25.
27. Kellam SG. Mental health and going to school: the Woodlawn program of assessment, early intervention, and evaluation. Chicago, IL: University of Chicago Press; 1975.
28. Armenian HK, Lilienfeld AK. Incubation period of disease. Epidemiol Rev. 1983;5:1–15.
29. Rothman KJ. Induction and latent periods. Am J Epidemiol. 1981;114:253–9.
30. Hafner H, Maurer K, Loffler W, an der Hediden W, Stein A, Konnecke R, et al. Onset and prodromal phase as determinants of the course. In: Gattaz WF, Hafner H, editors. Search for the causes of schizophrenia: Vol IV-- Balance of the century. Steinkopf/ Darmstadt: Springer; 1999. p. 35–58.
31. Golding J, Pembrey M, Jones R. ALSPAC—the Avon longitudinal study of parents and children. I Study methodology. Paediatr Perinat Epidemiol. 2001;15(1):74–87.
32. Eaton WW, Kalaydjian A, Scharfstein DO, Mezuk B, Ding Y. Prevalence and incidence of depressive disorder: the Baltimore ECA follow-up, 1981-2004. Acta Psychiatr Scand. 2007;116(3):182–8.
33. Poulton R, Moffitt TE, Silva PA. The Dunedin multidisciplinary health and development study: overview of the first 40 years, with an eye to the future. Soc Psychiatry Psychiatr Epidemiol. 2015;50(5):679–93.
34. Pedersen CB, Mors O, Bertelsen A, Waltoft BL, Agerbo E, McGrath JJ, et al. A comprehensive nationwide study of the incidence rate and lifetime risk for treated mental disorders. JAMA Psychiat. 2014;71(5):573–81.
35. Leboyer M, Berk M, Yolken RH, Tamouza R, Kupfer D, Groc L. Immuno-psychiatry: an agenda for clinical practice and innovative research. BMC Med. 2016;14(1):173.
36. Eaton WW, Anthony JC, Gallo J, Cai G, Tien A, Romanoski A, et al. Natural history of DIS/DSM major depression: the Baltimore ECA followup. Arch Gen Psych. 1997;54:993–9.
37. Alexopoulos GS. The vascular depression hypothesis: 10 years later. Biol Psychiatry. 2006;60(12):1304–5.
38. Zandi P, Wilcox H, Lin Y, Maher BS, Fallin MD. Genes as a source of risk for mental disorders. In: Eaton WW, Fallin MD, editors. Public mental health. 2nd ed. New York: Oxford University Press; 2019. p. 223–56.
39. Howard DM, Adams MJ, Clarke TK, Hafferty JD, Gibson J, Shirali M, et al. Genome-wide meta-analysis of depression identifies 102 independent variants and highlights the importance of the prefrontal brain regions. Nat Neurosci. 2019;22(3):343–52.
40. Eaton W. The sociology of mental disorders. 3rd ed. Westport, CT: Praeger Publishers; 2001.
41. Eaton WW, Chen C-Y. Epidemiology. In: Lieberman JA, Stroup TS, Perkins DO, editors. The American psychiatric publishing textbook of schizophrenia. Washington, DC: American Psychiatric Publishing, Inc.; 2006. p. 17–38.
42. Mednick S, Machon R, Huttunen M, Bonett D. Adult schizophrenia following prenatal exposure to an influenza epidemic. Arch Gen Psychiatry. 1988;45:189–92.
43. Brown AS, Derkits EJ. Prenatal infection and schizophrenia: a review of epidemiologic and translational studies. Am J Psychiatry. 2010;167(3):261–80.
44. Cannon M, Jones PB, Murray RM. Obstetric complications and schizophrenia: historical and meta-analytic review. Am J Psychiatr. 2002;159:1080–92.
45. Davies C, Segre G, Estrade A, Radua J, de Micheli A, Provenzani U, et al. Prenatal and perinatal risk and protective factors for psychosis: a systematic review and meta-analysis. Lancet Psychiatry. 2020;7:399–410.
46. Fatemi SH, Folsom TD. The neurodevelopmental hypothesis of schizophrenia, revisited. Schizophr Bull. 2009;35:528–48.
47. Ogendahl BK, Agerbo E, Byrne M, Licht RW, Eaton WW, Mortensen PB. Indicators of fetal growth and bipolar disorder: a Danish national register-based study. Psychol Med. 2006;36(9):1219–24.
48. Cannon TD, van Erp TG, Bearden CE, Loewy R, Thompson P, Toga AW, et al. Early and late neurodevelopmental influences in the prodrome to schizophrenia: contributions of genes, environment, and their interactions. Schizophr Bull. 2003;29(4):653–69.
49. Faris RE, Dunham W. Mental disorders in Urban areas. Chicago, IL: University of Chicago Press; 1939. p. 1939.
50. March D, Hatch SL, Morgan C, Kirkbride JB, Bresnahan M, Fearon P, et al. Psychosis and place. Epidemiol Rev. 2008;30(1):84–100.
51. Eaton W, Hayward C, Ram R. Schizophrenia and rheumatoid arthritis: a review. Schizophr Res. 1992;6:181–92.
52. Benros ME, Mortensen PB, Eaton WW. Autoimmune diseases and infections as risk factors for schizophrenia. Ann N Y Acad Sci. 2012;1262:56–66.
53. Eaton WW, Byrne M, Ewald H, Mors O, Chen C-Y, Agerbo E, et al. The association of schizophrenia and autoimmune diseases; linkage of Danish national registers. Am J Psychiatr. 2006;163:521–8.
54. Mechanic D. Medical sociology. 2nd ed. New York: The Free Press; 1978.
55. Kendler KS, Kessler RC, Walters EE, MacLean C, Neale MC, Heath AC, et al. Stressful life events, genetic liability, and onset of an episode of major depression in women. Am J Psychiatr. 1995;152:833–42.
56. Caspi A, Sugden K, Moffitt TE, Taylor A, Craig IW, Harrington H, et al. Influence of life stress on depression: moderation by a polymorphism in the 5-HTT gene. Science. 2003;301(5631):386–9.
57. Risch N, Herrell R, Lehner T, Liang KY, Eaves L, Hoh J, et al. Interaction between the serotonin transporter gene (5-HTTLPR), stressful life events, and risk of depression: a meta-analysis. JAMA. 2009;301(23):2462–71.
58. Karg K, Burmeister M, Shedden K, Sen S. The serotonin transporter promoter variant (5-HTTLPR), stress, and depression meta-analysis revisited: evidence of genetic moderation. Arch Gen Psychiatry. 2011;68(5):444–54.
59. Sharpley CF, Palanisamy SK, Glyde NS, Dillingham PW, Agnew LL. An update on the interaction between the serotonin transporter promoter variant (5-HTTLPR), stress and depression, plus an exploration of non-confirming findings. Behav Brain Res. 2014;273:89–105.
60. Chapman DP, Whitfield CL, Felitti VJ, Dubea SR, Edwards VJ, Andaa RF. Adverse childhood experiences and the risk of depressive disorders in adulthood. J Affect Disord. 2004;82:217–25.
61. Eaton WW, Muntaner C. Socioeconomic stratification and mental disorders. In: Scheid TL, Wright ER, editors. A handbook for the study of mental health: social contexts, theories, and systems. 3rd ed. New York: Cambridge University Press; 2016.
62. Eaton WW, Harrison G. Life chances, life planning, and schizophrenia: a review and interpretation of research on social deprivation. Int J Ment Health. 2001;30:58–81.

63. McCabe JH, Lambe MP, Chattinguis S, Sham PC, David AS, Reichenberg A, et al. Excellent school performance at age 16 and risk of adult bipolar disorder: national cohort study. Br J Psychiatry. 2010;196:109–15.
64. Agerbo E, Byrne M, Eaton W, Mortensen PB. Marital and labor market status in the long run in schizophrenia. Arch Gen Psychiatry. 2004;61:28–33.
65. Farah MJ. The neuroscience of socioeconomic status: correlates, causes, and consequences. Neuron. 2017;96(1):56–71.
66. Bhugra D, Hilwig M, Hossein B, Marceau H, Neehall J, Leff J, et al. First-contact incidence rates of schizophrenia in Trinidad and one-year follow-up. Br J Psychiatry. 1996;169:587–92.
67. Hutchinson G, Takei N, Bhugra D, Fahy TA, Gilvarry C, Mallett R, et al. Increased rate of psychosis among African-Caribbeans in Britain is not due to an excess of pregnancy and birth complications. Br J Psychiatry. 1997;171:145–7.
68. Kinney DK, Teixeira P, Hsu D, Napoleon SC, Crowley DJ, Miller A, et al. Relation of schizophrenia prevalence to latitude, climate, fish consumption, infant mortality, and skin color: a role for prenatal vitamin d deficiency and infections? Schizophr Bull. 2009;35(3):582–95.
69. Brown GW, Harris T. The social origins of depression: a study of psychiatric disorder in women. London: Tavistock; 1978. p. 1978.
70. Kendler KS, Myers J, Prescott CA. Sex differences in the relationship between social support and risk for major depression: a longitudinal study of opposite-sex twin pairs. Am J Psychiatry. 2005;162(2):250–6.
71. Eaton WW, Kessler RC, Mortensen PB, Rebok GW, Roth K. The population dynamics of mental disorders. In: Eaton WW, Fallin D, editors. Public mental health. 2nd ed. New York: Oxford University Press; 2019. p. 141–67.
72. Krueger RF, Markon KE. A dimensional-spectrum model of psychopathology: progress and opportunities. Arch Gen Psychiatry. 2011;68(1):10–1.
73. Mezuk B, Eaton WW, Albrecht S, Golden S. Depression and type 2 diabetes over the lifespan: a meta-analysis. Diabetes Care. 2008;31(12):2383–90.
74. Rugulies R. Depression as a predictor for coronary heart disease: a review and meta-analysis. Am J Prev Med. 2002;23(1):51–61.
75. Jorm A. History of depression as a risk factor for dementia: an updated review. Aust N Z J Psychiatry. 2001;35(6):776–81.
76. Alexopoulos GS, Meyers BS, Young RC, Campbell S, Silbersweig D, Charlson M. 'Vascular depression' hypothesis. Arch Gen Psychiatry. 1997;54(10):915–22.
77. Momen NC, Plana-Ripoll O, Agerbo E, Benros ME, Børglum AD, Christensen MK, et al. Association between mental disorders and subsequent medical conditions. N Engl J Med. 2020;382(18):1721–31.
78. Hoang U, Stewart R, Goldacre MJ. Mortality after hospital discharge for people with schizophrenia or bipolar disorder: retrospective study of linked English hospital episode statistics, 1999-2006. BMJ. 2011;343:d5422.
79. Eaton WW, Roth KB, Bruce M, Cottler L, Wu L, Nestadt G, et al. The relationship of mental and behavioral disorders to all-cause mortality in a 27-year follow-up of 4 epidemiologic catchment area samples. Am J Epidemiol. 2013;178(9):1366–77.
80. Berkson J. Limitations of the application of fourfold table analysis to hospital data. Biometrics. 1946;2:47–53.
81. Mora G. History of psychiatry. In: Kaplan HI, Sadock BJ, editors. Comprehensive textbook of psychiatry/IV. 4th ed. Baltimore, MD: Williams & Wilkins; 1985. p. 2034–54.
82. Panse F, Schmidt HJ. Pieter Bruegels Dulle Griet: Bildnis einer psychisch kranken. Bayer Lehrerkursen; 1967.
83. Torrey EF, Miller J. The Invisible Plague: the rise of mental illness from 1750 to the present. New Brunswick, NJ: Rutgers University Press; 2001. p. 2001.
84. Hare E. Schizophrenia as a Recent Disease. Br J Psychiatry. 1988;153:521–31.
85. Torrey E, Yolken R. At issue: coud schizophrenia be a viral zoonosis transmitted from house cats? Schizophr Bull. 1995;21:167–71.
86. Wickramaratne PJ, Weissman MM, Leaf PJ, Holford TR. Age, period and cohort effects on the risk of major depression: Results from five United States communities. J Clin Epidemiol. 1989;42(4):333–43.
87. Putnam R. Bowling alone: the collapse and revival of american community. New York: Simon & Schuster; 2000. p. 2000.
88. Guloksuz S, Rutten BPF, Pries LK, Ten Have M, de Graaf R, van Dorsselaer S, et al. The complexities of evaluating the exposome in psychiatry: a data-driven illustration of challenges and some propositions for amendments. Schizophr Bull. 2018;44(6):1175–9.
89. Redish AD, Gordon JA. Computational psychiatry: new perspectives on mental illness. New York: The MIT Press; 2017.

The Biopsychosocial Model of Evaluation and Treatment in Psychiatry

3

Luma Bashmi, Alexander Cohn, Shawna T. Chan, Gabriel Tobia, Yasmine Gohar, Nathalie Herrera, Raymond Y. Wen, Waguih William IsHak, and Katrina DeBonis

Introduction

The biopsychosocial (BPS) model was developed in 1977 by the late George L. Engel and psychiatrist John Romano, supported by the research of Adolf Meyer (1948) and Roy Grinker (1960s). It was established to address the shortcomings of the biomedical model that was dominating the mid-twentieth century [1–5]. Engel considered the biomedical model to be very problematic: it was reductionistic and dualistic in nature (the mind and body were treated as separate entities), where the patient was viewed as an object, and only biological factors were accounted for when addressing a patient's illness.

Through collaborating with Romano, Engel aimed to provide a more holistic view of evaluating and treating a patient's suffering and illness by placing value on the psychological and social factors related to the patient's subjective experience. As such, the BPS model defined disease as an interaction between biological, psychological, and social factors; similarly, treatment would also follow biological (medication and surgery), psychological (psychotherapy), and social (health policy changes) interventions [6]. According to Engel [5], the BPS model captured what was essentially lacking in the biomedical model, the humanistic and patient-centered care of viewing a patient and his/her attributes as a human being. As Engel viewed it, the BPS model would not only become a better "scientific model" for practice but also for education and medical research [7].

In the context of psychiatry, the introduction of a new biopsychosocial paradigm offered an opportunity for the discipline to take the forefront in advancing patient care and the relationship between physician and patient. It also allowed for more collaboration, communication, and complementarity among various healthcare professionals. However, much of its benefits were seen in advancing "bedside manner" rather than diagnosing and treating patients (Fig. 3.1) [8].

Ever since Engel and Romano proposed the BPS model, it has achieved wide acceptance in psychiatry including an endorsement from the American Psychiatric Association (APA) and the American Board for Psychiatry and Neurology

L. Bashmi (✉)
Department of Health Psychology, School of Medicine, Royal College of Surgeons in Ireland-Bahrain, Busaiteen, Kingdom of Bahrain
e-mail: Lbashmi@rcsi.com

A. Cohn · S. T. Chan · K. DeBonis
Department of Psychiatry and Biobehavioral Sciences, David Geffen School of Medicine at UCLA, Los Angeles, CA, USA
e-mail: ACohn@mednet.ucla.edu; STChan@mednet.ucla.edu; kdebonis@mednet.ucla.edu

G. Tobia
Department of Psychiatry, Brigham and Women's Faulkner Hospital, Boston, MA, USA
e-mail: gtobia@bwh.harvard.edu

Y. Gohar
Psychiatry Department, The Behman Hospital, Cairo, Egypt

N. Herrera
Cedars-Sinai Medical Center, Los Angeles, CA, USA

R. Y. Wen
San Diego Health, Skaggs School of Pharmacy and Pharmaceutical Sciences, University of California, San Diego, CA, USA
e-mail: Yowen@health.UCSD.edu

W. W. IsHak
Cedars-Sinai Health System, Department of Psychiatry and Behavioral Neurosciences, University of California Los Angeles, David Geffen School of Medicine, Los Angeles, CA, USA
e-mail: Waguih.IsHak@cshs.org

W. W. IsHak (ed.), *Atlas of Psychiatry*, https://doi.org/10.1007/978-3-031-15401-0_3

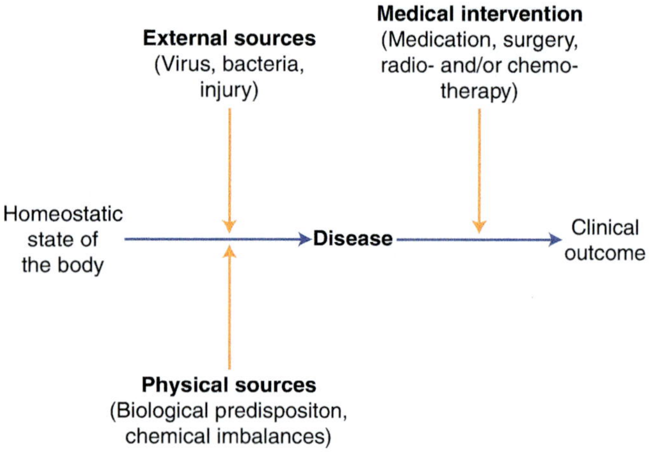

Fig. 3.1 The biomedical model

[9, 10]. Since its introduction, it has gained popularity in teaching and in clinical practice, coming to be viewed as the overarching framework of the field [11, 12]. Despite its following, the model is not without its critics. Its limitations include its vagueness, eclecticism, lack of coherence, and difficulty in measuring its components. Other critics claim that the BPS model has not succeeded in reducing the dominance of the biological approach in the past decades, especially in regard to clinical research [13, 14].

Despite these shortcomings, the BPS model is still regarded as a very useful tool in psychiatry teaching. It is recommended that the model may benefit from broadening its scope and conceptualization of cultural and structural factors, reflecting more on cross-cultural differences and conditions (social, economic, and political) rather than assuming homogeneity across community, culture, and society (Fig. 3.2) [15, 16].

Fig. 3.2 Contrasting the biomedical and biopsychosocial models for upper limbs disorders. (*Reprinted from* Burton et al. [16]; *with permission)*

	Biomedical model	Biopsychosocial model
Presentation	Focus is on physical causes of disease. Clinician asks questions about onset and cause, pain history, and other symptoms. However, empirical signs and symptoms of pain and tenderness are considered paramount.	Clinician aims to ascertain psychosocial and physical processes that may contribute to the arm pain. Clinician may ask for a history of recent life stressors and behaviours, in addition to conducting a clinical examination.
Diagnosis	Clinician examines the arm, and may consider x-ray and/or other lab tests (depending on signs and symptoms) and forms diagnosis.	Based on a combination of clinical examination of the arm, psychosocial factors, (probably without X-ray or other lab tests) the clinician forms an explanation for the symptoms.
Treatment	Medical plan prescribed for the patient based on biological aetiology and pathogenesis.	Clinician discusses available interventions with special attention to behaviours and lifestyles that could influence pain. The patient is involved in formulating and implementing the plan.

Landmark Theories, Concepts, and Key Contributors

Biomedical Model: Focus on Biological Factors and the Separation of Body and Mind

Medicine in the 1960s was dominated by the "biomedical" model. In this model, a classical factor-analytic approach was taken to treat patients' illnesses and suffering: physicians were focused only on biological factors limited to observations of the patient's body, specifically its cellular and physiological processes. The disease was strictly viewed as an organic malfunction; in turn, patients were viewed as symptoms that needed to be treated, where the caring aspect of the patient was substantially ignored (Table 3.1).

Limitations of the Biomedical Model: Dualism, Reductionism, and the Patient–Physician Relationship

Engel found several limitations to the biomedical model he pronounced over multiple published papers [1–5] that would later form the basis of the BPS model. First, the biomedical model was dualistic in its approach: it saw the body and mind as separate entities, where the body offered a more "scientific" and, therefore, accurate presentation of the disease because it only assessed biological factors. On the other hand, the mind was viewed more as a subjective, emotion-based narrative of how the patient was suffering. There was no attempt to bridge the two elements together to reflect a dynamic, integrated approach to how social and psychological processes such as stress or socioeconomic status can influence health and disease (Figs. 3.3, 3.4, 3.5, and 3.6) [17–20].

Second, the model took on a reductionist approach to disease, where a hierarchy based on biological systems fully accounted for any deviations from the biological norm, with no influence from other nonbiological systems. In this view, all diseases could be reduced to biological causes in the body and, as such, treatments for these diseases would also be biological in character [7, 21]. With the prominence of the biomedical approach, the field of psychiatry sought to assert itself as a medical discipline and so utilized reductionism in its approach. More specifically, it reduced mental health difficulties to brain diseases that would be treated with pharmacological interventions targeting biological abnormalities only, without taking into consideration psychosocial differences [22, 23]. Furthermore, factors such as anger, sadness, neglect, and attachment were discounted as they could not be verified and explained at the level of cellular and molecular processes. Further research in psychosomatics by Engel showed otherwise, noting the impact of psychological and social factors on the development and physiology of the whole organism (Figs. 3.7 and 3.8) [24–26].

Third, the biomedical model did not view the patient–physician relationship and healthcare system as potential factors influencing the accuracy of a diagnosis and the success of a chosen treatment. For example, factors such as a patient's adherence to medication and access to affordable, quality healthcare were aspects that were not considered within the scope of physician and patient care [21]. Engel's efforts to challenge and broaden the biomedical model helped give rise to the BPS model in practice, research, and education (Table 3.2; Figs. 3.9 and 3.10) [27, 28].

Table 3.1 Biomedical model characteristics

1. Dichotomy between health and disease
2. Duality of the body and mind
3. Disease is due to physical–biological causes
4. Observations through quantitative and quantitative measuring and analysis tools
5. Medical diagnosis does not depend on the patient–clinician relationship

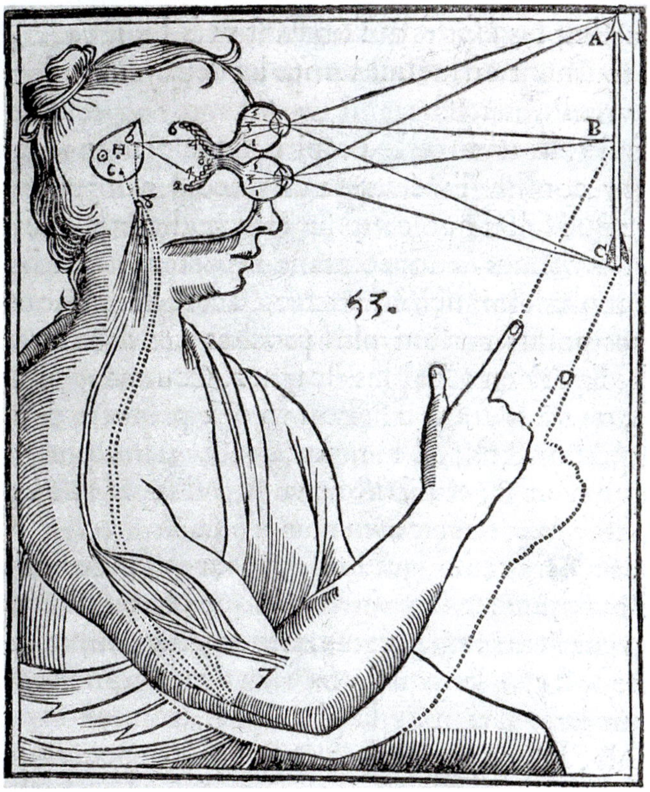

Fig. 3.3 Illustration of mind/body dualism, René Descartes (Creative Commons Attribution 4.0 International license) [17]

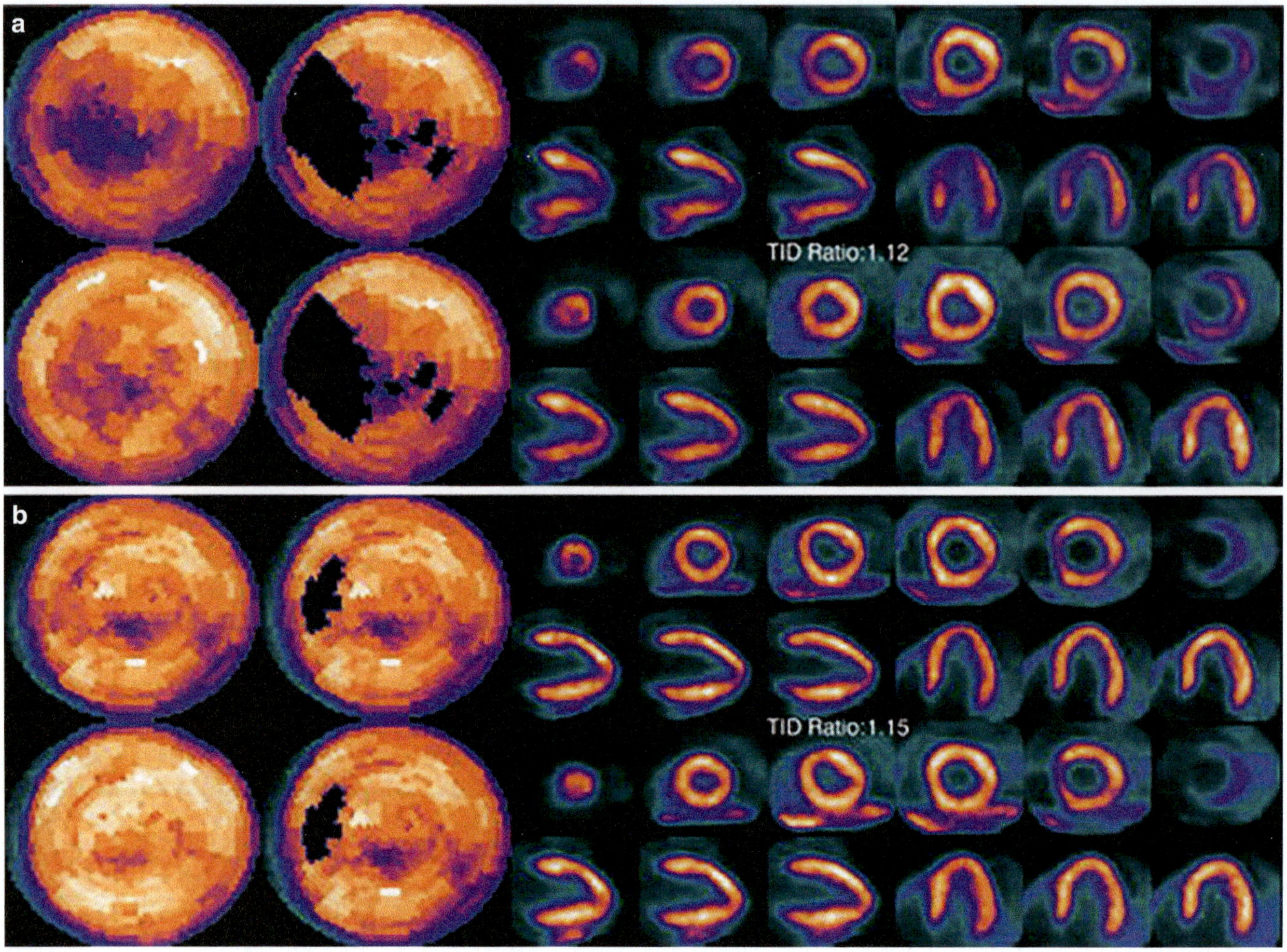

Fig. 3.4 Positron emission tomography (PET) myocardial perfusion scan in a twin pair. (**a**) Twin with PTSD. (**b**) Twin without PTSD. The hypofusion is shown as black, where the severity of hypofusion was quantified by a stress total severity score (STSS) indicating a casual relationship between PTSD and ischemic heart disease (IHD). (*From* Vaccarino and Bremner [18]; *with permission*)

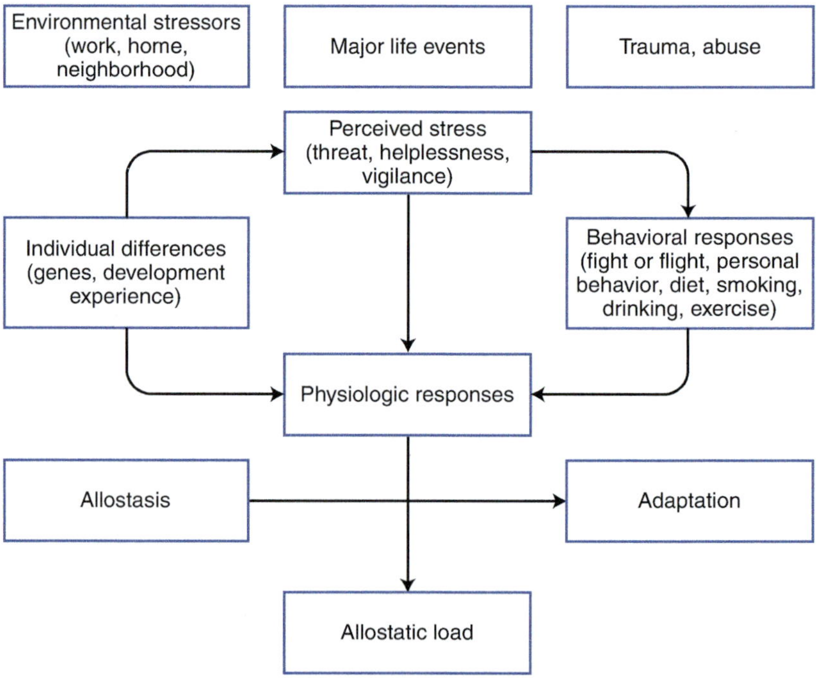

Fig. 3.5 The stress response and development of biological allostasis, which can be caused by physical or psychosocial burdens

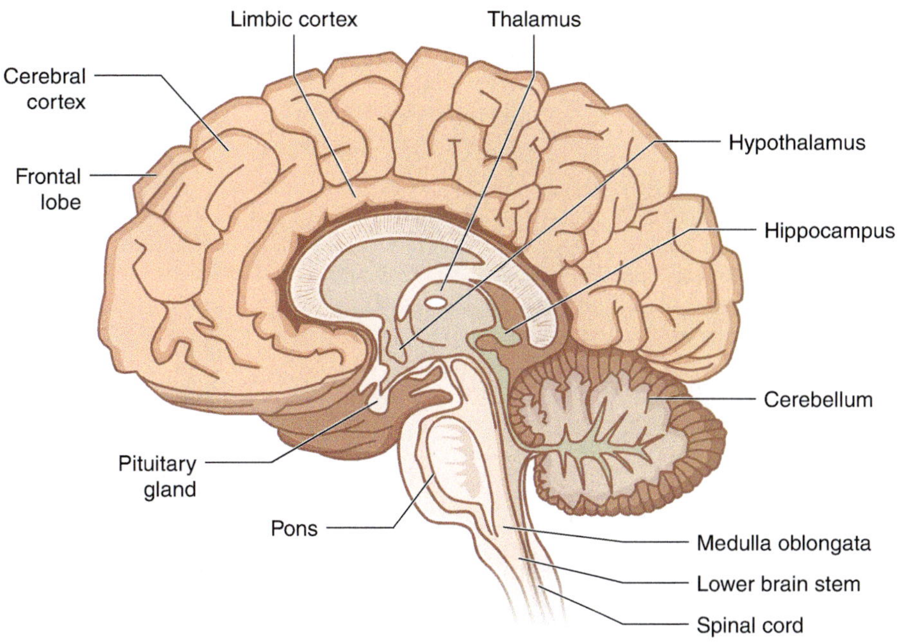

Fig. 3.6 The hypothalamus is the key structure in stress reactivity, which controls hormone balance, temperature, and dilation of blood vessels through the autonomic nervous system (ANS)

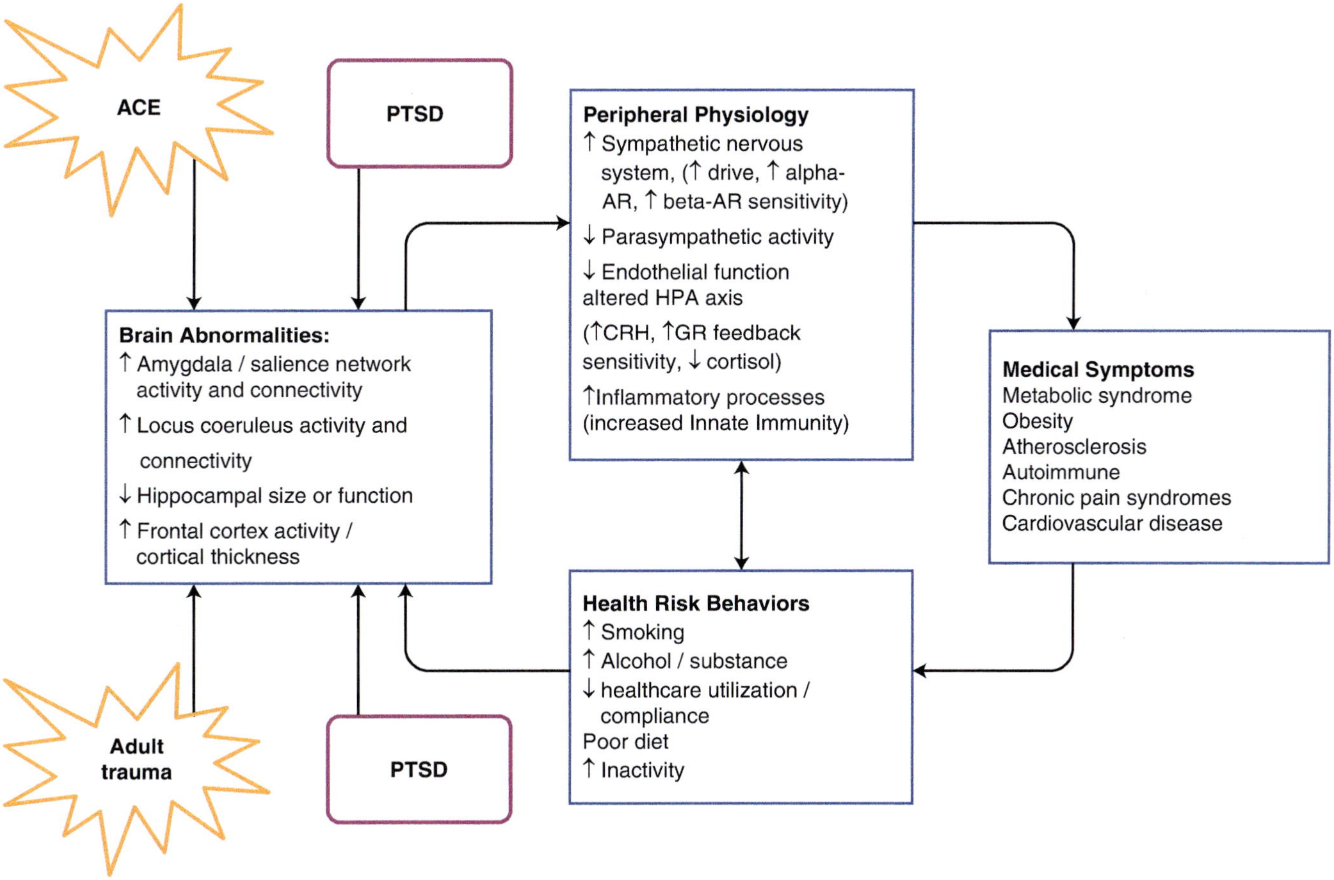

Fig. 3.7 Schematic diagram of childhood and adult trauma on brain and physiological systems. (*From* King [25]; *with permission*)

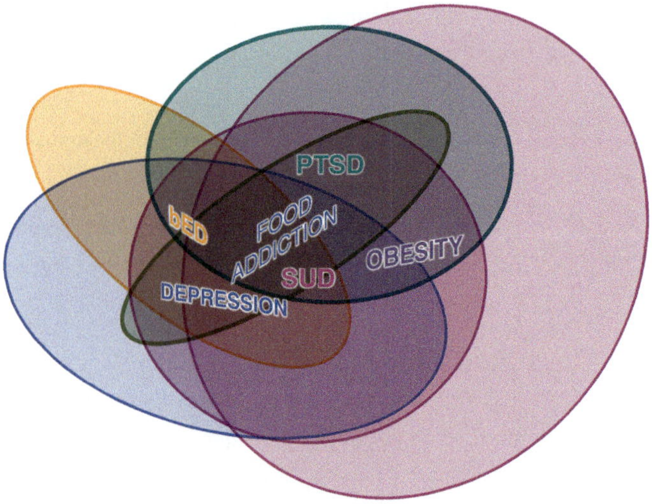

Fig. 3.8 Venn diagram displaying the overlapping associations between bulimic eating disorders (bED), substance use disorders (SUD), food addiction, posttraumatic stress disorder (PTSD), depression, and obesity. (*Adapted from* Brewerton [26]; *with permission*)

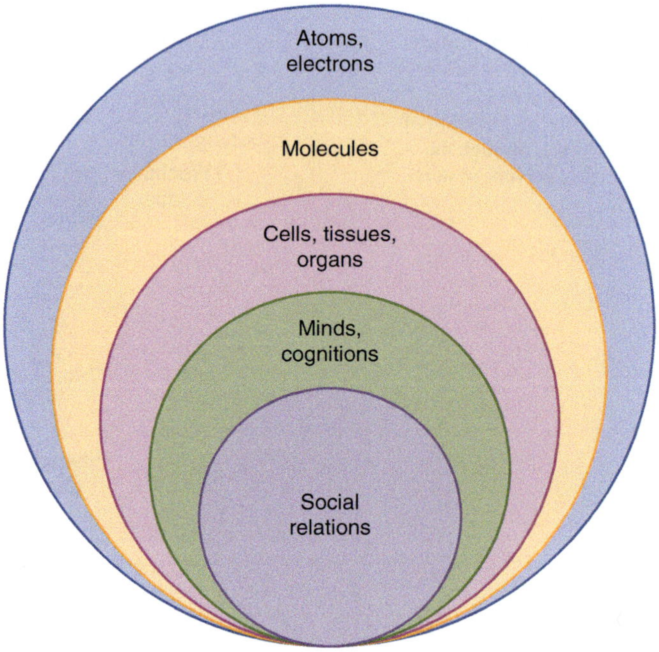

Fig. 3.9 A Venn diagram illustrating a reductionist ontology of wholes and parts. (From Rocca and Anjum [27]; Creative Commons Attribution 4.0 International License; http://creativecommons.org/licenses/by/4.0/)

Table 3.2 Engel's critique of biomedicine

1. A biochemical alteration does not translate directly into an illness. The appearance of illness results from the interaction of diverse causal factors, including those at the molecular, individual, and social levels. And the converse, psychological alterations may, under certain circumstances, manifest as illnesses or forms of suffering that constitute health problems, including, at times, biochemical correlates
2. The presence of a biological derangement does not shed light on the meaning of the symptoms to the patient, nor does it necessarily infer the attitudes and skills that the clinician must have to gather information and process it well
3. Psychosocial variables are more important determinants of susceptibility, severity, and course of illness than had been previously appreciated by those who maintain a biomedical view of illness
4. Adopting a sick role is not necessarily associated with the presence of a biological derangement
5. The success of most biological treatments is influenced by psychosocial factors, for example, the so-called placebo effect
6. The patient–clinician relationship influences medical outcomes, even if only because of its influence on adherence to a chosen treatment
7. Unlike inanimate subjects of scientific scrutiny, patients are profoundly influenced by the way in which they are studied, and the scientists engaged in the study are influenced by their subjects

The Biopsychosocial Model: An Overview

Engel's BPS model was seen as an approach to understanding health, illness, and health care delivery through the interactions between biological, psychological, and social factors [8]. These three domains were considered to be components of a continuum of natural systems that were basic to medical practice. The model helped explain that a person suffers not as isolated organs but rather as a whole [29]. This holistic perspective means that the person's personality, surrounding environment, emotional tone, and other social parameters influence the manifestation of an illness. Furthermore, the social and psychological factors could be understood on their own in a scientific manner or against biological correlates. Humanistic qualities became highly valued elements of the BPS model (Fig. 3.11) [12, 30].

In summary, all three domains: biological, psychological, and social, had to be taken into account. All three were relevant at all times in health care tasks [6]. Physicians also had the flexibility to choose to focus more on the "bio" domain with one patient and more on the "psycho" aspect with another. In a sense, the model was seen as an ode to additive eclecticism (more information is better), where physicians had the freedom to individualize treatment to the patient taking into consideration the patient's needs (Fig. 3.12) [21].

While the BPS theory was at the heart of modern psychiatry, Engel was not a psychiatrist and had never trained in psychiatry. He received training in internal medicine, specifically focused on gastrointestinal diseases, and only started taking an interest in the psychological aspects of gastrointestinal illness after meeting psychiatrist John Romano

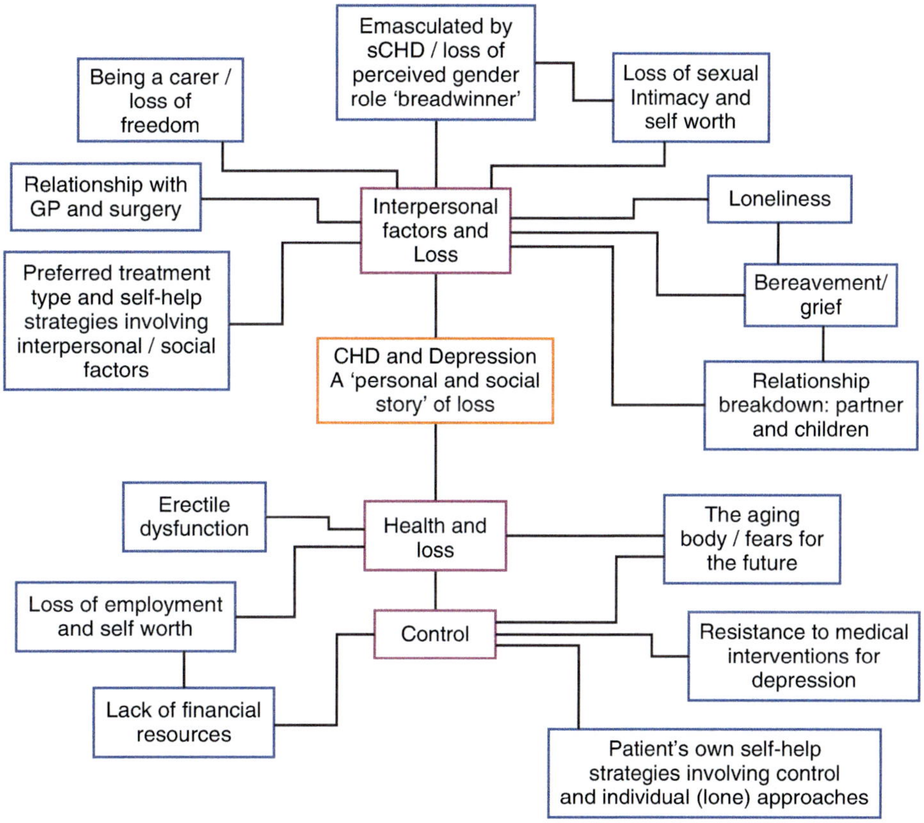

Fig. 3.10 Multifaceted perception of interpersonal factors and control in relation to patients' chronic heart disease and major depression. (*From* Simmonds et al. [28]; Creative Commons Attribution License; https://creativecommons.org/licenses/by/2.0)

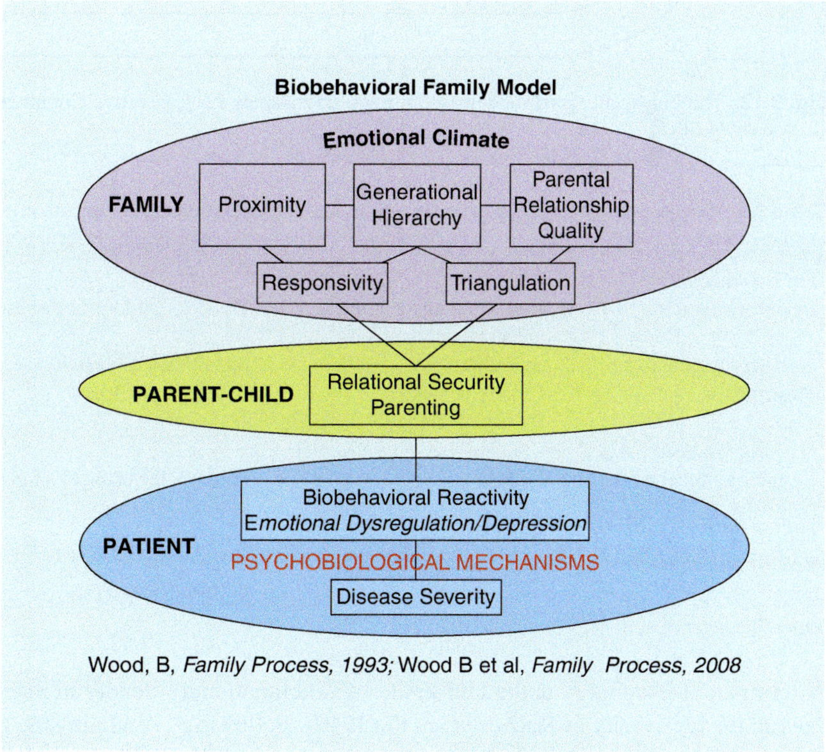

Fig. 3.11 Role of emotional climate in manifestation of disease severity. (*From* Wood et al. [30]; *with permission*)

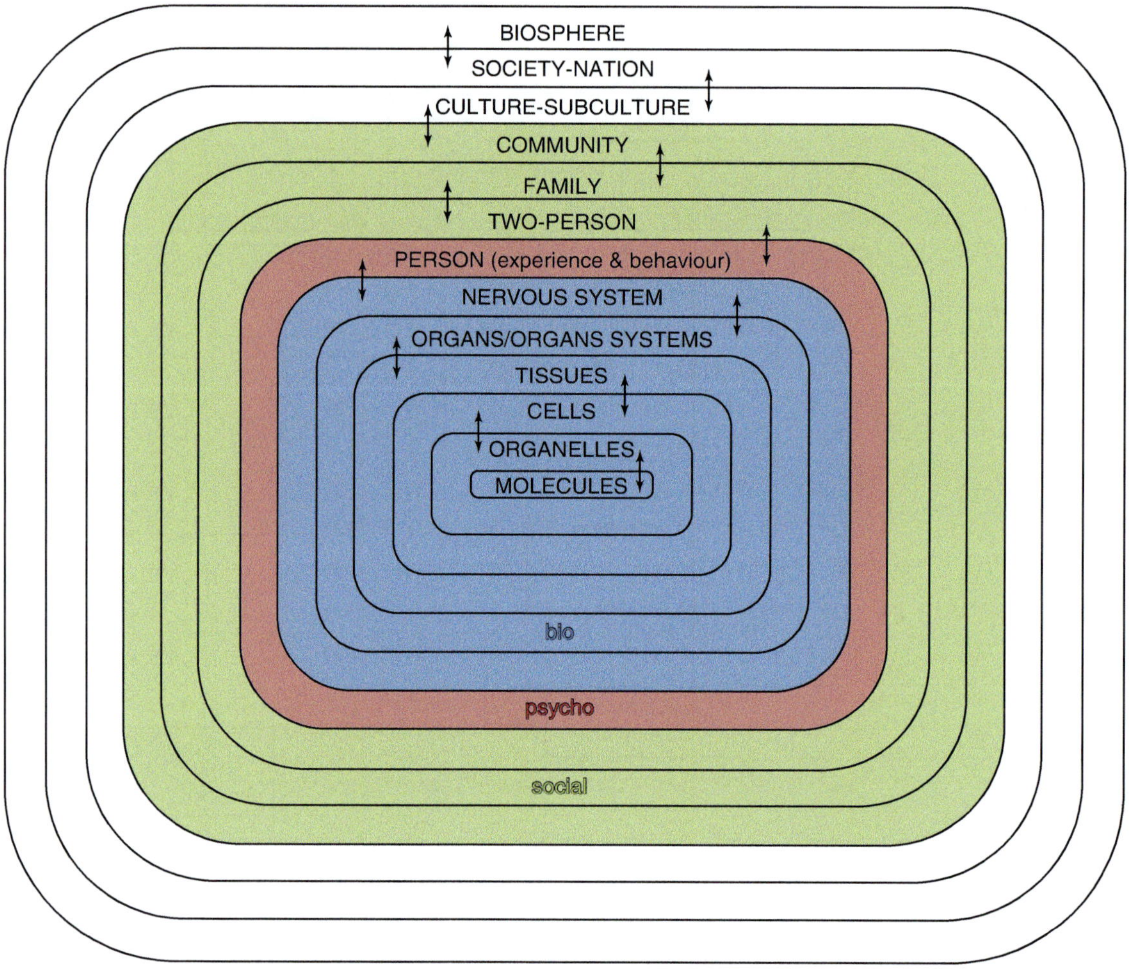

Fig. 3.12 The biopsychosocial model. (*From* Farre and Rapley [21]; Creative Commons Attribution 4.0 license [http://creativecommons.org/licenses/by/4.0])

Table 3.3 Comparison of stereotypical assumptions and interpretation of self-organizing processes within the three predominant frameworks

	Healing model	Biomedicine model	Biopsychosocial model
Key assumptions			
Key characteristics	Human beings within the universal order	Physical, biological disease	Multidimensional, biopsychosocial health
Auxiliary hypotheses	Spirituality	Specificity, objectivity	Productivity, collaboration
Treatment goals	Quality of shared transcendence	Symptom reduction	Psychosocial health and well-being
Framing of self-organization in mental health treatments			
Definition of mental health problems	Suffering	Disease, the primacy of physical–biological causes	Disorder, psychological strain, psychosocial functioning
Patient role	Ritualized	Passive/reactive	Proactive-collaborative
Role of self-organization	Transcendent effects	Placebo/nocebo effects of physiological effects	(partly) proactive, intended, and self-directed effects

From Flückiger et al. [31]; *with permission*

(Chairman of Psychiatry at the University of Cincinnati and later at the University of Rochester) in the 1940s. Following the meeting with Romano, he began training in Psychoanalysis under Franz Alexander (a student of Freud) and became a leader in Psychosomatic Medicine. When Engel started formulating the BPS model, he sought to psychologize medicine rather than medicalize psychiatry (Table 3.3; Figs. 3.13, 3.14, 3.15, and 3.16) [4, 31–34].

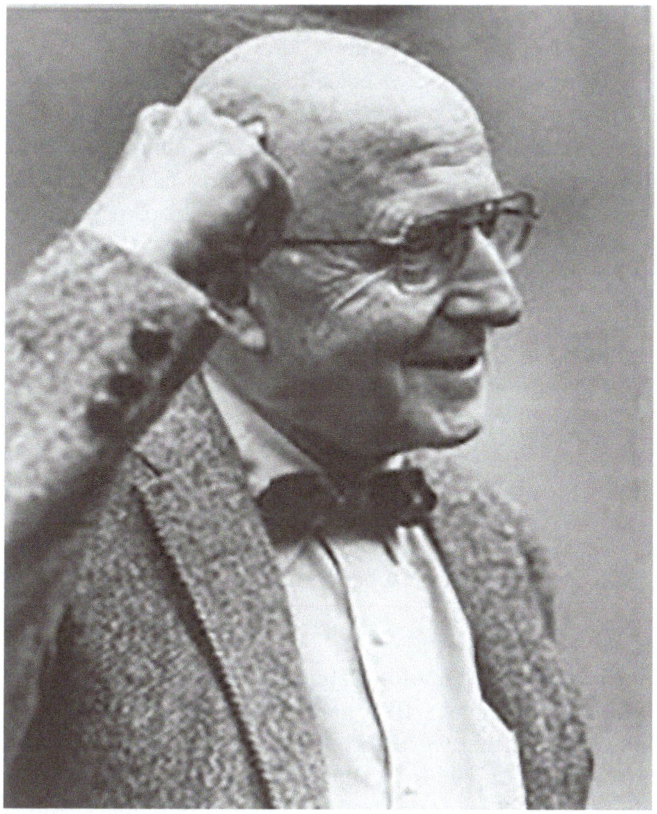

Fig. 3.13 Portrait of George Libman Engel (1913–1999)

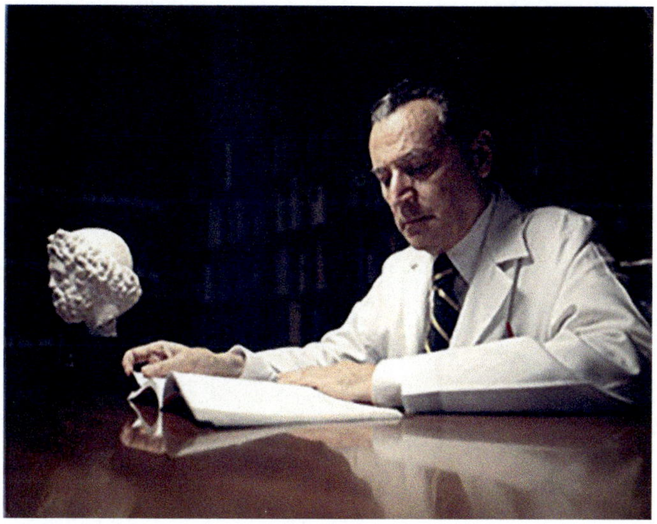

Fig. 3.14 Portrait of John Romano (1908–1994)

When Engel first submitted his paper on the BPS model to the *New England Journal of Medicine*, it was rejected but was quickly accepted by *Science*. The BPS model then began gaining attention in the 1980s, during the rise of the DSM-III and psychopharmacology and the decline of psychoanalysis.

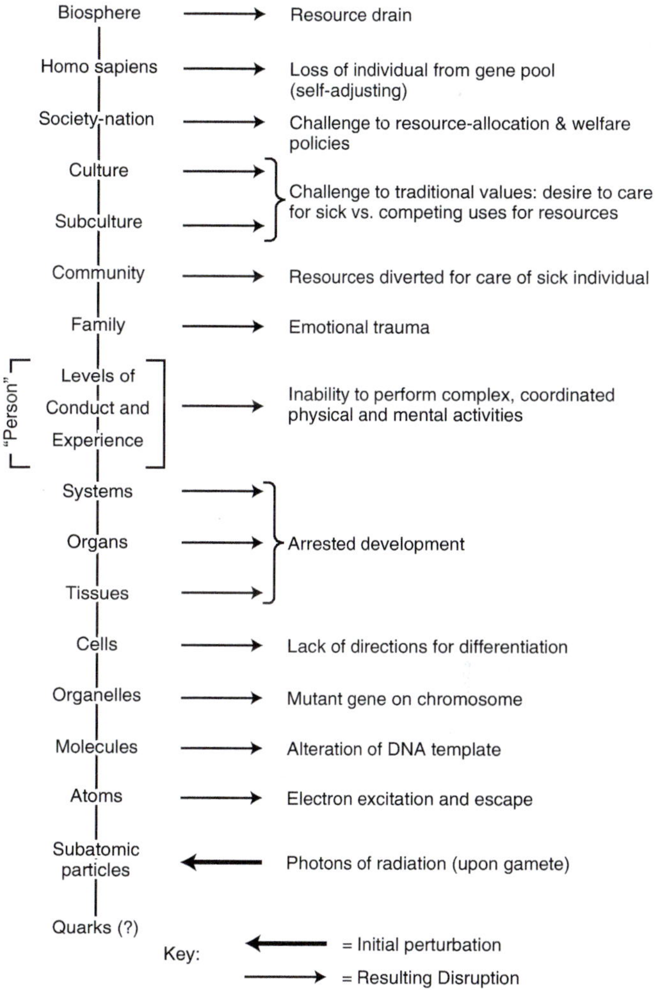

Fig. 3.15 Example of a biopsychosocial approach: severe physical and mental retardation caused by a radiation-induced mutation. (*From* Engel [4]; *with permission*)

Since then, it has been widely embraced and used internationally in multiple professions and academic disciplines, including religion, psychology, sociology, and philosophy (Fig. 3.17) [2].

Clinical Application of the BPS Model

The BPS model in clinical practice requires that several aspects be considered. First, the clinician must recognize that relationships are central to providing healthcare. Second, they must determine which aspects of the biological, psychological, and social domains are most important to understand and enhance a patient's health. Third, a clinician's use of self-awareness as a diagnostic and therapeutic tool can help develop a treatment plan that is more in line with the patient's

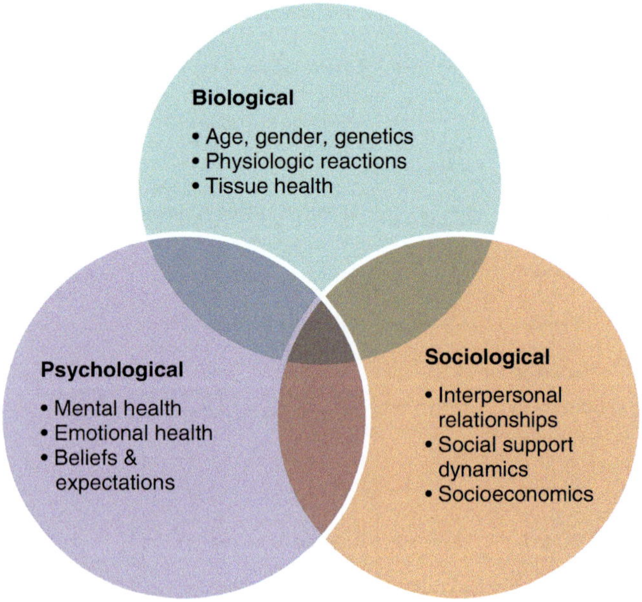

Fig. 3.16 Jorday A. Gliedt: Illustration of the biopsychosocial model comprised of biological, psychological and sociological influences. (*From* Gliedt et al. [34]; Creative Commons Attribution 4.0 license; http://creativecommons.org/licenses/by/4.0)

needs. Fourth, a patient's history should be obtained in the context of life circumstances. Finally, a multidimensional treatment reflecting the significant aspects of the three domains must be developed to address the patient's illness and suffering (Figs. 3.18, 3.19, 3.20, 3.21, 3.22, 3.23, and 3.24) [35–40].

Adolf Meyer and Roy Grinker: Key Contributors to the BPS Model

Several critics assert that while Engel may have formulated the BPS model, it was Adolf Meyer's "psychobiology" (1948) approach and Roy Grinker's work in the early 1960s that acted as precursors to the model.

Meyer, known to be an eclectic academic, may have been controversial in his thinking; he rejected the concept of disease and had a hostile view of biological approaches (one could not change biology), but ultimately had a profound impact on psychiatry. He founded the field of psychiatric epidemiology, coined the term mental hygiene, and acted as one of the first advocates for people who have mental illness [7]. In his psychobiology approach, Meyer outlined two assumptions, which were crucial stepping stones for the addition and integration of the psychosocial aspects to the BPS model:

1. Treatment involved an appreciation and study of the whole person in action.
2. The individual represented an integration of a hierarchy of functions that must be viewed together (Figs. 3.25 and 3.26) [41, 42].

Meyer's psychobiology approach ultimately led to the formation of Engel's BPS model, but there was a missing link between the two theories that were later cemented in the 1950s and 1960s by the prominent psychiatrist Roy Grinker. Grinker, a maverick of modern psychiatry, was a strong advocate for biopsychosocial eclecticism partly due to recognizing the dangers of the psychoanalytic doctrine. Some academics further claim that Grinker was the unrecognized founder of the BPS model and may have even coined the term "biopsychosocial" at least 25 years before Engel [7]. However, there was a clear distinction in the application of the model between the two doctors. While Grinker applied the concept to psychiatry to emphasize the "bio" aspect against psychoanalytic orthodoxy in the 1950s (prominent in the field at the time), Engel used the concept to emphasize the "psychosocial" element in medicine (Figs. 3.27 and 3.28) [43, 44].

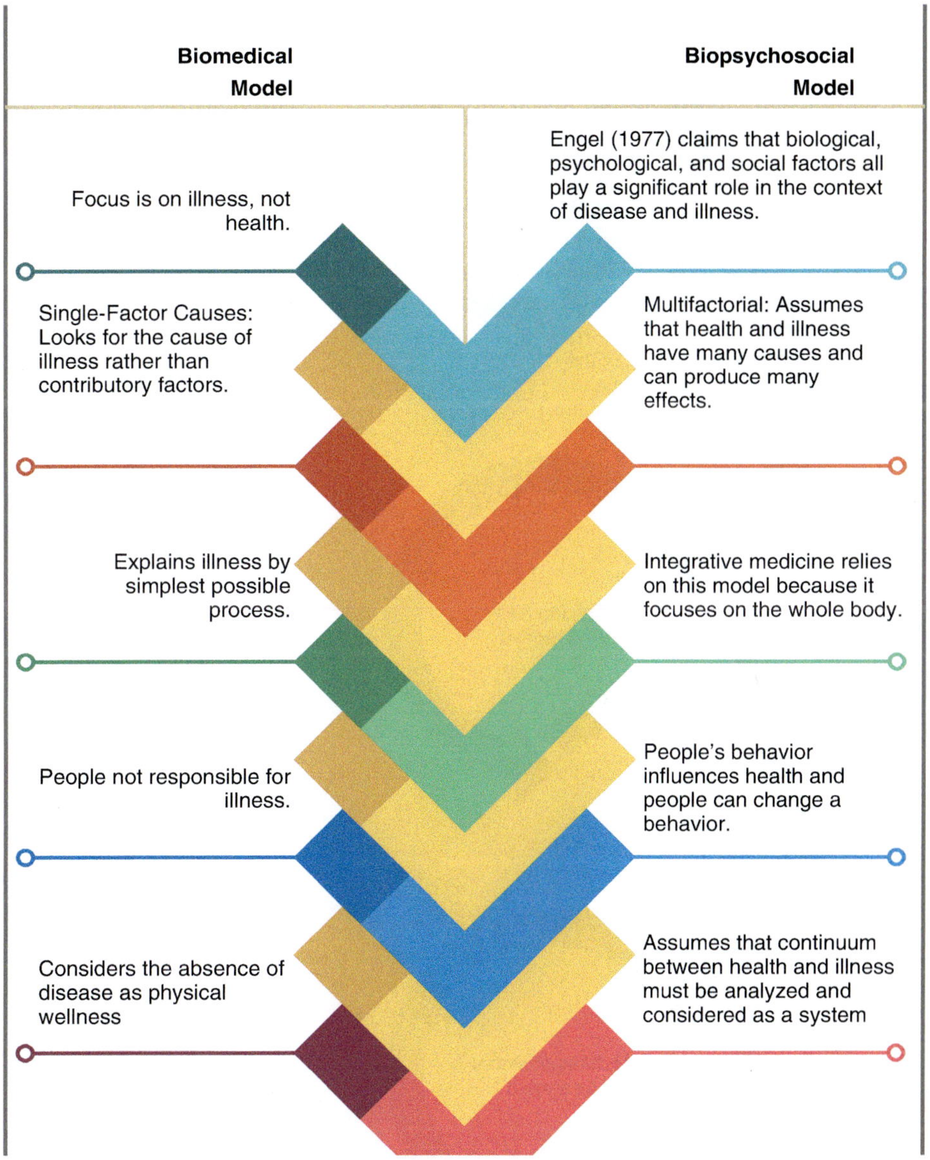

Fig. 3.17 Biomedical vs. biopsychosocial model

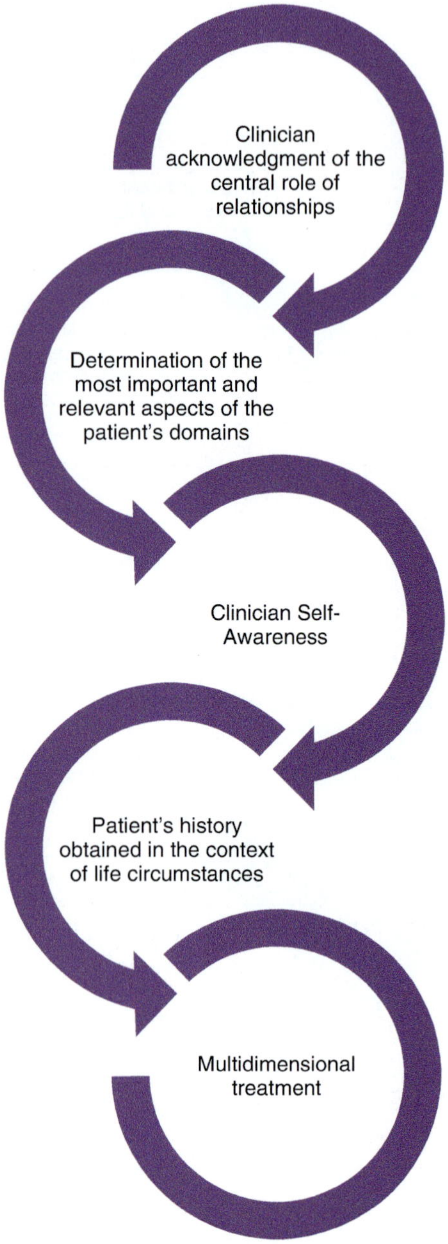

Fig. 3.18 Clinical application of the BPS model

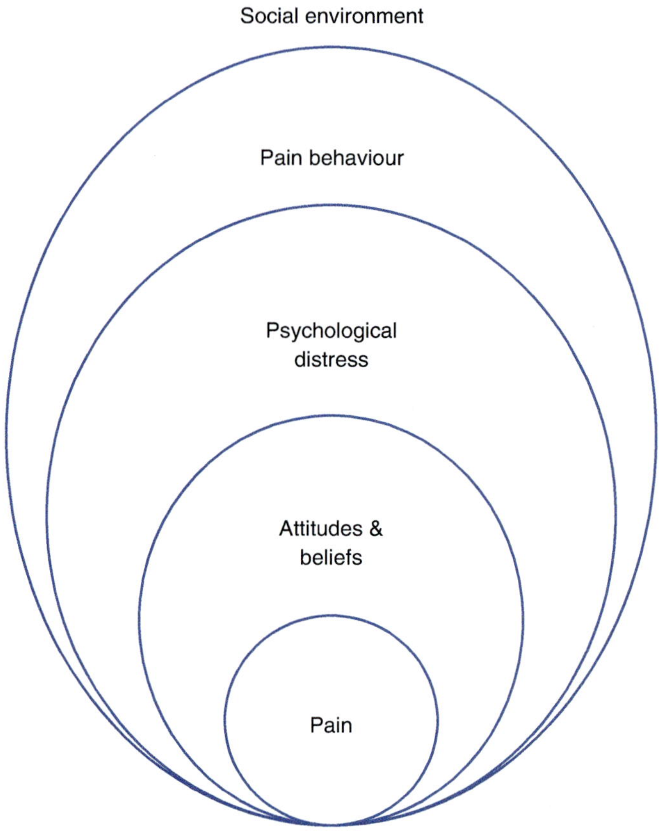

Fig. 3.19 Biopsychosocial model of pain behavior. (*From* Malpus [35]; *with permission*)

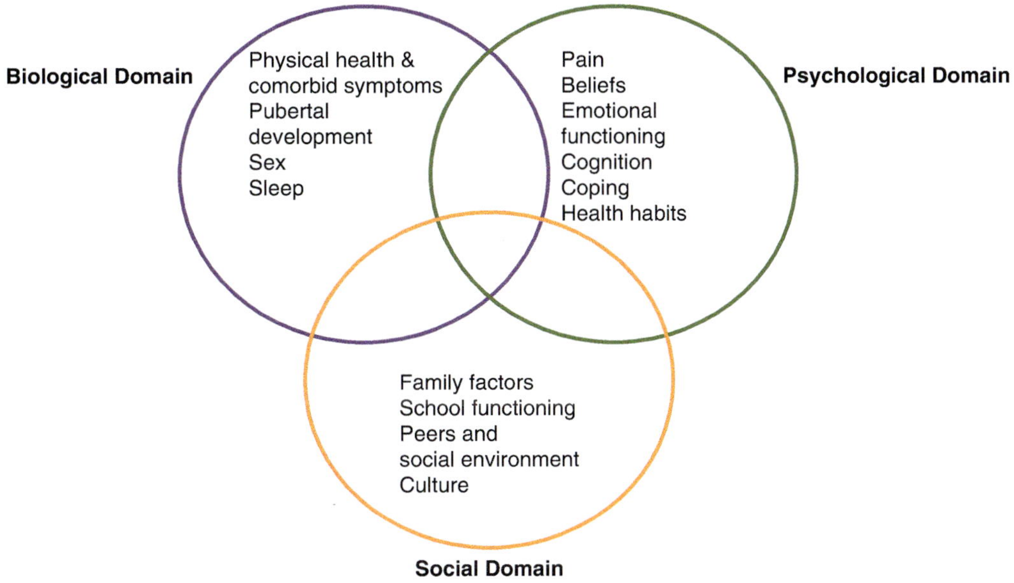

Fig. 3.20 A biopsychosocial conceptualization of pediatric chronic pain. (*From* Essner [36]; *with permission*)

Fig. 3.21 Role of social domains such as social status, self-empowerment, education, and income in epidemiology of cardiovascular disease. (*From* Reid and Owen [37]; *with permission*)

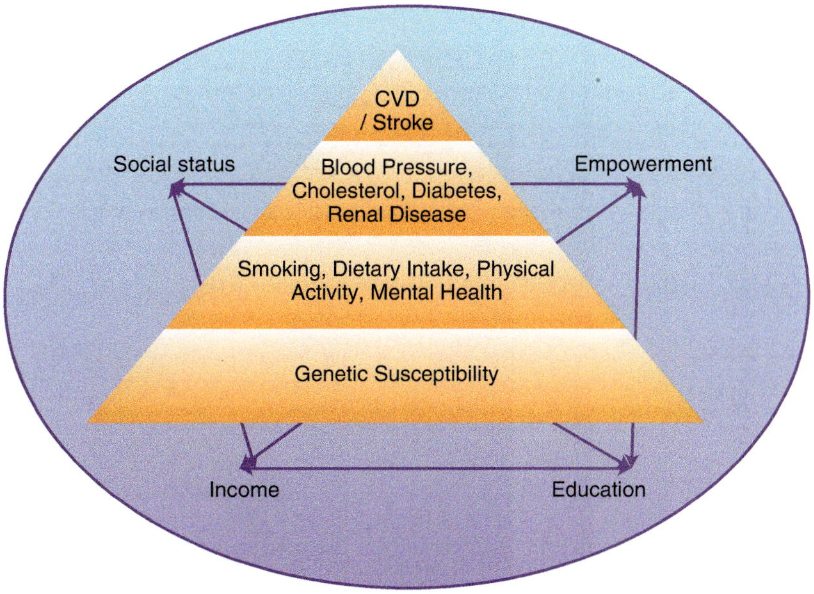

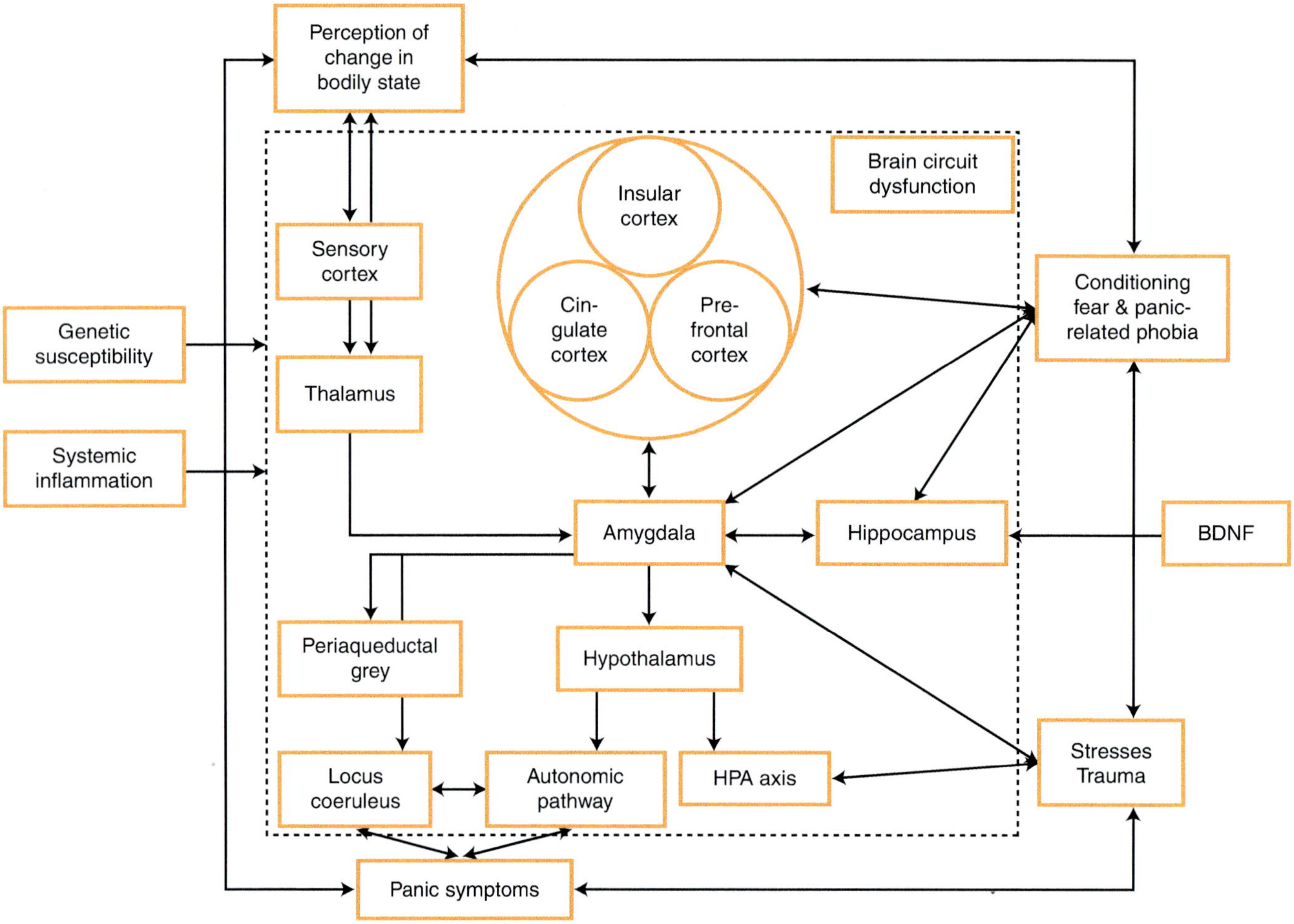

Fig. 3.22 Biopsychosocial and cognitive model for treatment resistant panic disorder. (*From* Chen and Tsai [38]; with permission)

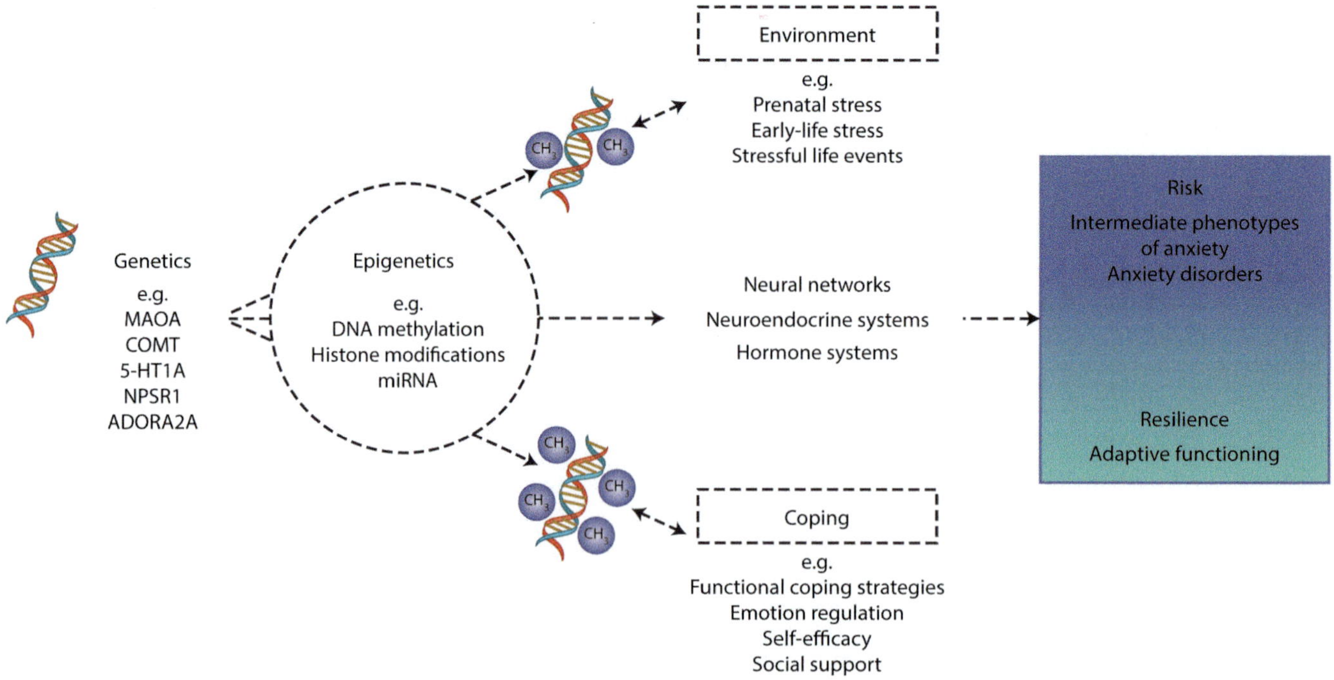

Fig. 3.23 Multilevel model of risk and resilience in anxiety disorders. Genetic factors interact with environmental stressors and coping-related protective factors in a risk- or resilience-increasing manner as governed by epigenetic mechanisms via the employment and regulation of neural networks, neuroendocrine systems, and hormone systems. (*From* Schiele and Domschke [39]; *with permission*)

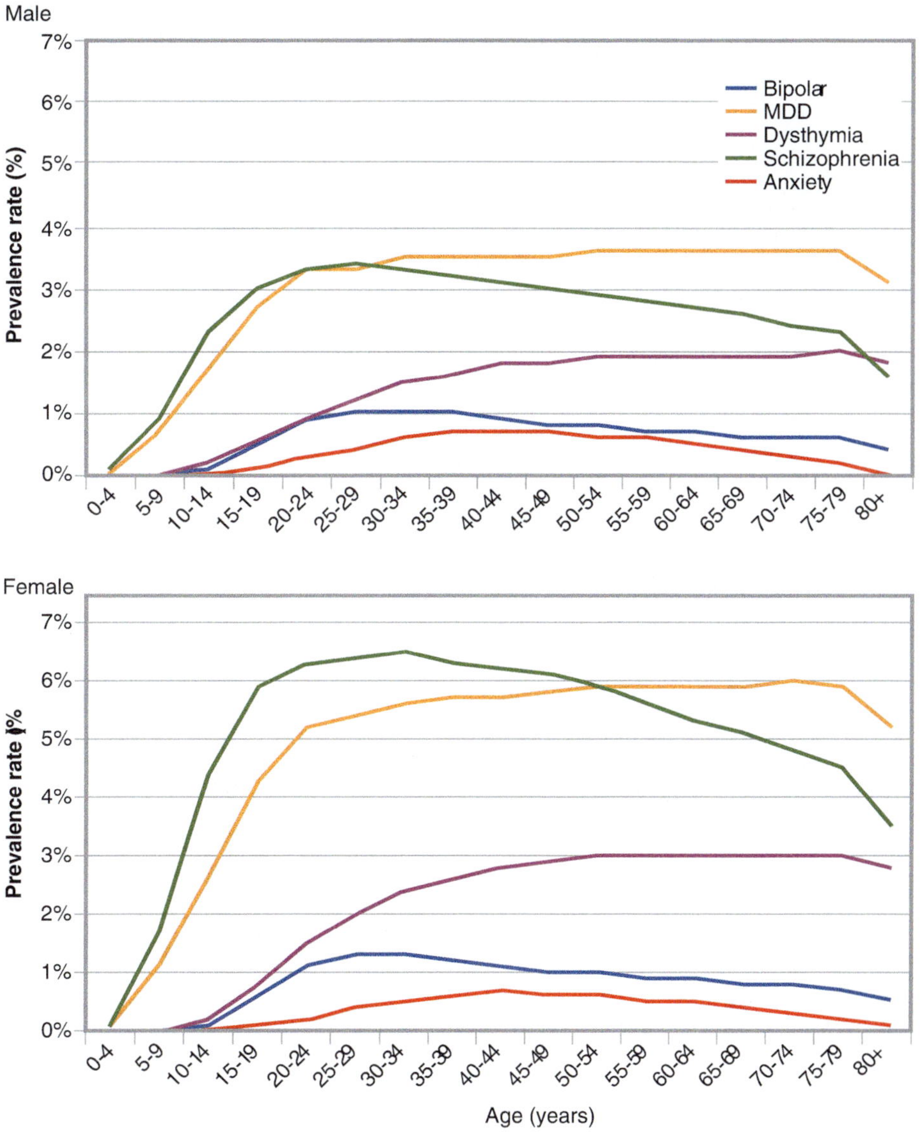

Fig. 3.24 Prevalence rates of bipolar disorder in 2013. (*From* Ferrari et al. [40]; *with permission*)

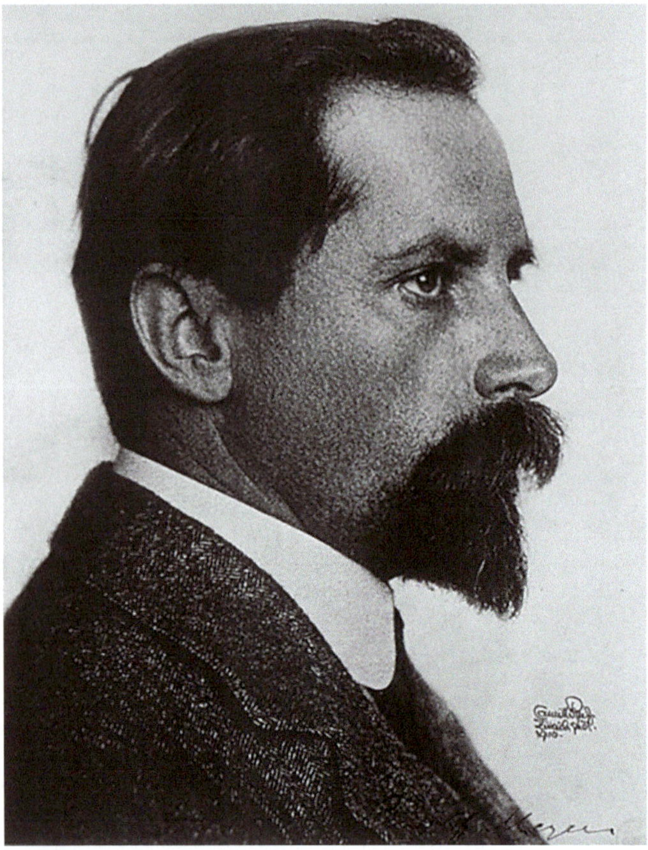

Fig. 3.25 Adolf Meyer

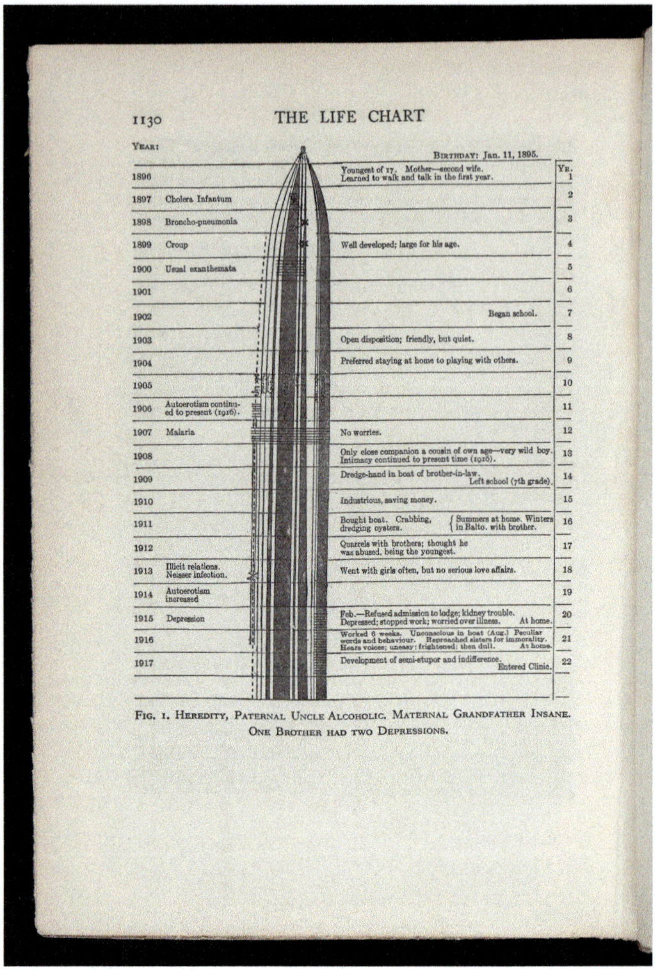

Fig. 3.26 Line drawing of the life chart by Adolf Meyer. (*From* Osler [42]; Welcome Collection; https://wellcomecollection.org/works/g7jrky99)

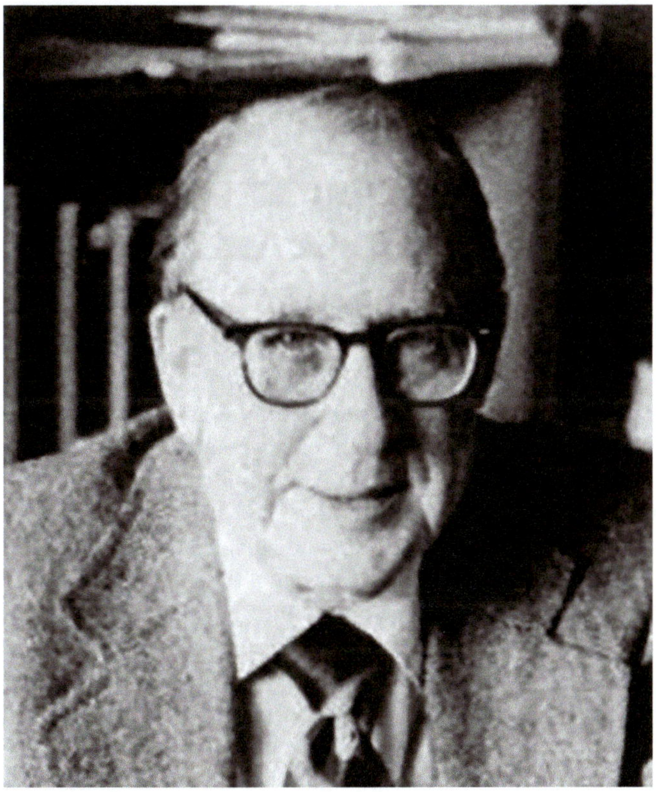

Fig. 3.27 Portrait of Roy Grinker (1900–1993)

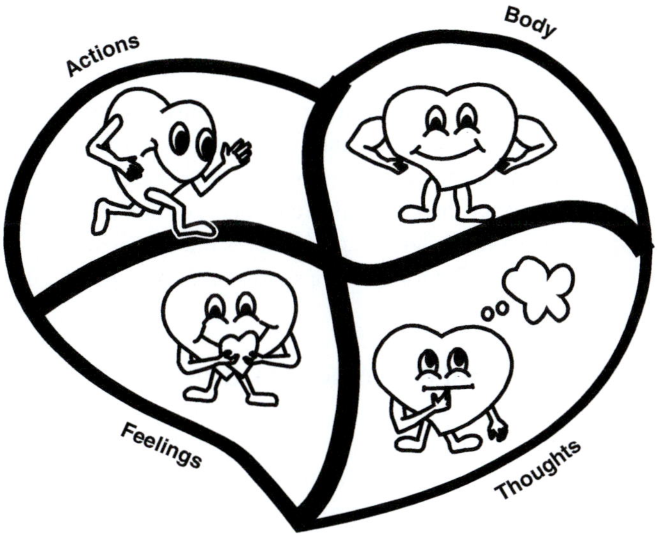

Fig. 3.28 Whole body model in chronic disease management. (*From* Clarke et al. [44]; *with permission*)

Components of the BPS Model

The Four P's

The biopsychosocial formulation grid (see Table 3.4) provides a useful structure for the model's application [45]. When information is gathered during the assessment, it is placed into a biopsychosocial framework to address the three domains (biological, psychological, and social) in the context of factors known as the "four P's" of case formulation [22–24, 46]:

1. **Predisposing** factors are those that increase the risk of the presenting problem. Examples of these are having a certain gene variation associated with a mental disorder

Table 3.4 Elements of a 4P case formulation matrix

	Biological	Psychological	Social
Predisposing	Genetics Birth complications Traumatic brain injury Medical comorbidities Medications Substance use	Personality traits Attachment style Defenses Coping mechanisms Self-esteem	Socioeconomic status, demographics Cultural identity History of trauma and/or abuse Social relationships Adversity Functional status
Precipitating (may become perpetuating factors)	Medication Substance use Acute illness	Grief Acute stressor Moral injury	Loss of employment Loss of housing Financial strain Relationship conflict Academic failure
Perpetuating	Medication nonadherence Poor response to or tolerability of medication Chronic illness	Personality traits Defenses Coping mechanisms Cognitive distortions	Housing instability Financial instability Social isolation Stigma regarding mental health treatment
Protective	Good physical health Diet and exercise Medication adherence	Psychological mindedness Insight, judgement Coping mechanisms Intellectual functioning	Social support Community involvement Access to mental health services

(biological), temperament (psychological), and socioeconomic status (social).

2. **Precipitating** factors are commonly known as external stressors or events (positive or negative) that are likely to trigger the onset of a presenting problem. Examples include childhood trauma, such as the loss of a loved one.
3. **Perpetuating factors** are factors that maintain the problem once it has become established. Such factors can be in the patient, family, community, or larger systems, such as unaddressed parental conflict or learning disabilities.
4. **Protective factors (strengths)** include any elements of the patient's characteristics (skills, talents, and interests) and external events (supportive elements within the family) that help enhance the adaptability and healthy functioning of the patient. Examples include a child that has a good relationship with a favorite elementary school teacher or a talent for art which may be used to engage the child in treatment and enhance self-esteem.
5. **Prognosis and potential for change** have been suggested as a fifth "P" for case formulation. These factors include any areas that are flexible to change or potential obstacles to successful treatment (Fig. 3.29).

The grid (Table 3.4) [46] presents a viable method to provide a comprehensive examination of the elements needed for a biopsychosocial formulation. To fully utilize this formulation, the first step is to provide a summary paragraph of the case, identify and assess the four P's in the patient's context using the formulation matrix, generate a problem list by connecting the data to presentation, and finally, develop a treatment plan that addresses the patient's individual needs. Thus, the ultimate aim of the biopsychosocial formulation is to provide a tailored, individualized, and specific intervention for the patient [47].

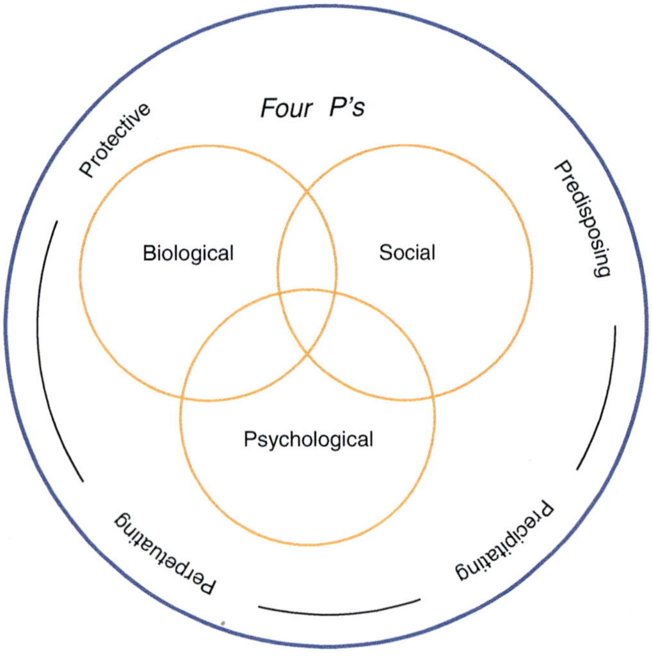

Fig. 3.29 The four Ps: components of the BPS Model

Clinical Application of the Biopsychosocial Model

Diagnosis Vs. Case Formulation

While *The Diagnostic and Statistical Manual of Mental Disorders* (DSM) attempts to identify clusters of signs and symptoms that make up discreet psychiatric diagnoses, it is frequently criticized for its oversimplification of the vast continuum of human psychology and behavior. It may be used as a clinical tool to help guide diagnosis, defined as the identification of an illness. However, the DSM offers minimal insight into the person behind the diagnosis and the experiences that led to his or her presentation at that specific moment in time. The term "diagnosis" may be particularly problematic in the realm of mental health if interpreted as a discrete epistemological label, given the dynamic and widely diverse nature of the human psyche. Meanwhile, the case formulation not only describes the rich phenomenology of the psychiatric presentation but also integrates key psychological, biological, and social factors to explore the etiologies of one's current mental condition and to guide patient-centered intervention and prognosis. It is important to note the fluid nature of the case formulation; for example, a perturbation in the psychological wing may lead to drastic alterations in the biological and/or social wing such that different approaches to risk assessment and/or treatment planning may be appropriate at different stages of one's life story [48]. The case formulation encapsulates the diagnosis and is what brings the diagnosis to life (Tables 3.5, 3.6, and 3.7).

Assessment and Outcome Measures

The rich data gathered through the lens of the biopsychosocial approach may be used to inform risk assessment and reduction, the level of care appropriate for the severity of the psychiatric condition, prognosis, and outcome measures. Risk factors for self-harm and harm to others must be considered from a holistic, patient-centered approach, as risk factors in themselves have been shown to be poor predictors of harmful behaviors in individual patients [48].

During risk assessment, it is especially crucial to recognize the various biological, psychological, and social forces at play at that moment in time. An effective risk assessment must weigh dynamic risk factors (e.g., substance use and intoxication, access to firearms) and protective factors (e.g.,

Table 3.5 Interview questions for the biological formulation

Biological formulation	
History of present illness	What physical symptoms are you experiencing? Medical review of systems
Predispositions	Is there a family history of mental illness? Do you have any psychiatric or medical comorbidities? What medications do you take? History of and/or current substance use? Are you up to date with physical and nutritional health maintenance?
Patient demographics and epidemiology of disorder(s) under consideration	What is your gender identity? What are your pronouns? What is your ethnic and/or racial identity?

Table 3.6 Interview questions for the psychological formulation

Psychological formulation		
General formulation	Predispositions	Was there anything unusual about your childhood? Have you ever experienced something traumatic that left a big emotional impact on you?
	Coping mechanisms	How do you deal with challenges? How do you respond to stressful situations?
Personality	Patterns of behavior, interpersonal style Characteristics of relationships with others Self-esteem	How would you describe your relationships with others? Have you ever had a serious romantic relationship? Close friendships? How would others describe you? What strengths and weaknesses do you perceive within yourself?
Cognitive perspective	Cognitive distortions • Do you get caught in negative feedback loops? • Do you tend to experience positive vs. negative emotions?	

Table 3.7 Interview questions for the social formulation

Social formulation	
Social history	Tell me about your: • Family • Friends, romantic partners • Educational background • Job • Living situation • Legal problems • Access to healthcare • Financial security or lack thereof
Cultural and spiritual background	What is your cultural identity? How does it shape your understanding of your illness? What is your family's understanding of your illness? Some people find a lot of comfort in religion. Do you have a faith that you practice?

creation of a safe environment, social support) against static risk factors to formulate a safe risk reduction plan. Planned interventions may include medication optimization, increased frequency of outpatient follow-up, placement in a drug rehabilitation program, or voluntary vs. involuntary psychiatric hospitalizations.

Similarly, outcome measures focused solely on symptom reduction, frequently documented via standardized patient-reported scales, may provide an incomplete clinical picture. As mental health professionals, we strive to enhance our patients' social functioning and psychological well-being rather than seek an end-all cure for mental afflictions, many of which may be considered chronic, recurring illnesses. Clinically relevant outcome measures must be meaningful to the patient and align with the patient's unique personal treatment goals (Table 3.8).

Collaborative Treatment Planning

The best treatment plans are co-created by patients with their clinicians; they are made for the person and not for the diagnosis. The clinician must correctly identify what the patient seeks, devise a pathway for intervention that aligns with the patient's strengths and skills and coping-response style, and, most importantly, the clinician must garner the patient's interest and motivation to follow through with the treatment plan. Recall that a change in a person's social circumstances may significantly impact one's biological and/or psychological situation, and so on and so forth. As therapy proceeds, new material may emerge to guide the patient–clinician dyad to modify their treatment approach or to integrate different styles of therapy and/or treatment modalities. This opens the door to a plethora of interventions for the thoughtful and creative clinician (Fig. 3.30).

Table 3.8 Measurement-based vs. person-centered outcome measures

Outcome measures		
	Measurement-based	Person-centered
Biological	Serum level of psychotropic medication or illicit substance Severity of metabolic syndrome (A1c, lipid panel, weight gain) Remission vs. relapse status	Functional status Activities of daily living
Psychological	Disorder-specific symptom rating scales Disorder-specific severity measures Personality inventories	Sense of purpose Self-esteem
Social	Disability measures (WHODAS 2.0) Rate of rehospitalization	Meaningful activities/relationships Steady employment Continuing education

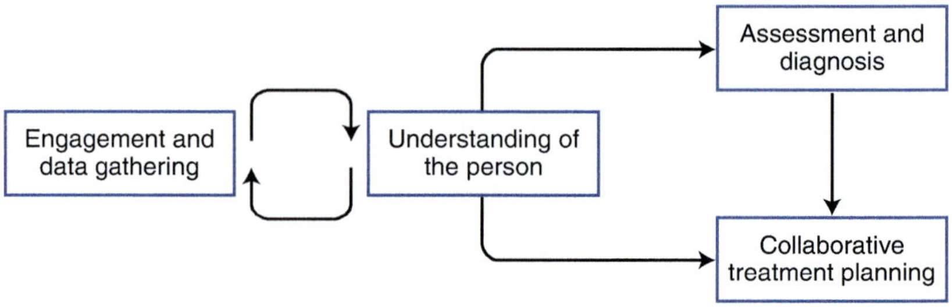

Fig. 3.30 The biopsychosocial engagement and data gathering process

Table 3.9 Biopsychosocial treatment plan

Biopsychosocial treatment plan		
	Treatment modalities	Inter-wing effects
Biological	Psychotropic medications Electroconvulsive therapy Transcranial magnetic stimulation Nutrition and exercise	Optimization of psychotherapy Increased financial strain Fear of social stigma
Psychological	Cognitive behavioral therapy Psychodynamic psychotherapy Mindfulness-based therapy Acceptance and commitment therapy	Changes in neuronal circuitry Interpersonal relationships
Social	Housing resources Social skills training Substance use cessation Support groups Family involvement	Medication adherence Decreased mood/ psychotic symptoms Improved distress tolerance

The understanding of the whole person enabled by the biopsychosocial formulation is the basis for continued engagement and data gathering in future encounters, assessment and diagnosis, and collaborative treatment planning. This process is dynamic and ever-evolving, and at its core lies the therapeutic alliance (Table 3.9).

Case Example

The power of the biopsychosocial model is its ability to take into account a patient in their entirety; they are more than their medical diagnoses. By crafting an assessment that encapsulates a patient's life more fully, clinicians can create a treatment plan that acknowledges how many facets of a patient's life impact their psychiatric health.

To help illustrate this, we can consider one patient from a purely biomedical perspective, then see how that reductive model could represent many different patients in the biopsychosocial model.

Biomedical Presentation

The patient is a 44-year-old woman with a past medical history of hypertension, hyperlipidemia, and major depressive disorder who presented to the emergency room with 2 months of insomnia, lack of concentration, decreased appetite, and 1 day of passive suicidal ideation without a plan. Discharged from the emergency room, she was referred to an outpatient psychiatrist for evaluation and treatment. She is currently taking lisinopril 10 mg daily, atorvastatin 40 mg daily, and sertraline 50 mg daily. She has no history of suicide attempts. She has only been on sertraline and has not trialed other psychiatric medications. She has never been in therapy. Her family history is notable for stroke in her father and ovarian cancer in her mother. No family history of suicide attempts.

Given the above information, a reasonable diagnosis would be a depressive episode as a recurrence of previously diagnosed major depressive disorder. With that diagnosis, a plan would be to switch antidepressants to escitalopram and refer for psychotherapy. We have a disease state and its corresponding treatment, the heart of the biomedical model (Fig. 3.31) [49].

Now, here is the same patient seen through a biopsychosocial lens:

Patient # 1

The patient is a 44-year-old woman with the same past medical history as seen earlier. She is currently unhoused and lives alone in her car, re-parking every few days when she has to leave an area. She had worked as an amusement park cast member but became unemployed 2 months ago because of the COVID-19 pandemic. She has originally prescribed sertraline from her primary care doctor, whom she can no longer see as her insurance was through her employer. She reported being scared about running out and only taking it "as needed." She can no longer afford the co-pay and has not been able to focus on filling out the paperwork for Medicaid.

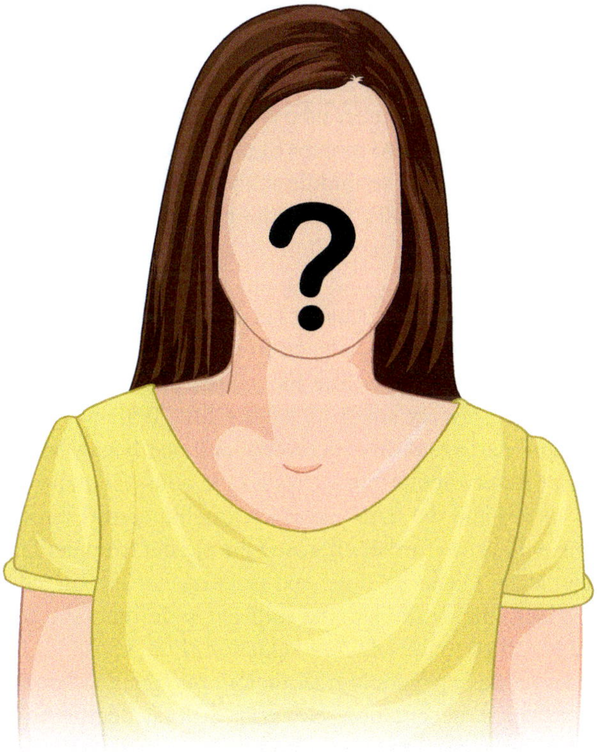

Fig. 3.31 44 years old woman, through the lens of the Biomedical model. Disease state and its corresponding treatment are the main focus

She began drinking wine to "quiet down" the negative thoughts she had been feeling about herself but switched to hard liquor as money became more and more scarce. She now drinks one handle of vodka a day. The stress of losing her job and apartment has led to a downward spiral in her mood, to the point where she identifies feeling completely hopeless about things getting better. She states she had to leave her former neighborhood to be in a more urban area with resources for homeless people. Because of the pandemic, she cannot stay with her friends or family and reports feeling very isolated. Feeling overwhelmed and suicidal, she self-presented to the emergency room, then was referred to an outpatient psychiatrist (Table 3.10; Fig. 3.32) [50].

With this patient, her social situation is a major factor in her psychiatric health. Not only did her unemployment serve as a stressor to push her into a depressive episode, but it also prevented her from getting the treatment she needed. Going back to the biomedical lens, only viewing the patient's disease state to guide treatment is not sufficient to help the patient overcome this depressive episode. She has not really failed a trial of sertraline since her social circumstances have prevented her from taking it regularly. Her treatment plan needs to include social work to help obtain insurance coverage. She also would benefit from further education about antidepressants and the need to take them regularly to be

Table 3.10 A comparison of a patient treatment plan according to the biomedical and biopsychosocial models

Patient 1	
Biomedical	Biopsychosocial
• Major depressive disorder—recurrent • Switch antidepressants to escitalopram • Psychotherapy	• Ensure safety from suicidal ideations • Social work for insurance • Psychoeducation • Talk therapy • Building a support network • Identify triggers for stress • Learn coping skills • Assess for possible inpatient care

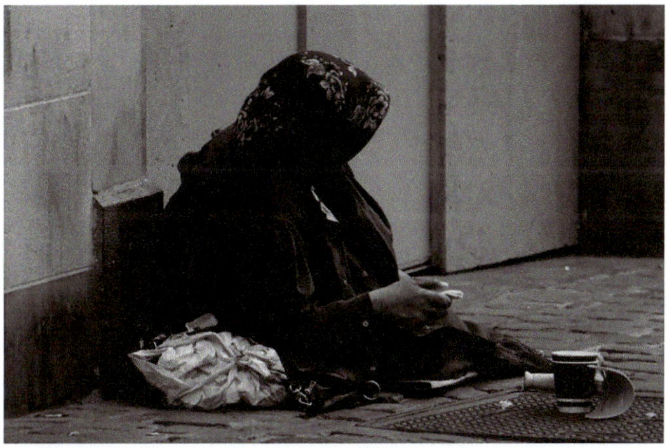

Figs. 3.32 44 years old woman, through the lens of the Biopsychosocial model. Focusing at the interconnection between biology, psychology, and social factors (public domain [51–53])

effective. Starting therapy would be ideal, but given the patient's circumstances, a thorough, flexible plan would be needed for her to attend regularly. Her use of alcohol to self-treat her symptoms of depression is reinforcing a use disorder that in turn is only perpetuating the depression. An alcohol use disorder program will be critical in helping her overcome her depression and overall mental health recovery. Most importantly, given her lack of a support network, significant burden of stressors, alcohol use disorder, and vague suicidal ideation, ensuring the patient's safety is critical. She may necessitate an inpatient admission (possibly to a dual diagnosis program) both for safety and to help put into place resources to help her receive treatment when discharged.

Patient #2

Patient #2 is a 44-year-old woman with the same past medical history and basic presentation. Here, she recently moved to the area to accept a position as a senior attorney at a prestigious law firm. She lives with her 17-year-old daughter from a previous marriage. As a Latinx woman, she finds her-

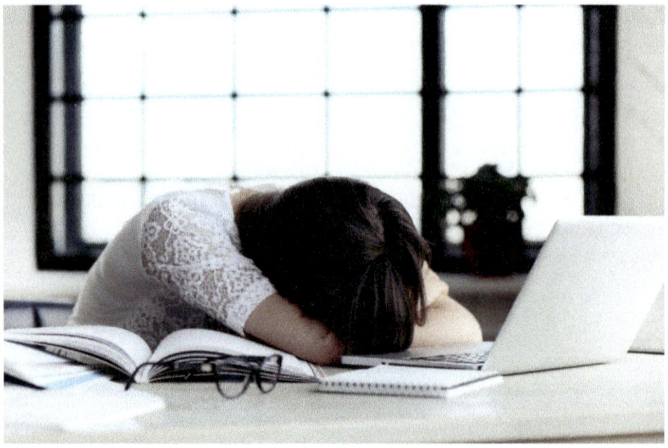

Fig. 3.33 44 years old woman, through the lens of the Biopsychosocial model. Focusing at the interconnection between biology, psychology, and social factors (public domain [51–53])

self the only person of color in an executive position at the firm. She is inundated with microaggressions every day. She now dreads going to work and feels more and more depressed. She has stopped exercising, her major form of stress management, because she is so exhausted from work. In addition, her daughter had a difficult time adjusting to her new school and is now applying for college. The patient has been trying to date and wants a romantic partner but finds it difficult because she has had feelings of low self-worth since childhood, particularly around her body image. Because of this, she does not want to take any new medications that will make her gain weight (Fig. 3.33) [51].

While patient #1's psychosocial stressors were primarily socioeconomic, patient #2's come from systemic racism, situational isolation, and psychologically ingrained conceptions of low self-worth. In understanding the patient's social and psychological concerns, we are able to better select a pharmacologic option, in this case, an antidepressant less likely to cause weight gain, given the patient's sensitivity to the issue. By seeing the patient's precipitating factors as more systemic in nature, supportive psychotherapy can be tailored towards addressing these stressors, possibly with a mental health provider with some background and expertise in those issues, which can make the patient feel comfortable and understood. In seeing some of the patient's psychological history of low self-worth and fear of rejection and criticism (a pattern established in childhood), psychodynamic therapy could prove a beneficial approach to exploring and understanding the root of these feelings. We also see how all three elements of the model impact each other. Socially, the patient's job and parenting duties are extremely time-consuming and emotionally draining. This impacts the biological part of her life by preventing her from exercising, which impedes her ability to improve her hypertension and hyperlipidemia.

Patient #3

Patient #3 is a homemaker and mother of three. Her wife is an executive computer engineer who is often away from the family on business trips. Two months ago, her eldest daughter did not make her competitive middle school's honor roll because she received a B+ in PE, which the patient took extremely personally as a sign of her failure as a mother. This led to a large argument between the patient, her daughter, and her partner, with the others accusing her of overreacting. Feeling ganged up on, the patient isolated from her family and began to feel her mood worsen. She has gotten upset by setbacks other people view as small all of her life. With worsening depression, her irritability increased, and she began lashing out at her family about things around the house, like uncompleted chores and the family dog tracking pawprints through the house. This has further alienated the patient from her family. She began to feel so alone and isolated that she started to think about suicide. When she told her wife this, she convinced her to go to the ED for evaluation (Fig. 3.34) [52].

Here, we have psychological factors playing a major role in the patient's presentation. Her poor distress tolerance and catastrophizing are impeding her ability to support or be supported by her family members. Her biological predisposition to depression makes her more vulnerable to an episode, but her psychological profile is allowing the episode to perpetuate and worsen. While an antidepressant may be helpful in her recovery, significant behavior-based psychotherapy may prove even more helpful. The patient needs to develop coping skills to better handle disappointments and setbacks in modulating her reaction to events; she can form better relationships with her family members, who in turn can support her and make her feel less isolated [53, 54]. Additionally, in looking at the patient's psychosocial factors, we see patterns of behavior concerning a possible personality disorder [55].

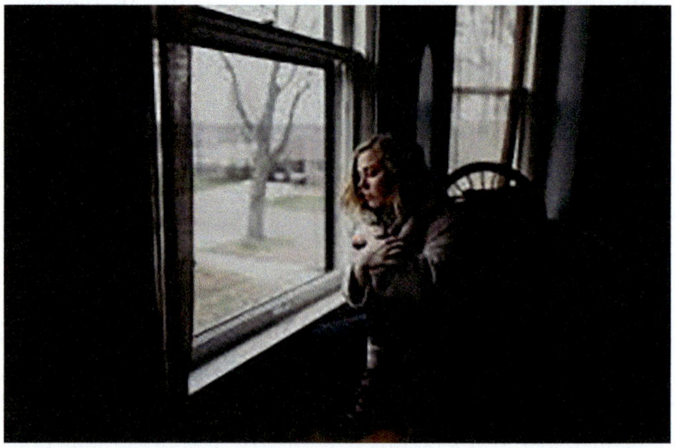

Fig. 3.34 44 years old woman, through the lens of the Biopsychosocial model. Focusing at the interconnection between biology, psychology, and social factors (public domain [51–53])

Had we only looked at her from a biomedical perspective, seeing her depression and previous diagnoses, we may have missed this. In finding comorbid conditions by considering the entire patient's life, we can further tailor the therapeutic modality, recommending Dialectical Behavioral Therapy (DBT) to help her work through some of her maladaptive defense mechanisms.

Limitations of the Biopsychosocial Model

Gabriel Tobia, Waguih William IsHak, and Yasmine Gohar

Ever since Engel and Romano proposed the BPS model, it has achieved wide acceptance in psychiatry. In the decades since its introduction, it has gained popularity both in teaching and in clinical practice, coming to be viewed as the overarching framework of the field. Despite its following, the model is not without its critics. The latter have been quick to point out its limitations, both in its scientific validity and in its usefulness in practice (Table 3.11) [56].

One criticism leveled against the BPS model is that it is, in fact, not a "model" in the rigorous scientific sense. The words "theory" and "model" are sometimes used interchangeably, but in the strict sense, while a theory can be defined as an "unbodied concept or abstract notion," a model should meet more exacting criteria. It is a "formal, working representation of an idea" that is "real," and its material consequences can be measured. In practice, while a theory is a useful tool to explain a phenomenon *post hoc*, it does not have the predictive value of a model [12]. Another shortcoming of the biopsychosocial model, some argue, is its vagueness and lack of coherence. Its inclusive approach has been criticized as unscientific and "fluffy," giving equal weight and merit to different perspectives. To one author [57], this is reminiscent of the dodo in Alice in Wonderland, who declared: "Everybody has won, and all must have prizes" (Fig. 3.35) [58].

Additionally, the BPS model has been criticized for its unbounded eclecticism. When the model was conceived, its creators sought to put an end to the strife that was brewing in psychiatry between the psychoanalytic and biomedical dogmas. The goal was to combat dogmatism in psychiatry by

Table 3.11 Summary of criticisms of the biopsychosocial model

1. Not a model: descriptive, not predictive
2. Vague, "fluffy," and lacks coherence
3. Vague conception of biology
4. Unclear boundaries between "bio," "psycho," and "social"
5. Fails to curtail the advance of biomedical psychiatry
6. Fails to appropriately account for the patient's subjective experience
7. Unsophisticated approach to cultural identity
8. Shortcomings as a teaching tool

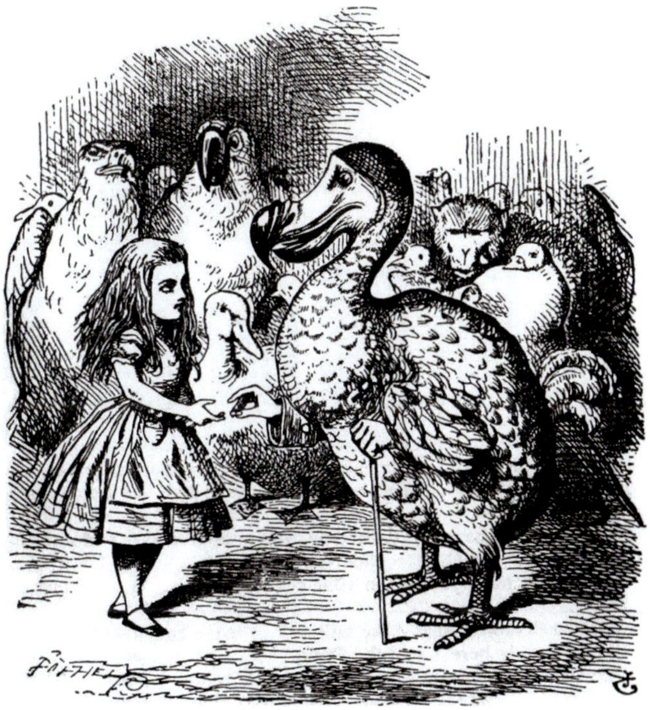

Fig. 3.35 Alice's Adventures in Wonderland by Lewis Carroll. Illustrating the "Dodo bird effect" as one of the limitations of the Biopsychosocial model

introducing some eclecticism into psychiatric practice and individualizing the treatment to the patient. Some argue that, in practice, this eclectic freedom has gone too far. Particularly, the boundaries and interrelationships of the "bio," "psycho," and "social" components become blurry at best when examined more closely [59]. Furthermore, in practice, practitioners choose to emphasize the "bio," the "psycho," or the "social," depending on their inclinations. If the goal of the proponents of the biopsychosocial model was to give an equal voice to the different approaches to treatment, then they have failed. Instead of overcoming dogmatism, it allowed each one to enact their own dogmas [60]. This can be seen in clinical practice, where the BPS model has failed to curb the dominance of the biological approach in the past decades, especially in the United States, where the vast majority of clinical research has been biomedically focused [61]. The proportion of biomedically focused articles in the American Journal of Psychiatry, for instance, has increased dramatically in the past half-century, in contrast to the British Journal of Psychiatry (Fig. 3.36) [62].

Another criticism leveled at the BPS model is that it does not give due attention to the patient's subjective experience of illness, such as in matters of personal meaning and spirituality. Furthermore, it fails in its conceptualization of psychopathology in larger social units, such as community, culture, and society [63]. Even when cultural factors are considered (pegged under the "social" domain), it is exclusively

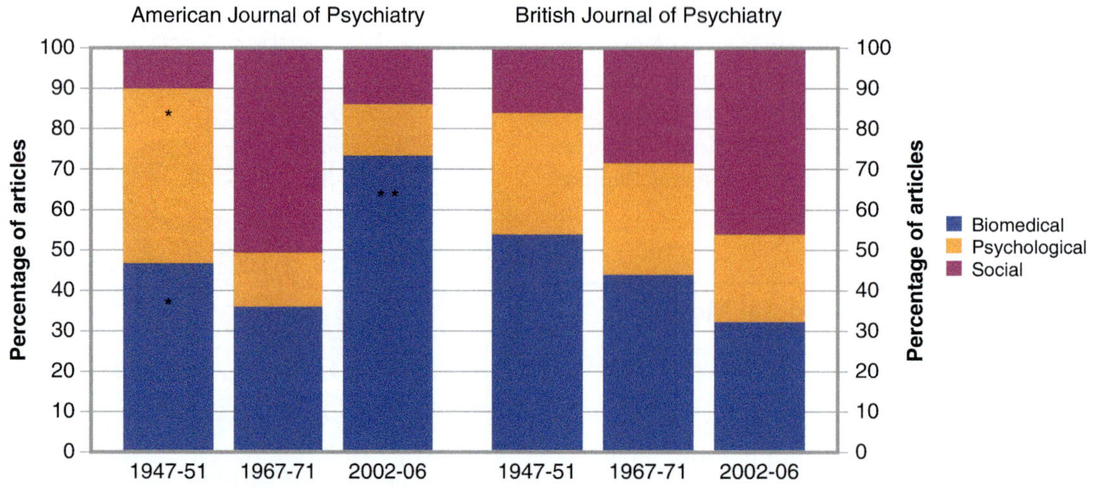

Fig. 3.36 Representation of dominant psychiatric models in psychiatric journals

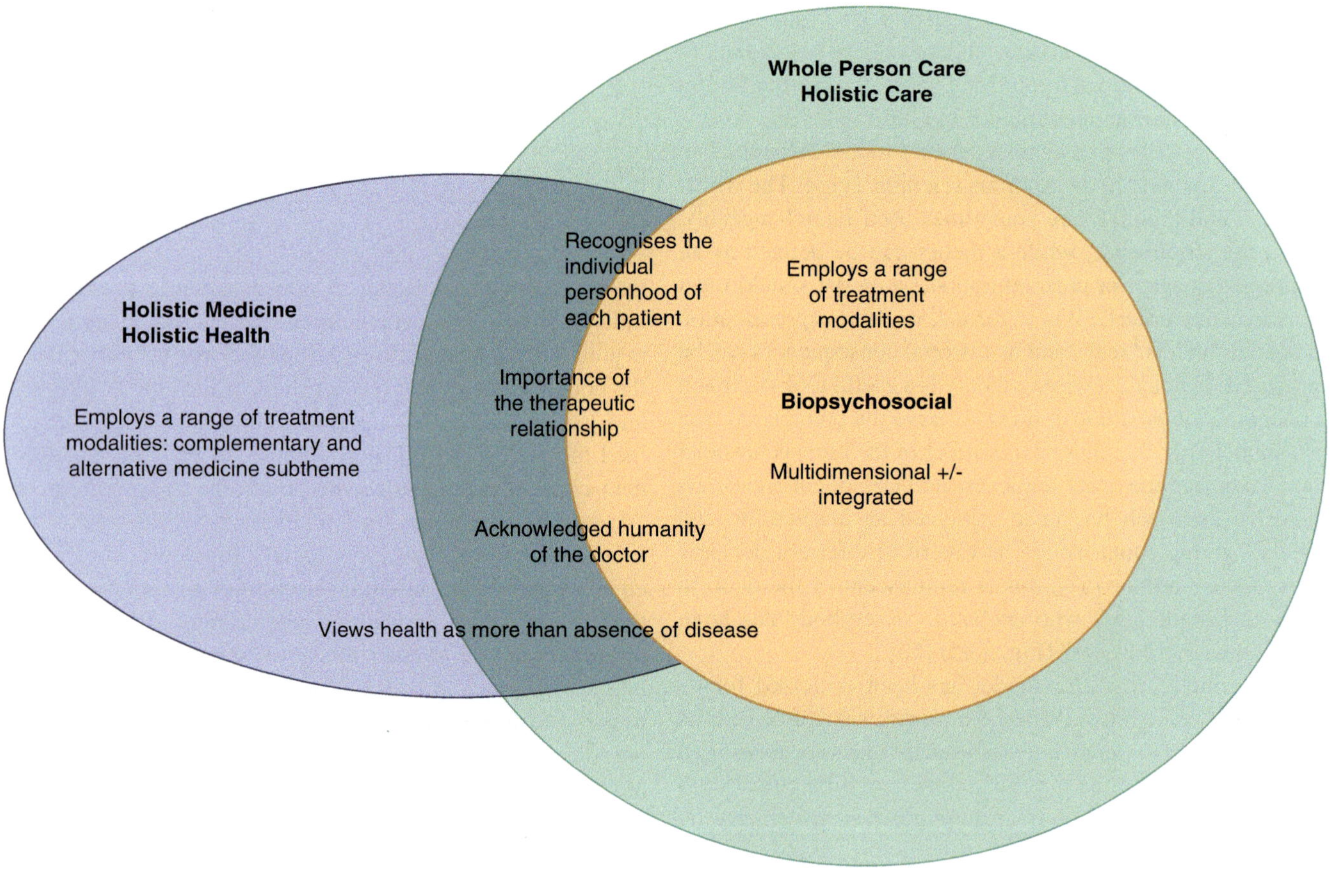

Fig. 3.37 The inter-relationship between biopsychosocial, whole person, and holistic terminology. (*From* Thomas et al. [68]; Creative Commons Attribution 4.0 license; http://creativecommons.org/licenses/by/4.0)

conceptualized through a positivistic lens that assumes that the groups are homogeneous, ignoring each individual's unique lived experience of the cultural identity [64].

The BPS model is still regarded as a very useful tool in the teaching of psychiatry [12]. Nevertheless, some have questioned its value in medical education, pointing out that its vagueness and eclecticism may baffle, if not repulse, medical students. As for psychiatry residents, they would be offered through their training a "confusing smorgasbord" of competing approaches to patient care [7].

Ultimately, critics argue the BPS model must move beyond the vague—albeit well-intentioned—inclusivity of its name and to become a true model that is predictive as well as explanatory (Fig. 3.37) [65–67].

Proposal for Future Consideration

Alexander Cohn, Shawna Chan, Katrina DeBonis, and Yasmine Gohar

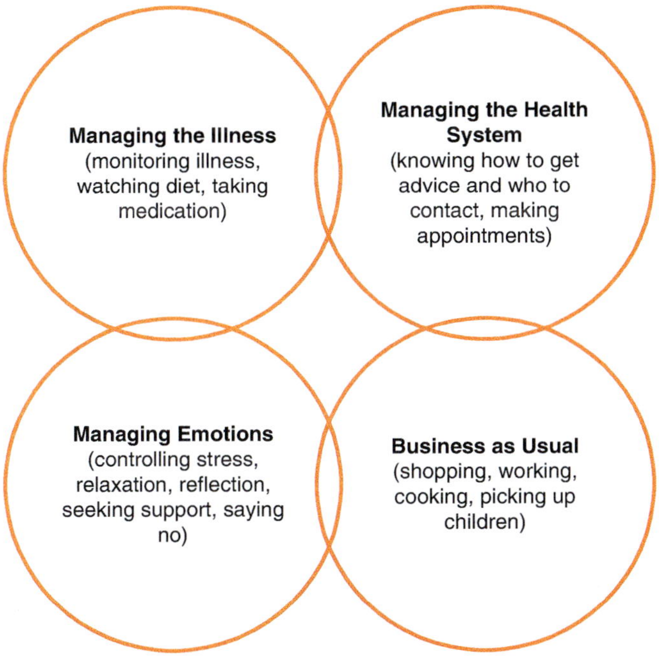

Fig. 3.38 Categories in self-management of illnesses requires active engagement with health-care practitioners. (*From* Clarke et al. [44]; *with permission*)

Use within the Health Care System and Potential Pitfalls

Our current healthcare system is one in which patients, in all of their complexity, are reduced to checkboxes of billable codes and diagnoses. Documentation is increasingly geared toward meeting the criteria for those billable services rather than providing an informative and meaningful account of the clinician's observations and assessment. Clinicians may find it hard to find the time to be thorough in history taking so as to include the factors that make up the BPS model. It may consequently lack the identification of potentially efficacious social or psychological interventions, which always leads to the ability to provide these to the patient due to the inequities in our system. Physicians must not only be trained in how to use the BPS model but how to advocate for its implementation within the systems in which they operate (Figs. 3.38 and 3.39) [43, 65].

Inclusion of Structural and Cultural Factors

If the intention of the BPS model is to conceptualize a patient holistically, with consideration of the factors that contribute to the development, expression, and progression of illness, then our knowledge of how cultural and structural factors contribute to health and disease naturally leads to their inclusion. Cultures are fluid systems of knowledge that can influ-

Fig. 3.39 Treatment structure of an interdisciplinary multimodal pain intervention approach. (*From* Jones et al. [66]; *with permission*)

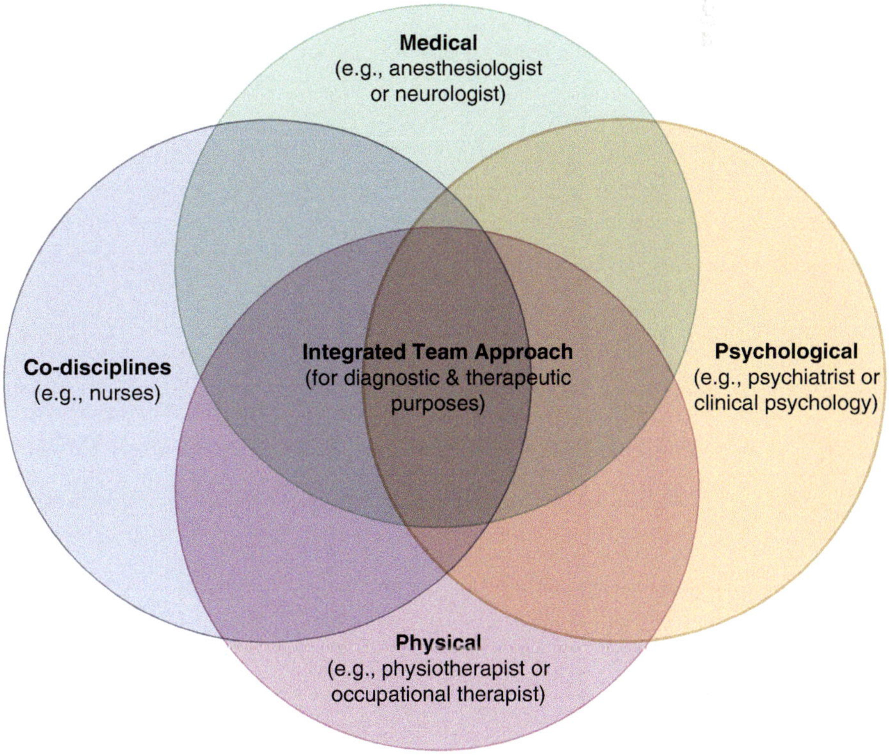

ence how illness is manifested and maintained [43]. Ample cross-cultural evidence has highlighted how illnesses such as depression are expressed and explained differently across the world [68]. Structural factors include the social, economic, and political conditions which contribute to a person's health and which, when considered in the conceptualization, can lead to interventions that target upstream forces on symptoms and diseases through advocacy and policy change [69]. For example, the inclusion of structural factors in the conceptualization of a patient with mental illness could lead to connecting that patient with a community organization that would help them afford their medications and greater advocacy efforts against unfair prescription drug pricing (Table 3.12; Figs. 3.40, 3.41, 3.42, 3.43, 3.44, 3.45, 3.46, and 3.47) [43, 62, 64–66, 68].

Table 3.12 Biopsychosocial model with inclusion of structural and cultural factors

Structural factors	Experience of discrimination Ability to pay for treatment Incarceration Housing insecurity Access to: • Educational opportunities • Employment opportunities • Nutritional food • Outdoor spaces
Cultural factors[a]	Language Spirituality and religion Family structures Customs and rituals Moral systems Explanatory models of illness Stigma resulting in barriers to treatment Cultural sources of strength and support Race/ethnicity
Biological	Age Sex Genetics/Family history Other medical conditions Nutritional status Medications Exposure to toxins History of substances
Social factors	Educational history Relationship history (romantic and platonic) Support system Occupation history Living situation Economic Status
Psychological factors	Personality traits Coping mechanisms Cognitive state (memory, negative thought patterns) Intrapersonal relationship Impulsivity History of treatment History of suicidal ideation/attempts Trauma history

[a]Can assess using the cultural formulation

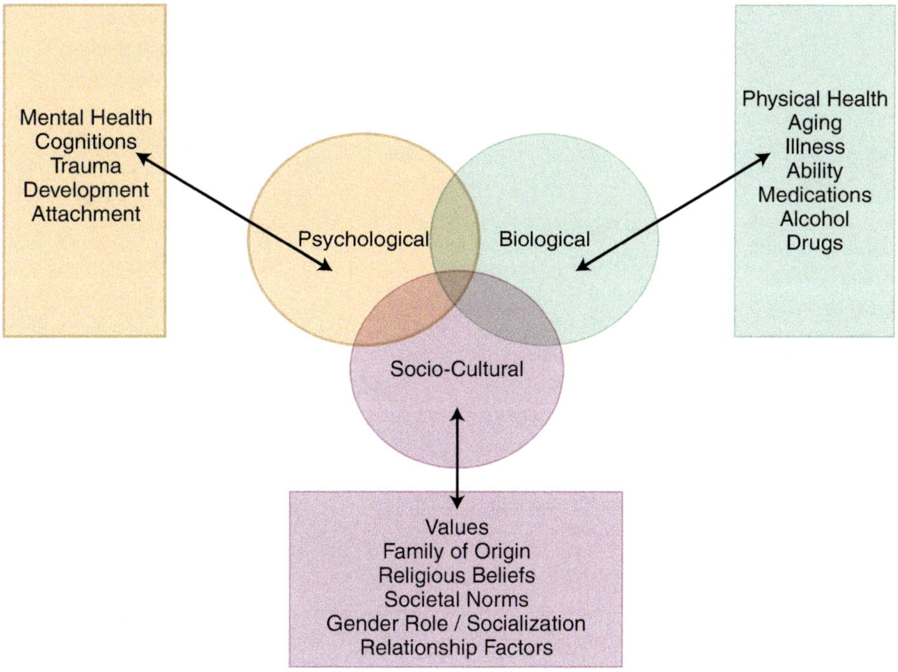

Fig. 3.40 A biopsychosocial model of sexual dysfunction with structural and social inclusions. (*From* Pahwa and Foley [67]; *with permission*)

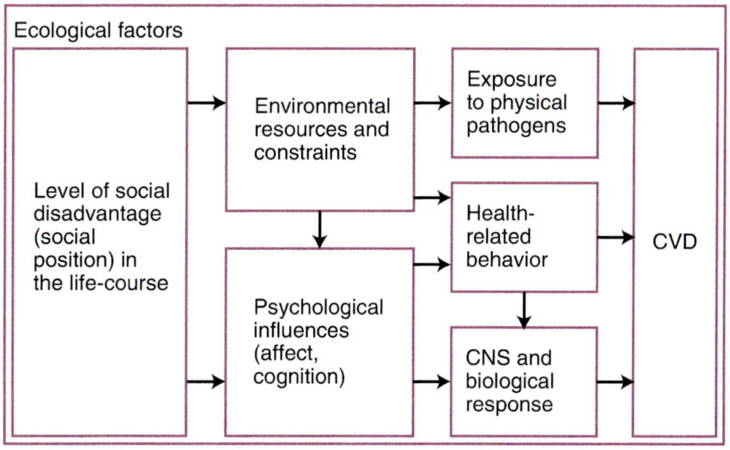

Fig. 3.41 Social and interpersonal factors in cardiovascular disease (CVD). (*From* Krokstad et al. [69]; *with permission*)

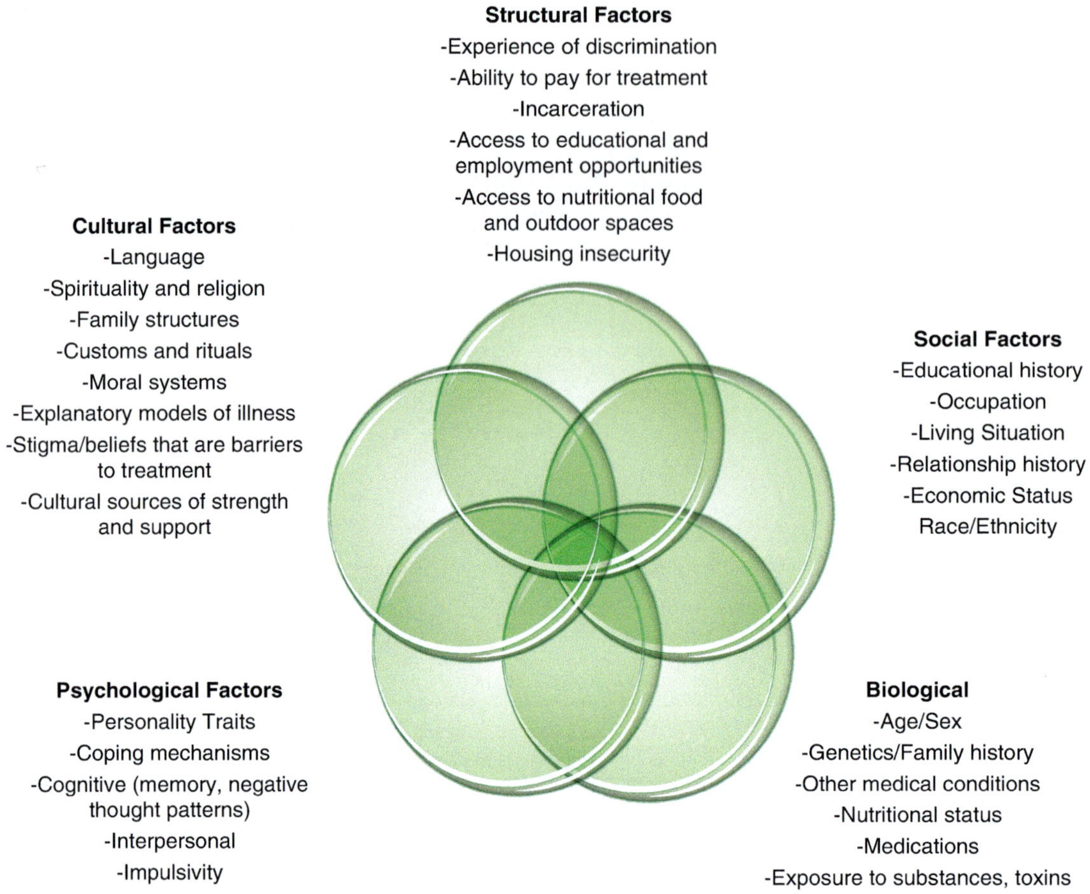

Fig. 3.42 Diagram of the biopsychosocial model with inclusion of structural and cultural factors

Fig. 3.43 The dynamic biopsychosocial model of health. This model incorporates to the biopsychosocial model a dynamic systems perspective, where each component includes a system that reciprocally influences other dynamics in the model and also has an impact in health [70]

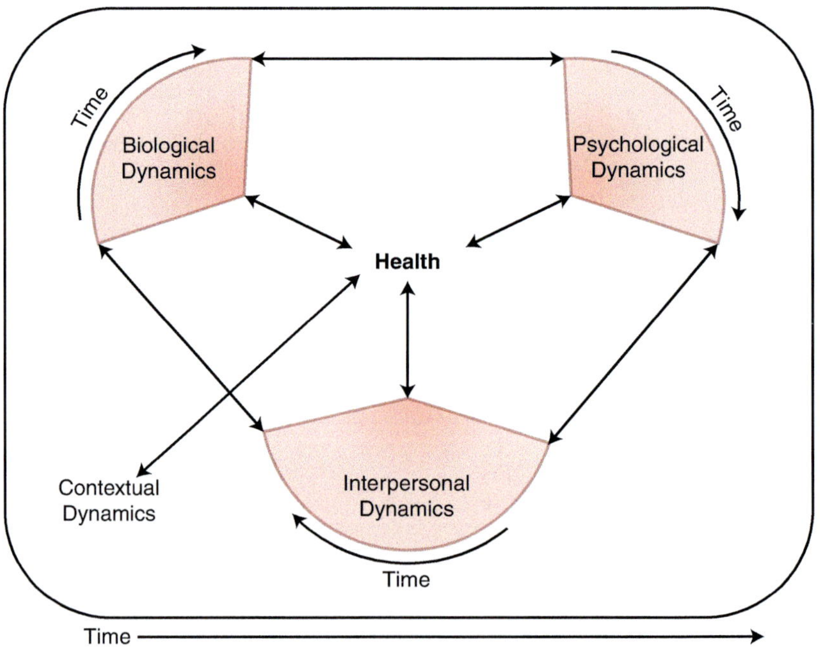

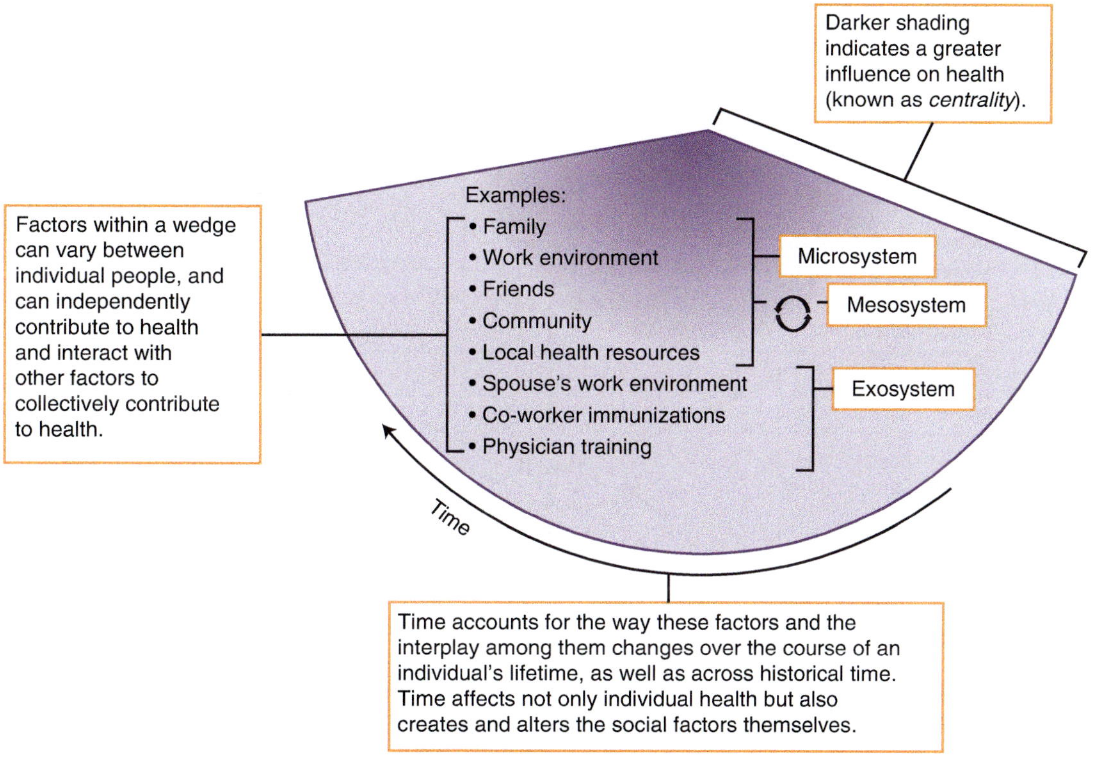

Figs. 3.44 Example of the interpersonal dynamic [70]

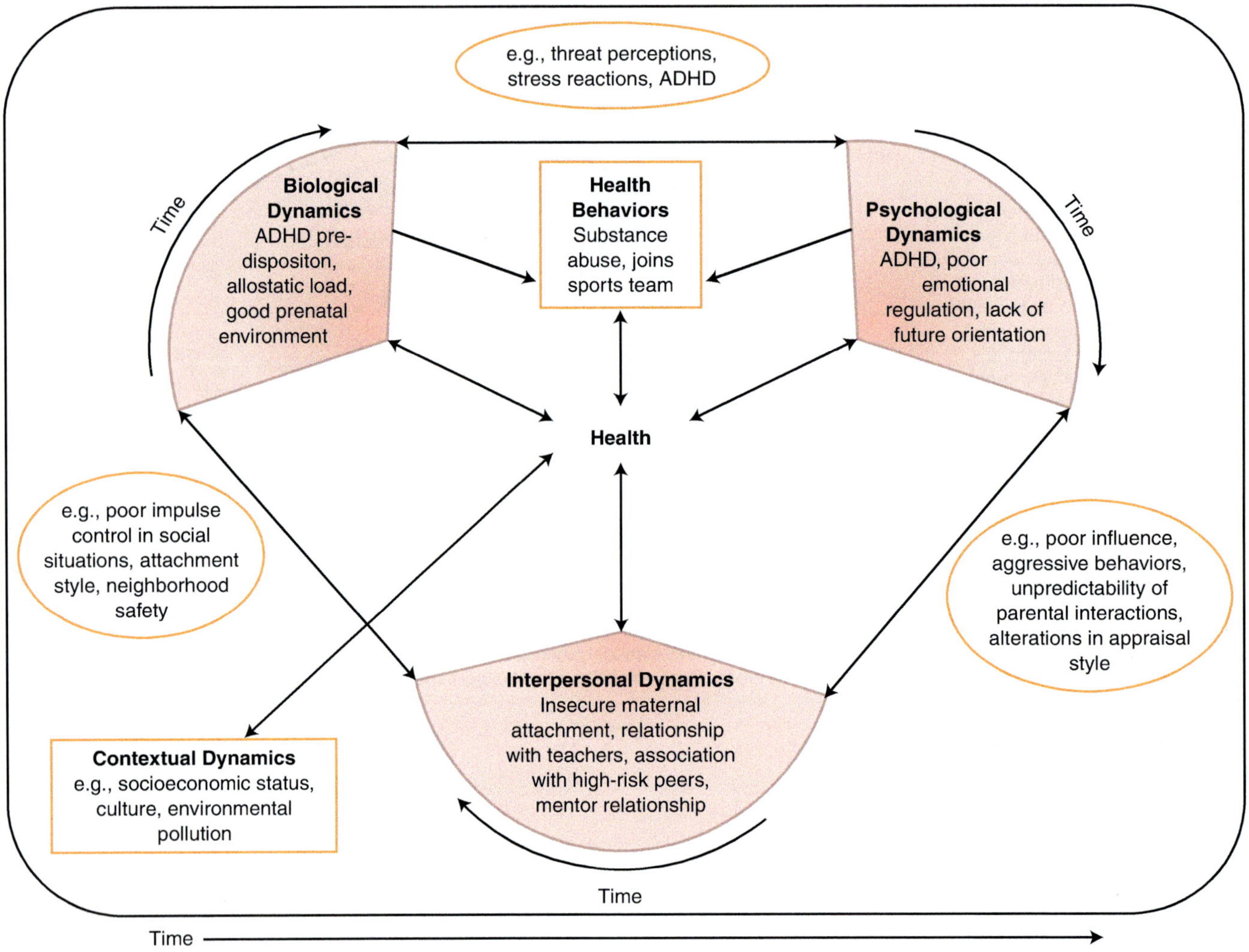

Fig. 3.45 Two hypothetical cases of study (Brandon and Ivvete), capturing and highlighting their singular dynamics that may change and mutually affect each other over time [70]

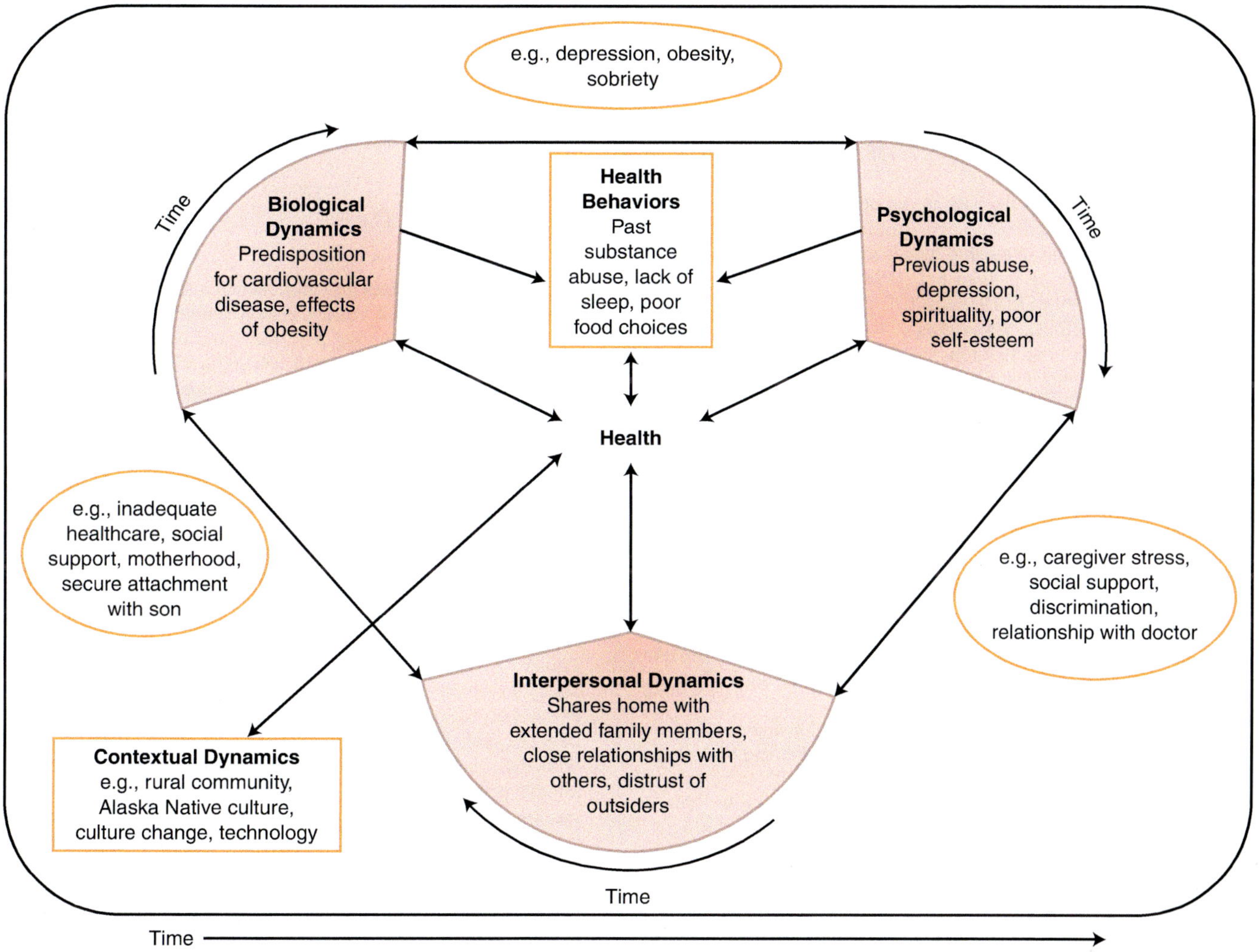

Fig. 3.46 Two hypothetical cases of study (Brandon and Ivvete), capturing and highlighting their singular dynamics that may change and mutually affect each other over time

Fig. 3.47 Moving from the static biopsychosocial Venn diagram (**a**) to a schematic of a dynamic person (**b**) (*From* Stilwell and Harman [65]; *with permission*)

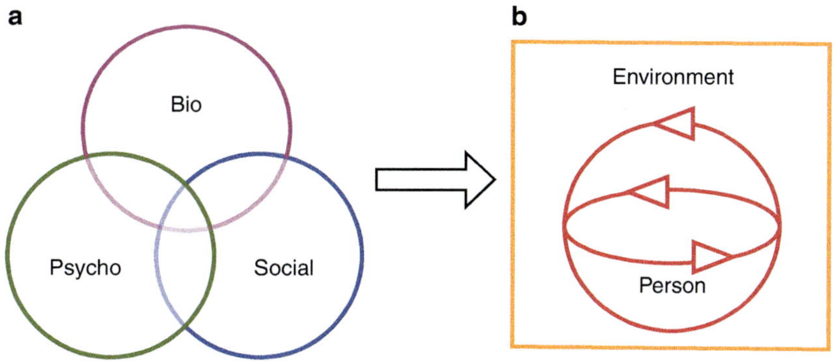

References

1. Engel GL. A unified concept of health and disease. Perspect Biol Med. 1960;3:459–85. https://doi.org/10.1353/pbm.1960.0020.
2. Engel GL. The need for a new medical model: a challenge for biomedicine. Science. 1977;196:129–36. https://doi.org/10.1126/science.847460.
3. Engel GL. The care of the patient: Art or science? Johns Hopkins Med J. 1977;140:222.
4. Engel GL. The biopsychosocial model and the education of health professionals. Ann N Y Acad Sci. 1978;310:169–81. https://doi.org/10.1111/j.1749-6632.1978.tb22070.x.
5. Engel GL. The clinical application of the biopsychosocial model. Am J Psychiatry. 1980;137:535–44.
6. Ghaemi SN. Biomedical reductionist, humanist, and biopsychosocial models in medicine. In: Schramme T, Edwards S, editors. Handbook of the philosophy of medicine. Dordrecht: Springer; 2017. https://doi.org/10.1007/978-94-017-8688-1_38.
7. Ghaemi SN. The rise and fall of the biopsychosocial model: Reconciling art and science in psychiatry. Baltimore, MD: Johns Hopkins University Press; 2010.
8. Hilty DM. Advancing science, clinical care and education: Shall we update Engel's biopsychosocial model to a biopsychosociocultural model? Psychol Cogn Sci Open J. 2015;1(1):e1–6. https://doi.org/10.17140/PCSOJ-1-e001.
9. Psychiatry Part II examination format, Patient Section. Buffalo Grove, IL: The American Board of Psychiatry and Neurology, Inc.; 2008.
10. McDermott JF, Sterilizer J, Lump KY, et al. Pilot study of explicit grading criteria in the American Board of psychiatry and Neurology Part II examination. Am J Psychiatry. 1996;153:1097–9.
11. Molina JA. Understanding the biopsychosocial model. Int J Psychiatry Med. 1983;13:29–36.
12. Adler RH. Engel's biopsychosocial model is still relevant today. J Psychosom Res. 2009;67(6):607–11. https://doi.org/10.1016/j.jpsy-chores.2009.08.008.
13. McLaren N. A critical review of the biopsychosocial model. Aust N Z J Psychiatry. 1998;32(1):86–92; discussion 93-6.
14. Tavakoli HR. A closer evaluation of current methods in psychiatric assessments: a challenge for the biopsychosocial model. Psychiatry (Edgmont). 2009;6(2):25–30.
15. Hilty DM, Ton H, Lu F, et al. Revising engel's biopsychosocial model to the biopsychosocialcultural model? Suggestions and implications. Keystone, CO: American Directors of Medical Student Education in Psychiatry; 2014.
16. Burton AK, Kendall NA, Pearce BG, Birrell LN, Bainbridge LC. Management of work-relevant upper limb disorders: a review. Occup Med (Lond). 2009;59(1):44–52.
17. Descartes, "L'homme et un traitte...". https://commons.wikimedia.org/wiki/File:Descartes,_%22L%27homme_et_un_traitte...%22_Wellcome_L0025506.jpg.
18. Vaccarino V, Bremner JD. Posttraumatic stress disorder and risk of cardiovascular disease. In: Alvarenga M, Byrne D, editors. Handbook of psychocardiology. Singapore: Springer; 2016. https://doi.org/10.1007/978-981-287-206-7_14.
19. Fritzsche K, Goli F, Dobos CM. What is psychosomatic medicine? In: Fritzsche K, McDaniel S, Wirsching M, editors. Psychosomatic medicine. Cham: Springer; 2020. https://doi.org/10.1007/978-3-030-27080-3_1.
20. Koh KB. Stress and illness. In: Stress and somatic symptoms. Cham: Springer; 2018. https://doi.org/10.1007/978-3-030-02783-4_5.
21. Farre A, Rapley T. The new old (and old new) medical model: four decades navigating the biomedical and psychosocial understandings of health and illness. Healthcare (Basel). 2017;5(4):88. https://doi.org/10.3390/healthcare5040088.
22. Borrell-Carrió F, Suchman AL, Epstein RM. The biopsychosocial model 25 years later: principles, practice, and scientific inquiry. Ann Fam Med. 2004;2(6):576–82. https://doi.org/10.1370/afm.245.
23. Racine NM, et al. Systematic review: predisposing, precipitating, perpetuating, and present factors predicting anticipatory distress to painful medical procedures in children. J Pediatr Psychol. 2016;41(2):159–81.
24. Winters NC, Hanson G, Stoyanova V. The case formulation in child and adolescent psychiatry. Child Adolesc Psychiatric Clin. 2007;16(1):111–32.
25. King AP. Somatic health issues in trauma-related disorders: effects on psychobiological axes affecting mental and physical health. In: Grassi L, Riba M, Wise T, editors. Person centered approach to recovery in medicine. Integrating psychiatry and primary care. Cham: Springer; 2019. https://doi.org/10.1007/978-3-319-74736-1_10.
26. Brewerton TD. Are eating disorders addictions? In: Brewerton T, Baker DA, editors. Eating disorders, addictions and substance use disorders. Berlin, Heidelberg: Springer; 2014. https://doi.org/10.1007/978-3-642-45378-6_13.
27. Rocca E, Anjum RL. Complexity, reductionism and the biomedical model. In: Anjum R, Copeland S, Rocca E, editors. Rethinking causality, complexity and evidence for the unique patient. Cham: Springer; 2020. https://doi.org/10.1007/978-3-030-41239-5_5.
28. Simmonds RL, et al. Patients' perceptions of depression and coronary heart disease: a qualitative UPBEAT-UK study. BMC Fam Pract. 2013;14:38.
29. Tripathi A, Das A, Kar SK. Biopsychosocial model in contemporary psychiatry: current validity and future prospects. Indian J Psychol Med. 2019;41(6):582–5. https://doi.org/10.4103/IJPSYM.IJPSYM_314_19.
30. Wood BL, et al. Testing the biobehavioral family model in pediatric asthma: pathways of effect. Fam Process. 2008;47(1):21–40.
31. Flückiger C, Vîslă A, Held J. Psychotherapeutic self-organization in the healing, biomedical and biopsychosocial model—An evidence-based practice perspective. In: Viol K, Schöller H, Aichhorn W, editors. Selbstorganisation – ein Paradigma für die Humanwissenschaften. Wiesbaden: Springer; 2020. https://doi.org/10.1007/978-3-658-29906-4_7.
32. George Libman Engel, M.D. Libraries: Edward G. Miner Library. 2020. https://www.urmc.rochester.edu/libraries/miner/rare-books-and-manuscripts/archives-and-manuscripts/faculty-collections/the-papers-of-george-allen-papers-engel.aspx. Accessed 10 Dec 2020.
33. Portrait of John Romano. https://www.urmc.rochester.edu/psychiatry/about/history.aspx
34. Gliedt JA, et al. The biopsychosocial model and chiropractic: a commentary with recommendations for the chiropractic profession. Chiropr Man Therap. 2017;25(16) https://doi.org/10.1186/s12998-017-0147.
35. Malpus Z. Pain as a biopsychosocial experience. In: Abd-Elsayed A, editor. Pain. Cham: Springer; 2019. https://doi.org/10.1007/978-3-319-99124-5_75.
36. Essner BS, Tran ST, Koven ML. Biopsychosocial approaches to pediatric chronic pain management. In: Shah R, Suresh S, editors. Opioid therapy in infants, children, and adolescents. Cham: Springer; 2020. https://doi.org/10.1007/978-3-030-36287-4_16.
37. Reid C, Owen A. Epidemiology of cardiovascular disease. In: Alvarenga M, Byrne D, editors. Handbook of psychocardiology. Singapore: Springer; 2016. https://doi.org/10.1007/978-981-287-206-7_5.
38. Chen MH, Tsai SJ. Treatment-resistant panic disorder. In: Kim YK, editor. Treatment resistance in psychiatry. Singapore: Springer; 2019. https://doi.org/10.1007/978-981-10-4358-1_13.
39. Schiele MA, Domschke K. Epigenetics at the crossroads between genes, environment and resilience in anxiety disorders. Genes Brain Behav. 2018;17:e12423. https://doi.org/10.1111/gbb.12423.

40. Ferrari AJ, Stockings E, Khoo JP, Erskine HE, Degenhardt L, Vos T, Whiteford HA. The prevalence and burden of bipolar disorder: findings from the Global Burden of Disease Study 2013. Bipolar Disord. 2016;18(5):440–50. https://doi.org/10.1111/bdi.12423.
41. Portrait of Adolf Meyer. https://collections.nlm.nih.gov/catalog/nlm:nlmuid-101423347-img
42. Osler, William, Sir, 1849-1919. Contributions to medical and biological research/dedicated to Sir William Osler, bart. M.D., F.R.S., in honour of his seventieth birthday, June 12, 1919, by his pupils and co-workers. https://wellcomecollection.org/works/g7jrky99.
43. Portrait of Roy Grinker. https://allanshowalter.com/2016/05/07/last-exit-from-michael-reese-hospital-the-final-days/.
44. Clarke DM, Perera DN, Casey MF. Psychological and behavioral contributions to rehabilitation and recovery in heart disease. In: Alvarenga M, Byrne D, editors. Handbook of psychocardiology. Singapore: Springer; 2016. https://doi.org/10.1007/978-981-287-206-7_49.
45. Weerasekera P. Formulation: a multiperspective model. Can J Psychiatry. 1993;38(5):351–8.
46. Selzer R, Ellen S. Formulation for beginners. Australas Psychiatry. 2014;22(4):397–401.
47. Campbell WH, Rohrbaugh RM. The biopsychosocial formulation manual: a guide for mental health professionals. London: CRC Press; 2006.
48. Shea SC. Assessment perspectives and the human matrix: bridges to effective treatment planning in the initial interview. In: Shea SC, editor. Psychiatric interviewing: the art of understanding: a practical guide for psychiatrists, psychologists, counselors, social workers, nurses, and other mental health professionals, with online video modules. 3rd ed. Philadelphia, PA: Elsevier - Health Sciences Division; 2016. p. 220–73.
49. Kirmayer LJ, Sartorius N. Cultural models and somatic syndromes. Psychosom Med. 2007;69(9):832–40. https://doi.org/10.1097/PSY.0b013e31815b002c. PMID: 18040090
50. https://images.app.goo.gl/Gi6wXccFV14cePHW8
51. https://bit.ly/2XRjEpw
52. https://pxhere.com/en/photo/1629581
53. https://pxhere.com/en/photo/93276
54. Kirmayer LJ. Cross cultural Variation in the response to psychiatric disorders and emotional distress. Soc Sci Med. 1989;29:327–39.
55. Metzl JM, Hansen H. Structural competency and psychiatry. JAMA Psychiat. 2018;75(2):115–6. https://doi.org/10.1001/jamapsychiatry.2017.3891. PMID: 29261822
56. American Psychiatric Association. Cultural formulation. In: Diagnostic and statistical manual of mental disorders. 5th ed. Washington, DC: American Psychiatric Association; 2013. p. 749–59.
57. Bolton D, Gillett G. The biopsychosocial model of health and disease. London: Palgrave Pivot; 2019.
58. Henriques G. The Biopsychosocial Model and Its Limitations. Psychology Today. https://www.psychologytoday.com/us/blog/theory-knowledge/201510/the-biopsychosocial-model-and-its-limitations. Published October 30, 2015. Accessed 29 Nov 2020.
59. Carroll L. Alice's adventures in Wonderland. New York: Macmillan; 1920.
60. Ghaemi N. The rise and fall of the bio-psychosocial model. Br J Psychiatry. 2009;195:3–4.
61. Benning TB. Limitations of the biopsychosocial model in psychiatry. Adv Med Educ Pract. 2015;6:347–52.
62. Hatala A. The status of the "biopsychosocial model" in health psychology: towards an integrated approach and a critique of cultural conceptions. Open J Med Psychol. 2012;1:51–62.
63. Kecmanovic D, Hadzi-Pavlovic D. Psychiatric journals as the mirror of the dominant psychiatric model. Psychiatry Bull R Coll Psychiatry. 2010;34:172–6.
64. McManus C. Engel, engels, and the side of the angels. Lancet. 2005;365:2169–217.
65. Stilwell P, Harman K. An inactive approach to pain: beyond the biopsychosocial model. Phenom Cogn Sci. 2019;18:637–65. https://doi.org/10.1007/s11097-019-09624-7.
66. Jones C, Kishino ND, Gatchel RJ. Biopsychosocial Rehabilitation approaches for older adults. In: Gatchel R, Schultz I, Ray C, editors. Handbook of rehabilitation in older adults. Handbooks in health, work, and disability. Cham: Springer; 2018. https://doi.org/10.1007/978-3-030-03916-5_3.
67. Pahwa PK, Foley SM. Biopsychosocial evaluation of sexual dysfunctions. In: IsHak W, editor. The textbook of clinical sexual medicine. Cham: Springer; 2017. https://doi.org/10.1007/978-3-319-52539-6_6.
68. Thomas H, Mitchell G, Rich J, et al. Definition of whole person care in general practice in the English language literature: a systematic review. BMJ Open. 2018;8:e023758. https://doi.org/10.1136/bmjopen-2018-023758.
69. Krokstad S, Sund ER, Ernstsen L, Holmen J. Social disadvantage and cardiovascular disease risk. In: Alvarenga M, Byrne D, editors. Handbook of psychocardiology. Singapore: Springer; 2016. https://doi.org/10.1007/978-981-287-206-7_35.
70. Lehman BJ, David DM, Gruber JA. Rethinking the biopsychosocial model of health: understanding health as a dynamic system. Soc Personal Psychol Compass. 2017;11:e12328. https://doi.org/10.1111/spc3.12328.

Neurobiological Sciences: Neuroanatomy, Neurophysiology, and Neurochemistry

4

Alexander J. Steiner, Leslie Aguilar-Hernandez, Rasha Abdelsalam, Krista Q. Mercado, Alexandra M. Taran, Lucas E. Gelfond, and Waguih William IsHak

Structural Neuroanatomy

Familiarity with the core structures that comprise the brain and central nervous system (CNS) is essential to an understanding of its function. In the subsections that follow, we provide select images and illustrations that review the most important neuroanatomical components of the CNS. These include the four cortical lobes, subcortical structures, cerebrovascular system, brainstem/spinal cord/cerebellum, and brain morphology as a whole.

A. J. Steiner (✉)
Executive Mental Health, Inc., Los Angeles, CA, USA
e-mail: asteiner@emhla.com

L. Aguilar-Hernandez · R. Abdelsalam
Department of Psychiatry and Behavioral Neurosciences, Cedars-Sinai Medical Center, Los Angeles, CA, USA
e-mail: aguilarlesliea@g.ucla.edu

K. Q. Mercado
Department of Ecology and Evolutionary Biology, University of California, Los Angeles, Los Angeles, CA, USA

A. M. Taran
Department of Integrative Biology, Oregon State University, Corvallis, OR, USA

L. E. Gelfond
Brown University, Providence, RI, USA
e-mail: lucas_gelfond@brown.edu

W. W. IsHak
Cedars-Sinai Health System, Department of Psychiatry and Behavioral Neurosciences, University of California Los Angeles, David Geffen School of Medicine, Los Angeles, CA, USA
e-mail: Waguih.IsHak@cshs.org

Neuron Cell Body, Axons, and Dendrite

Neurons consist of cell bodies, axons, and dendrites (see Fig. 4.1). Cell bodies contain most organelles; the nucleolus, mitochondria, rough and smooth endoplasmic reticulum, the golgi apparatus, and ribosomes. Dendrites receive excitatory or inhibitory signals from receptors within their synapses, and these signals generate an electrical potential. If the summation of signal potentials reaches the depolarization threshold, an action potential is generated at the axon hillock. Once generated, the electrical signal that results from an action potential travels down the axon, which is insulated by the myelin sheath. Upon arriving at the axon terminal of a neuron's synapse, vesicles containing neurotransmitters fuse with the synaptic membrane, causing the release and diffusion of the neurotransmitters into the synaptic cleft. These neurotransmitters are then available to bind to receptors on the synapses of the receiving dendrites in the proximal neuron.

Neuroglia Cells and Functions

Neuroglial cells function to support neuronal activity (see Fig. 4.2). Neuroglia is specific to either the central nervous system (CNS) or the peripheral nervous system (PNS). Astrocytes, ependymal cells, microglia, and oligodendrocytes are specific to the CNS. Astrocytes provide structural support, maintain ionic and nutrient concentrations in interstitial fluid, and play a role in the blood–brain barrier. Ependymal cells line ventricles and the central canal, in addition to producing and circulating cerebral spinal fluid. Microglia participate in phagocytosis. Oligodendrocytes produce the material that lines myelin sheath along axons, facilitating the electrical signal of action potentials. Satellite and Schwann cells are specific to the PNS. Satellite cells maintain nutrient concentrations and provide structural support for neurons in the PNS, while Schwann cells secrete myelin around axons of neurons in the PNS.

W. W. IsHak (ed.), *Atlas of Psychiatry*, https://doi.org/10.1007/978-3-031-15401-0_4

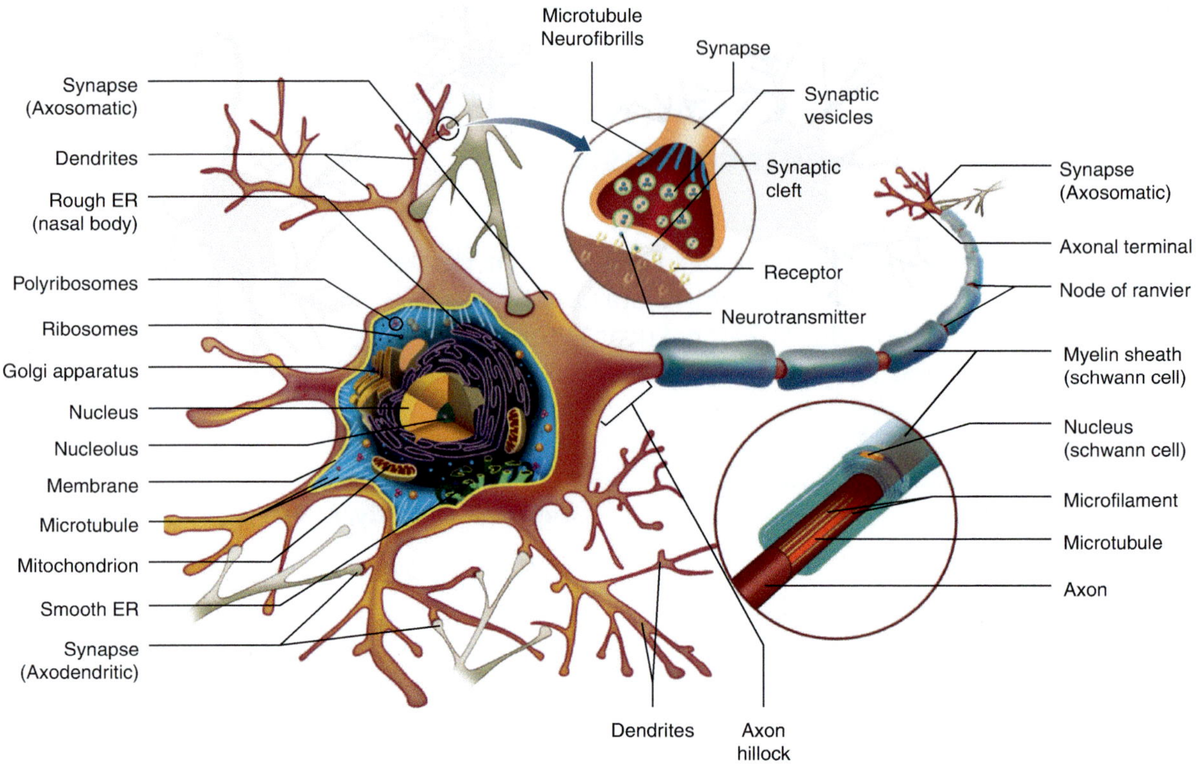

Fig. 4.1 Complete neuron cell

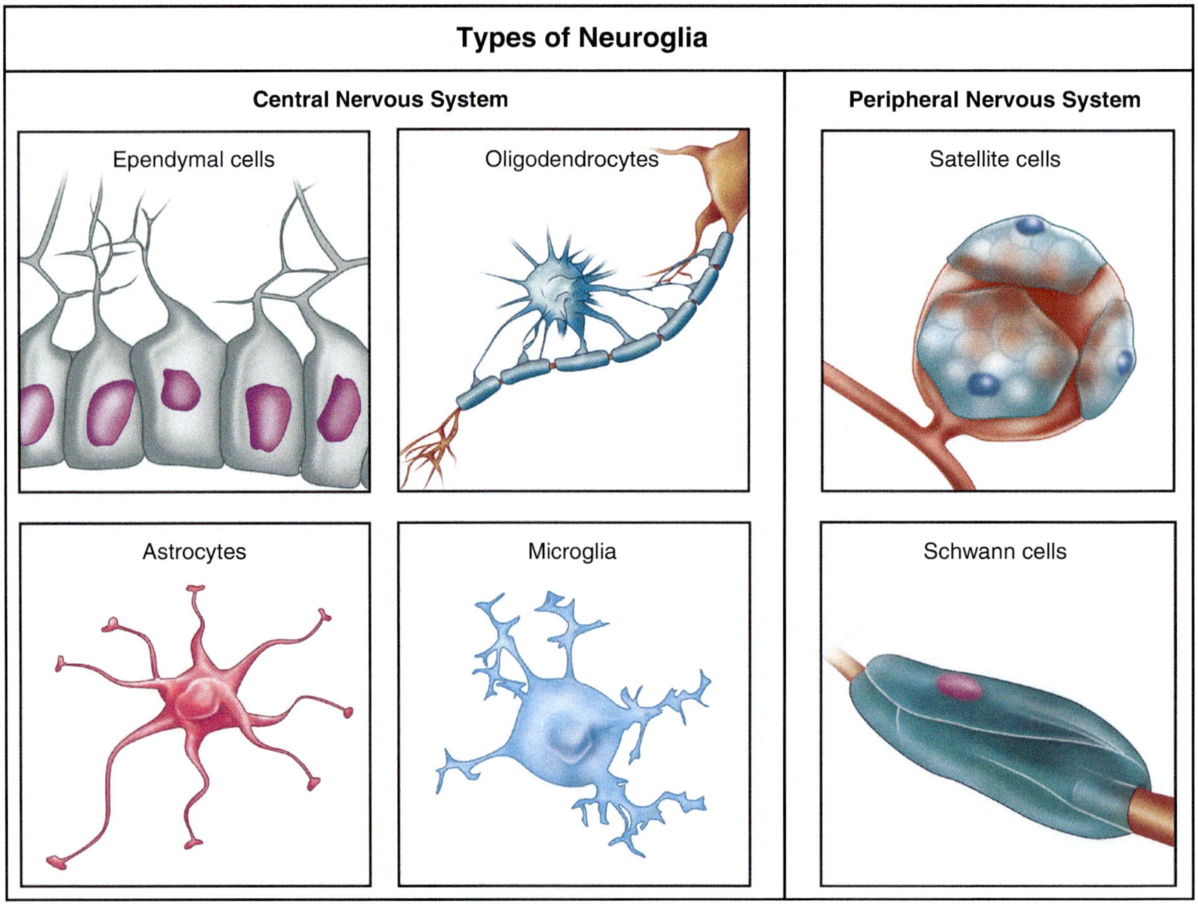

Fig. 4.2 Types of neuroglia

Grey and White Matter

Within the CNS, the term 'grey matter' is used to describe a collection of neuronal bodies. These are the cortical areas; they are located on both the surface of the brain and in deep cortical structures. In contrast, 'white matter' refers to the collection of axonal bodies from each cell. There are a plethora of large white matter tracts that allow different cortical regions to communicate with one another. Think of grey matter as cities within the brain, while white matter tracts are analogous to freeways that connect different cities (see Fig. 4.3).

Neuropathology, Proteins, and Stain Techniques

Neuropathologists are scientists who study dysfunction of the CNS and PNS on a cellular level. For example, in Alzheimer's disease, the two proteins associated with the devastating condition are collections of protein accumulations both intracellularly and extracellularly, namely Tau tangles and Amyloid plaques (displayed in Fig. 4.4).

There are a variety of techniques that these specialists employ, including various staining techniques to examine the cellular content and structure of brain tissue samples during post-mortem (after death) autopsy [2] (see Fig. 4.5).

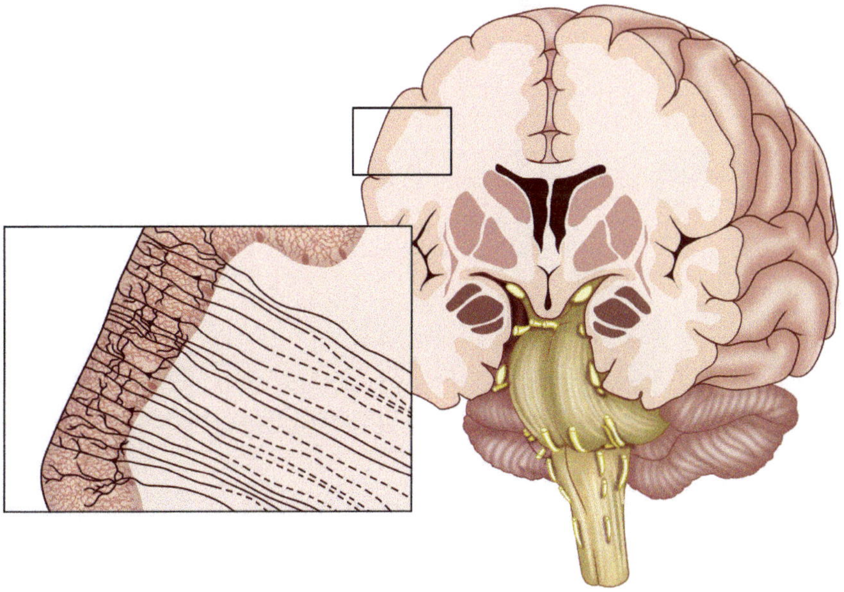

Fig. 4.3 Notice the distinction between the shading of the grey matter and the white matter beneath the surface of the neuronal cell bodies. Of importance, there are a significant number of grey matter structures located within the deep cortical regions as well, as illustrated in the figure. (*Reprinted from Bonilha* et al. [1]; Creative Commons Attribution License)

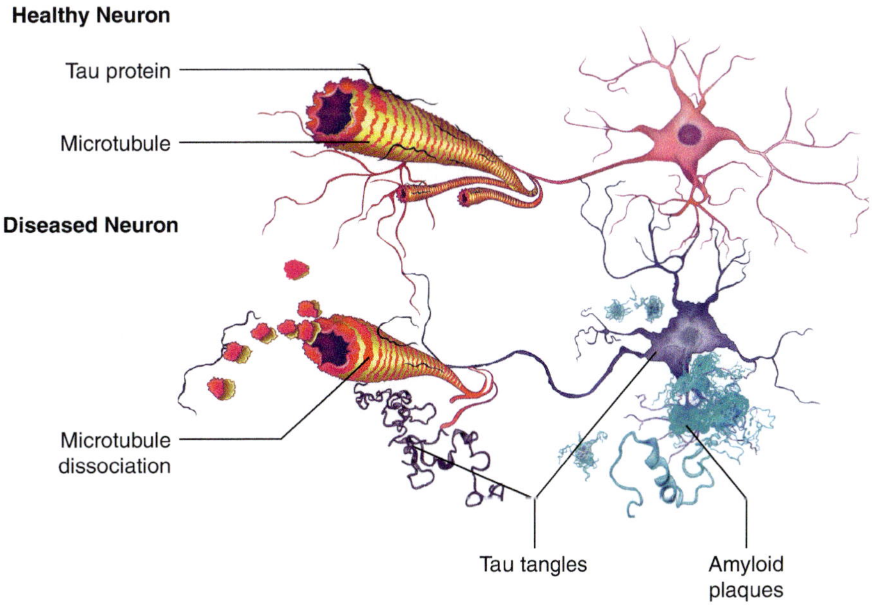

Fig. 4.4 A healthy neuron with intact Tau proteins and no amyloid plaques (above) compared to an Alzheimer's disease model, where Tau tangles and amyloid beta clusters accumulate

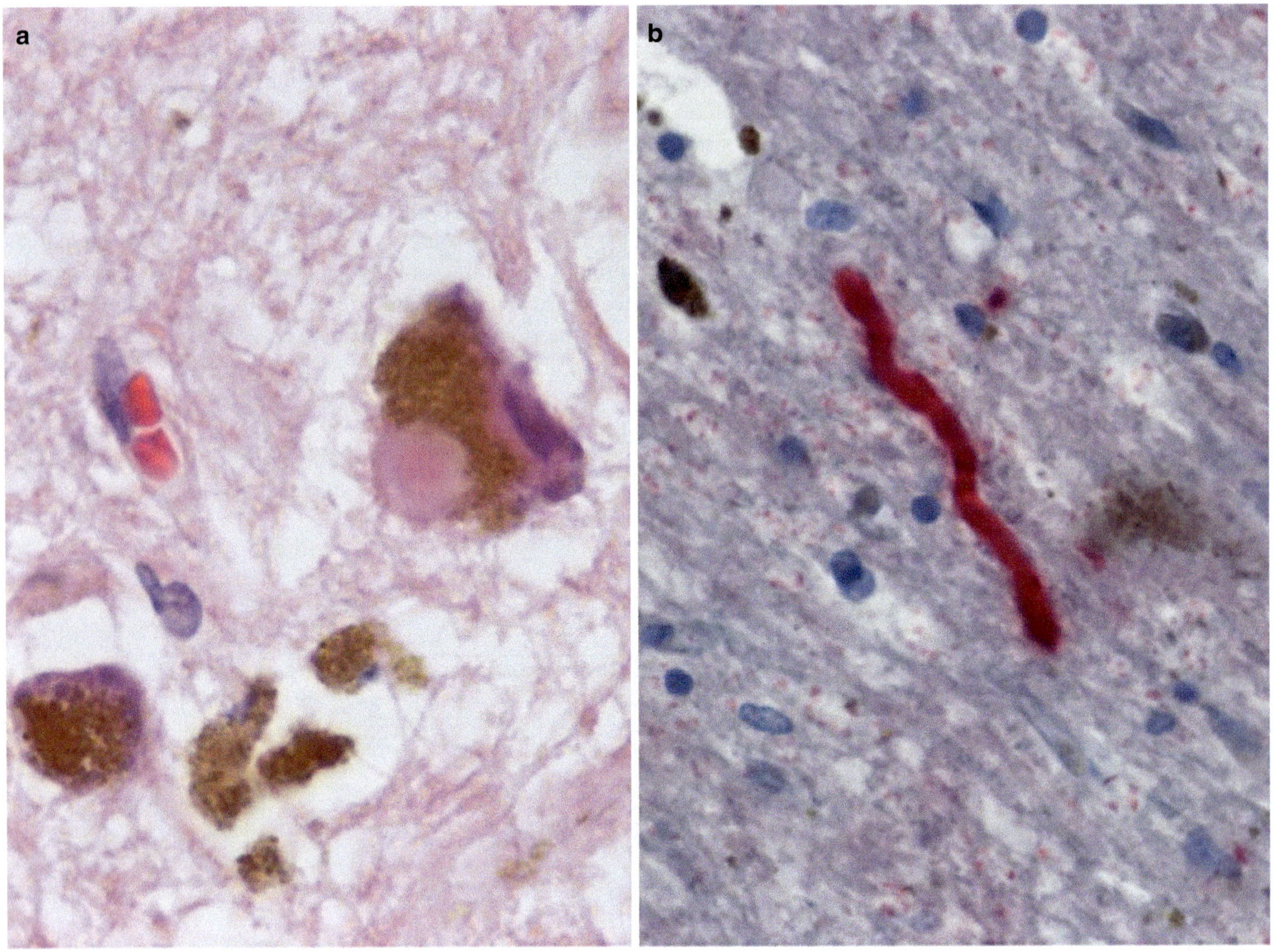

Fig. 4.5 Histological samples of the substantia nigra (SNpc) region in a patient with Parkinson's disease. (**a**) A neuron located in the SNpc with a Lewy body, which is an alpha-synuclein protein; extracellular neuromelanin and pigment-laden macrophages are also observed. (**b**) An alpha-synuclein-positive Lewy neurit at 400×. (*Reprinted from Werner* et al. [2]; Creative Commons Attribution License 2.0)

Cellular Morphology

Through the process of mammalian evolution, the cortical layers of differing species began to diverge. In comparison with other mammals, humans have an extensive number of cortical layers found in diverse regions of the brain (see Fig. 4.6). The natural consequence of such evolution, specifically with increases in brain mass and complexity of cortical circuitry, has allowed humans their high-order cognitive abilities [3].

The Four Lobes

The brain is divided into four cortical lobes, the frontal lobe, the temporal lobe, the parietal lobe, and the occipital lobe (see Fig. 4.7). These cortical regions are comprised of cell bodies of neurons, also known as grey matter. The extension of their axons, which represent nerve bundles (i.e., white matter fiber tracts), allow different cortical regions to communicate information and lay below the outer surface of the brain. Associated functions of each lobe will be discussed in the functional neuroanatomy sections that follow.

Gyri, Sulci, and Fissures

Gyri and sulci comprise the many folds and indentations of cortical tissue (see Fig. 4.8). Gyri represent the elevated ridges of cortical regions, while sulci are cortical surfaces that comprise the lowered indentations and groves of the brain's surface. Gyri are colloquially termed the "mountains" of the brain, where sulci are often referred to as the brain's "valleys." Fissures are long indentations of sulci that are neuroanatomical markers for the separations of different cortical lobes. Common fissures include the medial longitudinal fissure (the deep grove which separates the left lobe from the right lobe), the lateral fissure (a deep indentation that separates the temporal and parietal regions), the fissure of Rolando (also known as the Central Sulcus; it separates

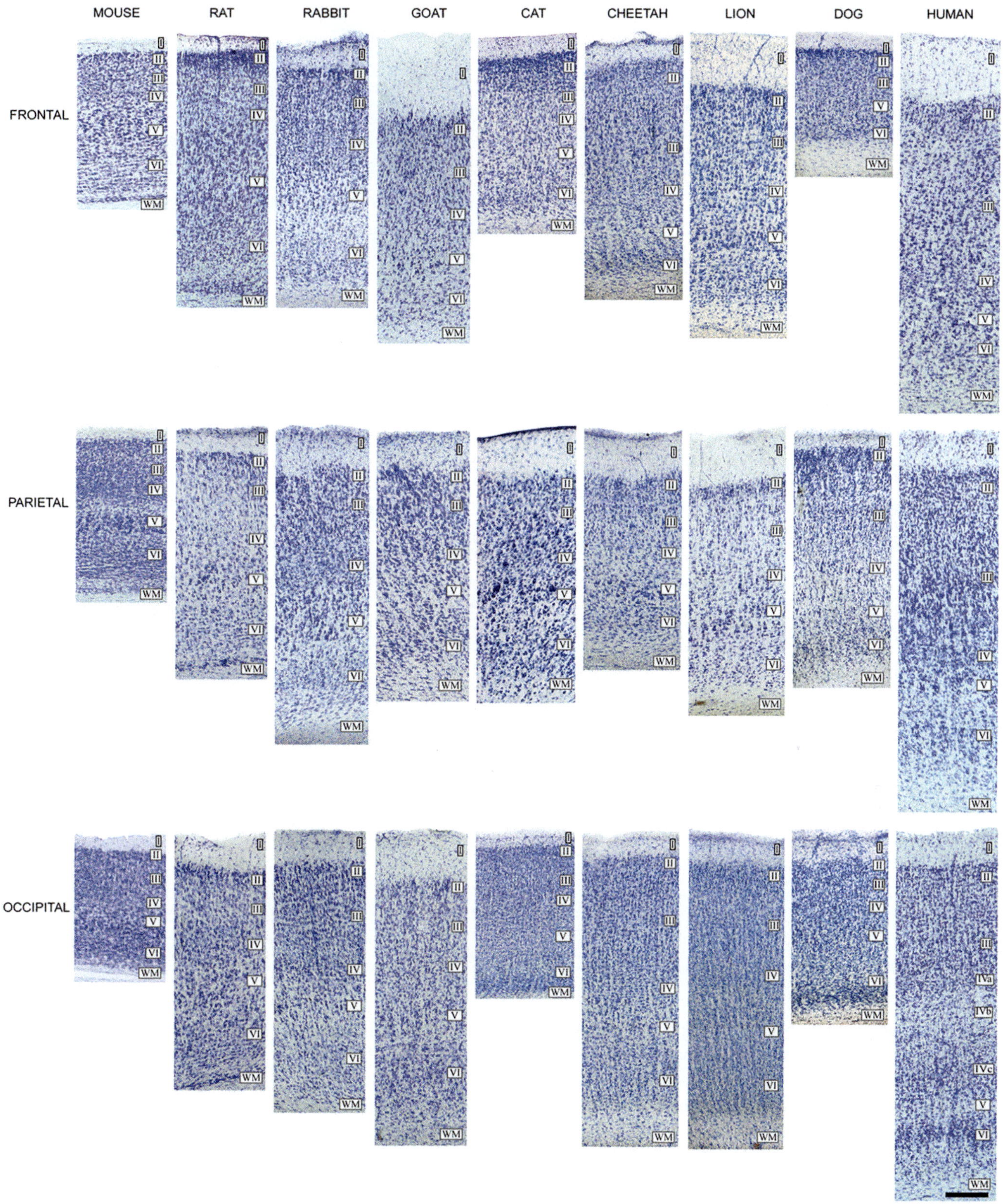

Fig. 4.6 The cytoarchitectonic differences in mammalian cortex across diverse cortical regions (e.g., frontal, parietal, and occipital) are displayed; the extraordinary number of cortical layers and concentration of cellular density across different regions in humans compared to other species is readily apparent. (*Reprinted from* Defelipe et al. [3]; Frontiers Media SA, under a non-exclusive license)

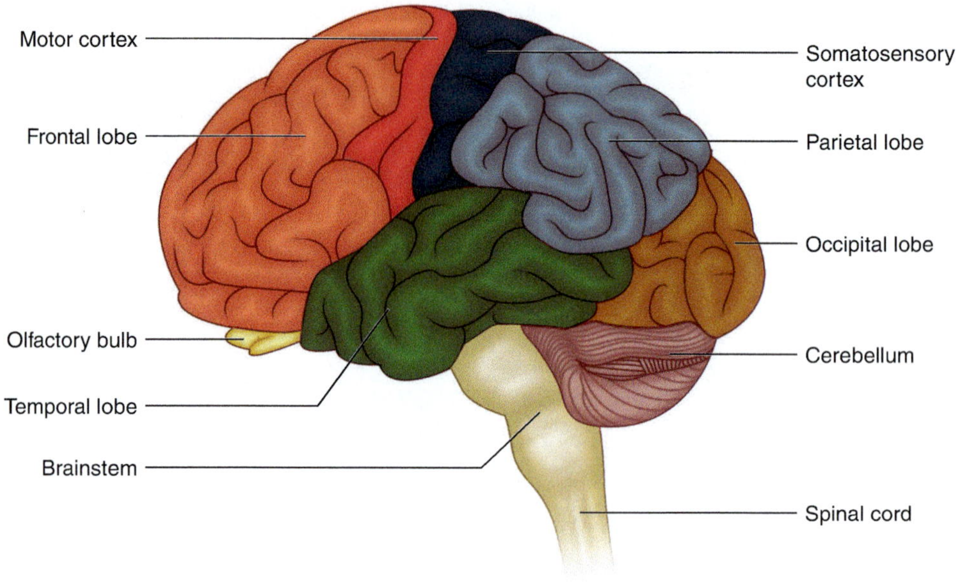

Fig. 4.7 The four lobes of the brain and accompanying structures (e.g., brainstem, cerebellum, and spinal cord). Of note, the motor cortex is located in the posterior region of the frontal lobe, while the somatosensory cortex is located in the anterior region of the parietal lobe

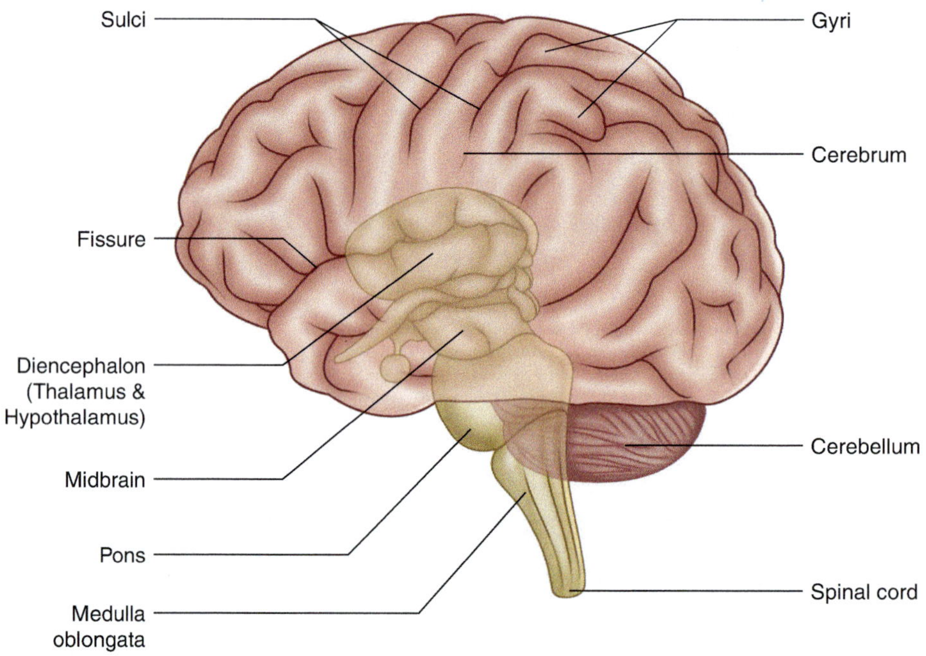

Fig. 4.8 Brain structures

the parietal and frontal lobes), and the parieto-occipital sulcus (a deep crater which separates the parietal lobe from the occipital lobe). Additional structures are displayed underneath the outer cortical layers (e.g., diencephalon, midbrain, pons, and medulla).

Radiological Orientation

Common terminology exists to describe the spatial orientation of the brain. Neuroradiologists utilize these terms to describe findings from various neuroimaging techniques during clinical and research procedures (see Fig. 4.9).

The Three Divisions of the Human Brain

Figure 4.10 displays a flow chart of the human nervous system. The brain is composed of three major divisions: the forebrain, the midbrain, and the hindbrain. The forebrain, which includes the hypothalamus, thalamus, and cerebrum, is associated with complex cognitive, perceptual, and motor activities. The midbrain, also known as the mesencephalon, is a portion of the brainstem involved in the reception and integration of sensory input, select motor control functions, alertness/arousal/consciousness, and regulation of select autonomic features (e.g., body temperature), among others. The hindbrain consists of the medulla, the pons, and the cerebellum. It facilitates the passage

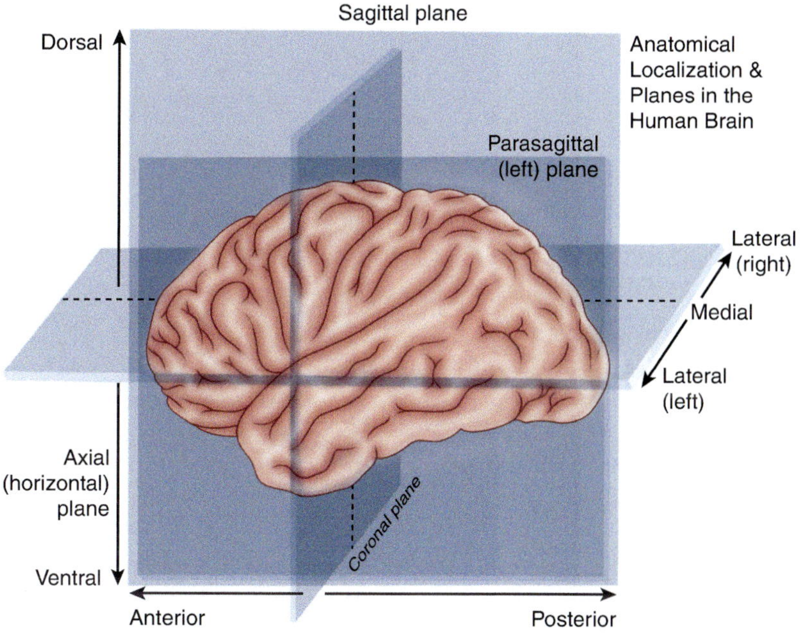

Fig. 4.9 The key radiological orientation terms

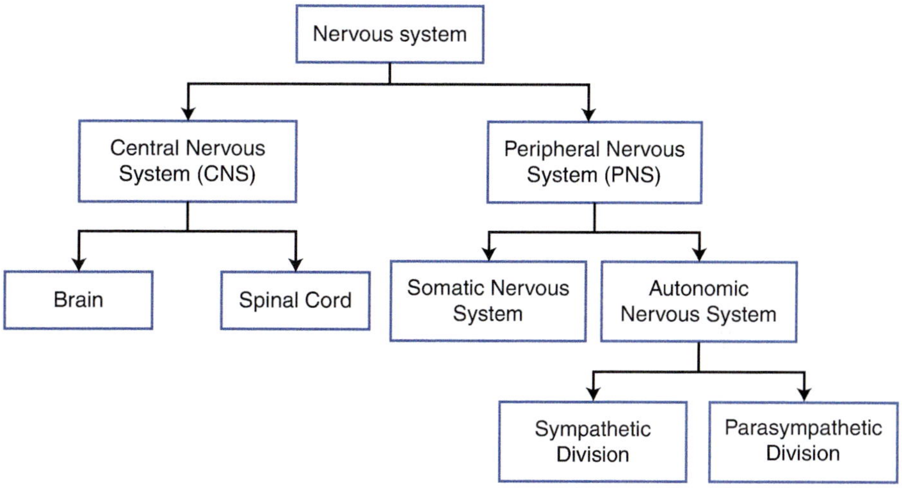

Fig. 4.10 Subdivisions of the human nervous system

of information from the cerebrum to the spinal cord, is critically involved in the regulation of fine motor control, and is associated with several other vital autonomic functions (i.e., respiratory rhythm, heart rate, sleep, and wakefulness).

Forebrain

The forebrain is divided into the diencephalon (i.e., hypothalamus, thalamus, subthalamus, and epithalamus) and the cerebrum. Within the forebrain is the limbic system—a group of structures that cooperate to regulate emotion, behavior, motivation, memory processing, and reward/motivation (see Fig. 4.11). The four main parts of the limbic system are the amygdala, which handles anger, fear processing, and stress response; the hippocampus, performing long-term memory consolidation; the hypothalamus, handling homeostatic maintenance and regulation of body temperature/motivation/hormones; and the thalamus, charged with relaying sensory and motor input to different cortical regions.

Brainstem

The brainstem consists of three different components: the midbrain, the pons, and the medulla oblongata (see Fig. 4.12). The midbrain plays a central role in the receipt and integration of sensory (i.e., auditory and visual) information as well as motor control, alertness, and temperature regulation. The pons relays information between the cerebrum and the cerebellum. In addition, the pons helps regulate breathing, sleep, hearing, taste, equilibrium, and facial sensory processing. The medulla controls many vital autonomic functions, including breathing, heart rate, swallowing, and digestion.

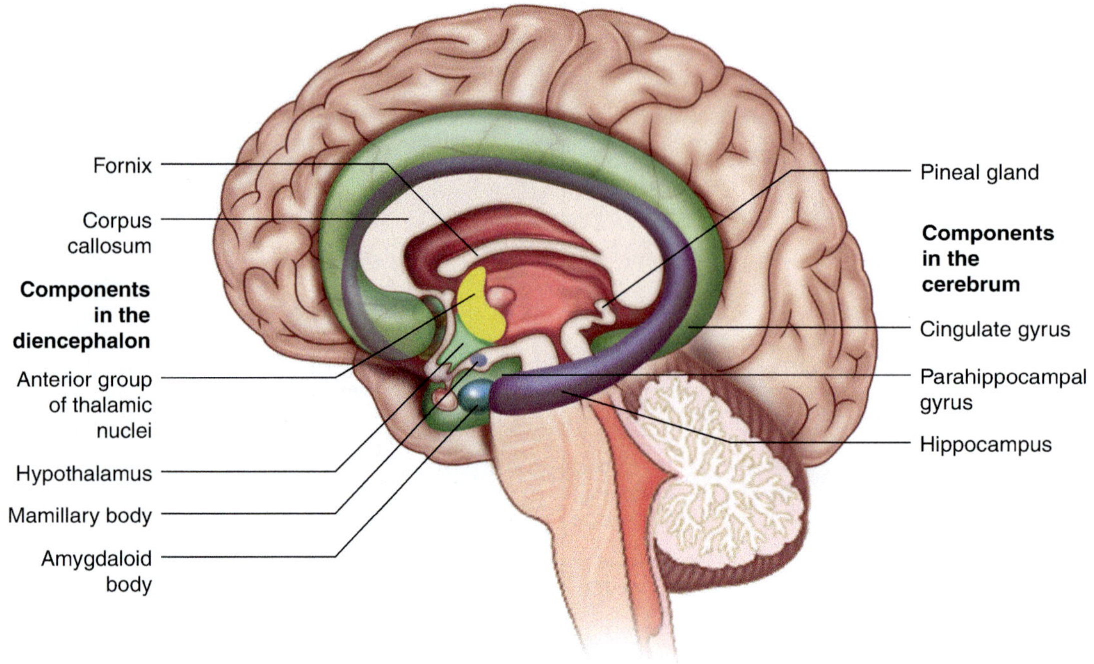

Fig. 4.11 The limbic system is a broad constellation of key cortical structures within the forebrain

Fig. 4.12 The components of the brainstem

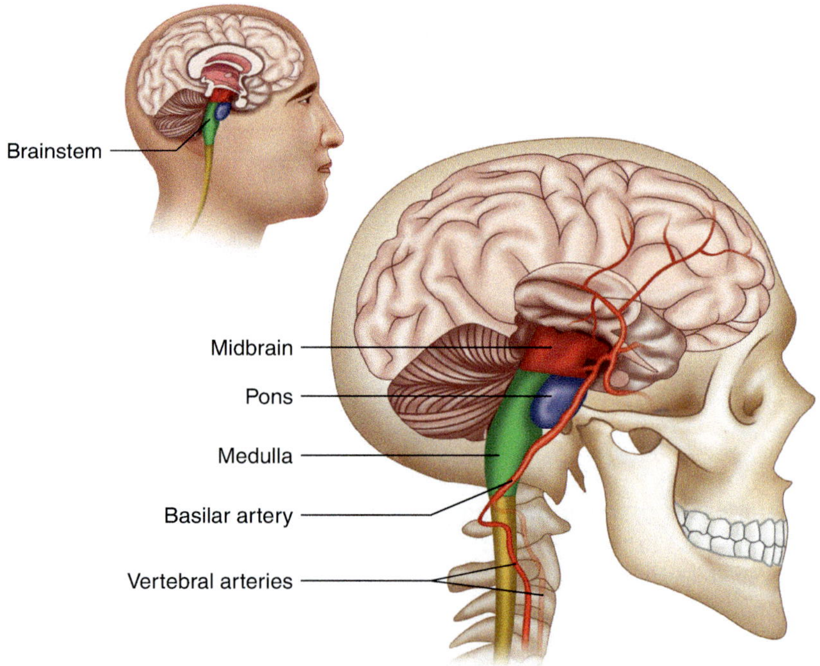

Spinal Cord

Figures 4.13 and 4.14 represent the ascending and descending pathways of the spinal cord, and Fig. 4.15 displays the two divisions of the autonomic nervous system.

Subcortical Structures

Subcortical structures represent a collection of grey matter beneath the cortical surface of the brain. Many of the most critical subcortical regions comprise the basal ganglia, which are located in the mesial (middle) and deep sections of the brain (see Figs. 4.16 and 4.17).

Ventricular System

Ventricles within the brain aid in the generation and circulation of cerebral spinal fluid. Three major ventricles perform this process, including the lateral, third, and fourth

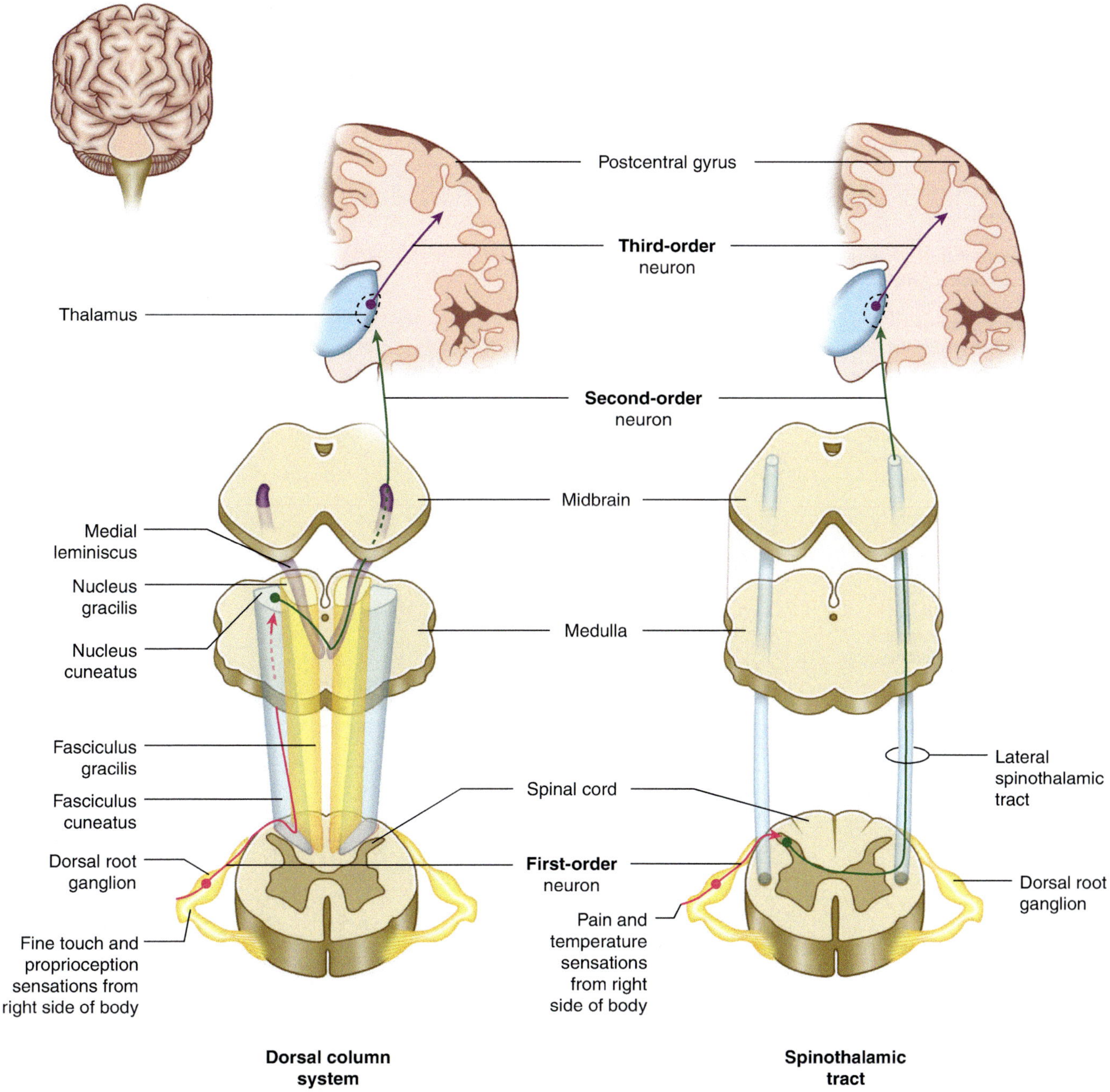

Fig. 4.13 The ascending (aka afferent) pathway of the spinal cord transmits sensory information to the brain. There are two major sensory pathways along the spinal cord: the dorsal column system (i.e., tactile stimuli input, sense of movement, body orientation feedback) and the spinothalamic tract (i.e., pain, temperature). The first-order neuron originates in the dorsal root ganglion for both of these pathways. In the dorsal column system (shown on the left), axons from the lower body enter the fasciculus gracilis, whereas axons from the upper body enter the fasciculus cuneatus. These axons terminate in the medulla, from which the second-order neuron projects and ascends to the thalamus for sensory relay processing. In the spinothalamic tract (shown on the right), the first-order neuron synapses with the second-order neuron in the dorsal horn. These axons ascend along the lateral spinothalamic tract and terminate in the thalamus. In both pathways, the third-order neuron extends from the thalamus and carries sensory information to the postcentral gyrus, located in the parietal lobe region

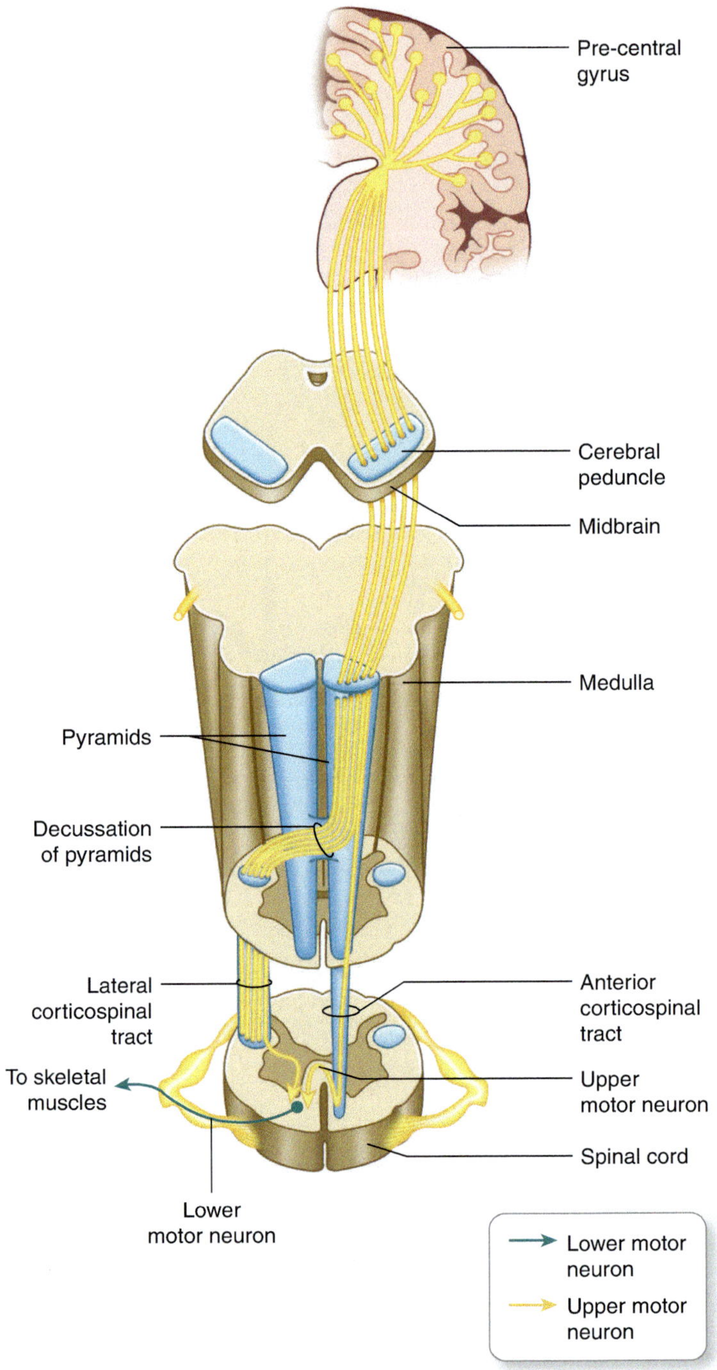

Fig. 4.14 The corticospinal tract (also known as the efferent pathway) is a major descending pathway of the spinal cord. It is responsible for transmitting motor output from the cerebral cortex to the skeletal muscles of the limbs and trunk to regulate and generate movement. The upper motor neuron descends from the primary motor cortex in the precentral gyrus (located in the frontal lobe) and passes through the midbrain and the pons. In the medulla, the axons form white matter tracts, famously termed the 'pyramid' tract. At the border of the medulla and the spinal cord, most of the axons cross over to form the lateral corticospinal tract, while the uncrossed axons comprise the anterior corticospinal tract. Once the upper motor neuron reaches the spinal cord, it synapses with the lower motor neuron, which carries motor signals to skeletal muscles to regulate movement. The corticobulbar tract is another descending pathway and is associated with the muscles of the face, head, and neck

ventricles, which are located in both cerebral hemispheres. Circulation of cerebral spinal fluid is critical for nutrient supply and removal of metabolic waste products. Several variants of hydrocephalus exist, including external hydrocephalus/hydrocephalus ex vacuo (i.e., excess CSF within the ventricles due to cortical atrophy), internal hydrocephalus (dilation of the ventricles from occlusion of circulation in the fourth ventricle) and communicating hydrocephalus (either external or internal CSF buildup that results from obstruction). Several regions regulate both production and flow of CSF within the brain, including the Choroid plexus, Cisterna magna, Foramen of Monro, Foramina of Luschka, and Foramen of Magendie. A visual image of the ventricular system is provided in Fig. 4.18.

If ventricle obstruction occurs or there is overproduction of CSF, fluid buildup and accumulation within the ventricles can occur, which often results in the necessity of neurosurgical intervention to reduce increasing intracranial pressure. Importantly, however, the suspected etiology or causes can be a contraindication for select surgical procedures (i.e., VP shunt/drain trial).

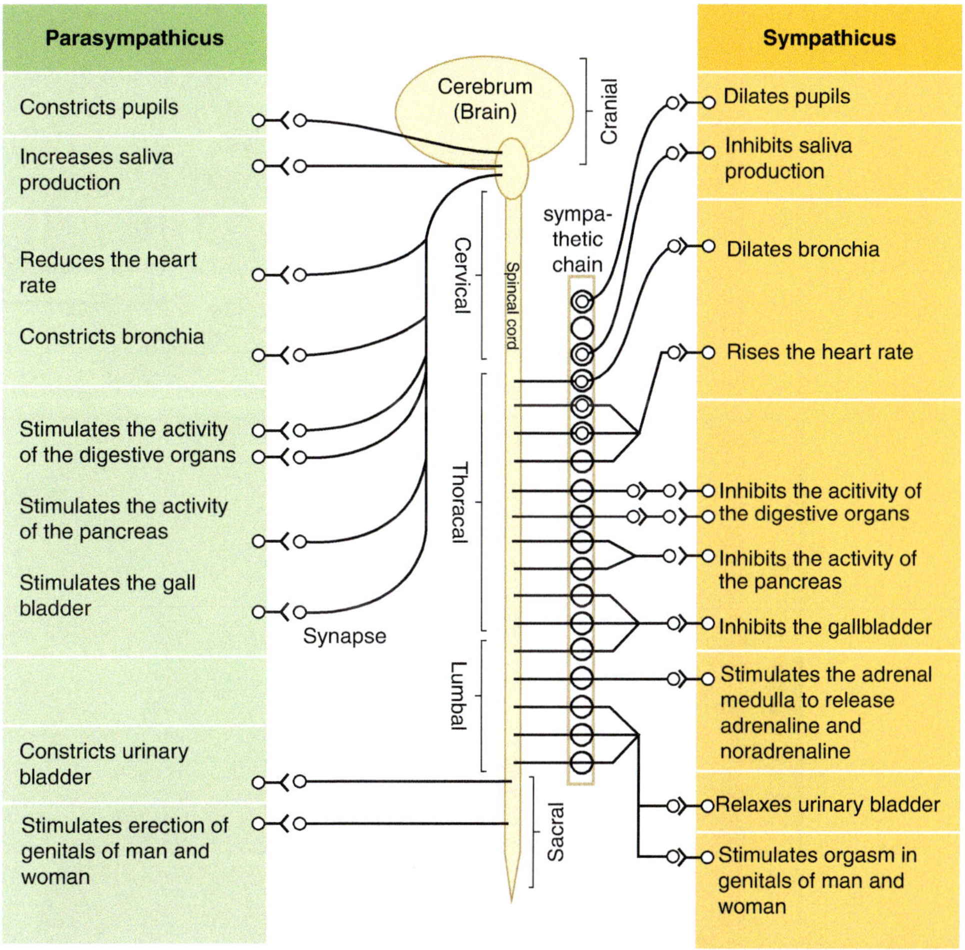

Fig. 4.15 The two divisions of the autonomic nervous system are displayed with their respective associated regions of the spine. The parasympathetic division is associated with the cranial, cervical, and sacral regions, while the sympathetic division corresponds to the thoracic and lumbar regions

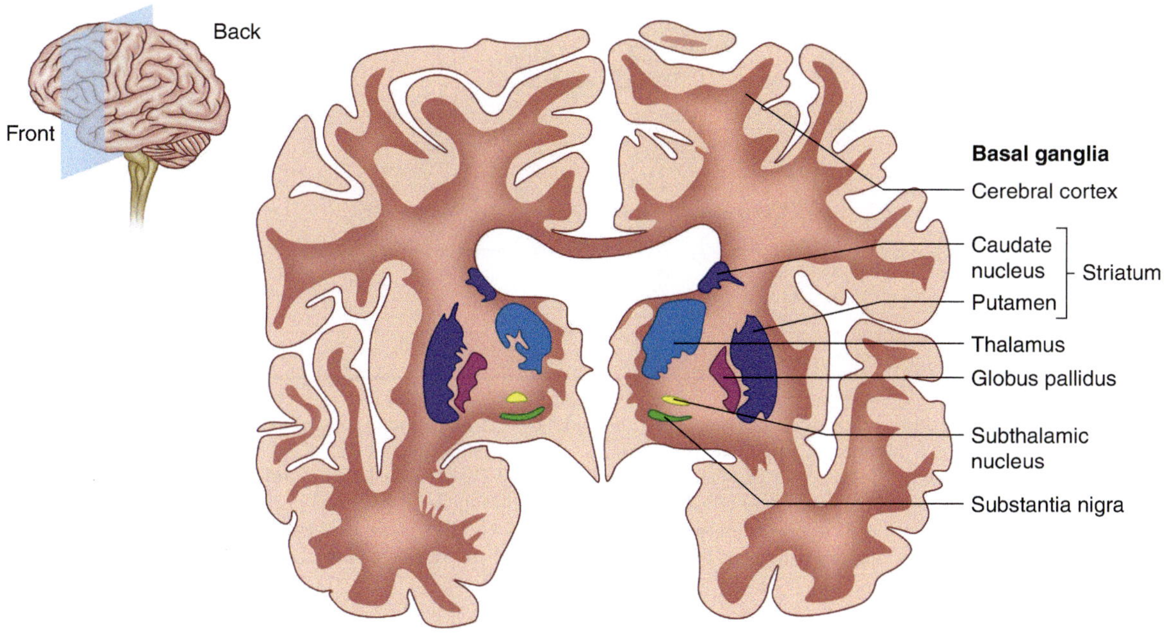

Fig. 4.16 The structures of basal ganglia in coronal plane orientation

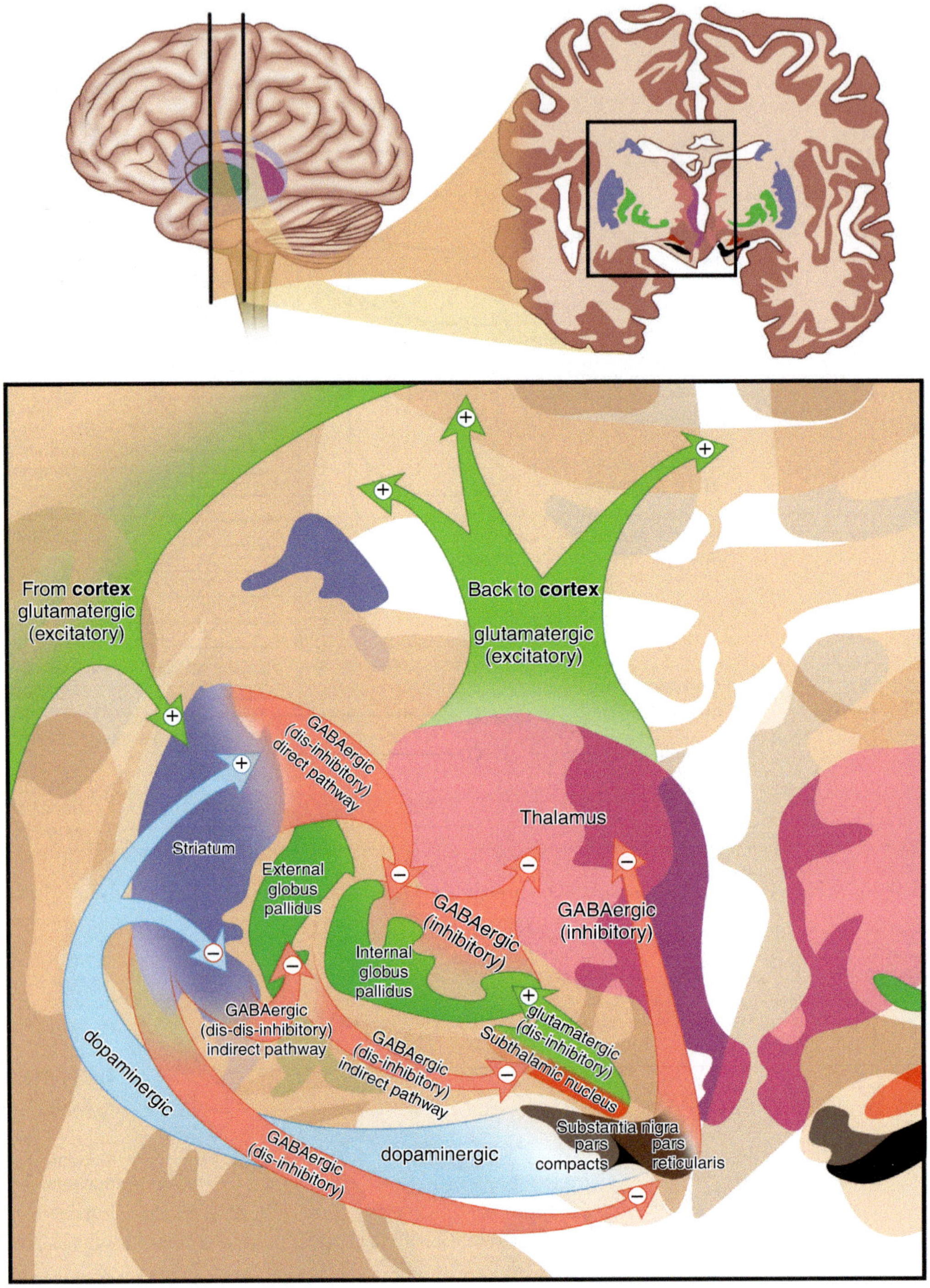

Fig. 4.17 The basal ganglia and other subcortical structures (i.e., the thalamus) play a critical role in a number of cognitive processes. Subcortical structures serve as a primary relay center that facilitates the reception and transmission of signals and the processing of information from neurochemical/electrical activity via select neurotransmitters (e.g., GABA, glutamate, and dopamine) that are comprised of feedback loops between various subcortical structures and other cortical regions via inhibitory/excitatory regulation/modulation to other cortical regions. This region helps maintain and regulate necessary feedback loops through inhibitory and excitatory regulation and modulation during various tasks like movement and motor planning, emotional regulation, and emotional, sensory, and cognitive processing

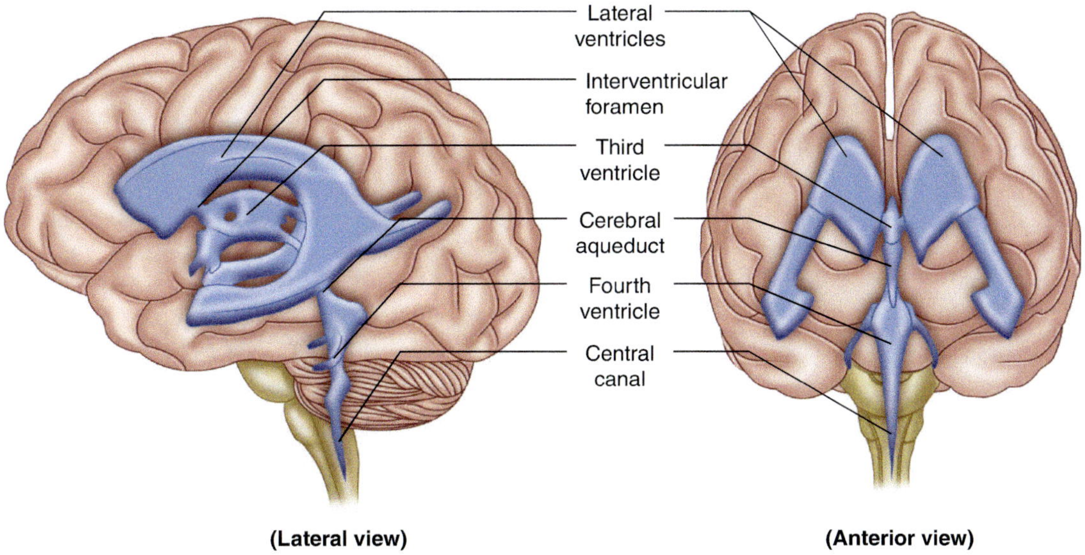

Fig. 4.18 Lateral and anterior views of the ventricles

Fig. 4.19 Meninges

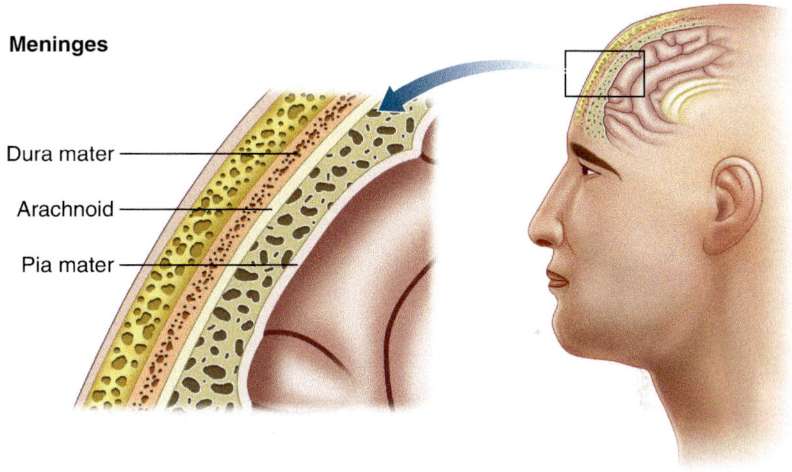

Protective Layers of the Brain

Surrounding the outer surface of the brain's grey matter are the protective layers of the brain including the meninges (e.g., dura matter, arachnoid matter, and pia matter), as well as thin areas of space between these divisions comprised of cerebral spinal fluid (CSF). Outside of the meninges are the skull bone and scalp. The meninges line the outer layer of the brain and help to protect vessels that provide the brain with blood. The meninges also contain CSF transmitted from the ventricular system between the pia matter and arachnoid matter (termed dural sinuses). One final protective layer of the brain is the blood–brain barrier, which is encompassed by endothelial cells that contain the least permeable capillaries because of tight junctions. The protective layers of the brain are displayed below (see Fig. 4.19).

Cerebrovascular System

The human brain contains a complex cerebrovascular system (see Fig. 4.20).

The ACA, MCA, and PCA provide oxygenated blood to various regions throughout the brain; occlusion of any of the major arteries for extended periods of time can result in anoxic/hypoxic injury to corresponding dependent cortical areas (see Figs. 4.21 and 4.22).

Cerebrovascular Accident and Stroke Mechanisms

Strokes can be categorized as one of two types, ischemic, which are the most common and comprise approximately 85–90% of strokes, and hemorrhagic. Ischemic stroke

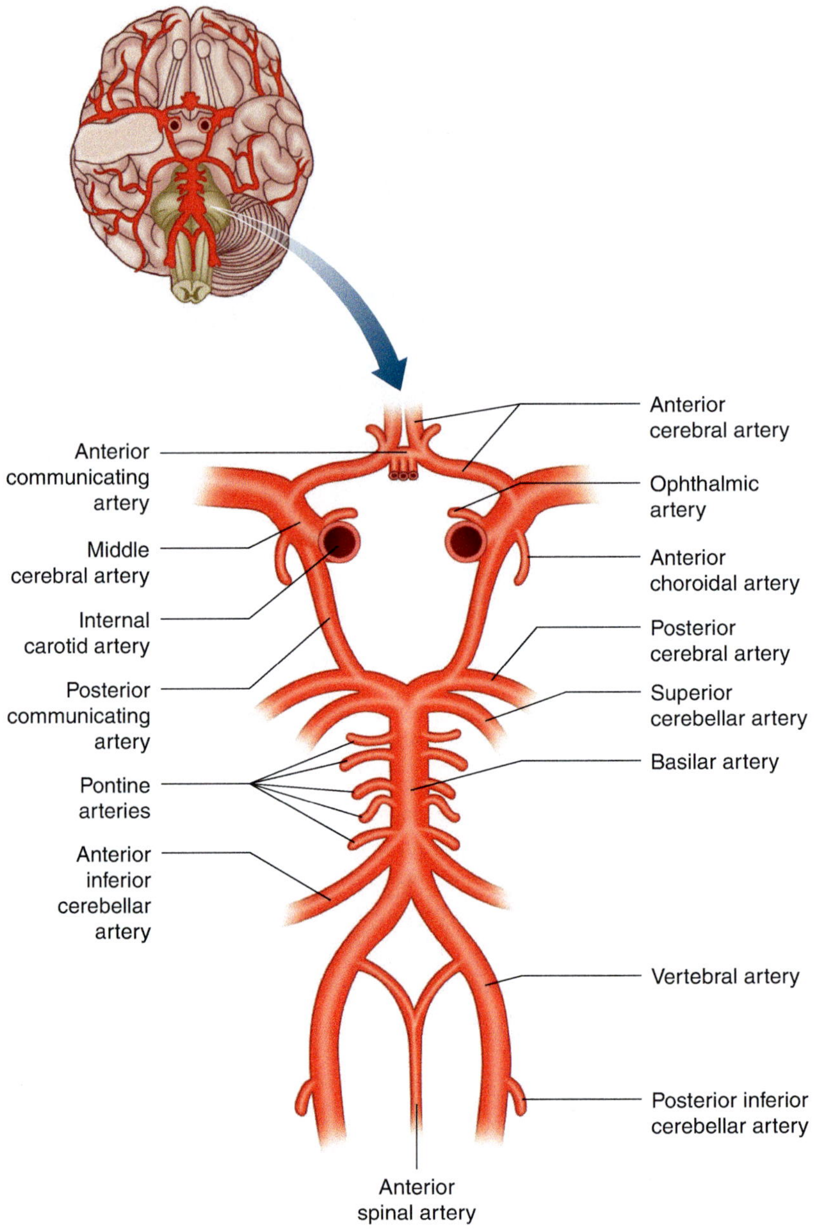

Fig. 4.20 The Circle of Willis is depicted with the different branches of the PCA, MCA, and ACA displayed, as well as their projections to different cortical regions. Blood flows to different cortical and subcortical regions through the Circle of Willis. Blood flows into the brain from the vertebral and carotid arteries and then enters the basilar artery. Notably, the possibility of locked-in syndrome, a devastating stroke condition, which can result in full paralysis aside from preserved eye movement, can result from occlusion of the basilar artery. Patients maintain eye movement because select cranial nerves are spared. The basilar artery is located before the posterior communicating artery (PCA), middle cerebral artery (MCA), and anterior communicating artery (ACA)

occurs when there is occlusion (blockage of an artery). There are two major subtypes of ischemic strokes. Thrombotic strokes occur when a blood clot that has developed inside the brain blocks blood flow. Embolic strokes result from either a blood clot or buildup of plaque debris that has developed outside the brain and traveled to one of the cerebral vessels. The other type of ischemic stroke is a lacunar infarct, which results from disruption of blood flow in microvascular vessels within the brain. Many lacunar strokes occur in subcortical regions because of the small size of the lenticulostriate arteries; major risk factors for lacunar infarct include hypertension, smoking, and hyperlipidemia. Conversely, hemorrhagic stroke occurs when a blood vessel ruptures within the brain and blood exits outside of the arterial wall (see Fig. 4.23).

When the ischemic injury occurs, a neurochemical cascade can occur (see Fig. 4.24).

Cranial Nerves

The human body contains 12 nerves with varying associated functions (see Fig. 4.25). The vagus nerve (cranial nerve 10) is of particular interest as it contains both efferent (motor)

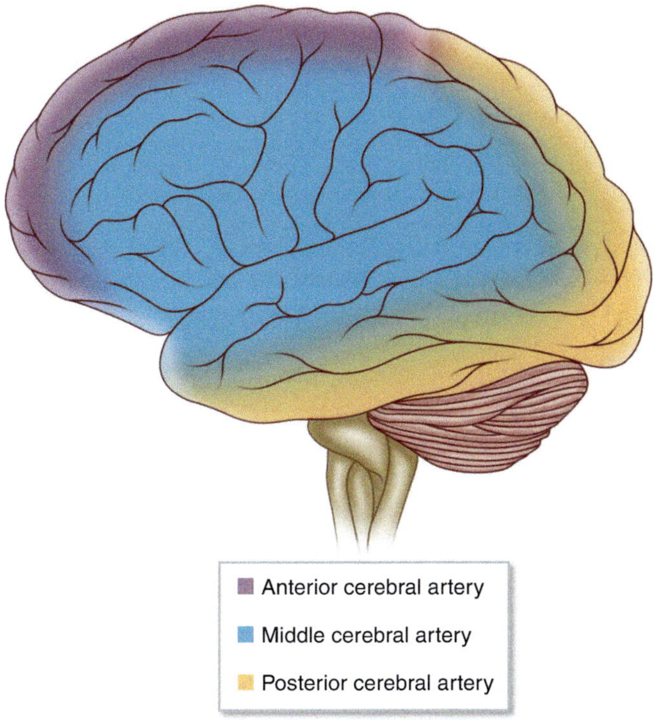

Fig. 4.21 The cortical vascular territories of the three major cerebral arteries

and afferent (sensory) fibers. Some efferent effects include thoracic and abdominal visceral parasympathetic responses and motor responses in upper airway components, as well as the pharynx, larynx, and trachea. Afferent effects include signaling from auditory and upper airway components.

Structural Neuroimaging

The reader is encouraged to reference Chap. 8 of the current textbook, which provides greater detail pertaining to the different structural neuroimaging techniques and their respective benefits/weaknesses. In brief, however, head computerized tomography (CT) scans are the quickest neuroimaging technique and are commonly utilized in emergency settings to monitor stroke/cerebrovascular accidents but provide low image resolution. Conversely, brain MRI imaging affords clinicians much higher resolution to detect structural abnormalities within the brain, but the procedure takes longer to administer relative to a CT scan. Diffuse tensor imaging (DTI) is commonly used in research settings to elucidate the location, orientation, and structural integrity of white matter pathways. A variety of other neuroimaging techniques are detailed in Chap. 8.

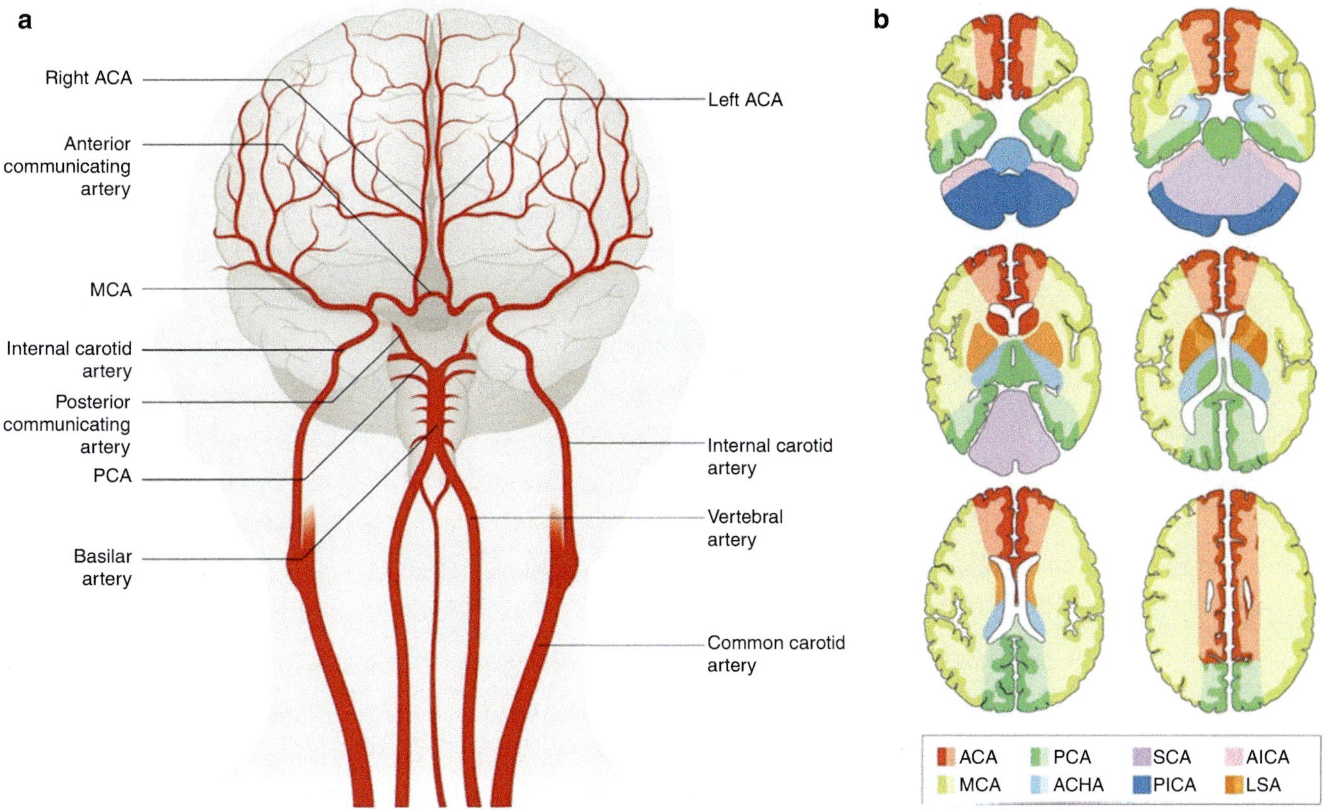

Fig. 4.22 The major arteries of the brain (**a**) and their vascular territories (**b**). Although simplified here for illustrative purposes, an ischaemic stroke in one of these vessels could cause tissue damage in the regions highlighted. *ACA* anterior cerebral artery, *ACHA* anterior choroidal artery, *AICA* anterior inferior cerebellar artery, *LSA* lenticulostriate artery, *MCA* middle cerebral artery, *PCA* posterior cerebral artery; *PICA* posterior inferior cerebellar artery, *SCA* superior cerebellar artery. (*From* Campbell et al. [4]; *with permission*)

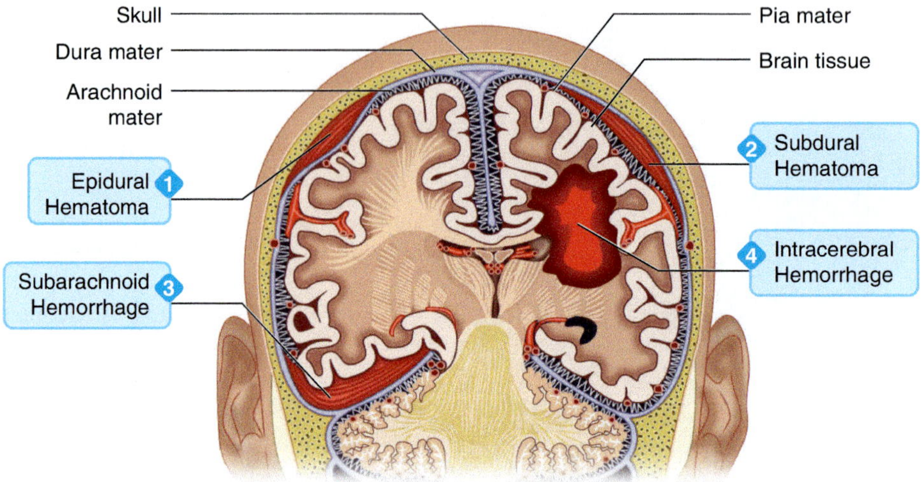

Fig. 4.23 Hemorrhagic strokes can occur intracranially (intracranial hemorrhage), within the subarachnoid space (subarachnoid hemorrhage), under the dura matter (subdural hematoma), or outside of the dura matter (epidural hematoma)

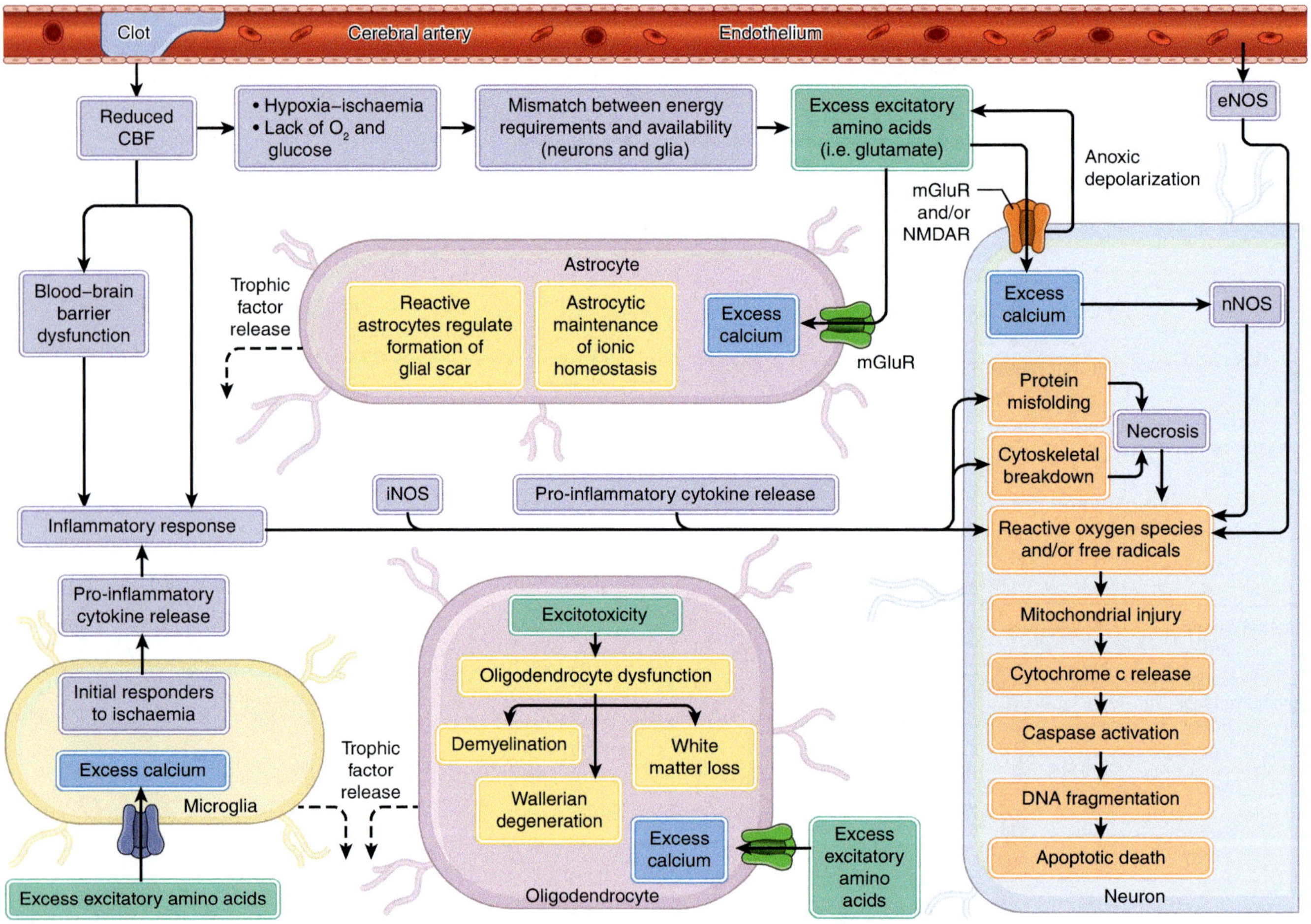

Fig. 4.24 Cellular effects of ischemia. Occlusion of a cerebral artery initiates a cascade of responses. Reduced cerebral blood flow (CBF) leads to reduced availability of glucose and oxygen and a mismatch in energy requirements and availability in neurons, glia, and endothelial cells. Anoxic depolarization and reduced activity of glutamate reuptake lead to increased extracellular levels of glutamate. This leads to neuronal calcium influx (through the *N*-methyl-D-aspartate (NMDA) ion receptor (NMDAR)) and release of calcium from intracellular stores in neurons and glia (mediated via metabotropic glutamate receptors (mGluRs)). Blood–brain barrier dysfunction and release of signaling molecules (for example, cytokines) from astrocytes, microglia, and oligodendrocytes lead to an inflammatory response. In neurons, the cumulative effect is cell death mediated through diverse pathways, including necrosis and apoptosis. *eNOS* endothelial nitric oxide synthase, *iNOS* inducible nitric oxide synthase, *nNOS* neuronal nitric oxide synthase. (*From* Campbell et al. [4]; *with permission*)

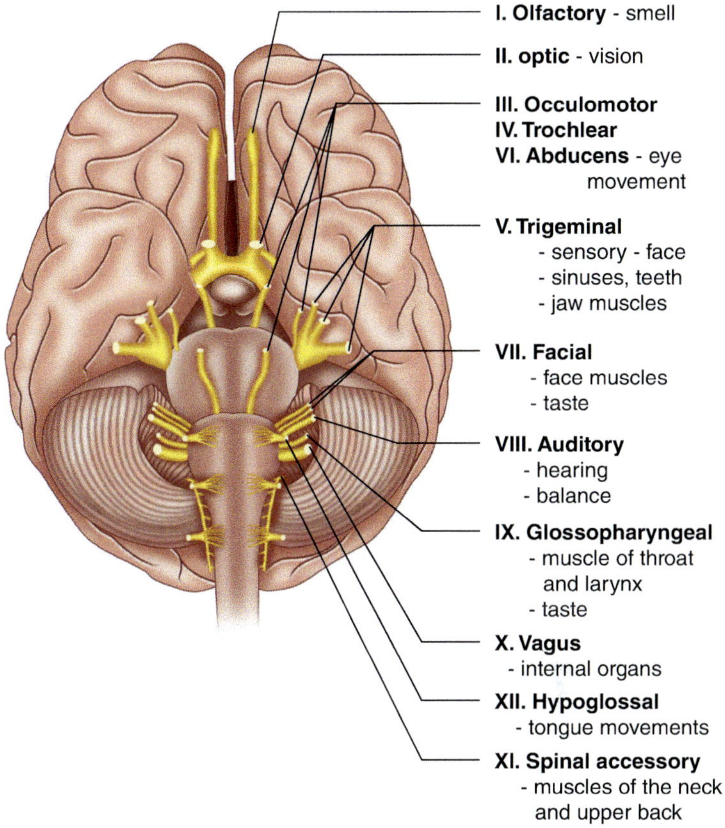

Fig. 4.25 The 12 cranial nerves, with their associated functions

Functional Neuroanatomy

Understanding the complex interactions between different cortical regions remains beyond the focus of this section in the current chapter (see Chap. 7), but select cortical regions are displayed in Figs. 4.26 and 4.27. However, the section will provide basic principles, and landmark theories will be provided.

In general, the frontal lobes are involved in motor planning, motor initiation, speech production, social cognition, and higher order executive skills. The lateral regions of the temporal lobes are involved in auditory processing, receptive language comprehension, confrontation naming, and object/facial recognition. The mesial temporal regions handle memory storage/consolidation and emotional processing. The parietal regions are heavily involved in spatial, sensory, and attentional processing, alongside aspects of reading, spelling, and mathematical computation. Injuries to the parietal regions can result in a number of neurological symptoms including agnosia, agraphia, acalculia, and apraxia (ideational and ideomotor). The occipital regions process visual stimuli.

The Frontal Lobes

Higher-order "executive" skills are discussed in greater detail in Chap. 7 of the current volume. For an exceptional review of executive control based upon the evolution of neuroanatomical trends in humans, the reader is referred elsewhere (see Bilder, 2012) [5]. Pioneering work by Fuster (2004) [6], which outlined the complex interactions between the frontal lobes and other cortical regions and detailed mechanisms of the '*perception-action cycle*' in cognitive processing, is also of note (see Figs. 4.28 and 4.29).

Motor and Somatosensory System

One of the most common misconceptions of neuroanatomy is the presumption that specific cortical regions are responsible for specific functions. In reality, a complex interlay of divergent cortical regions process (input) and communicate (output) information. This configuration allows humans to simultaneously process stimuli and pursues goal-directed movement through interdependent intention, facilitated by feedback loops (see Fig. 4.30). This said, broad processing of auditory, tactile, visual, and spatial information primarily occurs, at least initially, in circumscribed regions. Motor planning reflects a similar reality; distinct cortical regions are involved in the production/coordination of speech, initial planning of motor action, and execution of desired motor actions. Additional, specific parts of the brain assist with the processing of sensory and motor stimuli. In par-

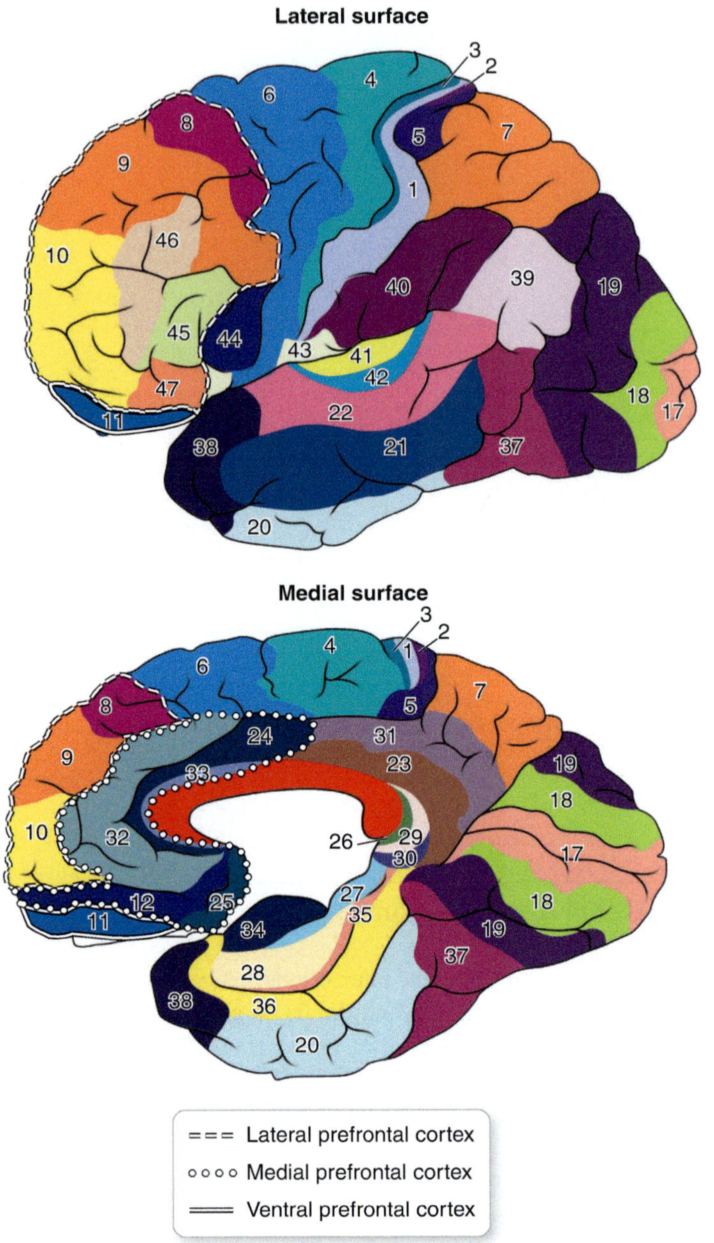

Fig. 4.26 Notable here is German anatomist Korbinian Brodmann, who published groundbreaking work on defining the organizations of neurons within the CNS based on the cytoarchitectural organization. He mapped distinct cortical regions based on his work, primarily with humans and monkeys. Brodmann's areas are displayed

ticular, the thalamus, located within the diencephalon, is a major relay center. The thalamus is comprised of a number of nuclei that relay information to downstream cortical regions. The reticular formation, a complex network of nerve bundles in the brainstem, regulates consciousness (arousal/alertness) and sleep-wake transitions via the reticular activating system (RAS). The reticular formation carries out this process in unison with the thalamus. The thalamus is extremely sensitive; in a clinical setting, even extremely small (but strategically placed) infarcts on the thalamus can have broad negative consequences on cognition.

Motor System

The motor system is extremely complex and is discussed in greater detail in the sections that follow.

Vestibular System

The vestibular system is responsible for monitoring motion, balance, and spatial orientation (see Fig. 4.31).

Somatosensory Processing Via the Thalamus

Several distinct nuclei within the thalamus receive input, process that information, and relay that information to other cortical regions (see Fig. 4.32) [7].

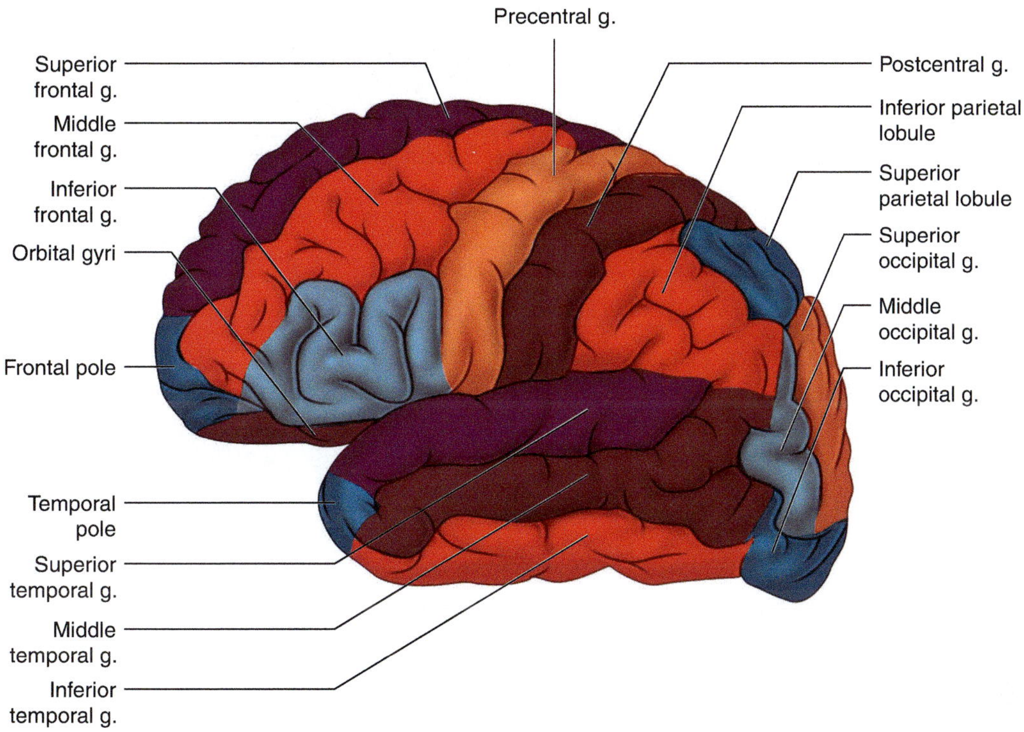

Fig. 4.27 The main cortical gyri

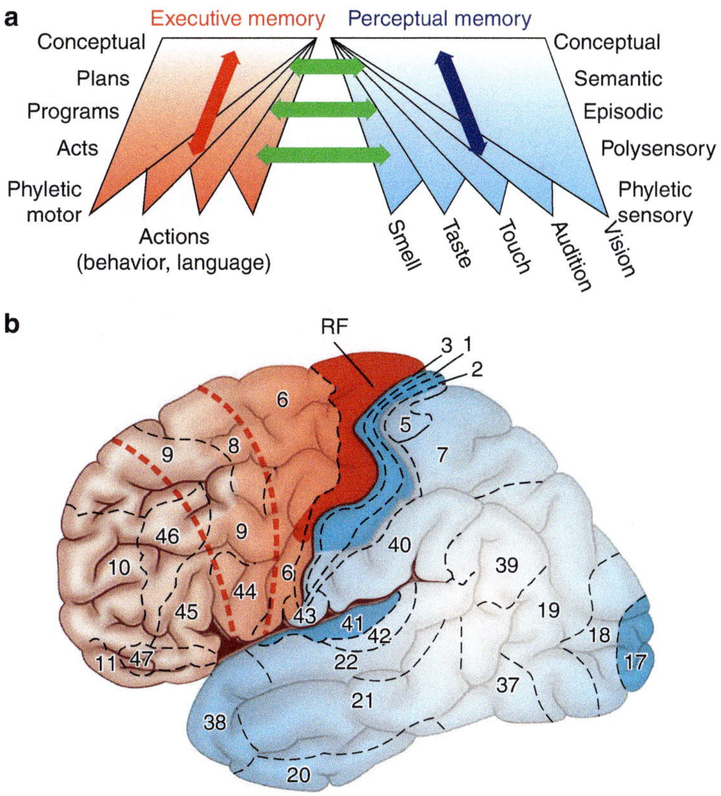

Fig. 4.28 Representational map of the human lateral cortex. (**a**) Schema of the hierarchical organization of memory and knowledge. (**b**) Approximate topographic distribution of memory networks, using the same color code as in (**a**). RF: Rolandic fissure. Red dashed lines demarcate the three frontal areas probed in the experiment by Koechlin et al. (*From* Fuster et al. [6]; *with permission*)

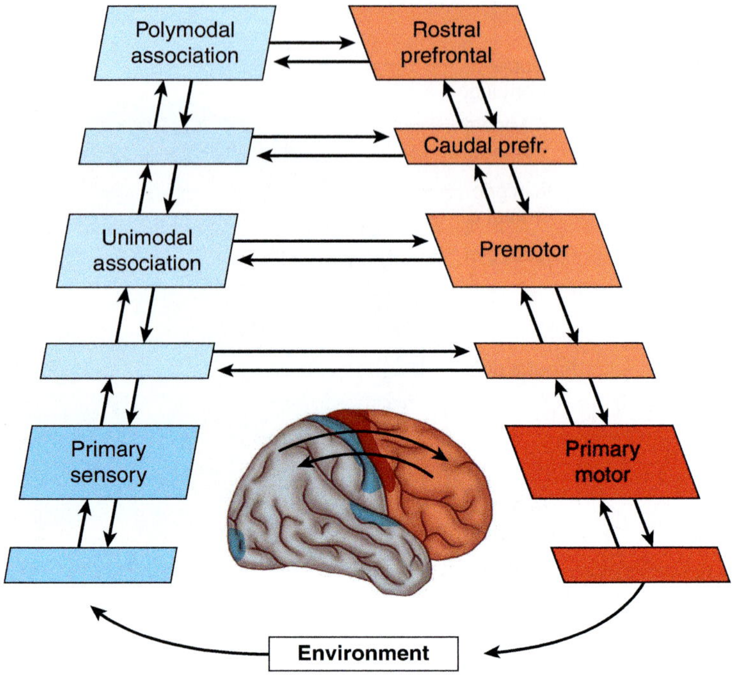

Fig. 4.29 The cortical substrate of the perception–action cycle. Blue represents the perception side of the cycle and red the action side. Unlabeled rectangles represent intermediate areas or subareas of the labeled cortex. *Prefr.* prefrontal). Arrows represent pathways anatomically identified in the monkey. The inset with the human brain highlights the reciprocal connectivity between the posterior and frontal cortices. (*From* Fuster et al. [6]; *with permission*)

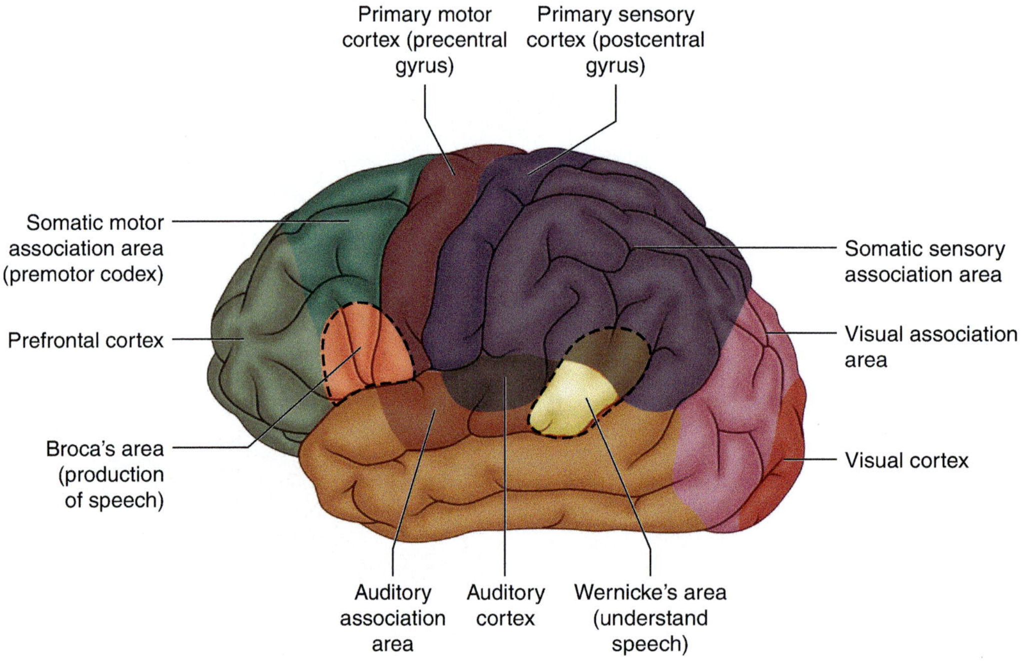

Fig. 4.30 The major motor and sensory region within the human brain

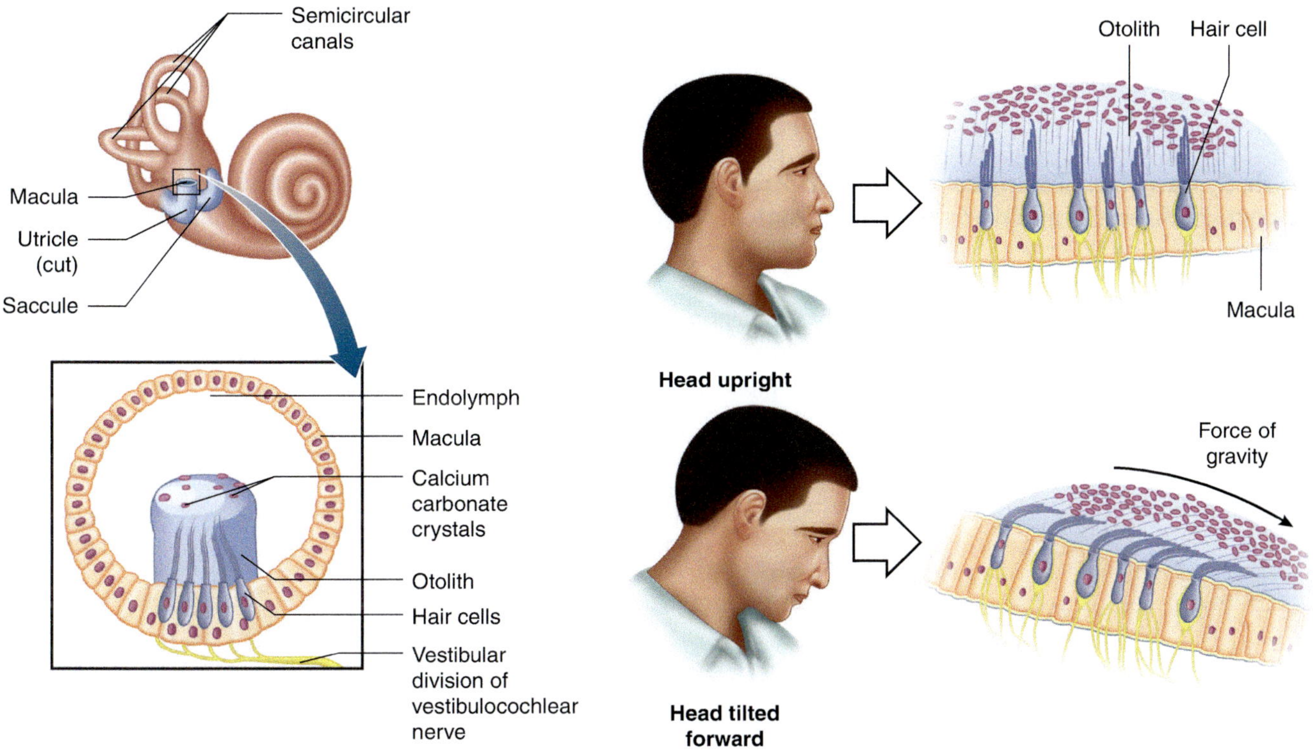

Fig. 4.31 The vestibular system consists of a group of structures within the inner ear that are essential for maintaining equilibrium, balance, normal movement, and spatial orientation. The three semicircular canals detect rotational head movements (i.e. angular acceleration), whereas the utricle and saccule inform the brain of changes in head position with respect to gravity (i.e. linear acceleration). When the head moves in a particular direction, the hair cells within these structures get displaced, and they respond by transmitting information about such movement to the brain

Fig. 4.32 The different nuclei within the thalamus and their associated projection areas to other cortical regions are displayed. *A1* primary auditory cortex, *S1* primary somatosensory cortex, *VA* ventral anterior nucleus, *VL* ventral lateral nucleus, *DL* dorsal lateral nucleus, *LP* lateral posterior nucleus, *VLP* ventral posterolateral nucleus, *VPM* ventral posteromedial nucleus.(*From* Granger & Hearn [7].; *with permission*)

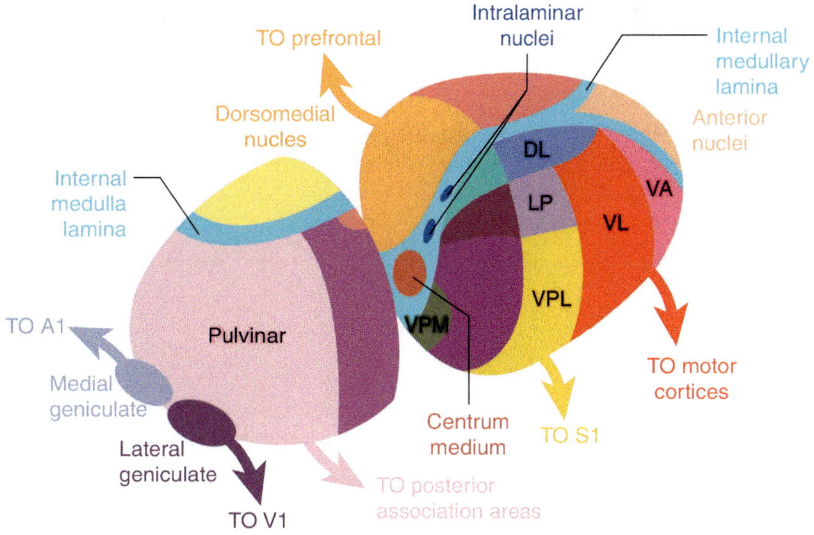

Taste and Smell

The mechanics of taste and smell are displayed in Figs. 4.33 and 4.34.

Limbic System, Basal Ganglia, and Additional Subcortical Area Connections to Other Cortical Regions

A number of key connections exist within the basal ganglia. Recently, researchers have discovered that original models of basal ganglia circuitry did not account for the complexity of the circuitry within the basal ganglia, as evidenced by more current anatomical investigations that have expanded upon previous models (see Fig. 4.35). This new research suggests that it is difficult to predict the transformations applied to inputs to generate outputs [8].

Likewise, there are an extensive number of connections and feedback loops between the basal ganglia and other cortical regions, as discussed in previous sections and demonstrated in Figs. 4.36 and 4.37 [8, 9]. The details of all circuits and connections remain beyond the primary focus of this introductory chapter but are provided for the readers' reference.

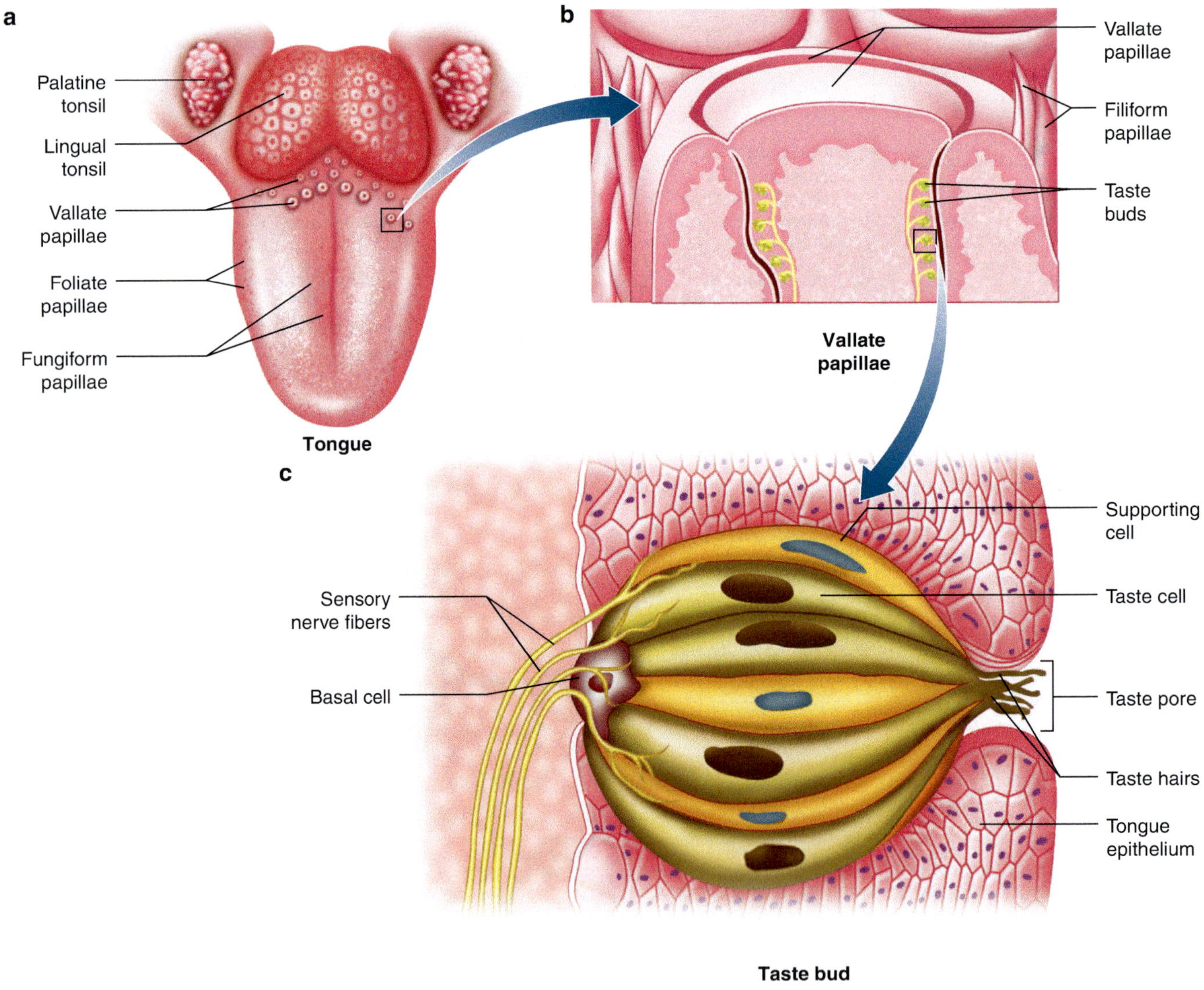

Fig. 4.33 Respective components of the human tongue. Human sense of taste arises from the interaction of taste buds (**b** and **c**) with dissolved food molecules. Taste buds are taste organs located within small bumps on the tongue called papillae. There are three different types of papillae, each associated with a different area of the tongue (**a**). When activated by dissolved molecules, taste cells within the taste buds transmit electrical impulses to the brainstem. This sensory information then travels to the thalamus, where it is integrated and relayed to higher regions of the brain for interpretation. The five taste perceptions are: sweet, sour, salty, bitter, and savory (umami)

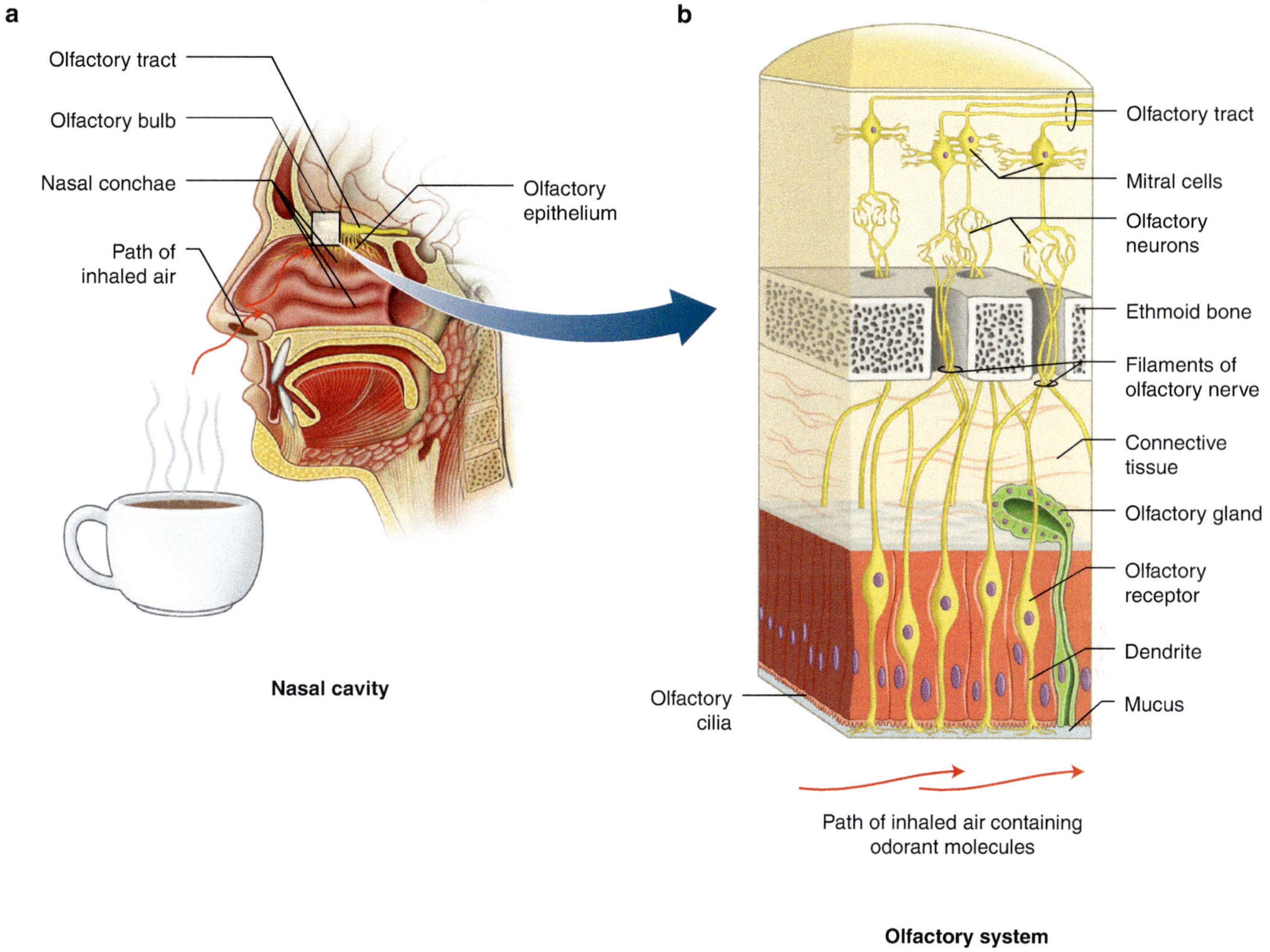

Fig. 4.34 Mechanics of olfactory processing. The olfactory receptors, olfactory bulb, and olfactory tract are structures that interact to produce the sense of smell. The olfactory pathway begins when odorant molecules enter the nasal cavity and bind to receptors embedded in the olfactory epithelium. Once activated, these receptors transmit electrical impulses along the olfactory nerve fibers toward the olfactory bulb in the brain, where the nerves synapse with mitral cells. The signals are then relayed through the olfactory tract via mitral cell axons "until such signals" reach the olfactory cortex for processing

Major White Matter Tracts

A number of key white matter tracts exist within the brain (see Fig. 4.38) [10].

With respect to the connections between the basal ganglia and other cortical regions, one of the initial models for movement proposed five basal ganglia-thalamocortical circuits: motor, oculomotor, dorsolateral prefrontal, lateral orbitofrontal, and anterior cingulate. The model proposed that these circuits engage specific regions of the human cortex, striatum, pallidum, substantia nigra, and thalamus [11]. A review of these complex circuits remains beyond the focus of this section, but the reader is strongly encouraged to review the pioneering work of Alexander, DeLong, and Strick (1986) [11].

Visual System

The visual system, like its sensory, motor, and auditory counterparts, is rather complex. A number of cortical regions are involved in the processing of visual stimuli. The subsections that follow provide a brief review of different aspects of visual processing.

Visual Pathway

The visual processing originates from incoming visual stimuli beginning at the optic nerve. These stimuli then travel through the optic chiasm and optic radiations to the visual cortex located within the occipital lobes. Any lesion to any part of the visual pathway can result in a number of visual field deficits (see Fig. 4.39).

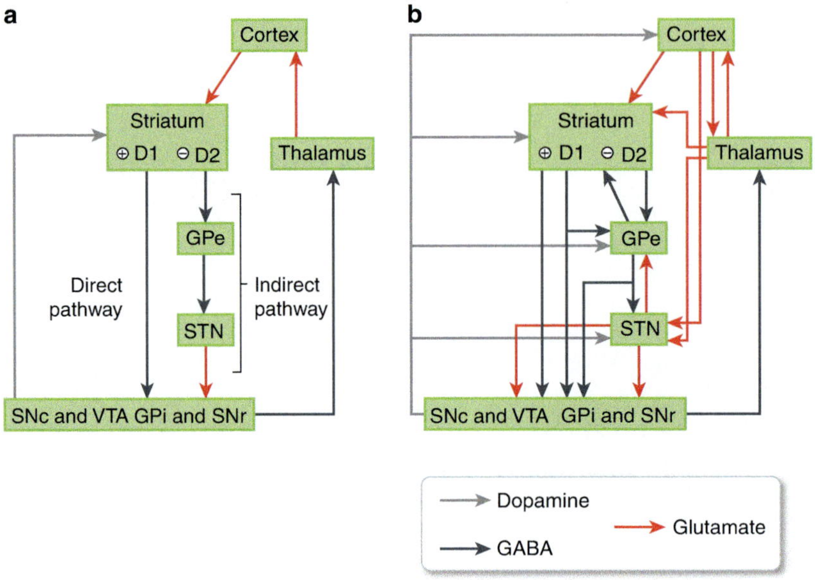

Fig. 4.35 Organization of intrinsic connections within the basal ganglia. (**a**) Model based on the influential proposal by Albin and colleagues, according to which the output of the basal ganglia is determined by the balance between the direct pathway—which involves direct striatonigral inhibitory connections that promote behavior—and the indirect pathway—which involves relays in the external globus pallidus (GPe) and subthalamic nucleus (STN), and suppresses behavior. The balance between these two projections was thought to be regulated by afferent dopaminergic signals from the substantia nigra pars compacta (SNc) and the ventral tegmental area (VTA) acting on differentially distributed D1 and D2 dopamine receptors. (**b**) Recent anatomical investigations have revealed a rather more complex organization in which the transformations that are applied to the inputs to generate outputs are less easy to predict. *GPe* globus pallidus pars externa, *GPi* globus pallidus pars interna, *SNr* substantia nigra pars reticulata. (*From* Redgrave et al. [8]; *with permission*)

Retinotopic Organization

The occipital lobes process information via retinotopic organization (see Fig. 4.40).

What Versus Where Visual Pathway

Once visual sensory information (i.e., color, motion) is processed in the occipital regions, other cortical areas make sense of what or where the information represents. This is known as the what-where pathway (see Fig. 4.41) [12]. Generally speaking, object recognition occurs in the temporal regions via the ventral pathway, while spatial processing happens in the parietal regions via the dorsal pathway, yet this is achieved by feedback loops of all cortical regions communicating with one another.

The ventral stream contains the fusiform gyrus, the primary cortical region involved in object recognition. This object identification is based on information received from the occipital regions (see Fig. 4.42).

Visuospatial Processing and Visual Neglect

Because of the complexity of object recognition (see Fig. 4.43), lesions to any part of the brain can result in visual deficits and a wide collection of syndromes (i.e., visual neglect and visual agnosia) [13].

Visual neglect can occur as a result of a neurodevelopmental or acquired injury. The neuroanatomical correlates of unilateral visuospatial neglect are displayed below (see Fig. 4.44).

Auditory Processing, Hearing, and Language

The reader is encouraged to review Fig. 4.30 again for a visual map of the locations of the primary auditory cortex (where auditory stimuli are initially processed), Broca's area (primary neuroanatomical region involved in speech production), and Wernicke's area (primary neuroanatomical region involved in auditory comprehension).

Auditory Processing Pathway

In brief, sound stimuli are first processed in the cochlea of the ear canal, and the signal is transmitted down the auditory nerve to the ventral and dorsal cochlear nuclei in the hindbrain. From there, information flows to the olivary complex, then to the trapezoid body, then to the inferior colliculus in the midbrain, then to the medial geniculate nucleus in the thalamus, and finally to the auditory cortex. Neurons in the primary auditory cortex process tonotopic organization from sound hertz and amplitude; this process is somewhat similar to the function and retinotopic organization within the primary visual cortex in the occipital regions. A "what" and "where" pathway also exists for auditory processing.

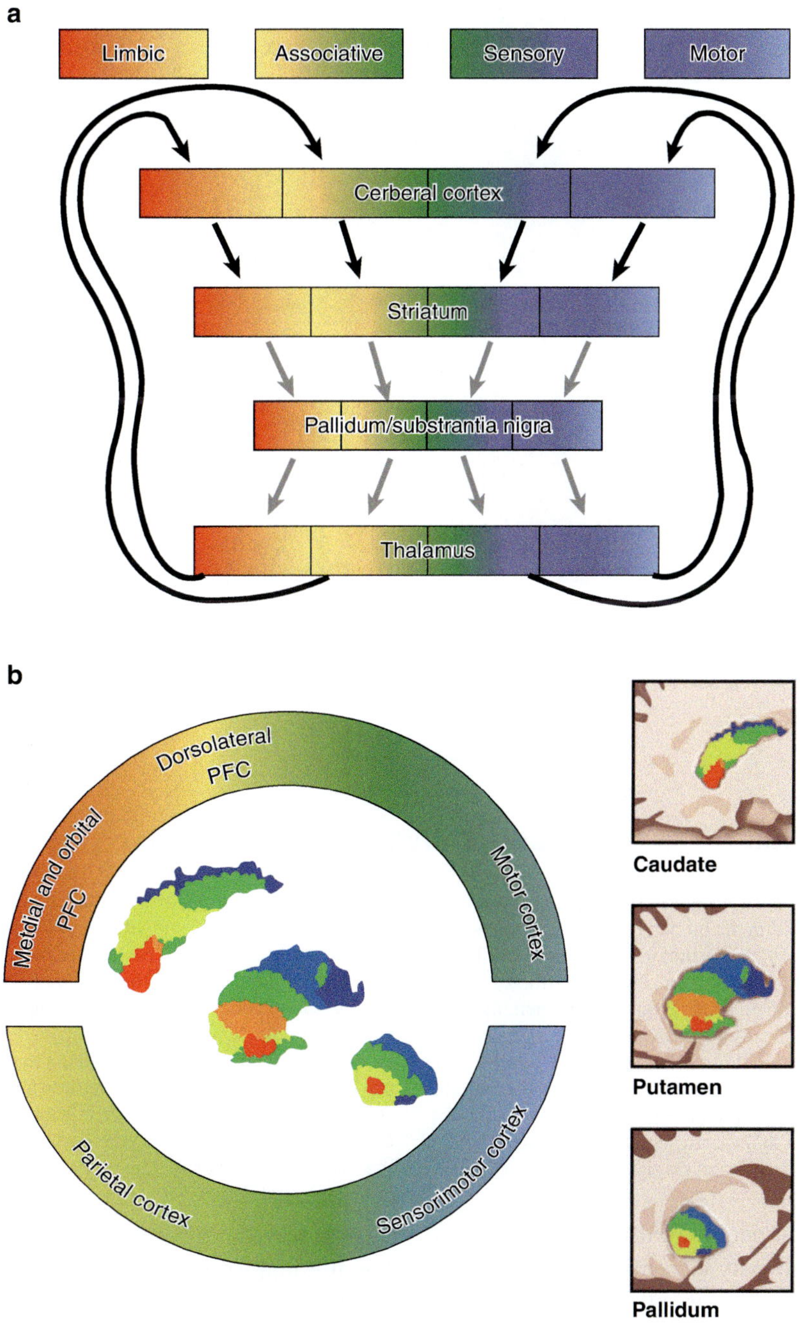

Fig. 4.36 Corticobasal ganglia–cortical loops in animals and humans. (**a**) The connections between the cerebral cortex and the basal ganglia can be viewed as a series of parallel-projecting, largely segregated loops or channels conveying limbic (shown in red), associative (shown in yellow-green), and sensorimotor (shown in blue-white) information. Functional territories represented at the level of the cerebral cortex are maintained throughout the basal ganglia nuclei and thalamic relays. Note, however, that for each loop the relay points in the cortex, basal ganglia, and thalamus offer opportunities for activity inside the loop to be modified or modulated by signals from outside the loop. Black arrows indicate glutamatergic projections; grey arrows indicate GABA (γ-aminobutyric acid)-ergic projections. (**b**) The spatially segregated 'rostral caudal gradient' of human frontal cortical connectivity in caudate, putamen, and pallidum. The color-coded ring denotes limbic (shown in red), associative (shown in yellow-green), and sensorimotor regions of the cerebral cortex in the sagittal plane (color coding after Haber). Using probabilistic tractography on magnetic resonance-diffusion weighted imaging data, Draganski et al. identified the regions of the striatum that receive the strongest input from the identified cortical regions (sagittal-oriented images contained within the ring). For better visualization, segmented basal ganglia nuclei are superimposed on T1-weighted structural images on the far right of the diagram (the rostral part is shown on the left and the caudal part is shown on the right). *PFC* prefrontal cortex. (*From* Redgrave et al. [8]; *with permission)*

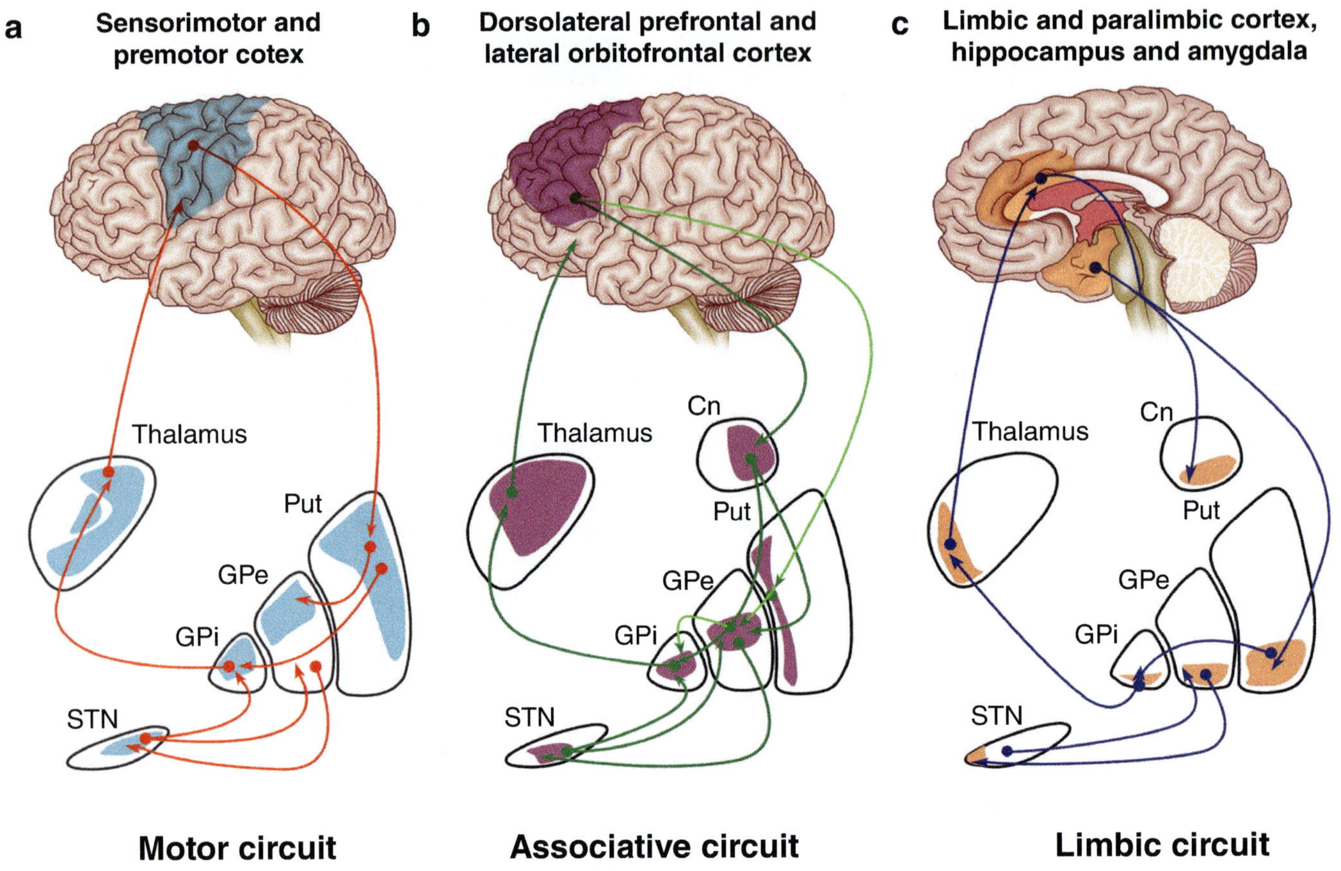

Fig. 4.37 Schematic diagram illustrating the main cortico-basal ganglia–thalamocortical circuits within the human brain. This figure shows a pseudo-anatomical arrangement of the motor, associative, and limbic pathways. (**a**) Motor circuit. Neurons from the sensorimotor cortex project to the posterolateral putamen (Put). From the putamen, there are two main projections topographically organized onto the posterolateral region of the target nuclei: (i) the direct circuit to the GPi and (ii) the indirect circuit connecting the posterior putamen to the globus pallidus pars externa (GPe), the STN, and the GPi. The GPi is the primary output nucleus of the basal ganglia to the cortex via the ventrolateral thalamus. (**b**) Associative circuit. This circuit originates in the dorsolateral prefrontal and lateral orbitofrontal cortices, which project to the caudate nucleus (Cn) and the anteromedial portion of the putamen. From the striatum (Cn + Put), it projects to the dorsomedial region of the GPi and anteromedial parts of the GPe and STN to converge onto the GPi and back to the cortex via the ventral anterior nuclei of the thalamus. (**c**) Limbic circuit. This loop starts in the hippocampus, amygdala, and paralimbic and limbic cortices and projects to the ventral striatum (ventral portion of the caudate and putamen, including NAcc). The ventral striatum projects to the limbic portion of the GPe and medioventral STN and ventral GPi and to the cortex via the mediodorsal nucleus of the thalamus. (*From* Krack et al. [9]; *with permission*)

Neurons work in unison to orient towards loudness and location. To convey the complexity of auditory processing, a model of musical processing is provided below (see Fig. 4.45).

Cortical Language Regions and Language Processing

The topic of the functional neuroanatomy of language processing deserves to be a whole volume in its own right. Hickok (2009) is an exceptional review of the functional neuroanatomy of language [15]. However, for the readers' reference, a schematic of the functional anatomy of language processing is provided below (see Fig. 4.46).

Likewise, two famous models of phonological short-term memory processing are included below (see Fig. 4.47) [15].

Language Reorganization

For the majority of individuals, expressive and receptive language processing is lateralized to the dominant (left) hemisphere, though there are several exceptions, such as a greater propensity for bilateral language representation among multilingual individuals. That said, strong justification exists regarding studied functional language reorganization in the human brain. This process can occur in individuals who have some sort of acquired injury very early in life, like hypoxic/anoxic injury, craniotomy, surgical resection in the context of brain tumors, or epilepsy. During this process, functional cortical reorganization of language can occur and "shift" to the contralateral side of injury if the process occurs early enough in an individual's life. As a rule, there is a gradient associated with recovery

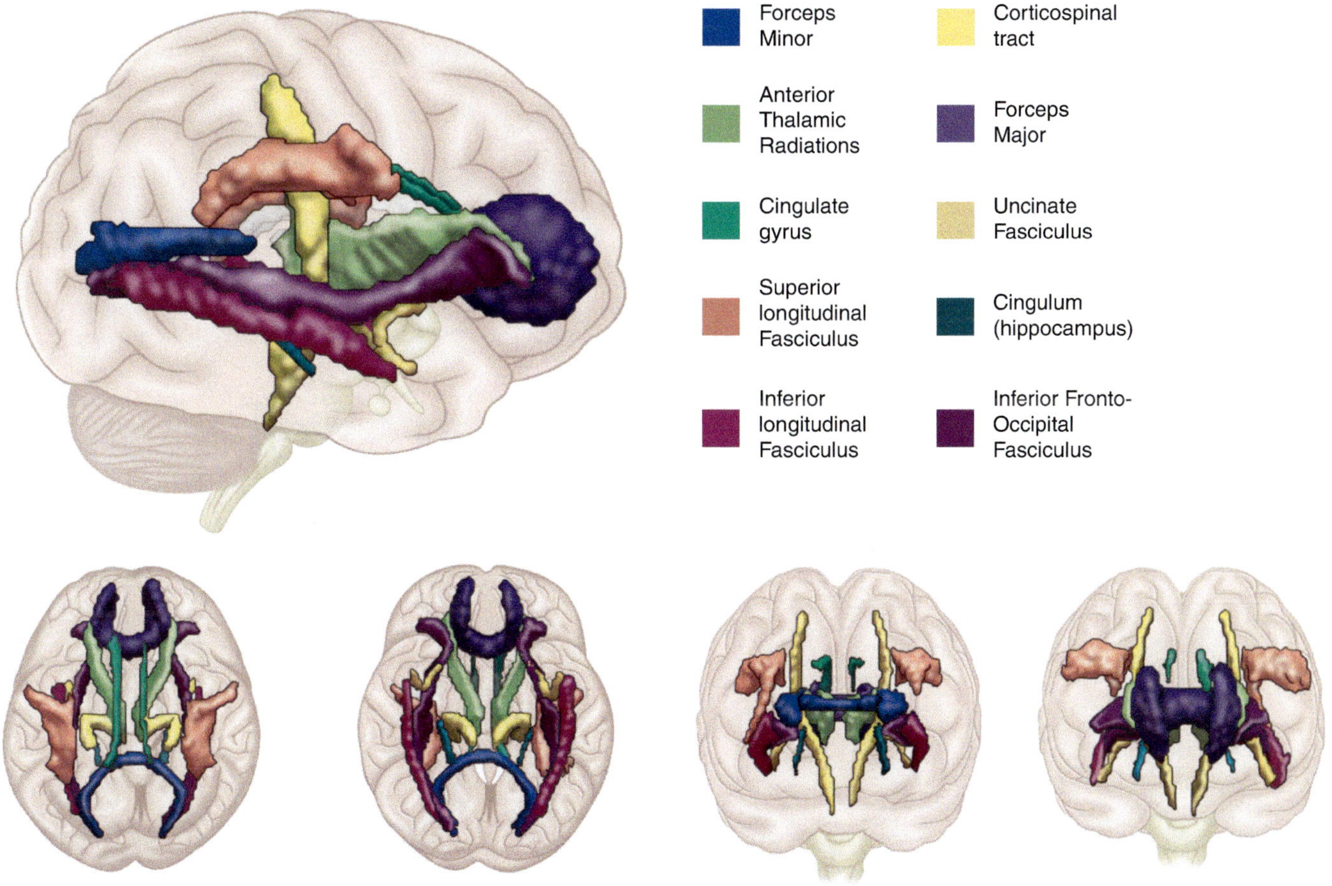

Fig. 4.38 Ten of the major white matter tracts within the human brain are displayed

of language abilities following any CNS injury, such that the younger an individual's age at the time of injury, the greater the likelihood of language reorganization/recovery because of greater plasticity. With that said, while patients can experience profound language impairment in the acute recovery phase following CNS insult, many can make real-world functional gains in language processing throughout the course of recovery (particularly with speech-language therapy intervention and implementation of compensatory strategies).

Memory Processing

Memory processing is arguably one of the broadest and most complex systems within the brain and represents a complexly orchestrated process of diverse cortical and subcortical regions within the brain. It is greatly attenuated by other cortical regions responsible for additional neurocognitive abilities, like frontal "executive" abilities, processing speed, language processing, and visual processing.

Types of Memory

Long-term memory can be characterized as declarative memory or non-declarative memory. For a comprehensive and thorough review of memory processing systems, the reader is encouraged to read the work of Henke (2010) [16]. The neuroanatomical correlates of the subdivisions of declarative versus non-declarative memory are displayed below (see Fig. 4.48).

The Hippocampal Formation and Projections to Other Cortical and Subcortical Regions

Furthermore, one of the more 'famous' cortical structures within the human brain is the hippocampus, the area of the brain responsible for the consolidation and storage of information. The hippocampus circuitry has a number of connections *within* its structural zones and *between* other neocortical regions (see Fig. 4.49) [16].

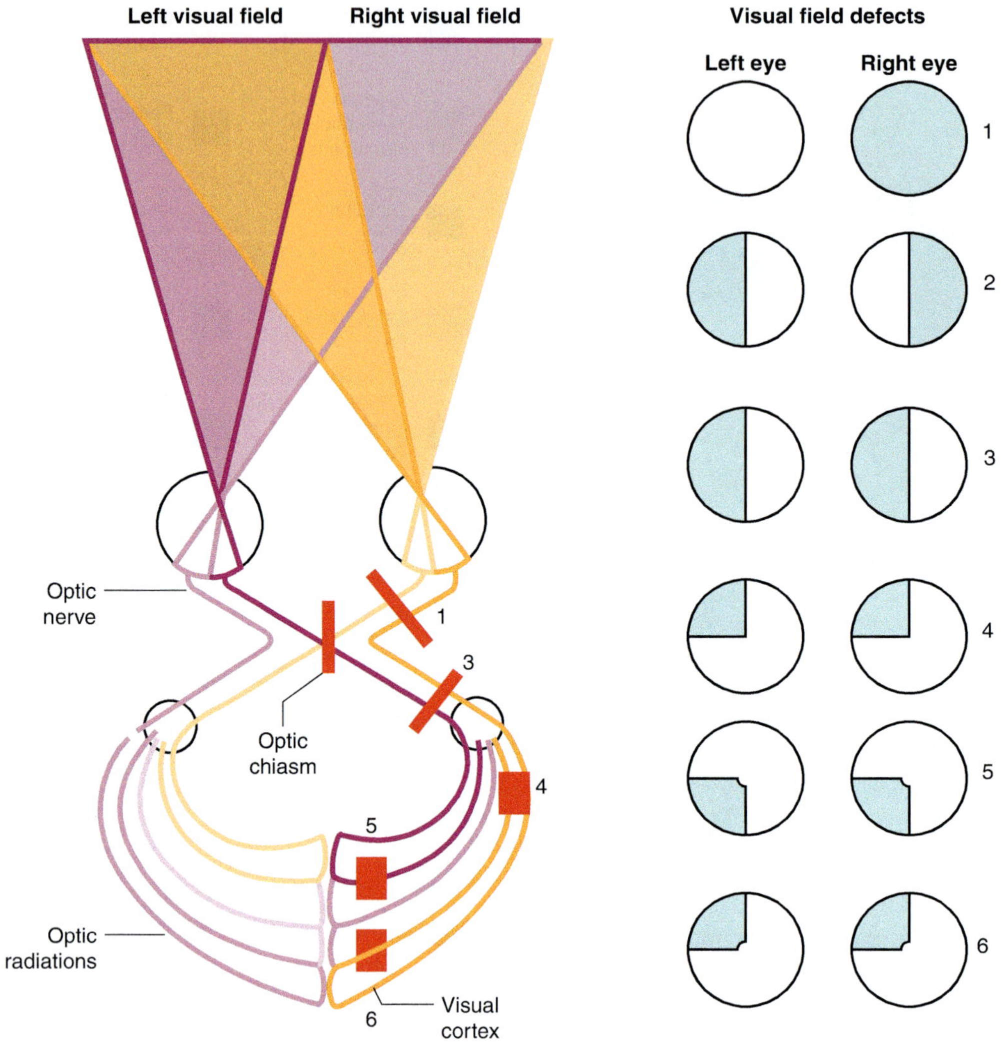

Fig. 4.39 The visual pathway is displayed with associated lesions and consequential visual field deficits

A Processing-Based Model of Memory Systems

A number of theoretical models of memory processing exist. A review of such models extends beyond the boundaries of this chapter. However, one proposed model is included below, which conceptualizes the processing-based divisions within memory systems (see Fig. 4.50) [16].

Long-Term Potentiation

One of the greatest findings in the field of neuroscience is the work of Bliss and Lomo (1973), who discovered that high-frequency stimulation of hippocampal neurons could result in persistent increases in synaptic strength, a process termed long-term potentiation (LTP) [17]. We now know that this process is modulated by the *N*-methyl-D-aspartate receptor (NMDA), which is one of the three ionotropic glutamate receptors. Of particular clinical relevance, researchers have begun investigating the clinical utility of NMDA antagonists. Specifically, as NMDA plays a role in LTP, the administration of NMDA antagonists may provide therapeutic benefits for a wide range of psychiatric disorders. In particular, NMDA receptor antagonists may optimize behavioral sensitization for individuals afflicted with PTSD.

Spatial and Emotional Memory Processing

The scientific community is currently investigating the neuroanatomical correlates of specific types of memory. We know that the hippocampus plays a crucial role in the formation and storage of memory, yet more recent research efforts have initiated the investigation of what subregions within the hippocampus are responsible for different modes of information. For example, with respect to encoding and retrieval of spatial information, one study demonstrated that increased activity (using an *f*MRI paradigm) was observed during the encoding of spatial information in the right CA2, CA3, and dentate gyrus (CA23DG) regions, whereas activity in the right subicular region was greater during retrieval of spatial

Fig. 4.40 A schematic of retinotopic organization

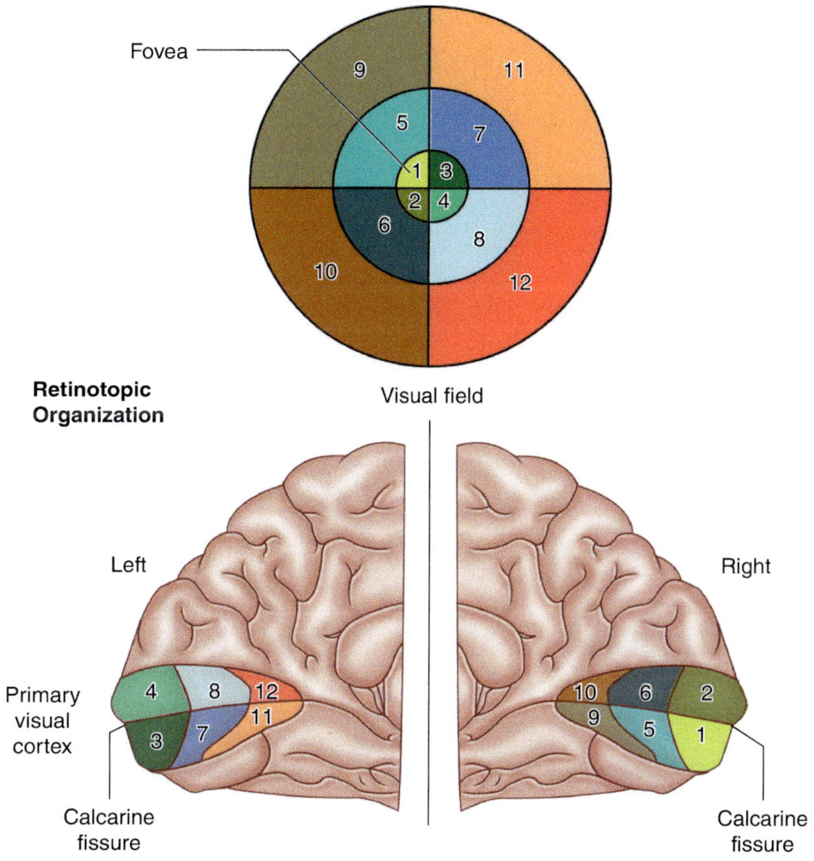

Fig. 4.41 Neural pathways are involved in visuospatial processing. The dorsal stream, which includes the parietal cortex and its projections to the frontal cortex, is involved in the processing of spatial information. The ventral stream, which includes the inferior and lateral temporal cortex and their projections to the medial temporal cortex, is involved in the processing of categorical or semantic information. The parieto-medial temporal (PMT) integrates information from both pathways and is involved in the encoding of landmarks in spatial navigation and in the integration of objects into contextual frames. (*From* Martins et al. [12]; *with permission*)

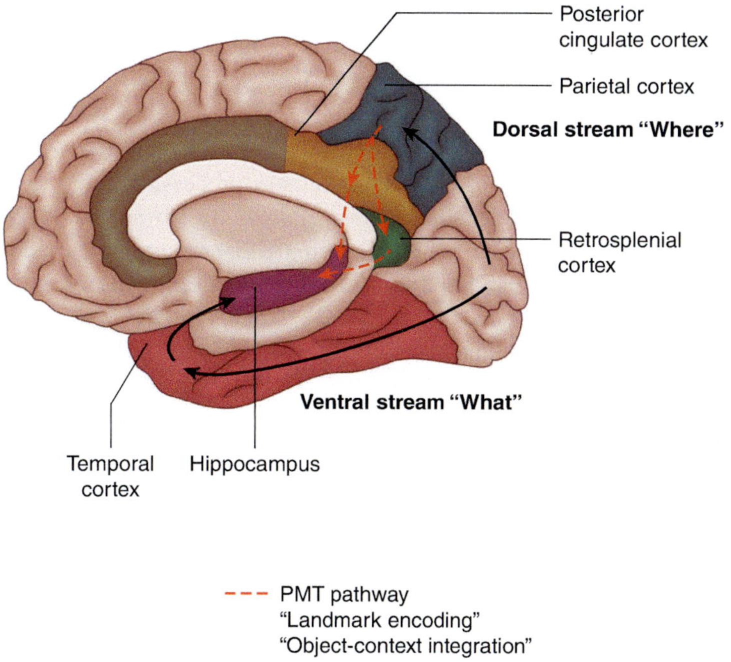

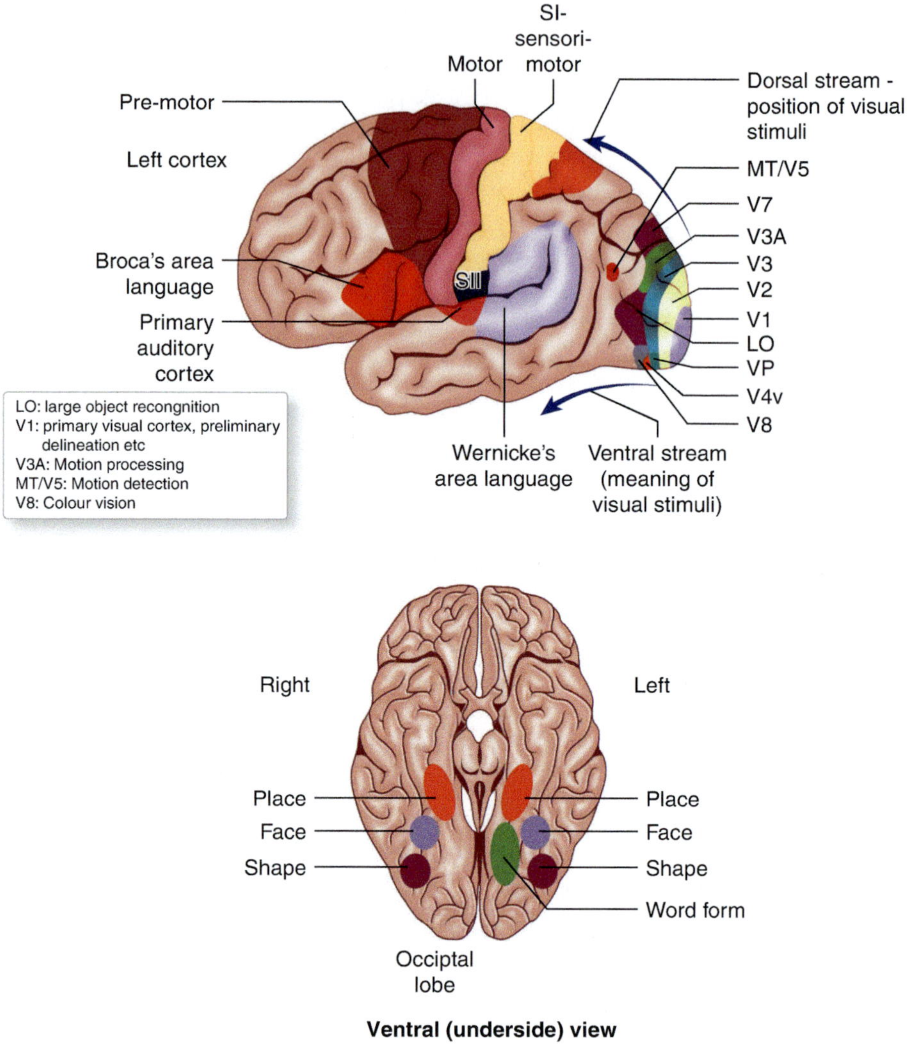

Fig. 4.42 **Top**: various cortical regions and their respective functions for visual processing. **Bottom**: the fusiform gyrus and select subregions that process different aspects of incoming visual stimuli to derive the meaning of such stimuli

information [18]. Other efforts have focused on identifying the neural substrates of emotional memory processing and refining existing models in this area of study. In particular, the amygdala has received an increasingly disproportionate yet scientifically sound and logically warranted amount of investigation for its role in emotional memory processing relative to other anatomical structures (see Fig. 4.51) [19].

Behavior, Emotional Processing, and Social Cognition

Neuroanatomical correlates of select behavioral features are often difficult to clarify, as human behavior is a complex phenomenon comprised of broad criteria. Other chapters in the current volume will review the neuroanatomical correlates of distinct neurological and psychiatric disorders in greater detail. However, social cognition as a broad construct has received increasing research interest within the past two to three decades. Figures 4.52 and 4.53, courtesy of Van Overwalle (2009), provide a map of distinct brain regions and their associated roles in the functions of a number of behavioral characteristics, emotional abilities, and constructs within the category of social cognition [20].

Functional Neuroimaging

The reader is encouraged to reference Chap. 8 of the current textbook, which provides greater detail pertaining to the different functional neuroimaging techniques employed in research in clinical settings, as well as their applicable use among different etiologies that result in neurocognitive disorders (detailed in Chap. 13). Nonetheless, broadly speaking, functional MRI (*f*MRI), which measures brain activity via cerebral blood flow and neuronal activity, is commonly

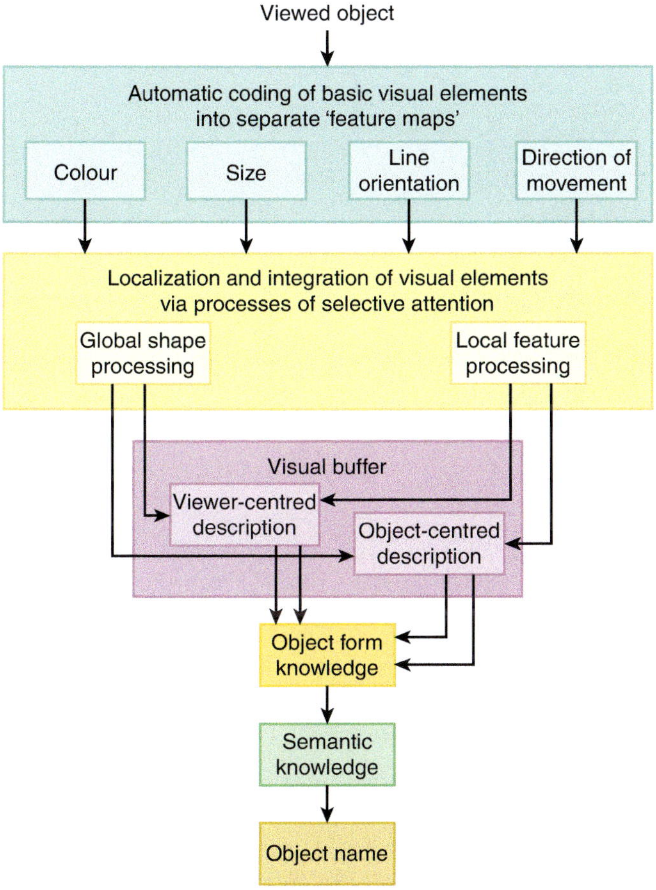

Fig. 4.43 A schematic information-processing model of object recognition. (*From* Halligan et al. [13]; *with permission*)

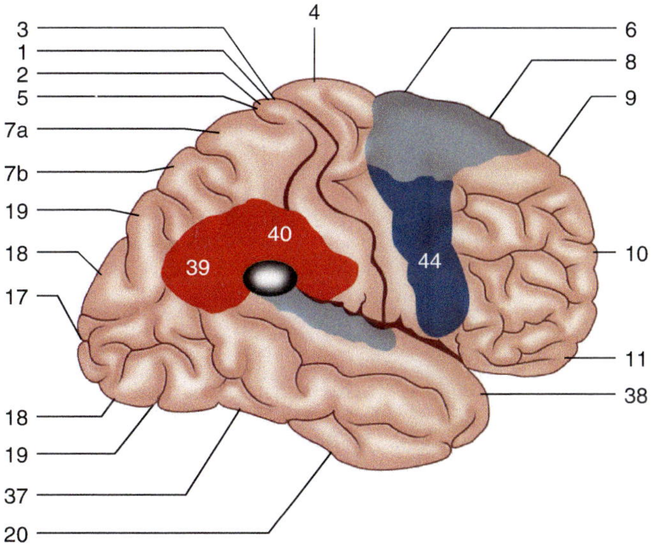

Fig. 4.44 Cortical anatomical correlates of unilateral visuospatial neglect. Most anatomo-clinical correlation studies show that the lesion responsible involves the right inferior parietal lobule (Brodmann areas, BA 39 and 40, highlighted in red), particularly the supramarginal gyrus, at the temporo-parietal junction (black-grey area). Neglect after right frontal damage is less frequent and usually associated with lesions to the frontal premotor cortex, particularly to the more ventral parts (BA 44 and ventral BA 6, dark blue area). Neglect can also be associated with damage to the more dorsal and medial regions of the frontal premotor cortex and to the superior temporal gyrus (lighter blue areas). (*From* Halligan et al. [13]; *with permission*)

used to detect the localization of language, memory, and motor functions in presurgical candidates among patients living with epilepsy or brain tumors. Another functional neuroimaging technique, positron emission tomography (PET) scanning, relies on a radioactive tracer to measure and visualize metabolic or other physiological changes that occur in the brain, including blood flow, chemical or protein composition, and uptake/absorption. There are numerous radioactive tracers that have been validated for medical use, including fluorodeoxyglucose (FDG), which is commonly used in the detection and diagnostic work-up of neurodegenerative conditions or malignant tumors. Single-photon emission computed tomography (SPECT) is another technique of note. More specialized scans, like the DaTscan and Flourodopa F18 F-Dopa scan, are forms of SPECT and PET imaging techniques, respectively, that measure dopamine transporter levels/uptake in various brain regions (see Fig. 4.54) [21].

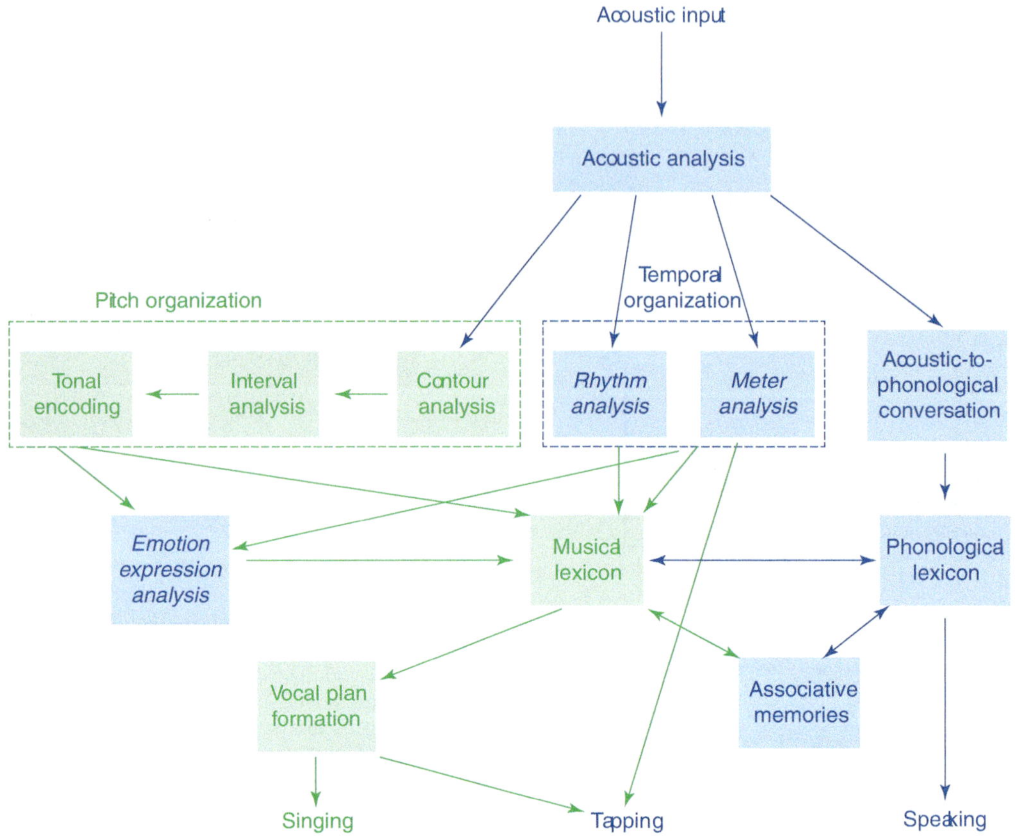

Fig. 4.45 A modular model of music processing. Each box represents a processing component, and arrows represent pathways of information flow or communication between processing components. A neurological anomaly may either damage a processing component (box) or interfere with the flow of information between two boxes. All components whose domains appear to be specific to music are in green; others are in blue. There are three neutrally individuated components in italics—rhythm analysis, meter analysis, and emotion expression analysis—whose specificity to music is currently unknown. They are represented here in blue, but future work may provide evidence for representing them in green. (*From* Peretz et al. [14]; *with permission*)

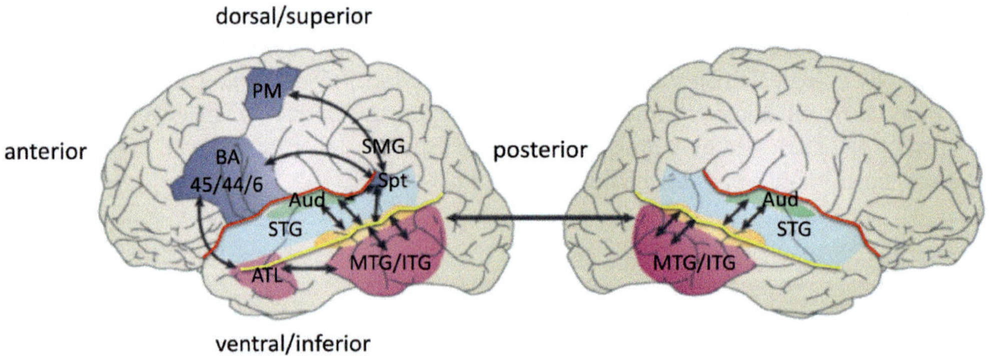

Fig. 4.46 Two broad processing streams are depicted, a ventral stream for speech comprehension that is largely bilaterally organized, and which flows into the temporal lobe, and a dorsal stream for sensory-motor integration that is left dominant and which involves structures at the parietal- temporal junction and frontal lobe. *ATL* anterior temporal lobe, *Aud* auditory cortex (early processing stages), *BA 45/44/6* Brodmann areas 45, 44, and 6, *MTG/ITG* middle temporal gyrus, inferior temporal gyrus, *PM* premotor, dorsal portion, *SMG* supramarginal gyrus, *Spt* Sylvian parietal temporal region (left only), *STG* superior temporal gyrus, *red line* Sylvian fissure, *yellow line* superior temporal sulcus (STS). (*From* Hickok [15]; *with permission*)

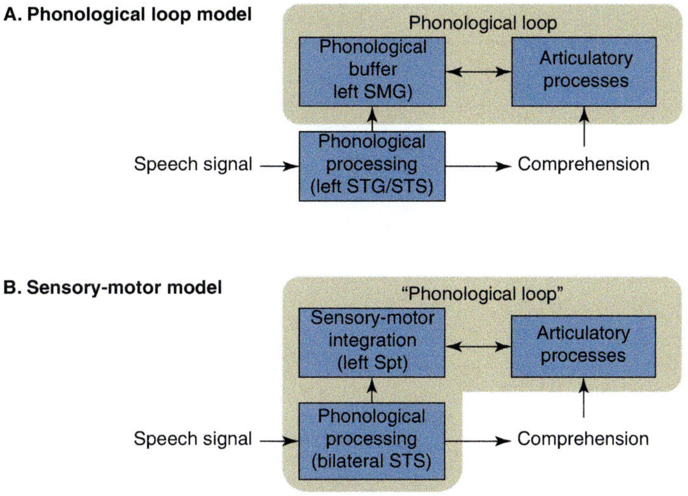

Fig. 4.47 (**a**) Baddeley's phonological loop model (tan box) is embedded in a simplified model of speech recognition. In this model, the phonological buffer (or "phonological store") is a dedicated storage device separate from phonological processing as it is applied in speech recognition. The contents of the buffer are passively stored for 2–3 s but can be refreshed via articulatory rehearsal. (**b**) A reinterpretation of the "phonological loop" within the context of a sensory-motor circuit supporting speech functions. Articulatory processes are the same across both models, but in the sensory-motor model, the phonological "store" is coextensive with phonological processes involved in normal speech recognition, and a sensory-motor translation system is interposed between the "storage"/phonological system and the articulatory system. (*Reprinted from* Hickok [15]; *with permission*)

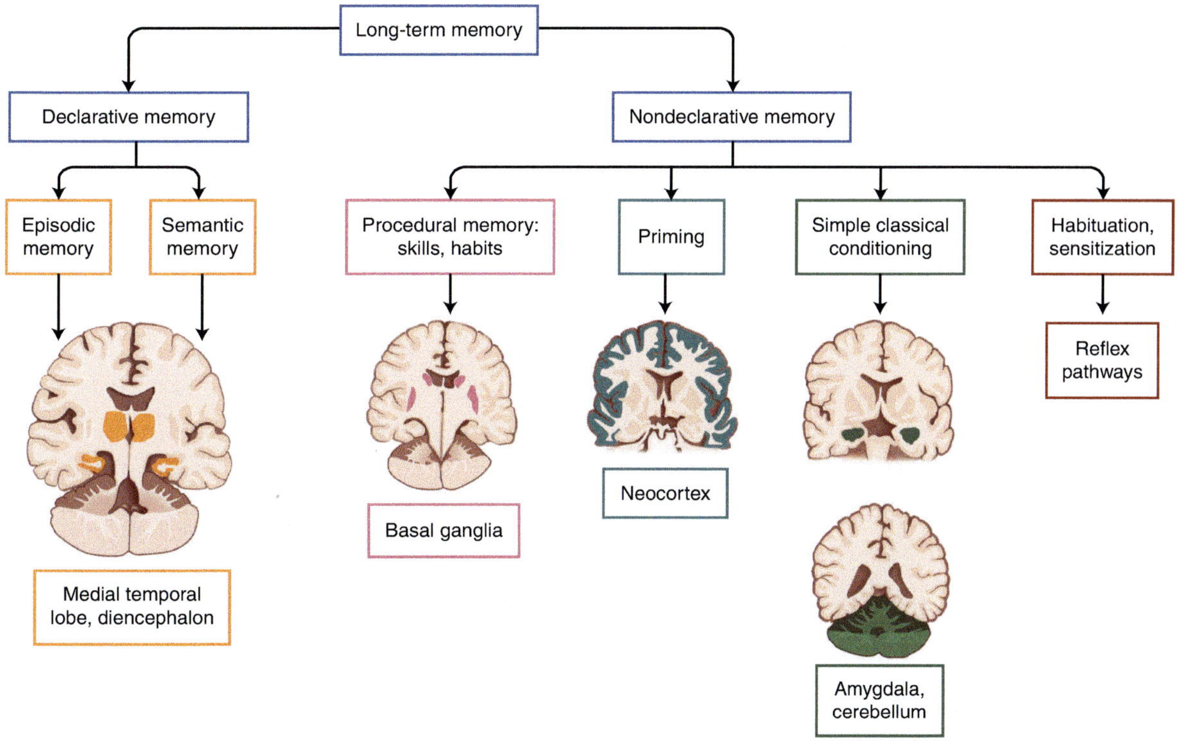

Fig. 4.48 In this model, long-term memory is divided into two broad classes. One class is characterized by the capacity for conscious recollection and is called declarative memory. The other class encompasses diverse unconscious learning and memory abilities and is referred to as nondeclarative memory. Declarative memory consists of two subclasses: episodic memory, which consists of memories of autobiographical events; and semantic memory, which consists of facts and general knowledge. Semantic memories are impersonal and devoid of autobiographical context, whereas episodic memories are personal. These include where and when episodes happened and are accompanied by a feeling of retrieving personally experienced episodes (autonoetic consciousness). In this model, both episodic and semantic memories are dependent on the medial temporal lobe and diencephalon. Nondeclarative memory in this model includes procedural learning of sensorimotor and cognitive skills and habits, priming, simple conditioning, and habituation and sensitization, all of which are expressed in behavioral changes and are independent of the medial temporal lobe. (*From* Henke [16]; *with permission*)

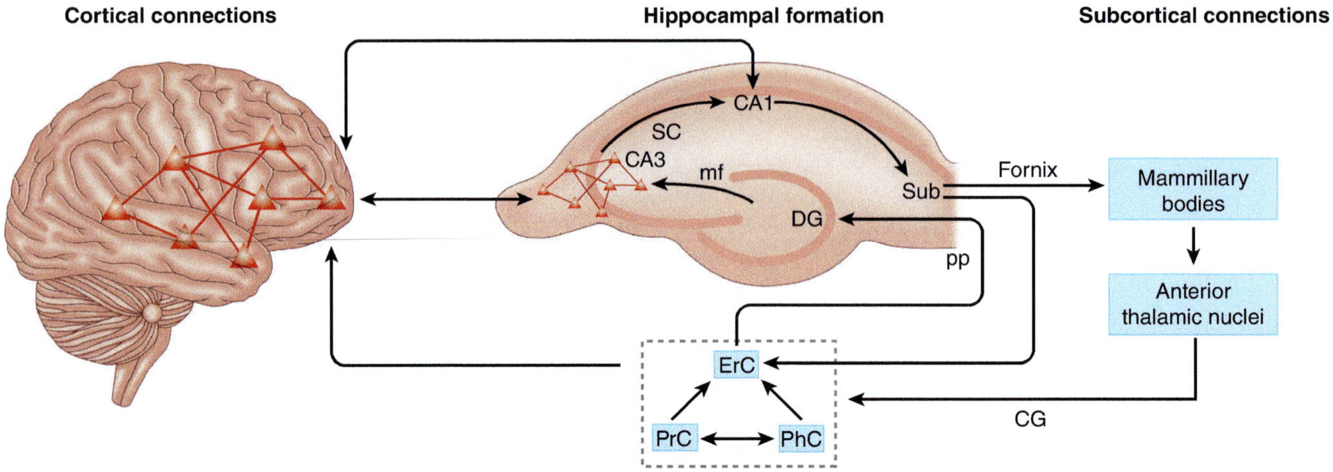

Fig. 4.49 The primate hippocampal formation is reciprocally connected with all neocortical association areas either directly or through the parahippocampal cortex (PhC), perirhinal cortex (PrC), and entorhinal cortex (ErC). Projections from the ErC reach the granule cells of the dentate gyrus (DG) through the perforant path (pp). The DG cells project to the CA3 subfield through the mossy fibers (mf), which provide convergent input to CA3 pyramidal cells (around 50 mf per CA3 cell). The largest number of synapses on CA3 neurons is provided by axon collaterals of other CA3 neurons (forming associational connections) throughout the entire hippocampal formation. The CA3 system, with its many widespread associational fibers, thus allows each CA3 neuron to transmit information rapidly to every other CA3 neuron. This is suggestive of an auto-associative network (represented by the schematic network in CA3 and neocortex) that can recreate the whole event from its parts. CA3 neurons in turn give rise to the major Schaffer collateral (sc) projection to CA1. Unlike CA3 neurons, CA1 neurons do not project significantly to other levels of CA1 but to the subiculum (Sub). From the Sub, the information is funneled back to the ErC, from where it is redistributed to neocortical areas. The information flow through the hippocampal formation is mostly unidirectional. Some hippocampal efferents also travel in the fornix to the mammillary bodies, the anterior thalamic nuclei, the septal nuclei, and through the cingulate gyrus (CG) to the retrosplenial cortex and back to the parahippocampal gyrus. (*From* Henke [16]; *with permission*)

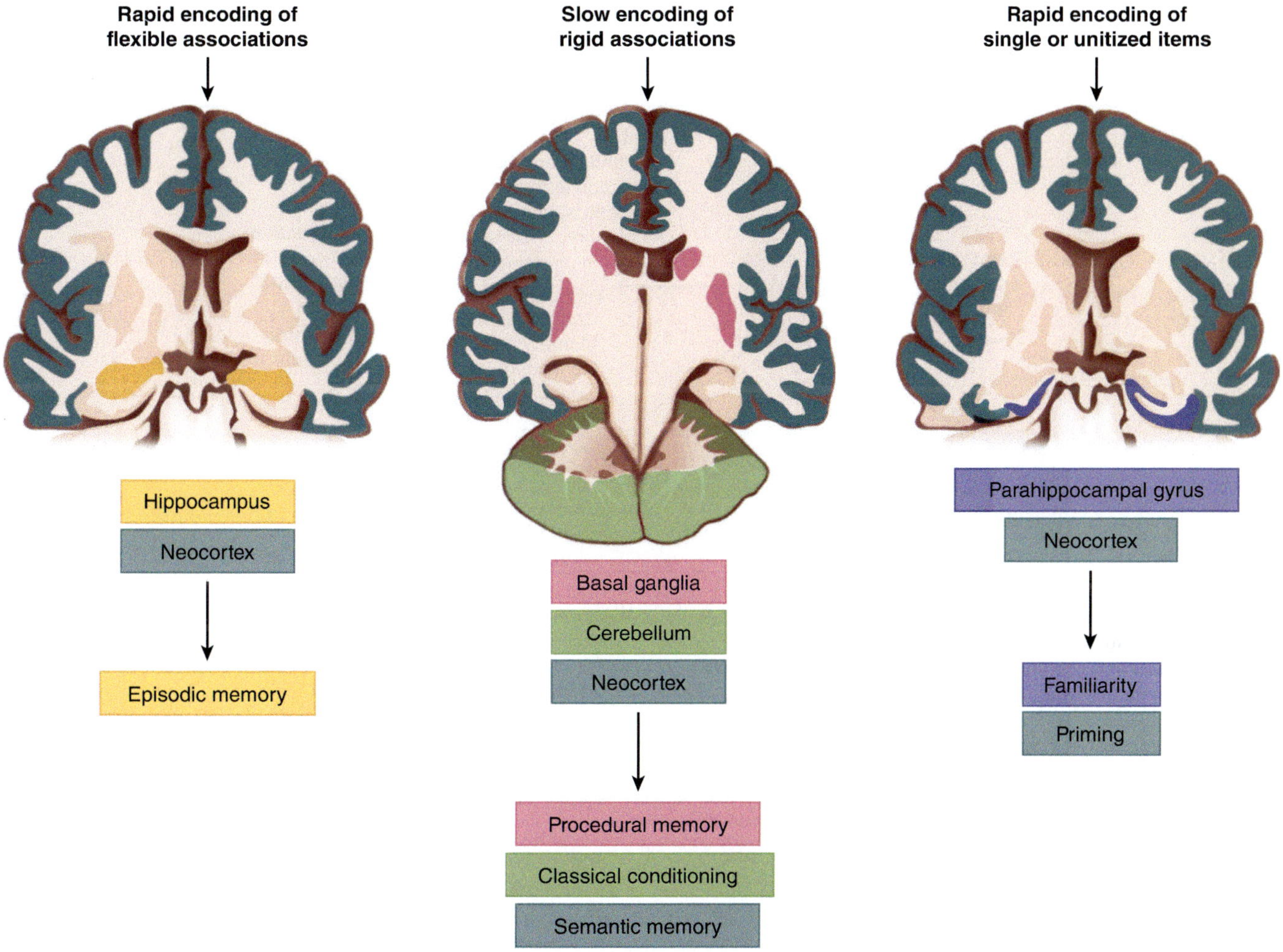

Fig. 4.50 The model distinguishes three basic processing modes that differ with respect to three variables: rapid versus slow encoding, associative versus single item encoding, and flexible and compositional versus rigid and unitized representation. The three processing modes select specialized brain systems, which in turn generate qualitatively distinct memories that can be classified in traditional terms. The consciousness of encoding and retrieval does not select memory systems and hence does not feature in this model. Episodic memory refers to rapidly encoded and flexibly represented associations of any kind and relies on the hippocampus and neocortex. The slow encoding of rigid associations engages the basal ganglia, cerebellum, and neocortex for classical conditioning for the creation of new procedural or semantic memories. The rapid encoding of single or unitized items involves the parahippocampal gyrus and neocortex to afford priming and familiarity. (*From* Henke [16]; *with permission*)

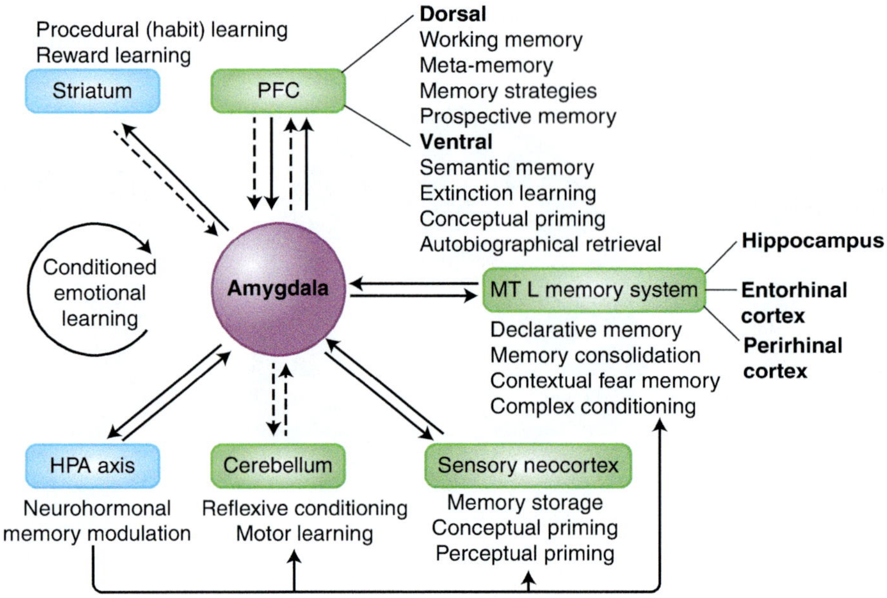

Fig. 4.51 Potential mechanisms by which the amygdala mediates the influence of emotional arousal on memory. In addition to emotional learning that takes place intrinsically in the amygdala, direct and indirect neural projections target several memory systems in the brain, including those that subserve working memory, declarative memory, and various nondeclarative forms of memory (for example, procedural learning, priming, and reflexive conditioning). Complex conditioning refers to various higher-order conditioning procedures that are hippocampal-dependent, including trace conditioning and conditional discrimination learning. The amygdala also triggers the release of stress hormones by way of the hypothalamic–pituitary–adrenal (HPA) axis, which feeds back onto memory consolidation and storage sites as well as the amygdala itself to enhance memory over longer time intervals. Solid arrows indicate direct connections; dashed arrows indicate indirect connections. Blue labels indicate connections with subcortical structures. *MTL* medial temporal lobe, *PFC* prefrontal cortex. (*From* LaBar and Cabeza [19]; *with permission*)

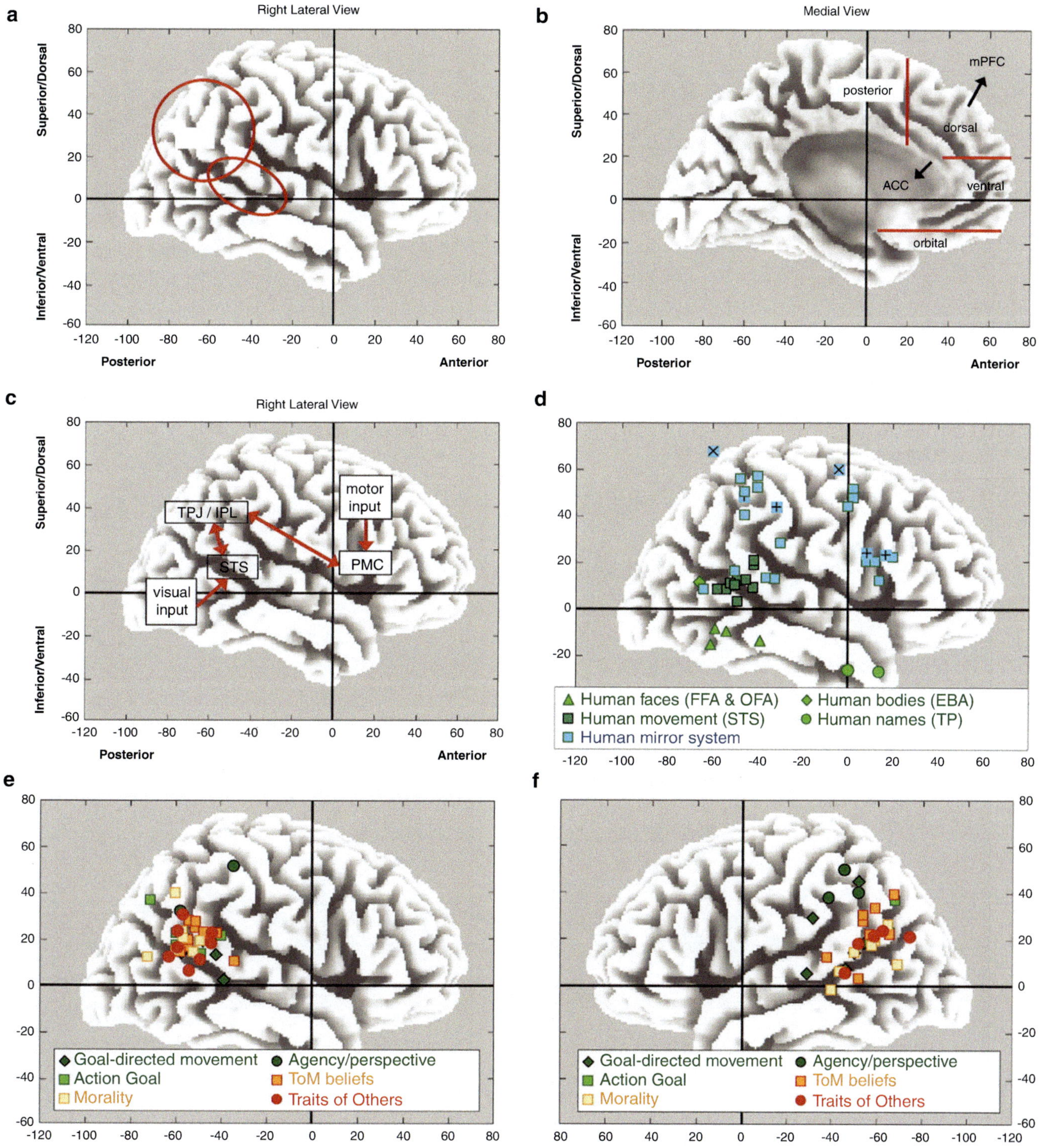

Fig. 4.52 (**a**, **b**) The anatomy of the human brain and the major areas involved in social cognition are placed in *x*-*y*-*z* stereotactic atlas. Left-right (not shown) reflects the anatomical x-axis, posterior-anterior at the bottom reflects the anatomical *y*-axis, and inferior-superior (or ventral-dorsal) on the left reflects the anatomical z-axis. (**c**) The mirror system: Visual input in the STS is propagated to the TPJ/IPL and further to the PMC, where it is compared with its own action schemas and associated goals. The matched goal behind the action detected at the PMC is sent back to the TPJ/IPL (for goal identification) and STS (for agency identification). (**d**) How a human, its body (parts), movements, and name are represented in the brain in the FFA (Fusiform Face Area), OFA (Occipital Face Area), EBA (Extrastriate Body Area), STS (Superior Temporal Sulcus), and the anterior Temporal Pole, and how the mirror system is recruited for observing (posterior areas) and executing (anterior areas) movements of mouth/face [+], hand/arm [□], or foot [×]. (**e**, **f**) The TPJ is involved in social inferences of intentionality and traits; right and left lateral view, respectively. (*Reprinted from* Van Overwalle [20]; *with permission*)

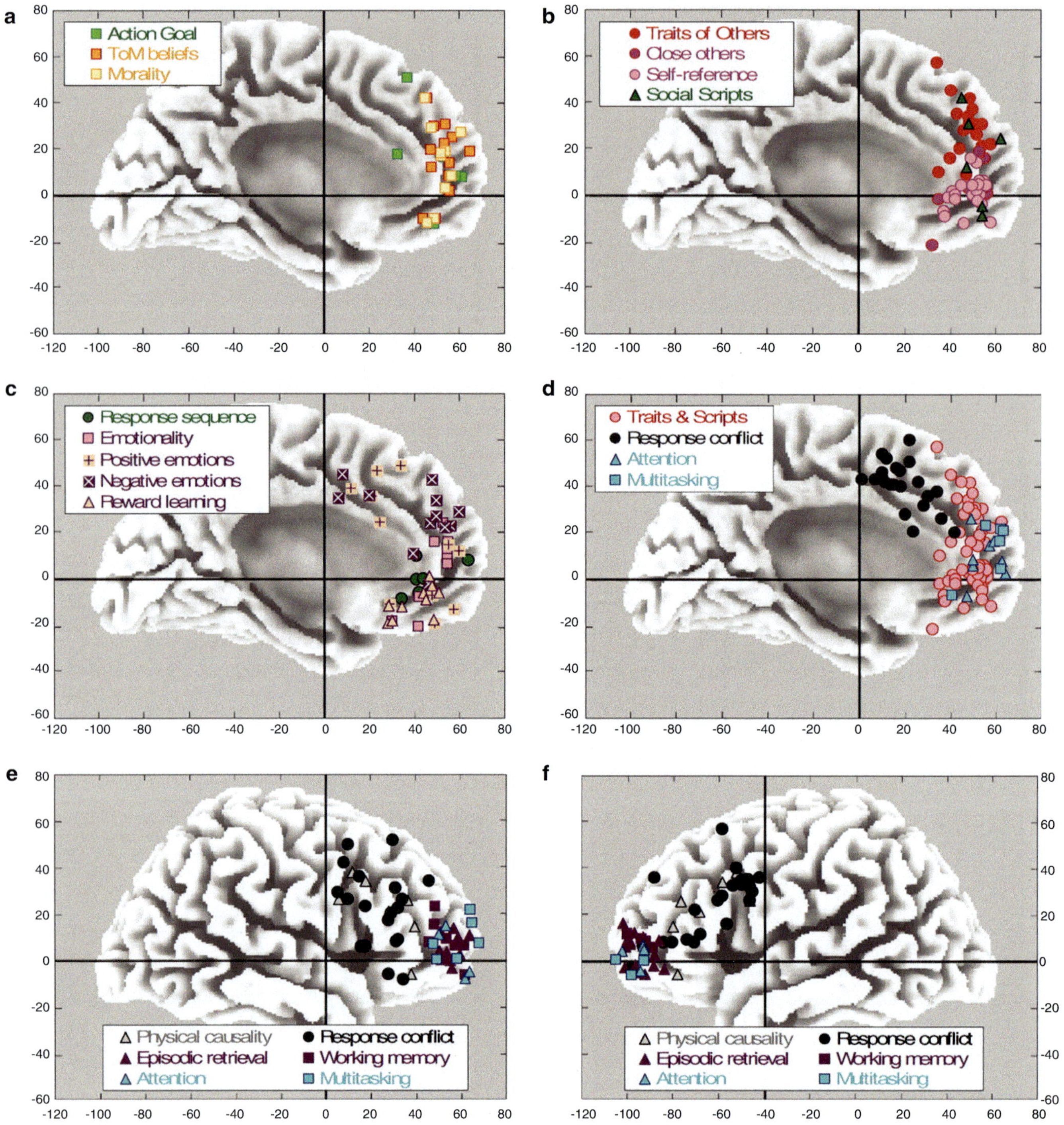

Fig. 4.53 (**a**) The mPFC involved in social inferences of intentionality. (**b**) The mPFC involved in social inferences of traits (other and self) and scripts. Social inferences during interpersonal games are included in the trait inferences of others. (**c**) The mPFC involved in sequence learning and emotional responses. (**d**) The medial PFC involved in executive functions, in comparison with social inferences of traits and scripts (copied from Fig. 4.2b). (**e**, **f**) The lateral PFC involved in causal learning and executive functions; right and left lateral view, respectively. (*Reprinted from* Van Overwalle [20]; *with permission*)

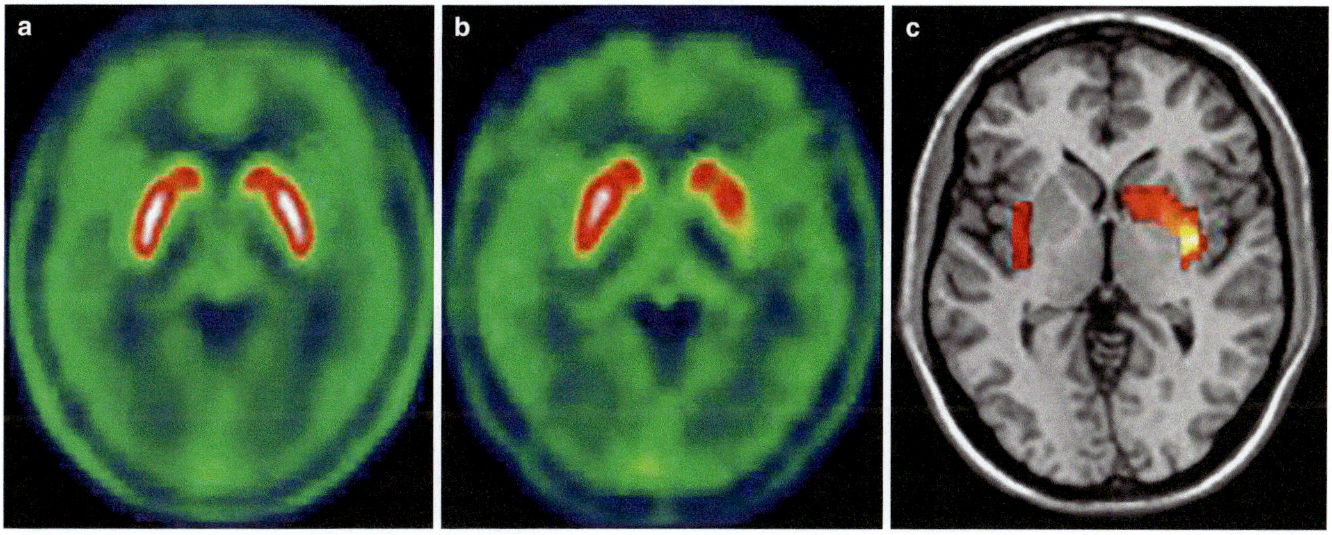

Fig. 4.54 This image displays striatal dopamine innervations using F-Dopa PET. (**a**) represents mean values from eight healthy control subjects, while (**b**) represents markedly reduced dopamine uptake in the left posterior putamen and mildly reduced uptake in the anterior putamen and caudate of the left hemisphere from a patient with Parkinson's disease. (**c**) represents the statistical difference between the difference in mean dopamine uptake values of the healthy control group (**a**) and the reduced uptake in the patient with Parkinson's disease, which is rendered over MRI for anatomical localization purposes. (*Reprinted from* Obeso et al. [21]; *with permission*)

Neurophysiology

Neurophysiology, as a discipline, centers on the physiology of the brain. It frequently intersects with neuroscience, including the study of the properties and functions of cellular and electrical activity within the CNS. Many techniques used in the field of neurophysiology are reviewed in Chap. 8 of this volume.

Single Cell Recordings

Single-cell recording is a measurement of voltage changes over time in a single neuron (see Fig. 4.55) [22].

Electroencephalograms

An electroencephalogram (EEG) is an electrophysiological clinical method that is used to monitor electrical activity in the brain; it measures the sum of the excitatory and postsynaptic potentials across neuron membranes in different cortical regions. An EEG is displayed as waveforms depicting measured frequency, amplitude, and voltage levels (see Fig. 4.56).

On the screen, you first look for:

1. *Montages*: The combinations of information from the electrodes.
2. *Sensitivity*: The voltage that allows you to see the waveforms the best.
3. *Filter*:

   LF (Low Frequency) Filter: EEG will not amplify any frequencies below the number you set it to read (commonly set to 1.0 Hz).

   HF (High Frequency) Filter: EEG will not show any frequencies above the established level.

Then you look for:

1. *Background activity*: This represents the overall electrical activity of an individual (robust readings occur in the posterior channel, usually the occipital regions).
2. *Stage of alertness*.
3. *Symmetry*: Determine whether there are any lateralizing or focal abnormalities.
4. *Abnormality*: Investigate whether any ictal activity, sharp wave spikes, or slowing have occurred.

The recording system of an EEG:

There are many different configurations of EEG in use with variable electrode counts. Regardless, the electrodes are named according to the corresponding region of the brain that the electrodes are measuring (see Fig. 4.57):

- A = Auricular (ear electrode).
- C = Central.
- F = Frontal.
- O = Occipital.
- P = Parietal.
- Fp = Frontopolar.
- T = temporal.

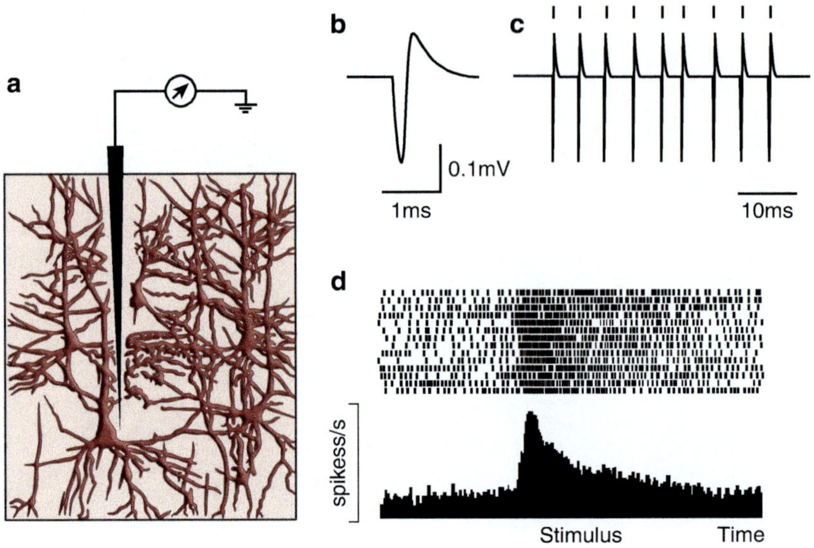

Fig. 4.55 (**a**) An electrode tip is placed close to but outside a nerve cell body. (**b**, **c**) Display of a single action potential (**b**) train of spikes. (**c**) The extracellular space recordings with biphasic shapes and small amplitude. A marker above the spike train shows the time of occurrence of spikes. (**d**) The top image shows spike trains in response to multiple stimulus presentations; each dash shows a single potential, and each row, aligned on the time of the stimulus, shows a separate trial. The bottom represents a peri-stimulus time histogram to show the average activity through all trials. (*From* Ludvig et al. [22]; *with permission*)

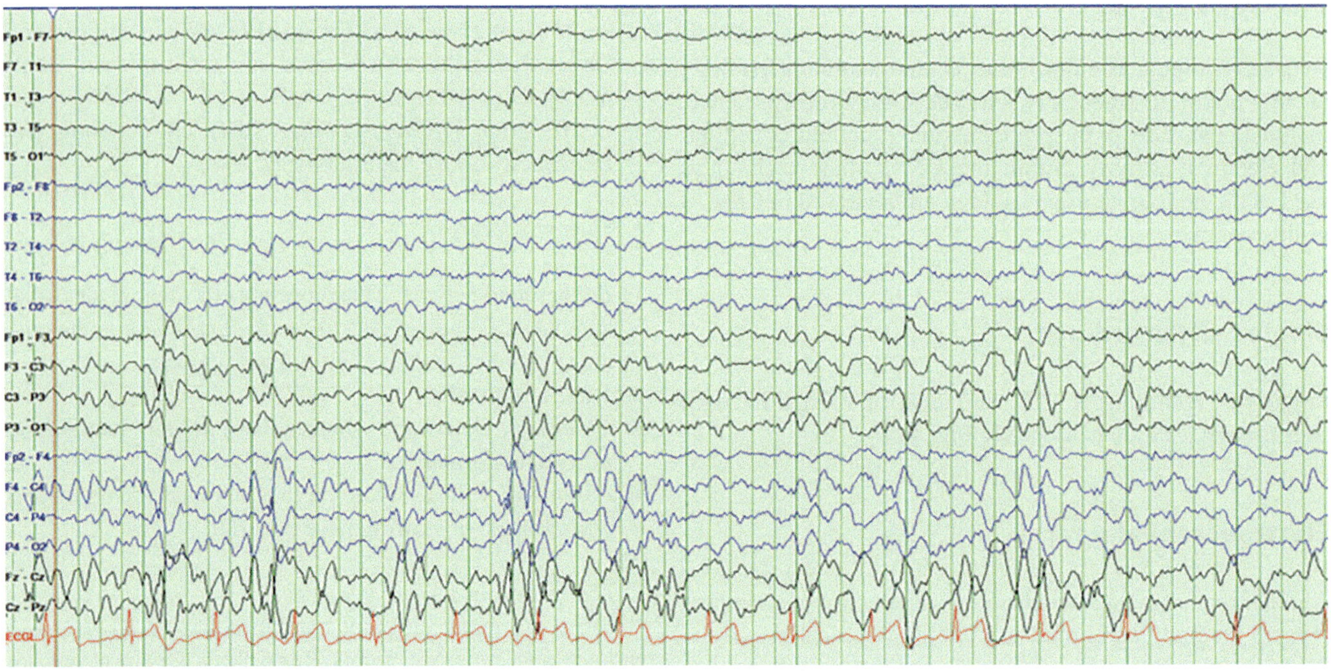

Fig. 4.56 Vertex waves on EEG. (Creative Commons Attribution-ShareAlike 4.0 International; https://commons.wikimedia.org/wiki/File:Vertex_waves_EEG.png)

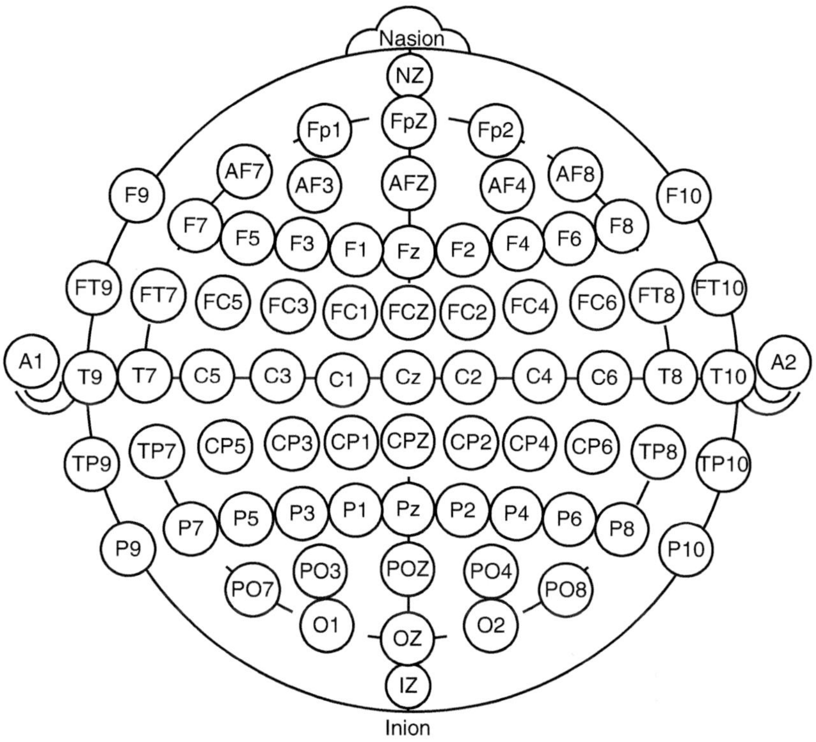

Fig. 4.57 The placement of electrodes on the human scalp using the International 10–20 system

Normal EEG Patterns

Characteristics of normal EEG patterns include:

- Normal background activity.
- No asymmetry.
- No changes in the EEG were provoked by hyperventilation or photic stimuli.
- No abnormalities were observed in the background.

In general, brain wave frequencies range from 0.5–500 Hz. The following classifications of brain wave frequencies are the most common:

- Alpha waves: 8–13 Hz.
- Beta waves: Over 13 Hz.
- Delta waves: 3 Hz or less.
- Theta waves: 3.5–7.5 Hz.

Alpha waves: These are the most common waves in adults. Eye closing and relaxation states elicit them, and they are more common in posterior regions than anterior regions.

Beta waves: These are symmetric small amplitude patterns that commonly occur in greater frequency in anterior regions. Of note, select sedative/hypnotic/anxiolytic classes of drugs (i.e., benzodiazepines and barbiturates) result in beta wave patterns.

Delta waves: These are slow waves that occur in deep sleep states and are infrequent/rare in wakeful adults. They generally have the largest amplitude and can be either focal or diffuse.

Theta waves: Most commonly observed during sleep state across the lifespan.

In addition to the aforementioned wave patterns earlier, several additional waveforms exist. K complex waves are high-amplitude delta frequency waves. V waves are sharp wave patterns occurring during the sleep state. Sleep spindles is a generic term that refers to a collection of waves that occur during sleep, particularly in the stage 2 sleep cycle. Lambda waves are positive waves commonly observed in bilateral posterior sections, namely occipital cortical regions, which are triangular in form and symmetric; Lambda waves are commonly elicited during awake states with limited visual stimuli exposure. Positive occipital sharp transients of sleep or POSTS are triangular and symmetric waves that occur in bilateral occipital sections, most commonly during stage 2 sleep. Mu waves are asymmetric rhythmic waves with a rounded shape in one direction and a sharp contour in the other direction, which often disappear during motor activity on the contralateral side of the body and are frequently observed in the posterior frontal sections). Finally, sharp waves and spikes can be identified based on their narrow base, sharp top, and height, all of which are indicative of abnormal electrical activity. For additional information pertaining to the wide range of normal and abnormal EEG patterns, the reader is encouraged to review the work of Stern (2013) [23].

Seizures and Epilepsy

A seizure is a phenomenon of abnormal electrical activity in the brain. The term epilepsy infers a history of multiple seizures in a given individual, seizures that are, by definition, "unprovoked." For example, an individual can have a single isolated seizure secondary to a number of extraneous factors that affects the brain's electrical activity. However, in an individual with a diagnosis of epilepsy, the seizures are presumably the result of structural abnormalities within the brain rather than external environmental influences (e.g., pharmacological agents). The duration of seizure activity is variable, often lasting for several seconds to a few minutes. Critically, seizures that occur for longer than 5 min in duration with continuous electrographic seizure activity or recurrent seizure activity without inter-ictal recovery indicate a grave medical emergency, termed status epilepticus. There are many origins or etiological causes of the broad spectrum of seizures, but they are classified based on whether they are congenital or acquired. Congenital forms of epilepsy generally indicate that seizures occur in a child with a predisposition to epilepsy (i.e., familial) or are restricted to individuals that have experienced seizures at or prior to birth. In contrast, acquired epilepsy represents seizures resulting from acquired brain injury (e.g., anoxic/hypoxic injury, traumatic brain injury, brain tumors, and neurodegenerative processes).

Common mechanisms of seizure formation include:

- *Increased nerve excitation*: Results from an influx of Na or Ca and the electrical outcome of excitatory neurotransmitters (i.e., glutamate, aspartate).
- *Decreased inhibition*: GABA is the major inhibitory neurotransmitter found in the mammalian CNS. GABA mediates ion channels for negatively charged chloride ions. Disruption of the modulating role GABA plays in the CNS can result in increased excitatory activity because of a lack of influx of negatively charged chloride ions that serve to lower the internal charge within a cell.
- *Hypersynchronization, hyperexcitability, and epileptogenesis*: A hyperexcitable neuron cannot generate a seizure in unison. Rather, it is the abnormal synchronization of a collection of neuronal electrical activity that kindles the spread of abnormal electrical spikes.

There are two general types of seizures. Primary (generalized) seizures are those which indicate abnormal electrical activity across all brain regions and, most importantly, in both hemispheres. In contrast, a partial (focal) seizure represents an abnormal electrical activity that is restricted to one localized region. Partial seizures are subdivided into simple focal seizures (no major loss of alertness/conscious activity) and complex focal seizures (usually indicating loss of conscious activity/alertness). Complex focal seizures commonly occur in the temporal lobes. To clarify, complex focal seizures do not infer that a person has "passed out." Rather, an individual may be observed as displaying an extended staring spell or "blank look," which can indicate an absence of seizure. Such seizures are often preceded by feelings of Déjà vu or auras. Likewise, the post-ictal stage (activity following a seizure event) can vary depending on the specific location of abnormal electrical activity.

While the common behavioral, affective, and motor/sensory abnormalities preceding, occurring during, or following seizure activity remain beyond the scope of this chapter (see Rossetti & Kaplan, 2010 [24]), the term 'seizure semiology' refers to the actual manifestation of abnormal electrical activity. Epileptologists are neurologists with a specialty in the study and treatment of epilepsy. Epileptologists routinely use video EEG recordings (the interplay of reading EEG patterns while observing video and audio recordings) of patients experiencing a seizure. Their ability to see the stages and sequences of electrical activity while observing the patient during pre-ictal, ictal, and post-ictal phases allows them to develop a working hypothesis of the origin of seizure focus (see Fig. 4.58).

Background Slowing, Metabolic Effects, or Coma

EEG background can indicate the general health of an individual's brain. Normal background activity is characterized by symmetric findings with no significant distinctions in amplitude or laterality. A posterior dominant rhythm (PDR) should be present (see Fig. 4.59) [25]. This rhythm is a pattern of anterior to posterior gradient frequencies; anterior regions should include faster frequencies in the beta range, while posterior sections should demonstrate slower, higher amplitude frequencies [23, 26, 27]. Furthermore, spontaneous variability and reactivity to stimulation or action (i.e., opening/closure of eyes) should be present [26, 27]. In addition, a "state of consciousness" should be observed regardless of whether or not a patient is awake, drowsy, or sleepy [26, 27].

When the PDR is slower than the normative lower range for a patient's age, it is considered background slowing, which is a nonspecific finding, often indicative of mild encephalopathy. Common examples of nonspecific background slowing can be the result of a number of scenarios, including a superimposed neurodegenerative process, prior anoxic/hypoxic injury, or effects of different pharmacological agents (particularly sedative/hypnotic medications); the latter example is quite common in acute medical settings during which time patients may be experiencing toxic metabolic abnormalities or receiving sedative or analgesic medications. In relation, intermittent slowing can occur, which is the observed activity of bursts of slowing in the background (commonly in the theta and delta ranges within anterior regions of the brain). Diffuse slowing is characteristic of

Clinical feature	Anatomical origin	Lateralization	Reliability
Well-defined somatosensory symptoms	parietal (primary sensory cortex)	contralateral	high
Unilateral elementary visual phenomena	occipital	contralateral	high
Ascending visceral feelings	mesiotemporal, insula, supplementary motor area	none	moderate
Forced thinking	frontal or mesiotemporal	dominant hemisphere	moderate
Ictal fear	amygdala, hippocampus	none	high
Forced head version	frontal, temporal	contralateral	high
Nonversive head turning	temporal	ispilateral	moderate
Focal clonic activity	frontal (primary motor cortex)	contralateral	high
Unilateral dystonia	temporal or frontal (basal ganglia)	contralateral	high
Nystagmus	frontal eye field or parieto-temporal junction	contralateral to fast component	high
Ictal laughing	hypothalamus, temporal, mesiofrontal	none	moderate
Ictal eye closure	nonepileptic seizure	none	high
Asymmetric termination of cloni	temporal, frontal	ipsilateral (to the last cloni)	high
Postictal paresis	frontal, temporal	contralateral	high
Postictal nose wiping	temporal, frontal	ipsilateral	high
Postictal aphasia/dysnomia	frontal, temporal, parietal	dominant hemisphere	high

Fig. 4.58 Overview of some ictal or postictal clinical features with regard to the anatomical origin and their reliability. (*From* Rossetti and Kaplan [24]; *with permission*)

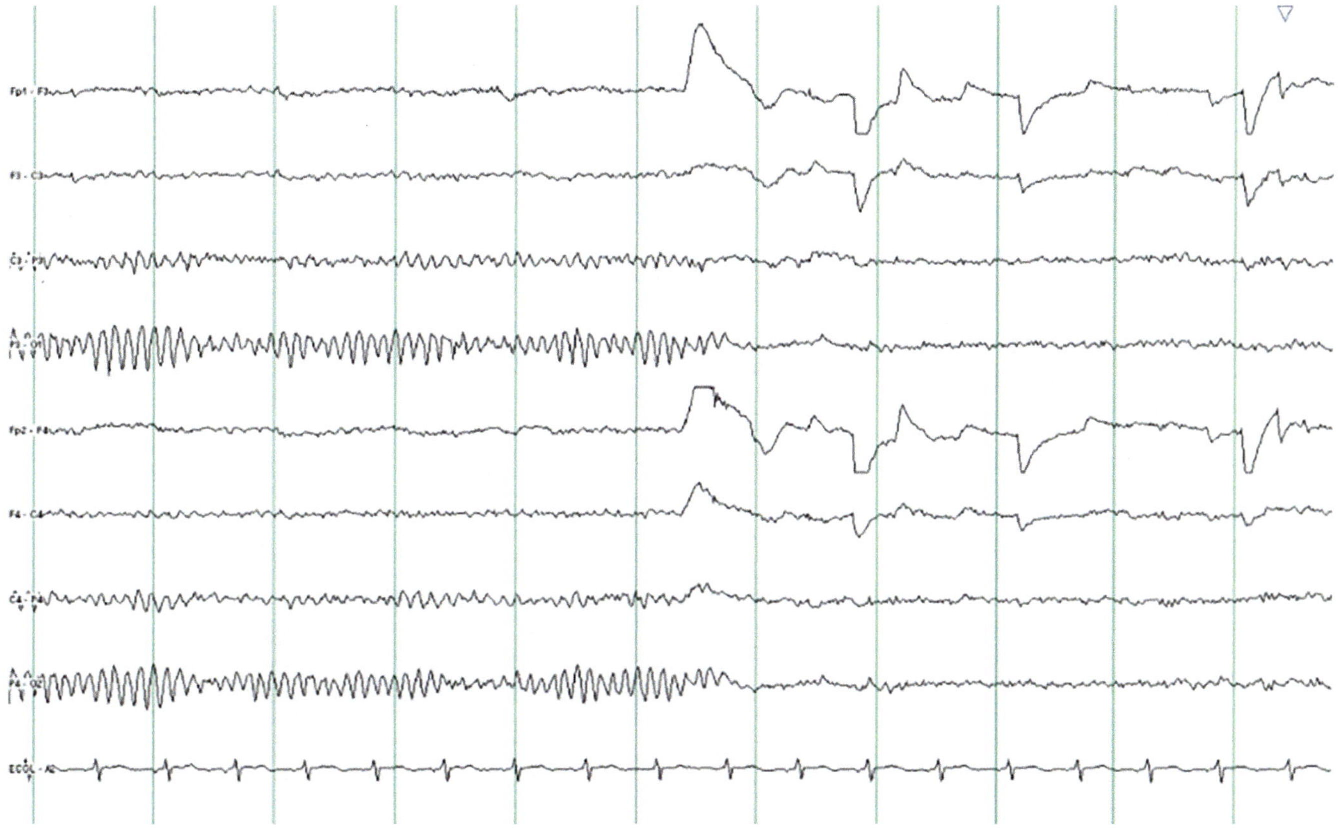

Fig. 4.59 The posterior dominant alpha rhythm. The normal background EEG during wakefulness contains posteriorly dominant, symmetrical, and reactive alpha rhythms. Alpha activity is more prominent in amplitude during relaxed, eyes-closed wakefulness and demonstrates reactivity by decreasing in amplitude and presence during eye-opening and mental alerting. (*From* Britton et al. [25] *with permission)*

theta and delta patterns in anterior regions and is indicative of diffuse moderate to severe brain abnormalities (i.e., in patients with coma, during post-ictal seizure activity, when a patient is sedated) or can be indicative of static encephalopathy related to developmental delay, anoxic injury, or diffuse axonal injury [23, 26, 27]. There are other abnormal patterns of slowing detailed elsewhere, including but not limited to alpha coma (non responsive EEG activity to stimulation), spindle coma (diffuse spindles occurring in the absence of an anterior-posterior gradient that is continuous in space/time), burst suppression (a common finding in patients experiencing deep coma or towards the end of a status epilepticus event), and background suppression (a finding of minimal or absolute absence of EEG signal) [23, 26, 27].

Neurochemistry

Broadly speaking, neurochemistry is the concentrated study of chemicals within the brain, including small molecules, neuropeptides, and neurotransmitters, which regulate and control the nervous system's physiology.

Electrical Activity in Neurons

Electrical activity is determined by the ionic gradient between the extracellular and intracellular sides of the neuron's plasma membrane. This ionic gradient is determined by ion channels and pumps (see Fig. 4.60).

Resting Potentials

Resting potential mechanics are depicted below (see Fig. 4.61).

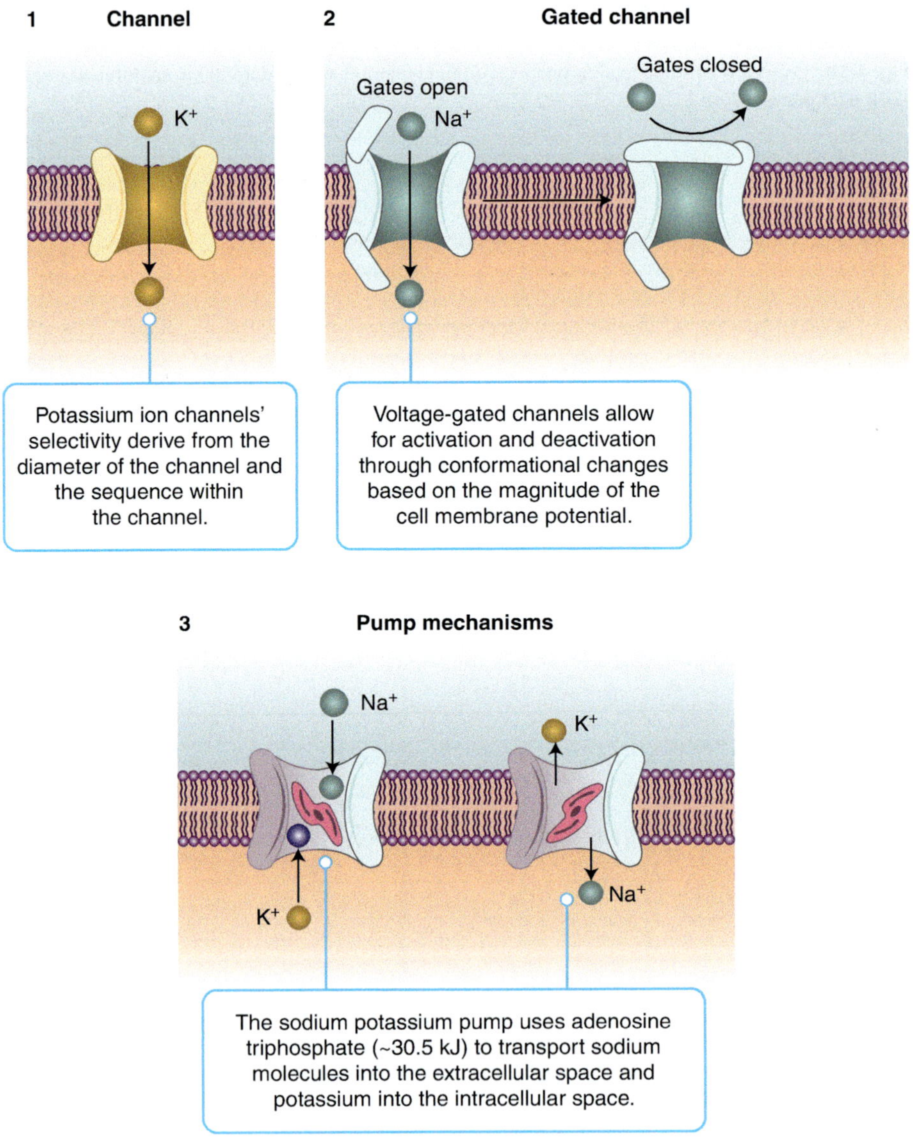

Fig. 4.60 (1) Channels permit select ions to pass through the membranes of each cell. (2) Gated channels change conformation to facilitate or inhibit the passage of select ions. Gated channels can also be deactivated by pore occlusion. (3) Pumps can change shape and use energy to transport molecules against their electrochemical gradients between the membrane of each cell

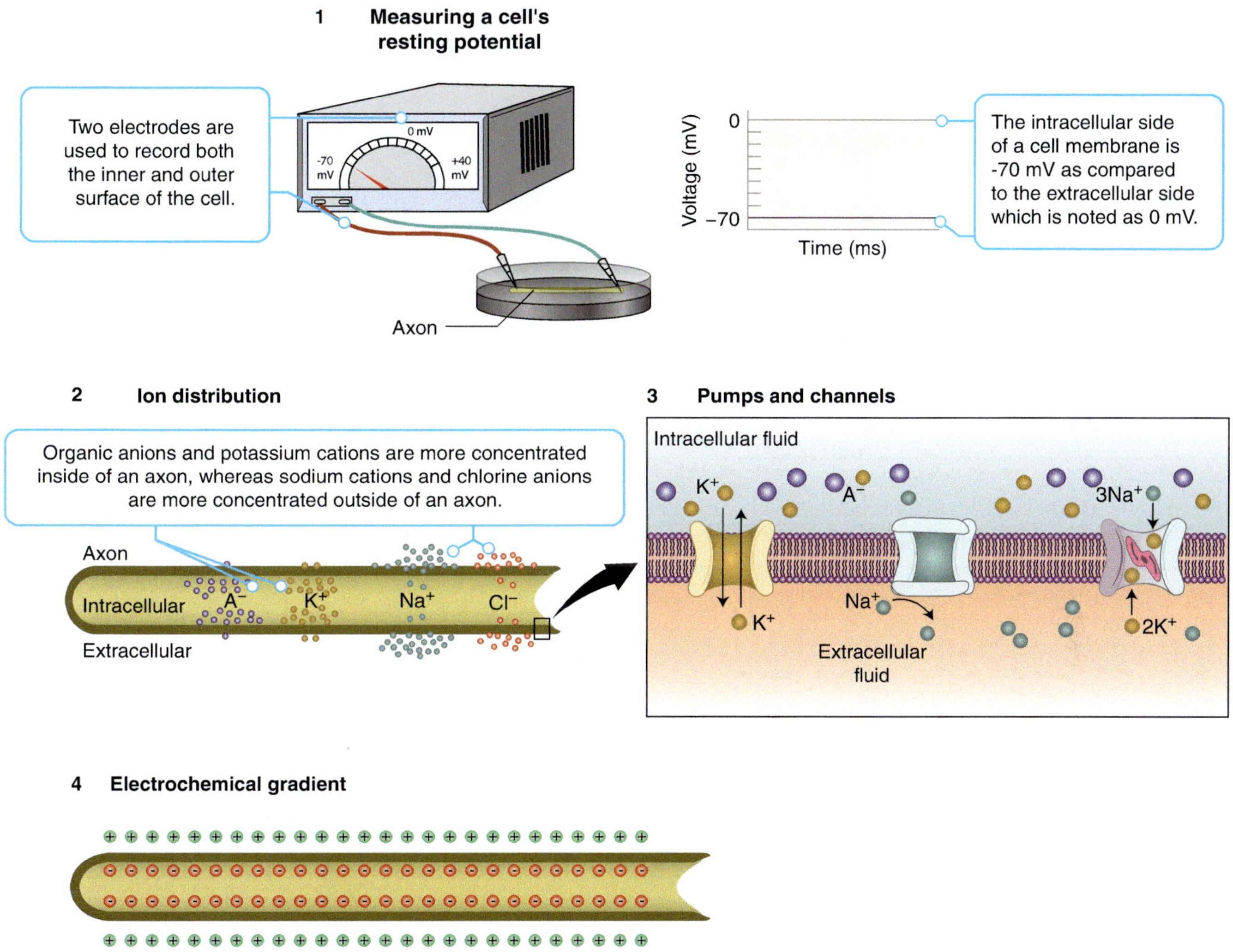

Fig. 4.61 (1) During resting potential, the membrane potential is determined by the ionic gradient between the intracellular and extracellular surfaces of the cells' axon. (2) The ionic gradient is caused by the concentration gradient of both anions and cations. (3) The intracellular and extracellular concentrations of these anions and cations are maintained by potassium channels, closed sodium-gated channels, and sodium-potassium pumps. (4) The unequal intracellular and extracellular distribution of these anions and cations creates the electrochemical gradient indicated by the −70 mV resting potential

Graded Potentials

Graded potentials represent a change in the membrane potential. At rest, it is at a polarized state or resting membrane potential of −70 mV (see Fig. 4.62).

Action Potentials

The cycle and mechanisms of an action potential are displayed below (see Fig. 4.63).

Saltatory Conduction and Myelin Sheaths

Saltatory conduction is the process through which nerve impulses or action potential signals pass through a myelinated axon. Myelination is possible through the growth of glial cells, which create the myelin sheath surrounding the axon, thus providing a layer of electrical insulation to flow down an axon. Without the complete formation of the myelin sheath, saltatory conduction will be slowed or stopped, leading to unfortunate consequences. This is the case in multiple sclerosis (MS), in which one's nerves are hindered from

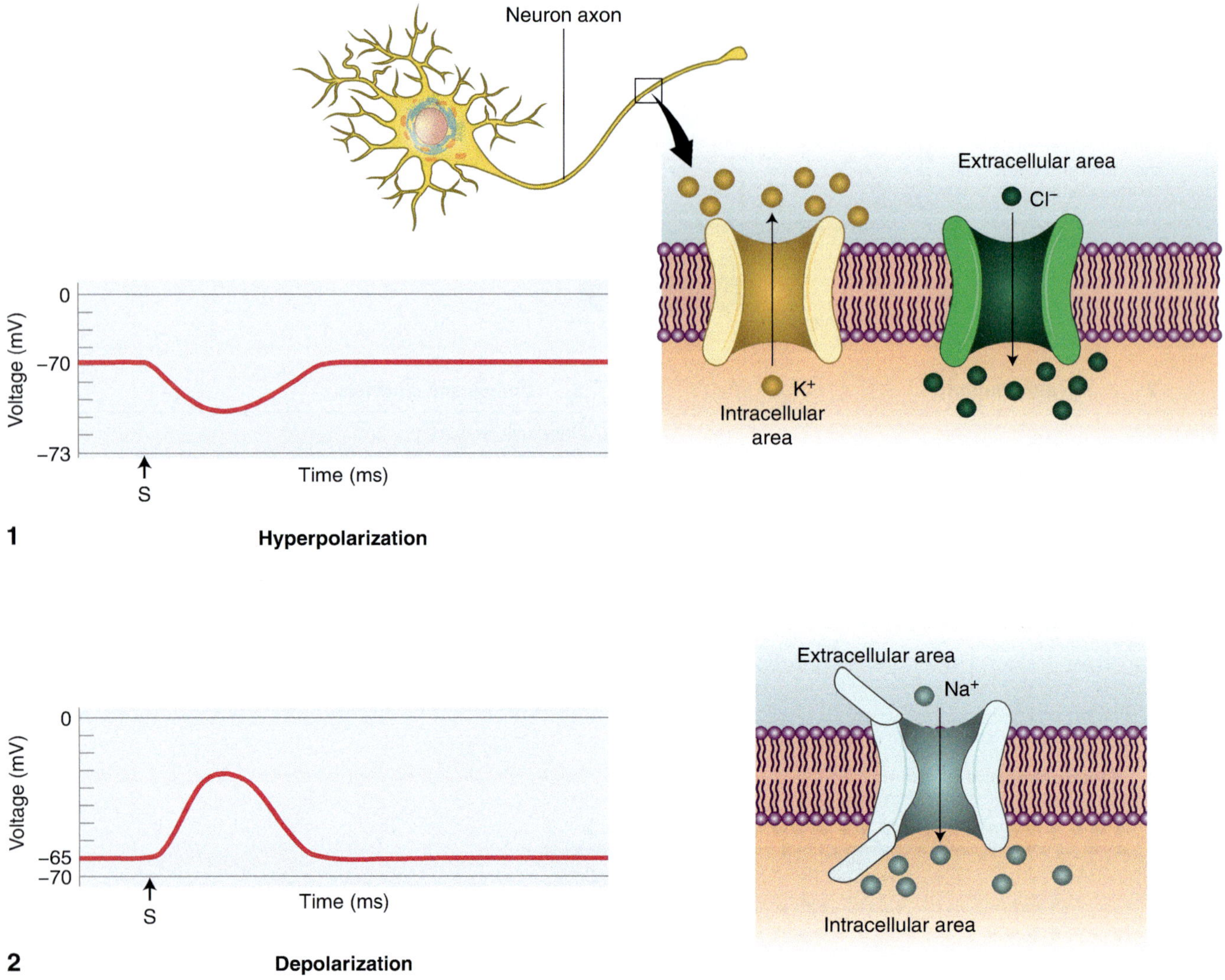

Fig. 4.62 (1) Hyperpolarization (inhibitory potential) represents an increase of the membrane potential caused by the efflux of positively charged potassium through potassium channels and the influx of negatively charged chlorine ions through chlorine channels. (2) Depolarization (excitatory potentials) represents a decrease in membrane potential caused by the influx of sodium ions through gated sodium channels

sending and receiving strong signal conduction because of white matter injury (see Fig. 4.64) [28].

Neurotransmitters

Neurotransmitters are fast-acting but short-term response chemical substances that transmit signals between neurons, across a synapse. Neurotransmitters fall into two categories, excitatory and inhibitory. Excitatory neurons lead to an increase in ion flow. Inhibitory neurons lead to a decrease in ion flow. A variety of neurotransmitters exist within the brain. Each neurotransmitter has a number of general functions, reactions from elevated amounts, and consequences from depleted levels, as displayed in Table 4.1.

Small Molecule Transmitters

There are many small organic molecules that are derived from the foods we eat and are synthesized and packaged in the axon terminal (see Fig. 4.65). They are fast-acting molecules that include acetylcholine (Ach), amines, such as dopamine (DA), norepinephrine (NE) or noradrenaline (NA), epinephrine (EP), serotonin (5-HT), and histamine, as well as amino acids such as glutamate (Glu), gamma-aminobutyric acid (GABA), and glycine.

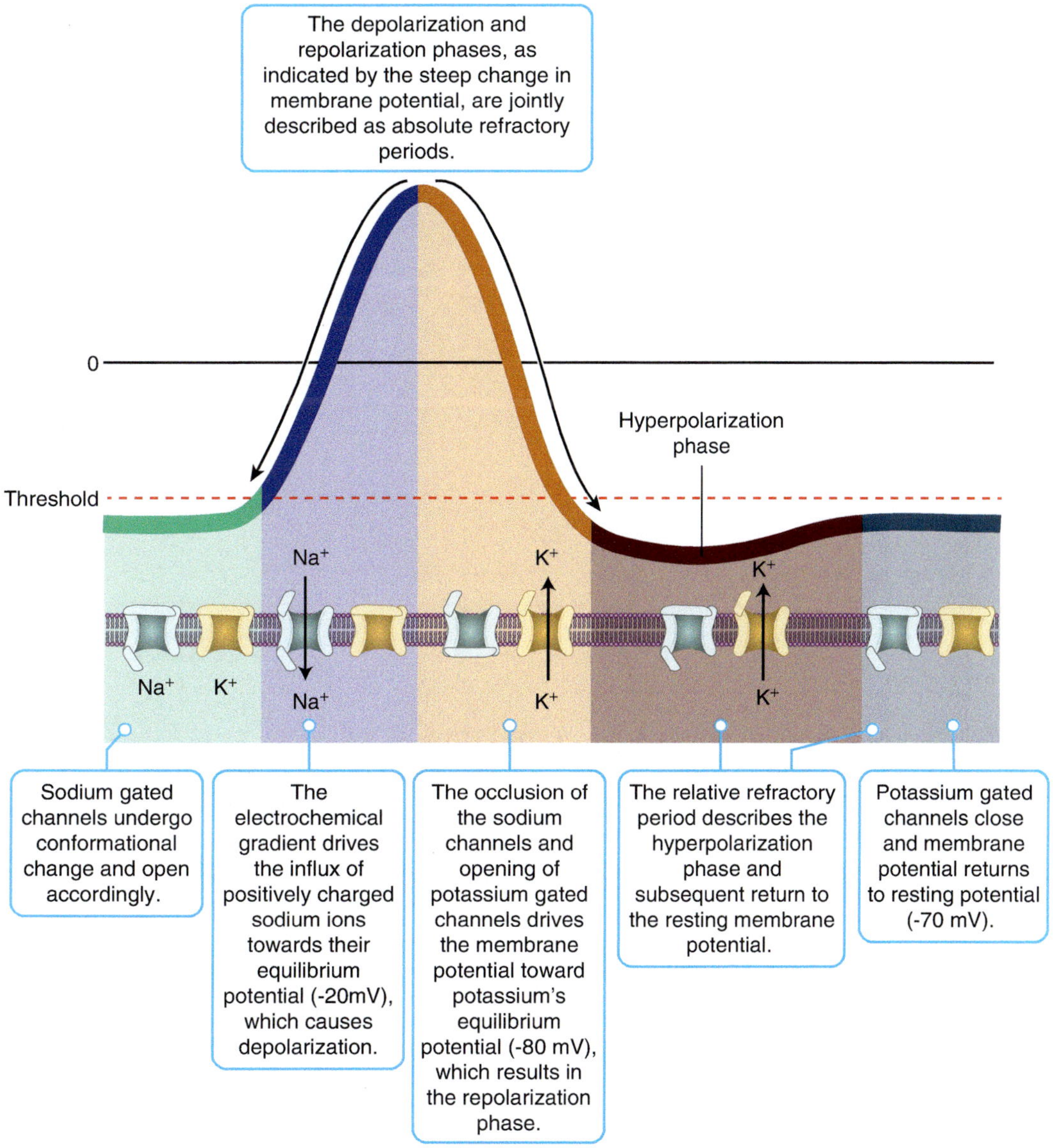

Fig. 4.63 When input signals' summation reaches the threshold potential (−50 mV), it triggers an action potential. An action potential results in the depolarization and subsequent repolarization of the membrane potential, followed by a hyperpolarization before a return to the resting potential. Both voltage-gated channels and channels occluded by a cytoplasmic unit can influence the membrane potential. Voltage-gated channels change conformational upon membrane voltage changes, while occlusion by a cytoplasmic unit takes place after conformational changes. The residues in the cytoplasmic unit interact with complementary sites, sites that are exposed only after the conformational change to open the channel has occurred

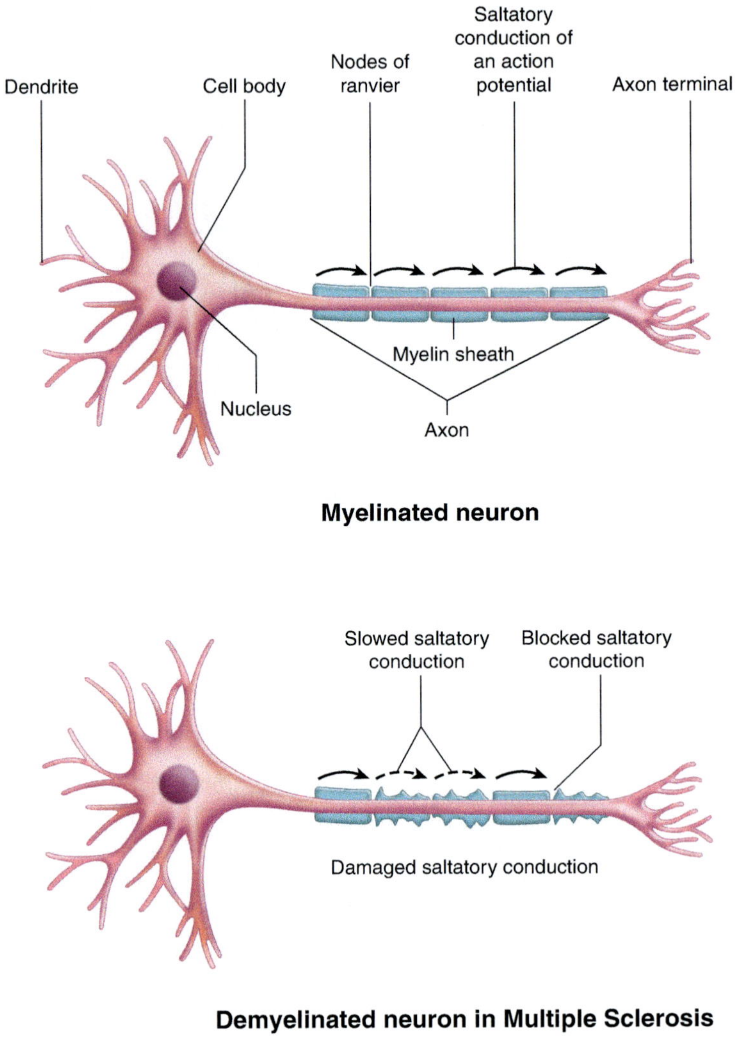

Fig. 4.64 In MS, the immune system attacks the body's CNS, specifically attacking and damaging the myelin sheath. As such, MS is considered a demyelinating disease. Neuroradiological findings of individuals with MS often reveal multifocal white matter lesions on T2 MRI sequences, commonly occurring in the periventricular, juxtacortical, infratentorial, or spinal cord regions. (*From* Christogianni et al. [28]; *with permission*)

Table 4.1 Summary of the known major neurotransmitters

Type of neurotransmitter	Neurotransmitter	General function	Surplus relations	Deficit relations
Acetylcholine	Acetylcholine (ach)	Muscle control, memory formation, learning	Muscle contractions	Paralysis, memory impairment (as in Alzheimer's disease)
Monoamines	Epinephrine (EP)	Adrenaline, defense mechanism against stress, activates autonomic system		
Monoamines	Norepinephrine (NE)/ noradrenaline (NA)	Involved in arousal and mood, responds to low blood pressure and stress, promotes vasoconstriction	Anxiety	Depression, may lead to development of attention deficit hyperactivity disorder
Monoamines	Serotonin	Regulates mood, sleep, eating and aggressive behavior		Anxiety, mood disorders
Monoamines	Dopamine	Muscle movements, cognition, reward pathways	Psychotic symptoms (e.g., perceptual disturbances, mania, addiction/compulsion)	Parkinsonian features
Amino acids	GABA	Inhibitory neurotransmitter, balances and offsets excitatory messages, reduces CNS activity	Sleep and eating disorders	Anxiety
Amino acids	Glutamate	Excitatory neurotransmitter, enhances transmission of information, memory, neuroplasticity	Seizures	

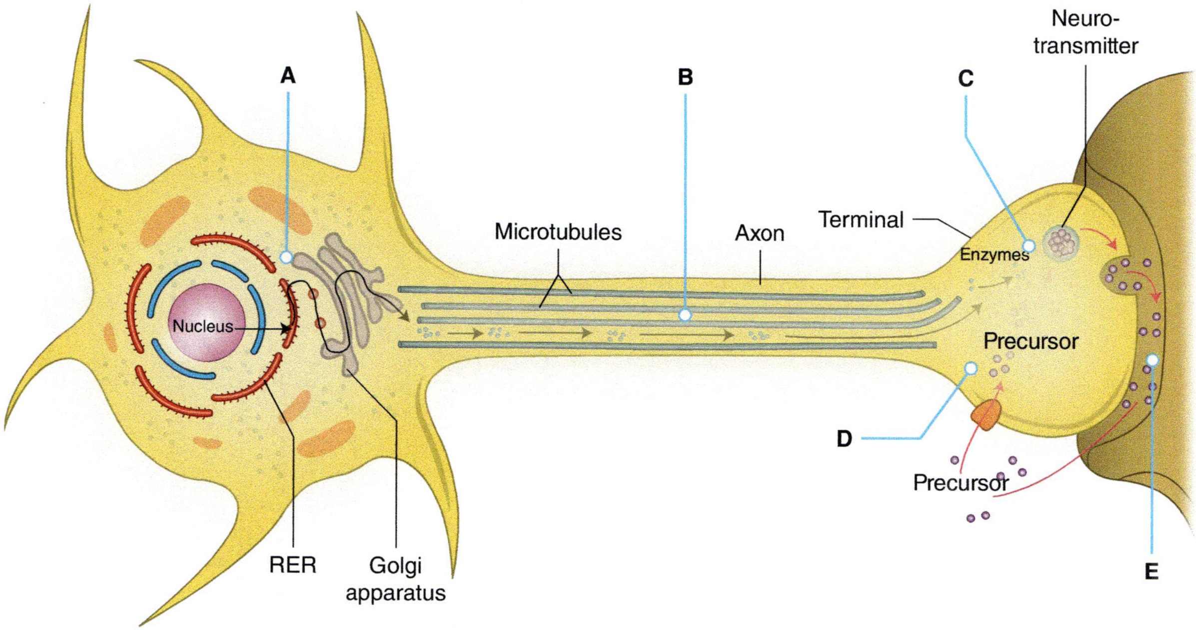

Fig. 4.65 This illustration depicts the process of (**a**) small-molecule neurotransmitter enzymes being synthesized at the presynaptic nerve terminal, (**b**) followed by the transport of such enzymes down the axon, (**c**) then being synthesized and packaged as small-molecules and (**d**) the integration of precursors into the terminal section, (**e**) while concluding with the eventual distribution and release of small-molecule neurotransmitters

Neuropeptides

Neuropeptides are chains of amino acids connected by peptide bonds that serve as slow-acting but prolonged action neurotransmitters. Neuropeptides are produced in the cell body and contain certain receptor proteins. Peptides have a variety of functions (displayed in Table 4.2).

Transmitter Gases

Gas neurotransmitters or gasotransmitters, such as nitric oxide (NO) and carbon monoxide (CO), act by diffusion and play roles in the central nervous system (see Fig. 4.66). Through the use of metabotropic and ionotropic receptors, they help maintain synaptic plasticity; metabotropic receptors prolong slow changes of cellular excitability, and ionotropic receptors serve in fast-acting neurotransmission [29].

The Process of Neurotransmission

Neurotransmission or synaptic transmission refers to communication at the synapse between neurons in the form of chemical or electrical signals. These signals may excite or inhibit the postsynaptic neuron (see Fig. 4.67).

Inhibitory and Excitatory Messaging

There are two types of synapses, Type I and Type II. Type I synapses are found on the dendritic spine and shaft. They are excitatory, meaning they polarize and stimulate neurotransmitters in the postsynaptic membrane, which increases the likelihood of the action potential. For example, when acetylcholine is released at the neuromuscular junction by a presynaptic neuron, it causes postsynaptic Na+ channels to open. Na+ enters the postsynaptic cell, leading to depolarization, also known as an excitatory postsynaptic potential (EPSP).

Type II synapses are found in the cell body. They are inhibitory, meaning they depolarize and inhibit neurotransmitters, decreasing the likelihood of the action potential. For example, when GABA is released by a presynaptic neuron, it causes Cl^- channels to open, leading to hyperpolarization of the presynaptic membrane, also known as inhibitory postsynaptic potentials (IPSP).

Reuptake Inhibition

In reuptake, neurotransmitters that were released into the synaptic cleft are returned to the terminal button so that the postsynaptic neuron only has brief exposure, thus regulating the synapse (see Fig. 4.68). Reuptake inhibitors are drugs that interfere with this process, increasing neurotransmission. There are five classes of reuptake inhibitors; norepinephrine reuptake inhibitors (NRIs), norepinephrine-dopamine reuptake inhibitors (NDRIs), selective serotonin reuptake inhibitors (SSRIs), serotonin-norepinephrine reuptake inhibitors (SNRIs), and serotonin-norepinephrine-dopamine reuptake inhibitors (SNDRIs).

Table 4.2 Classes of neuropeptides, locations of action, and general functions

Neuropeptide	Location of action	General function
Enkephalin	Inhibits afferent pain fibers/ opioid receptors	Main functions include analgesia, stress response regulation, and peristalsis modulation
Substance P	Transmission of pain from peripheral receptors to the CNS	Diminishes pain sensation
LHRH/GnRH	Acts on the pituitary → release of luteinizing hormone (LH) + follicle-stimulating hormone (FSH)	Functions on growth modulatory factor, acts on the ovaries, hypothalamic anovulation, and reproductive maturation
Vasopressin	Located within the paraventricular nuclei, ed. nucleus of the stria terminalis (BNST), medial amygdala (MeA), and suprachiasmatic nucleus (SCN)	Involved in metabolism and maintenance of metabolic rate Potential with stress-related states, evidence of role in regulation of the HPA axis
CKK	Involved in gastric enzyme secretion.	Promotes feeling of satiety
VIP	Immunoregulatory neuropeptide, distributed in the CNS and PNS	Increases gastric motility
Endorphin	Peptide hormones are released into the circulatory system by the pituitary gland.	Reduces pain sensation, promotes feeling of euphoria
Neurotensin	Found in the CNS, and in the gastrointestinal tract	Analgesia, hypothermia, and increased locomotor activity. Also involved in regulation of dopamine pathways
TRH	Exerts the hormonal control of thyroid-stimulating hormone levels	Regulation of metabolic and hormonal functions.
Angiotensin-II	Part of the renin–angiotensin system	Central regulation of blood pressure and stress response
Somatostatin	Regulates the endocrine system, affects neurotransmission and cell proliferation	Significantly contributes to emotionality, stress behaviors.
Oxytocin	Produced in the hypothalamus and released by the posterior pituitary	Role in social bonding, reproduction, and childbirth

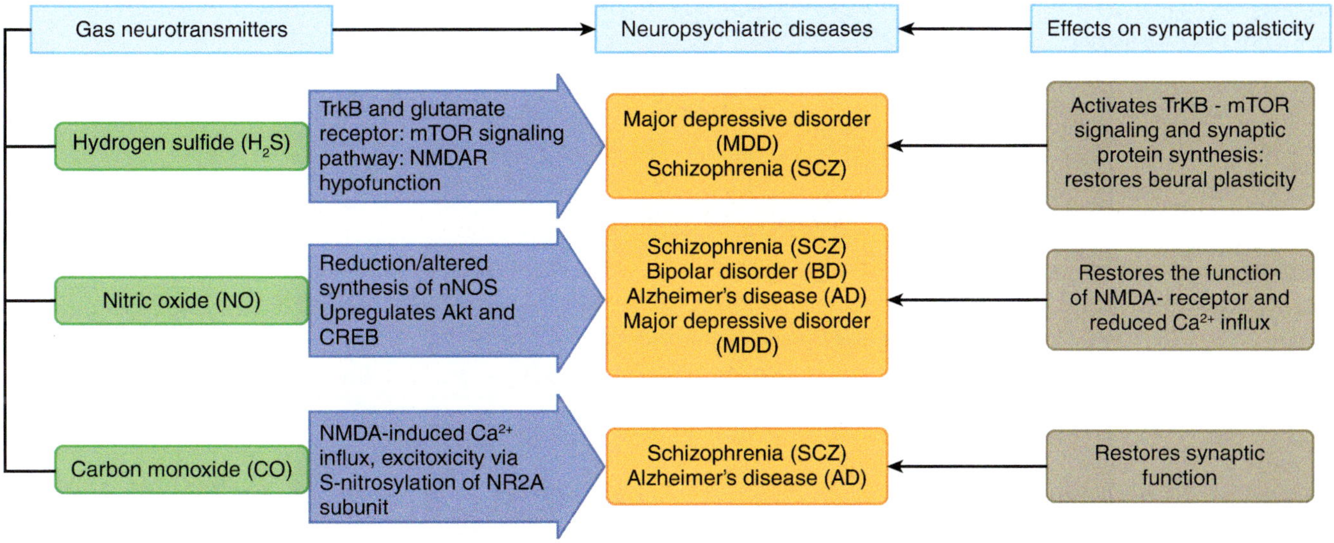

Fig. 4.66 Role of gas neurotransmitters in neuropsychiatric diseases. The three gas neurotransmitters such as hydrogen sulfide (H2S), nitric oxide (NO), and carbon dioxide (CO) have a role in neuropsychiatric conditions such as major depressive disorder (MDD), schizophrenia (SCZ), bipolar disorder (BD), and Alzheimer's disease (AD) to maintain proper synaptic plasticity as well as neural homeostasis. H2S has a role in tropomyosin receptor kinase B (TrKB) and glutamate as well as mechanistic targets of rapamycin (mTOR) signaling pathways, and it activates the TrKB-mTOR signaling pathway as well as synaptic protein in MDD. NO has a role in the regulation of altered synthesis of nNOS as well as upregulates Akt and cyclic AMP (cAMP) response element binding (CREB) protein which restores function in *N*-methyl-D aspartate (NMDA) receptor and reduces Ca^{2+} influx in schizophrenia, MDD, and AD. CO has a role in NMDA-induced calcium ion (Ca^{2+}) influx or excitotoxicity via S-nitrosylation of antiglutamate receptor NMDAR2A (NR2A) subunit and restores synaptic function in AD and SCZ. However, these gas neurotransmitters work in various ways to maintain or restore synaptic plasticity in these neuropsychiatric diseases. (Reprinted from Shefa et al. [29]. Creative Commons Attribution License)

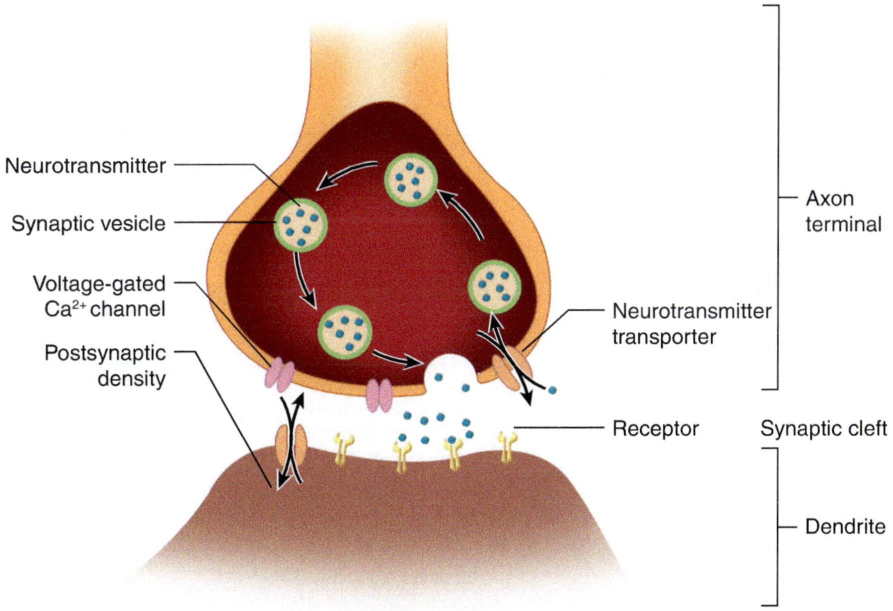

Fig. 4.67 The process of neurotransmission

Fig. 4.68 The process of how SSRIs block the reuptake of serotonin

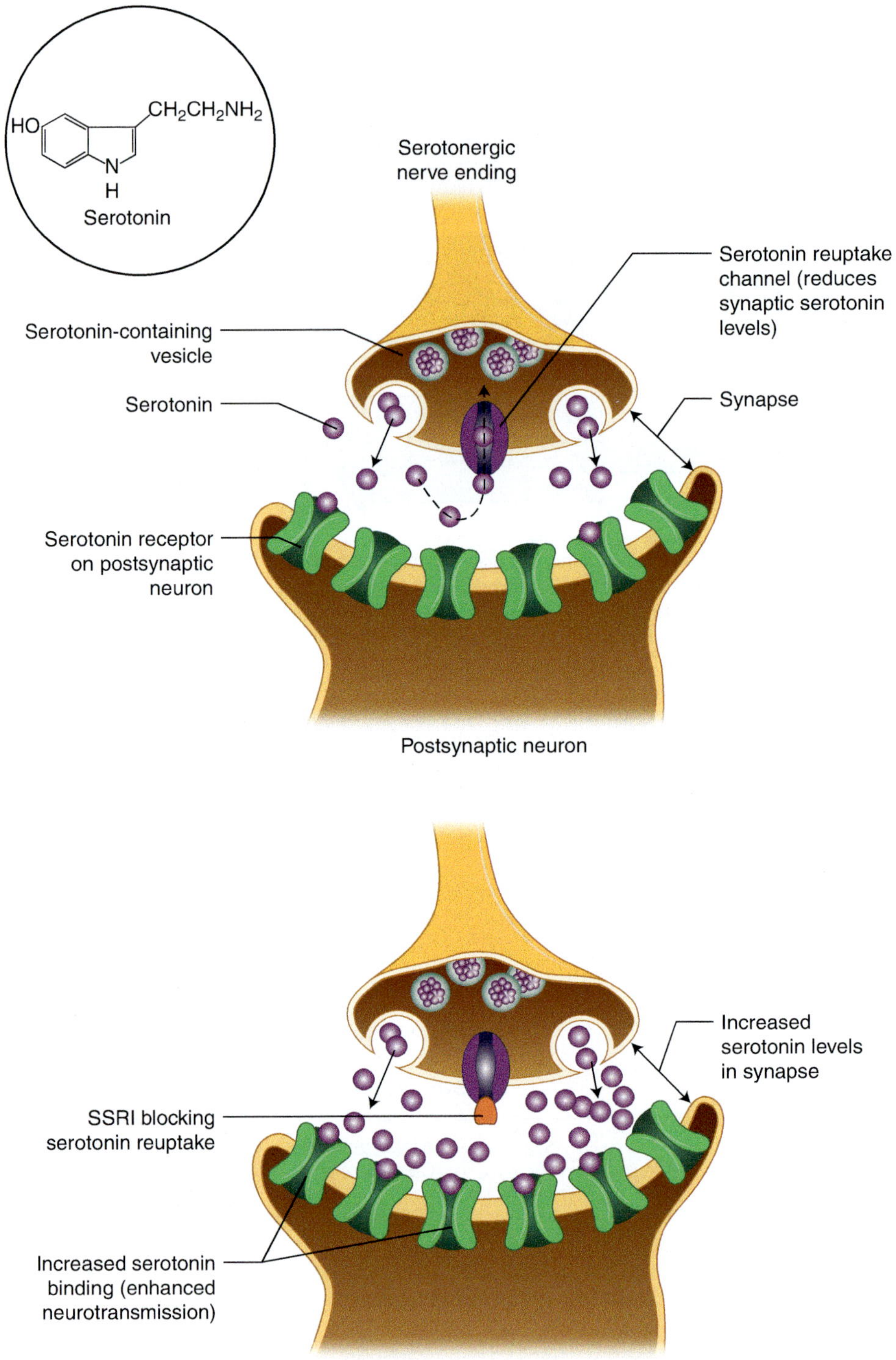

Activating Systems

Within the CNS, the primary activation systems include the serotonergic, cholinergic, dopaminergic, and noradrenergic systems (see Table 4.3 and Fig. 4.69).

Classification of Psychoactive Drugs and Review of Clinical Applications

Psychoactive drugs are chemical substances that alter brain function, leading to changes in behavior, perception, and mood. The distinctions between different types of psychoactive drug classes are displayed in Table 4.4. The mechanistic pathway through which these drugs influence the brain also has implications for the therapeutic uses of these drugs. For example, depressants can be used to treat anxiety, and opioids are used as analgesics for acute pain.

In relation, there are a number of hormones that control and coordinate homeostasis. These hormones also influence reproduction, growth, and metabolism, among other functions (see Fig. 4.70).

Table 4.3 Activating systems

Cholinergic system	Dopaminergic system	Noradrenergic system	Serotonergic system
Acetylcholine	Dopamine	Noradrenaline/norepinephrine	Serotonin
Maintains neuron excitability, important for learning and memory Note: Death of ach neurons believed to be related to Alzheimer's disease	Associated with motivation, pleasure, and motor behavior Note: Hyperfunction of dopaminergic cells may lead to manic behavior. Hypofunction may lead to depression.	Regulates arousal and anxiety Note: Altered noradrenergic function may explain pathogenesis of depression, PTSD, anxiety disorders	Role in decision based functions, reward, impulsivity, modulates mood, sleep, appetite Note: Linked to anxiety disorders, depression and Parkinson's disease

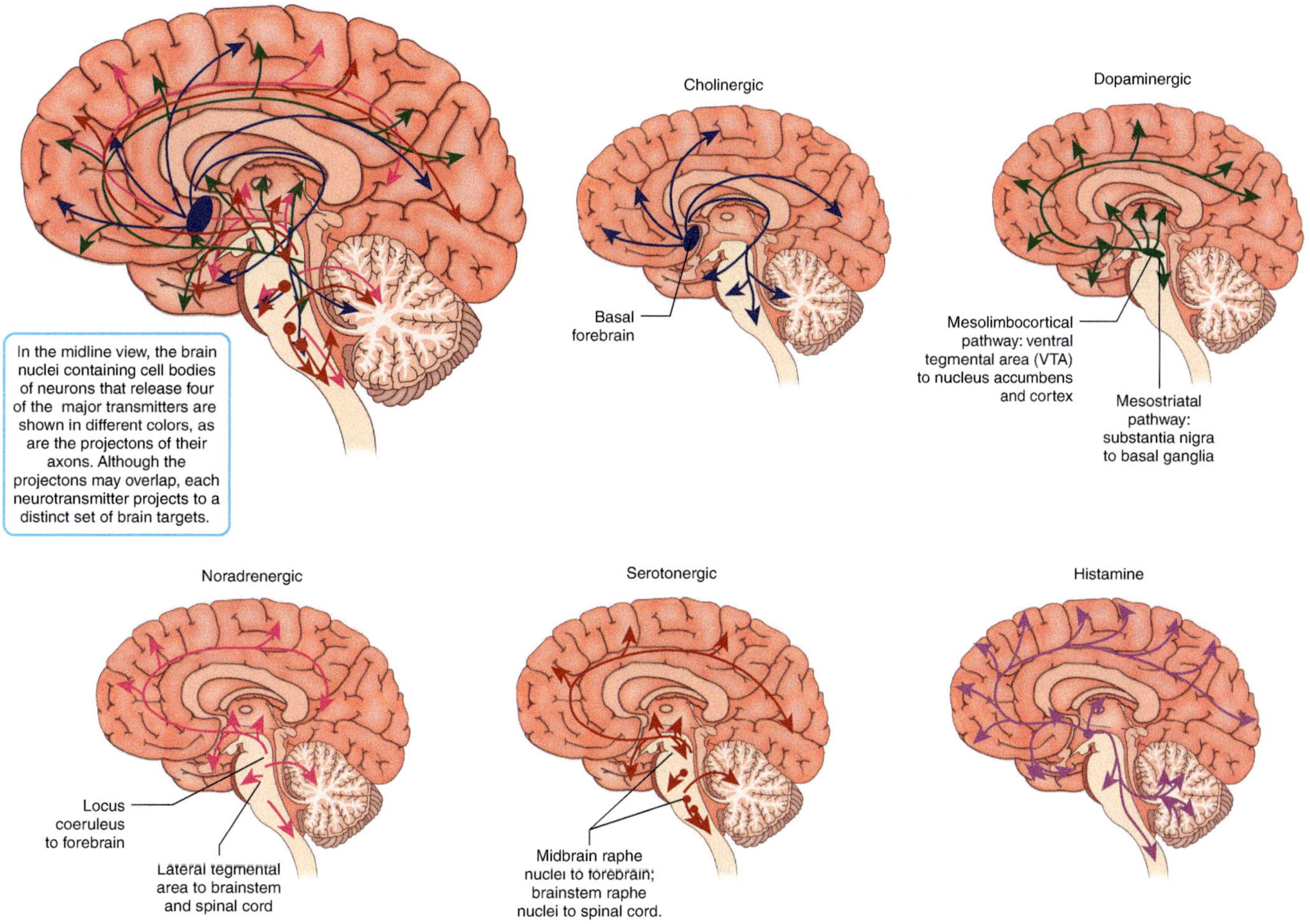

Fig. 4.69 Neurotransmitter systems within the brain. (*From* Watson and Breedlove [30]; *with permission*)

Table 4.4 Psychoactive drugs and their functions

Psychoactive drugs					
Depressants	Stimulants	Hallucinogens	Narcotic and analgesics	Inhalants	Cannabis
Increases GABA:	Blocks the reuptake of dopamine/ serotonin	Mimics effects of serotonin and epinephrine	(Opioids) stimulates endorphins	Enters the lungs and enters brain through bloodstream. Depending on the type of inhalant, may depress the CNS, nitrites dilate and relax blood vessels	Activates cannabinoid receptors, increases dopamine activity
Decreases CNS activity: Less alert, slow breathing, heart rate, drowsiness	Increases CNS: Alert, aroused	Makes one see, hear, small and feel things that are not there	Reduces pain sensation or creates sense of euphoria	Produces short-lived, mind-altering effects	Changes in sensory perception, euphoria, relaxation, appetite
Alcohol, benzodiazepines, barbiturates, valium	Amphetamines, cocaine, Benzedrine, caffeine, nicotine	LSD, psilocybin, mescaline, peyote, ayahuasca	Morphine, heroin, codeine, Percodan, Demerol	Laughing gas, solvents, aerosols, gases, nitrites	Marijuana & THC extracts

GABA gamma aminobutyric acid, *CNS* central nervous system, *LSD* lysergic acid diethylamide, *THC* tetrahydrocannabinol

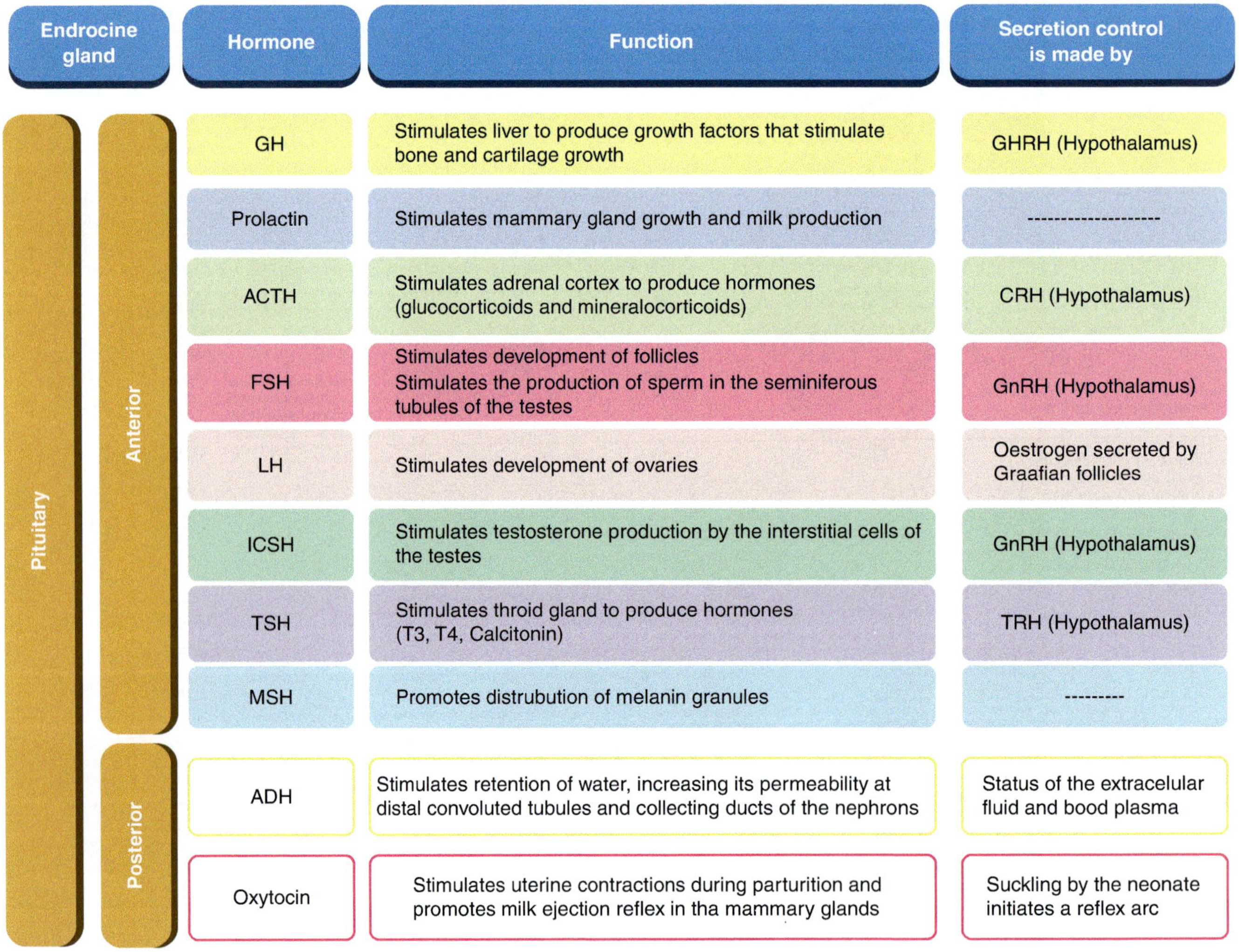

Fig. 4.70 Select hormones, their respective functions, and the origin of secretion control

Metabolic Disorders and Infection

In metabolic disorders, abnormal chemical reactions disrupt the body's metabolic process to create and store energy from ingested substances. Metabolic disorders are most commonly caused by genetic defects and environmental factors. These disorders can lead to hormone or enzyme deficiencies and abnormal neurochemical activity. For example, abnormally low blood sugar levels associated with hypoglycemia can cause severe confusion, loss of consciousness, or seizures. Abnormally low glucose values can lead to a number of adverse conditions (i.e., stroke, epilepsy, cognitive impairment, behavioral changes) because the brain requires glucose to function. In hyponatremia, low sodium levels can result in additional phenomena, including short-term memory impairment or in severe cases, osmotic demyelination syndrome.

Furthermore, pathogens (i.e., bacteria, fungi, viruses) can infiltrate the CNS via a crossing of the blood–brain barrier or via the blood–cerebrospinal fluid barrier [31]. When an individual has a weak or compromised immune system, such as in patients with HIV/AIDS or those taking immunosuppressants (i.e., organ transplants or MS patients), they are at substantially increased risk of opportunistic infection. More commonly, viral or bacterial meningitis can occur in patients with preserved immune function. Meningitis is an inflammation of the meninges and a serious condition that requires immediate medical care. One rare opportunistic infection is progressive multifocal leukoencephalopathy (PML), resulting in multifocal and diffuse but widespread white matter injury (see Fig. 4.71).

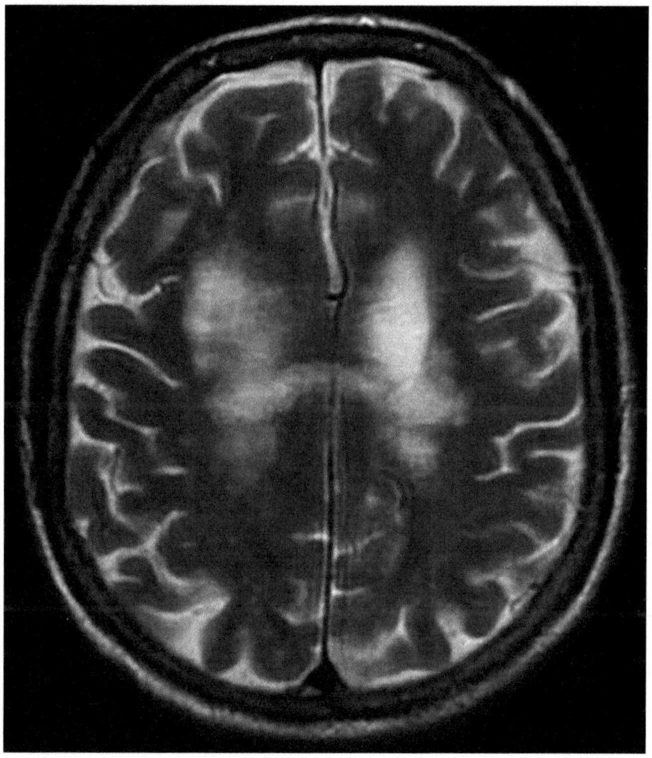

Fig. 4.71 Symptoms of PML are dependent on the focal regions within the CNS. Residual cognitive, behavioral, and motor deficits are common among patients who survive. Displayed is an MRI slice of a patient with progressive multifocal leukoencephalopathy. (Creative Commons Attribution 3.0 Unported; https://commons.wikimedia.org/wiki/File:Progressive_multifocal_leukoencephalopathy_002.jpg)

Conclusion

We hope you have found this chapter to be useful as you persevere in your pursuit to understand neuroanatomy, neurophysiology, and neurochemistry. Brief summaries of seminal scientific studies and landmark theories have been reviewed earlier. As such, we encourage the reader to reference the original sources listed below and related chapters in the current volume.

References

1. Bonilha L, Gleichgerrcht E, Nesland T, Rorden C, Fridriksson J. Gray matter axonal connectivity maps. Front Psych. 2015;6:35.
2. Werner CJ, Heyny-von Haussen R, Mall G, Wolf S. Proteome analysis of human substantia nigra in Parkinson's disease. Proteome Sci. 2008;6(1):1–14.
3. Defelipe J. The evolution of the brain, the human nature of cortical circuits, and intellectual creativity. Front Neuroanat. 2011;5:29.
4. Campbell BC, De Silva DA, Macleod MR, Coutts SB, Schwamm LH, Davis SM, Donnan GA. Ischaemic stroke. Nat Rev Dis Primers. 2019;5(1):1–22.
5. Bilder RM. Executive control: balancing stability and flexibility via the duality of evolutionary neuroanatomical trends. Dialogues Clin Neurosci. 2012;14(1):39.
6. Fuster JM. Upper processing stages of the perception–action cycle. Trends Cogn Sci. 2004;8(4):143–5.
7. Granger RH, Hearn RA. Models of thalamocortical system. Schlepped. 2007;2(11):1796.
8. Redgrave P, Rodriguez M, Smith Y, Rodriguez-Oroz MC, Lehericy S, Bergman H, Obeso JA. Goal-directed and habitual control in the basal ganglia: implications for Parkinson's disease. Nat Rev Neurosci. 2010;11(11):760–72.
9. Krack P, Hariz MI, Baunez C, Guridi J, Obeso JA. Deep brain stimulation: from neurology to psychiatry? Trends Neurosci. 2010;33(10):474–84.
10. Kievit RA, Davis SW, Griffiths J, Correia MM, Henson RN. A watershed model of individual differences in fluid intelligence. Neuropsychologia. 2016;91:186–98.
11. Alexander GE, DeLong MR, Strick PL. Parallel organization of functionally segregated circuits linking basal ganglia and cortex. Annu Rev Neurosci. 1986;9(1):357–81.
12. Martins MJ, Fischmeister FP, Puig-Waldmüller E, Oh J, Geißler A, Robinson S, Beisteiner R. Fractal image perception provides novel insights into hierarchical cognition. NeuroImage. 2014;96:300–8.
13. Halligan PW, Fink GR, Marshall JC, Vallar G. Spatial cognition: evidence from visual neglect. Trends Cogn Sci. 2003;7(3):125–33.

14. Peretz I, Coltheart M. Modularity of music processing. Nat Neurosci. 2003;6(7):688–91.
15. Hickok G. The functional neuroanatomy of language. Phys Life Rev. 2009;6(3):121–43.
16. Henke K. A model for memory systems based on processing modes rather than consciousness. Nat Rev Neurosci. 2010;11(7):523–32.
17. Bliss TV, Lømo T. Long-lasting potentiation of synaptic transmission in the dentate area of the anaesthetized rabbit following stimulation of the perforant path. J Physiol. 1973;232(2):331–56.
18. Suthana N, Ekstrom A, Moshirvaziri S, Knowlton B, Bookheimer S. Dissociations within human hippocampal subregions during encoding and retrieval of spatial information. Hippocampus. 2011;21(7):694–701.
19. LaBar KS, Cabeza R. Cognitive neuroscience of emotional memory. Nat Rev Neurosci. 2006;7(1):54–64.
20. Van Overwalle F. Social cognition and the brain: a meta-analysis. Hum Brain Mapp. 2009;30(3):829–58.
21. Obeso JA, Rodriguez-Oroz MC, Goetz CG, Marin C, Kordower JH, Rodriguez M, et al. Missing pieces in the Parkinson's disease puzzle. Nat Med. 2010;16(6):653–61.
22. Ludvig EA, Bellemare MG, Pearson KG. A primer on reinforcement learning in the brain: psychological, computational, and neural perspectives. In: Alonso E, Mondragón E, editors. Computational neuroscience for advancing artificial intelligence: models, methods and applications; 2011. p. 111–44. https://www.igi-global.com/chapter/primer-reinforcement-learning-brain/49232. https://doi.org/10.4018/978-1-60960-021-1.ch006.
23. Stern JM. Atlas of EEG patterns. 2nd ed. Philadelphia, PA: Lippincott Williams & Wilkins; 2013.
24. Rossetti AO, Kaplan PW. Seizure semiology: an overview of the 'inverse problem'. Eur Neurol. 2010;63(1):3–10.
25. Britton JW, Frey LC, Hopp JL, et al. The Normal EEG. In: St. Louis EK, Frey LC, editors. Electroencephalography (EEG): an introductory text and atlas of Normal and abnormal findings in adults, children, and infants. Chicago, IL: American Epilepsy Society; 2016.
26. Kaplan PW. The EEG in metabolic encephalopathy and coma. J Clin Neurophysiol. 2004;21(5):307–18.
27. Westmoreland BF, Klass DW, Sharbrough FW, Reagan TJ. Alpha-coma: electroencephalographic, clinical, pathologic, and etiologic correlations. Arch Neurol. 1975;32(11):713–8.
28. Christogianni A, Bibb R, Davis SL, Jay O, Barnett M, Evangelou N, Filingeri D. Temperature sensitivity in multiple sclerosis: an overview of its impact on sensory and cognitive symptoms. Temperature. 2018;5(3):208–23.
29. Shefa U, Kim D, Kim MS, Jeong NY, Jung J. Roles of gasotransmitters in synaptic plasticity and neuropsychiatric conditions. Neural Plast. 2018;2018:1824713.
30. Watson NV, Breedlove SM. The Mind's machine: foundations of brain and behavior. 2nd ed. Sunderland, MA, Sinauer Associates; 2016.
31. Dando SJ, Mackay-Sim A, Norton R, Currie BJ, John JAS, Ekberg JA, et al. Pathogens penetrating the central nervous system: infection pathways and the cellular and molecular mechanisms of invasion. Clin Microbiol Rev. 2014;27(4):691–726.

5 Psychosocial Sciences: Theories and Applications

Paloma Garcia, Michael W. Ishak, and Manuel Trujillo

Introduction

This chapter provides an overview of the major theories of behavior and their applications, beginning with the first mention of mental illness in Egyptian records in 1550 BC (see Fig. 5.1). In the millennium preceding 1 AD, philosophers such as Plato, Aristotle, and Hippocrates speculated about the source of thought and temperament. By 900 AD, Al-Razi began practicing a primitive form of psychotherapy. In the following decades and centuries, mentions of depression and mental illness began to increase, creating a rich lode for further developments as societies became more advanced and could utilize more resources for healthcare. Despite centuries of criminalization, exile, and subjugation of the mentally ill, in the middle of the eighteenth century, through the efforts of many (though symbolically personified in the actions of the French psychiatrist Phillipe Pinel) the mentally ill were freed from their chains, and—if initially only in theory—obtained the rights of citizenship, the dignity of the equality afforded all citizens, and the entitlement to medical care as humane and as (limitedly) effective as the general medical care of the times.

In 1879, the first experimental psychology laboratory was founded. A basic biopsychosocial conceptual framework of care grew unevenly over the years, as scientific discovery and political winds both accelerated its progress and slowed it down. The beginning of the twentieth century bore witness to great conceptual progress in biological psychiatry under the taxonomic diagnostic principles enunciated by Kraepelin and through the radical innovation regarding the science of the unconscious brought about by Freud's discovery of Psychoanalysis. Furthermore, the social dimension of the biopsychosocial model started to gain ascendancy, manifesting itself, when available, through more humane care and pragmatic access to protected rehabilitative work activities, which took place in the facilities (asylums) where patients were housed. At that time, such facilities were often located in remote areas of most states, at a safe distance from the growing urban areas perceived as too stressful for vulnerable people. In the 1920s, Piaget developed the first systematic account of developmental psychology. Freud and Piaget were followed by a myriad of other psychological theories, including behaviorism, classical conditioning, Gestalt psychology, and attachment theory. Mid-century, in the aftermath of World War II, returning military psychiatrists contributed valuable psychosocial insights that they learned from the long war. These insights included providing prompt treatment in close proximity to the patient's unit and comrades, encouraging rest, emotional support, re-moralization, and appropriate medication. These techniques were reworked and repurposed to treat patients in crisis in their communities through interventions such as psychoeducation, crisis intervention, family and community engagement, supportive psychotherapies, and the emerging (and increasingly more effective) new psychiatric medications.

Three major waves of new psychotherapies and psychosocial interventions capable of producing reasonably good outcomes and increasingly supported by solid scientific evidence emerged in the second half of the twentieth century. The first wave consisted of behavioral therapies that evolved to promote a more scientific approach to therapy grounded in experimental behavioral science. A second wave, equally committed to clinical scientific rigor, and where Beck is seen as a leading figure, focused on cognitive distortions as a driver of pathology, leading to the development of cognitive behavioral therapy (CBT). The third wave of therapies has emerged in the last two decades partly in response to the concern that, though CBT tech-

P. Garcia (✉)
Brown University, Providence, RI, USA
e-mail: paloma_garcia@brown.edu

M. W. Ishak
Princeton University, Princeton, NJ, USA
e-mail: mi1933@princeton.edu

M. Trujillo
Department of Psychiatry, New York University School of Medicine, New York, NY, USA
e-mail: Manuel.Trujillo@nyulangone.org

W. W. IsHak (ed.), *Atlas of Psychiatry*, https://doi.org/10.1007/978-3-031-15401-0_5

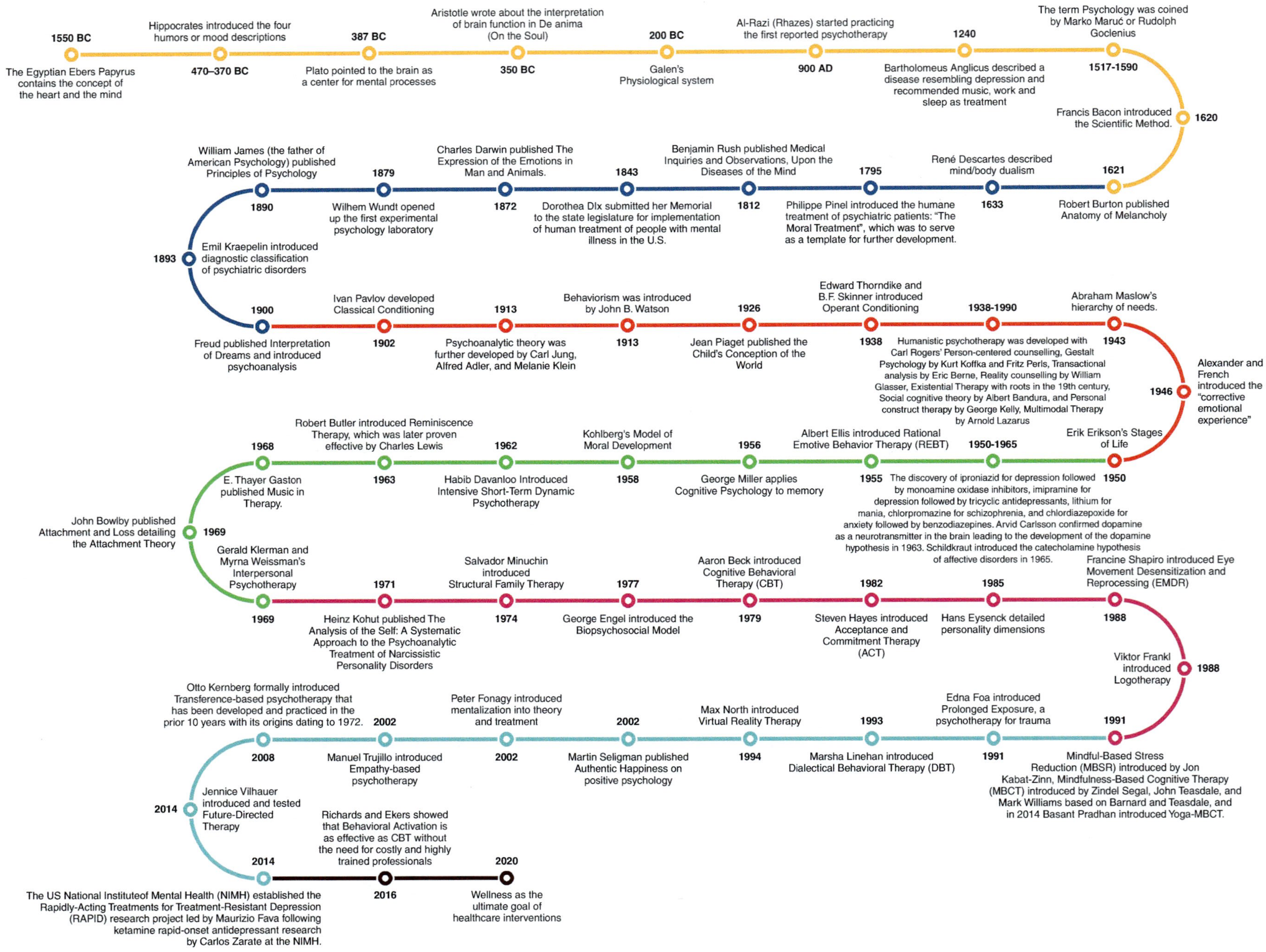

Fig. 5.1 Timeline of the psychosocial theories of behavior and development of psychotherapy

niques are fairly well validated, the link between cognitive therapy and cognitive science continues to be weak. Mindfulness-based interventions, for example, rather than challenge the validity of automatic thoughts, seek to help the patient achieve a state of present focus and to acknowledge and accept the flow of sensations, emotions, and thoughts without avoidance or negative judgment. Acceptance is aided by meditation exercises such as deep breathing, which further reduce distress by achieving a better sympathetic-parasympathetic balance. The supported work activities of yore gave rise to the now expanded principles of psychiatric rehabilitation and to professional vocational services and interventions. In the more recent decades, other therapeutic modalities, such as interpersonal psychotherapy, dialectical behavioral therapy, and behavioral activation, have gained prominence Fig. 5.1. summarizes the timeline of the psychosocial theories of behavior and the development of psychotherapy.

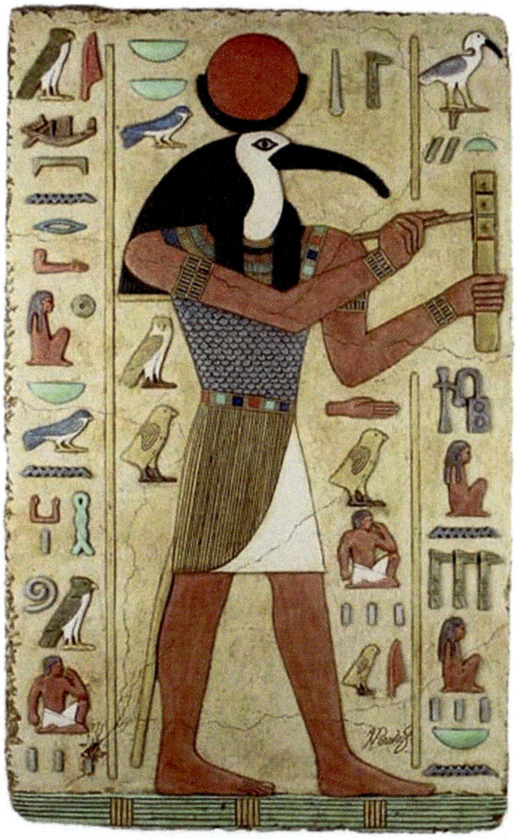

Fig. 5.2 Thoth the god of healing who also created religion, magic, philosophy, law, writing, and science. (*From* Okasha [1]; *with permission*)

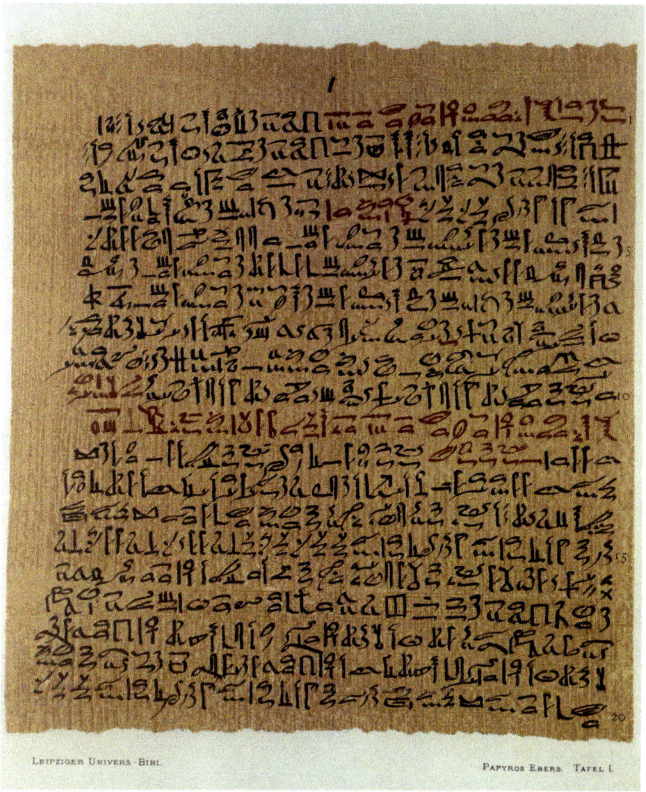

Fig. 5.3 The Egyptian Ebers Papyrus mentions depression for the first time

Theories of Behavior and Development of Psychotherapy

In early history, psychosocial behavior theories flowed from their views of mankind and attempted to understand the mind, the body, and its relationship to the cosmos (eternity). In ancient Egypt, a person was made of three parts: Khat (the body), Ka (the soul), and Ba, which transitioned the body to eternity. The Akh is the immortal self. There is no symbol in hieroglyphics to represent death. Thus, the art of healing became part and parcel of ancient Egyptian religion, and it is conceived as supporting an optimum transition to eternal life. Thoth was the god of healing (see Fig. 5.2) [1].

(1550 BC) The first mention of depression: The Egyptian Ebers Papyrus describes mood disorders as disorders of the heart and cardiovascular system. This document is a record of ancient Egyptian medicine, suggesting these mental disorders were viewed similarly to physical ones (see Fig. 5.3) [2].

(470–370 BC) Hippocrates' four humors: Hippocrates introduced the four humors, each of which corresponds to a season, natural element, and bodily fluid, to account for people's temperamental disposition. He believed that the balance of these four humors was critical for physical and mental health. The four humors were choleric (angry), sanguine (joyful), melancholic (sad), and phlegmatic (relaxed) (see Fig. 5.4) [3].

(387 BC) Plato and the brain: Plato believed that the soul contained an individual's essence and that there were three parts of the soul in the body. He believed that rationality and voluntary movement resided in the brain (Logos) and that this aspect of the soul was immortal. This part of the soul maintains its capacity to think and live after death and is continually reborn into different bodies. Anger (Thymos) and desire (Eros) were thought to

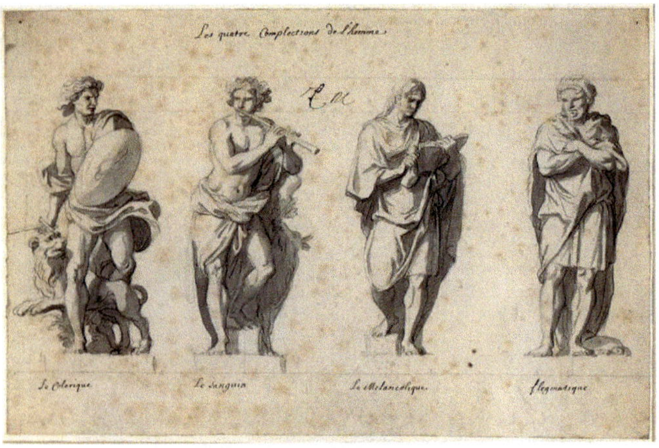

Fig. 5.4 Hippocrates' four humors (moods or temperaments): choleric (angry), sanguine (joyful), melancholic (sad), and phlegmatic (relaxed) as drawn by Charles Le Brun, part of the Grande Commande, the Palace of Versailles

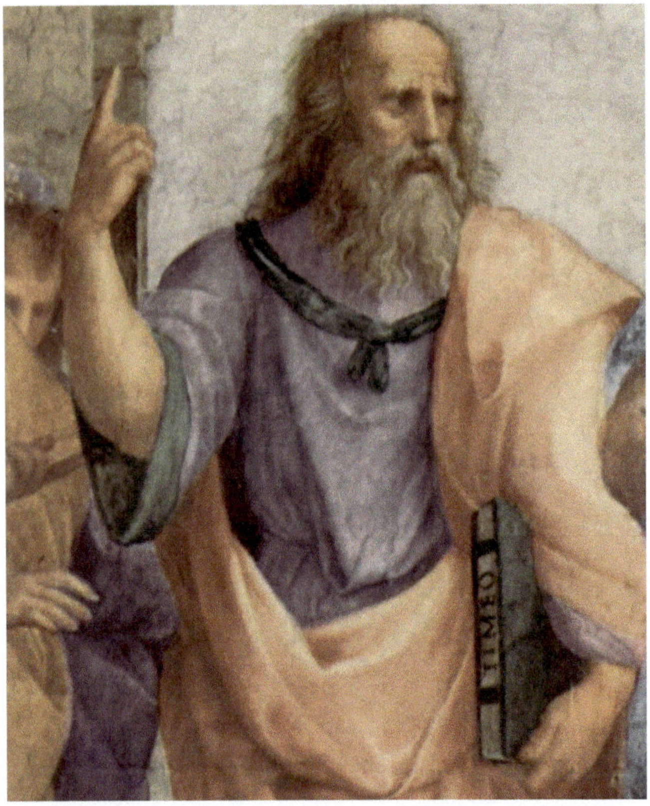

Fig. 5.5 Plato is depicted in Raphael's *The School of Athens* carrying a bound copy of Timaeus. Plato pointed to the brain as a center for mental processes and defined thought as a "dialogue of the soul with itself"

reside in the chest and stomach, respectively. This is an early rendition of Freud's conception of the mind as tripartite: with the ID being the equivalent of Plato's Eros and Thymos, and Ego (Self) and Superego would be akin to Logos (see Fig. 5.5) [4].

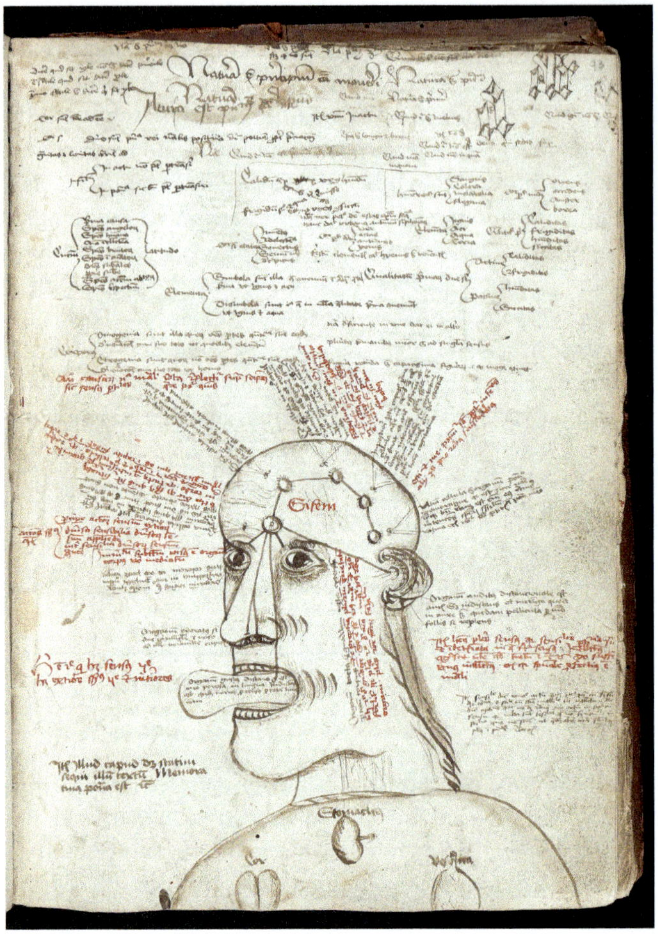

Fig. 5.6 Aristotle's De anima (On the Soul) depicts the interpretation of brain function

(350 BC) Aristotle and the brain: In *De Anima* (On the Soul), Aristotle posits that the soul serves as the true essence of any living being. He argued that only humans possess the rational soul, and he further divided the rational soul into two categories: one that contains all the mind's ideas and concepts (possible intellect) and the other that contains what the mind is currently thinking about (agent intellect). He describes agent intellect as immaterial, able to exist without the body, and immortal (see Fig. 5.6) [5].

(200 BC) Galen and the physiological system: Building upon the teachings of Hippocrates and other influential ancient Greeks, Galen asserted that four humors originated from the four bodily fluids (blood, yellow bile, black bile, and phlegm), and an imbalance of these humors would cause poor temperament or physical disease. He also posited a theory of the cardiopulmonary system, in which blood was imbued with natural spirit in the liver, vital spirit in the heart, and animal spirit in the brain (see Fig. 5.7) [6].

(900 AD) The first psychotherapist: Al-Razi was a widely known physician during the tenth century. He believed that psychological well-being was a critical factor

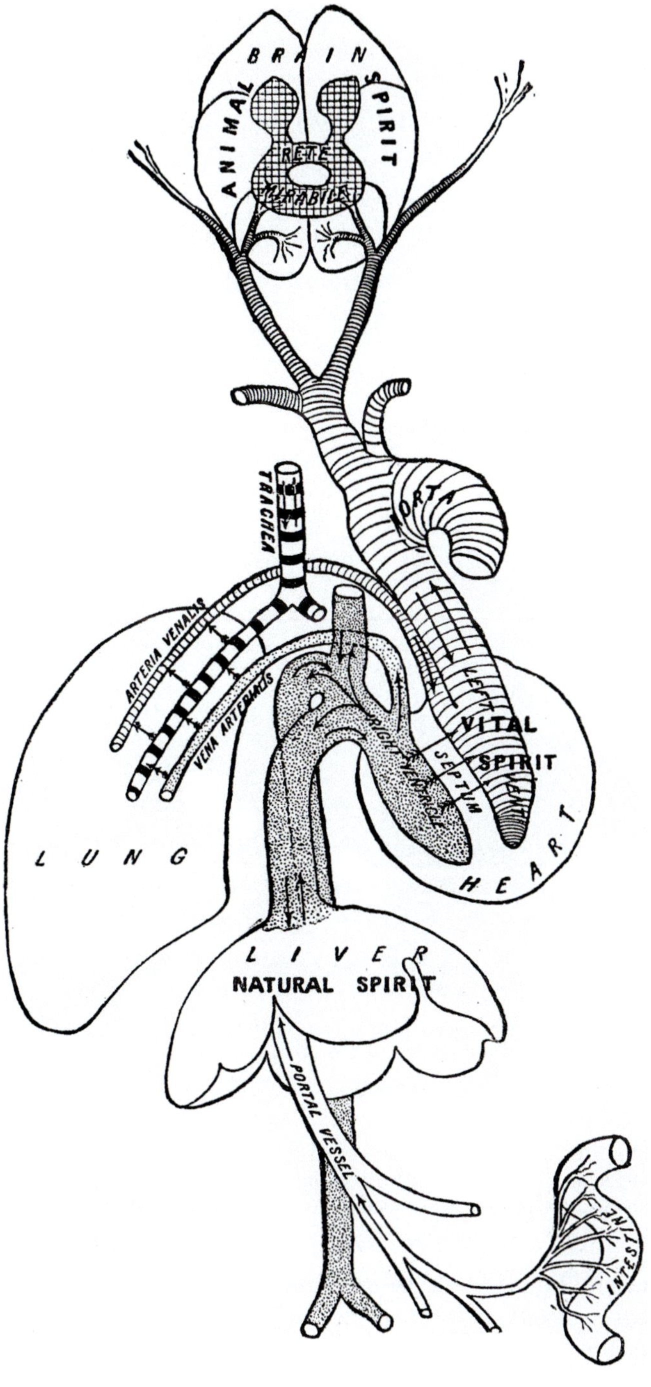

Fig. 5.7 Galen's view of the human "Physiological system"

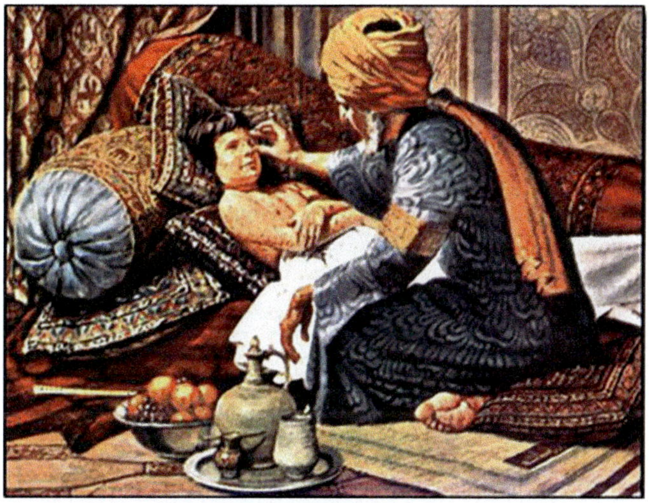

Fig. 5.8 Al-Razi (Rhazes) practiced the first reported psychotherapy. Notice the uncanny similarity of this scene to Freud's couch and the touching of the patient's forehead, which Freud used as a way to promote free associations after he abandoned hypnosis. The difference is that Freud placed himself behind the patient's couch

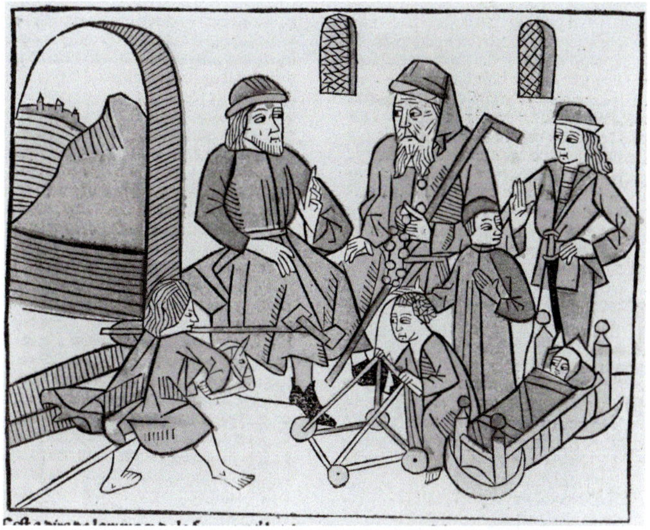

Fig. 5.9 Bartholomeus Anglicus' Stages of Life from infancy to old age woodcut from De proprietatibus rerum (On the Properties of Things). Later, he recommended music therapy, work, and sleep for depression

in physical health and understood mental illness as a medical condition. He introduced the concept of psychiatric wards and practiced some forms of psychotherapy, including a primitive form of cognitive therapy for obsessive behaviors (see Fig. 5.8) [7].

(1240) Depression described: Bartholomeus Anglicus was a monk who described a disease resembling modern-day depression in one of his many encyclopedias. He recommended music as a treatment for this mental illness (see Fig. 5.9) [8].

(1517–1590) Marculić coins the term "psychology": While the origin of the term "psychology" is often attributed to Glocenius, the term was used by Marculić over 60 years earlier. The word comes from the Greek word "psyche," which has been translated to "soul" or "life" in English (see Fig. 5.10) [9].

(1620) Knowledge is power: In his book *Novum Organum*, Francis Bacon proposed the Scientific Method, which laid the groundwork for modern scientific experi-

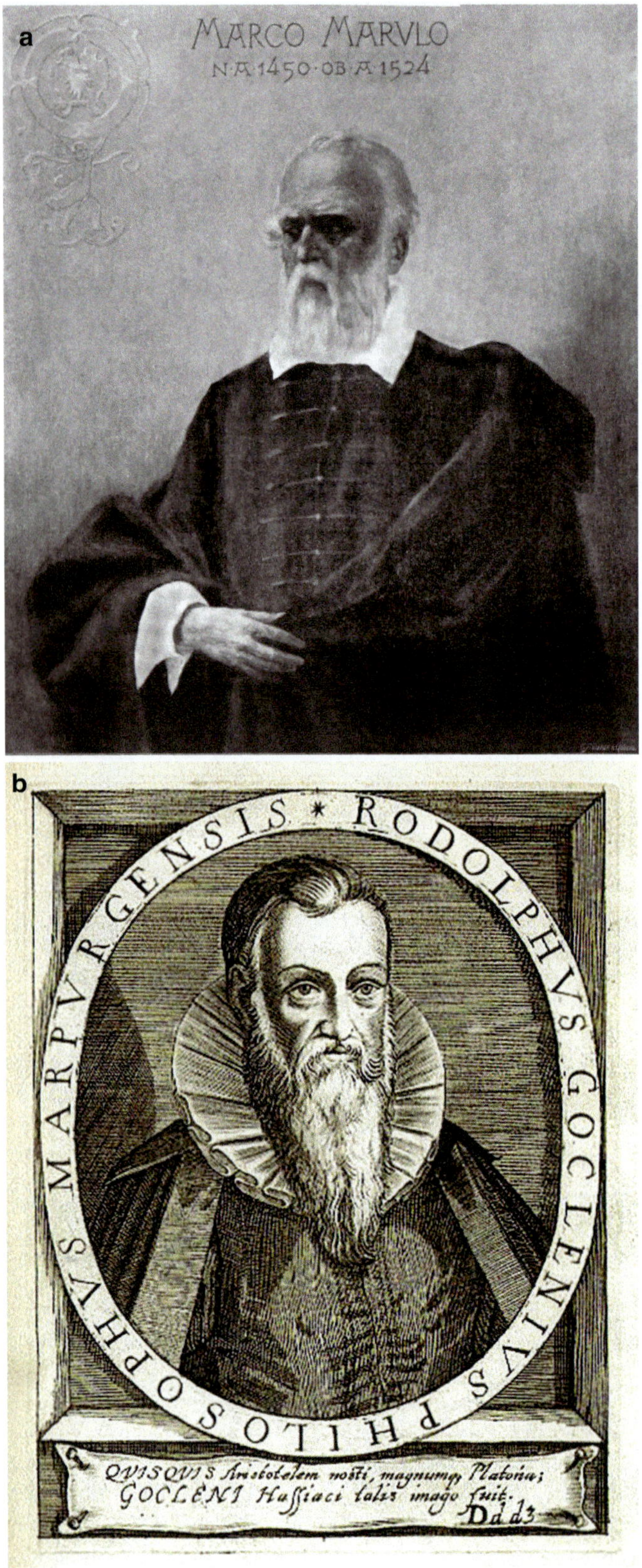

Fig. 5.10 (**a** and **b**) The term Psychology was coined by a. Marko Marulić in *Psichiologia de ratione animae humanae* (1517) or b. Rudolph Goclenius in *Yucologia hoc est de hominis perfectione, anima, ortu* (1590)

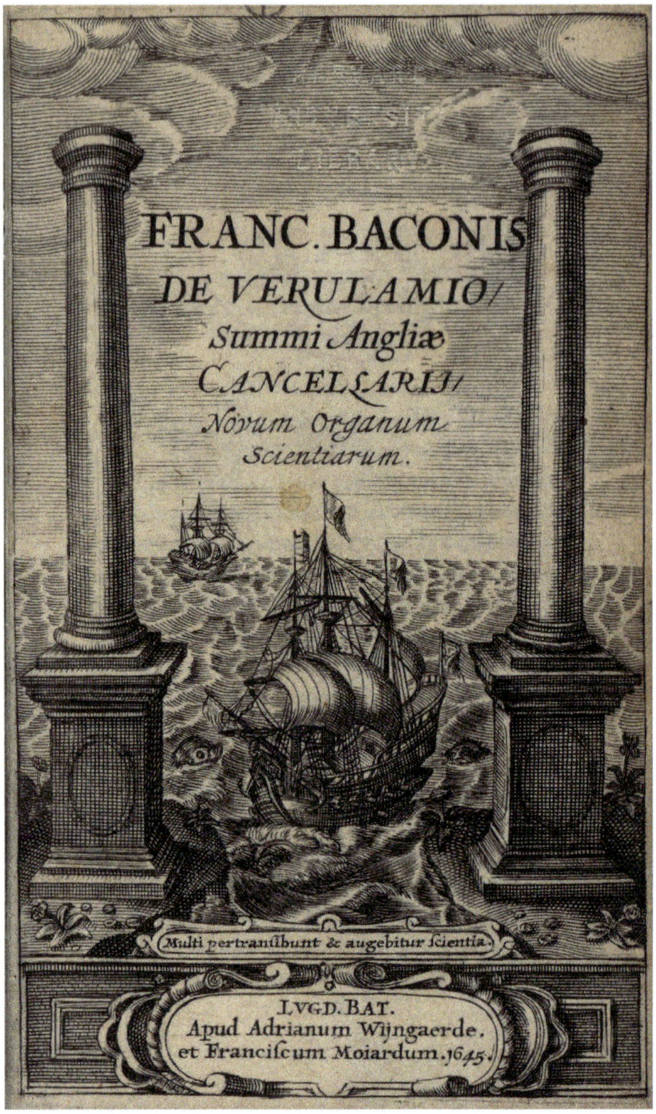

Fig. 5.11 Francis Bacon introduced the Scientific Method in Novum Organum (1620), discussed memory, imagination, and reason, and is credited with the phrase "ipsa scientia potestas est" or knowledge is power

ments. In this work, he criticized previous knowledge discovery methods for their lack of rigor and objectivity. His method emphasized systematic experimentation that included the manipulation of variables, replication, and careful observation to induce accurate facts (see Fig. 5.11) [10].

(1621) The Anatomy of Melancholy: Robert Burton published the *Anatomy of Melancholy*, which discussed melancholy (now known as, but not limited to, depression) in a highly interdisciplinary manner. He proposed possible treatments for melancholy, including exercise, nutrition, and marriage. While the book was intended to be a medical textbook, it discussed melancholy more broadly and emphasized its relationships with a wide variety of disciplines (see Fig. 5.12) [11].

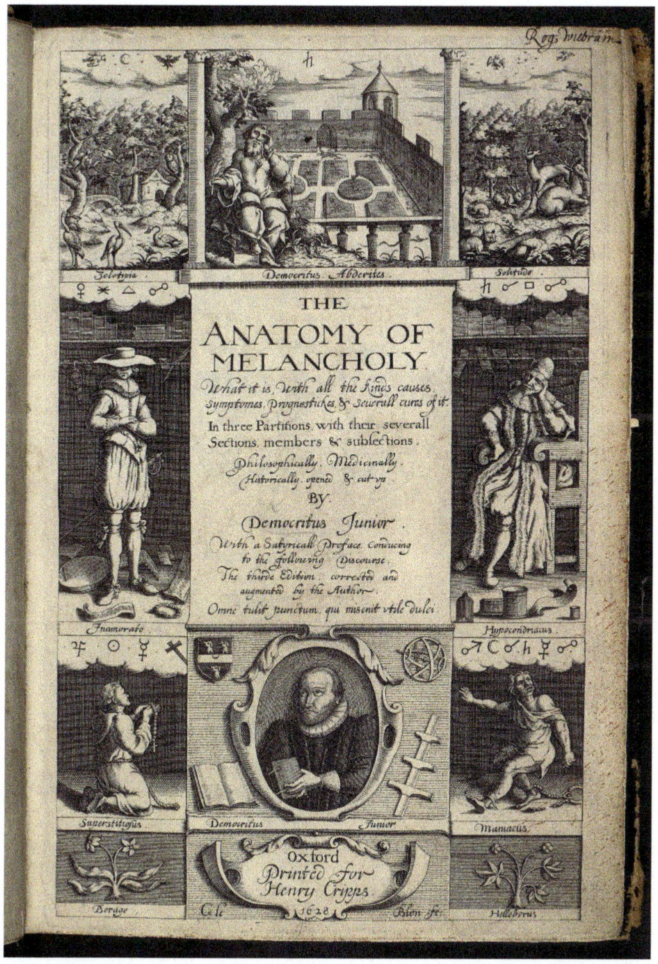

Fig. 5.12 Robert Burton's *Anatomy of Melancholy* describes the psychosocial factors in depression, such as social isolation and poverty, and recommends exercise, nutrition, herbs, travel, music, and marriage as treatment

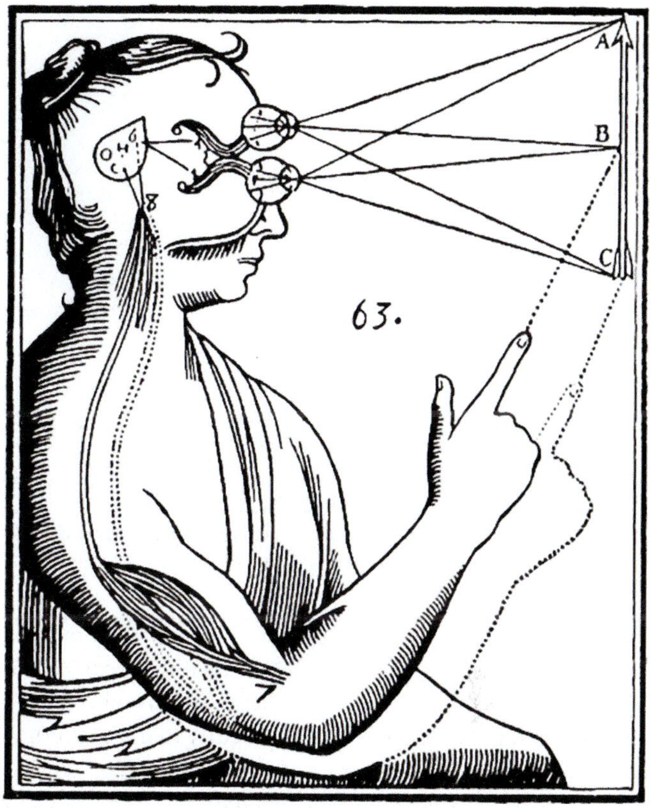

Fig. 5.13 René Descartes' illustration of mind/body dualism. Descartes believed inputs were passed on by the sensory organs to the epiphysis in the brain and from there to the immaterial spirit

(1633) René Descartes and the mind/body: Descartes proposed Cartesian dualism, a theory that states that it is possible for the mind and the body to exist without each other. He argued that the mind is immaterial and does not exist in space, and thus the mind and the body are composed of two distinct substances (see Fig. 5.13) [12].

(1795) Philippe Pinel introduces the humane treatment of psychiatric patients: In tandem with the primitive physical care available for mental disorders in the 1790s, the concept of "moral" treatment emerged. The name moral treatment lends itself to historical misinterpretation. In the philosophical context of the enlightenment where it developed, the word "moral" alludes to the psychological functions of the mind, not just to the narrow conformance of behavior to existing "moral rules." The moral treatment of the eighteenth century is the equivalent of the psychological treatment of today. In the context of the enlightenment-era focus on social welfare and people's rights, the moral treatment concept consisted of three critical components: (1) the recognition and respect of the patient's dignity, (2) a rudimentary form of humane psychological treatment, and (3) few social interventions, beyond improved living conditions and access to work activities (see Fig. 5.14) [13].

Pinel's moral treatment combined the key elements of new psychiatry (biopsychosocial psychiatry), as it included the essential components of this movement. Pinel did away with treatments such as bleeding, purging, and blistering and instead promoted a therapy program that included discussion of personal difficulties with the patient and the cultivation of an ongoing therapeutic dialogue that provided the patients with support, encouragement, and with enough trust to dare to discuss the distortions of their own thinking. By creating such an atmosphere, Pinel opened the door to what later was named the "milieu" therapy movement, the purposeful modification of features of the patient's living environment to achieve therapeutic goals.

Philippe Pinel's essay "Memoir on Madness" in 1794 explains his "psychological treatment," the principles and values of the humane method that made him a de facto founder of psychiatry as a legitimate medical specialty in France. In fact, Memoir of Madness has been recently described in the American Journal of Psychiatry as a fundamental text of modern psychiatry [13]. Pinel discarded

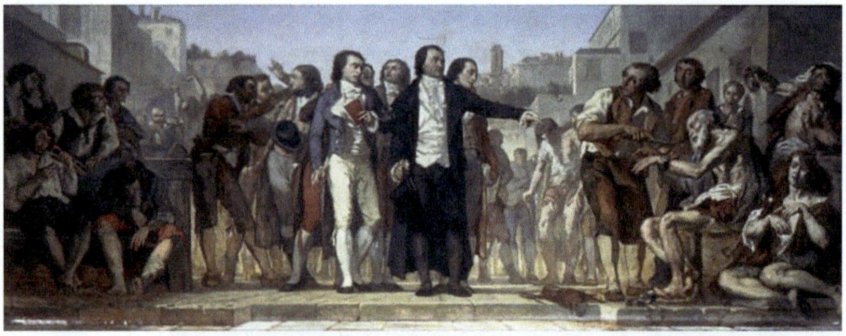

Fig. 5.14 French psychiatrist Philippe Pinel releasing the mentally ill from their chains at the Bicêtre asylum in Paris. Painting by Charles-Louis Muller

Table 5.1 The conceptual triad that moves psychiatry forward

1. **A theory of man**: A philosophical view about **what it means to be human**
2. **A theory of mind** and behavior which includes theories and **methods the study healthy and correct ill behaviors**
3. **A theory of therapy**: **Practices, technologies, and institutions** to care for people suffering from behavioral disorders

the long-popular equation of mental illness with demoniacal possession; instead, he regarded mental illness as the result of excessive exposure to social and psychological stresses and, in some measure, of heredity and physiological damage.

In *Nosographie philosophique* (Philosophical Classification of Diseases, 1798), he distinguished various psychoses and described, among other phenomena, hallucinations, withdrawal, and a variety of other symptoms. Pinel's writings convey the importance of each patient as a special person, a person endowed with a reason that can be appealed to, with sensitive and deep personal feelings, and with a unique life history, often full of tragedy and trauma. Pinel's book had an enormous influence on both French and Anglo-American psychiatrists during the nineteenth century. Going forward, all therapeutic proposals seemed to have followed the same methodological sequence, a foundational conceptual triad.

Pinel believed strongly in the primacy of liberty and equality of all citizens and the value of the individual as the subject of such rights. From that base, a theory of mind followed, based on the moral (psychological subjective) domain that gave rise to a new clinical concept: the moral treatment, which in turn gave birth to new institutions and practices that could implement such values (see Table 5.1).

(1812) Benjamin Rush, the 'Father of American Psychiatry': Rush adopted many of Pinel's principles and extended his influence. He published the first descriptions of mental illness and its treatment in his 1812 book Medical Inquiries and Observations, Upon the Diseases of the Mind (see Fig. 5.15) [14].

(1843) Dorothea Dix advocated for better treatment of people with mental illness: Dix, an influential social reformer of the Second Great Awakening, advocated with passionate energy for the improvements of the living conditions and treatment of the mentally ill (see Fig. 5.16) [15].

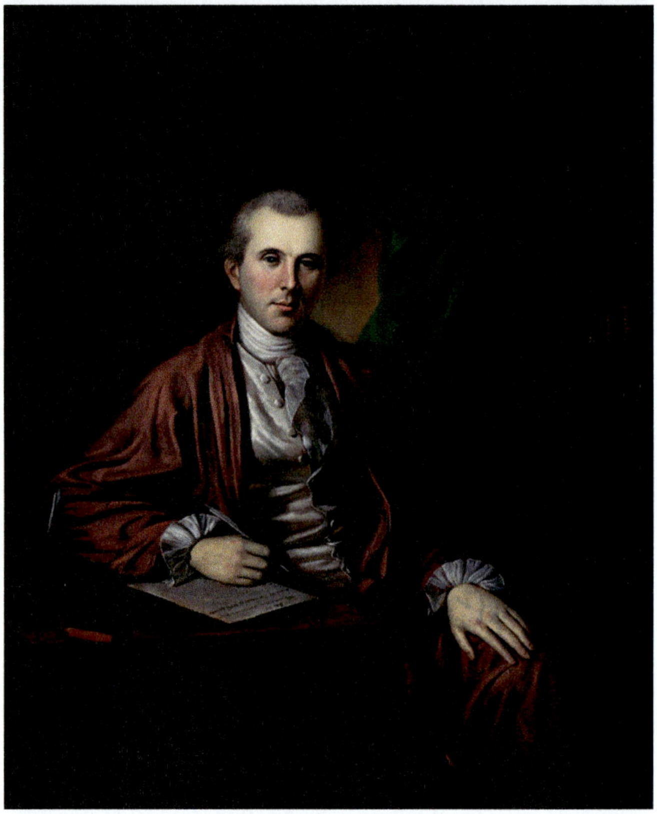

Fig. 5.15 Dr. Benjamin Rush was painted by Charles Willson Peale in 1783

(1872) Charles Darwin and the major scientific theories of emotional behavior: In 1872, Darwin published *The Expression of the Emotions in Man and Animals*, which inspired most scientific theories of emotional behavior (see Fig. 5.17) [16].

(1879) The first experimental psychology laboratory: Wilhelm Wundt is regarded as the father of experimental psychology after founding the first experimental psychology laboratory. This was particularly significant because it established psychology as an independent field of study (see Fig. 5.18) [17].

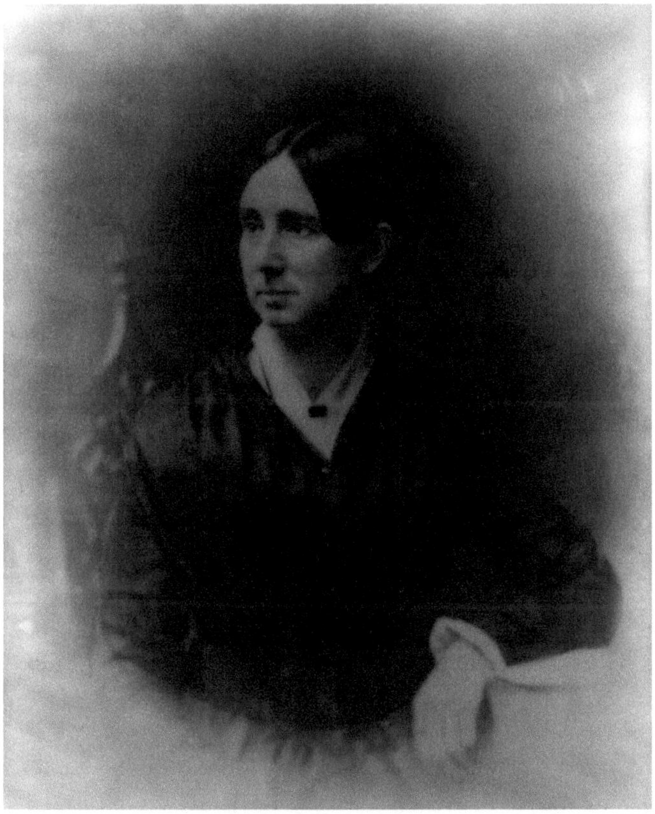

Fig. 5.16 Dorothea Lynde Dix persuaded numerous legislatures throughout the United States to develop humane facilities to treat mental illness. Based on her systematic observations and vivid descriptions of the abhorrent conditions in which mentally ill people were housed and treated, Dix petitioned to create Asylums in her 1843 Memorial to the state legislature. She posited that Asylums would be spaces where moral treatment could be implemented so that hope, kindness, and therapeutic ministrations would make a recovery possible for many formerly deemed hopeless patients

(1890) William James, the father of American psychology: James described in detail the stream of consciousness, emotion, habit, and will in his book *The Principles of Psychology* in 1890, which contains his most famous quote about attention *"My experience is what I agree to attend to"* (see Fig. 5.19) [18].

(1893) Emil Kraepelin introduced a diagnostic classification of psychiatric disorders: He is often considered the founder of modern scientific psychiatry, psychopharmacology, and psychiatric genetics. Kraepelin theorized much ahead of his time that mental illness largely originates from genetics (see Fig. 5.20) [19].

(1887) Psychoanalysis and psychoanalytic psychotherapies: Early treatment of mental illness was based on either a religio-magical or a naturalistic view of disease. The religious and magical era, which still bears significant influence in vast areas of the world today, saw certain forms of personal suffering, personal isolation, or of alienation from family or group as caused by an evil spirit that had gained entrance into the sufferer. Treatment was based on having the subject participate in suitable rites under the guidance of a tribe elder, a priest–physician, or a shaman.

By contrast, the naturalistic tradition viewed mental illness as a phenomenon that could be understood using the same methods of biology or general medicine. Although these enlightenment-era naturalistic ideas often lacked a theory of the mind, they formally expressed interest in the patient's emotional lives and initiated the systematic exploration of the patient's life narrative and inner subjective experiences and feelings. The next big step in the conceptual development of psychotherapy was using hypnosis. A leading figure in that movement was the French physician Jean-Martin Charcot who used hypnosis to treat the behavioral and conversion symptoms of Parisian females under his care (see Fig. 5.21) [20].

(1900) Freud's take on psychotherapy: Learning from Charcot, the Viennese physician Sigmund Freud, first working with his contemporary Josef Breuer and later on his own, modified the hypnotic procedure. He applied light pressure on the patient's forehead while the patient, adopting a recumbent position on the iconic psychoanalytic couch (Fig. 5.22), was encouraged to allow the free flow of thoughts without exercising censorship. That procedure (a precursor of the classical psychoanalytic free association) allowed Freud to make seminal discoveries about the relationship between adult emotional illness and certain emotionally charged, damaging childhood experiences that had undergone some degree of suppression or repression. Out of these discoveries grew the theory and practice of the first modern "talking cure": classical psychoanalysis that made possible the subsequent development of the many forms of psychoanalytic psychotherapies practiced today (see Fig. 5.22) [21].

(1900–1915) Freud's unconscious mind: Freud emphasized the importance of unconscious thought, and a central tenet of his theory was the belief that children had an unconscious sexual desire for their opposite-sex parent and unconscious hatred for their same-sex parent. Furthermore, he believed that dreams represented repressed desires and could be used to study the unconscious mind (see Fig. 5.23) [22].

(1902) Pavlov's dog and classical conditioning: Pavlov demonstrated that dogs could learn to associate two unrelated stimuli when they were regularly presented together. In one experiment, he rang a bell before feeding the dogs to condition them to associate the sound of the bell with food. After the conditioning phase, the dogs would salivate upon hearing the bell ring, even if they were not presented with food (see Fig. 5.24) [23].

(1913) Jung's analytical psychology: After working closely with Freud on psychoanalysis, Carl Jung separated from Freud and coined the term analytical psychology. Jung's views concerning the human unconscious differed significantly from Freud's, specifically in regard to Jung's

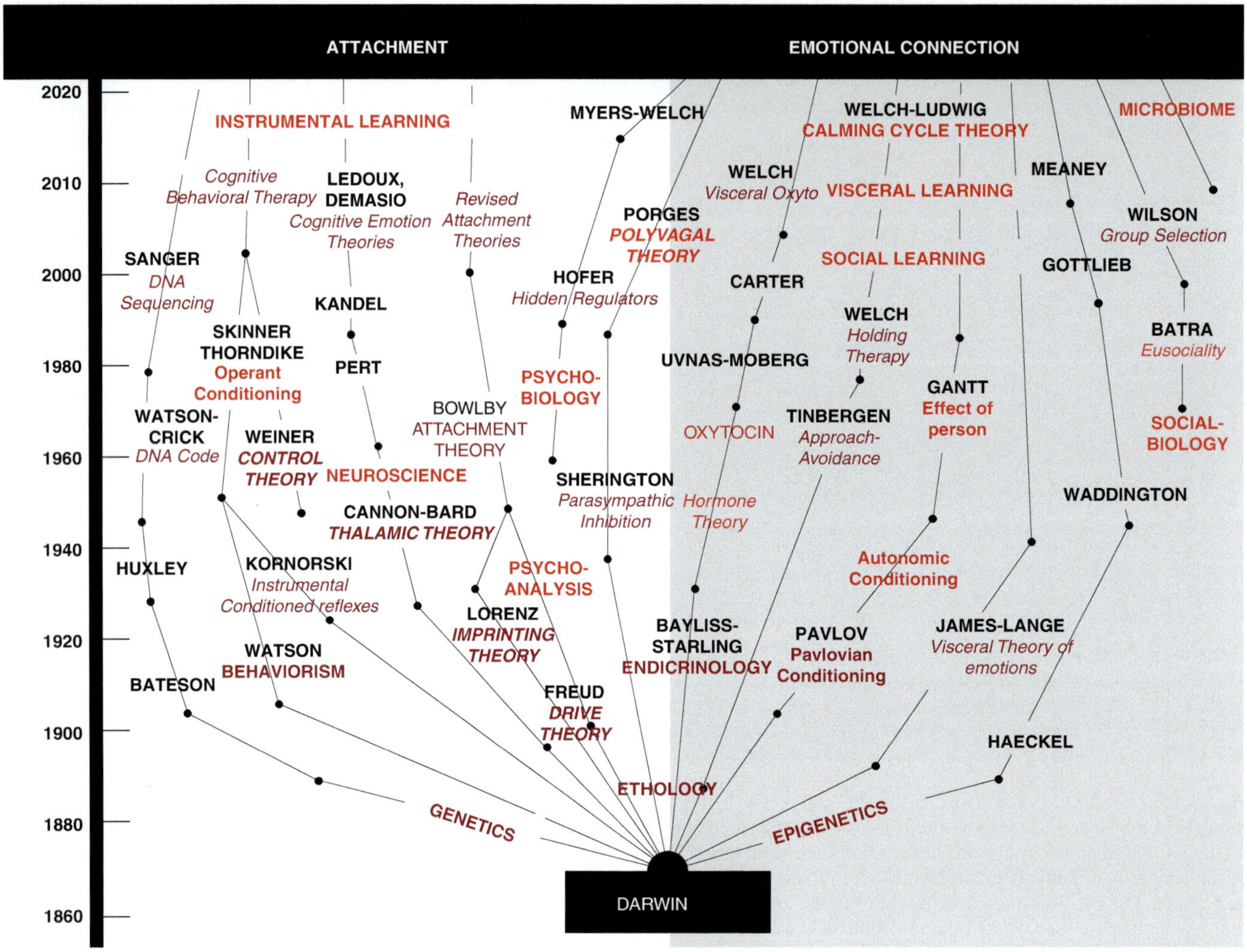

Fig. 5.17 A diagram showing the contrasting development of theories related to the dilemmas of instincts and heart rate control since Darwin. On the left are theories leading to the behavioral construct of attachment. On the right are theories leading to the behavioral construct of emotional connection. The two sides highlight scientific arguments and theoretical conflicts in multiple fields. (*From* Ludwig and Welch [16]; Attribution 4.0 International (CC BY 4.0). https://creativecommons.org/licenses/by/4.0)

indifference toward the influence of sexual development and his emphasis on the collective unconscious. Jung believed that our psyche was partially constituted by the collective unconscious, the part of the unconscious mind that is shared amongst all human beings and passed down through generations. He posited that the primary goal of life was self-actualization, which is achieved through merging personal consciousness with the collective unconscious through symbols (Jungian archetypes). Jungian archetypes originate from the collective unconscious and are underlying forms—shaped by sociocultural factors—that govern conscious behavior (see Fig. 5.25) [24].

(1913) Adler's individual psychology: Alfred Adler founded individual psychology, a subdiscipline that focuses on the unity and indivisibility of each individual's personality [25].

His theories of behavior emphasized the importance of feelings of inferiority and resulting overcompensation. Melanie Klein was among the first psychologists to use psychoanalysis with children. She was also critical in the development of object relations theory, which highlights the importance of interpersonal relationships and the environment in child development (see Fig. 5.26) [26].

(1913) Watson's behaviorism: John B. Watson proposed behaviorism, which states that behavior can be understood by observing external events without requiring introspection or study of internal states. He posited that psychology must focus on objective, observable behaviors to accurately predict and control behavior because introspection is unreliable. According to his theory, all behaviors are learned through environmental conditioning. Furthermore, he believed that there was little difference between human and animal behav-

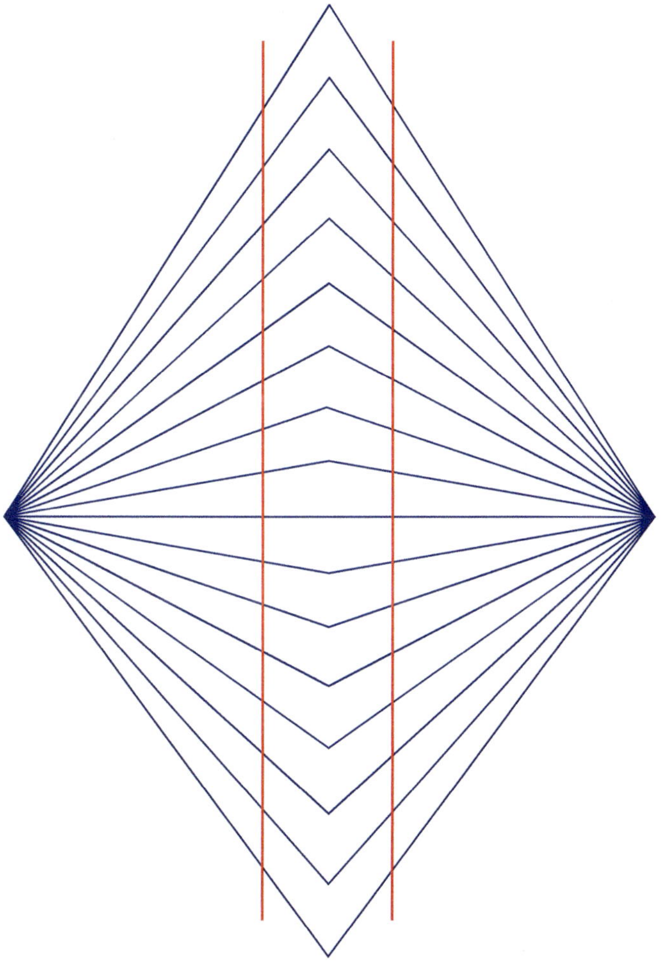

Fig. 5.18 The Wundt Illusion shown above characterizes the advanced study of perception that took place in this laboratory. While the two red lines are actually straight and parallel, they appear as though they are curved to many observers. (Creative Commons Attribution-Share Alike 3.0 Unported; https://creativecommons.org/licenses/by-sa/3.0/deed.en)

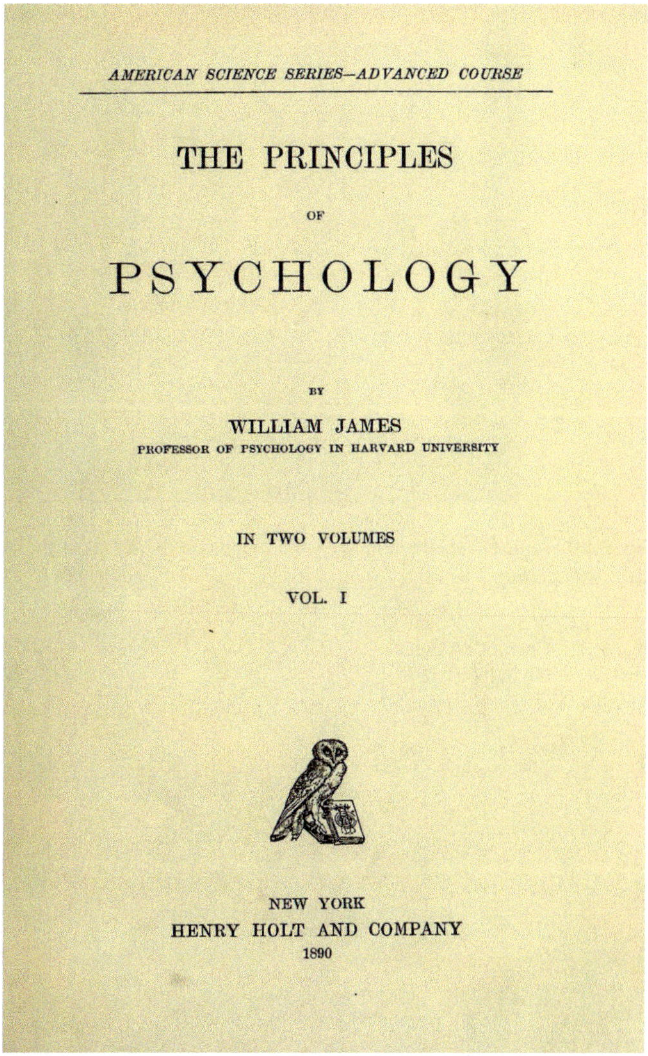
AMERICAN SCIENCE SERIES—ADVANCED COURSE

THE PRINCIPLES

OF

PSYCHOLOGY

BY

WILLIAM JAMES

PROFESSOR OF PSYCHOLOGY IN HARVARD UNIVERSITY

IN TWO VOLUMES

VOL. I

NEW YORK

HENRY HOLT AND COMPANY

1890

Fig. 5.19 William James' 1890 The Principles of Psychology was a breakthrough text for this developing field: "Millions of items of the outward order are present to my senses which never properly enter into my experience. Why? Because they have no interest in me. My experience is what I agree to attend to. Only those items which I notice shape my mind—without selective interest, experience is utter chaos. Interest alone gives accent and emphasis, light and shade, background and foreground intelligible perspective in a word. It varies in every creature, but without it, the consciousness of every creature would be a chaotic gray indiscriminateness, impossible for us even to conceive" [18]

ior, so research conducted on animals could be easily applied to humans (see Fig. 5.27) [27].

(1926) Piaget's stages of cognitive development: Through observations of his own children, Jean Piaget recognized that children think in a fundamentally different way than adults. He believed that children were born with innate reflexes but acquire most of their skills and knowledge from their environments. He proposed four stages of cognitive development (see Fig. 5.28), which illustrate the developmental progression of skills and complex thought in children [28].

(1938) Operant conditioning: Operant conditioning rests on the basic tenet that the consequences of an action determine the likelihood that it is repeated. After extensive work with animals, Thorndike proposed the law of effect, which states that behaviors followed by a positive reward are more likely to be repeated, and behaviors followed by a negative consequence are less likely to be repeated. Skinner derived operant conditioning from Thorndike's law of effect and further studied different types and schedules of reinforcement (see Fig. 5.29) [29].

(1935) Gestalt psychology: Gestalt psychology is a theory of perception that seeks to explain perception in terms of patterns or configurations rather than individual constituents. This theory delineated the Gestalt principles of perceptual grouping and organization, including the proximity principle, the similarity principle, the closure principle, the symmetry principle, and the continuity principle, among others.

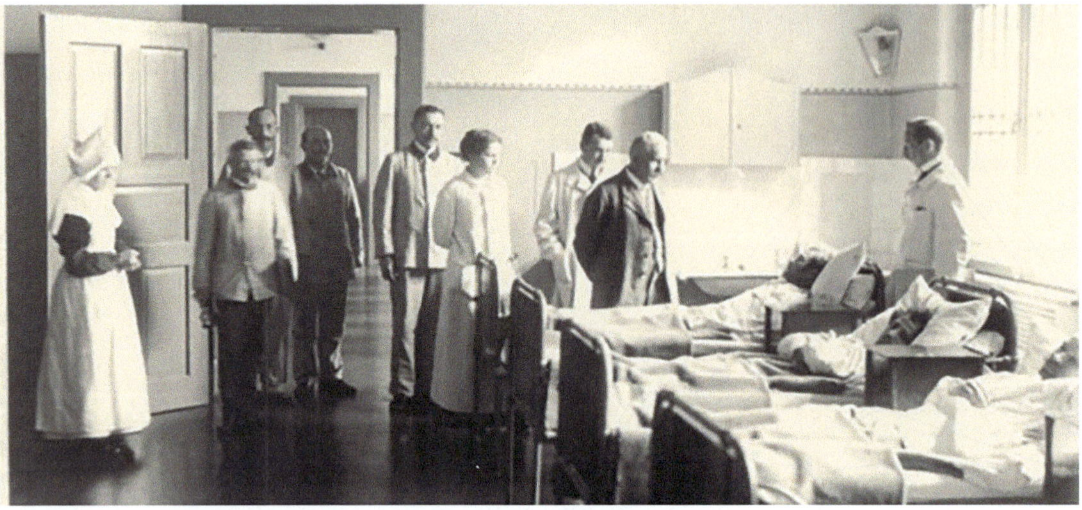

Fig. 5.20 Emil Kraepelin completes his rounds on the wards at the Munich clinic. (*From* The University Department of Psychiatry in Munich [19]; *with permission*)

Fig. 5.21 Charcot's Clinical Lessons at the Salpêtrière in Paris in 1887

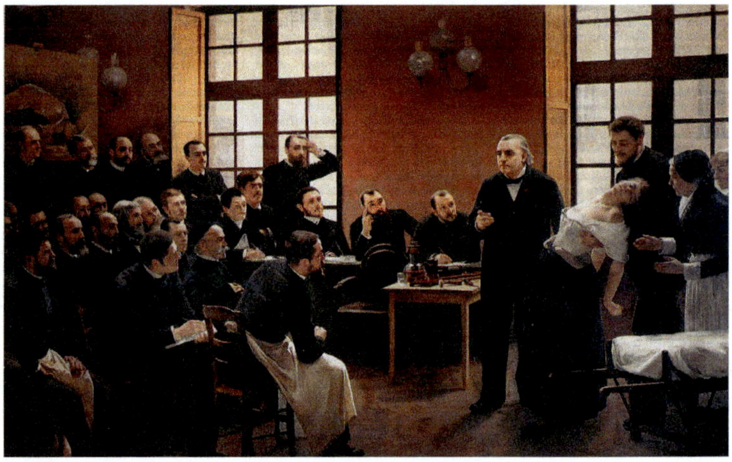

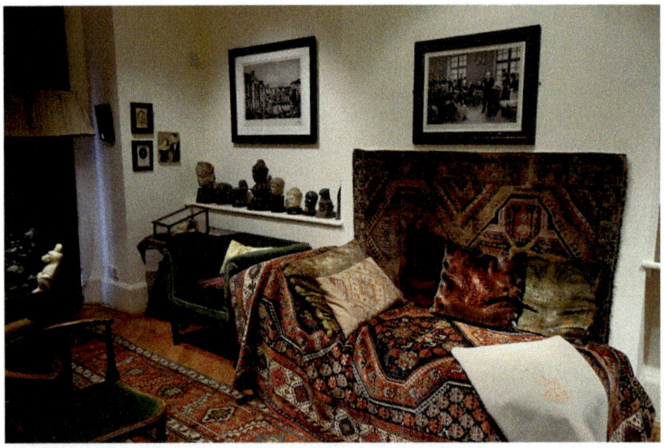

Fig. 5.22 Sigmund Freud introduced psychoanalysis. The patient would lie down on the couch while Freud sat on the chair behind the patient, encouraging the free expression of thoughts and feelings (free association), taking notes, and ultimately making interpretations leading to the development of insight into one's behavior

The similarity principle (see Fig. 5.30) states that objects are perceptually grouped together if they share similar qualities such as a color or shape [30].

(1957) Berne's theory of transactional analysis: Eric Berne developed the concept of transactional analysis, in which the therapist evaluates social transactions to classify the ego state of the patient. The transactional analysis proposes three potential ego states: parent, adult, and child. The parent ego state consists of behaviors, feelings, and thoughts that unconsciously mimic parental figures. The child's ego state consists of behaviors, feelings, and thoughts similar to childhood. The adult ego state is a state in which individuals view reality objectively and rationally, and the goal of transactional analysis is to strengthen this ego state (see Fig. 5.31) [31].

(1943) Maslow's hierarchy of needs: Abraham Maslow's hierarchy of needs is a theory of behavioral motivation intended to illustrate the pattern of human motivation. Starting from the bottom of the pyramid, Maslow proposed that individuals must satisfy the needs of each level before

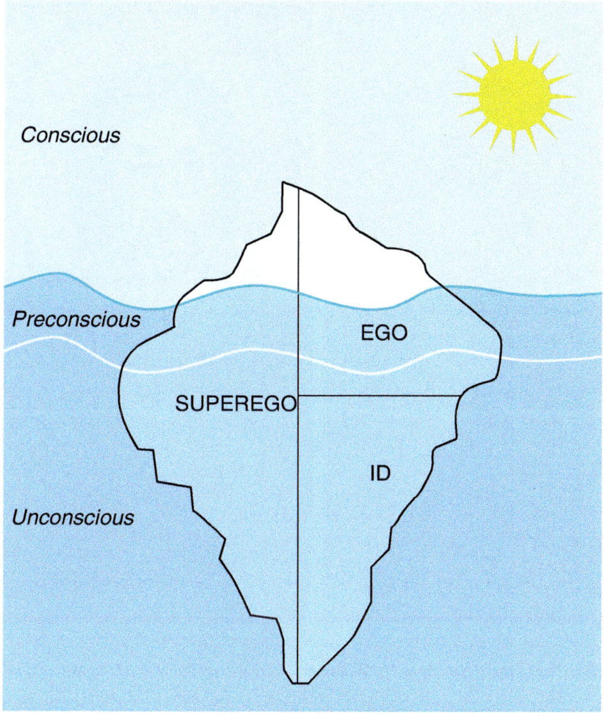

Fig. 5.23 Freud believed the personality could be divided into three components: the Id, the Ego, and the Superego. The Id is the most primal, driven by pleasure and desire, and is fully subconscious. The ego, partially conscious, attempts to satisfy the desires of the Id in a socially acceptable and realistic manner. The superego, also only partially conscious, serves as a moral regulator

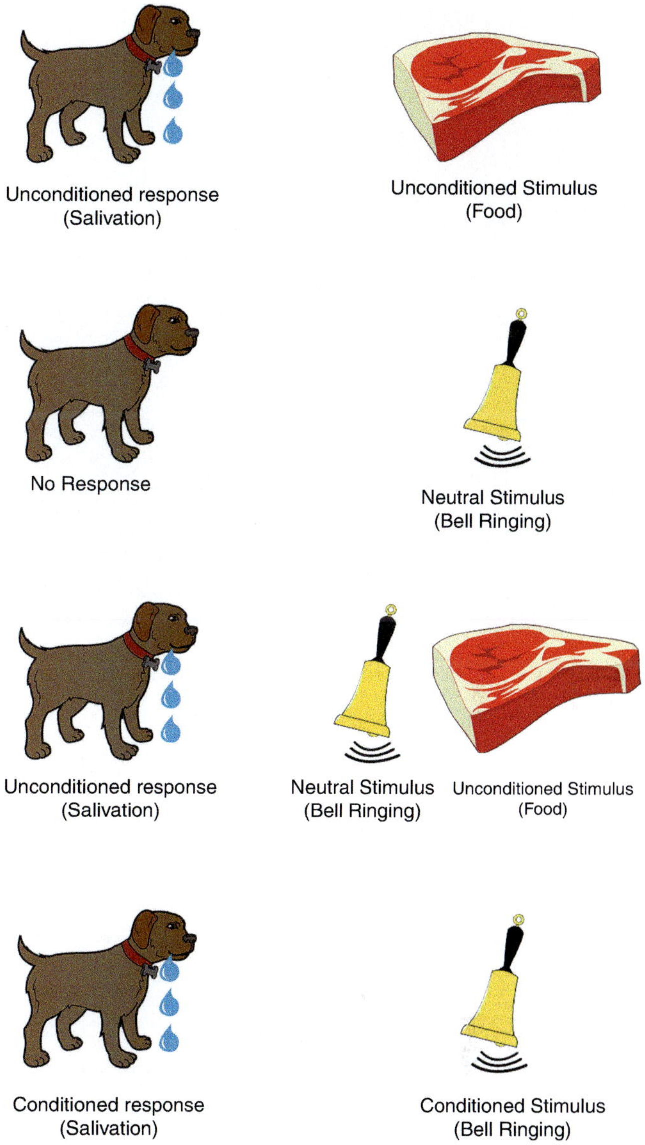

Fig. 5.24 Ivan Pavlov's Classical Conditioning is still enormously relevant to the field of psychology

motivation arises for the next one. The lowest level, physiological needs, consists of basic needs such as food, water, and shelter. The second level is safety, and the third level includes intimate relationships and friendships. The fourth level concerns self-esteem and feeling of accomplishment, and the final level is self-actualization (see Fig. 5.32) [32].

(1946) The corrective emotional experience: Alexander and French proposed the "corrective emotional experience," in which patients reexperience previously repressed thoughts and emotions about their parents. Patients are instructed to redirect the emotions they felt as a child toward their therapist, and the therapist must assume an active role and respond in a way that is opposite to the patient's expectations. Importantly, Alexander posits that it is not enough for the patient to gain insight into their previously repressed emotions solely—they must actually experience a new outcome to instill the idea that a new resolution is possible (see Fig. 5.33) [33].

(1950) Erikson's stages of life: Erik Erikson's stages of psychosocial development consist of eight sequential stages, each of which is characterized by two opposing tendencies, one positive and one negative (see Fig. 5.34) [34].

(1950–1965) The golden age of psychopharmacology: The 1950s were rich with discovery of new psychiatric drugs. Iproniazid was introduced as a treatment for depression, followed by monoamine oxidase inhibitors, imipramine, and tricyclic antidepressants. Other drugs discovered included lithium for mania, chlorpromazine for schizophrenia, and chlordiazepoxide for anxiety, followed by benzodiazepines. Arvid Carlsson confirmed dopamine as a neurotransmitter in the brain, leading to the development of the dopamine hypothesis in 1963. Schildkraut introduced the catecholamine hypothesis of affective disorders in 1965 [35].

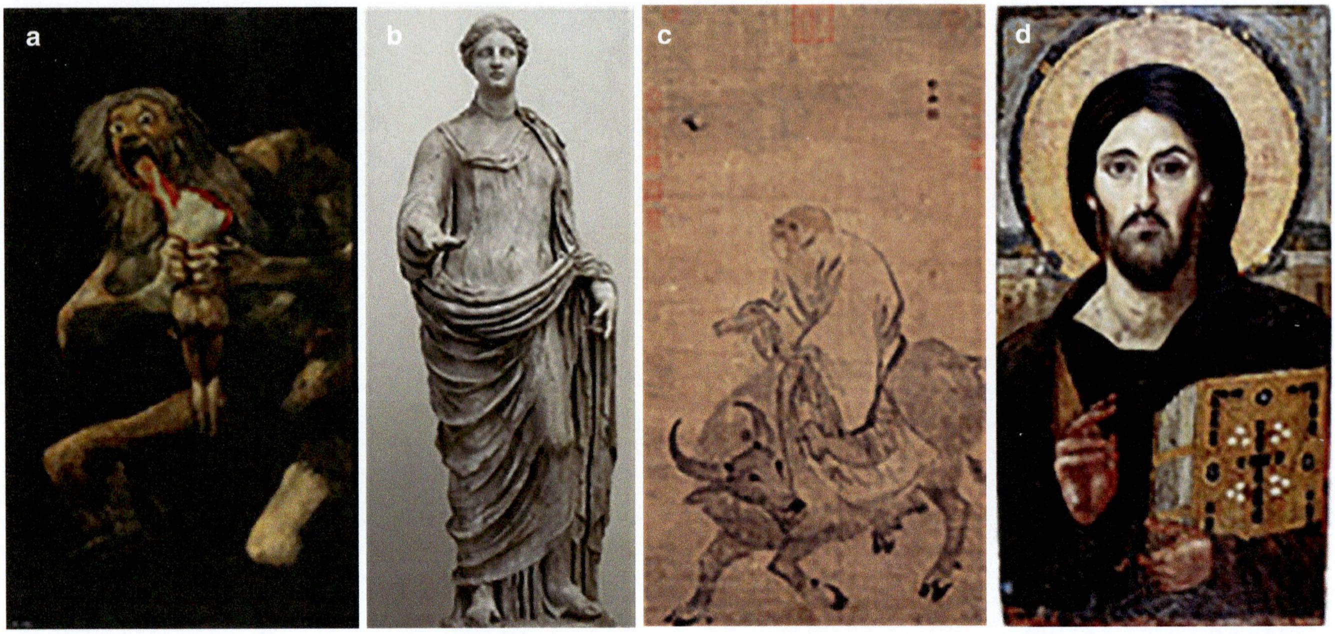

Fig. 5.25 Carl Jung's Common archetypal motifs include (**a**) *The Devourer*, (**b**) *The Great/Benevolent Mothe*r, (**c**) *The Wise Old Man*, and (**d**) *The Hero/Self*

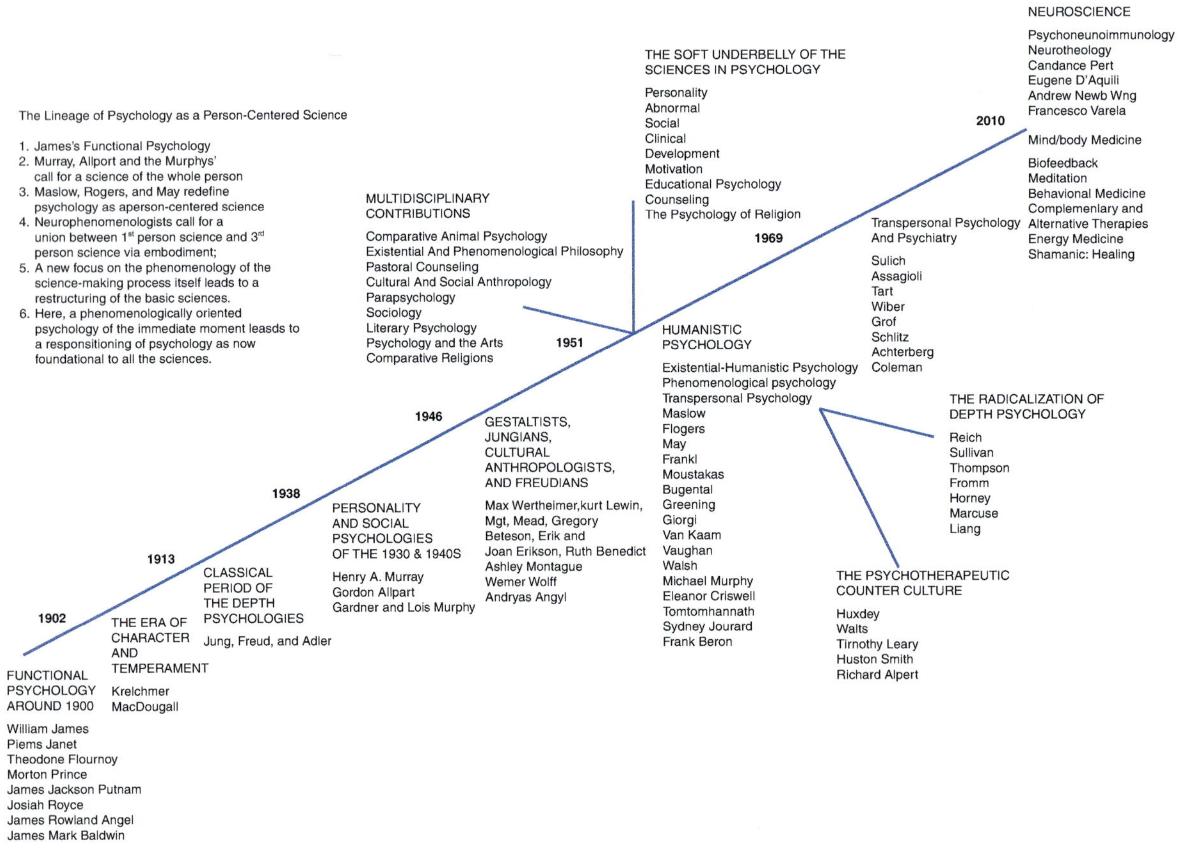

Fig. 5.26 The lineage of theories of 'Individual-based' psychology and psychotherapy. (*From* Rieber [77]; *with permission*)

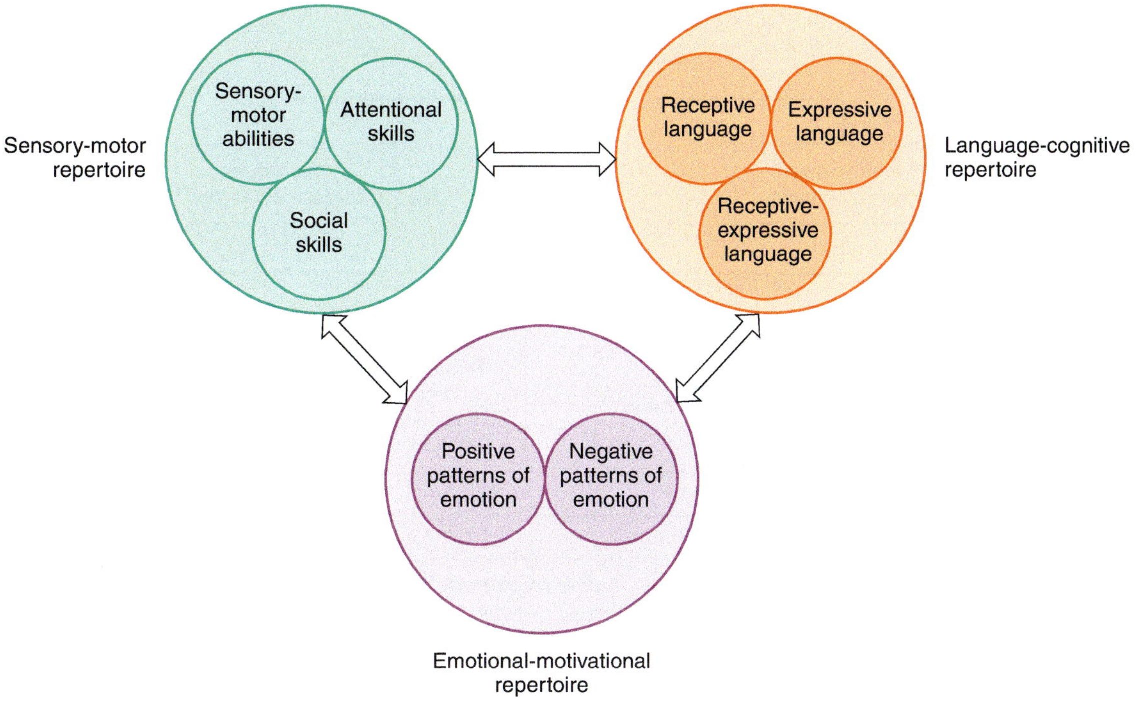

Fig. 5.27 Behaviorism was introduced by John B. Watson. Behavioral repertoires of personality are shown here based on information from Staats' Behavior and personality: psychological behaviorism

Fig. 5.28 Key features of Piaget's stages of cognitive development. *(Reprinted from* Oogarah-Pratap et al. [78]; *with permission)*

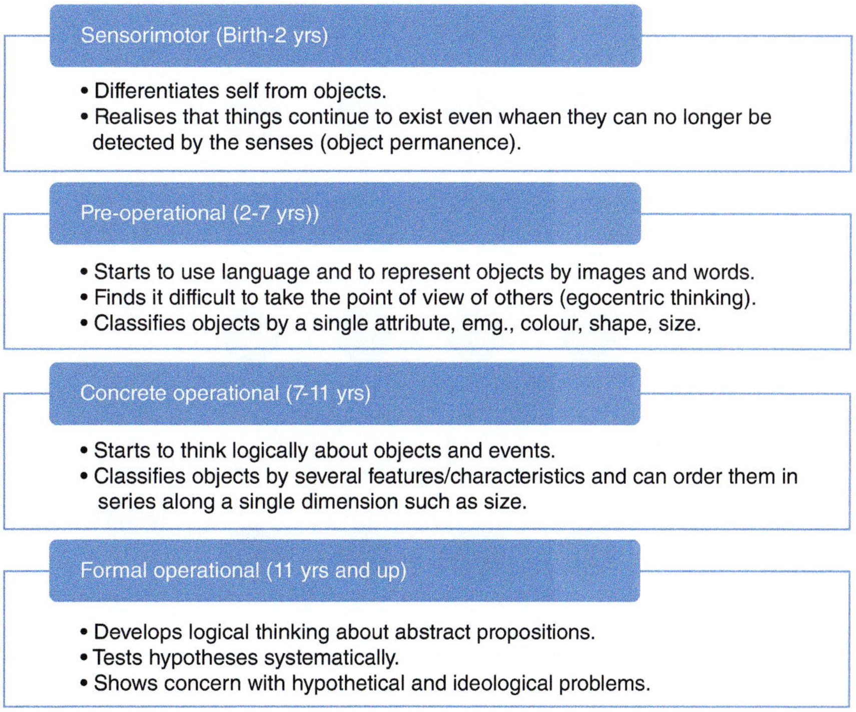

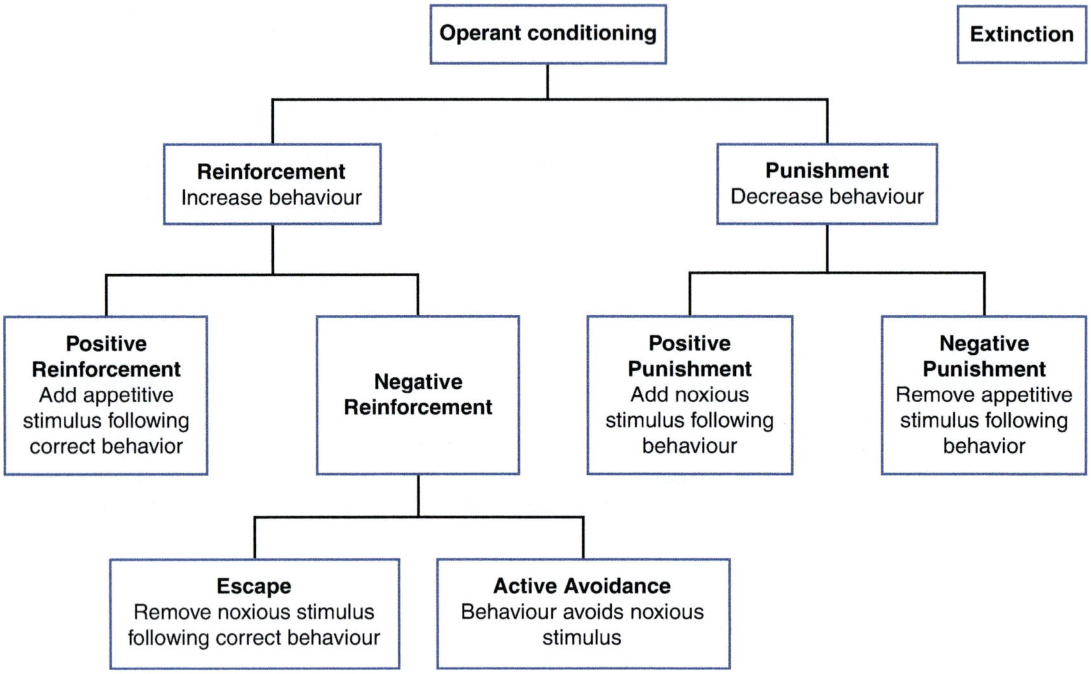

Fig. 5.29 Edward Thorndike and B.F. Skinner introduced Operant Conditioning

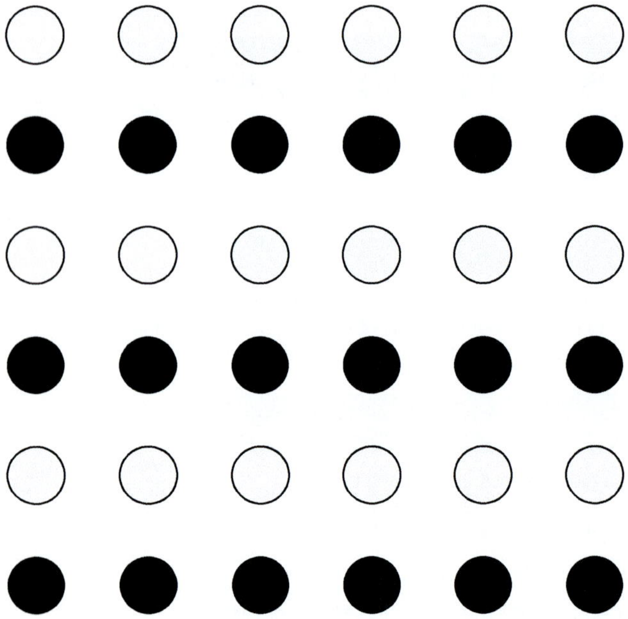

Fig. 5.30 Kurt Koffka published *Principles of Gestalt Psychology* with a number of principles, including the principle of similarity shown here

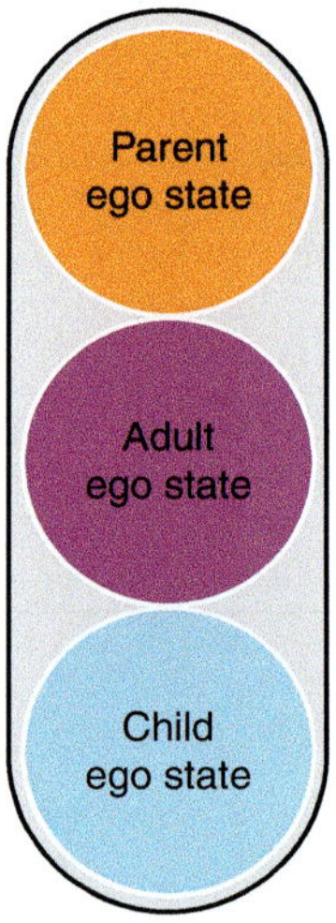

Fig. 5.31 Structural diagram of personality, created by Eric Berne

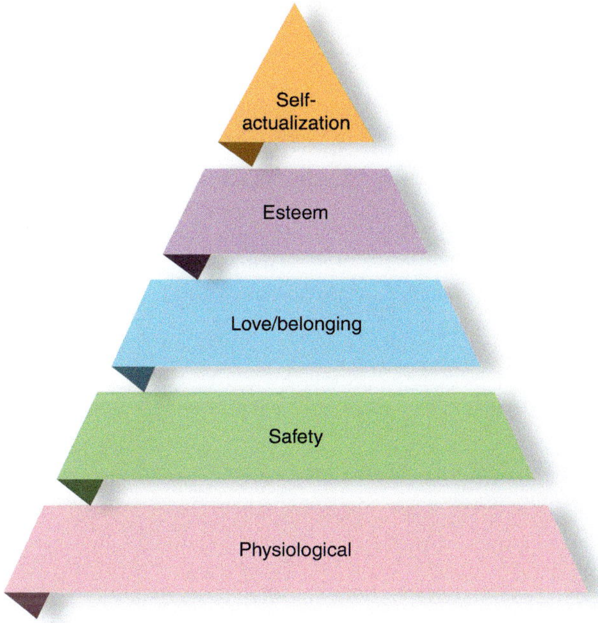

Fig. 5.32 Abraham Maslow's hierarchy of needs started humanism as a force in psychology

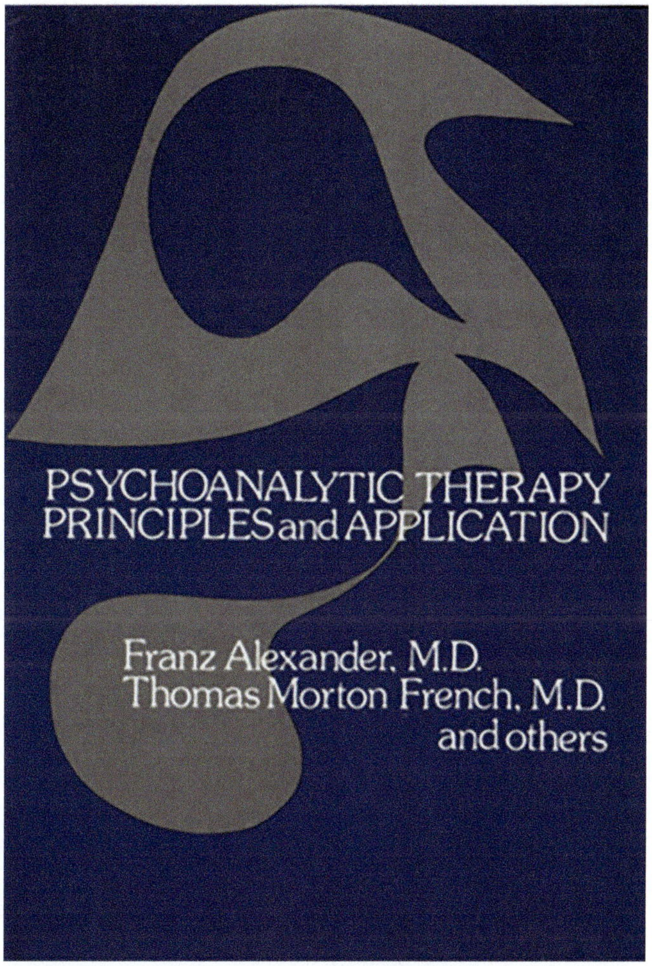

Fig. 5.33 Alexander and French introduced the corrective emotional experience

The dopamine hypothesis, which postulated that symptoms of schizophrenia are related to hyperactive dopamine transmission, was introduced following Arvid Carlsson's discovery of dopamine as a neurotransmitter in the brain and his joint discovery with Margit Lindqvist that dopamine receptors are blocked by chlorpromazine and haloperidol (see Fig. 5.35) [36].

(1965) The catecholamine hypothesis of affective disorders: This hypothesis was introduced by Schildkraut [37] and continued by Bunney and Davis [38]. It turned into the monoamine hypothesis implicating serotonin, norepinephrine, and dopamine leading to the development of newer antidepressants (see Fig. 5.36) [39].

(1955) Rational emotive behavior therapy (REBT): REBT relies on Ellis's insight that individuals have a choice between healthy and unhealthy negative emotions in the face of adversity, but they often self-train to choose unhealthy coping strategies. His theory consists of the "ABCs of REBT": when goals are hindered and adversity (A) is encountered, individuals use either useful, rational beliefs or irrational and dysfunctional beliefs (B) to construct consequences (C) (feelings and actions). REBT employs three main techniques, each corresponding to one of the ABCs. Problem-solving techniques are taught to address adverse events (A), cognitive restructuring techniques address dysfunctional and irrational beliefs, and coping strategies are taught to help the patient manage the consequences (C) of the adverse events and their dysfunctional attitudes about them (see Fig. 5.37) [40].

(1956) Miller's magical number: George Miller's 1956 article "The magical number seven plus or minus two…" functionally introduced the concept of working memory into the field of psychology. In this experiment, he found that humans can effectively use five to nine categories (with an average of seven) when classifying stimuli. He also demonstrated that humans, on average, could remember a chronological list of roughly seven random words. Finally, he found that people can estimate the number of objects presented to them without counting if there are seven objects or fewer (see Fig. 5.38) [41].

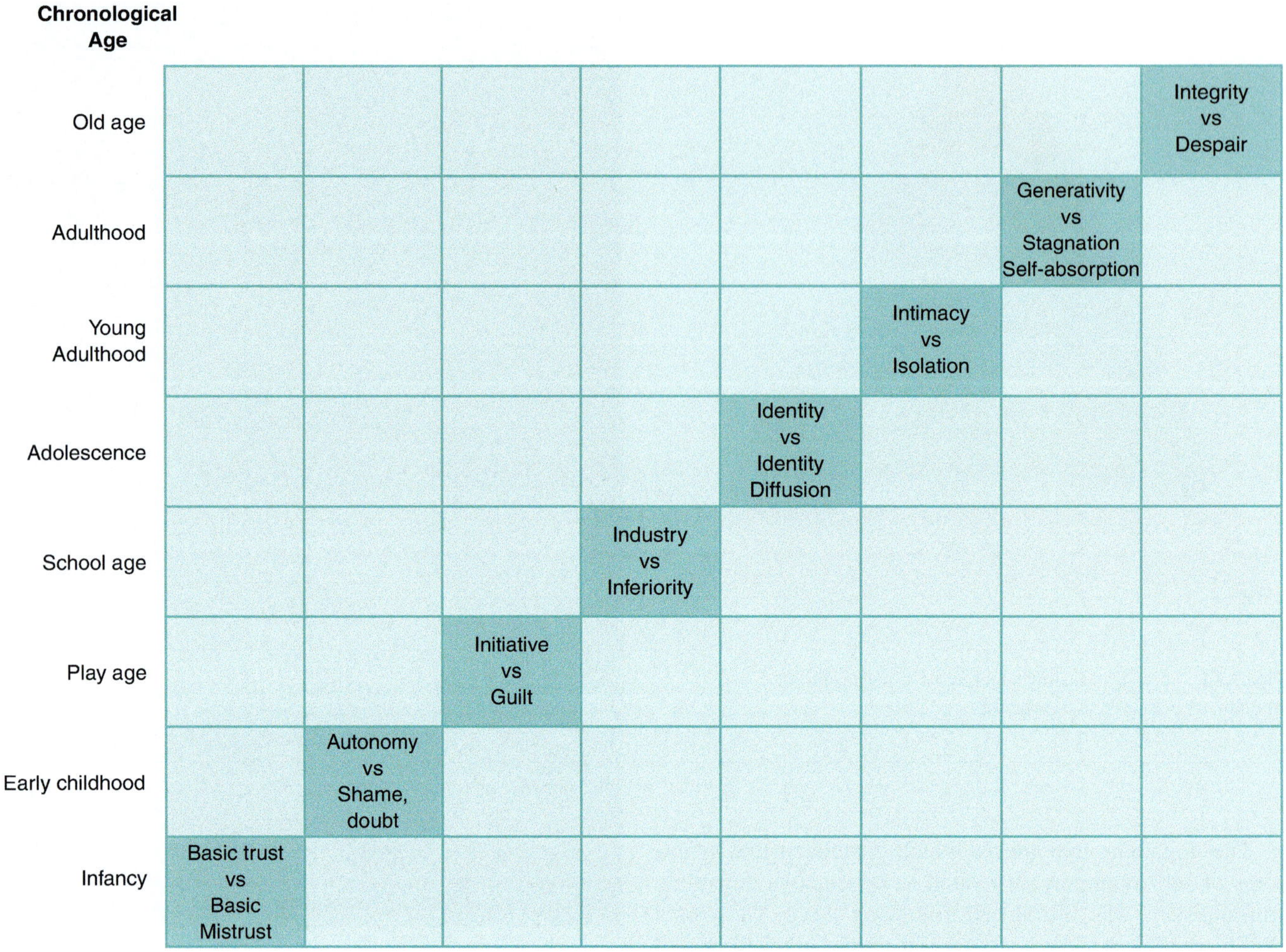

Fig. 5.34 Erik Erikson's Stages of Psychosocial Development. Erikson posits that each of these stages leads to the development of a virtue or a maldevelopment—a virtue in the case of the positive tendency and maldevelopment in the case of the negative tendency. For example, in stage 2, the potential virtue is a will, and the potential maldevelopment is the compulsion (*Reprinted from* Marcia [79]; *with permission*)

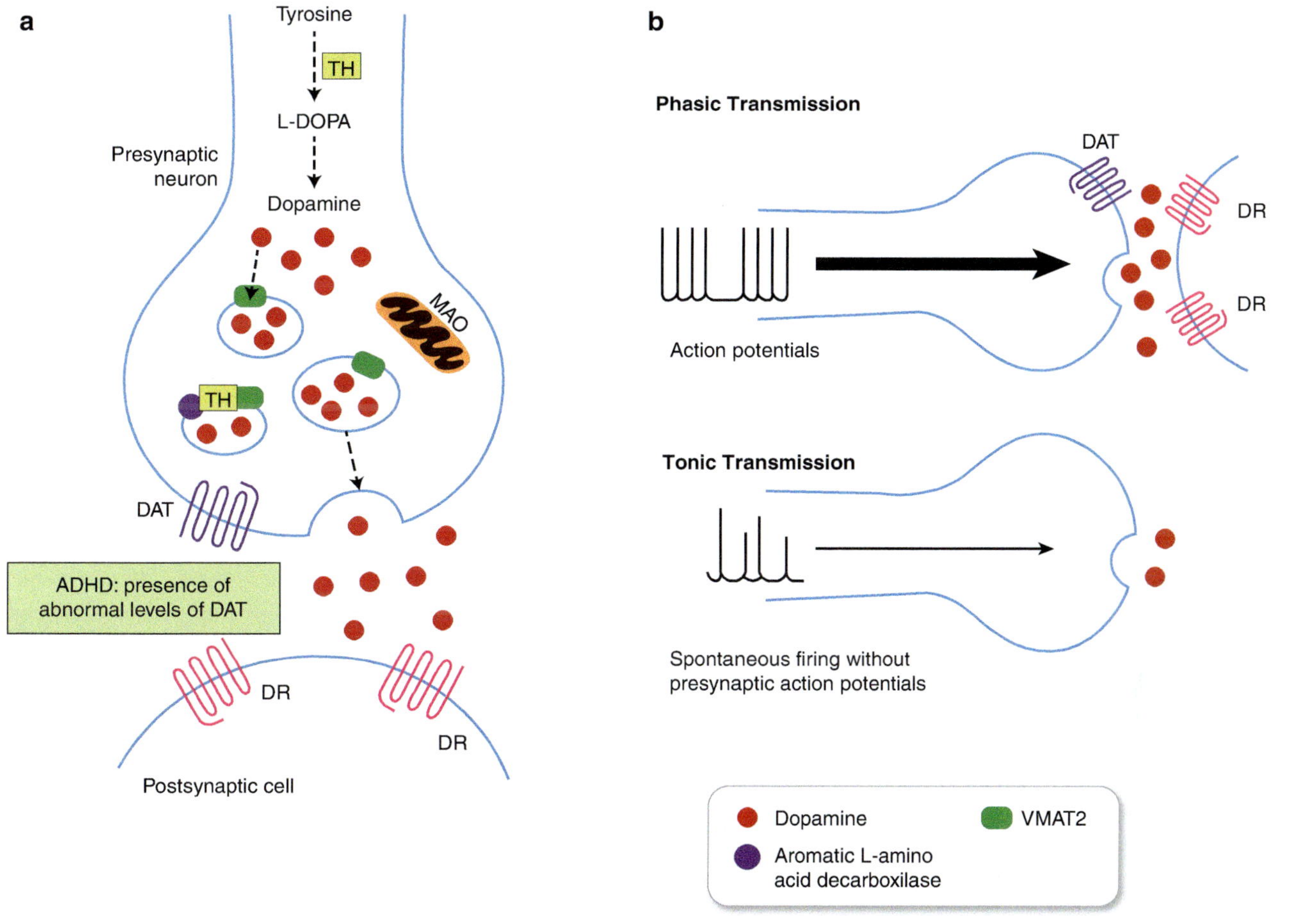

Fig. 5.35 Dopamine synthesis and phasic/tonic transmissions. (**a**) Primary metabolic route involving a two-step synthesis: First, tyrosine hydroxylase (TH) converts tyrosine to L-DOPA, which can then be converted to dopamine. Dopamine is transported from the cytosol by a vesicular monoamine transporter (VMAT2) into synaptic vesicles, where it is stored until released into the synaptic cleft. Dopamine degradation pathways with monoamine oxidase (MAO) are present in the outer mitochondrial membrane. Dopamine receptors are present in both post and presynaptic neurons (including dopamine transporter, DAT). Moreover, there is an association between the presence of atypical levels of DAT and the onset of ADHD. (**b**) Dopamine phasic transmission is triggered by action potentials that reach the dopaminergic neuron synapse, resulting in a fast and transient dopamine release in the synaptic cleft due to synchronized burst firing. Tonic transmission occurs by slow and irregular firing in the neuron without presynaptic action potentials, being regulated by the activity of other neurons and neurotransmitter reuptake or degradation. (*From* Klein et al. [80] and Bilder et al. [81]; *with permission*)

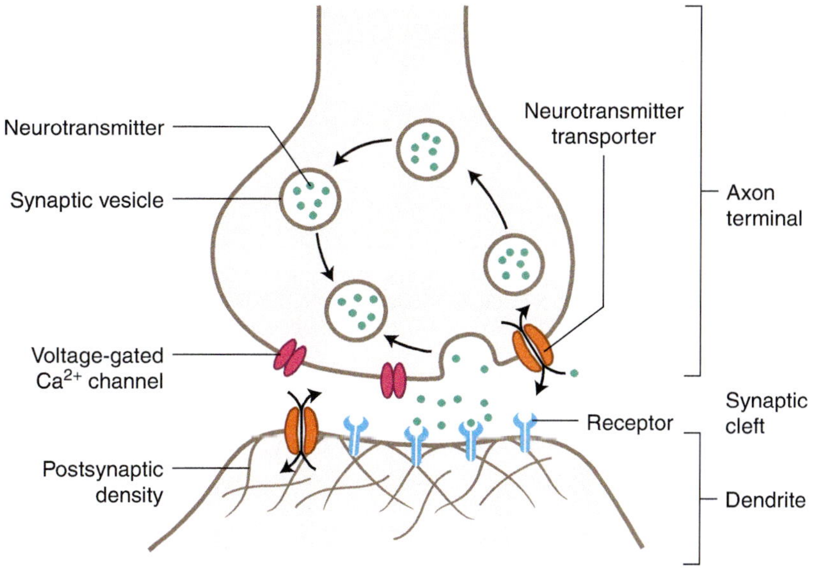

Fig. 5.36 A breakthrough neurobiological hypothesis. A deficiency of norepinephrine (NE) was hypothesized to produce major depression based on the antidepressant effects of monoamine oxidase inhibitors, which reduced NE metabolism, thus increasing NE, and response to imipramine, which increased NE. Furthermore, the effects of reserpine were found to cause depression by depleting NE

(1958) Kohlberg's model of moral development: This model is concerned with the thought process that occurs during moral decision-making rather than the actual decision or action. He proposed six stages of moral development, which can be divided into three levels (see Fig. 5.39) [42].

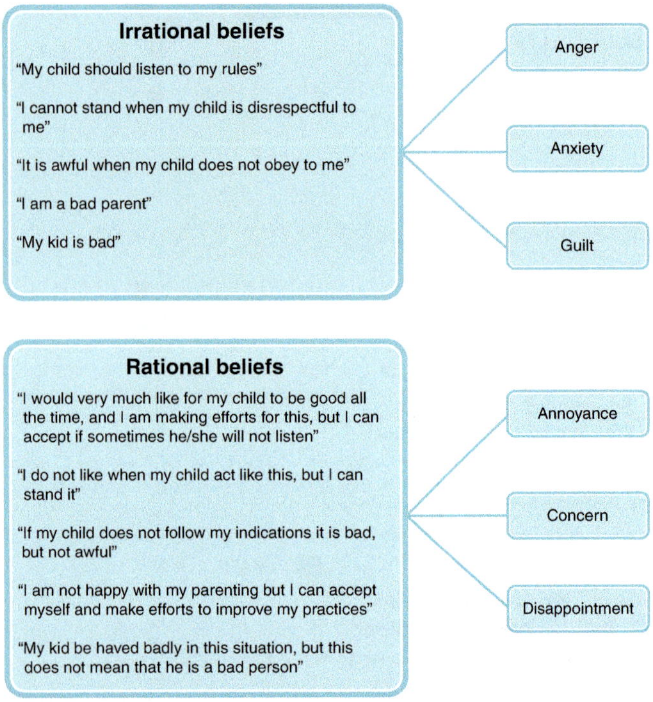

Fig. 5.37 Rational emotive behavior therapy involves the relationship between irrational/rational beliefs and dysfunctional/functional emotions. (*From* David et al. [82]; *with permission*)

(1962) Intensive short-term dynamic psychotherapy (ISTDP): ISTDP is a short-term, intensive form of psychotherapy that encourages patients to experience and address previously repressed or unconscious negative emotions. Davanloo posited that previous trauma and disruptions in attachment could cause anxiety, and patients must overcome their own internal resistance and experience these negative feelings to address their current symptoms (see Fig. 5.40) [43].

(1963) Reminiscence therapy (RT): RT was originally developed by Robert Butler in 1963 as a therapeutic modality for older adults. In sessions, patients are encouraged to reflect on previous experiences, often with the aid of photos or other memorabilia. It is often held in group sessions and can be used as a treatment for older adults with dementia or cognitive decline. In 1973, Charles Lewis conducted an experiment demonstrating its efficacy for improving cognitive symptoms [44].

(1968) Music therapy: Music therapy was established by E. Thayer Gaston, a psychologist and the father of music therapy, based on three principles: (1) the establishment or re-establishment of interpersonal relationships; (2) the bringing about of self-esteem through self-actualization; and (3) the utilization of the unique potential of rhythm to energize and bring order (Thayer EG. Music in Therapy. New York: Macmillan; 1968). Music therapy has a significant role in the treatment of psychiatric disorders, given the emerging evidence of the impact of music on the brain (see Fig. 5.41) [45].

(1969) Bowlby's attachment theory: John Bowlby proposed attachment theory, which posits that children are born with the innate motivation to form attachments to their caregivers as an evolutionary mechanism for survival. Bowlby

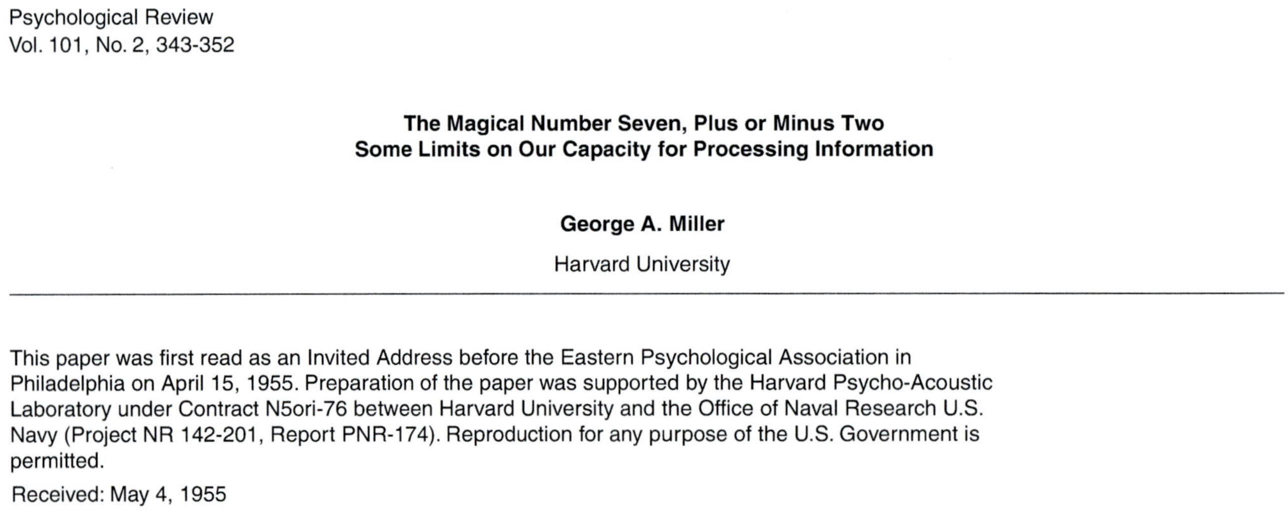
Psychological Review
Vol. 101, No. 2, 343-352

The Magical Number Seven, Plus or Minus Two
Some Limits on Our Capacity for Processing Information

George A. Miller

Harvard University

This paper was first read as an Invited Address before the Eastern Psychological Association in Philadelphia on April 15, 1955. Preparation of the paper was supported by the Harvard Psycho-Acoustic Laboratory under Contract N5ori-76 between Harvard University and the Office of Naval Research U.S. Navy (Project NR 142-201, Report PNR-174). Reproduction for any purpose of the U.S. Government is permitted.

Received: May 4, 1955

Fig. 5.38 George Miller applies cognitive psychology, concluding that the average number of objects a human can hold in short-term memory is 7 plus or minus 2

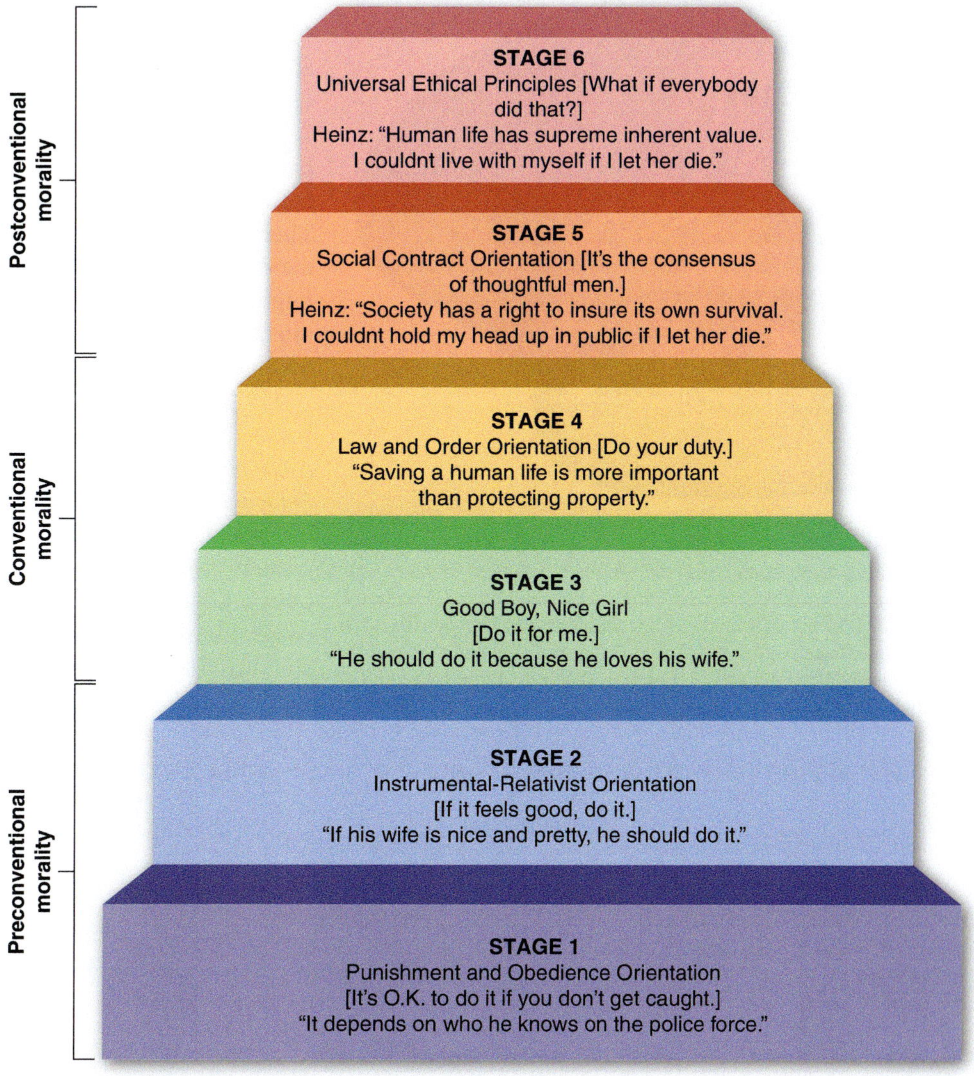

Fig. 5.39 Kohlberg's model of moral development. In the first level, morality is controlled by authority figures, so moral decision-making is determined by the potential consequences of the action. In the second level, moral decision-making is driven by social approval and adherence to social norms and rules. Finally, in the third level, moral reasoning is determined by consideration of individual rights and universal ethical principles

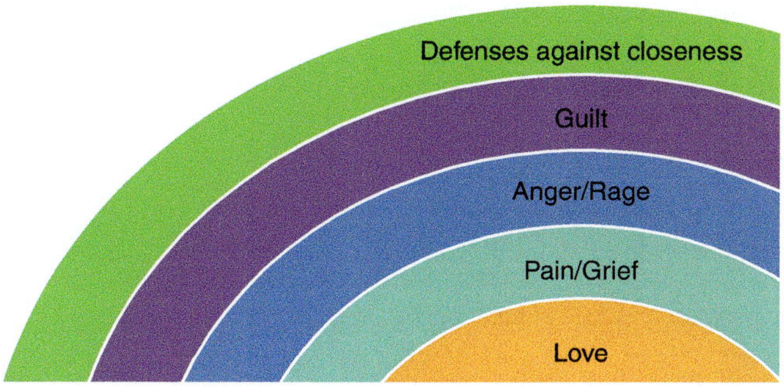

Fig. 5.40 Theory of short-term dynamic psychotherapy. (*From* Eppel [83]; *with permission*)

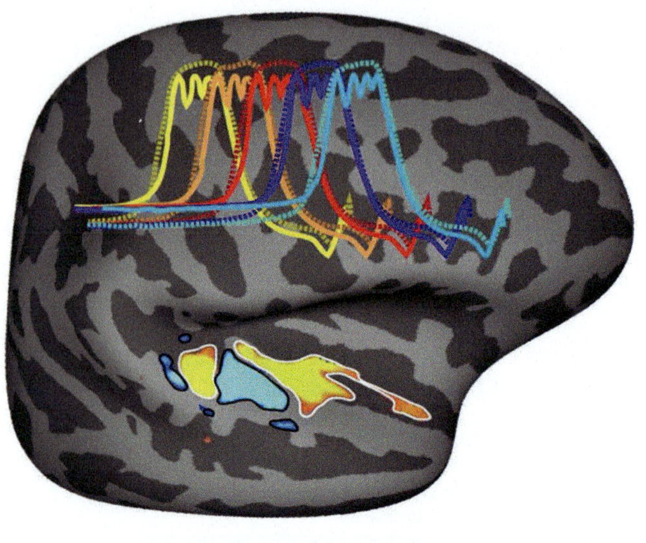

Fig. 5.41 Human brain responding to musical pitch. NIH-funded scientists found that our brains may be uniquely sensitive to pitch, the harmonic sounds we hear when listening to speech or music. The study highlights the promise of Sound Health, a joint project between the NIH and the John F. Kennedy Center for the Performing Arts, in association with the National Endowment for the Arts, that aims to understand the role of music in health

claims that a strong infant–caregiver attachment is necessary for the child to form strong relationships and trust others. He also proposed four stages of attachment that occur throughout development (see Fig. 5.42) [46].

(1969) Interpersonal psychotherapy (IPT): In IPT, the patient is encouraged to examine the reinforcing cycle between their symptoms and interpersonal difficulties. Therapists assist patients in breaking this cycle to improve their symptoms and interpersonal relationships through improved communication skills and engagement with their interpersonal network. IPT is designed as a brief, focused treatment for depression (see Fig. 5.43) [47].

(1971) Heinz Kohut and *The Analysis of Self*: In 1971, Kohut published *The Analysis of the Self: A Systematic Approach to the Psychoanalytic Treatment of Narcissistic Personality Disorders* [48]. He described the self as an agency that maintains a dynamic representation of the person's perception of their value as a person and manages bonds with others. Kohut introduced the term 'narcissistic rage' and discussed the psychoanalytic technique modifications for patients with narcissistic personality disorders (see Fig. 5.44) [48].

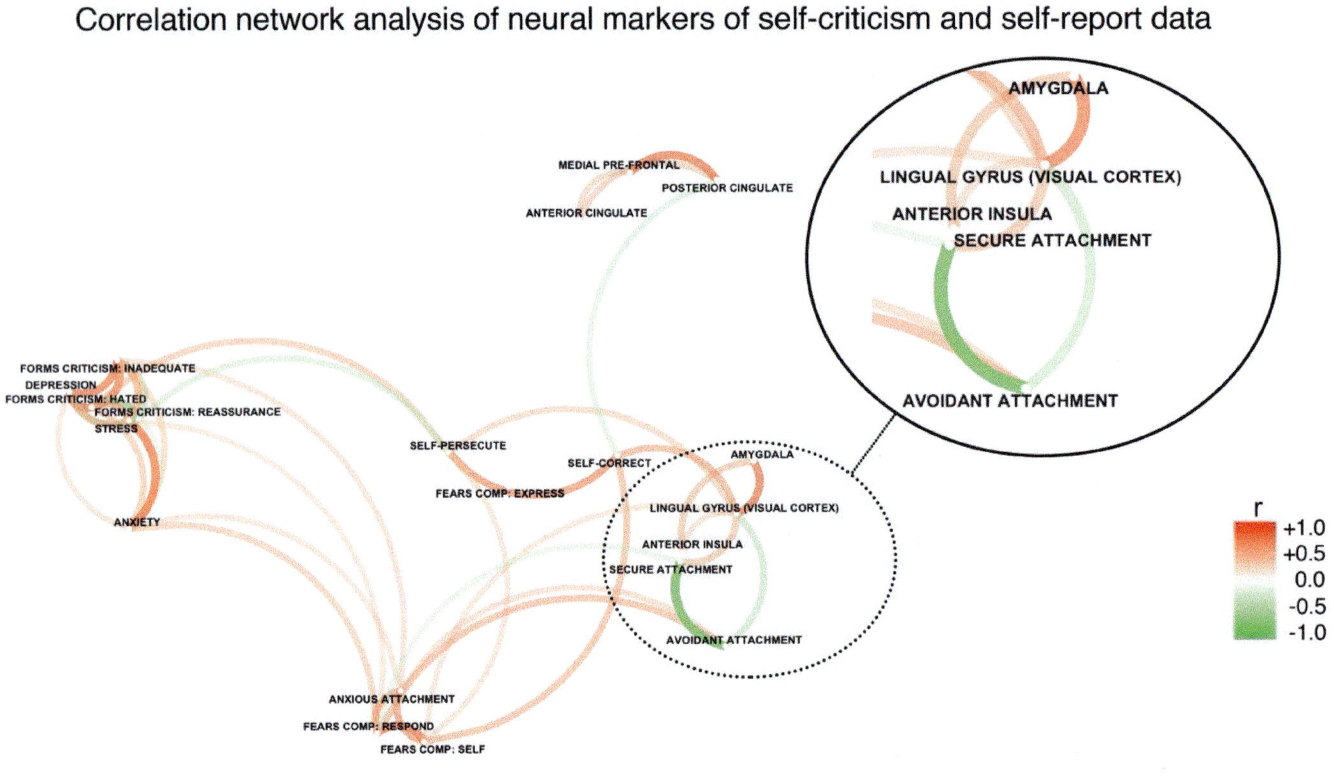

Fig. 5.42 Attachment styles and neural markers. A correlation network approach that visualizes the correlation matrix between neural markers of self-criticism and self-report data. Each dot corresponds to a variable, and each line corresponds to a path between correlated variables. Clusters of variables highlight constructs that are interrelated. Greater width and less transparency of a path indicate the presence of a stronger correlation. Scale bar: red color and luminance depict a strong positive correlation, and green color and luminance depict a strong negative correlation. Variable positioning is created from multidimensional scaling of the correlation absolute values. Figure inset (solid black-lined circle) depicts the relationship between neural markers of self-criticism and self-report attachment style. $N = 40$ for all measures except attachment styles, where $N = 38$, accounting for listwise deletion. Pearson correlation formula was used. (*From* Kim et al. [84]; Creative Commons CC BY license http://creativecommons.org/licenses/by/4.0/)

(1974) Salvador Minuchin's structural family therapy: In 1974, Minuchin based this practice on the theory that working to improve relational patterns first will eventually lead to improving individual behaviors and experiences [49]. The therapy starts by identifying the different relations in the family map, as shown in the figure below, tracking interactions between family members in the room, and using enactment to promote relational changes (see Fig. 5.45) [50].

(1977) George Engel's biopsychosocial model: Engel introduced this model with the following quote: *'the existing biomedical model does not suffice. To provide a basis for understanding the determinants of disease and arriving at rational treatments and patterns of health care, a medical model must also take into account the patient, the social context in which he [*sic*] lives, and the complementary system devised by society to deal with the disruptive effects of illness, that is, the physician role and the health care system. This requires a biopsychosocial model'* [51]. Based on general system theory, the patient is part of the hierarchy and continuum of natural systems that are structurally and functionally interconnected as shown below (see Fig. 5.46) [52].

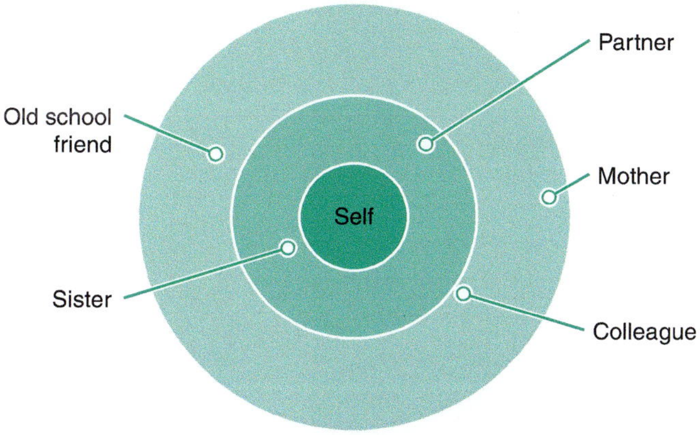

Fig. 5.43 Interpersonal psychotherapy inventory diagram of a patient's interpersonal network. (*From* Law [85]; *with permission*)

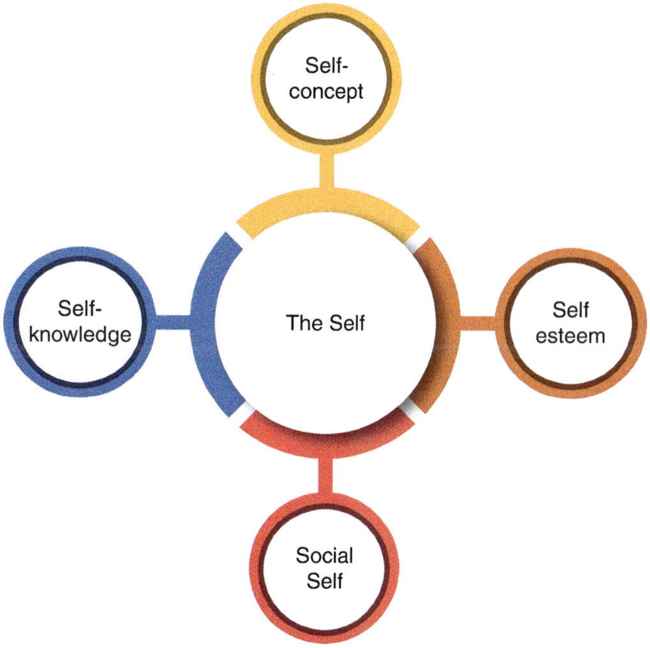

Fig. 5.44 One's self-perception is defined by their self-concept, self-knowledge, self-esteem, and social self

Fig. 5.45 Symbols represent different relations in the family map. The map below is a case example of Jessica, the identified patient (IP). Fourteen-year-old Jessica had been repeatedly suspended from school due to her fighting with schoolmates and disrespect for her teachers. Jessica lived with her mother, Barbara; her stepfather, Anthony; and her 16-year-old sister, Angela (*From* Colapinto [50]; *with permission*)

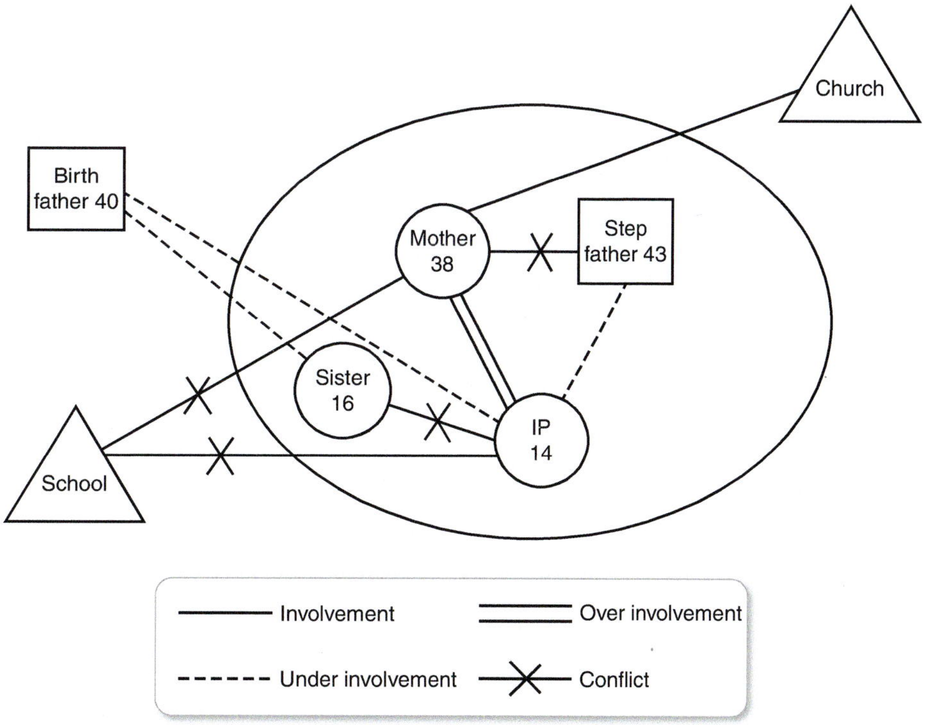

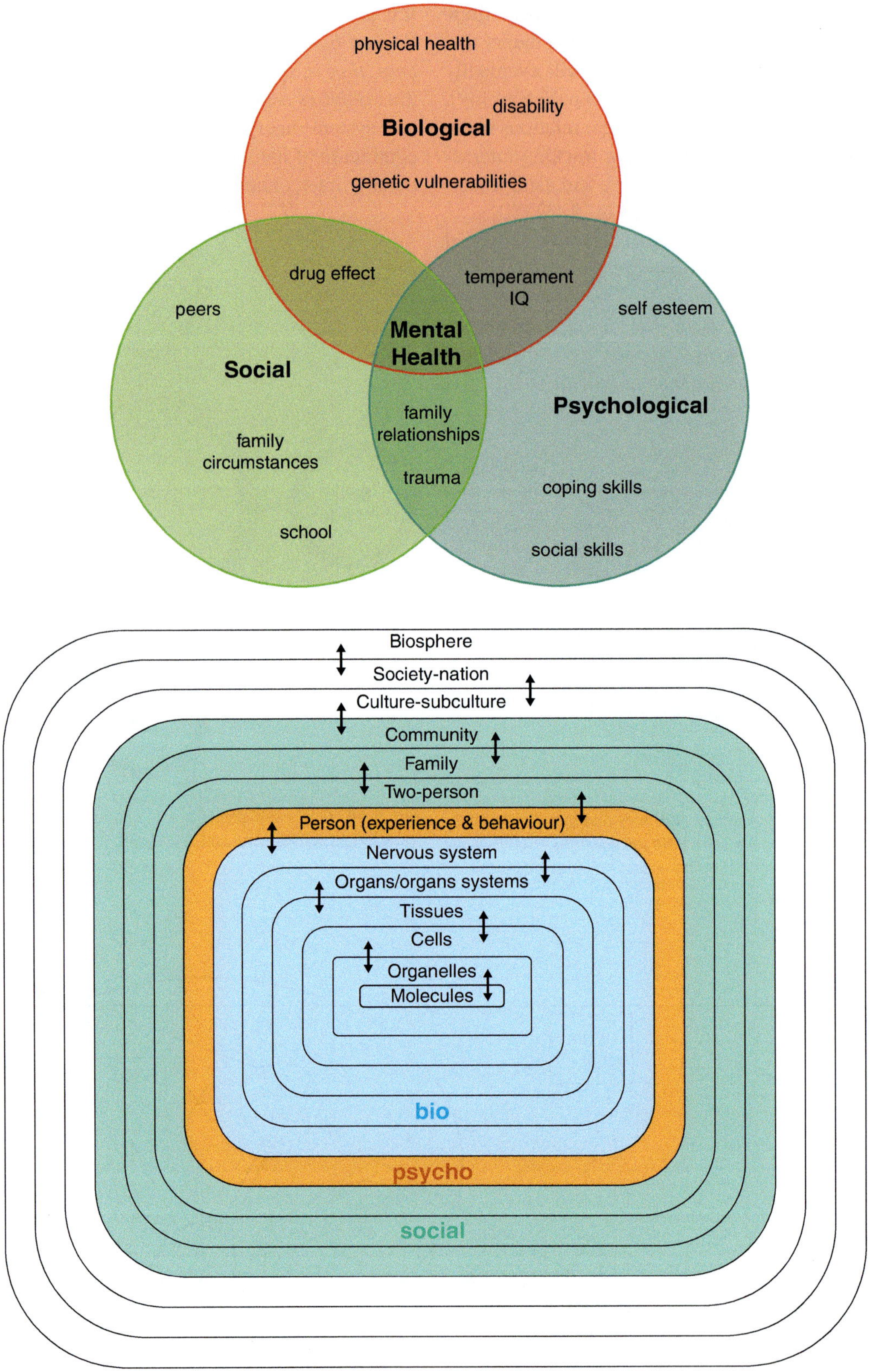

Fig. 5.46 The biopsychosocial model. (*From* Mehta and Kapoor [86]; with permission)

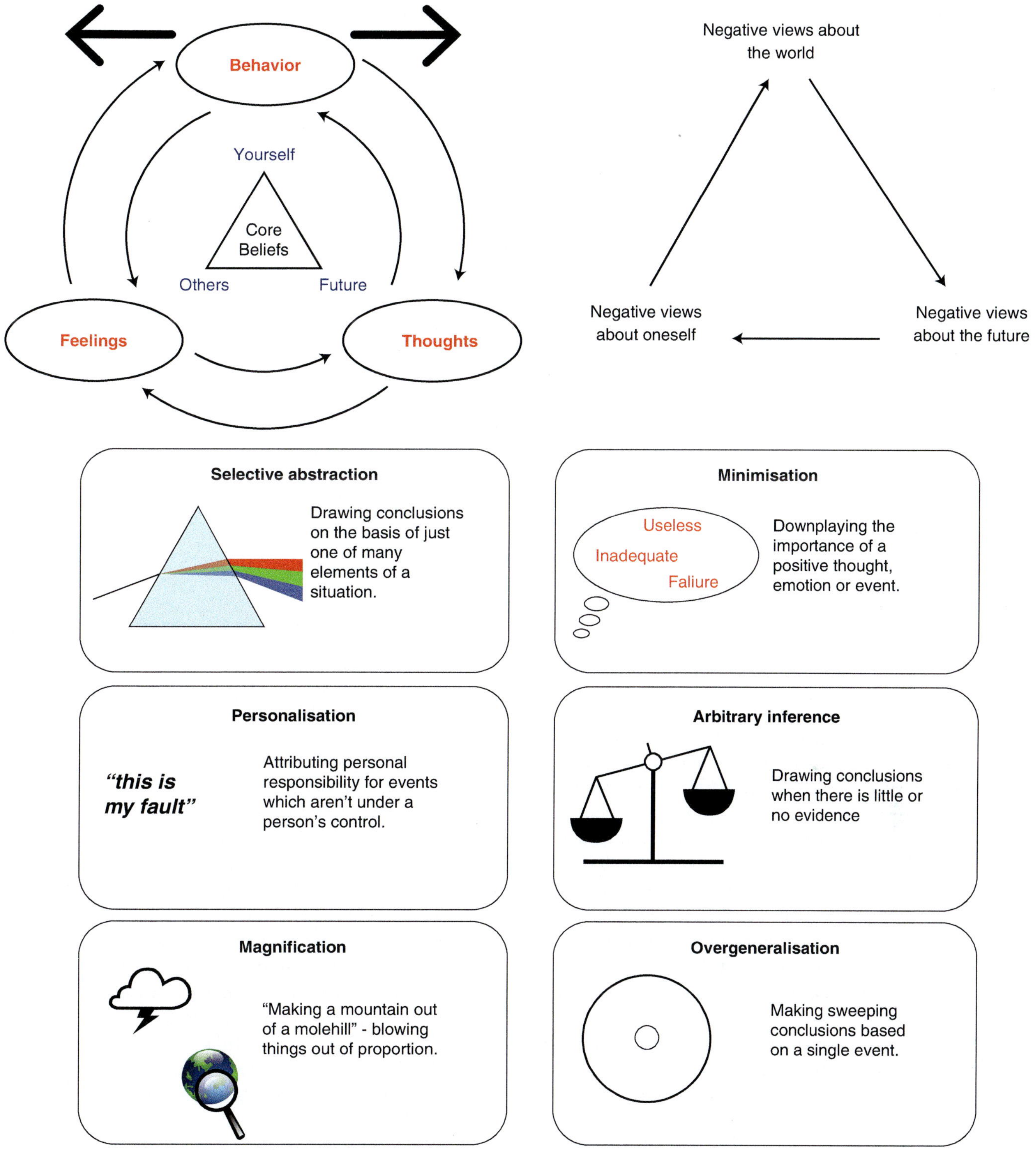

Fig. 5.47 Cognitive behavioral therapy was largely influenced by Aaron Beck's Cognitive Theory

(1979) Cognitive behavioral therapy (CBT): CBT focuses on how a patient perceives a situation rather than the situation itself. CBT seeks to help patients identify and reevaluate "automatic" negative thoughts and distorted thinking to foster a more positive cognitive and behavioral habits. By ameliorating these unhelpful thoughts and behaviors, patients are better able to cope with psychological symptoms and achieve their goals (see Fig. 5.47) [53].

(1982) Acceptance and commitment therapy (ACT): ACT combines mindful acceptance strategies with commit-

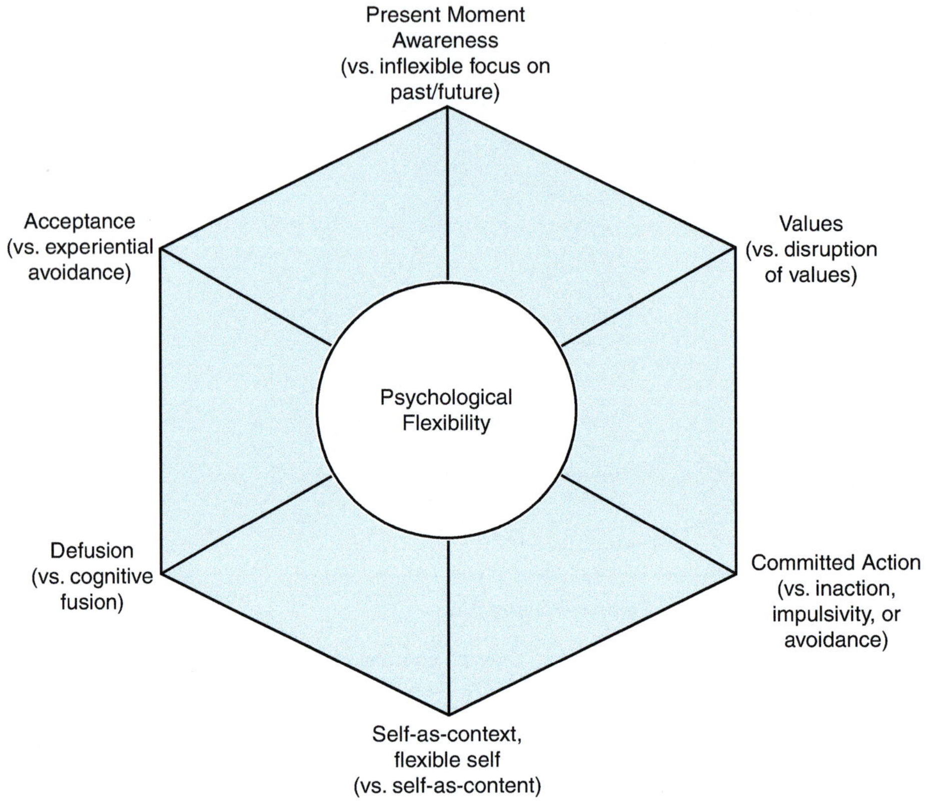

Fig. 5.48 Processes of change in acceptance and commitment therapy as depictured in the hexaflex. (Morgan and Aljabari [87]; with permission)

ment and behavioral change strategies. ACT was developed by Steven Hayes in 1982 with the main goal of improving psychological flexibility, which is the ability to be present and alter behavior within different contexts in accordance with one's chosen values (see Fig. 5.48) [54].

(1985) Eysenck's introversion/extraversion and neuroticism/stability: Eysenck suggested that variability in personality could be largely attributed to two major dimensions: introversion/extraversion and neuroticism/stability. These two dimensions create four dimensions: choleric (stable extroverts), melancholic (unstable introverts), sanguine (stable extroverts), and phlegmatic (stable introverts) (see Fig. 5.49) [55].

(1988) Eye Movement Desensitization and Reprocessing (EMDR): EMDR is a trauma-focused approach that is based on the adaptive information processing model, which postulates that traumatic memories may be physiologically stored in unprocessed form, leading to problems in day-to-day functioning (see Fig. 5.50) [56].

(1988) Viktor Frankl's logotherapy: This psychotherapy uses de-reflection (focusing away from self), paradoxical intention (pursuing actions that normally produce the most fear), and socratic dialogue (identifying own actions and words and interpreting them) [57]. Logotherapy (from the Greek word *logos*, meaning "reason" or "truth") stemmed from Frankl's theory that humans are motivated by the desire to find meaning in life, thus indicating a new Meaning-Seeking Model (see Fig. 5.51) [58].

(1991) Mindfulness-based stress reduction therapy (MBSR): MBSR involves mindful meditation and yoga with additional practice of these techniques at home. While originally designed by Jon Kabat-Zinn for stress and pain management, it can be used to treat a number of medical and psychological disorders [59]. MBSR impact on physiological responses to stress is shown in the figure below from a systematic review of the evidence (see Fig. 5.52) [60].

(2002) Mindfulness-based cognitive therapy is an evidence-based 8-week psychotherapy based on CBT and mindfulness meditation for the treatment of depression and anxiety, among other disorders [61].

(2014) Yoga and mindfulness-based cognitive therapy (Y-MBCT): Y-MVCT involves a combination of physical exercises, cognitive therapy, and mindful meditation. The five-factor model of mind serves as the theoretical framework, and there is a significant focus on traditional meditation and yoga techniques and practice. Mindfulness techniques such as attention, empathy, compassion, and mentalization are emphasized. This method can be used as a brief therapy for psychosis or in an extended form (see Fig. 5.53) [62].

(1991) Prolonged exposure (PE): PE is an evidence-based psychotherapy for trauma and PTSD that involves

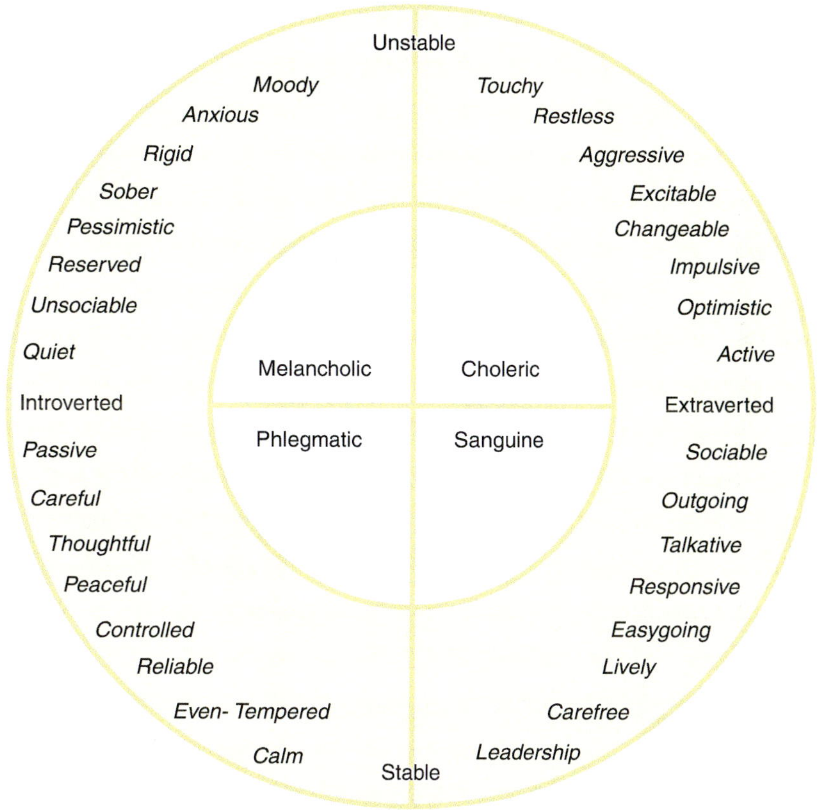

Fig. 5.49 Relation between the four temperaments and the neuroticism-extraversion dimensional system. Eysenck believed that these qualities were largely genetically and biologically based. (*From* Strelau [88]; *with permission*)

imaginal exposure as well as in vivo exposure to the situations and objects related to trauma in a safe setting, thus enabling corrective learning and integration of information. Extinction of fear and avoidance response enhances the sense of mastery over past traumatic experiences (see Fig. 5.54) [63].

(1993) Dialectical behavioral therapy (DBT): DBT was introduced by Marsha Linehan as a treatment for patients with a borderline personality disorder. In DBT, the therapist accepts and validates the patient's feelings while also teaching the patient a set of skills to improve their quality of life. DBT treatment typically consists of individual therapy sessions, group therapy, and phone coaching (see Fig. 5.55; Table 5.2) [64].

(1994) Virtual reality therapy (VR): VR can be used in desensitization therapy for patients with phobias. This therapeutic modality allows for the generation of anxiety-inducing stimuli in safe and private environments for patients who have difficulty visualizing or may not be ready to experience real situations (see Fig. 5.56) [65].

(2002) Positive psychology: Martin Seligman proposed that happiness could be divided into three parts, all of which we choose for their own sake: positive emotion (pleasurable feelings), engagement, and meaning (see Fig. 5.57) [66].

(2002) Mentalization-based therapy (MBT): Mentalization is the ability to generate and employ mental representations of one's own emotional states and the emotional states of others. Peter Fonagy and Anthony Bateman proposed mentalization-based treatment as a treatment for borderline personality disorder. This treatment focuses on improving mentalization skills, specifically achieving a balance among each of the four dimensions of mentalizing (see Fig. 5.58) [67].

(2002) Manuel Trujillo's empathy-based psychotherapy. In 2002, Trujillo developed this treatment based on how attachment bond disruptions become severely traumatic, leading to pain, rage, guilt, and layers of defenses (see Fig. 5.59) [68].

This therapy utilizes empathy, transference, activation of primitive self-states, imaginary reconstruction, working through rage, reactivation, and integration of self to free the person up to utilize their emotional and intellectual assets and pursue joyful living with a sense of purpose (see Fig. 5.60) [68].

(2008) Otto Kernberg's transference-based psychotherapy: This treatment was developed and practiced in the 1990s with its origins dating to 1972 [69]. This therapy is based on modern object relations theory, with the goal of achieving improvement through changing mental representations of self and others [69]. Kernberg viewed the level of

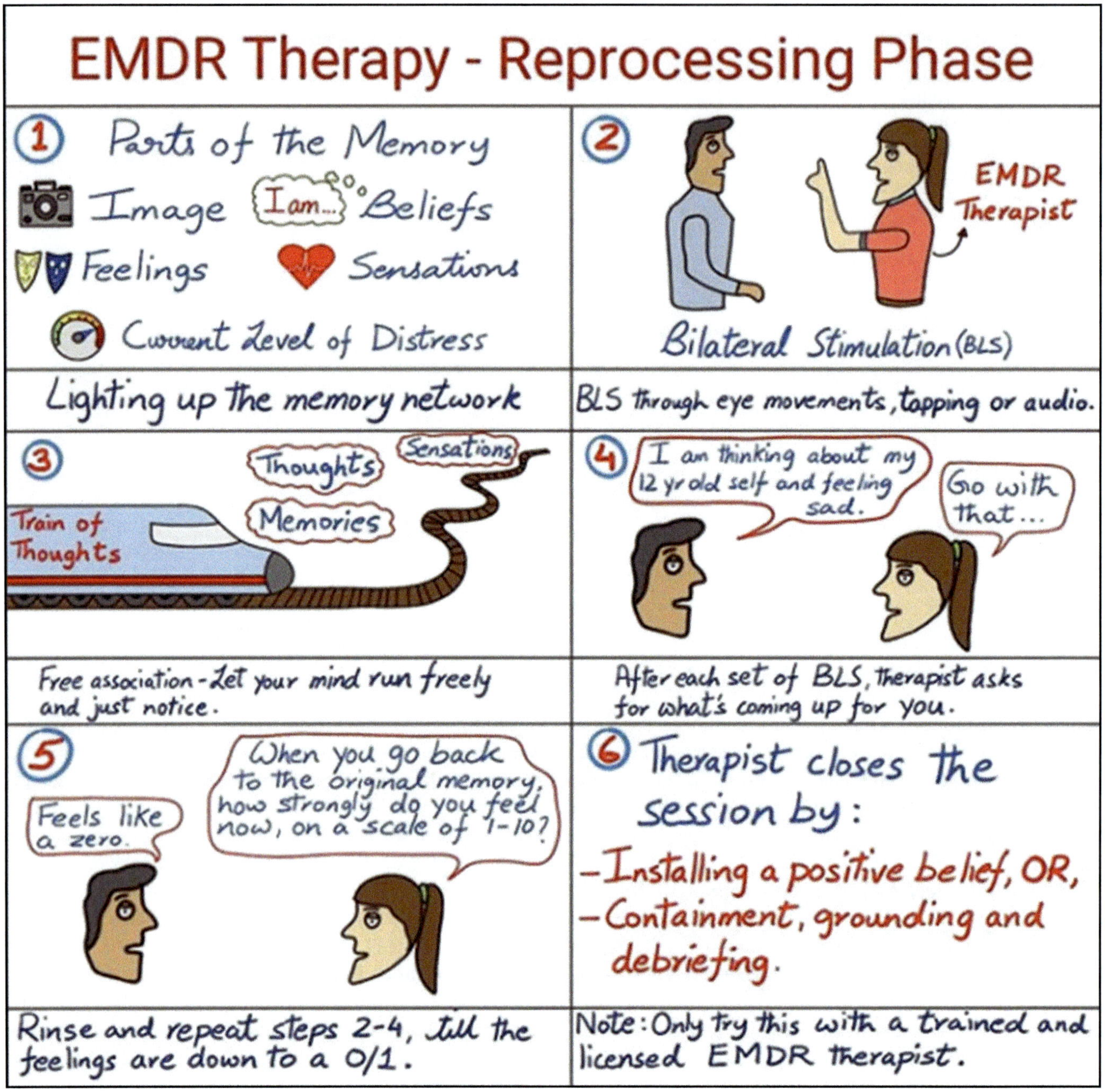

Fig. 5.50 Eye movement desensitization and reprocessing: EMDR therapy. EMDR focuses on target memories for processing using bilateral sensory stimulation, e.g., bilateral eye movements following the clinician's finger or hand or other visual or auditory stimuli according to the patient's comfort level. (*From* O'Shea Brown [89]; with permission)

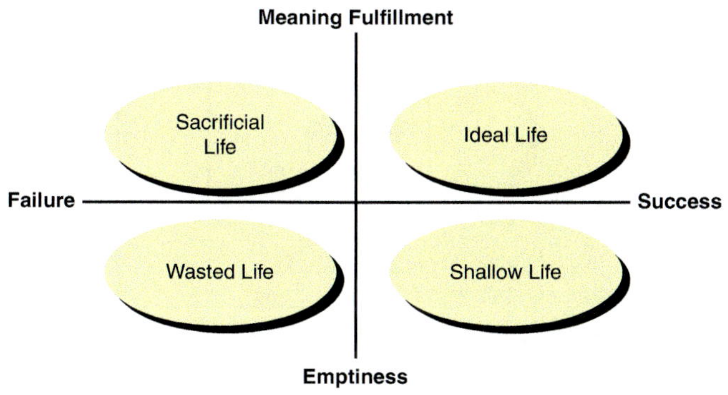

Fig. 5.51 Meaning mindset versus success mindset. (*From* Wong PTP [90]; *with permission*)

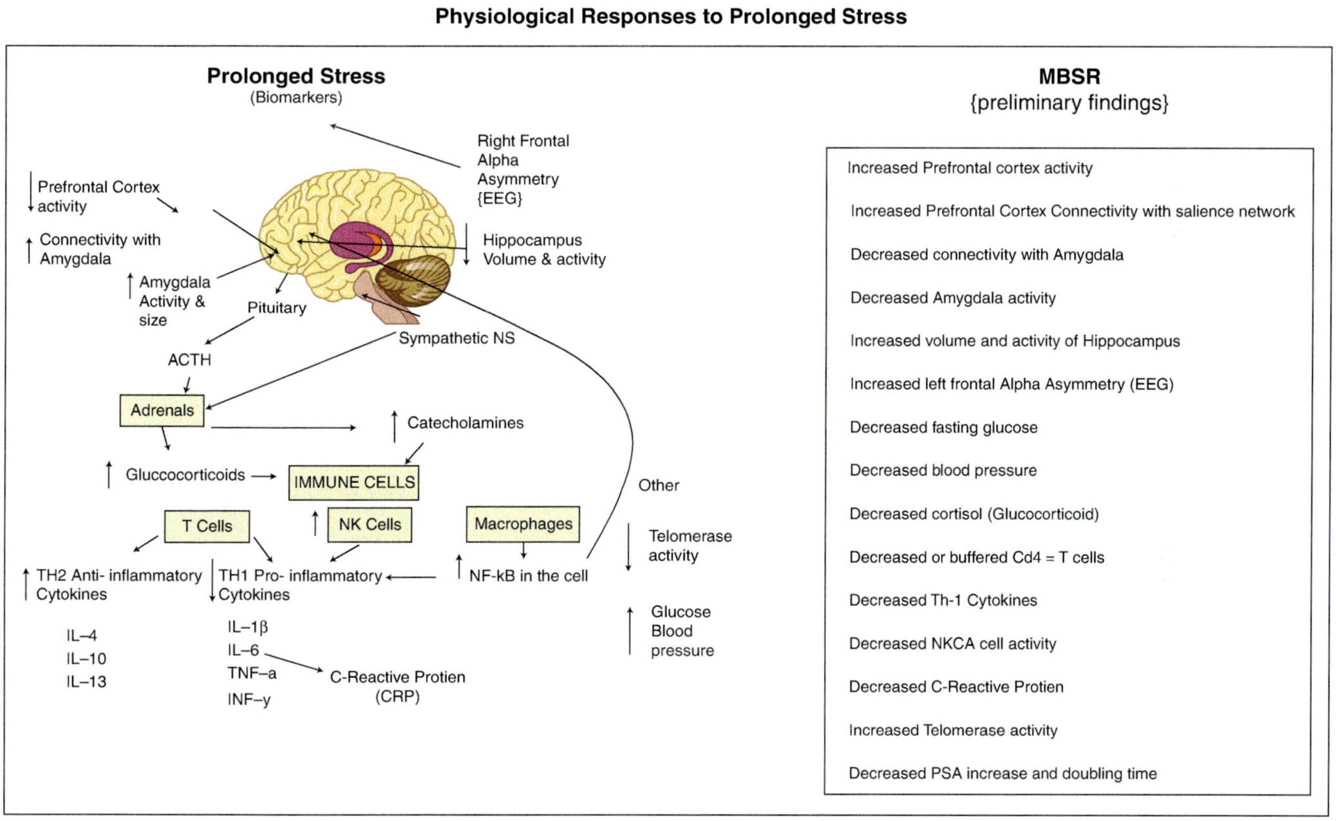

Fig. 5.52 Impact of mindfulness-based stress reduction (MBSR) on physiological responses to stress. (*From* Reive [60]; *with permission*.) https://doi.org/10.1016/j.explore.2019.01.001

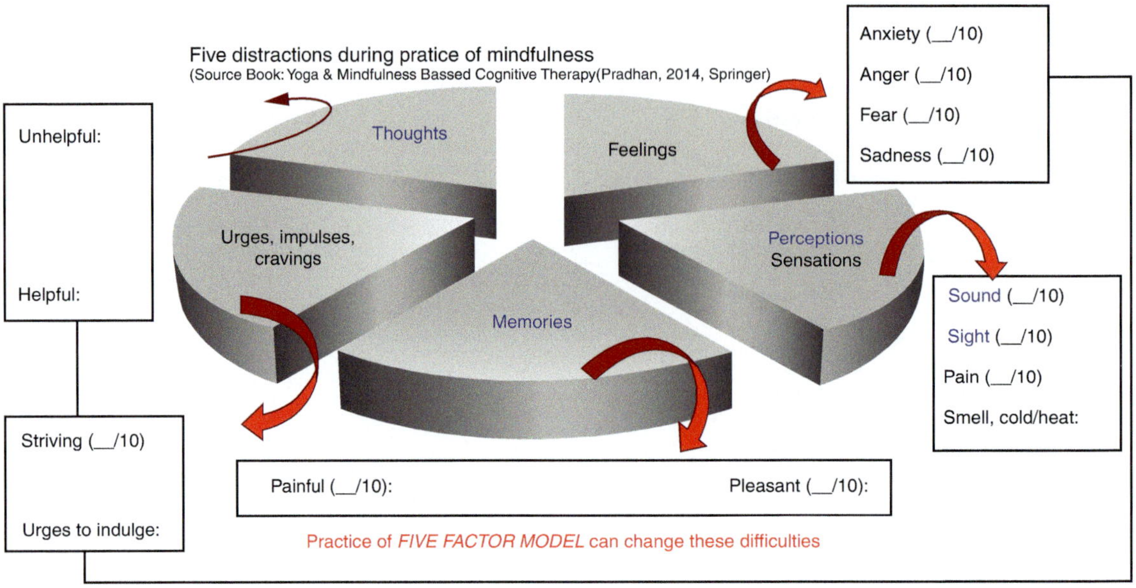

Fig. 5.53 The *five-factor inventory* developed by Pradhan (2014) based on the five-factor model is the main tool in yoga and mindfulness-based cognitive therapy for psychosis (*Y-MBCT*$_p$©). (*From* Pradhan and Pinninti [91]; *with permission*)

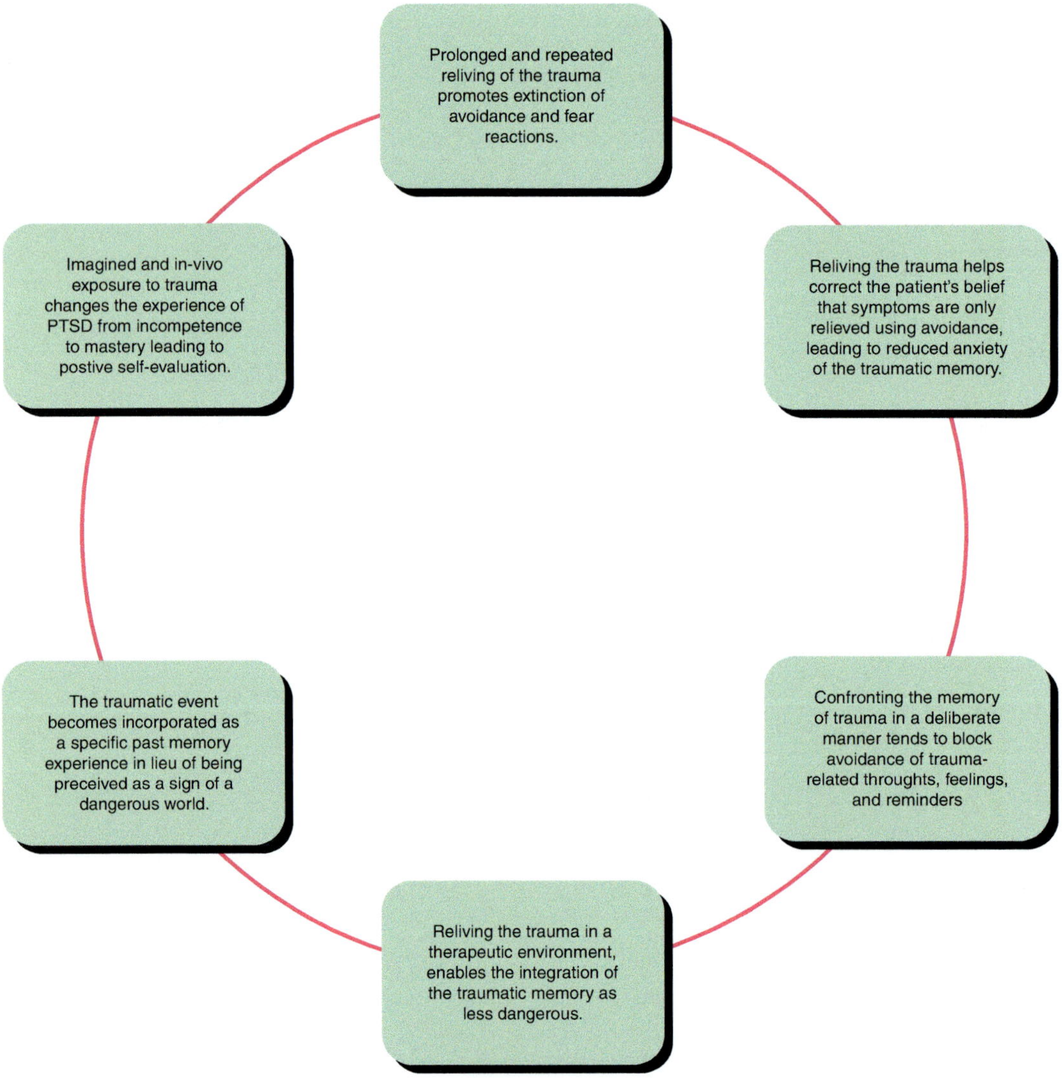

Fig. 5.54 Theoretical underpinnings of prolonged exposure (PE). (From Pagel [92]; with permission)

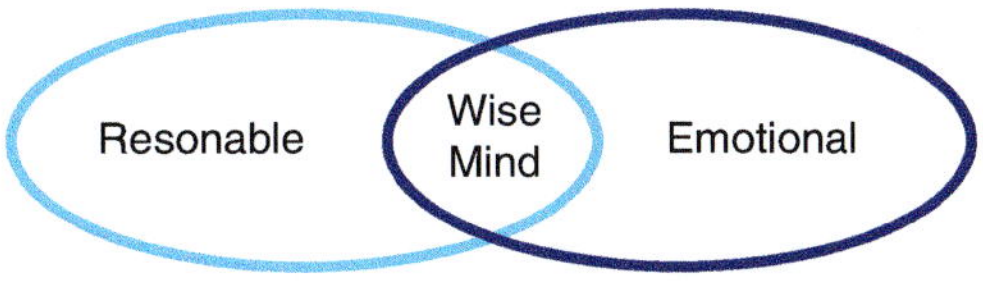

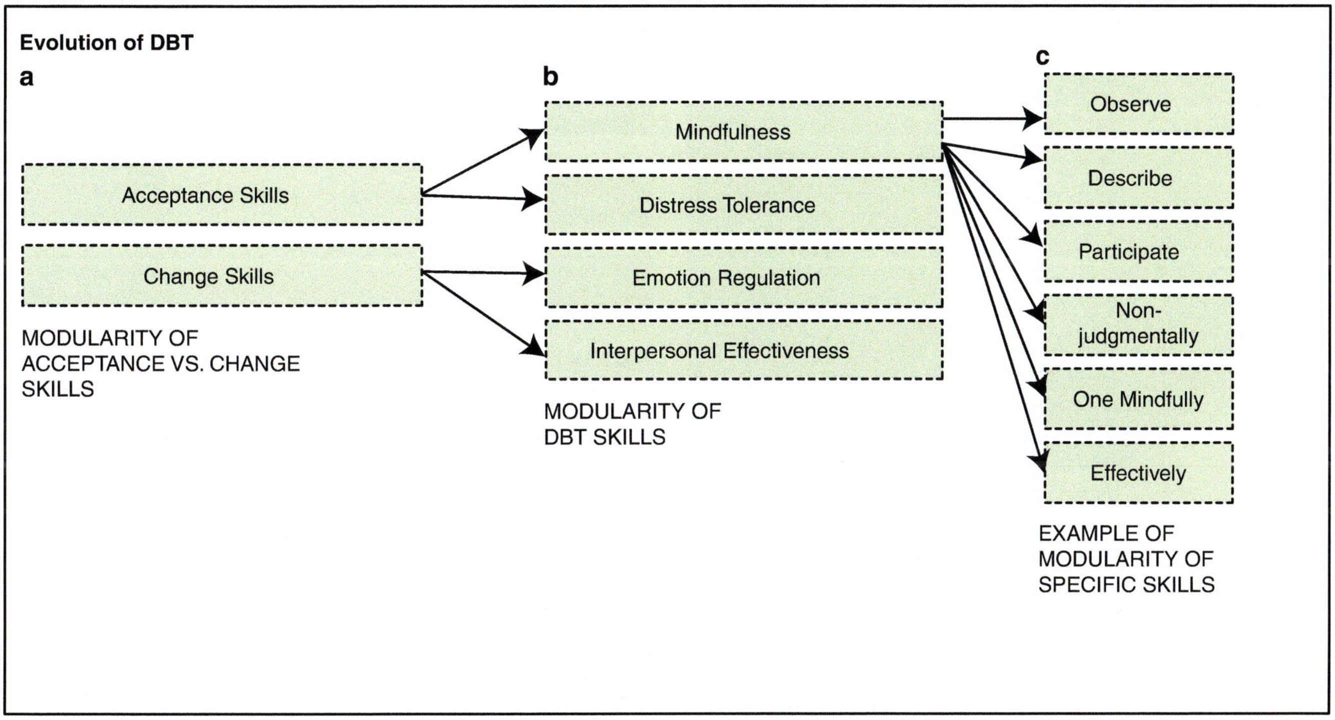

Fig. 5.55 (**a**) Dialectical behavioral therapy (DBT) consists of four skill modules: mindfulness, emotion regulation, distress tolerance, and interpersonal effectiveness. (**b**) Mindfulness skills are focused on radical acceptance of the present situation, and emotion regulation focuses on managing maladaptive emotional responses. Distress tolerance encourages the patient to tolerate and manage their negative emotions, and interpersonal effectiveness helps improve one's communication skills with others. (**c**) Examples of specific skills within the mindfulness module

Table 5.2 The hierarchy of primary targets in DBT

Stage of treatment	Targets addressed	Strategies
Pretreatment	1. Orientation to treatment and agreement upon goals	1. Psychoeducation on: (a) DBT model, history, and research (b) Biosocial model (c) Stage 1 targets of behavior (d) Patterns of dysregulation (secondary targets) (e) Behavior chain analysis (f) Expectations for treatment 2. Commitment strategies 3. Gaining commitment from client to treatment and taking suicide and/or self-injury off the table for 1 year
Stage 1	1. Decreasing suicidal behaviors 2. Decreasing therapy interfering behaviors 3. Decreasing quality of life interfering behaviors 4. Increasing behavioral skills (a) Core mindfulness skills (b) Interpersonal effectiveness (c) Emotion regulation (d) Distress tolerance (e) Self-management	1. Behavioral chain analysis 2. Diary card 3. Validation 4. Problem solving 5. Location perspective 6. Coaching
Stage 2	1. Decreasing posttraumatic stress	1. Deployment of additional evidence-based treatments and strategies related to client's remaining symptoms
Stage 3	1. Increasing respect for self 2. Achieving individual goals	1. Deployment of additional evidence-based treatments and strategies related to client's remaining symptoms

From Bailey [76]; *with permission*

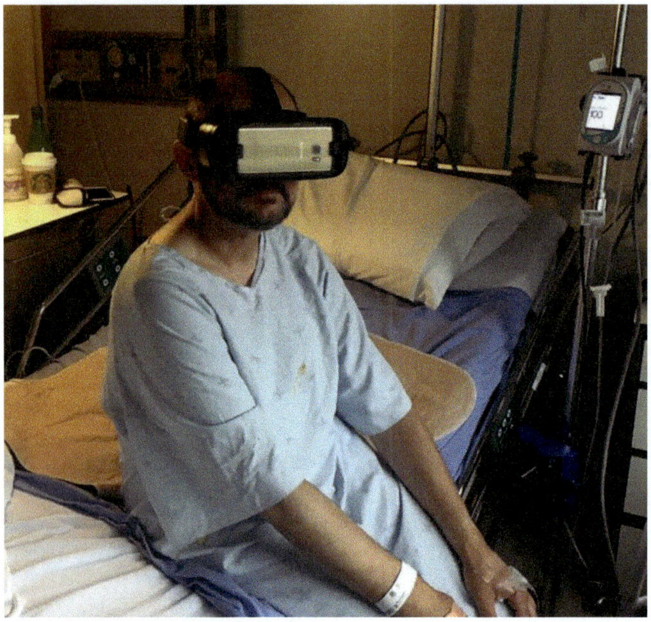

Fig. 5.56 Example of a participant being treated with virtual reality therapy. A nurse, informal caregiver, or RC helped the participants sit up in their hospital room bed, and the RC helped them put on and remove the HMD and headphones. Written, informed consent was obtained from the individuals for the publication of this image. (*From* Appel et al. [93]; Creative Commons Attribution 4.0; http://creativecommons.org/licenses/by/4.0/)

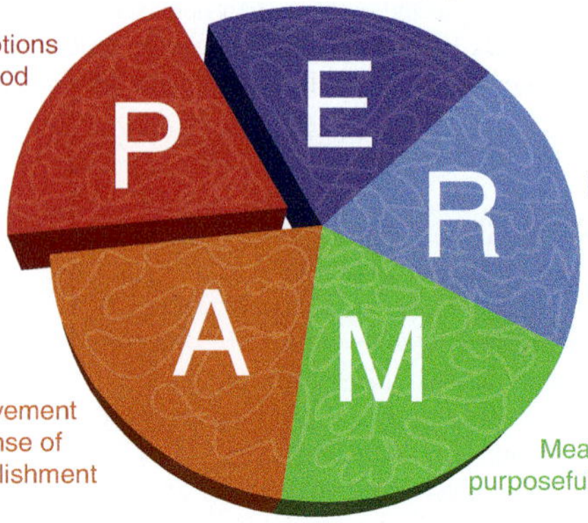

Fig. 5.57 Martin Seligman's positive psychology PERMAN model of life satisfaction. Positive psychology encourages individuals to go beyond simple pleasures and to identify and employ their existing strengths in order to create a more satisfying and enjoyable life. These strengths can be used to engage in activities that promote flow (engagement) and discover self-purpose and contribute to something larger than oneself (meaning). (*From* Pociask and Stefanowicz-Kocoł [94]; *with permission.*)

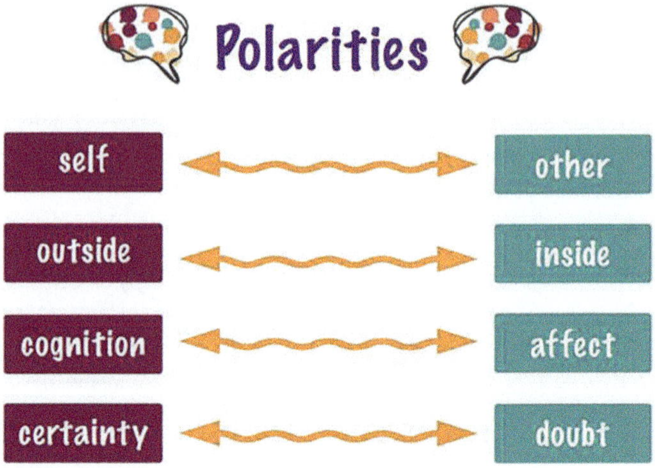

Fig. 5.58 Mentalization dimensions or "polarities" according to Peter Fonagy and Anthony Bateman in Mentalization-based treatment. Ultimately, mentalization-based therapy aims to help patients develop new attachment styles, improve emotional regulation, and increased stability in interpersonal relationships. (*From* McLaren and Sharp [95]; *with permission*)

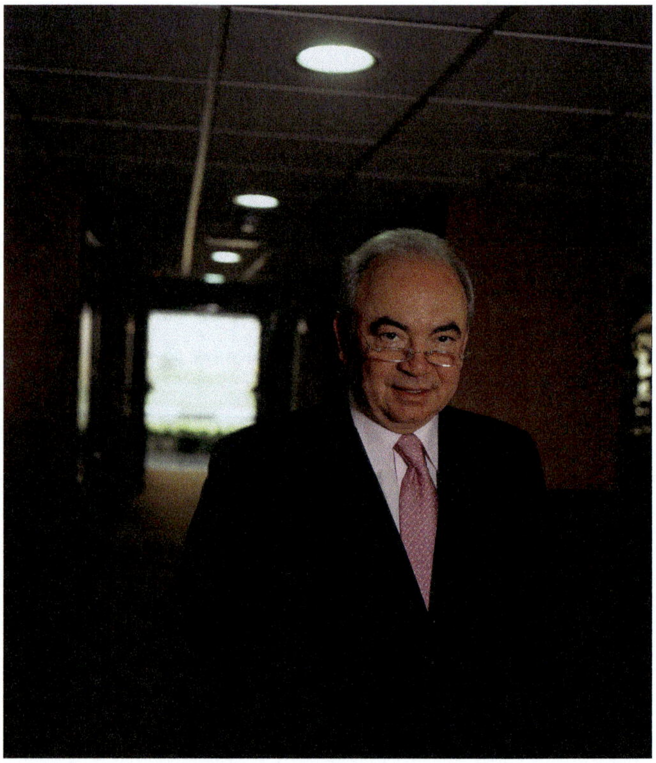

Fig. 5.59 Manuel Trujillo, M.D., Professor of Psychiatry, New York University

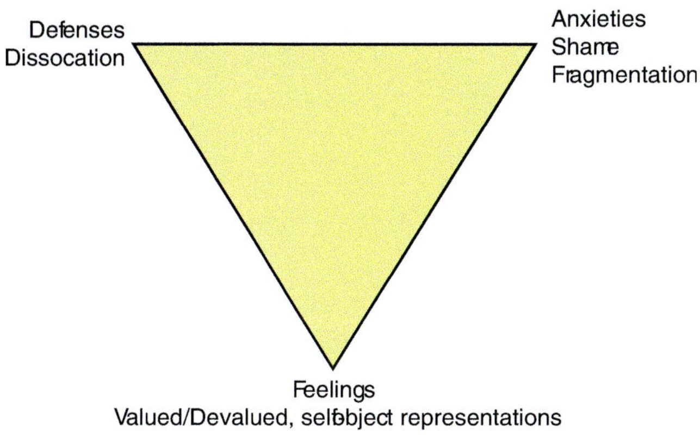

Fig. 5.60 Triangle of the self (Trujillo)

borderline personality organization as a function of severity and introversion/extraversion, as seen in the figure below (see Fig. 5.61). The treatment model includes the following components: verbal contract, focusing on interpersonal behaviors with the therapist and others, using interpretations, and making changes in interpersonal behaviors [70].

(2014) Future-directed therapy (FTD): FTD is a treatment for depression developed based on the understanding that the brain is future-oriented. This therapeutic method focuses on managing negative expectations and helps patients plan and anticipate more positive future outcomes (see Fig. 5.62) [71].

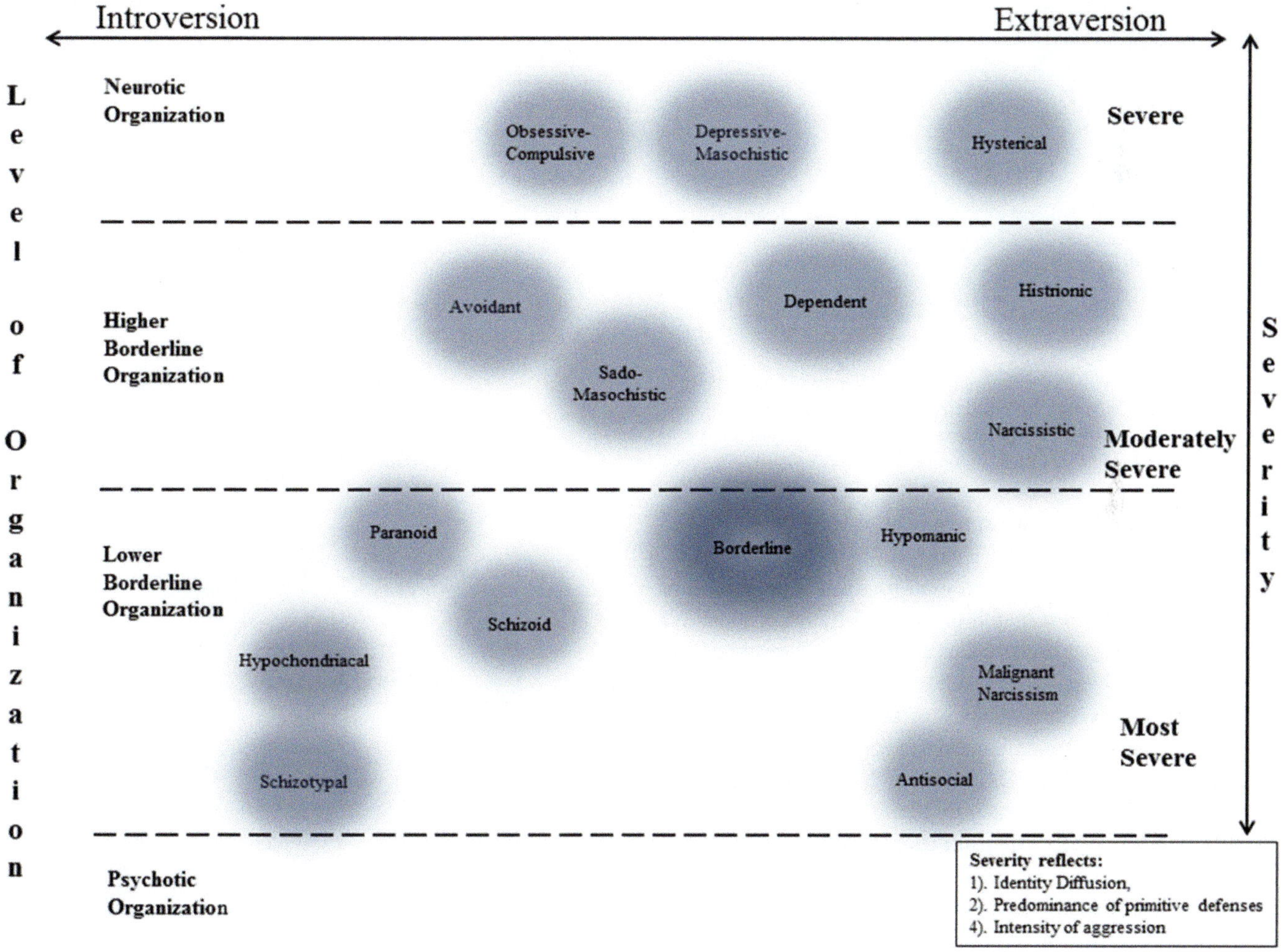

Fig. 5.61 Level of personality organization by Otto Kernberg. The severity dimension reflects the joint impact of identity diffusion, predominance of developmentally primitive psychological defenses, and the intensity of aggression present in the individual. The DSM-5 personality disorders and other conditions (e.g., malignant narcissism) are positioned in this hypothetical conceptual space. The shaded cloud surrounding each disorder's name reflects the hypothetical potential range of clinical expression. (*From* Clarkin et al. [70]; *with permission*)

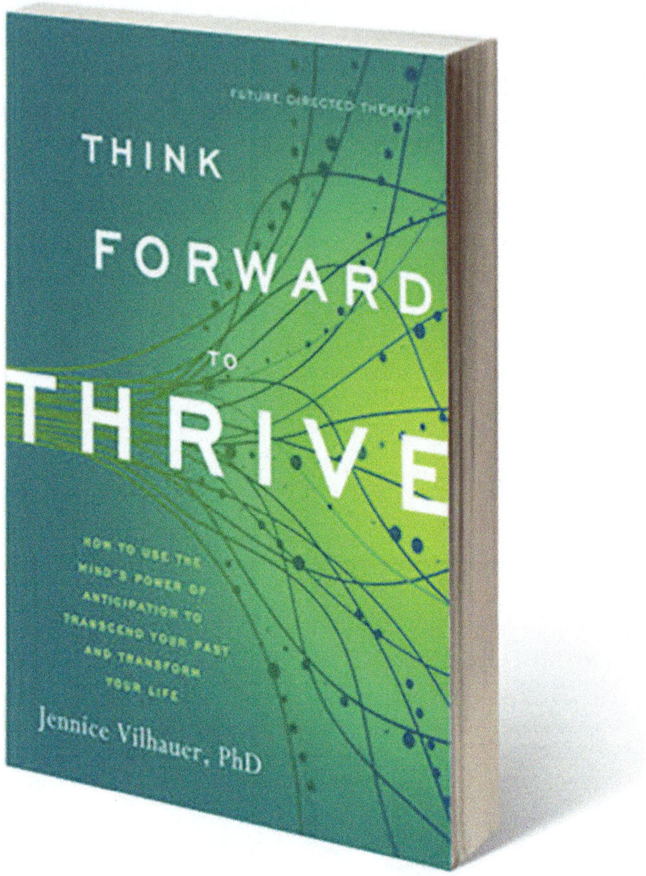

Fig. 5.62 Jennice Vilhauer's Future Directed Therapy. Shown above is Vilhauer's groundbreaking book titled *Think Forward to Thrive: How to Use the Mind's Power of Anticipation to Transcend Your Past and Transform Your Life*. (*From* https://jennicevilhauer.com/book)

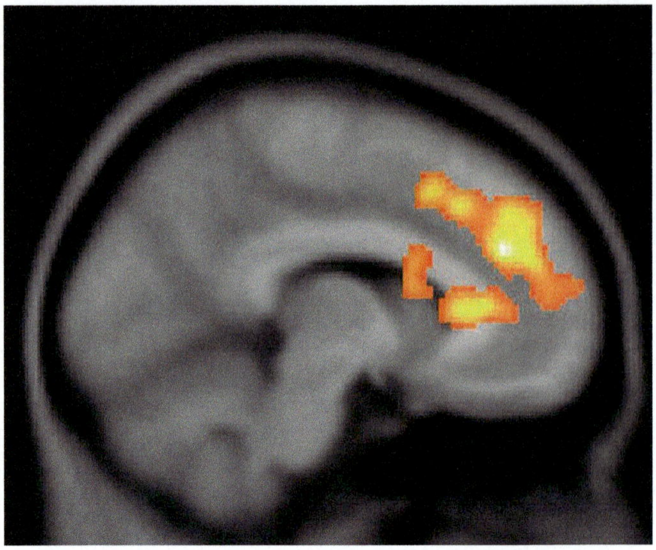

Fig. 5.63 PET scan of ketamine rapid-onset antidepressant effect. PET scans revealed that ketamine rapidly restored bipolar depressed patients' ability to anticipate pleasurable experiences by boosting activity in the dorsal anterior cingulate cortex (yellow) and related circuitry. The picture shows PET scan data superimposed on an anatomical MRI image. (*From* National Institute of Health)

(2014) Ketamine as a rapid-onset antidepressant: The National Institute of Mental Health (NIMH) in 2014 established the Rapidly-Acting Treatments for Treatment-Resistant Depression (RAPID) research project led by Maurizio Fava at Harvard's Massachusetts General Hospital. Rapidly acting antidepressants were discovered a few years earlier, and research efforts by Carlos Zarate of the NIMH showed that ketamine could improve depressive symptoms within hours (see Fig. 5.63) [72]. The FDA approved Ketamine nasal spray for the treatment of depression in 2019.

(2016) Behavioral activation therapy (BA): BA is based on the idea that depressed behavior (e.g., apathy) is a coping strategy to avoid aversive environments. Thus, this therapeutic modality focuses on helping the patient identify triggers and maladaptive coping mechanisms that serve to maintain their negative affect (see Fig. 5.64) [73].

Behavioral activation is significantly less costly than CBT but is similarly effective (see Fig. 5.65) [74].

(2020) Wellness medicine: The ultimate goal of healthcare interventions could be achieved with the help of wellness medicine, a field that focuses on improving overall

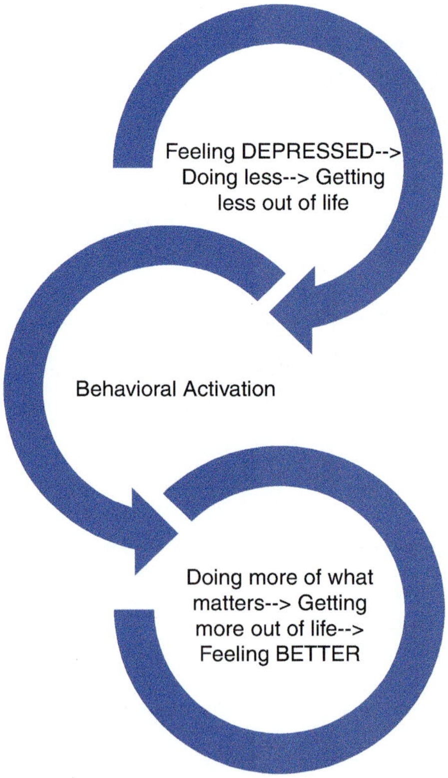

Fig. 5.64 Behavioral activation to improve depression. After the patient's triggers are identified, the patient is encouraged to evaluate their own behavior and choose to engage in healthy behaviors rather than continuing the cycle of avoidance

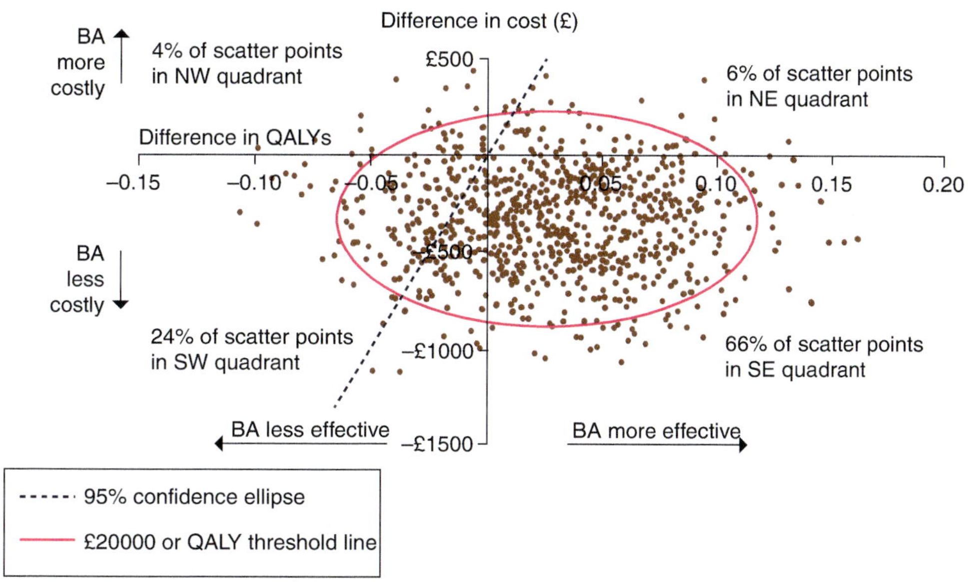

Fig. 5.65 Behavioral activation therapy vs. cognitive behavioral therapy. Richards and Ekers showed that BA, a simpler psychological treatment than CBT, can be delivered by junior mental health workers with less intensive and costly training, with no lesser effect than CBT. Effective psychological therapy for depression can be delivered without the need for costly and highly trained professionals. The figure shows bootstrapped mean differences in costs and effects of BA compared with CBT. *BA* behavioral activation, *CBT* cognitive behavioral therapy, *NE* northeast, *NW* northwest, *SE* southeast. *SW* southwest, *QALY* quality-adjusted life-year. (*From* Richards et al. [96]; Creative Commons Attribution (CC BY 4.0); https://creativecommons.org/licenses/by/4.0)

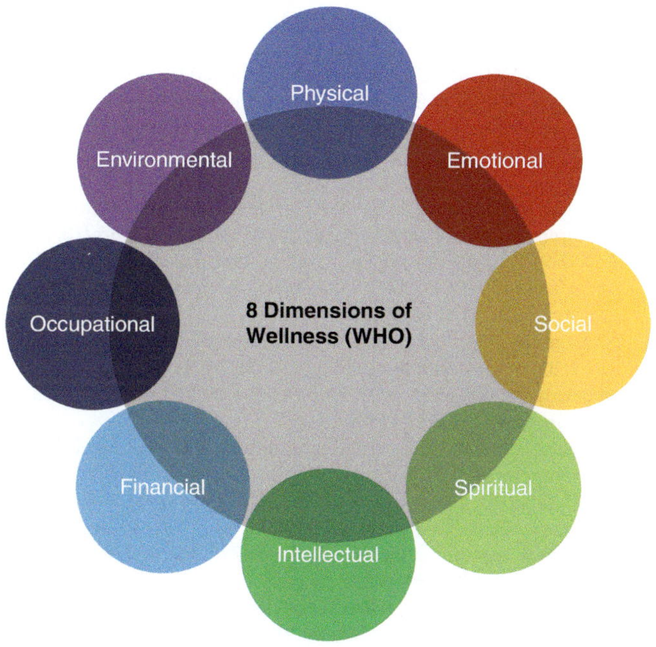

Fig. 5.66 World Health Organization (WHO) eight dimensions of wellness

functioning, quality of life, and well-being, beyond symptom management of medical illness, leading to restoration and maintenance of health [75].

Developing a personalized wellness life plan involves setting the plan, scheduling activities, getting support, tracking, measuring the impact, and updating the plan. The personalized wellness life plan involves scheduling wellness activities from each of the eight dimensions of wellness: physical, emotional, social, spiritual, intellectual, financial, occupational, and environmental, as seen in the figure below, on a daily, weekly, monthly, and yearly basis (see Fig. 5.66) [75].

Conclusion

From spiritual healing exercises to advanced psychotherapies, from mysteries of the unconscious to detailed models of neurological processes, from exile to the legitimate treatment of mental illness, the field of psychiatry has clearly come a long way yet still has significant potential to grow. The conceptual and technical development of psychiatry as a scientific discipline and the parallel growth of the institutions and practices of psychiatric care is a fascinating—if at times tortuous—story with many heroes and heroines who promoted the liberation of the mentally from the triple bondage of deviance (of being considered deviants and sinners), exclusion (not entitled to the rights of citizenship), and abandonment (not worthy of receiving community support and treatment). Thus, an ongoing struggle facing the field is the question of how society can unlearn centuries worth of deviance, exclusion, and abandonment in a continuing battle to increase the acceptance and accessibility of mental healthcare. Mental illness is sometimes even refuted as a legitimate issue, especially in school systems and workplaces, where poor mental health is often trivialized or disregarded as a common struggle. With the rise of wellness and positive psychology in the last several decades, the field has expanded tremendously as more people realize that attention to mental health is not something reserved for "the sick." The discoveries of recent years have shown that mental health likely exists on a spectrum, where some people may require more care than others, but all are welcome to improve—an idea that will remain relevant to this field. From mindfulness to virtual reality to music therapy, recent innovations have demonstrated that the possibilities are truly endless when it comes to psychiatric diagnosis and treatment.

References

1. Okasha TA. Major trends of psychosomatic medicine in North Africa and Middle East. In: Leigh H, editor. Global psychosomatic medicine and consultation-liaison psychiatry. Cham: Springer; 2019. https://doi.org/10.1007/978-3-030-12584-4_8.
2. Bou Khalil R, Richa S. When affective disorders were considered to emanate from the heart: the Ebers papyrus. Am J Psychiatry. 2014;171(3):275. https://doi.org/10.1176/appi.ajp.2013.13070860.
3. Kalachanis K, Michailidis IE. The Hippocratic view on humors and human temperament. European journal of Soc Behav 2015;2 (2):1-5. https://www.researchgate.net/profile/Konstantinos-Kalachanis/publication/283119853_The_Hippocratic_View_on_Humors_and_Human_Temperament/links/562b6d7d08ae22b170335331/The-Hippocratic-View-on-Humors-and-Human-Temperament.pdf. Accessed 1 May 2021.
4. Hendrik. Stanford encyclopedia of philosophy. 2009. https://plato.stanford.edu/entries/ancient-soul/#3. Accessed 1 May 2021.
5. Shields C. 2020. https://plato.stanford.edu/entries/aristotle-psychology/
6. West JB. Galen and the beginnings of Western physiology. Am J Physiol Lung Cell Mol Physiol. 2014;307(2):L121–8. https://doi.org/10.1152/ajplung.00123.2014.
7. Musa Y. Muhammad ibn Zakariya al-Razi and the First Psychiatric Ward. Published Online:1 Sep 2018. https://doi.org/10.1176/appi.ajp-rj.2018.130905.
8. Garrido S, Davidson J. Music and mood regulation: a historical enquiry into individual differences and musical prescriptions through the ages. Aust J Music Ther. 2013;24:89–109. https://www.researchgate.net/publication/259440453_Music_and_mood_regulation_A_historical_enquiry_into_individual_differences_and_musical_prescriptions_through_the_ages. Accessed 1 May 2021.
9. Klempe SH. The first use of the term "psychology". In: Tracing the emergence of psychology, 1520–1750. Theory and history in the human and social sciences. Cham: Springer; 2020. https://doi.org/10.1007/978-3-030-53701-2_2.
10. Klein J. 2020. https://plato.stanford.edu/entries/francis-bacon/#SciMetNovOrgTheInd. Accessed 1 May 2021.
11. Burton R. Anatomy of melancholy. Mary Ann Lund. 2010. https://books.google.com/books?hl=en&lr=&id=6FTrO_Ev4ewC&oi=fnd&pg=PR9&dq=Robert+Burton+published+Anatomy+of+Melancholy&ots=YpdFztf7z2&sig=by3tRLgYF-E-CH4sZ47PezVN2A0#v=onepage&q=Robert%20Burton%20published%20Anatomy%20of%20Melancholy&f=false. Accessed 1 May 2021.
12. Robinson H. Dualism. 2020. https://plato.stanford.edu/entries/dualism/. Accessed 1 May 2021.
13. Weiner DB. Philippe Pinel's "memoir on madness" of December 11, 1794: a fundamental text of modern psychiatry. Am J Psychiatry. 1992;149(6):725–32. https://doi.org/10.1176/ajp.149.6.725.
14. Ellis H. Benjamin Rush: American physician and statesman. Br J Hosp Med (Lond). 2013;74(4):234. https://doi.org/10.12968/hmed.2013.74.4.234.
15. Dix D. Memorial to the state legislature, 1843. http://www.teachushistory.org/second-great-awakening-age-reform/resources/memorial-legislature-massachusetts. Accessed 1 May 2021.
16. Ludwig RJ, Welch MG. Darwin's other dilemmas and the theoretical roots of emotional connection. Front Psychol. 2019;10:683. https://doi.org/10.3389/fpsyg.2019.00683.
17. Kim A. Wilhelm Wundt. 2016. https://plato.stanford.edu/entries/wilhelm-wundt/. Accessed 3 May 2021.
18. James W. The principles of psychology. New York: Henry Hold and Company; 1890.
19. The University Department of Psychiatry in Munich. The Munich Hospital Managed by Emil Kraepelin. In: The University Department of Psychiatry in Munich. Berlin, Heidelberg: Springer; 2008. https://doi.org/10.1007/978-3-540-74017-9_7.
20. Walusinski O, Bogousslavsky J. Charcot, Janet, and French models of psychopathology. Eur Neurol. 2020;83(3):333–40. https://doi.org/10.1159/000508267. Epub 2020
21. Meissner WW. Freud's methodology. J Am Psychoanal Assoc. 1971;19(2):265–309. https://doi.org/10.1177/000306517101900203.
22. Sigmund Freud. 1926. https://www.britannica.com/topic/Sigmund-Freud-on-psychoanalysis-1983319
23. Rehman I. Classical conditioning. 2020. https://www.ncbi.nlm.nih.gov/books/NBK470326/. Accessed 15 May 2021.
24. Yung CG. The essential Jung: selected and introduced by Anthony Storr. Princeton, NJ: Princeton University Press; 1983.
25. Adler A. The practice of individual psychology. London: Routledge; 1924.
26. Klein M. The Psycho-Analysis of Children, The Psycho-Analysis of Children. First Published October 1, 1933. https://doi.org/10.1111/j.1467-954X.1933.tb01887.x. https://journals.sagepub.com/doi/abs/10.1111/j.1467-954X.1933.tb01887.x?journalCode=soraKlein. Accessed 15 May 2021.
27. Watson JB. Psychology as the behaviorist views it. Psychol Rev. 1913;20(2):158–77. https://doi.org/10.1037/h0074428.
28. Sugarman S. Piaget's construction of the child's reality. Chicago, IL: Princeton University Press; 1987.
29. Sproatt D, Navab A. Operant conditioning. In: Volkmar FR, editor. Encyclopedia of autism spectrum disorders. New York, NY: Springer; 2013. https://doi.org/10.1007/978-1-4419-1698-3_127.
30. Todorovic D. Gestalt principles. 2008. http://www.scholarpedia.org/article/Gestalt_principles?__hstc=77520074.36a0ddae8e24bce7. Accessed 15 May 2021.
31. Berne E. Transactional analysis: a new and effective method of group therapy. Am J Psychother. 1958;12(4):735–43. https://doi.org/10.1176/appi.psychotherapy.1958.12.4.735.
32. Maslow AH. A theory of human motivation. Psychol Rev. 1943;50(4):370–96. https://doi.org/10.1037/h0054346.
33. Christian C, Safran JD, Muran JC. The corrective emotional experience: a relational perspective and critique. In: Castonguay LG, Hill CE, editors. Transformation in psychotherapy: corrective experiences across cognitive behavioral, humanistic, and psychodynamic approaches. Washington, DC: American Psychological Association; 2012. p. 51–67. https://doi.org/10.1037/13747-004.

34. Ornestein G. Eriksons stages of psychosocial development. 2020. https://www.ncbi.nlm.nih.gov/books/NBK556096/. Accessed 15 May 2021.
35. Moriarty KM, Alagna SW, Lake CR. Psychopharmacology. An historical perspective. Psychiatr Clin North Am. 1984;7(3):411–33.
36. Carlsson A, Lindqvist M. Effect of chlorpromazine or haloperidol on formation of 3methoxytyramine and normetanephrine in mouse brain. Acta Pharmacol Toxicol (Copenh). 1963;20:140–4. https://doi.org/10.1111/J.1600-0773.1963.Tb01730.X. Pmid: 14060771
37. Schildkraut JJ. The catecholamine hypothesis of affective disorders: a review of supporting evidence. Am J Psychiatry. 1965;122:509–22.
38. Bunney WE Jr, Davis JM. Norepinephrine in depressive reactions. A review. Arch Gen Psychiatry. 1965;13:483–94.
39. Gold PW, Wong ML. Re-assessing the catecholamine hypothesis of depression: the case of melancholic depression. Mol Psychiatry. 2021; https://doi.org/10.1038/s41380-021-01133-x.
40. Encyclopedia of psychotherapy. https://www.sciencedirect.com/referencework/9780123430106/encyclopedia-of-psychotherapy. Accessed 15 May 2021.
41. Cowan N. George Miller's magical number of immediate memory in retrospect: observations on the faltering progression of science. Psychol Rev. 2015;122(3):536–41. https://doi.org/10.1037/a0039035.
42. Sanders CE. Stages of moral development. 2016. https://www.britannica.com/science/Lawrence-Kohlbergs-stages-of-moral-development. Accessed 15 May 2021.
43. Buller S. Understanding Davanloo's intensive short–term dynamic psychotherapy: a guide for clinicians. Psychodyn Pract. 2018;24(3):281–8. https://doi.org/10.1080/14753634.2018.1435301.
44. Lewis MI, Butler R. Life review therapy. 1974. https://books.google.com/books?hl=en&lr=&id=bsRrAAAAMAAJ&oi=fnd&pg=PA199&dq=lewis+reminiscence+therapy&ots=GjmQUS4Gfr&sig=2tW1zIDjzr2mD7sCTL5oGN0wC4s#v=onepage&q=lewis%20reminiscence%20therapy&f=false. Accessed 15 May 2021.
45. Norman-Haignere SV et al., fMRI responses to harmonic tones and noises reveal divergence in the functional organization of human and macaque auditory cortex. Nat Neurosci 2019; 22(7):1057-1060. DOI: 10.1038/s41593-019-0410-7.
46. Bowlby J. Attachment and loss. New York: Basic Books; 1969.
47. Gerald L, Klerman GL, Weissman M. Interpersonal psychotherapy of depression: a brief, focused, specific strategy. Maryland: Rowan and Littlefield; 1984.
48. Kohut H. The analysis of the self: a systematic approach to the psychoanalytic treatment of narcissistic personality disorders. Chicago, IL: University of Chicago Press; 1971.
49. Minuchin S. Families and family therapy. Cambridge, MA: Harvard University Press; 1974.
50. Colapinto J. Structural family therapy. In: Lebow JL, Chambers AL, Breunlin DC, editors. Encyclopedia of couple and family therapy. Cham: Springer; 2019. https://doi.org/10.1007/978-3-319-49425-8_334.
51. Engel GL. The need for a new medical model: a challenge for biomedicine. Science. 1977;196(4286):129–36. https://doi.org/10.1126/science.847460.
52. Farre A, Rapley T. The new old (and old new) medical model: four decades navigating the biomedical and psychosocial understandings of health and illness. Healthcare. 2017;5(4):88. https://doi.org/10.3390/healthcare5040088.
53. Beck AT, Rush AJ, Shaw BF, Emery G. Cognitive therapy of depression. New York: Guilford Press; 1979.
54. Hayes SC, Luoma JB, Bond FW, Masuda A, Lillis J. Acceptance and commitment therapy: model, processes and outcomes. Behav Res Ther. 2006;44(1):1–25. https://doi.org/10.1016/j.brat.2005.06.006.
55. Eysenck SB, Eysenck HJ. Impulsiveness and venturesomeness: their position in a dimensional system of personality description. Psychol Rep. 1978;43(3 Pt 2):1247–55. https://doi.org/10.2466/pr0.1978.43.3f.1247.
56. Shapiro F, Wesselmann D, Mevissen L. Eye movement desensitization and reprocessing therapy (EMDR). In: Landolt MA, Cloitre M, Schnyder U, editors. Evidence-based treatments for trauma related disorders in children and adolescents. Cham: Springer International Publishing; 2017. p. 273–97. https://doi.org/10.1007/978-3-319-46138-0_13.
57. Frankl VE. The will to meaning;: foundations and applications of logotherapy. New York, NY: World Pub. Co; 1984.
58. Frank VE. Man's search for meaning. Boston, MA: Beacon Press; 1984.
59. Kabat-Zinn J. Full catastrophe living: using the wisdom of your body and mind to face stress, pain, and illness. New York: Delta Trade Paperbacks; 1991.
60. Reive C. The biological measurements of mindfulness-based stress reduction: a systematic review. Explore (NY). 2019;15(4):295–307. https://doi.org/10.1016/j.explore.2019.01.001.
61. Segal Z, Teasdale J, Williams M. Mindfulness-based cognitive therapy for depression. New York: Guilford Press; 2002.
62. Pradhan B. Yoga and mindfulness-based cognitive therapy (Y-MBCT©): use of yoga in its entirety. In: Yoga and mindfulness based cognitive therapy. Cham: Springer; 2015. https://doi.org/10.1007/978-3-319-09105-1_7.
63. Foa EB, McLean CP, Brown LA, Zang Y, Rosenfield D, Zandberg LJ, Ealey W, Hanson BS, Hunter LR, Lillard IJ, Patterson TJ, Rosado J, Scott V, Weber C, Wise JE, Zamora CD, Mintz J, Young-McCaughan S, Peterson AL, STRONG STAR Consortium. The effects of a prolonged exposure workshop with and without consultation on provider and patient outcomes: a randomized implementation trial. Implement Sci. 2020;15(1):59. https://doi.org/10.1186/s13012-020-01014-x.
64. Chapman AL. Dialectical behavior therapy: current indications and unique elements. Psychiatry (Edgmont). 2006;3(9):62–8.
65. North MM, North SM, Coble JR. Virtual reality therapy: an effective treatment for psychological disorders. Stud Health Technol Inform. 1997;44:59–70.
66. Seligman M. The original theory: authentic happiness. 2011. https://www.authentichappiness.sas.upenn.edu/learn/wellbeing. Accessed 31 May 2021.
67. Fonagy P. 2016. https://www.youtube.com/watch?v=MJ1Y9zw-n7U
68. Trujillo M. Intensive short-term dynamic psychotherapies. In: Sadock BJ, Sadock VA, Ruiz P, editors. Kaplan & Sadock's comprehensive textbook of psychiatry. 10th ed. Philadelphia, PA: Wolters Kluwer; 2017. p. 2796–815.
69. Kernberg OF, Yeomans FE, Clarkin JF, Levy KN. Transference focused psychotherapy: overview and update. Int J Psychoanal. 2008;89(3):601–20. https://doi.org/10.1111/j.1745-8315.2008.00046.x.
70. Clarkin JF, Cain NM, Lenzenweger MF. Advances in transference-focused psychotherapy derived from the study of borderline personality disorder: clinical insights with a focus on mechanism. Curr Opin Psychol. 2018;21:80–5. https://doi.org/10.1016/j.copsyc.2017.09.008.
71. Vilhauer J. 2014. https://www.futuredirectedtherapy.com/
72. Lally N, Nugent AC, Luckenbaugh DA, Ameli R, Roiser JP, Zarate CA. Anti-anhedonic effect of ketamine and its neural correlates in treatment-resistant bipolar depression. Transl Psychiatry. 2014;4(10):e469. https://doi.org/10.1038/tp.2014.105.
73. Hopko DR, Lejuez CW, Ruggiero KJ, Eifert GH. Contemporary behavioral activation treatments for depression: procedures, principles, and progress. Clin Psychol Rev. 2003;23(5):699–717. https://doi.org/10.1016/s0272-7358(03)00070-9.
74. Richards DA, Ekers D, McMillan D, Taylor RS, Byford S, Warren FC, Barrett B, Farrand PA, Gilbody S, Kuyken W, O'Mahen H,

Watkins ER, Wright KA, Hollon SD, Reed N, Rhodes S, Fletcher E, Finning K. Cost and outcome of behavioural activation versus cognitive behavioural therapy for depression (COBRA): a randomised, controlled, non-inferiority trial. Lancet. 2016;388(10047):871–80. https://doi.org/10.1016/S0140-6736(16)31140-0.

75. IsHak WW. The handbook of wellness medicine. Cambridge: Cambridge University Press; 2020.
76. Bailey RM. Dialectical behavioral therapy: the case of Moses. In: Dealey RP, Evans MR, editors. Discovering theory in clinical practice. Cham: Springer; 2021.
77. Rieber RW. Encyclopedia of the history of psychological theories. New York: Springer; 2012.
78. Oogarah-Pratap B, Bholoa A, Ramma Y. Stage theory of cognitive development—Jean Piaget. In: Akpan B, Kennedy TJ, editors. Science education in theory and practice. Springer Texts in Education. Cham: Springer; 2020. https://doi.org/10.1007/978-3-030-43620-9_10.
79. Marcia JE. Life transitions and stress in the context of psychosocial development. In: Miller T, editor. Handbook of stressful transitions across the lifespan. New York, NY: Springer; 2010. https://doi.org/10.1007/978-1-4419-0748-6_2.
80. Klein MO, Battagello DS, Cardoso AR, et al. Dopamine: functions, signaling, and association with neurological diseases. Cell Mol Neurobiol. 2019;39:31–59. https://doi.org/10.1007/s10571-018-0632-3.
81. Bilder R, Volavka J, Lachman H, et al. The catechol-O-methyltransferase polymorphism: relations to the tonic–phasic dopamine hypothesis and neuropsychiatric phenotypes. Neuropsychopharmacology. 2004;29:1943–61. https://doi.org/10.1038/sj.npp.1300542.
82. David OA, Oltean HR, Cardoş RAI. REBT and parenting interventions. In: Bernard M, Dryden W, editors. Advances in REBT. Cham: Springer; 2019. https://doi.org/10.1007/978-3-319-93118-0_15.
83. Eppel A. The emergence of short-term psychodynamic psychotherapy. In: Short-term psychodynamic psychotherapy. Cham: Springer; 2018. https://doi.org/10.1007/978-3-319-74995-2_1.
84. Kim JJ, Kent KM, Cunnington R, et al. Attachment styles modulate neural markers of threat and imagery when engaging in self-criticism. Sci Rep. 2020;10:13776. https://doi.org/10.1038/s41598-020-70772-x.
85. Law R. Interpersonal psychotherapy for depression. Adv Psychiatr Treat. 2011;17(1):23–31.
86. Mehta M, Kapoor S. Role of psychosocial factors in the management of health problems. In: Misra G, editor. Psychosocial interventions for health and well-being. New Delhi: Springer; 2018. https://doi.org/10.1007/978-81-322-3782-2_2.
87. Morgan TA, Aljabari R. Using acceptance and commitment therapy in the treatment of borderline personality disorder: rationale, preliminary evidence, and future directions. Curr Treat Options Psych. 2019;6:271–83. https://doi.org/10.1007/s40501-019-00185-9.
88. Strelau J. Temperament. In: Zeigler-Hill V, Shackelford TK, editors. Encyclopedia of personality and individual differences. Cham: Springer; 2020. https://doi.org/10.1007/978-3-319-24612-3_446.
89. O'Shea BG. An overview of psychotherapy modalities for the treatment of complex trauma. In: Healing complex posttraumatic stress disorder. Essential clinical social work series. Cham: Springer; 2021. https://doi.org/10.1007/978-3-030-61416-4_8.
90. Wong PTP. Viktor Frankl's meaning-seeking model and positive psychology. In: Batthyany A, Russo-Netzer P, editors. Meaning in positive and existential psychology. New York, NY: Springer; 2014. https://doi.org/10.1007/978-1-4939-0308-5_10.
91. Pradhan B, Pinninti NR. Yoga and mindfulness-based cognitive therapy for psychosis (Y-MBCT$_p$©): a pilot study on its efficacy as brief therapy. In: Pradhan B, Pinninti N, Rathod S, editors. Brief interventions for psychosis. Cham: Springer; 2016. https://doi.org/10.1007/978-3-319-30521-9_5.
92. Pagel JF. Prolonged exposure therapy. In: Post-traumatic stress disorder. Cham: Springer; 2021. https://doi.org/10.1007/978-3-030-55909-0_11.
93. Appel L, Kisonas E, Appel E, et al. Introducing virtual reality therapy for inpatients with dementia admitted to an acute care hospital: learnings from a pilot to pave the way to a randomized controlled trial. Pilot Feasibility Stud. 2020;6:166. https://doi.org/10.1186/s40814-020-00708-9.
94. Pociask M, Stefanowicz-Kocoł A. Language activities aimed at social competencies for nursing students in practice. In: Kenny N, Işık-Taş E, Jian H, editors. English for specific purposes instruction and research. Cham: Palgrave Macmillan; 2020. https://doi.org/10.1007/978-3-030-32914-3_7.
95. McLaren V, Sharp C. What is mentalizing? In: Williams L, Muir O, editors. Adolescent suicide and self-injury. Cham: Springer; 2020. https://doi.org/10.1007/978-3-030-42875-4_1.
96. Richards DA, Ekers D, McMillan D, Taylor RS, Byford S, Warren FC, et al. Cost and outcome of behavioural activation versus cognitive behavioural therapy for depression (COBRA): a randomised, controlled, non-inferiority trial. Lancet. 2016;388(10047):871–80. https://doi.org/10.1016/S0140-6736(16)31140-0. Epub 2016 Jul 23. PMID: 27461440; PMCID: PMC5007415

Assessment: Interview, History, Physical, and Mental Status Examination

6

Rob Poole, Robert Higgo, and Tom Lorenz

Introduction

All medicine is practiced through interaction with patients. This is particularly obvious in psychiatry, where we consciously make use of the doctor–patient relationship as a therapeutic tool.

Initial assessment of patients involves collecting systematic information about them whilst at the same time forming a helpful therapeutic relationship. Failure to pay attention to the latter task can have adverse effects (such as distrust or misunderstandings) that can be difficult to overcome.

Although it is sometimes implied that making a diagnosis involves weighing up information about the patient and comparing it with DSM-5 [1] criteria, this is not the process that experienced clinicians follow. Patients are assessed in a variety of circumstances. The information available before the interview starts will inevitably suggest diagnostic possibilities (Fig. 6.1).

Consequently, although a thorough and systematic collection of information is important, this occurs within an interview process where the doctor already has a hypothesis. It is helpful to recognise what this is and to consciously assess what information tends to support it and what tends to refute it. This active process within the interview allows a new, better, hypothesis to form which can be tested in turn.

In this chapter, we set out a number of lists, including headings for history taking and the mental state examination. These templates help with the methodical collection and recording of information, but they are not programmes for interviews. Good psychiatric interviews are conversational in tone, not machine-like or formulaic (Fig. 6.2).

Interpersonal empathy is a key tool. Psychiatrists are not only interested in what patients say. They need to understand what the patient has experienced and the likely causes. The social and psychological context in which the problem has arisen is always important, even where the disorder appears to have been caused by clear-cut organic pathology (Fig. 6.3).

R. Poole (✉) · R. Higgo
Centre for Mental Health and Society, Prifysgol Bangor University, Wrexham, Wales, UK
e-mail: r.poole@bangor.ac.uk; robert.higgo@wales.nhs.uk

T. Lorenz
Department of Child and Adolescent Psychiatry, Betsi Cadwaladr University Health Board, Flintshire, Wales, UK
e-mail: tom.lorenz@wales.nhs.uk

W. W. IsHak (ed.), *Atlas of Psychiatry*, https://doi.org/10.1007/978-3-031-15401-0_6

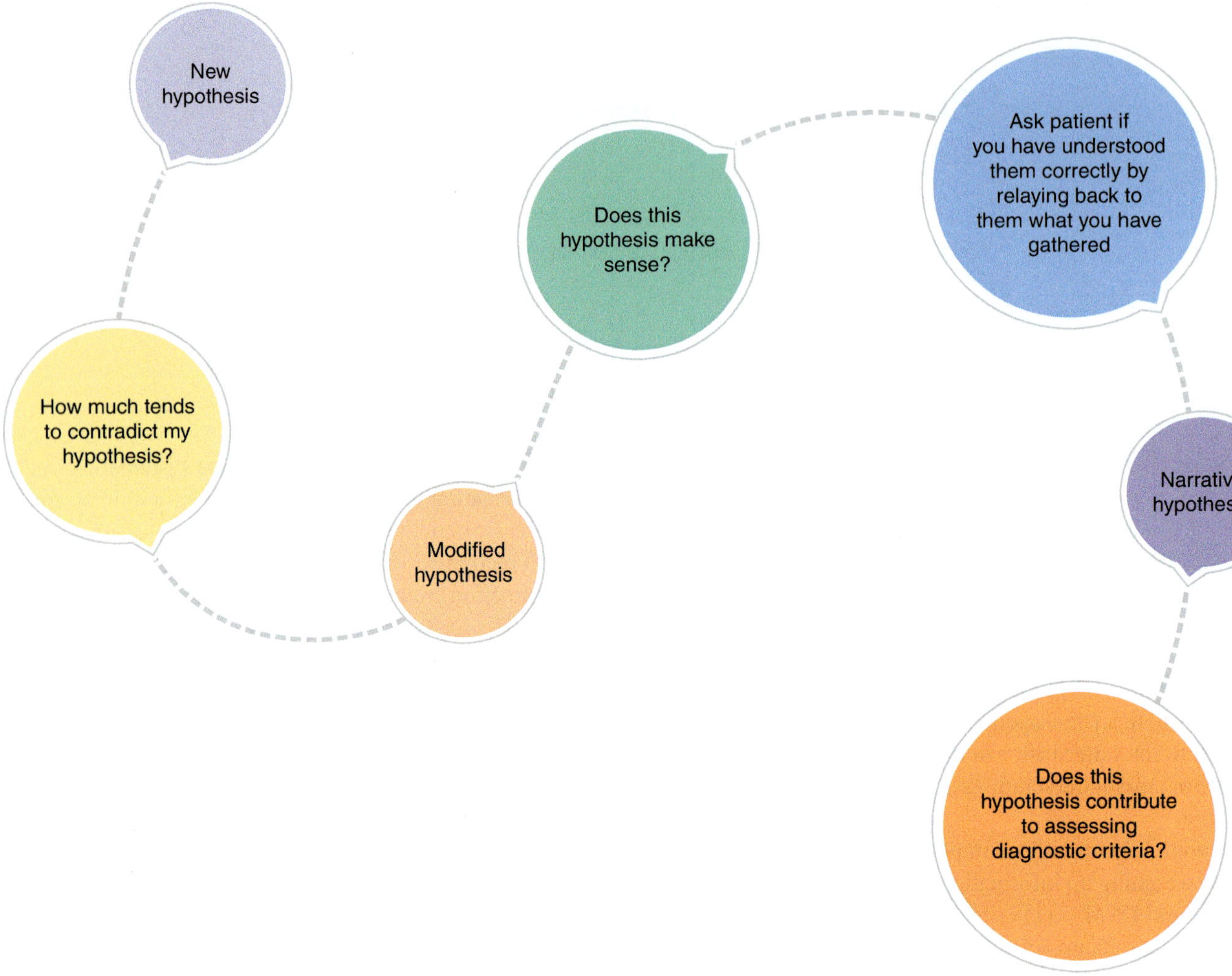

Fig. 6.1 Clinical hypothesis formation and elaboration

Fig. 6.2 Understanding the patient is the key

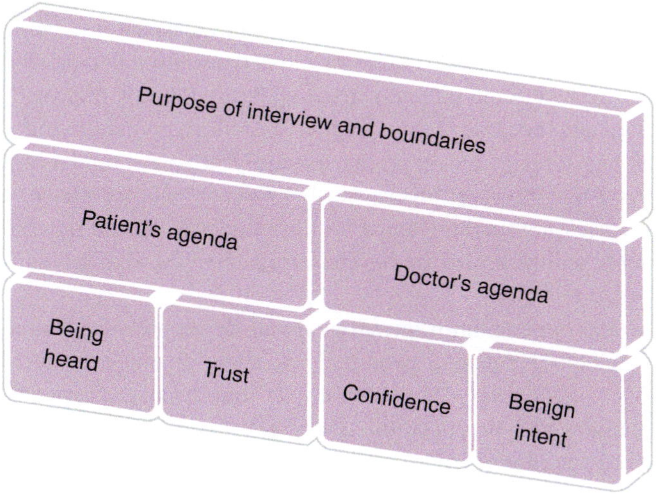

Fig. 6.3 Relational aspects of assessment

Purpose of Assessment

Although initial assessments include making a provisional diagnosis or formulation of the patient's problem, these interviews can have a variety of other purposes. They include initiating or suggesting treatments, taking action to reduce risk, review of medications, exclusion of organic causes for psychiatric symptoms, etc. You should be clear at the outset about the purpose of the interview and other people's expectations of it.

The setting affects how the interview is conducted. Assessments in the psychiatrist's office are different from those conducted in hospital wards or in the community. There are differences in emphasis according to the patient's age and evident mental state.

It is frequently useful to speak to family or other informants. In part, this is to help understand the person more fully but is also often to understand the impact that their problem has had on those around them, including partners and dependent children (Fig. 6.4).

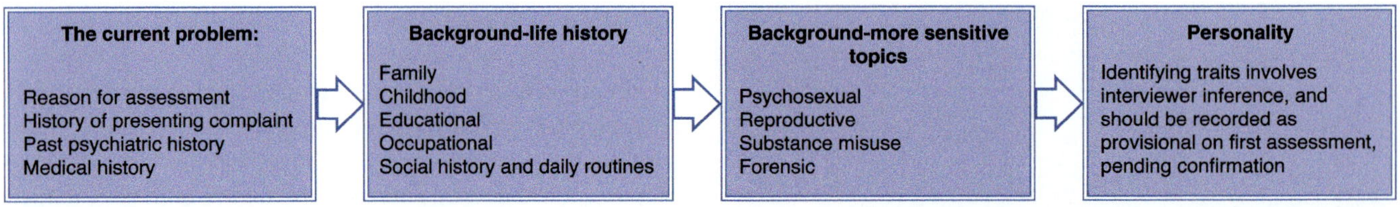

Fig. 6.4 Main structure of psychiatric history taking

History

When history-taking, ask about which year things happened. This allows events in different domains to be linked so that you can understand the chronology properly. The main headings are as follows.

Reason for Assessment

What has happened that has led to this assessment? What facts are known at the outset about preceding events (for example, what led up to the patient been assessed urgently).

History of Presenting Complaint

What is bothering the patient (irrespective of whether they attribute that to a mental health problem, the behaviour of others, or something else)? How did it start? How has it developed? How does it affect the patient's behaviour and daily activities? What do they think causes the problem? What have they done to relieve their distress, and has it worked? What does any informant say about these issues (Fig. 6.5)?

Psychiatric History

Has the patient ever felt like this before? What did they do about it? What helped? Have they ever seen a psychiatrist before? What did the psychiatrists say and do about the problem? Record dates and locations of interventions and hospital admissions wherever possible.

Family History

This includes whether family members have had similar problems or other mental health difficulties. Equally important, it involves detail about family structure, family occupations, bereavements (with dates), and the quality of relationships. A family diagram can be helpful. People often have complex family structures involving half-sibships (where one parent is shared) and step-sibships (where people are part of the same family group but are not genetically related). The distinction is important.

Childhood History

Childhood adversity has an enduring impact on physical and mental health throughout the life course. It is important to know about key childhood events, as well as the social and emotional environment in which the patient grew up. This includes the quality of their relationship with each parent and siblings, childhood illness and accidents, frequent changes of address, and episodes of being looked after away from their parents. Physical and emotional abuse is usually mentioned in response to these questions. Childhood sexual abuse, if it is not volunteered here, is best asked about when discussing psychosexual history. It is conventional to ask the age at which the patient started walking, talking, and reading, and became dry at night (the 'developmental milestones') but in our experience, hardly anyone ever knows. Persistent bed-wetting is worth knowing about because it involves continuing shame and humiliation. We do not ask about nail-biting, as we have never understood what it is supposed to signify.

More meaningful questions about developmental factors focus on evidence of hyperactivity, attention and concentration difficulties (daydreaming), impulsivity, forward-planning/self-organisation skills, and social communication (for example, use of gestures and metaphors).

There is a general rule that you should ask patients to describe tangible events and what actually happened. Most people find this easier than describing how they felt. For example, when a patient says that they had a poor relationship with a parent, it is helpful to ask what the parent *did.* There is a general rule in history-taking: *Ask what happened.*

Fig. 6.5 General interviewing tips

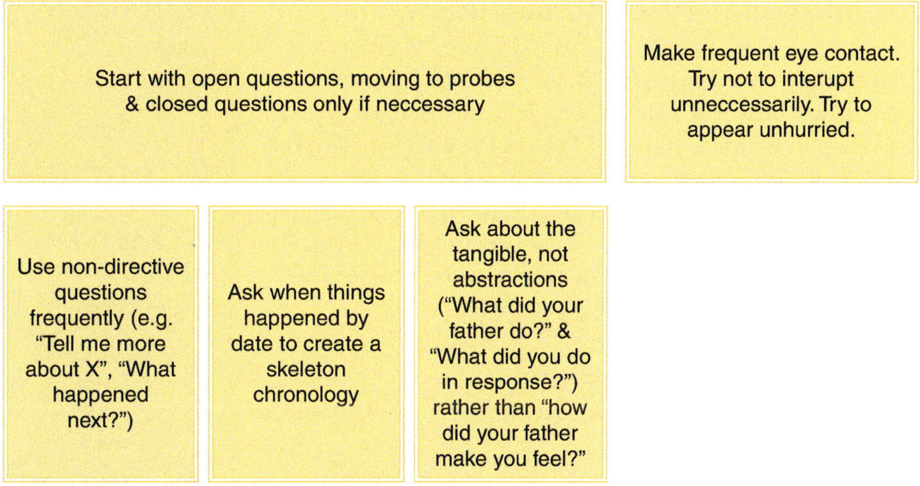

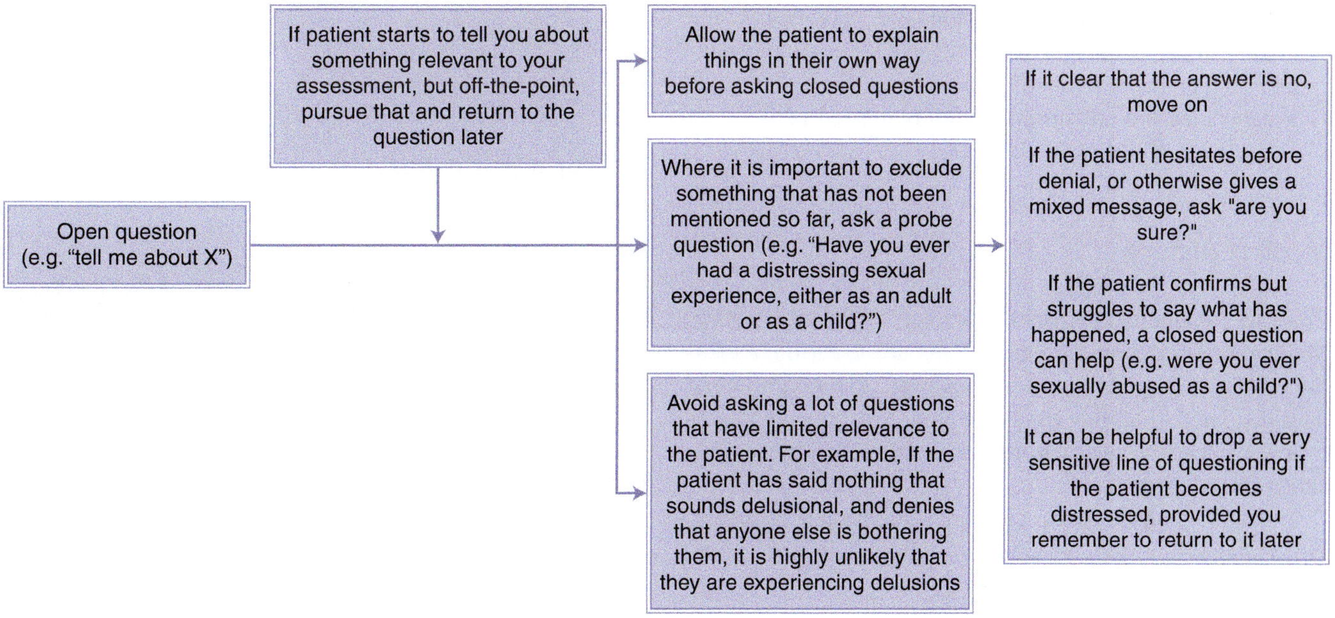

Fig. 6.6 Using probes to elicit information

Educational History

Which schools did the patient attend, and between what dates? Were there problems with peer relationships and academic attainment? You should ask about their relationships with teachers, disciplinary problems, exclusions, and their experience of bullying (as perpetrator and victim, bearing in mind that these often co-exist). Ask what age they finished school, whether this was early, and the reasons. Complaints that they felt let down or misunderstood by the educational system are common in people with (at the time) undiagnosed neurodevelopmental problems, irrespective of their eventual educational attainment.

A similar approach should be followed for college and higher educational history. Details of qualifications are useful to know, including non-university and vocational qualifications as well as grade of degree.

Occupational History

Most people know the dates when they started and left jobs, and the reasons. However, some occupations are very irregular, such as construction work or entertainment. In these cases, understanding patterns of employment, and lengthy periods of unemployment are more important than precise dates of long-forgotten engagements (Fig. 6.6).

Psychosexual and Reproductive History

Patients vary considerably in the ease with which they discuss their sexual lives. For patients who feel awkward, it may be necessary to return to the topic later in the interview, or at a later date. Discomfort usually indicates that the subject is important, so it is not an indication that the subject should be permanently avoided. Good interviewers must be relaxed about these subjects themselves, because unease will affect patients.

Relevant questions include:

- Age of earliest sexual experience.
- Length of relationships and reasons for relationships ending.
- Promiscuity.
- Unwelcome sexual experiences as a child or as an adult.
- Current partner, their occupation and personality, and quality of the relationship.
- Children and contact with them.
- Pregnancies and outcomes, including miscarriages.
- Experience of domestic violence.

Medical History

Physical and mental health interact with each other. Medications for long-term conditions are often only mentioned if you ask about *all* medications. Ask people what they take, not what they are prescribed. Most people do not follow prescribing instructions very well, and some significantly deviate from them.

Ask about current illness and medications, as well as previous major illnesses, treatments, and surgical operations, with dates (Fig. 6.7).

Social History and Daily Routine

This refers to how people live every day. In gathering this information, you learn a good deal about the patient's personality as well as their lifestyle.

Ask about friendships. Does the patient have many friends, just a few, or none? Are their relationships stable and enduring, or turbulent and transient?

How do they spend their time? What is their current pattern of activity through a typical weekday/weekend? Was it different before they started to feel unwell? Ask about patterns of eating and sleeping.

Patients' hobbies and interests are important. Are they still pursued or have they given up lately?

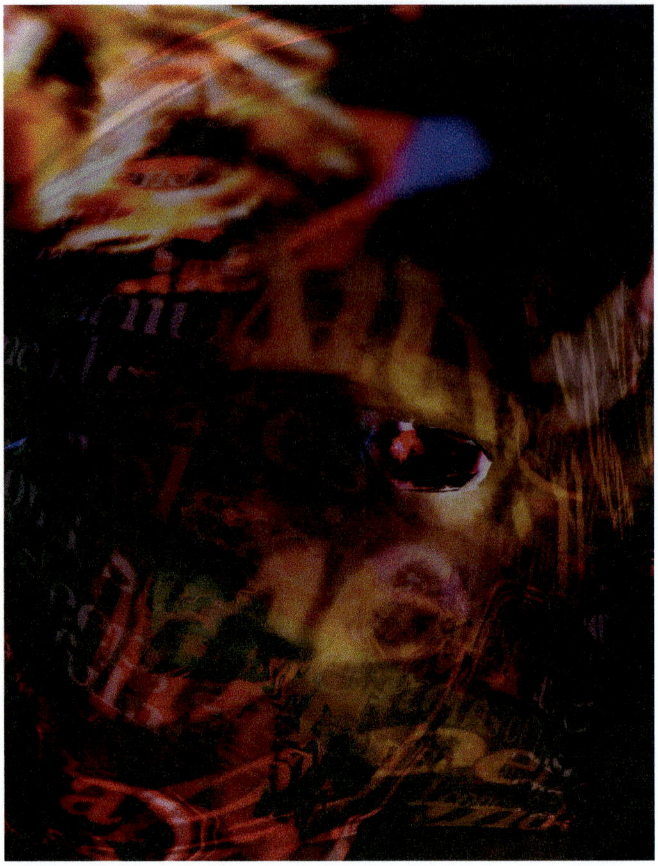

Fig. 6.7 A good assessment is not just words; it is a map of the patient's life

Substance Misuse History

All patients should be asked about substance misuse, irrespective of whether they appear to be stereotypical drug users or drinkers. For example, alcohol and drug abuse are common in the elderly and are easily overlooked (Fig. 6.8).

There are three broad types of common substance misuse: alcohol misuse, street drug misuse, and misuse of prescription or over-the-counter medications. In our experience (and somewhat counter-intuitively), street drug users tend to be more forthcoming about their behaviour than either drinkers or prescription drug misusers.

The principles are to ask:

- What do you take?
- What strength?
- What happens if you do not take it?
- What do you see as the benefits and adverse consequences?

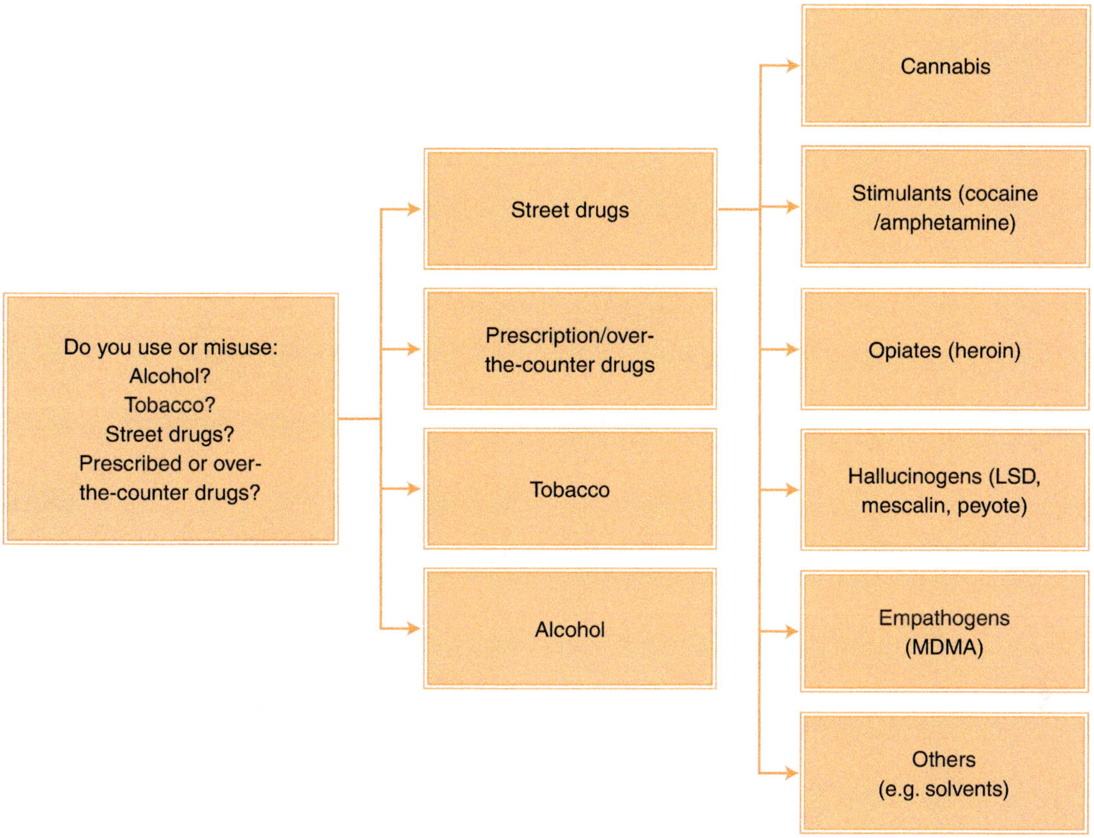

Fig. 6.8 Substance misuse history

Look out for signs of substance misuse such as constant runny nose (snorting cocaine), burns to the end of the nose (crack cocaine), or the smell of alcohol. When you spot these things, ask the patient about them.

Where substance misuse is confirmed, ask if they had withdrawal symptoms, including delirium and seizures, and whether they use drugs/alcohol to avoid or relieve withdrawal symptoms. Do they lie to partners, conceal their use, steal, or otherwise prioritise substance misuse (Fig. 6.9)?

Forensic History

It can be embarrassing to ask an ostensibly law-abiding citizen whether they have ever been in trouble with the law, but if you do not ask, it is unlikely to be volunteered. A high proportion of men have some offending history before the age of 25 years, but you are also interested in more serious offences and penalties. Even trivial adolescent offences can be associated with surprising levels of shame that last into late middle age and beyond (Fig. 6.10).

Questions include:

- Have you ever been prosecuted and if so, were you convicted?
- What was the offence? What was the penalty?
- Have you had any problems in the civil justice system?

Premorbid Personality

All assessments should include consideration of the patient's personality, which is usually evident from patterns of behaviour that they have described. It is worth running your impressions past the patient, saying that you have noticed that, for example, they seem to be someone for whom orderliness and regular routines are important. Initial impressions can be quite misleading (Fig. 6.11).

Fig. 6.9 Principle questions about substance misuse

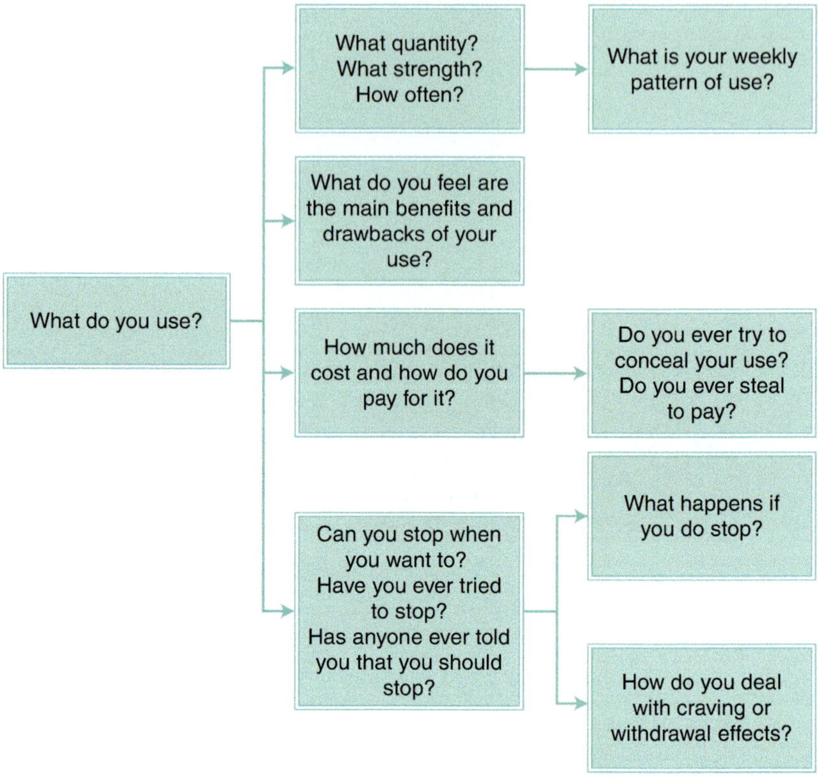

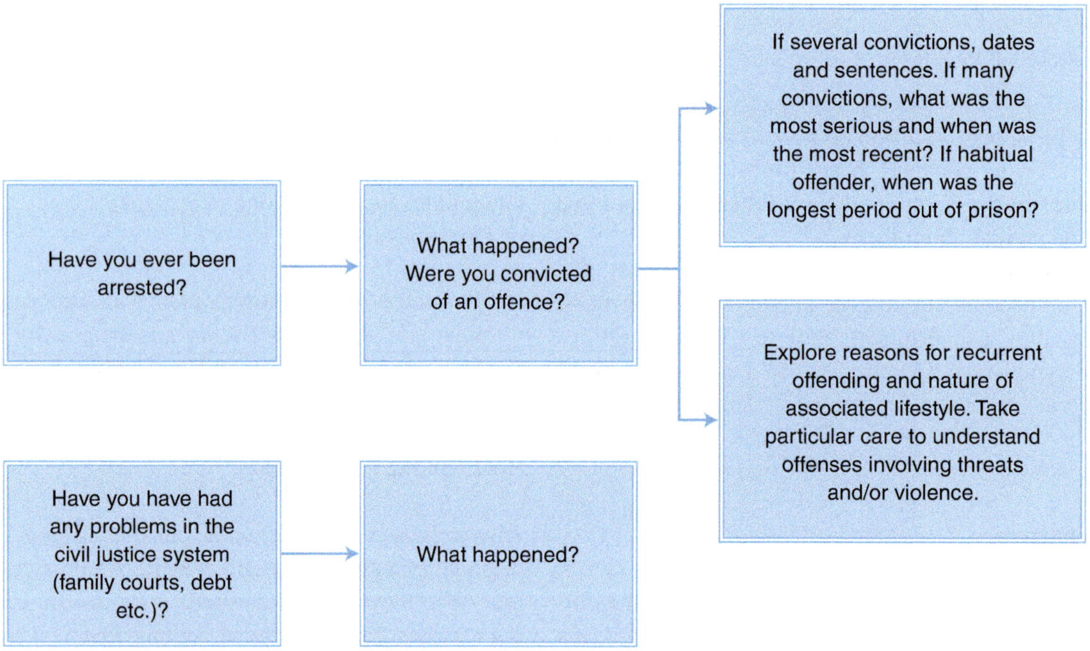

Fig. 6.10 Forensic history questions

Personality disorder is the most contested of psychiatric diagnoses, and assessment should be cautious. It should be based upon information from several sources, gathered over time. Short-term behaviours caused, for example, by episodes of an affective disorder can lead to behaviours reminiscent of personality disorder, which then disappear when the mood disorder is treated.

You should be familiar with the main personality traits and DSM-5 personality diagnoses and clusters (Fig. 6.12).

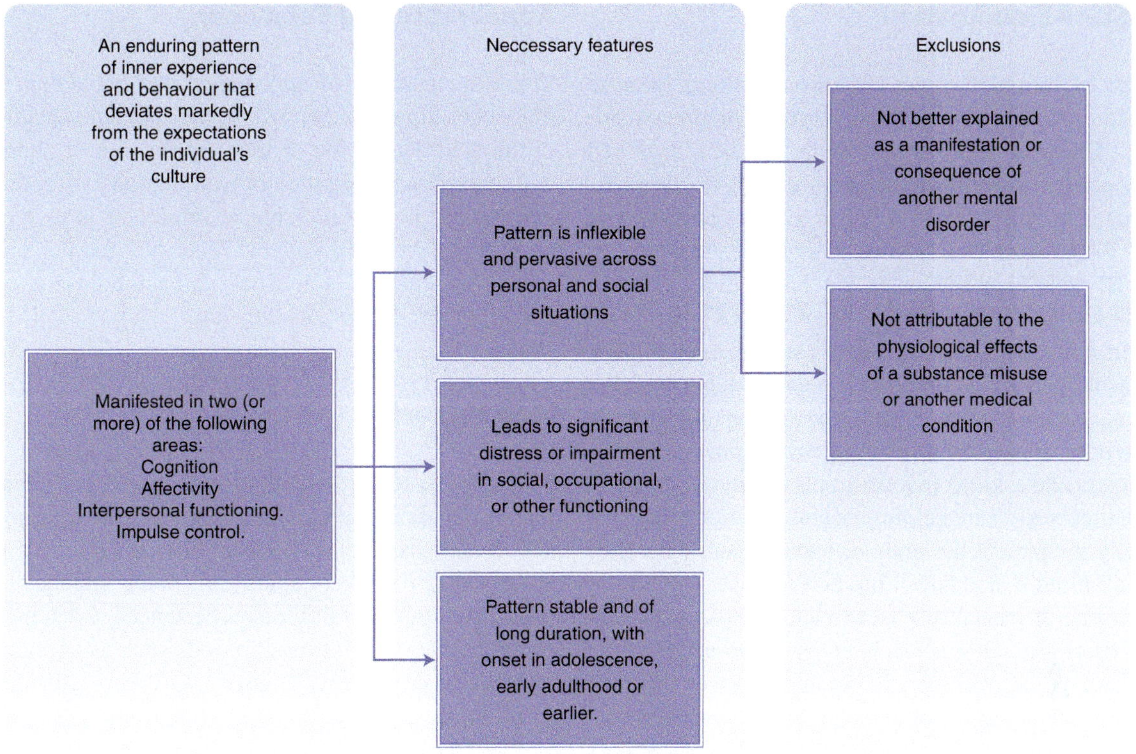

Fig. 6.11 General criteria for personality disorder

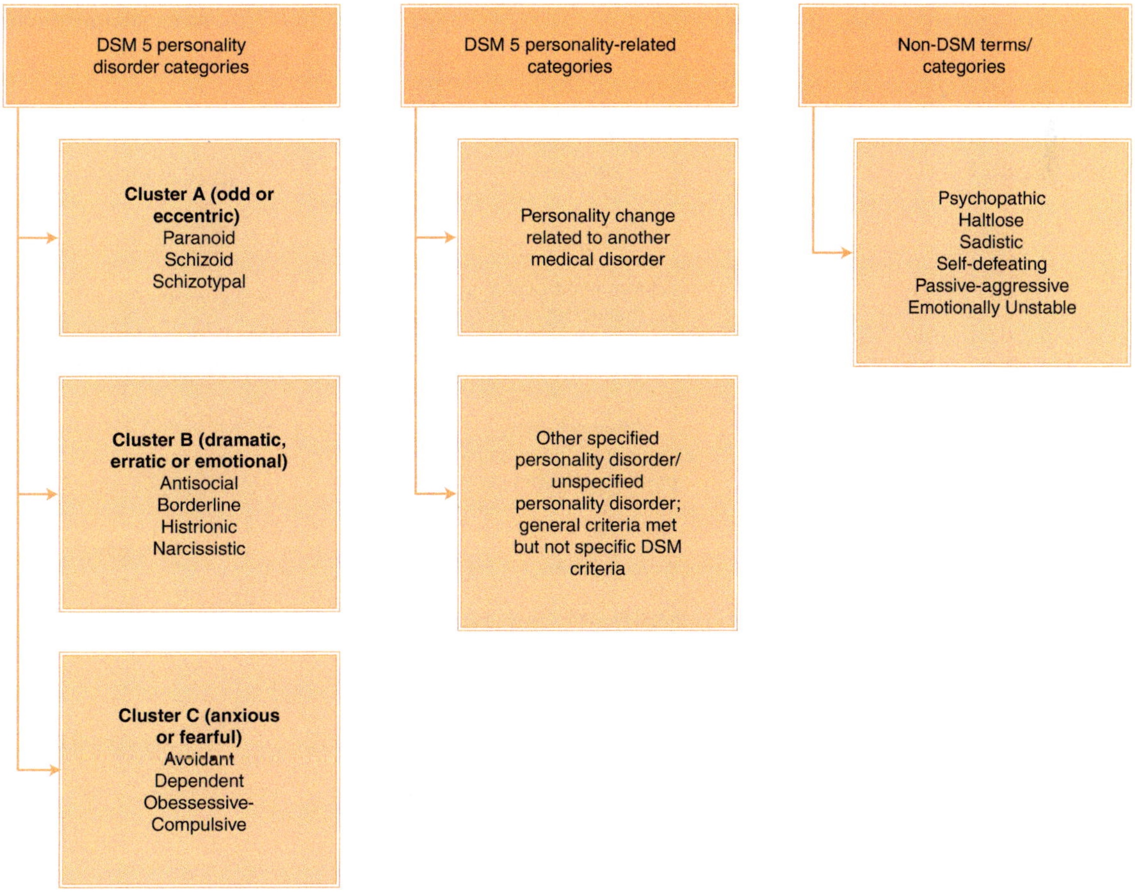

Fig. 6.12 Personality disorder typologies

Mental State Examination

Mental state examination comes after history taking, because the context in which symptoms arise is crucial to understanding them. However, specific symptoms are best explored when they are first mentioned, often quite early in the interview. If this is not possible, "I'd like to go back and ask you about….." feels natural and conversational when raised later.

A mental state examination is not just a description of what the patient says. It is an interactive process. Experienced interviewers get better accounts from patients than beginners. Knowing what you are looking for is important, but so is the ability to make patients comfortable when disclosing distressing experiences. Firing off a lot of questions does not work well. Curiosity and asking obvious simple questions ("why?," "how does that work") are helpful. Useful questions focus on what exactly the patient has done or experienced, what they believe has caused it, and how it has come about.

The structure of mental state examination helps to organise and order observations. It is not an interview schedule. You need a repertoire of probe questions, for example, "Does anything interfere with your ability to concentrate?," which can elicit both anxiety symptoms or experiences of thought interference. Probes must come conversationally from the interviewer (Fig. 6.13).

Appearance and Behaviour

There are patterns of appearance and behaviour that carry diagnostic significance, such as the anguished hand wringing of agitated depression or the combination of abnormal gait and inconsolable agitation in Huntingdon's disease. They are not terribly common. What is important is to record what you notice about the patient. Whenever the person's behaviour or appearance is unusual, you should ask why they are acting, or are dressed, as they are.

Mood/Affect

Mood refers to persistent patterns, and affect means manifest mood state, but they are essentially used as synonyms. Mood states are multifaceted rather than simple points on a happiness-to-misery spectrum. Some nuances and variations distinguish individual experiences, as well as 'classic presentations' of abnormal moods such as euphoric mania, or retarded depression. Figure 6.14 was originally intended to illustrate that certain 'basic emotions' are recognisable across cultures [2]. From the point of view of a clinical psychiatrist, however, the photographs have a cartoonish

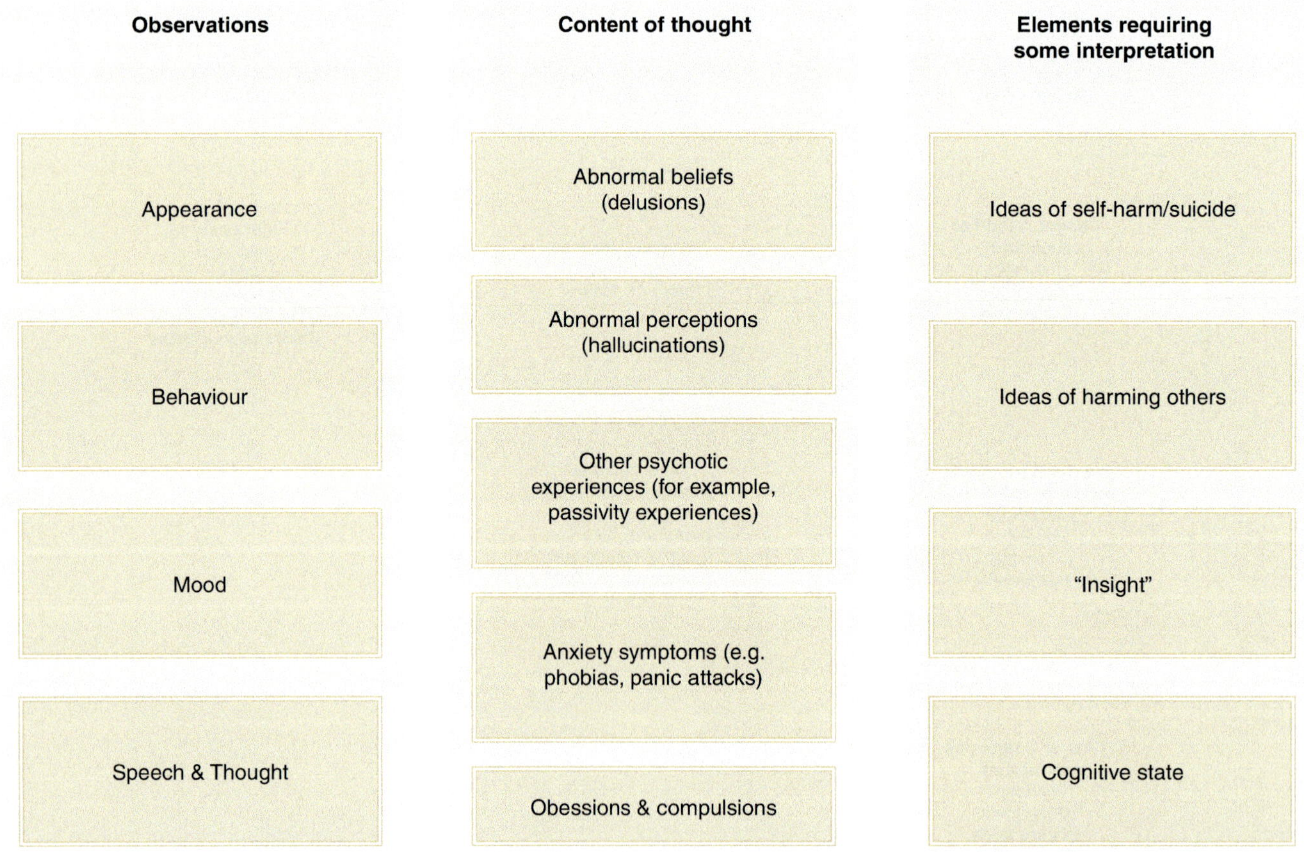

Fig. 6.13 Formal structure of mental state examination

Fig. 6.14 Percentage agreement in how a photograph was judged across cultures. (*From* Ekman 1973 [2]; *with permission from Elsevier*)

	Percentage Agreement in How Photograph Was judged Across Cultures				
	United States (*N*=99)	Brazil (*N*=40)	Chile (*N*=119)	Argentina (*N*=168)	Japan (*N*=29)
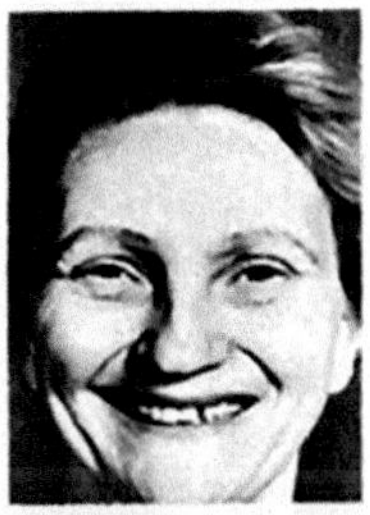	97% Happiness	95% Happiness	95% Happiness	98% Happiness	100% Happiness
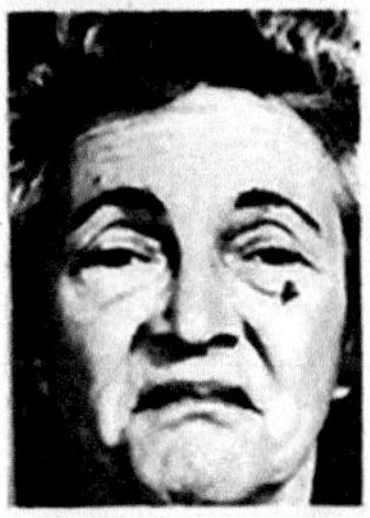	92% Disgust	97% Disgust	92% Disgust	92% Disgust	90% Disgust
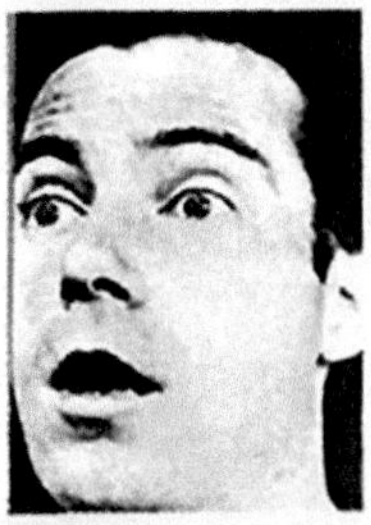	95% Surprise	87% Surprise	93% Surprise	95% Surprise	100% Surprise
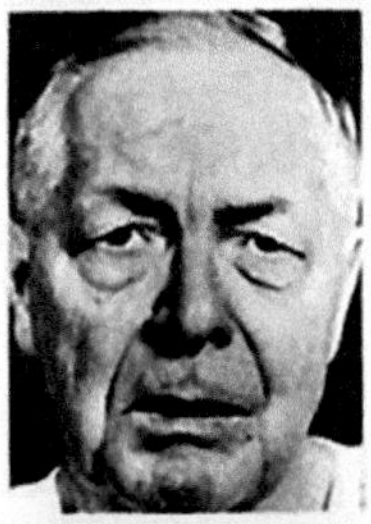	84% Sadness	59% Sadness	88% Sadness	78% Sadness	62% Sadness
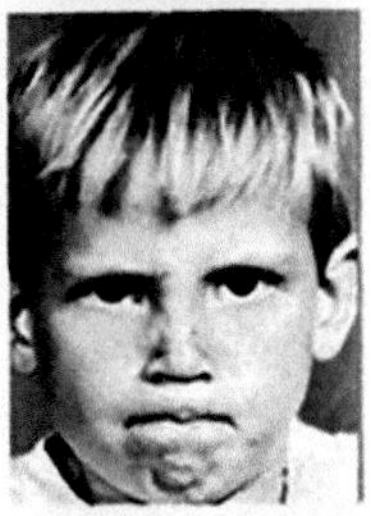	67% Anger	90% Anger	94% Anger	90% Anger	90% Anger
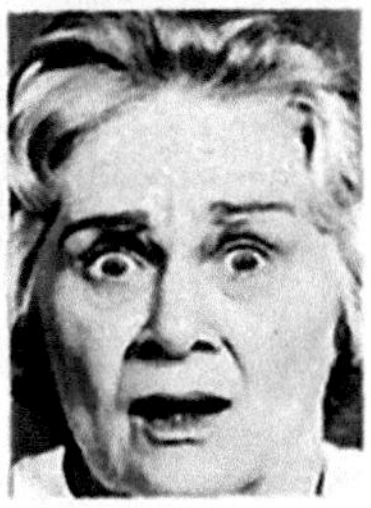	85% Fear	67% Fear	68% Fear	54% Fear	66% Fear

quality. They freeze expressions that in life are part of a dynamic sequence. They illustrate that, in trying to understand people in emotional distress, complexity is the rule, not the exception.

The major mood states of interest are depression, euphoria, anger, and perplexity. These can co-exist in all combinations. Some items of history, such as patterns of sleep, appetite, diurnal variation of mood, tearfulness, and concentration are relevant to assessing mood.

There are four major abnormalities of mood reactivity: labile mood, flattened affect, irritability, and incongruous affect. The latter is a mood state that does not have a close link to either the patient's situation or their thought content. It is a schizophreniform phenomenon. It is not easy to identify correctly, as some people who are disdainful or very anxious can appear superficially similar. True incongruous affect is usually accompanied by marked perplexity.

Hopelessness and despair are important, as they have implications for suicide risk. Ask what people think will happen to them and whether there is a possibility that things could improve.

Speech and Thought

This section concerns the fluency, or form of speech and thought. It is important to exclude disorders of speech first. Thought can only be assessed through the medium of speech. The commonest disorders of speech are dysphasia, impaired fluency due to poor education, stuttering and efforts to control this, and verbal tics.

The major abnormalities of the form of thought are set out in Fig. 6.15.

Elation:

- Rapid pace of thought (pressure of speech/thought).
- Excessive digression (prolixity/circumstantiality).
- Loss of direction of thought due to punning, alliteration, rhyming, and linking words rather than ideas.

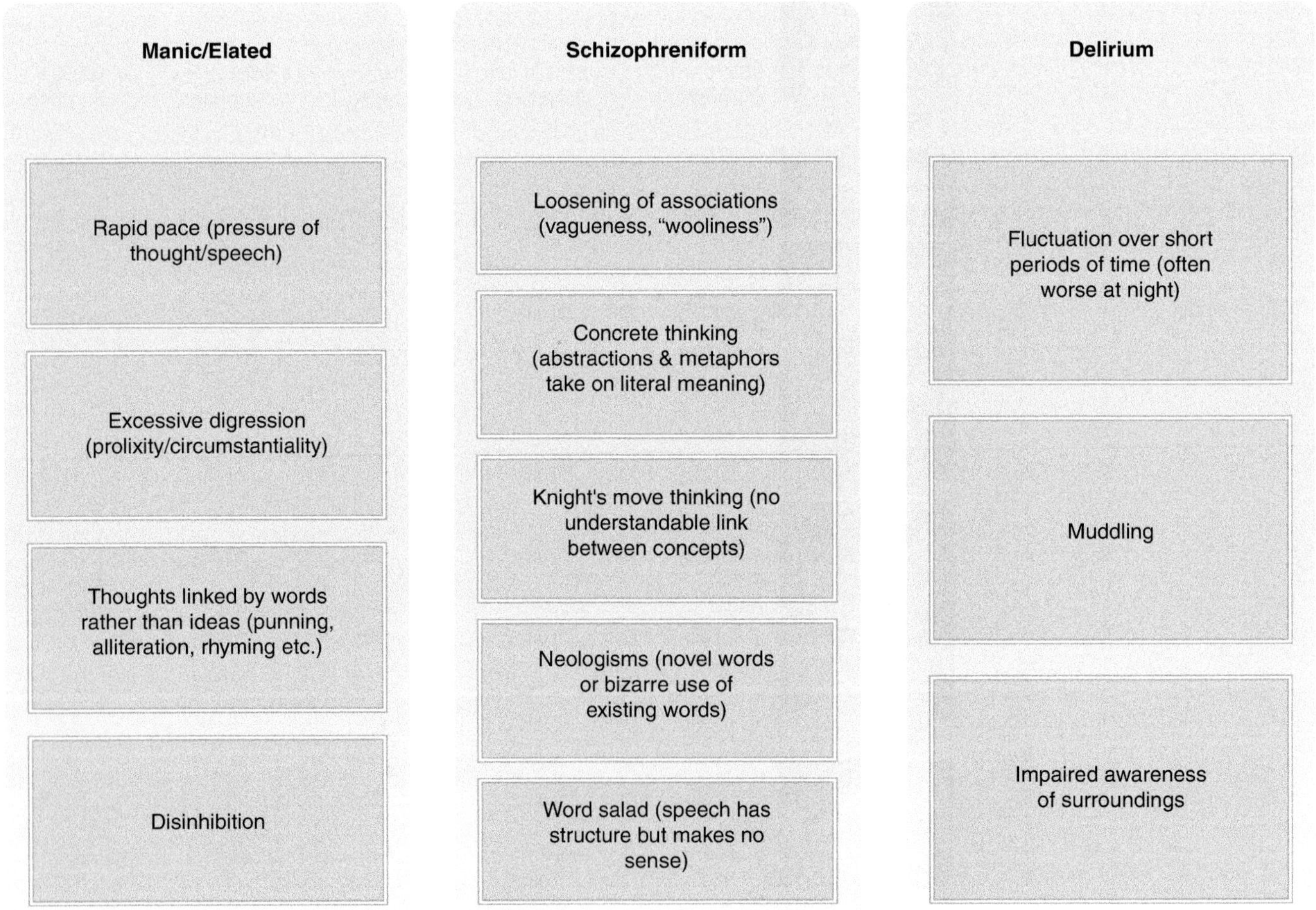

NB there are no pathognomic features in thought disorder

Fig. 6.15 Abnormalities of form of thought (thought disorder)

Schizophreniform thought disorder:

- Loosening of associations (vagueness/"woolly thinking").
- Concrete thinking (abstractions and metaphors take on literal meaning).
- Knight's move thinking (ideas lurch without a logical link).
- Use of neologisms (novel word forms or bizarre use of existing words).
- Word salad (speech that has structure but makes no sense).

Delirium and dementia.

- Muddling and confusion (can also occur in psychosis).

All of these are observed and cannot be elicited by questioning. You must be certain that the abnormality is persistent and prominent. It is a mistake to decide on the basis of a small fragment of speech which you do not understand, as the problem may be with you, not the patient.

Delusions

Delusions are fixed false beliefs that are not culturally congruent. Their salience and their fixity are as important as the content. These distinguish them from unusual opinions or widely held conspiracy theories. They may arise as sudden realisations (primary delusions), or they may arise as a consequence of an abnormality of mood or perception (secondary delusions). Delusions may be bizarre (more likely as primary delusions) or mood-congruent (by definition, secondary delusions).

The preponderances of delusions are paranoid, grandiose, depressive, or referential. Paranoid delusions are the belief that you are being victimised, usually in implausible ways. Grandiose delusions are expansive beliefs about identity and personal powers, often involving extreme wealth or messianic identity. Depressive delusions are usually centred on ruination or the belief that the person's body is diseased or even already dead. Delusions of reference are where neutral stimuli, such as the content of television programmes, are believed to be personally directed. They are common.

Other common types of delusion include jealous delusions (that a partner is unfaithful) and delusions of infestation. Some authorities recognise *forme fruste* delusions called "overvalued ideas," but these are very hard to define and reliably identify.

Some types of delusion carry an intrinsic risk of self-harm or violence. For example, depressive delusions of inadvertently causing harm to loved ones carry a risk of self-harm, and paranoid delusions about specific individuals in the immediate environment carry a risk of violence.

Hallucinations and Related Experiences

The commonest hallucinations are auditory, but they are not the same as "hearing voices." Hearing voices is common and includes a wide range of different experiences, many of which are understood by the person to be internal and private. Pseudo-hallucinations are an example, although the concept is contested. The key quality of hallucinations is that the patient believes they have been caused by someone else, and does not believe that they are truly internal experiences. However, hallucinations do not necessarily have the same quality as true perceptions, especially in people with persistent psychosis.

The apparent locations of hallucinations (for example, inside or outside the head) is less important than the patient's belief about the cause, specifically whether the voice is thought to be ego alien. "Voices" may talk directly to the patient (second person) or about them (third person).

Hallucinations caused by physical illness are usually vivid, and the patient often reacts to them, for example, by arguing with them. Major behavioural reactions to hallucinations should raise the suspicion of a physical cause (including intoxication or a withdrawal state).

Visual and tactile hallucinations can occur in psychosis but are most commonly due to organic factors (for example, the feeling of bugs creeping under the skin following cocaine misuse). Olfactory hallucinations raise the suspicion of an epileptic aura or prodrome.

Vivid, intrusive imageries related to painful memories are known as flashbacks. Although they often occur in post-traumatic stress disorder, they can occur in the absence of severe trauma. They are unpleasant experiences that are not hallucinations but have some features in common with them.

Other Psychotic Symptoms

There is a range of less common psychotic symptoms, many of which can be difficult to elicit. The most important are passivity experiences (the experience that thoughts, movements or feelings are under direct external control), and disorders of possession of thought (the belief that your thoughts are not private, but can be read or are being broadcast, or that thoughts are being inserted or removed).

Anxiety Symptoms

Anxiety is intense apprehension, accompanied by autonomic changes such as tachycardia, rapid shallow breathing, sweating, and light-headedness. Intense anxiety can turn into a panic attack, a state of terror that something awful, such as your death, is happening here and now. Panic attacks are commonly, but not always, accompanied by hyperventilation. An overwhelming desire to escape from whatever situation you are in is an intrinsic feature. Panic attacks are short-lived, rarely longer than 20 min, but they can come in clusters.

Phobias involve anxiety related to particular objects or circumstances, accompanied by avoidance of the feared stimulus.

Obsessions and Compulsions

Obsessions are repetitive thoughts that you experience as irrational and are resisted. They tend to focus on themes of loss of control, contamination, violence, and sexuality. They are often accompanied by actions aimed at neutralising the thoughts, such as repetitive handwashing or counting rituals. These actions are compulsions.

Low-grade obsessions and compulsions are common throughout the population, but when severe they are amongst the most distressing of psychiatric symptoms. Questions about orderliness and repetitive rituals will often elicit them when they have not been volunteered.

Ideas of Harming Self or Others

No psychiatric evaluation is complete without an exploration of ideas of self-harm and, although less commonly held, ideas of harming others. Asking people whether they have felt that they did not want to carry on or that life is not worth living are reliable probe questions. They are often best asked when patients talk about their mood. If the patient has entertained ideas of taking their own life, it is important to find out whether they have thought about what they would do and whether they have taken active steps to secure the means of acting. Putting their affairs in order, for example, by writing a will or giving away a loved pet, is particularly ominous. You should also ask what effect they expect their death will have on those around them; many depressed people recognise that their loved ones would be distressed, but also believe that this will be outweighed by shedding an emotional or material burden.

Ideas of harming others are more difficult to broach and may arise out of an exploration of forensic history. More often, when a patient is angry or paranoid about specific individuals or groups of people, it is helpful to ask whether they have thought of doing anything about it, and if so, what. Both fantasies and tangible plans are relevant.

'Insight'

The concept of insight in psychiatry is complex and contested. Traditionally, people in psychotic states who do not believe that there is anything wrong with them (that is, they locate the problem entirely outside of themselves) have been considered 'insightless'. However, insight can also refer to psychological mindedness or the extent to which the patient

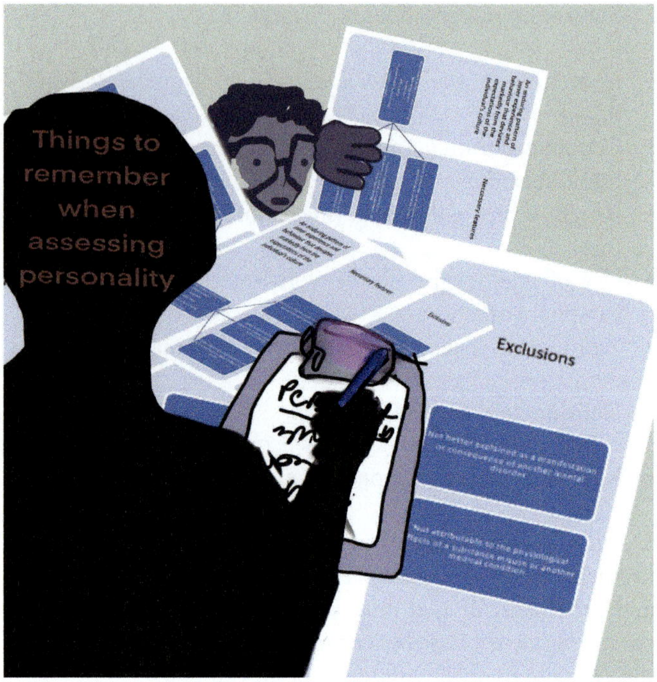

Fig. 6.16 Insight

agrees with the psychiatrist (who can, of course, be wrong). Where people have long-term psychotic symptoms, they often come to recognise that they are ill but continue to hold delusional beliefs. The degree of insight is then hard to define. We recommend that under this heading should be recorded the patient's belief about the nature of their problem, without attribution of the degree of 'insight' or otherwise (Fig. 6.16).

Cognitive State

Basic clinical screening of cognitive function includes tests of attention and concentration (serial 7 s or 3 s) and tests of short-term memory (by asking the patient to remember some words or some names, and then asking them to recall them sometime later).

There are several validated clinical cognitive tests available, none of which is entirely satisfactory for all purposes. Some specific schedules are recommended for specialist areas of practice. In the ordinary clinical setting, a suspicion of cognitive impairment may arise, but proper assessment requires systematic exploration of a range of cognitive abilities. This is neither necessary nor appropriate for all patients.

There is a major pitfall about clinical impressions of cognitive function where the patient's attention and concentration are impaired through anxiety or depression. Severe depression can cause depressive pseudo-dementia that resolves with adequate treatment of the underlying mood disorder.

Physical Examination

Psychiatrists are doctors for a reason. They often have to use their medical knowledge to make judgements about investigations for possible physical problems. The extent to which a physical examination and specific tests are necessary varies with the setting and the nature of the problem. Patients admitted to psychiatric inpatient units should certainly have a physical examination and routine blood tests, such as full blood count, renal, liver, and thyroid function tests, all of which are relevant to diagnosis and treatment. If a patient is to be commenced on a drug that can cause cardiac problems, an electrocardiogram is indicated. However, in a fit young patient assessed in an office with a problem that has no likely physical cause, a physical examination may be superfluous. We emphasise that this is a matter of clinical judgement for each patient (Fig. 6.17).

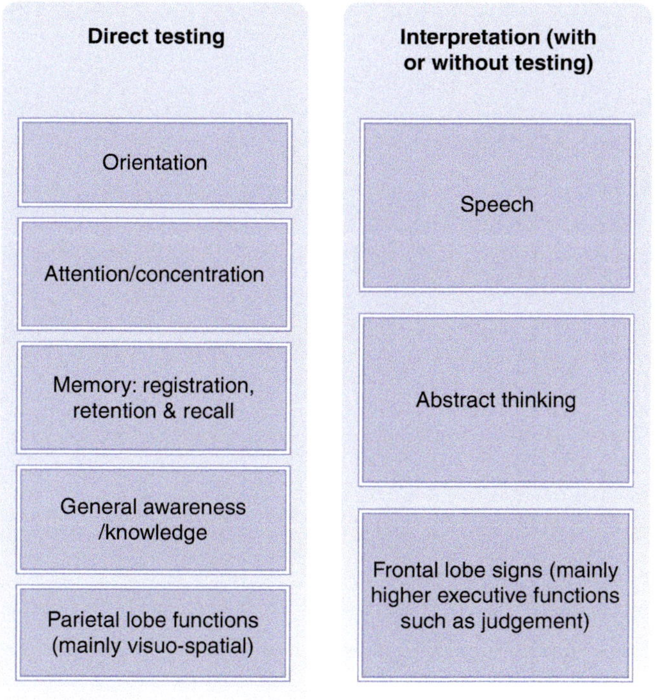

Fig. 6.17 Cognitive functions that may require specific assessment

References

1. American Psychiatric Association. Diagnostic and statistical manual of mental disorders. 5th ed. Arlington: American Psychiatric Publishing; 2013.
2. Ekman P. Cross-cultural studies of facial expression. In: Ekman P, editor. Darwin and facial expression. New York: Academic Press; 1973. p. 169–222.

Further Reading

Casey P, Kelly B. Fish's clinical psychopathology: signs and symptoms in psychiatry. 4th ed. Cambridge: Cambridge University Press; 2019.

Oyebode F. Sims' Symptoms in the mind: textbook of descriptive psychopathology 6th Edition London: Elsevier; 2018.

Poole R, Higgo R. Psychiatric interviewing and assessment. 2nd ed. Cambridge: Cambridge University Press; 2017.

Shea SC. Psychiatric interviewing: the art of understanding. New York: Elsevier; 2017.

Diagnostic Testing: Rating Scales and Psychological and Neuropsychological Tests

7

Shane S. Bush and Noah K. Kaufman

Introduction

Mental health professionals are trained interviewers and astute observers of human behavior, applying such skills for diagnostic and treatment purposes, and for the promotion of health and functioning. Through careful questioning, mental health professionals gain an understanding of the thoughts and feelings of those they serve. The information obtained from patients is considered in the context of the professional's understanding of psychological and neuropsychological theory and scholarly research. Such information allows for an evidence-based approach to the understanding and care of others. The professional's experience provides an additional rich source of information for understanding the thoughts, feelings, and behaviors of others. Ultimately, diagnoses, recommendations, and treatment plans are based on the professional's informed judgment. However, such judgment, regardless of the knowledge and experience of the professional, is subject to limitations, including biases. Supplementing the qualitative information obtained through interviews and observations with quantitative data improves the professional's ability to understand, diagnose, and care for patients. The purpose of this chapter is to provide an overview of psychological and neuropsychological diagnostic testing. An initial overview of sources of bias that can threaten the professional's objectivity helps to illustrate the importance of adding objective, quantitative assessment to the more subjective, qualitative component of the diagnostic process.

Biasing Influences in Assessment

> We see what we look for, and we look for what we know—Goethe (Roberts, 1999, p. 209).

S. S. Bush (✉)
Long Island Neuropsychology, PC, Lake Ronkonkoma, NY, USA

N. K. Kaufman
Center for Neuropsychological Studies, Las Cruces, NM, USA
e-mail: noah71@pm.me

Personal biases exist in healthcare professionals, as they do in all people, and routinely influence professional activities and decision-making. To help understand complex and/or ambiguous information and facilitate decision-making, mental shortcuts (heuristics) are often used; however, the selection and application of such shortcuts are subject to bias. Biasing influences can operate during data collection and/or during data interpretation [1] and can result in misdiagnoses, inappropriate treatments, misallocation of resources, inaccurate expert opinions, and exacerbation of a patient's problems.

Like clinicians, patients present with biases that may be intentional or unintentional. Biases can be idiographic and unique to a given patient or nomothetic reflections of human diversity issues. Factors associated with age, gender, gender identity, race, ethnicity, culture, national origin, religion, sexual orientation, disability, language, socioeconomic status, and other relevant individual and cultural differences may affect how patients approach the world, including how they view and respond to mental health services. Patient bias may take the form of subtle, unintentional influences on the manner in which they present or respond to professionals (e.g., guardedness), or they may be marked, intentional misrepresentation of information (e.g., factitious disorder, malingering). Clinicians who understand such biases and strive to minimize their impact on clinical decision-making are best positioned to provide effective services. Simply being aware that bias exists and can be a threat to clinical judgment is not sufficient to avoid falling prey to such biases. Figure 7.1 illustrates differences in performance on an intelligence test according to race.

Proactive efforts, including the use of disconfirmation strategies and self-examination questions, can help minimize biases and their effects. Additionally, the use of objective psychometric tests provides a powerful, evidence-based supplement to clinical judgment that facilitates sound decision-making and effective treatment. A sample of biases that tend to be encountered in mental health practice is listed in Table 7.1.

W. W. IsHak (ed.), *Atlas of Psychiatry*, https://doi.org/10.1007/978-3-031-15401-0_7

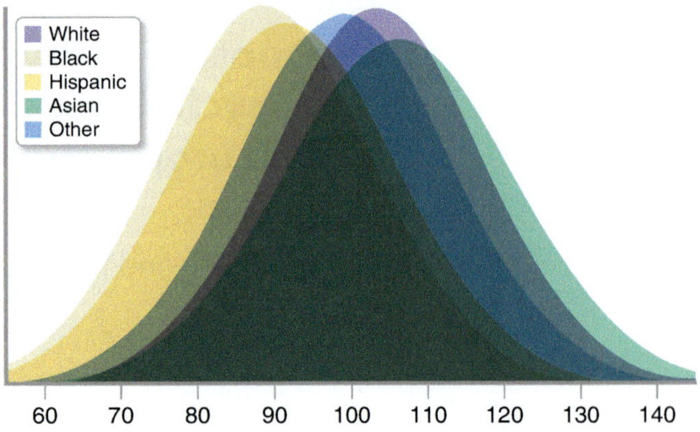

Fig. 7.1 Wechsler adult intelligence scale, fourth edition (WAIS-IV) full scale intelligence quotient (FSIQ) by race

Table 7.1 Sample of biases

• Confirmation bias
• Attribution error
• Self-referencing
• Stereotyping biases
• Rosy retrospection (good old days) bias
• Expectancy effects
• Availability heuristic
• Representative heuristic
• Framing effect
• Anchoring effect
• Prior knowledge and labeling effects
• Confirmatory hypothesis testing
• Reconstructive memory
• Hindsight bias
• Intentional blindness
• Illusory correlations

Debiasing Techniques

"Debiasing" is a process in which the clinician systematically applies strategies to minimize flawed judgment and reasoning. For example, one practical debiasing strategy for understanding the cause of a low psychological test score involves listing all relevant causes for a low test score and then systematically eliminating the causes that are unsupported by objective data. Examples of potential causes of low cognitive test scores, other than a neurological injury or illness, that should be considered in the debiasing process are listed in Table 7.2.

Table 7.2 Possible causes of low cognitive test scores, other than neurological injury or illness

• Premorbid educational or intellectual limitations
• Poor effort/malingering
• Environmental distractions, including the presence of a third party
• Intoxication or medication effects
• Fatigue
• Anxiety, psychotic symptoms, or other acute psychological distress
• Physical pain
• Other medical cause
– Dietary, vitamin, and mineral deficiency (A, C, B-12, folate)
– Hormonal dysfunction (thyroid dysregulation)
– Delirium

Illusory Correlations

To illustrate an objective method of controlling for illusory correlations in diagnostic decision making, the postconcussional syndrome is used as an example. Physical, cognitive, emotional, and behavioral problems, which are commonly experienced by people following a concussion, are nonspecific symptoms; that is, they are experienced frequently by people who have not sustained a concussion [2–4]. However, because they commonly occur in those who have sustained a concussion, there can be a tendency among some clinicians to draw an *illusory correlation* between the symptoms and a history of concussion, whereby the symptoms are misattributed to brain damage. If the relationship between a set of symptoms (e.g., physical, cognitive, emotional, and behavioral complaints) and a given diagnosis (e.g., postconcussional syndrome) truly exists, the symptoms must occur significantly more often among those with the diagnosis than they do among those who do not have the diagnosis.

An *analysis of covariation* between a cluster of symptoms and a diagnosis believed to represent that cluster of symptoms requires the creation of a 2 × 2 matrix. With such a matrix, the clinician crosses the diagnosis variable comprising two levels (i.e., diagnosis present versus diagnosis absent) with the sign or symptoms variable comprising two levels (i.e., symptoms present versus symptoms absent). In doing this, the result is four cells in the matrix. Evidence of a true relationship between the symptoms and the diagnosis comes from filling in *all four* of the cells: A, B, C, and D. See the covariation example, using concussion, in Table 7.3.

If, as is the case with the postconcussional syndrome, many people experience the constellation of physical, cognitive, emotional, and behavioral symptoms who have never had a concussion (Cell C), it is hard to assert a causal relationship between concussion and the symptoms of the postconcussional syndrome. Conversely, if the only people with the symptoms have a recent history of suffering a concussion (Cell A), it is easier to assert a causal relationship between concussion and the symptoms of the postconcussional syndrome. In practice, healthcare workers have a biased sample, meaning that most of the people they encounter have symptoms. It is, therefore, a short, convenient jump from having the symptoms to being given the diagnosis. An awareness of this tendency among mental health professionals can reduce diagnostic errors, iatrogenic problems, and misallocation of resources. Thus, the appropriate use of objective, statistically based, psychometric testing reduces biases and promotes sound patient care.

Table 7.3 Covariation table

	Symptoms present	Symptoms absent
Concussion present	A (50)	B (50)
Concussion absent	C (450)	D (450)

Note: Clinicians naturally over focus on Cell A, without considering Cells B–D

Landmark Theories and Concepts

Measuring Function and Change

People typically present to mental health professionals for evaluation and treatment because there is a problem or change from a prior level of functioning. Determining whether the reported problem represents a significant deviation from what is considered normal is key to making accurate diagnoses and providing beneficial care (see Fig. 7.2). Therefore, selecting the appropriate point of comparison is an essential task for the clinician.

For emotional and personality constructs (e.g., depression, extraversion), normative comparison standards are typically used. That is, an individual's test score or profile is compared to population averages, both normal/healthy populations and groups with known psychiatric disorders. The degree to which a given score or profile departs from the normal population and reflects that of a known psychiatric group increases the confidence that can be placed in a given clinical diagnosis. Similarly, for some developmental disorders (e.g., learning disorders), deviation from population norms is considered.

For neurocognitive disorders, deficit measurement in the form of change from a previously higher level is employed. Deficit comparisons can be made against population norms and/or estimates of a given patient's premorbid cognitive functioning. Using a given patient's estimated pre-injury or pre-illness level of functioning is particularly important when the patient's abilities diverge from the population norm; that is when their prior cognitive ability was much higher or lower than average. Such individual comparisons are important for diagnostic determinations and assessment of change (improvement or decline) over time. Statistical methods (e.g., Reliable Change Index) can be used to determine whether observed change differs in a meaningful way (i.e., statistically significant) from prior scores. Methods used to estimate premorbid intellectual/cognitive functioning are described later in this chapter.

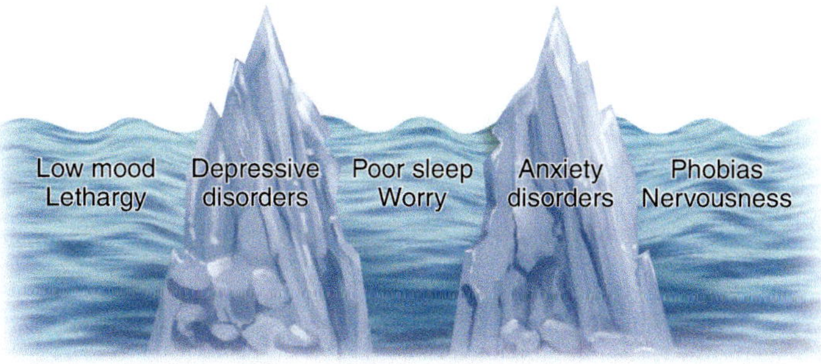

Fig. 7.2 Symptoms versus diagnosis. (*Modified from* Stevens and Rodin [31]; *with permission*)

Neuropsychological Assessment Process, Procedures, and Methods

The assessment of cognitive and emotional functioning involve obtaining both qualitative information and quantitative data. Such data provide information about the etiology of the condition of interest (see Fig. 7.3).

Mental health education and training generally focus more on qualitative information, such as information obtained from patient self-report, interviews of collateral sources, records produced by other healthcare providers, and observations of the patient's behavior. Some of these sources of information, particularly behaviors, can be quantified. However, the ability to obtain data in the form of responses or performances on standardized tests and then compare these data, statistically, to various normative groups adds a degree of objectivity and quantification not available from other methods (see Fig. 7.4).

Clinicians can select tests or batteries of tests in a variety of ways, such as always using the same measures with all patients (i.e., fixed approach), using different measures or batteries with different patients based on the needs of that patient (i.e., flexible approach), or, as is most common among neuropsychologists, using what is generally a core battery of tests for a certain patient population while adding or subtracting measures based on the needs of the specific patient (i.e., flexible battery approach). Regardless of the specific approach, there are multiple components to a neuropsychological evaluation (see Table 7.4). Additional skills, functions, and abilities (e.g., academic achievement, adap-

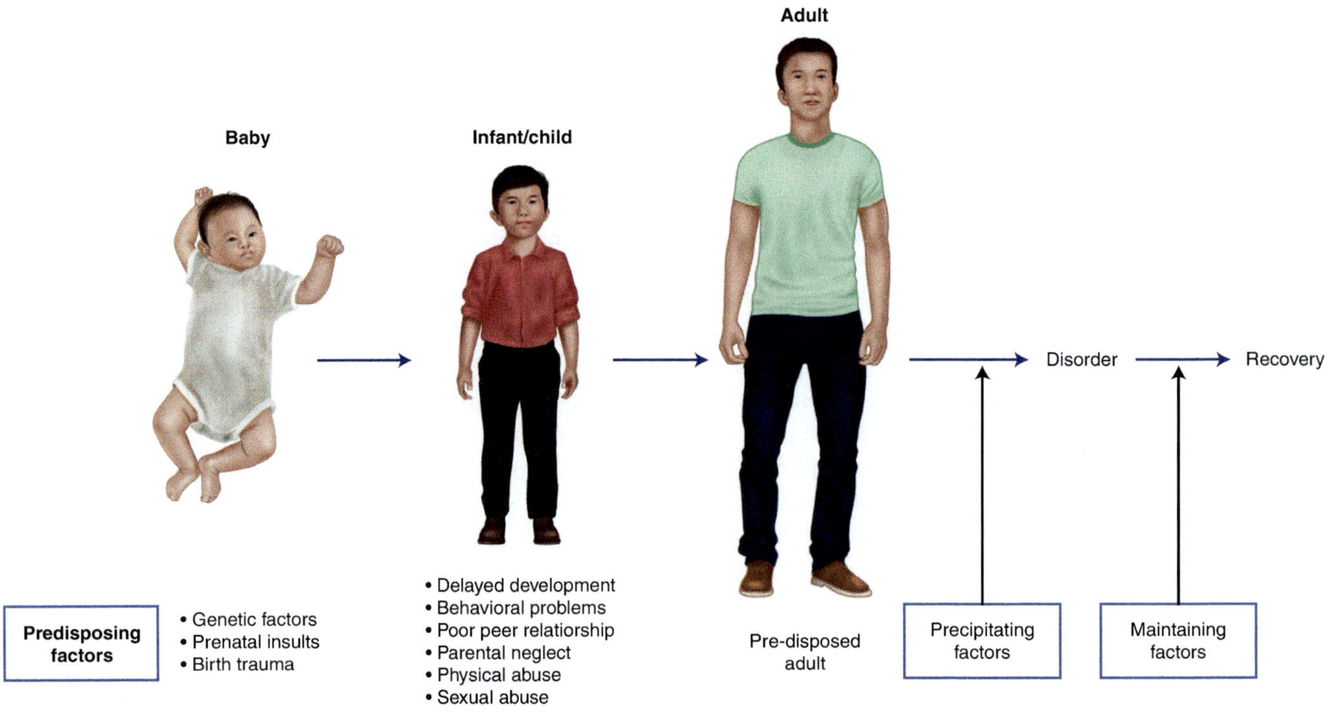

Fig. 7.3 Etiological factors in psychiatric illness. (*Modified from* Stevens and Rodin [31]; *with permission*)

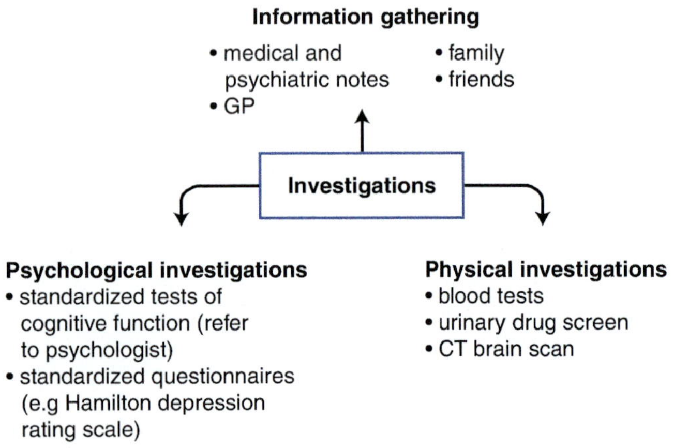

Fig. 7.4 Methods of investigation in diagnostic assessment. (*Modified from* Stevens and Rodin [31]; *with permission*)

Table 7.4 Neuropsychological evaluation components

1. Estimate of premorbid ability
2. Symptom and/or performance validity
3. Intelligence
4. Language
5. Visuospatial and constructional skills
6. Attention/concentration
7. Learning and memory
8. Executive functions
9. Motor/sensory functions
10. Emotional state/personality traits

tive behavior) may also be assessed depending on the purposes of the evaluation.

In test selection, the examiner considers many factors, including the statistical properties of the tests. Basic statistical properties to consider include the test's reliability, validity, and predictive values (positive and negative). *Reliability* refers to the consistency of measurement; that is, a person should obtain a very similar score on a test if taken more than once. Additional statistics (e.g., standard error of measurement; reliable change index) are used to determine whether performance on a subsequent administration deviates significantly from a prior administration. *Validity* refers to the extent to which a test measures what it is supposed to measure. There are multiple types of reliability and validity and much more to know about each, but such a description is beyond the scope of this chapter. Test users are responsible for understanding the psychometric properties of the tests that they select and for basing their test selection in part on such properties.

Positive predictive accuracy is the proportion of those said by the clinician to have a condition who truly has the condition. A clinician who always correctly diagnoses a given condition is going to have perfect positive predictive accuracy, represented by a positive predictive value (PPV) of 1.0. A clinician who always *in*correctly diagnoses the given condition is going to have no positive predictive accuracy, represented by a value of 0.

Negative predictive accuracy is the proportion of those patients said by the clinician to *not* have a given condition who truly do *not* have the condition. A clinician who always correctly does *not* diagnose the condition is going to have perfect negative predictive accuracy, represented by a negative predictive value (NPV) of 1.0. A clinician who always incorrectly does *not* diagnosis the condition is going to have no negative predictive accuracy, represented by a value of 0. Table 7.5 provides the formulas for calculating positive and negative predictive values.

Once a test or battery of tests has been selected, it must be used correctly; that is, it must be administered in the same manner in which it was administered when it was developed and standardized. Deviation from standardized instructions can affect the results and lead to inaccurate conclusions and inappropriate treatments or other recommendations. However, in some instances, such as with patients who have significant (a) sensory or motor limitations, (b) problems with speech or language, or (c) arousal/fatigue issues, modifications to standard administration or other accommodations must be made. In such instances, the examiner considers the potential impact of such deviations on the test data and tempers the conclusions accordingly.

Table 7.5 Formulas for positive and negative predictive values

PPV = A/(A + B)
NPV = D/(D + C)

Pretesting Considerations

All involved parties, including the examiner, referral source, patient, and any involved family members, should have a clear understanding the nature of the evaluation process before testing is begun. Typically, orientation to the evaluation process occurs at the outset of the service, at which point the patient, if a competent adult, provides consent. During the informed consent process, the patient is informed about the purpose of the testing (e.g., the specific referral question), the nature of the testing, the anticipated benefits and risks, and confidentiality issues, including who will receive the results. Logistics are discussed and agreed upon, such as whether a third-party observer (e.g., family member, attorney) will be allowed to be present during the testing. In nearly all instances of cognitive testing, having a third party, including a recording device, present should be avoided because such a presence (a) affects the patient's performance and can invalidate the test results and (b) threatens the security of the tests [5, 6]. Any cultural issues that could affect the testing process or the ability to measure the constructs of interest in a valid manner should also be considered and addressed as needed. Illustration 7.1 offers a sample consent form for use with neuropsychological evaluations in forensic contexts.

When patients lack the capacity to make healthcare decisions, the clinician can follow a structured process to determine the patient's best interests (see Fig. 7.5). When the patient's decisional capacity is lacking or in question, following the Five Principles of Capacity helps clinicians advocate for the patient's best interests (see Fig. 7.6).

Estimating Premorbid Intellectual/Cognitive Functioning

As statistics tell us, and mental health professionals understand, different people naturally have widely varying cognitive abilities. Diagnostic testing in some contexts, such as with those who have developmentally based disorders, provides a depiction of one's mental abilities. In contrast, in contexts in which one's current abilities reflect a change (i.e., decline) from a previously higher level (e.g., after acquired brain injury or dementia onset), the patient's premorbid level of functioning must be estimated to determine whether the current scores reflect the change. Thus, for a given cognitive test score to be meaningful, the examiner must have an idea of what the optimal score would be, or would have been.

There are multiple empirical methods available to the examiner for determining or estimating premorbid intellectual or cognitive functioning (see Table 7.6). The best indication of determining prior ability is pre-injury or pre-illness test scores. Some patients have undergone prior testing for a reason unrelated to their decline, such as in academic contexts. The availability of such records, although not particularly common, tends to provide the clearest evidence of premorbid cognitive functioning.

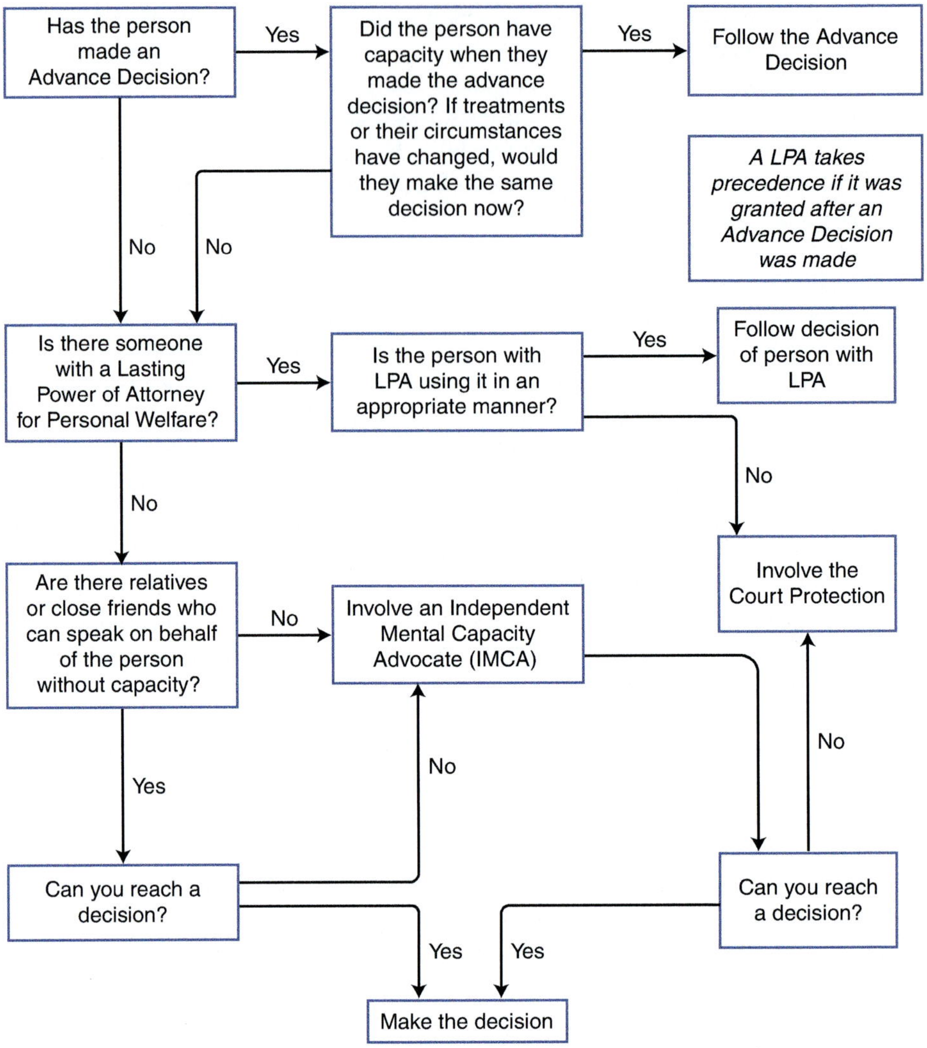

Fig. 7.5 Determining the patient's best interests in medical decision making. (*Modified from* Stevens and Rodin [31]; *with permission*)

A second method for estimating premorbid cognitive functioning is the use of so-called "hold tests." For most people, certain mental abilities tend to be fairly resilient to the effects of neurological injury and illness and thus hold up well in the context of such conditions. Reading single words is one such ability. Tests involving reading single words, particularly words that do not sound as they are spelled (e.g., "debt") are either commonly employed for this purpose or have been developed primarily for this use. These tests are described here as "so-called" hold tests because some factors can affect performance on these tests, resulting in a score that can underrepresent the patient's true overall cognitive abilities; a developmental history of a verbal learning disorder and an acquired brain injury that affects areas of the brain involved in reading are two such examples. Consider the case of a patient who obtains a Reading Efficiency Index of 75 (borderline range) on the Test of Irregular Word Reading Efficiency (TIWRE) but has a history of a verbal learning disorder. The unsophisticated examiner would conclude that other cognitive test scores falling in or near the borderline range are normal for this person. However, because of the history of verbal learning disorder, the borderline range would underestimate premorbid cognition, and important declines in ability would be missed (false negative/type II error). Vocabulary also tends to be fairly resilient to the effects of many types of neurological disorders but has similar limitations.

A third method for estimating premorbid cognitive functioning involves the use of demographic variables. Some demographic groups tend to perform better than others on cognitive tests. For example, people with higher levels of education, as a group, tend to perform better on measures of cognitive ability than do groups of people with lower levels of education. Research has shown that actuarial formulas can be developed by combining such variables, providing an estimate of premorbid functioning. The Barona Index [7] and a formula provided as part of the Wechsler Advanced Clinical Solutions [8] are two examples. A primary limitation of this approach is that there tends to be a large standard error of estimate; that is, any given individual's abilities may not be reflective of the group. For example, a patient's demographics result in a Barona Index of 120 (superior range). The examiner might be tempted to conclude that cognitive test scores now falling in the average or high average ranges reflect a decline for this patient. However, with a standard error estimate of 12.14, there is a 68% chance that the

Fig. 7.6 Five principles of capacity. (*Modified from* Stevens and Rodin [31]; *with permission*)

DO	PRINCIPLE	DON'T
Formally assess capacity	Assume people have capacity unless proved otherwise	Assume someone lacks capacity on the basis of factors such as their age or diagnosis
Take the time to help people understand and make decisions. If they may regain capacity and it is possible to wait, then do so	Help people make their own decisions	View capacity as a static phenomenon – it will change over time and will be affected by the way in which you communicate information
Base your assessment of capacity on how the person arrives at their decision, not on what they decide	People have the right to make what you think are unwise decisions	Conclude that someone doesn't have capacity because you disagree with their decision
Use whatever means available to decide what the person would have wanted for themselves if they had capacity	When someone lacks capacity, act in their best interests	Assume you know what is best for other people
Think about the least intrusive and restrictive means of achieving what is in the person's best interests	When someone lacks capacity, do not restrict their liberty more than is necessary	Do more than is necessary

Table 7.6 Methods of estimating premorbid/optimal intellectual/cognitive functioning

- Records—Prior test results
- "Hold tests"
  - Single word reading tests
    - Test of premorbid functioning (TOPF)
    - Test of irregular word reading efficiency (TIWRE)
    - Wechsler test of adult reading (WTAR)
  - Vocabulary
- Demographic variables
  - Actuarial formulas
    - Barona index
    - Wechsler advanced clinical solutions
- Highest test scores
  - Clusters (not a single score)

patient's true ability level is between 108 and 132. In general, true ability levels are typically closer to the mean (the mean for standard scores is 100). Therefore, a BI of 120 likely overestimates this patient's true ability level; therefore, stating that scores in the average and high average ranges reflect impaired performance results in false positive determinations (type I error).

A fourth method for estimating premorbid cognitive functioning involves considering the highest scores obtained from a battery of tests. From a battery of tests, having some scores cluster in a certain higher range than other scores may indicate that the lower scores have declined. However, a certain degree of within-person variability is common and expected, so care must be taken not to overstate the importance of one or two high scores. The pattern of high and low scores should also make neuropsychological sense given what is known about the suspected or known etiology of the decline.

Validity Assessment

As described in the Landmark Theories and Concepts section of the present chapter, for test data to be accepted as an accurate reflection of the construct of interest (e.g., depression, memory), the patient must have validly approached the evaluation; that is, they must have responded truthfully to questions and put forth a good effort on tests of cognitive ability. It is the examiner's task to determine whether the patient's approach to the evaluation and thus the test data, are valid for clinical interpretation. A multimodal approach to validity assessment that includes standardized tests is needed for making such determinations; clinical judgment alone is insufficient. Patterns of deceptive responding also emerge in functional neuroimaging (see Fig. 7.7).

Three types of validity that are considered when making determinations about whether the patient's approach to the evaluation was genuine: Response validity, symptom validity, and performance validity. *Response validity* [9] refers to whether the patient responded to interview questions in a valid manner. Although there are no psychometric measures for assessing response validity, a comparison of self-reported information with medical, education, legal, or other records can help establish the accuracy of the information provided by the patient.

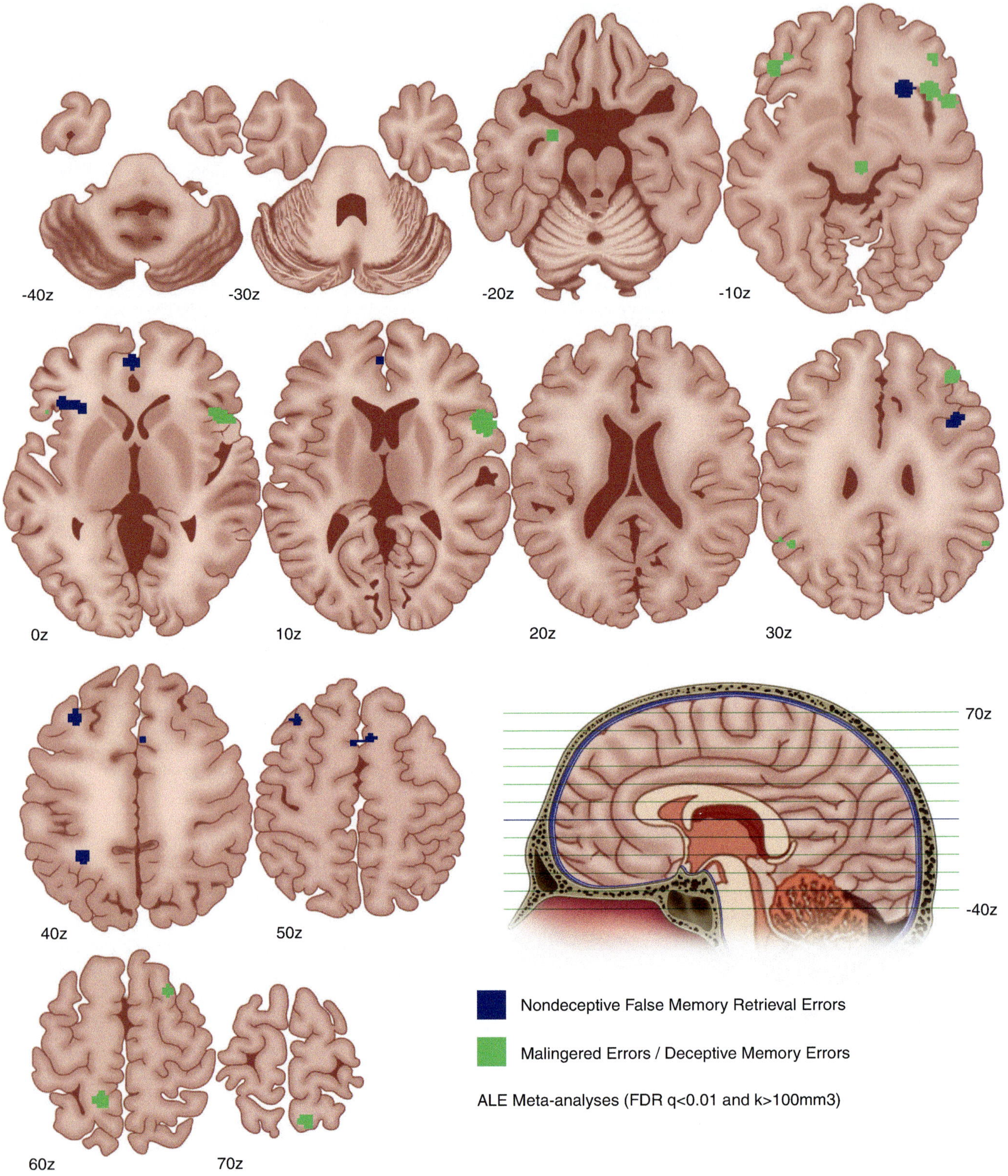

Fig. 7.7 Prototypical regions of brain activation associated with the production of purposefully deceptive and unintentional false responses, evident on fMRI. *ALE* activation likelihood estimation, *FDR* false discovery rate. (*From* Browndyke [32]; *with permission*)

Symptom validity [10] refers to the accuracy of the patient's reported symptoms. Depending on conscious or unconscious motivations, patients may minimize problems and common human frailties or exaggerate or fabricate symptoms. Comprehensive psychological questionnaires, such as the MMPI family of tests, have well-established validity scales that help clinicians characterize the patient's approach to the test (Fig. 7.8 provides a sample MMPI-2-RF validity scale profile). Some free-standing measures (e.g., Structured Inventory of Malingered Symptomatology), known as symptom validity tests (SVTs), have been created specifically for determining symptom validity.

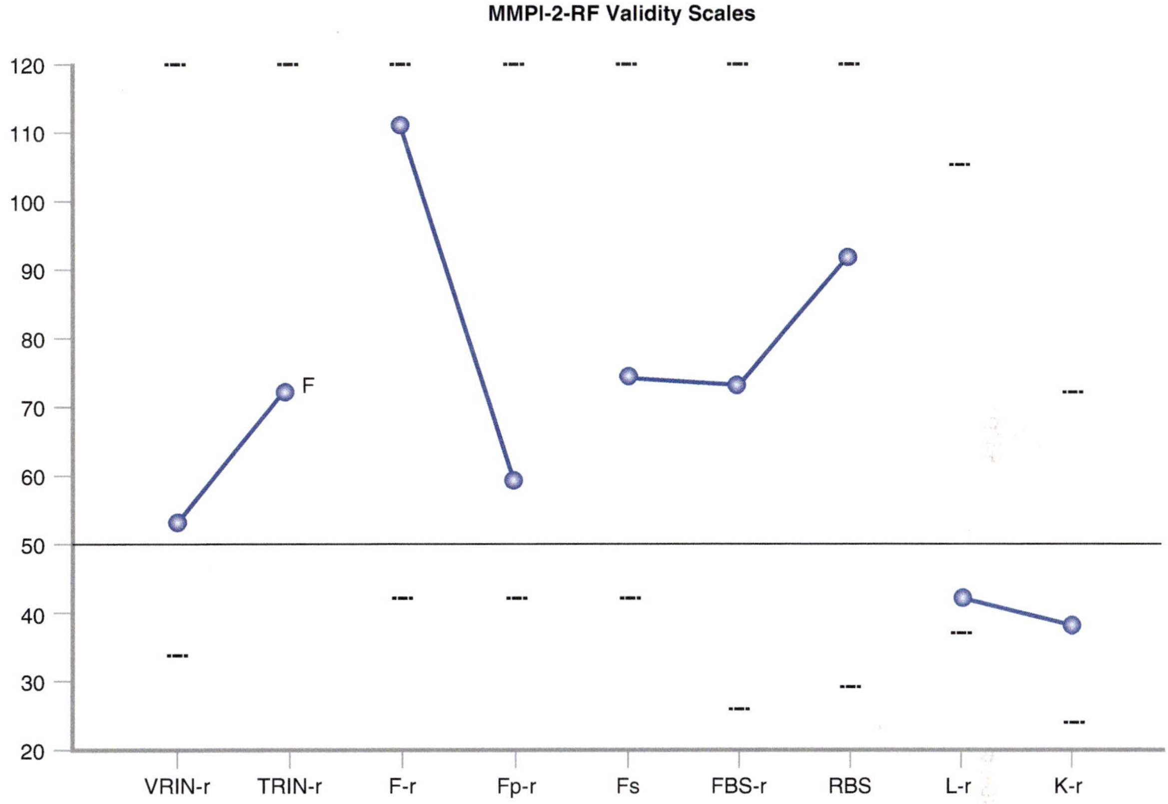

	VRIN-r	TRIN-r	F-r	Fp-r	Fs	FBS-r	RBS	L-r	K-r
Raw Score:	4	8	15	2	4	15	15	1	4
T Score:	53	73 F	111	59	74	73	92	42	38
Response %:	100	100	100	100	100	100	100	100	100
Cannot Say (Raw):	0				Percent True (of items answered):				47%

The highest and lowest T scores possible on each scale are indicated by a "---"; MMPI-2-RF T scores are non-gendered.

VRIN-r Variable Response Inconsistency
TRIN-r True Response Inconsistency
F-r Infrequent Responses
Fp-r Infrequent Psychopathology Responses
Fs Infrequent Somatic Responses
FBS-r Symptom Validity
RBS Response Bias Scale
L-r Uncommon Virtues
K-r Adjustment Validity

Fig. 7.8 Sample MMPI-2-RF validity scale profile

Although the initial publication of symptom and performance validity tests provides cutoff scores or norms, improved and preferred normative data or cutoff scores are often published subsequent to the initial publication of a test. Clinicians should be familiar with the various validity assessment options and choose those that are best suited for a given patient.

Performance validity [10] refers to effort put forth on tests of cognitive ability (e.g., memory) and physical functioning (e.g., motor skills). Abnormally low scores compared to what is known for given conditions raise questions of suboptimal performance. For example, much poorer performance on a memory test by someone with a remote history of a single mild traumatic brain injury (mTBI), compared to groups of patients who sustained severe TBIs or have advanced Alzheimer's disease, is suggestive of suboptimal performance. Many commonly used neuropsychological tests have variables for which a patient's scores can be compared to groups of patients with various known conditions to help determine performance validity. In addition, numerous free-standing performance validity tests (PVTs) have been developed for this sole purpose.

A common PVT format consists of a forced choice paradigm. That is, the patient is shown a stimulus (e.g., a picture) and is then asked to identify the stimulus from among two options. There is a 50/50 chance of responding correctly just by chance (e.g., guessing) alone. When this is done over many trials, the examiner can determine whether the number of correct responses is above or below chance. Most healthy persons and patient groups score well above chance, typically near perfect. PVTs have various norms and cutoff scores for poor performance. Excluding scenarios where, for example, a patient is severely demented or acutely psychotic, patients typically perform well on PVTs. The only way for a patient to score *significantly below chance* is to know the correct answers and intentionally provide the incorrect answers over multiple trials. Such a performance is very informative and invalidates the patient's approach to the test, and likely to the overall evaluation. Specific criteria for diagnosing suboptimal performance and malingering, using probabilistic language, have been developed and refined [11]. It is important for clinicians to remember that severe psychiatric conditions can result in patient's misperceiving stimuli (see Fig. 7.9) or misspeaking responses due to abnormalities of thought (see Fig. 7.10), which are valid representations of their psychiatric condition but will not lead to an accurate understanding of cognitive constructs of interest (e.g., memory).

Figure 7.11 illustrates how older adults presenting in a valid manner typically perform on Trials 1 and 2 of the Test of Memory Malingering (TOMM) [12]. These ranges can be used for comparison for these and other patient groups. For example, if a middle age adult with a remote history of mTBI who functions independently were to obtain a score of 35 on Trial 2, which is lower than older adults with dementia, the clinician could conclude that the person's performance was likely invalid. Figure 7.12 illustrates how various groups perform on the Word Memory Test (WMT) [13]. Determinations about the validity of a patient's performance can be made by comparing their scores to those of the known groups. Using the same mTBI example, if that person obtained a delayed recognition (DR) score of 70% correct, that would be lower than groups of children with extremely low intellectual and adaptive functioning ("mental retardation"), which is inconsistent with what is known about cognitive functioning following a single, remote mTBI and is indicative of invalid performance. Such information is essential for important clinical decisions (e.g., diagnosis), making routine use of SVTs and PVTs a required part of diagnostic testing in most situations [9].

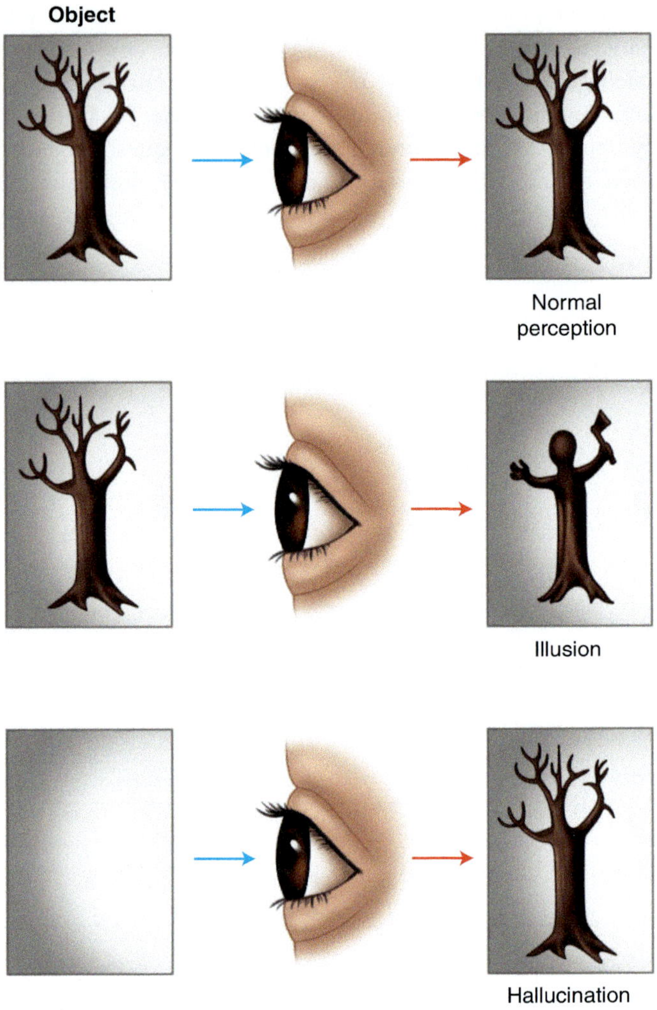

Fig. 7.9 Perception, illusion, and hallucination. (*Modified from* Stevens and Rodin [31]; *with permission*)

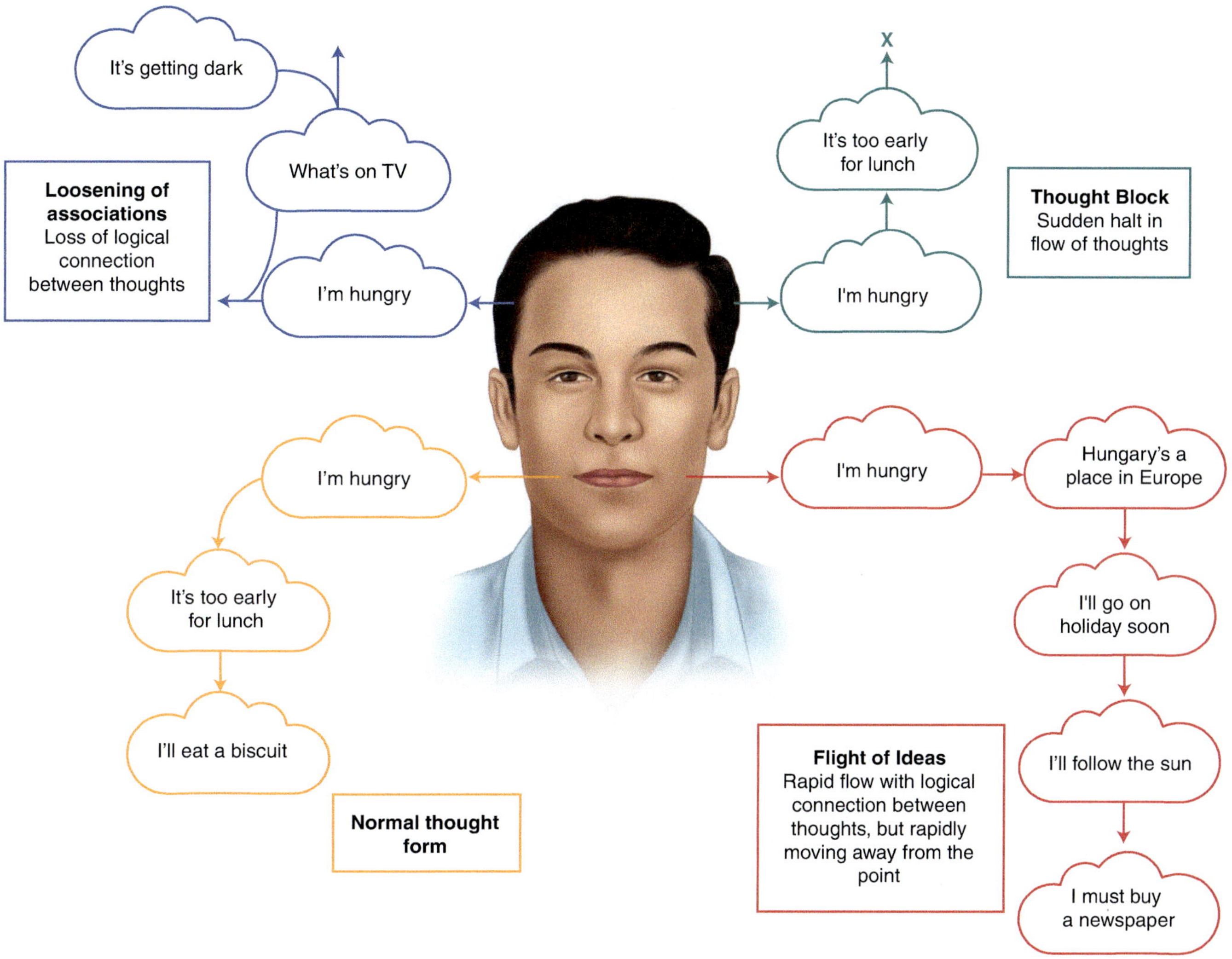

Fig. 7.10 Abnormalities of thought. (*Modified from* Stevens and Rodin [31]; *with permission*)

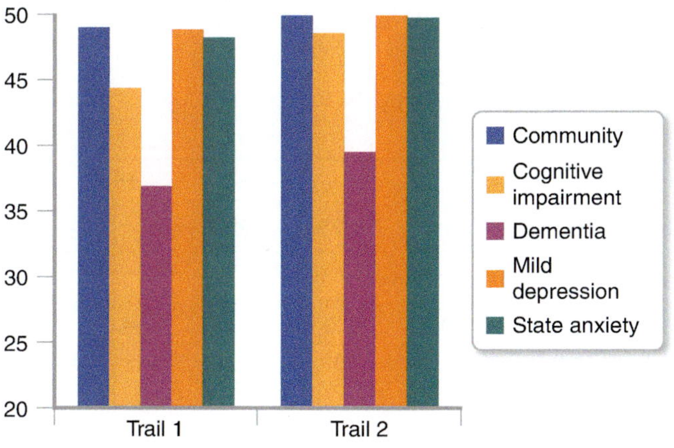

Fig. 7.11 Test of memory malingering performance by older adults. (*Data from* Iverson et al.[33]; *with permission*)

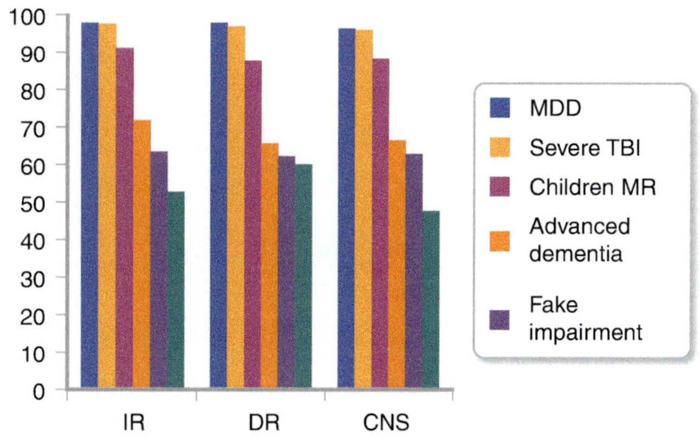

Fig. 7.12 Word memory test performance comparisons

Data Interpretation

The primary value of diagnostic testing lies in its empirical foundations. Statistics are considered and applied not only in the development of tests but also in the interpretation of test data. Examiners must be familiar with basics statistical concepts and calculations, including means, standard deviations, *T* scores, and *z* scores. Norm-referenced measurement, which is useful for diagnostic purposes, is distinguished from criterion-referenced measurement, which is more useful for determining whether a person can perform a specific function. Norm-referenced measurement compares a given patient's scores to large groups of subjects representing healthy persons and, sometimes, those with various disorders. If the person's scores deviate significantly (which can be defined in different ways) from the mean of the healthy group, the clinician can determine that pathology exists. If the score is similar to a particular type of disorder, and the other obtained information is also consistent, then that diagnosis can be made.

Most psychological and neuropsychological test results do not use specific cutoff scores to determine impairment or pathology; rather, deviation from the normal range is considered. To make such determinations, raw scores are converted to standardized scores (e.g., *T* scores, *z* scores, percentiles, standard scores), and the distance from the mean is determined via standard deviations. Different tests use different standardized scores, and different clinicians have different preferences for how they report the scores; therefore, mental health professionals who perform diagnostic testing need a working knowledge of what the various scores mean. Figure 7.13 is the bell curve (normal distribution) with corresponding values for each of the primary standardized scores. Figures 7.14 and 7.15 provide the formulas for calculating z scores and *T* scores, respectively.

Because persons with different demographic characteristics tend to perform differently, it is typically important for diagnostic purposes to compare a given patient's scores to the score patterns of demographically similar persons. For example, comparing a person with a low education level to someone with an advanced degree on a test of ver-

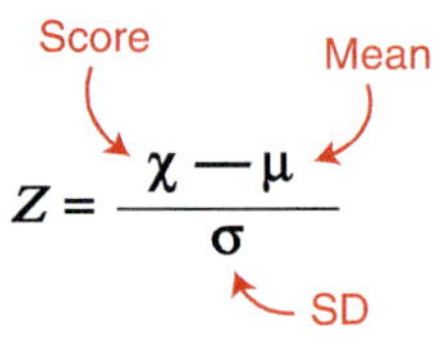

Fig. 7.14 z-score formula

$$t = \frac{\bar{X} - \mu}{S / \sqrt{n}}$$

or, if z-score has already been calculated,
T = 10 (z-score) + 50

Fig. 7.15 *T* score formula

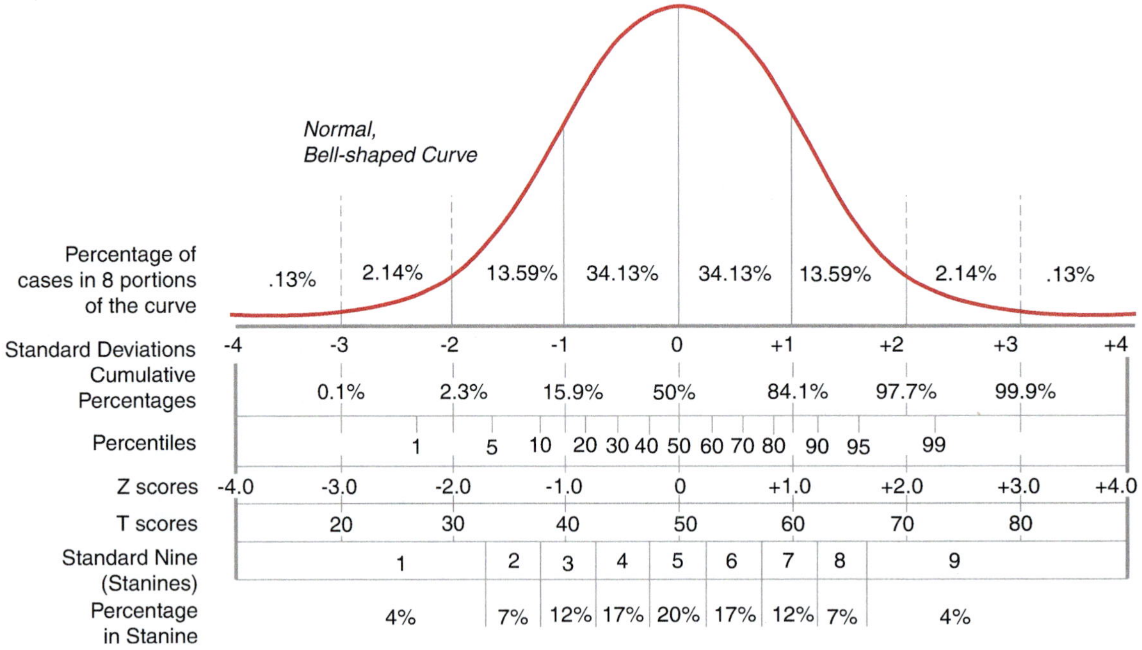

Fig. 7.13 Bell curve / Normal Distribution. (*Modified from* https://psychology.wikia.org/wiki/Bell_curve_grading. Creative Commons Attribution-Share Alike License 3.0 (Unported) (CC-BY-SA). https://creativecommons.org/licenses/by-sa/3.0)

bal reasoning can result in an inaccurate determination of impairment for the person with a lower education. However, controlling for years of education can be nuanced, since there is a bidirectional relationship between years of schooling and cognitive abilities. For example, if a person has limited schooling, such as an eighth-grade education, because of learning difficulties, controlling for education may hide important cognitive deficits. In contrast, if the person only has an eighth-grade education because they were forced to quit school to work, and there is no early history of learning difficulties, controlling for years of schooling would be more justified.

For questions of overall functioning, such as whether someone is safe to live independently, comparisons are best made to the general population. For example, it might be quite common (i.e., normal) for a 95-year-old person to remember no words from a list of words that was previously presented to the person. However, despite being normal for the person's age, the considerable lack of memory would reflect significant impairment compared to the general population and would be very problematic for daily functioning. This point is easily appreciated if an elderly person's IQ is calibrated in comparison to what is normal for much younger adults. Thus, selecting the right normative comparisons for the given patient and the specific goals of the evaluation is essential for concluding that benefit the parties involved. Tables 7.7 and 7.8 provide examples of the importance of using appropriate normative data sets.

Table 7.7 Normative data case illustration for trail making test, part B

- 60-year-old white male
- TBT B: 130″ (Heaton et al., 2004 demographically corrected norms)
  - 7–8 years of education, *T* score = 47
    - Failure to use demographically corrected norms would over-pathologize this person (type I/false positive error)
  - 18–20 years of education, *T* score = 30
    - Failure to use demographically corrected norms would fail to identify a deficit (type II/false negative error)

Table 7.8 Normative data case illustration for montreal cognitive assessment (MoCA)

- Suggested normal range is 26–30, based on initial norms
  - 90 healthy Canadian participants
  - Mean age = 72.84 years
  - Mean education level = 13.33 years
- Demographically corrected norms (Rossetti et al. 2011)
  - 2653 ethnically diverse participants
  - Corrected for age and education
- 60-year-old with <12 years of education
  - MoCA raw score = 19
  - Demographically correct mean = 19.94 (SD = 4.43)
  - Score of 19 is entirely within normal limits
- Failure to use the demographically correct norms in this case would result in a false positive finding

Determining Impairment

Compared to subjective clinical judgment alone, psychometric testing has the advantage of providing a statistical means of determining when a patient's scores reflect cognitive or emotional pathology. However, there is no single level of performance or pattern of performance that reflects impairment or psychopathology for all patients and all tests. Various test manuals offer different recommendations for classifying scores that deviate from normal in a meaningful way. Similarly, different clinicians may have different preferences for determining when a given score or combination of scores reflects pathological performance or response. Typically, a given deviation from the mean (i.e., arithmetic average) is used to determine when a given score is statistically different from normal, healthy populations. Common values include 1 standard deviation from the mean, 1.5 standard deviations from the mean, or 2 standard deviations from the mean. Sometimes, for clinicians preferring to use percentiles, the tenth percentile is used. Selection of the value used to determine a statistically significant deviation from the mean occurs before test interpretation and is applied consistently across tests or subtests.

Significant problems can arise when different clinicians utilize different qualitative descriptions for quantitative test scores. This problem occurs in large part because different test publishers use different terms to describe performance ranges. In an attempt to rectify this problem, the American Academy of Clinical Neuropsychology [14] provided a consensus statement on uniform labeling of performance test scores, both for tests with normal distributions and those with non-normal distributions (see Tables 7.9 and 7.10). Including such a chart in the test report can allow readers to more readily understand what the reported terms and numbers mean.

Clinicians who use psychometric tests must understand the consequences of each of these cutoff levels, most importantly the fact that the more liberal the cutoff point (i.e., the less distance from the mean), the more likely that scores will fall in that range due to normal variation in ability or chance (e.g., random factors in the testing process that cannot be controlled). There is a risk of overdiagnosing pathology when one standard deviation

Table 7.9 Recommended test score labels based on standard scores and percentiles for tests with normal distributions

Standard score	Percentile	Score label
>130	>98	Exceptionally high score
120–129	91–97	Above average score
110–119	75–90	High average score
90–109	25–74	Average score
80–89	9–24	Low average score
70–79	2–8	Below average score
<70	<2	Exceptionally low score

From Guilmette et al. [14]; *with permission*

Table 7.10 Recommended test score labels based on percentiles for tests with non-normal distributions

Percentile	Score label
>24	Within normal expectations score or within normal limits score
9–24	Low average score
2–8	Below average score
<2	Exceptionally low score

From Guilmette et al. [14]; *with permission*

from the mean is used, and a risk of failing to identify pathology when two standard deviations are used. This issue is discussed in greater detail in the following section on base rates.

Base Rates of Low Scores

It is common to have some low scores in any battery of cognitive tests, even for persons with no neurocognitive disorder. Research has found that tests scores falling more than one standard deviation below the mean occur in 10–15% of healthy adults; that is, in a battery that generates 20 scores, two or more scores falling more than one standard deviation below the mean is considered normal [15].

Consider specifically WAIS-IV and Wechsler Memory Scale, Fourth Edition (WMS-IV) which are among the most commonly used cognitive tests. Together, these tests generate 10 index scores and 20 primary subtest scores. Fifty percent of the standardization sample had at least one Index score fall one standard deviation or more below the mean (i.e., ≤16th percentile, standard score ≤ 85), and one out of five healthy people had at least one Index score at or below the fifth percentile (standard score ≤ 75). When the 20 primary subtest scores were considered simultaneously, over 75% of the sample had one or more subtest scores at or below the sixteenth percentile, and more than 40% of the sample had at least one score at or below the fifth percentile [16].

In addition to base rates of low test scores, clinicians must consider the base rates of a given disorder. For example, when considering diagnosing progressive dementia, it is advantageous for the clinician to be aware of the most common forms of dementia (see Fig. 7.16).

Clinicians can use the base rates of a given condition or symptoms statistically to help arrive at a correct diagnosis. Using postconcussive syndrome as an example, the base rate is the percentage of those who sustained a concussion who truly have a postconcussive syndrome. The base rate

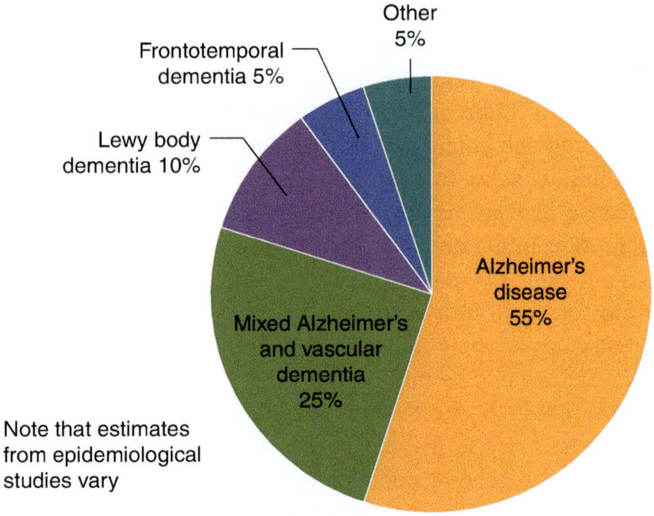

Fig. 7.16 Prevalence of the most common types of dementias. (*Modified from* Stevens and Rodin [31]; *with permission*)

Table 7.11 Base rate X diagnosis

	Disorder truly present	Disorder truly absent
Test positive	A (true positives)	B (false positives)
Test negative	C (false negatives)	D (true negatives)

Note: Cross-tabulating base rate information (columns) with diagnostic information (rows) yields sensitivity, specificity, and overall diagnostic accuracy statistics (e.g., Youden's J index [23] [sensitivity + specificity – 1] or a diagnostic odds ratio [A/B]/[C/D])

is theoretically represented by a 2 × 2 matrix. In this 2 × 2 matrix (see Table 7.11), the clinician crosses a diagnosis variable comprising two levels (i.e., diagnosis given versus diagnosis *not* given) with a reality variable comprising two levels (i.e., disorder truly present versus disorder truly absent). In doing this, the following four cells are created in the matrix:

The base rate is computed as follows: (A + C)/(A + B + C + D). Put simply, the base rate is the percentage of those truly known to have the disorder. The lower the base rate for a disorder, the harder it is to *correctly* give the diagnosis. That is, if very few people in the population ever get postconcussive syndrome, the methods used to diagnose postconcussive syndrome may not be effective. Under these circumstances, using the base rate as the primary guide for decision making is preferred to other decision-making guides (e.g., unstructured clinical judgment), which are likely to be less accurate.

Assessing Change

A variety of patient, situational, and test factors can affect a given patient's test performance from one test administration to another. Efforts should be made to reduce environmental distractors and other situational factors to the extent possible. Test variables (e.g., the novelty of the task) and statistical variables (e.g., regression to the mean) can also affect test scores from one administration to another. Additionally, the experience of having previously undergone psychometric testing tends to result in higher scores on subsequent testing for some abilities and tests; this is known as *practice effects*. All sources of error should be considered in the analysis of the results. Table 7.12 provides examples of sources of measurement error.

Although the possible impact of many of the sources of error tends to be subjective and impressionistic, there are statistical methods for determining whether an observed change in test scores from one administration to another is within the expected standard error of measurement or reflects a greater change than may be expected. The Reliable Change Index (RCI) is one such method for determining whether observed changes in test scores exceed what would be expected based on measurement error alone. A commonly used formula for calculating the RCI is provided in Table 7.13. The use of alternative forms of the same test can help control for practice effects to some degree. Additional statistical methods are available for assessing the meaningfulness of a given patient's changes in test scores from one administration to another; clinicians should select the methods that best meet their needs.

Table 7.12 Sources of measurement error: examples

Patient factors
• Fatigue
• Anxiety, frustration, and other emotional states
• Hunger
• Physical health
– Pain
– Infections
– Thyroid function
– Vitamin B12 level
– Blood glucose levels)
• Intoxication
• Expected improvement
– Recovery following TBI
• Expected decline
– Alzheimer's disease and other progressive neurocognitive disorders
• Secondary gain
Situational factors
• Distractions in the testing environment
• Poor lighting
• Uncomfortable furniture
• Presence of third parties in the testing room (if allowed)
Test/statistical factors
• Novelty of the task
• Regression to the mean

Table 7.13 Reliable change index formula [24]

RCI = $T_2 - T_1$ / SED
• SED = SD$\sqrt{2 - r_1 - r_2}$
• If $\lvert RCI \rvert > 1.64$, then the change is significant

Data Integration and Analysis

Once the test data have been obtained, all sources of information are integrated and analyzed. The clinician arrives at a diagnosis and offers a prognosis and recommendations.

Diagnosis

Establishing or ruling out psychopathy or neuropathology based in part on psychometric test scores involves comparing obtained scores to patterns of psychological characteristics or strengths and weaknesses of healthy populations and groups known to have various disorders. Patterns of strengths and weaknesses are compared to established patterns for various psychiatric and neurological disorders. Possible explanations other than psychopathology or a neurocognitive disorder must be considered (e.g., the patient and situational variables previously described). For neurocognitive disorders, determinations are generated regarding underlying brain integrity and functional abilities. Clinicians must understand the pathological processes underlying various disorders and how those processes manifest behaviorally. For example, Fig. 7.17 illustrates the basic mechanisms of CNS damage in HIV/AIDS, while Fig. 7.18 provides neuroimaging evidence of the damage caused to brain structures, and Fig. 7.19 illustrates the link between HIV and mental illness.

However, attention is also given to nonspecific non-neurological factors that can impact test performance and the understanding of the constructs of interest (see Fig. 7.20).

Fig. 7.17 Mechanisms of CNS damage in HIV-AIDS. (*From* Hilsabeck and Huckans [34]; *with permission*)

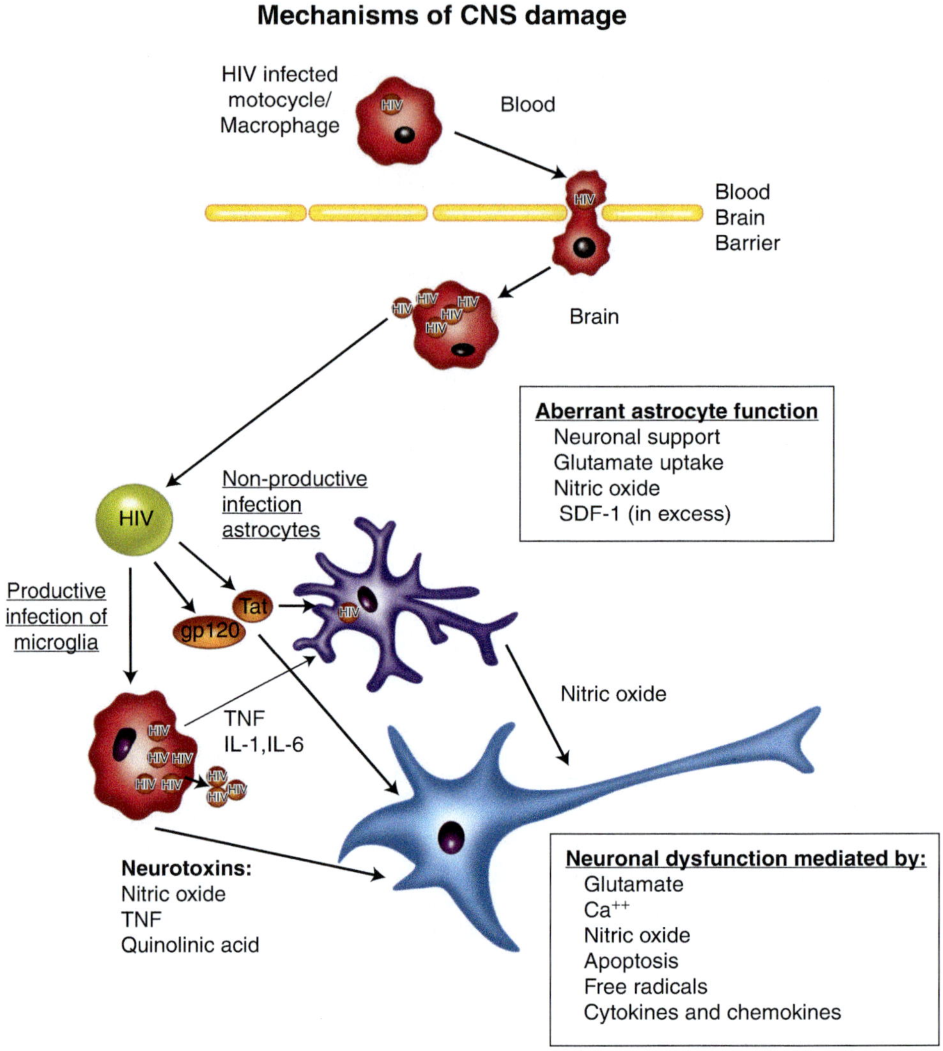

Diagnostic determinations are informed by the patient's level of performance and pattern of performance on cognitive testing. For example, Fig. 7.21 provides examples of various performances on the Clock Drawing Test, a commonly used cognitive screening measure, and Fig. 7.22 illustrates information that can be gleaned from impaired performance on the Rey-Osterrieth Complex Figure Test. The nature or pattern of the patient's performance on the test can provide valuable clinical information about a possible neurocognitive disorder.

The test data are an important, but insufficient, piece of information to consider in making a diagnosis and must be integrated with information obtained through interviews, observations, and review of records. Where uncertainty remains, caveats are offered to appropriately limit the confidence that is placed in the conclusions.

Prognosis

Based on what is known about (a) the disorder that has been diagnosed, (b) the various treatment options, and (c) the characteristics of the specific patient and the patient's support system, the clinician offers a prognosis. Such information helps the patient and the referral source anticipate of the course of the disorder and what to expect in terms of interventions and support. An emphasis is placed on avoiding iatrogenic effects that needlessly add distress and complicate the clinical picture.

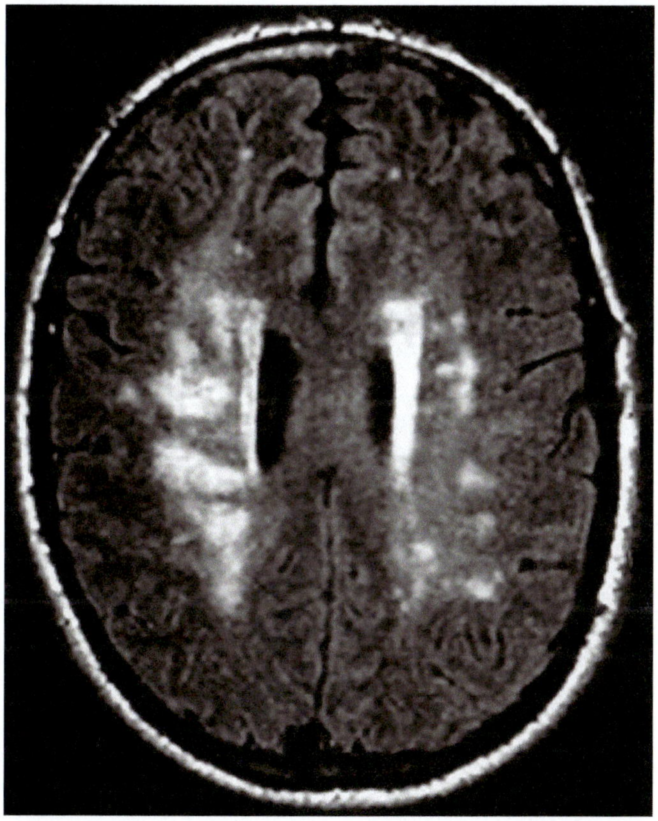

Fig. 7.18 MRI T2 FLAIR image of HIV. (*From* Hilsabeck and Huckans [34]; *with permission*)

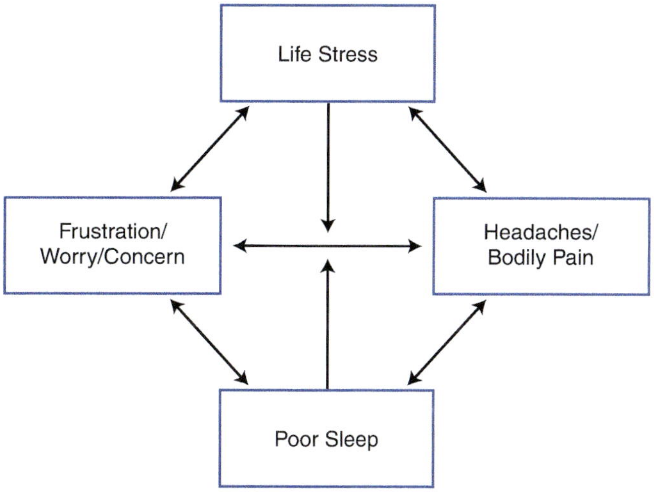

Fig. 7.20 Interwoven and mutually reinforcing factors that can cause or maintain nonspecific neurological symptoms. (*Adapted from* Carone et al. [35]; *with permission*)

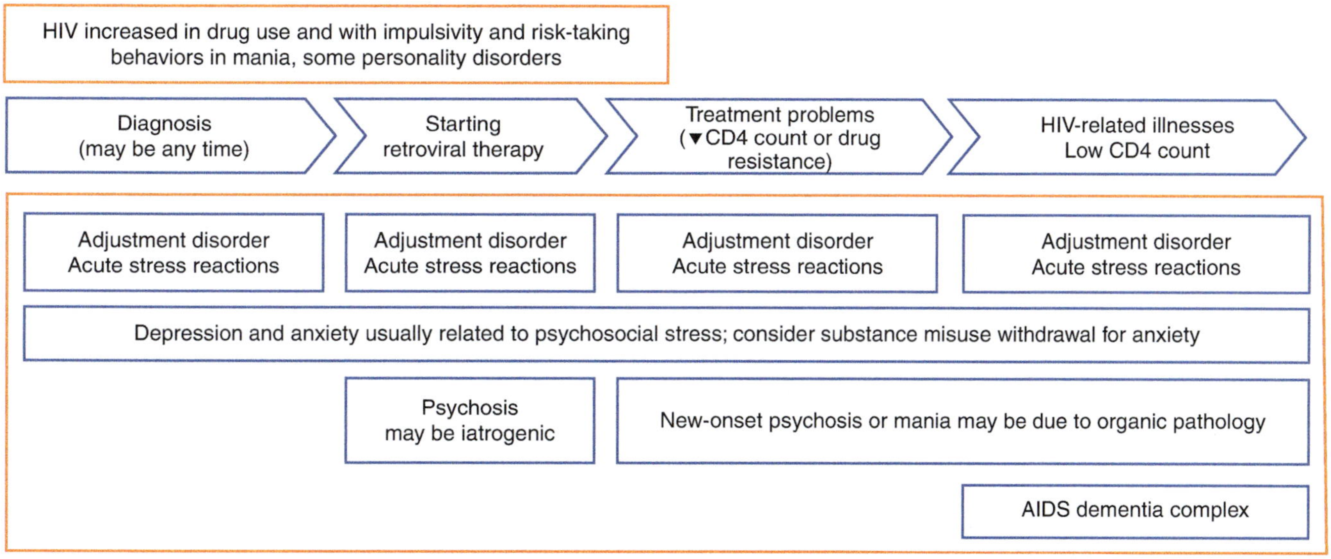

Fig. 7.19 Links between HIV and mental illness. (*Modified from* Stevens and Rodin [31]; *with permission*)

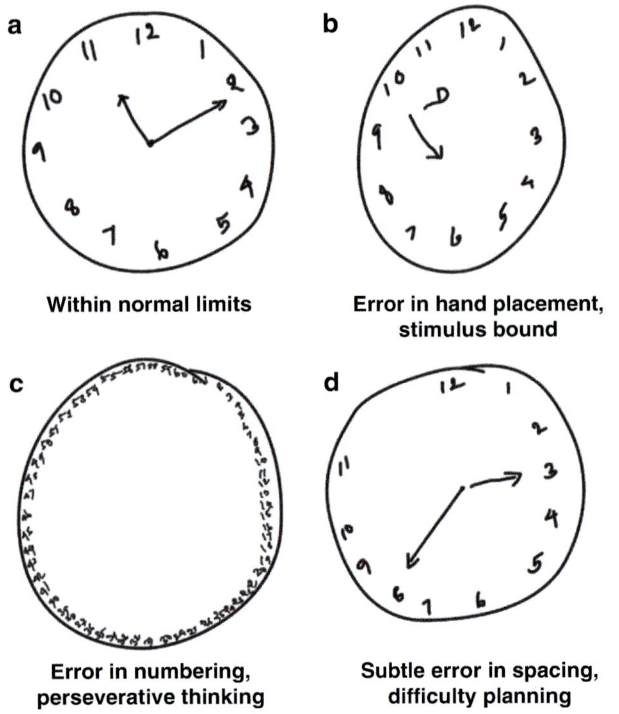

Fig. 7.21 Client clock drawing examples, demonstrating varying cognitive status and ability. (**a**) A client response within normal limits, accurately depicting "10 min after 11." (**b**) A client response with an error in hand placement (11:10), demonstrating stimulus-bound behavior. (**c**) A client response with an error in numbering, demonstrating perseverative thinking. (**d**) A client response with an error in spacing of the numbers (depicting "20 min to 4"), demonstrating planning difficulties. (*Modified from* Renn and John [36]; *with permission*)

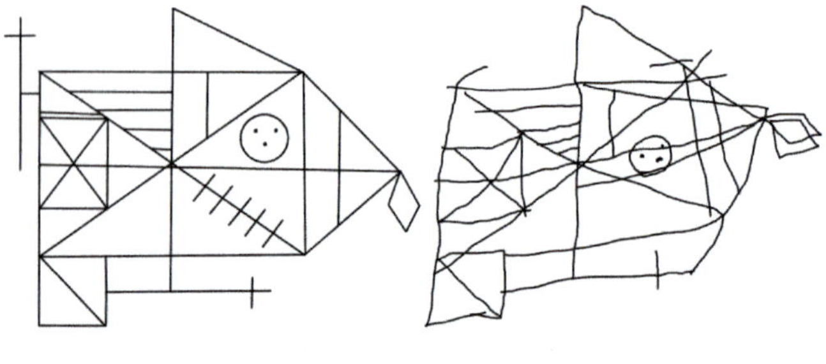

Fig. 7.22 Rey-osterrieth complex figure test. The figure on the left is the stimulus to be copied by patients. A perfect score is a maximum of 36 points. The figure on the right was copied by a person diagnosed with age-associated memory impairment (MMSE score 24/30). Although copying the figure does require memory processes, the reproduction reveals impairment in other cognitive domains, including visuospatial skills, planning, organization, and attention to detail. This pattern of performance provides information regarding underlying cerebral systems. *MMSE* folstein mini-mental state examination. (*Modified from* Kimiko et al. [37]; *with permission*)

Recommendations

The ultimate goal of diagnostic testing is to provide conclusions that are of benefit to the referral source and, in clinical (versus forensic) contexts, the person being tested, their family members or other caregivers, and treatment teams. Such conclusions commonly involve recommendations for maximizing the well-being, safety, and functioning of the patient. Although recommendations that are generic to given patient populations can be of value, recommendations that are individually tailored and specific to a given patient tend to be the most helpful. Table 7.14 provides a sample of recommendations for a patient who has a neurocognitive disorder.

Care should be taken not to overstate the evidence base for a particular recommendation. For example, a poor perfor-

Table 7.14 Sample recommendations for patients with neurocognitive disorders

- Tests
  - Neuroimaging
  - Medical laboratory tests
  - Sleep studies
  - Psychological/neuropsychological re-evaluation (specify time frame)
- Treatment
  - Psychotherapy
  - Psychotropic medication
  - Substance abuse rehabilitation
  - Cognitive rehabilitation
  - Pain management
  - Interdisciplinary rehabilitation (e.g., PT, OT, SLP)
  - Physician-approved physical exercise (e.g., yoga, strength training, aerobic activity)
  - Dietary changes, overseen by a dietician
  - Bibliotherapy
- Educational
  - Special education services
  - Tutoring
  - Individual attention—1:1
  - Extra time for assignments/tests
  - Separate location with reduced distractions for tests
  - Multiple choice tests
  - Preferential classroom seating
  - Record lectures
  - Frequent breaks
  - Present material and test in the verbal/visual (preferred) domain
  - Present information in brief amounts, with repetition
  - Present information in a contextual/meaningful format
- Vocational
  - Accommodations as needed
  - Job coach
  - Discontinue working if necessary
  - Return to work when appropriate
  - Engage in volunteer work
- Compensatory
  - Devices
    - Calendar
    - Alarms
    - Notes
    - Recording

Table 7.14 (continued)

– Strategies
Categorizing and chunking information
Use of key words to facilitate recall
Meaningful associations
Processing information through multiple sensory modalities
• Social/leisure/spiritual
– Engage in relaxing and meaningful activities to the extent possible (individually tailored)
– Interact with family and peers who are supportive and enrich life
– Join groups with common interests
– Engage in spiritually meaningful activities
– Participate in religious events
• Safety
– Supervision
– Discontinue driving
– Discontinue use of stove/oven

Table 7.15 Features of effective reports

• Clearly labeled sections
• Clear statement of purpose for the evaluation / referral question(s)
• Limited use of professional jargon (or technical terms are defined)
• Diagnosis
– Avoid use of "rule out" diagnoses unless specific information (e.g., additional testing, consultation with a collateral source of information, unclear clinical picture due to inchoate neurodevelopment) is needed to make or rule out the diagnosis; the needed information should be stated. If multiple diagnoses are being considered, the reasoning for, and degree of confidence in, each diagnosis can be described
• Prognosis
• Recommendations
• Referral question answered

mance on a given cognitive test may not translate into a functional limitation in real-world activities. That is, the test may not have strong ecological validity [17].

The Report

Psychological and neuropsychological reports vary widely in terms of format, length, and use of terminology. Effective reports share certain features (see Table 7.15).

Limitations and Pitfalls in Diagnostic Testing

The ability to quantify cognitive, emotional, and behavioral functioning and compare the results to large normative populations is a considerable benefit of diagnostic testing. However, diagnostic testing is not without its limitations (see Table 7.16).

Table 7.16 Diagnostic testing limitations

• No direct observation of patients performing daily tasks
• Reliance on self-report or information from invested parties
– May be incomplete or inaccurate
Intentionally or unintentionally
• Measurement error

Table 7.17 Common pitfalls in diagnostic testing

• Failure to appropriately assess symptom and performance validity
• Failure to use appropriate normative data
• Failure to interpret tests in an evidence-based manner
• Failure to adequately consider the potential impact of the multiple personal, environmental, and test-related factors that can affect test scores
• Letting the desire to please the referral source, or not upset patient, affect diagnostic determinations

All examiners, particularly those who are unqualified, are vulnerable to pitfalls that can affect diagnostic accuracy and subsequent recommendations and treatment decisions (see Table 7.17). Making a concerted effort to avoid common pitfalls can maximize the effectiveness of the diagnostic testing process for everyone involved.

Ethical Considerations

Psychodiagnostic testing provides valuable information for promoting the care and well-being of patients, which is consistent with the bioethical principle of *beneficence*. Clinicians using such testing who strive to avoid harming patients by using appropriate methods and arriving at evidence-based conclusions are practicing in a manner consistent with the ethical principle of *nonmaleficence*. A primary consideration in the avoidance of harming patients involves practicing in a manner that is consistent with one's professional competence. Years of education, supervised training, and experience in psychodiagnostic testing are needed for the service to benefit, and not harm, patients. The appropriate selection, use, and interpretation of diagnostic tests depend on having the appropriate knowledge and skills. Clinicians who employ such methods without the requisite knowledge and skill are practicing outside the bounds of ethical requirements. Such ethical misconduct can be easily avoided through collaboration with interdisciplinary colleagues, such as by referring patients who need testing to qualified clinicians.

Consistent with the ethical principle of respect for patient autonomy, an appropriate informed consent process is needed to allow patients (or their representatives) to determine whether to undergo the testing. For patients who lack the capacity to make such decisions, the clinician should nevertheless seek the patient's assent and obtain consent from the patient's legal decision maker. Also consistent with patient autonomy is the right of the patient to be informed of the results of the testing. It may be tempting for clinicians to withhold the results of an evaluation when the conclusions involve a diagnosis that could be upsetting to patients or their families (e.g., a progressive neurocognitive disorder). Despite the desire to protect patients from such information, they have a right to know, and compassionately presenting such results can help patients and their families begin to address the symptoms and limitations and prepare for the anticipated course of the condition. Bush (2009) reviewed and advanced the understanding of these issues in the context of mental health practice with older adults (see Fig. 7.23).

Bush, Russo, and Cuesta (2012) [18] proposed a systematic approach to ethical decision-making through which clinicians arrive at sound solutions to ethical issues and challenges (see Fig. 7.24).

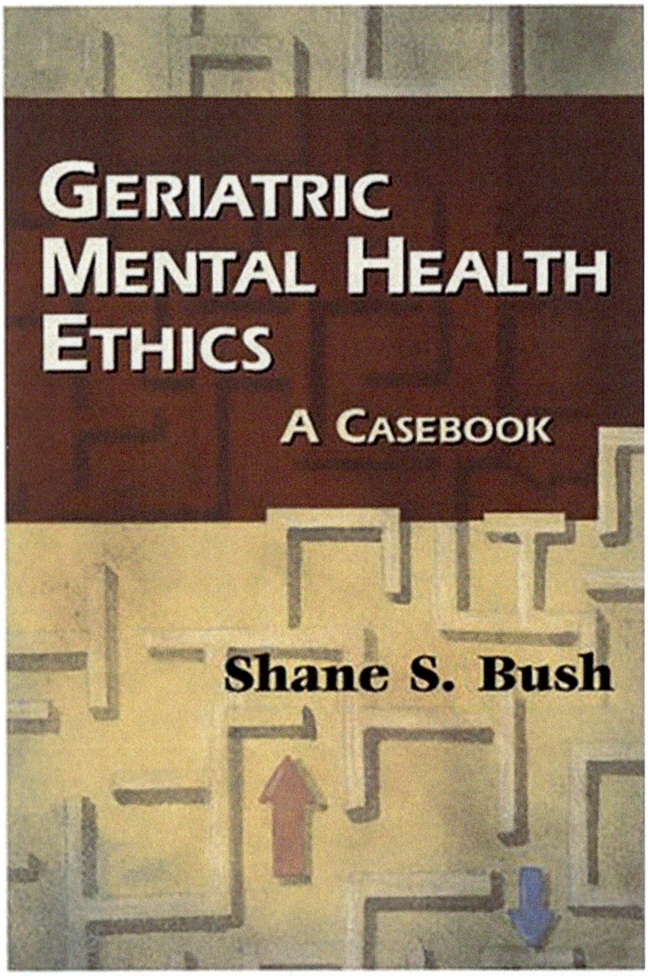

Fig. 7.23 Geriatric mental health ethics: a casebook. (From Bush [38]; *with permission*)

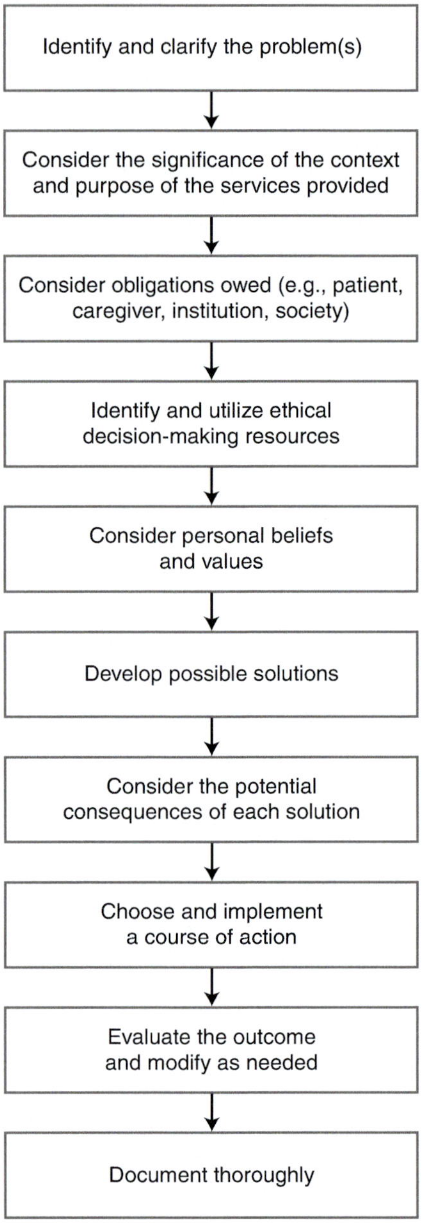

Fig. 7.24 Ethical decision-making model. (*Adapted from* Bush et al. [9]; *with permission*)

Key Contributors and Contributions

The recorded history of testing mental abilities has its origins in 2200 B.C. during the first dynasty of traditional Chinese history (Xia dynasty). The Chinese emperor King Yu (see Fig. 7.25) had his officials examined every 3 years to determine their fitness for office. The grueling testing was modified and refined over the centuries until written exams were introduced during the Han dynasty.

Rating scales are widely used as a means of quantifying subjective psychological variables. An early, crude form of

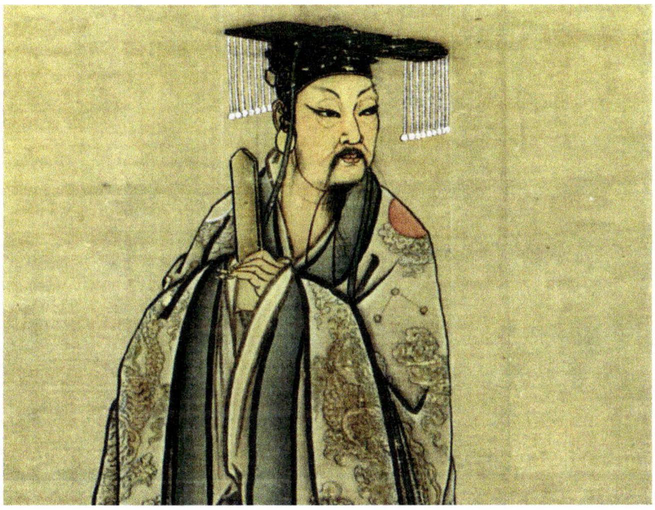

Fig. 7.25 King Yu of Xia dynasty

rating scale can be traced back to the second-century Greco-Roman physician Galen. However, Christian Thomasius (1655–1728) is credited with being the first person to devise and apply rating scales for measuring psychological variables.

During the fourth century, interest in judging inner character from one's outward (especially facial) appearance emerged. This methodology, *physiognomy*, despite being invalid, remained popular for centuries and led to the development by Francis Joseph Gall of *phrenology*, another methodology involving the practice of reading bumps on the head to understand the underlying brain functions and associated thoughts and abilities. In 1931, Henry C. Lavery created the psychograph (see Fig. 7.26) as a device used in the practice of phrenology.

In late nineteenth century Europe and Great Britain, experimental psychology began employing objective methods to test human abilities, particularly sensory functions. Brass instruments were used to measure sensory thresholds and reaction times, which were then equated with intelligence (see Fig. 7.27). Wilhelm Wundt founded the first psychological laboratory in 1879 in Leipzig. He proposed the novel idea that the speed of processing information might differ among people.

In the late nineteenth century and early twentieth century, Francis Galton, James McKeen Cattell, and others (e.g., Wilhelm Wundt) pioneered the new experimental psychology, with a focus on objective, standardized measurement of individual differences in physical and behavioral domains. J. M. Cattell (1860–1944) established at testing laboratory at the University of Pennsylvania in 1888 and helped to establish the foundations of mental measurement in the U.S. Efforts begun in Europe were brought to the U.S. Cattell coined the term "mental test." In 1904, Spearman (1863–1936) introduced a two-factor theory of intelligence consisting of a general factor (g) and specific factors(s).

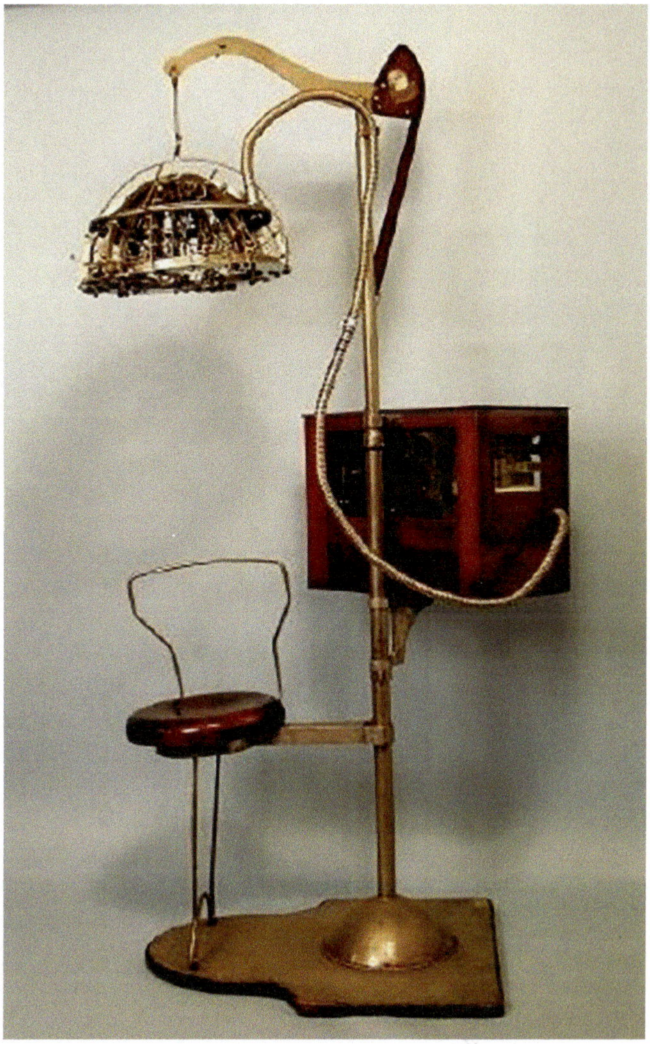

Fig. 7.26 Psychograph

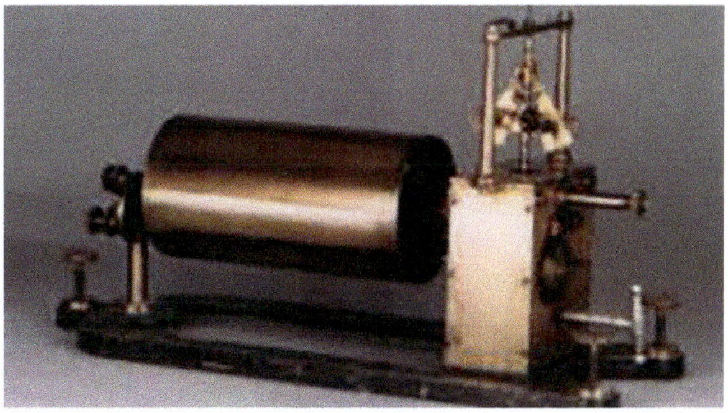

Fig. 7.27 Brass instrument

Alfred Binet (1857–1911) and his co-investigator in 1905 developed a test of intelligence (Binet–Simon Scale) for

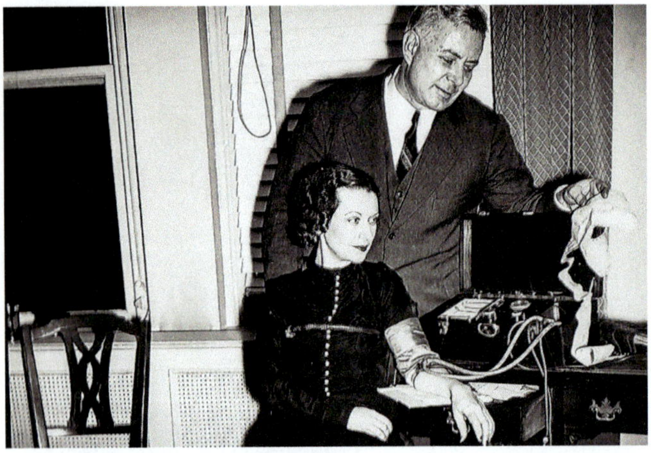

Fig. 7.28 William Maulton Marston using lie detector test

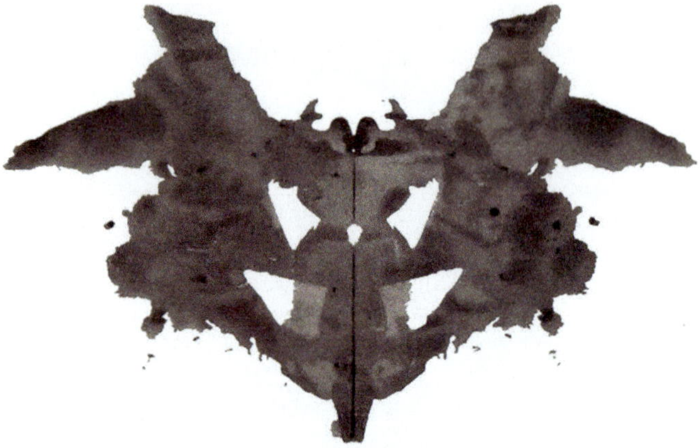

Fig. 7.29 Sample Rorschach Inkblot card

screening school children. Binet believed that intelligence could be better measured through higher psychological processes rather than more basic sensory and motor functions. One of the earliest uses of IQ tests was testing for giftedness in children to assist with academic placement. Stanford professor Lewis M. Terman (1857–1956) popularized IQ testing with his substantial revision of the Binet scales in 1916. The Stanford–Binet was a substantial revision. The Stanford–Binet remained the standard of intelligence testing for decades. Also occurring during this period of IQ test development was the work of William Maulton Marston, creator of the lie detector test and the comic strip, Wonder Woman (see Fig. 7.28).

Group testing of intelligence became popular when the USA entered WWI and Robert M. Yerkes convinced the US government and the Army that all recruits should be given intelligence tests (Army alpha and Army beta tests) for purposes of weeding out those with substandard mental abilities and assigning the rest to positions for which they were well suited. Group testing was then applied in educational settings, and the introduction of machine scoring in the 1930s allowed for objective group testing to be carried out even more efficiently than it had been.

Tests of aptitude, achievement, and personality traits evolved after WWI to more closely reflect their present form. Projective tests emerged. In 1921 Swiss psychiatrist Hermann Rorschach published his famous monograph, *Psychodiagnostics*, which led to the development of the Rorschach Inkblot Test [19] (see Fig. 7.29 for a sample of the Rorschach Inkblot cards).

Thurstone (1887–1955) proposed in 1933 a multiple factor analytic approach to the study of human abilities. By 1938, mental tests had reached the status of big business; according to the *1938 Mental Measurements Yearbook*, at least 4000 psychological tests were in print at that time. In 1939 David Wechsler (1896–1981) published the Wechsler–Bellevue Intelligence Scale (later to become the Wechsler Adult Intelligence Scale, with multiple revisions). The

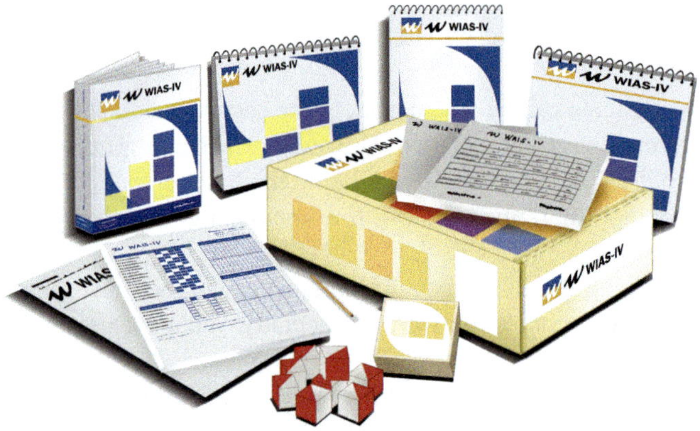

Fig. 7.30 Wechsler adult intelligence test

Wechsler Intelligence Scale for Children was published in 1949, with multiple revisions since then. Today, multiple versions of the Wechsler family of tests are available for children and adults and are the most popular instruments used for the measurement of cognition in general and intelligence in particular (see Figs. 7.30 and 7.31).

Table 7.18 contains multiple definitions of what IQ tests measure.

In 1943, the objective Minnesota Multiphasic Personality Inventory (MMPI) was developed to quantify the emotional states and personality traits and introduced the use of validity scales to determine whether the patient's responses were a true reflection of the constructs of interest [20]. The MMPI has grown into a family of measures for various patient populations and practice needs, and numerous additional brief and comprehensive measures of emotional and personality variables have emerged, offering practitioners options to best serve their patients.

Raymond B. Cattell (1905–1998) proposed a theory of fluid and crystalized intelligence in 1963. Aaron T. Beck (1921–), regarded as the father of both cognitive therapy and cognitive behavioral therapy, developed self-report measures of depression and anxiety which have become widely used. Theodore Millon (1928–2014) developed diagnostic ques-

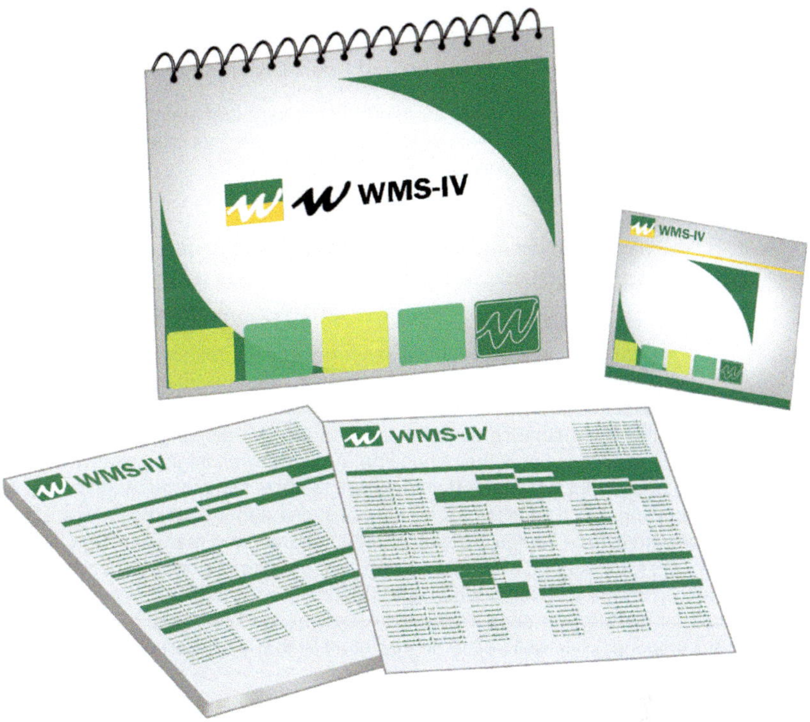

Fig. 7.31 Wechsler memory scale

Table 7.18 Definitions of Intelligence

1. "The tendency to take and maintain a definite direction; the capacity to make adaptations for the purposes of attaining a desired end; and the power of autocriticism" (Binet [25])
2. "…the ability to undertake activities that are characterized by • Difficulty • Complexity • Abstractness • Economy • Adaptiveness to a goal • Social value • The emergence of originals, and to maintain such activities under conditions that demand a concentration of energy and a resistance to emotional forces" (Stoddard [26])
3. "The aggregate or global capacity of the individual to act purposefully, to think rationally and to deal effectively with his [or her] environment." (Wechsler [27])
4. "…the ability to plan and structure one's behavior with an end in view" (Das [28])
5. "Intelligence is a collective term that refers to the possession of useful knowledge and special information-processing capabilities." (Hunt [29])
6. "Intelligent behavior reflects the survival skills of the species, beyond those associated with basic physiological processes." (Sattler [30])

tionnaire tools such as the Millon Clinical Multiaxial Inventory (currently in its fourth edition) and contributed to the development of earlier versions of the *Diagnostic and Statistical Manual of Mental Disorders*.

Ralph Reitan (1922–2014), one of the fathers of clinical neuropsychology in the USA, in 1955 published a seminal paper entitled *Certain Differential Effects of Left and Right Cerebral Lesions in Human Adults* and, with Ward Halstead, developed the Halstead–Reitan Neuropsychological Battery. Charles Golden in 1981 published the Luria–Nebraska Neuropsychological Battery.

The ability of any measure to be of value to mental health professionals rests on the belief that the patient responded honestly to test questions and put forth a good effort on tests of cognitive abilities; that is, they approached the assessment process in a valid manner. Patients in various contexts have incentives to provide inaccurate information or put forth suboptimal effort (e.g., avoiding stressful or dangerous environments, such as war or prison; obtaining financial awards or benefits). Although mental health professionals are trained to assess human behavior, and many believe they are good at detecting dissimulation, a body of research suggests that this is not an area of strength for clinicians [21]. Therefore, objective methods and procedures are needed [9]. The MMPI validity scales were among the first to quantify (in)valid responding on a psychological test. For measures of cognitive and motor functioning, Swiss psychologist Andrey Rey led the efforts with a dot counting test in 1941 and a 15-item memory test in 1964. In the 1970s, a forced-choice paradigm was developed, and the term "symptom validity assessment" was coined by Pankratz (1979) [22], significantly advancing and forever changing the nature of cognitive assessment.

Tests of normal and pathological cognitive, emotional, and behavioral functioning, informed by evidence-based theory, have continued to be developed and updated to (a) reflect the evolving science, (b) address the requirements of a changing society, and (c) meet the needs of clinicians in various practice settings (see Fig. 7.32). Clinicians must remain abreast of developments in the field in order to effectively serve those in need.

Sample Informed Consent Form

Independent and Court-Ordered Forensic Neuropsychological Examinations

This is a general template for informed consent that may not apply to one's particular circumstances or jurisdiction. It is recommended that psychologists seek advice from personal counsel to determine if this consent is appropriate for their circumstances and jurisdiction.

Referral Source:

You have been referred for an independent forensic neuropsychological examination (i.e., evaluation of your thinking abilities) by ______________________________ (name of referral)

Nature and Purpose:

The goal of neuropsychological assessment is to determine if any changes have occurred in your attention, memory, language, problem solving or other thinking skills. The current examination has been requested because of your claim of neuropsychological injury. It is common when someone is in an accident, is injured, and sees doctors for evaluation and treatment, that the insurance carrier or an attorney representing the defense in a law suit will request an examination by an expert neuropsychologist of their choosing. A neuropsychological examination will include an interview, where questions will be asked about your background and current medical symptoms. Additionally, standardized tests and other techniques my be used, including, but not limited to, asking questions about your knowledge of certain topics, reading, drawing figures and shapes, learning word lists or stories, viewing printed material, and manipulating objects. Your task is to answer questions as accurately as you can; for example, when discussing your problems, do not minimize significant problems, but also do not exaggerate lesser concerns. You are to give your best effort during the testing. This does not mean that you have to get every answer or problem correct, for no one ever does. However, you do have to give your best effort. Part of the examination will address the accuracy of your responses, as well as the degree of effort that you exert on the tests.

Foreseeable Risks, Discomforts, and Benefits:

For some individuals, neuropsychological examinations can cause fatigue, frustration, and anxiousness. An attempt will be made to help you minimize these factors. The results of this examination may either support or not support your claim.

Limits of Confidentiality:

The results of this examination will be forwarded to ______________________________ ______________. If your claim involves a lawsuit, at minimum, the defense attorney and staff and your attorney and staff will have access to the results of this examination. Should your case proceed to trial, those involved in the trial will be exposed to the results of the examination, and the court record will be available for anyone to review. Beyond the above, confidential information about you obtained during the examination can ordinarily be released only with your written permission. There are some special circumstances that can limit confidentiality, which include, but are not limited to, (a) a statement of intent to harm yourself or others, (b) statements indicating harm or abuse of children or vulnerable adults, and (c) a subpoena from a court of law.

I have read and agree with the nature and purpose of this examination and to each of the points listed above. I have had an opportunity to clarify any questions and discuss any points of concern before signing.

______________________________ ________/________/________

Examinee Signature Date

______________________________ ________/________/________

Parent/Guardian or Authorized Surrogate (if applicable) Date

______________________________ ________/________/________

Witness Signature Date

From: Bush, S.S., and National Academy of Neuropsychology Policy & Planning Committee (2005). Independent and court-ordered forensic neuropsychological examinations: Official statement of the National Academy of Neuropsychology. Archives of Clinical Neuropsychology, 20 (8), 997-1007.

Fig. 7.32 Sample consent form for forensic neuropsychological examinations. (*Modified from* Bush [38] and National Academy of Neuropsychology Policy and Planning Committee [39]; *with permission*)

Conclusions

Diagnostic testing plays a valuable role in the understanding of the cognitive, emotional, and behavioral symptoms with which many psychiatric patients present. Such testing provides an objective, quantifiable, evidence-based addition to the more subjective and qualitative components of mental health evaluations. Diagnostic testing can help limit the effects of biases that are inherent in clinical activities. Diagnostic testing is a complex process and is not without its limitations and pitfalls. Years of education, supervised training, and experience in psychodiagnostic testing are needed for the service to benefit, and not harm, patients. Interdisciplinary collaboration is often a very effective approach to understanding and treating patients with psychiatric disorders.

References

1. Kaufman NK, Bush SS. Validity assessment in military psychology. In: Kumar U, editor. The Routledge international handbook of military psychology and mental health. New York, NY: Routledge Taylor & Francis Group; 2020. p. 211–23.
2. Hung R, Carroll LJ, Cancelliere C, Côté P, Rumney P, Keightley M, et al. Systematic review of the clinical course, natural history, and prognosis for pediatric mild traumatic brain injury: results of the international collaboration on mild traumatic brain injury prognosis. Arch Phys Med Rehabil. 2014;95(3):S174–91.
3. Lees-Haley PR, Brown RS. Neuropsychological complaint base rates of 170 personal injury claimants. Arch Clin Neuropsychol. 1993;8:203–9.
4. Lagarde E, Salmi L-R, Holm LW, Contrand B, Masson F, Ribéreau-Gayon R, et al. Association of symptoms following mild traumatic brain injury with posttraumatic stress disorder vs postconcussion syndrome. J Am Med Assoc Psychiatry. 2014;71(9):1032–40.
5. American Academy of Clinical Neuropsychology. Policy statement on the presence of third party observers in neuropsychological assessment. Clin Neuropsychol. 2001;15:433–9.
6. National Academy of Neuropsychology. Presence of third party observers during neuropsychological testing: official statement of the National Academy of Neuropsychology. Arch Clin Neuropsychol. 2000;15:379–80.
7. Barona A, Reynolds CR, Chastain R. A demographically based index of premorbid intelligence for the WAIS—R. J Consult Clin Psychol. 1984;52(5):885.
8. Pearson. Advanced clinical solutions for WAIS-IV and WMS-IV: Administration and scoring manual. San Antonio, TX: Pearson; 2009.
9. Bush SS, Heilbronner RL, Ruff RM. Psychological assessment of symptom and performance validity, response bias, and malingering: official position of the Association for Scientific Advancement in Psychological Injury And Law. Psychol Injury Law. 2014;7(3):197–205.
10. Larrabee GJ. Performance validity and symptom validity in neuropsychological assessment. J Int Neuropsychol Soc. 2012;18(04):625–30.
11. Sherman EMS, Slick DJ, Iverson GL. Multidimensional malingering criteria for neuropsychological assessment: a 20-year update of the malingered neuropsychological dysfunction criteria. Arch Clin Neuropsychol. 2020;35(6):735–64. https://doi.org/10.1093/arclin/acaa019.
12. Tombaugh TN. Test of memory malingering (TOMM). New York: Multi-Health Systems; 1996.
13. Green P. Manual for the word memory test for windows (Rev. ed.). Edmonton, AB: Green's Publishing; 2005.
14. Guilmette TJ, Sweet JJ, Hebben N, Koltai D, Mahone EM, Spiegler BJ, Stucky K, Westerveld M, Conference Participants. American Academy of clinical neuropsychology consensus conference statement on uniform labeling of performance test scores. Clin Neuropsychol. 2020;34(3):437–53. https://doi.org/10.1080/13854046.2020.1722244. Epub 2020 Feb 10. PMID: 32037942
15. Binder LM, Iverson GL, Brooks BL. To err is human: "abnormal" neuropsychological scores and variability are common in healthy adults. Arch Clin Neuropsychol. 2009;24:31–46.
16. Brooks BL, Iverson GL, Holdnack JA, Feldman HH. Potential for misclassification of mild cognitive impairment: a study of memory scores on the Wechsler memory scale-III in healthy older adults. J Int Neuropsychol Soc. 2008;14:463–78.
17. Sbordone RJ, Long C. Ecological validity of neuropsychological testing. Boca Raton, FL: St. Lucie Press; 1996.
18. Bush SS, Russo AC, Cuesta GM. Ethical considerations in the neuropsychological evaluation and treatment of veterans. In: Bush SS, editor. Neuropsychological practice with veterans. New York: Springer Publishing Company; 2012. p. 333–56.
19. Rorschach H. Psychodiagnostics. 5th ed. Berne: Verlag Hans Huber; 1942. (original work published 1921)
20. Hathaway SR, McKinley JC. A multiphasic personality schedule (Minnesota): I. construction of the schedule. J Psychol. 1940;10:249–54.
21. Faust D, Hart KJ, Guilmette TJ, Arkes HR. Neuropsychologists' capacity to detect adolescent malingerers. Prof Psychol Res Pract. 1988;19(5):508–15.
22. Pankratz L. Symptom validity testing and symptom retraining: procedures for the assessment and treatment of functional sensory deficits. J Consult Clin Psychol. 1979;47:409–10.
23. Youden WJ. Index for rating diagnostic tests. Cancer. 1950;3(1):32–5.
24. Jacobson NS, Truax P. Clinical significance: a statistical approach to defining meaningful change in psychotherapy research. J Consult Clin Psychol. 1991;59(1):12–9.
25. Terman LM. The uses of intelligence tests. In: Terman ILM, editor. The measurement of intelligence. Mifflin and Company: Houghton; 1916. p. 3–21. https://doi.org/10.1037/10014-001.
26. Stoddard GD. The meaning of intelligence. New York: The Macmillan Company; 1943.
27. Wechsler D. The measurement and appraisal of adult intelligence. 4th ed. Oxford: Williams & Wilkins; 1958.
28. Das JP. Structure of cognitive abilities: evidence for simultaneous and successive processing. J Educ Psychol. 1973;65(1):103–8. https://doi.org/10.1037/h0034744.
29. Hunt E. The role of intelligence in modern society. American Scientist. July-August 1995. http://www2.psych.utoronto.ca/users/reingold/courses/intelligence/cache/Hunt-full.html.
30. Sattler JM. Assessment of children: cognitive applications. 4th ed. San Diego, CA: Jerome M. Sattler Publisher, Inc.; 2001.
31. Stevens L, Rodin I. Psychiatry: an illustrated colour text. 2nd ed. London: Churchill Livingstone; 2010.
32. Browndyke JN. Functional neuroanatomical bases of deceptive behavior and malingering. In: Carone DA, Bush SS, editors. Mild traumatic brain injury: symptom validity assessment and malingering. New York: Springer Publishing Company; 2013. p. 303–21.
33. Iverson GL, Le Page J, Koehler BE, Shojania K, Badii M. Test of memory malingering (TOMM) scores are not affected by chronic pain or depression in patients with fibromyalgia. Clin Neuropsychol. 2007;21:532–46.
34. Hilsabeck RC, Huckans M. Human immunodeficiency virus and hepatitis. In: Bush SS, editor. Neuropsychological practice

with veterans. New York: Springer Publishing Company; 2012. p. 201–26.
35. Carone DA, Bush SS, Iverson GL. Providing feedback on symptom validity, mental health, and treatment in mild traumatic brain injury. In: Carone DA, Bush SS, editors. Mild traumatic brain injury: symptom validity assessment and malingering. New York: Springer Publishing Company; 2013. p. 101–18.
36. Renn BN, John SE. Mental status examination. In: Segal DL, editor. Diagnostic interviewing. Cham: Springer; 2019. p. 77. https://doi.org/10.1007/978-1-4939-9127-3_4.
37. Kimiko D-R, Flanagan ME, Grabowski TJ Jr. Dementias. In: Rosenberg RN, editor. Atlas of clinical neurology. Cham: Springer; 2019. p. 287. https://doi.org/10.1007/978-3-030-03283-8_6.
38. Bush SS. Geriatric mental health ethics: a casebook. New York: Springer Publishing Company; 2009.
39. National Academy of Neuropsychology Policy & Planning Committee. Independent and court-ordered forensic neuropsychological examinations: Official statement of the National Academy of Neuropsychology. Arch Clin Neuropsychol. 2005;20(8):997–1007.

Diagnostic Neuroimaging and Laboratory Tests

8

Nian Liu, Fei Li, Zhiyun Jia, Taolin Chen, Haoyang Xing, Ying Chen, Su Lui, and Qiyong Gong

Introduction

Psychiatric disorders are heterogeneous and have integrations of varied alterations in emotion, cognition, motor activity, and social function, which has increased the challenges in delivering an accurate diagnosis and effective treatment. The primary diagnosis of psychiatric disorder is based on its symptom dependent on the experience and subjective judgment of clinicians. Detection of subtle clinical abnormalities in the early course of psychiatric disorders requires skilled doctors who are highly specialized in mental health services. There is a pressing need to identify objective biomarkers to assist the individual diagnosis, classification of different bio-subtypes, and prediction of disease prognosis. Psychoradiology is an emerging field that applies medical imaging technologies to the analysis of mental health, neurophysiology, and psychiatric disorders [1]. A prominent advantage of psychoradiology is that it relies on imaging data analysis rather than visual inspection of images [2]. Magnetic resonance imaging (MRI), together with other medical imaging techniques such as positron emission tomography and electroencephalogram, is the mainstay of psychoradiology. Using psychoradiological methods, structural and functional cerebral alterations have been identified in psychiatric disorders. With the application of artificial intelligence, psychoradiology may not only advance the understanding of pathological mechanisms of psychiatric disorders but also translate the observations into clinical practice, the findings of which have shown promise as neuroimaging biomarkers for classification, subtyping, and prediction [3–5]. The biomarkers found by psychoradiology also showed promises in biologically redefining psychiatric disorders and in optimizing drug treatment selection, thus paving the way to personalized and precision medicines for patients with psychiatric disorders.

In addition to imaging biomarkers, the dysfunction of immune-inflammatory process is also associated with the pathogenesis of psychiatric disorders, suggesting that combined neuroimaging and laboratory biomarkers may be helpful to make connections between molecular basis, neural pathophysiology, and behavioral symptoms in psychiatric disorders, and may boost diagnostic sensitivity and specificity.

In this chapter, we summarize various approaches to identifying biomarkers in psychoradiology. Specifically, we will discuss image data acquisition and quality control, the diagnostic neuroimaging and laboratory tests for psychiatric disorders, and the status of psychoradiology in clinical practice with a specified focus on its translational potentiality. The published clinical applications for different MRI modalities were introduced according to their role in disorder classification, subtyping, and prediction. The use of innovative biomarkers, beyond clinical symptoms, may be a way forward to improve differential diagnoses and individualized patient cares for psychiatric disorders. With the emerging multi-

N. Liu
Huaxi MR Research Center (HMRRC), Department of Radiology, West China Hospital of Sichuan University, Chengdu, China

Department of Radiology, Affiliated Hospital of North Sichuan Medical College, Nanchong, China

F. Li · T. Chen
Huaxi MR Research Center (HMRRC), Department of Radiology, West China Hospital of Sichuan University, Chengdu, China

Functional and Molecular Imaging Key Laboratory of Sichuan Province, West China Hospital of Sichuan University, Chengdu, China

Z. Jia
Department of Nuclear Medicine, West China Hospital of Sichuan University, Chengdu, China

H. Xing · Y. Chen
Huaxi MR Research Center (HMRRC), Department of Radiology, West China Hospital of Sichuan University, Chengdu, China

Research Unit of Psychoradiology, Chinese Academy of Medical Sciences, Chengdu, China

S. Lui · Q. Gong (✉)
Huaxi MR Research Center (HMRRC), Department of Radiology, West China Hospital of Sichuan University, Chengdu, China

Department of Radiology, West China Xiamen Hospital of Sichuan University, Xiamen, China
e-mail: qiyonggong@hmrrc.org.cn

W. W. IsHak (ed.), *Atlas of Psychiatry*, https://doi.org/10.1007/978-3-031-15401-0_8

center studies and the development of advanced statistical analyses, considerable interdisciplinary collaborations that involve radiologists, psychiatrists, psychologists, and computer scientists could foster an optimized psychoradiological examinations flow for patients with psychiatric disorders and set up prospective clinical studies to identify and validate the accuracy and reliability of previous findings.

The application of emission computed tomography (ECT) using radioactive tracing technique has considerably advanced understanding of the pathophysiology of psychiatric disorders. ECT's unique superiorities and developments in the study of psychiatric disorders were described in the third section of this chapter with a focus on imaging of regional cerebral blood flow, neurotransmitter, and neuroreceptor. These advances, together with improvements in scanner resolution, enable ECT to play an increasingly important role in clarifying causes and pathological mechanisms of psychiatric disorders based on molecular level.

As an important complement to fMRI and ECT techniques, eletroencephalography (EEG) are becoming more and more popular because of its low cost and excellent temporal resolution. The fourth section first described the neural basis and measurement of quantitive EEG and then focused on recent advances arising from event-related potential (ERP) studies in identifying objective and reliable biomarkers for the diagnosis of mental disorders. It is promising that considerable physiological evidence accumulated by EEG research and multicenter databases can be used to develop the "gold standard" of neuroelectrophysiological markers for clinical practice, and combine machine learning and multi-modality imaging indicators to further enhance the reliability and effectiveness of biomarkers for mental disorders. Another brain functional imaging tool, magnetoencephalography (MEG) featured with high spatial and temporal resolutions offers a unique view of psychiatry diagnosis. The new insights that MEG studies have provided into searching for biomarkers of psychiatric disorders were discussed in the fifth section. Developing new devices possessing lower prices and higher performance will greatly promote the clinical research and application of MEG.

Laboratory tests is also an effective and indispensable approach to identifying biomarkers of psychiatric disorders. We focally discussed the value of genetic testing and plasma-targeted metabonomic method in diagnosing mental disorders and predicting treatment response and/or adverse events in the last part of this chapter.

Data Acquisition and Quality Control

Anatomical MR Acquisition and Quality Control

T1-Weighted Anatomical MR Acquisition

Three-dimensional fast inverse recovery gradient-echo (GE) sequences, with field of view (FOV) covering the entire head, are useful for brain structure segmentation and cortical surface reconstruction. They are commonly acquired in the sagittal plane with 1-mm isotropic voxel size. Moreover, fat suppression is usually employed to reduce signal from bone marrow and scalp fat. The resolution can be further increased to 0.8 mm for most 3 T clinical scanners by using a 32-channel head coil. It is also recommended to acquire a pair of phase-encoding reversed spin-echo scans to construct a field map for readout distortion correction.

T2-Weighted Anatomical MR Acquisition

It is also recommended to acquire high-resolution anatomical T2 weighted images for psychiatric research. By calculating the T1w/T2w ratio, a myelin content map may be generated across the cortical surface and used to distinguish many architectonic areas non-invasively [6]. High-resolution T2 scans are commonly acquired with a slab excited 3D fast spin echo sequence with the same FOV and resolution of the T1w scan.

Quality Control

Artifacts in anatomical images may bias the outcome of structure segmentation and further statistical inference [7]. Despite head coverage and intensity inhomogeneity, quality control of anatomical images is mainly focused on the visual inspection and evaluation of motion artifacts, such as blurring and ringing (Fig. 8.1). Large motion artifacts have been shown to affect automated segmentation and parcellation techniques implemented in FreeSurfer [7, 8]. However, there is currently no established software package or criteria to determine the threshold of motion artifact. Based on our own experience, the recommended method is to send the data to the automatic segmentation process and then overlay the segmentation results on the original image for visual inspection. It is recommended to exclude volumes from further processing if motion artifacts significantly affect the segmentation.

Diffusion MR Acquisition and Quality Control

Diffusion MR Acquisition

Diffusion MR can measure subtle movement of water molecules within their local tissue environment. Diffusion MR is able to provide two types of metrics as potential biomarkers for psychiatric disorders. Voxel-wise metrics of diffusion properties, like fractional anisotropy (FA), mean diffusivity (MD) and NODDI measures, reflect the local status of tissue microstructure. Global metrics based on deterministic or probabilistic tractography reflect structural connectivity between pairs of brain regions. To fit a simple tensor model, at least one diffusion-weighted shell ($b = 1000$) and 30 diffusion-encoding directions should be acquired. For more complicated diffusion models or structural connectome estimation,

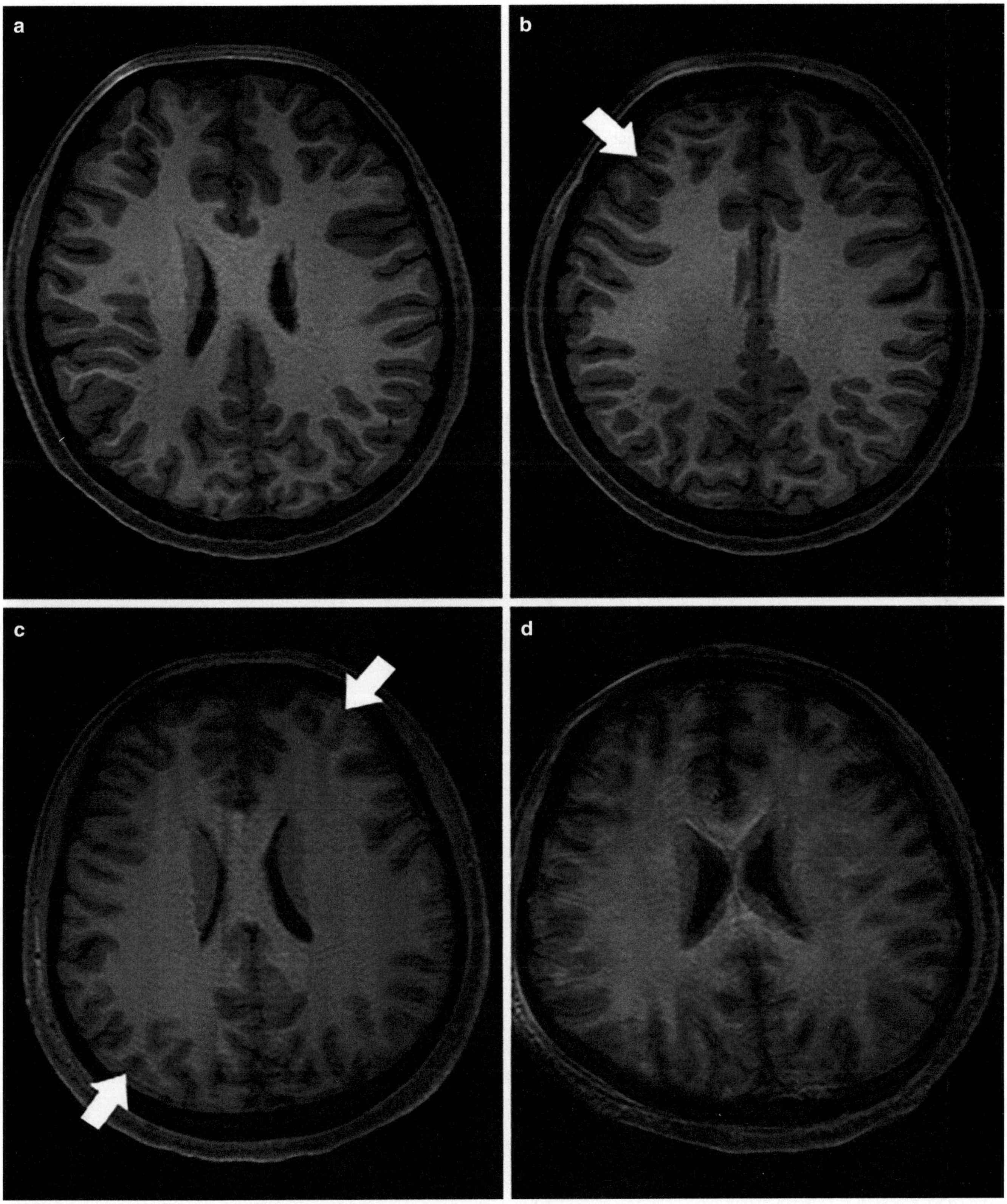

Fig. 8.1 T1 weighted image with excellent quality (**a**) and with mild (**b**), moderate (**c**), and severe (**d**) motion artifact. White arrows indicate the ring and blur effect

two or more diffusion-weighted shells and 60 diffusion-encoding directions for each shell are recommended. Isotropic voxel size is required for any analysis based on fiber tractography. In order to generate appropriate fieldmap to perform EPI specific distortion correction, two acquisition strategies can be chosen depending on the patient's tolerance. In the first option, all diffusion volumes are acquired with identical phase encoding direction and one additional b0 with opposite phase encoding direction is acquired to estimate the inhomogeneity fieldmap. In the other option, two volumes are captured with the opposite phase encoding direction for each b-value and diffusion direction. This allows the combination of the two volumes of each diffusion direction and shells into a single volume to increase SNR.

Quality Control

The quality of diffusion-weighted images is evaluated from the following aspects: (1) Geometric distortion. Distortion is unavoidable for EPI sequence but should be within acceptable limits. For images with opposite phase encoding directions, the distortion should also be opposite (Fig. 8.2a); (2) Head motion. Head motion in diffusion MRI is mainly reflected by signal loss in certain slices of a volume, which can easily be detected through visual inspection (Fig. 8.2b); and (3) Signal-to-noise ratio (SNR). The SNR can only be calculated quantitatively and should be consistent within a range for a given b value. If large fluctuation happens, the radio frequency emission and receiver parts of the imaging system should be checked.

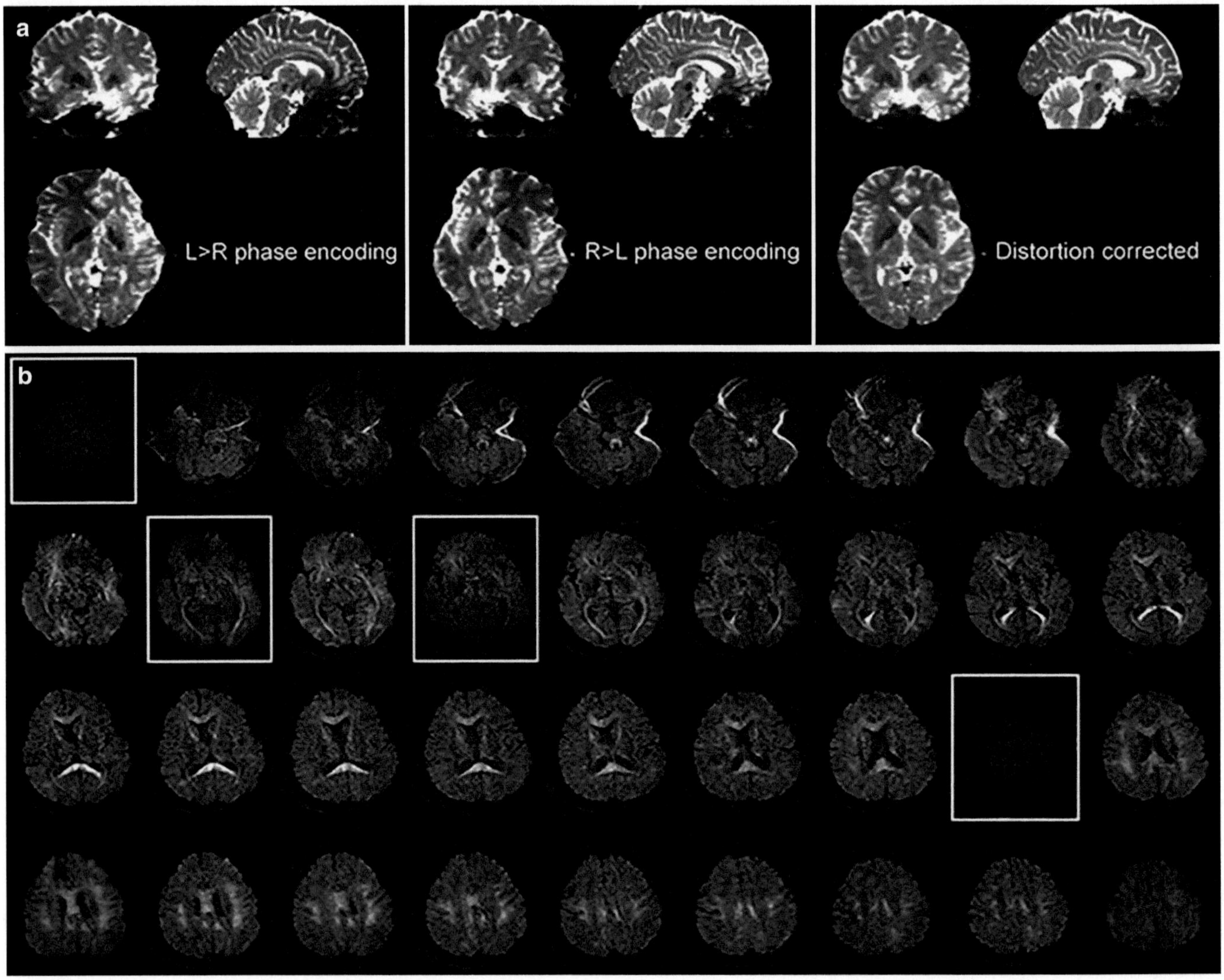

Fig. 8.2 Diffusion volumes with opposite phase encoding directions and the distortion free volume after correction (**a**). Head motion in diffusion MRI is mainly manifested by partial or complete signal loss in certain slices (indicate by white rectangle) of a volume (**b**)

Geometric distortion. Distortion is unavoidable for EPI sequence but should be within acceptable limits. For images with opposite phase encoding directions, the distortion should also be opposite (Fig. 8.2a) Head motion. Head motion in diffusion MRI is mainly manifested by signal loss in certain slices of a volume, which can easily be detected through visual inspection (Fig. 8.2b) Signal to noise ratio (SNR). The SNR can only be calculated quantitatively and should be constant within a range for a given *b* value, if large fluctuation happens, the radio frequency emission and receiver parts of the imaging system should be checked (Fig. 8.3).

Functional MR Acquisition and Quality Control

Functional MR Acquisition

Resting-state functional MRI ("rfMRI") measures the changes in signal intensity caused by blood oxygenation levels associated with cerebral intrinsic activity. It can provide a valuable estimation of functional connectivity between pairs of brain regions. The rfMRI images can be acquired by a gradient echo formation followed by an EPI readout. The spatial resolution is around 3 mm and the temporal resolution is about 2 s for conventional single-shot GE-EPI sequence at 3 T. More than 5 min of scan duration is recommended for stable and effective signal series. The spatial and temporal resolution can be further improved by adopting the multi-band technique, which permits sub-second whole brain coverage at about 2 mm isotropic resolution. This is achieved by acquiring multiple slices in the time of a single EPI echo train with multiple receiver coils and a multi-band excitation pulse sequence. A pair of phase-encoding reversed spin-echo scans with identical geometry as rfMRI volumes are also needed to generate a field map for distortion correction.

Quality Control

The quality control points of fMRI are similar to those of diffusion MR, focusing on image distortion, signal-to-noise ratio, and motion artifacts. Since the TR of fMRI is much smaller than that of diffusion MR, motion artifacts on fMRI are mainly represented by head displacement rather than signal loss. There are several open source software available for quantitative QC, such as fsl, fMRIPrep, etc. In general, data with absolute head displacement greater than 2 mm or absolute rotation angle greater than 5° should be excluded in further analysis (Fig. 8.4).

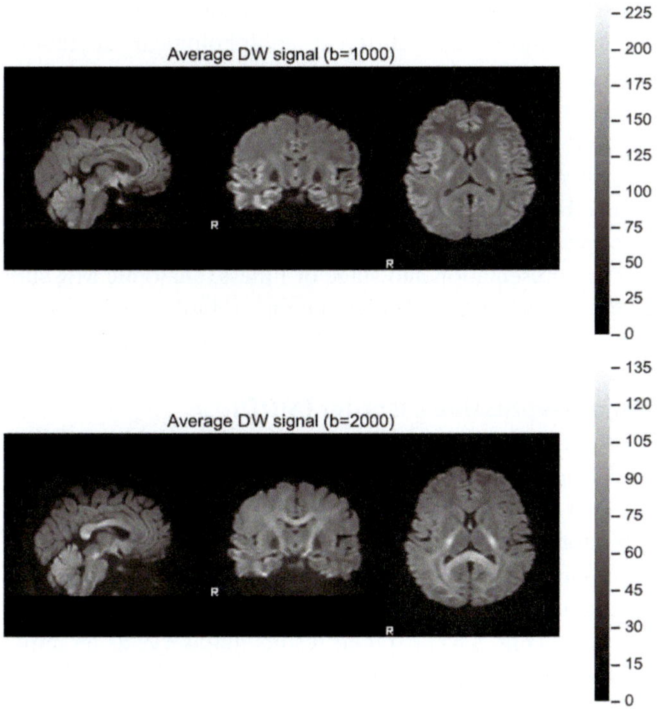

Fig. 8.3 Average signal intensity of diffusion weighted images at $b = 1000$ and $b = 2000$

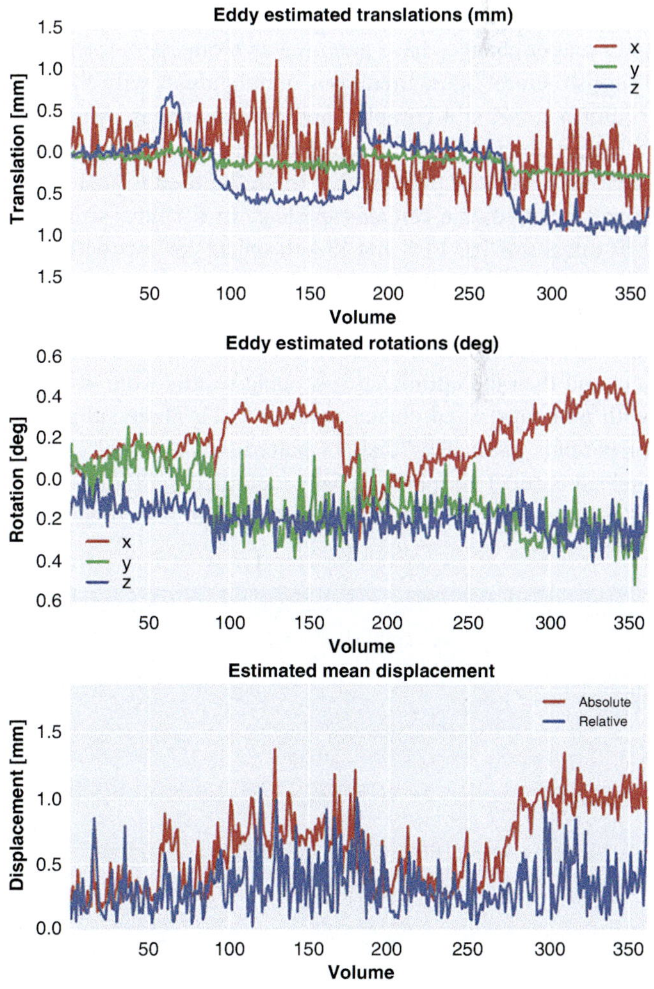

Fig. 8.4 Quantitative plot of head motion during a scan session. Motions in translation, rotation, and displacement are showed, respectively

Diagnostic Neuroimaging Tests

Classification and Subtyping

Schizophrenia

Although regional brain deficits have been well documented in schizophrenia (SZ), one important question that remains largely unanswered is whether those deficits revealed by MRI could be used as individual biomarkers to discriminate patients from healthy controls. In a study, 163 drug-naïve first-episode SZ (FES) patients and 163 demographically matched healthy controls were recruited. Support Vector Machine was used to explore the potential utility of neuroanatomic measurements in the differentiation of individual patients and healthy controls [9]. The accuracy of the classification was 85.0% (specificity 87.0%, sensitivity 83.0%) for surface area and 81.8% (specificity 85.0%, sensitivity 76.9%) for cortical thickness. Regions contributing to classification accuracy mainly included the default mode, central executive, salience, and visual networks (Fig. 8.5, Table 8.1). These findings suggest that the patterns of illness-related gray matter changes have potential as biomarkers for identifying structural brain alterations in individuals with SZ.

Further, SZ is a complex and heterogeneous syndrome. Whether quantitative imaging biomarkers can identify discrete subgroups of patients that might be used to foster personalized medicine remains unclear. In a study, structural MR images of 163 FES and 133 chronical patients with mid-course SZ and a total of 403 healthy controls were recruited [10]. Morphometric measures (cortical thickness, surface area and subcortical structures) were extracted for each subject and then the optimized subtyping results were obtained with non-supervised cluster analysis [11]. Three subgroups of patients defined by distinct patterns of regional cortical and subcortical morphology were identified in FES (Fig. 8.6) [12]. A similar three subgroup pattern was identified in the

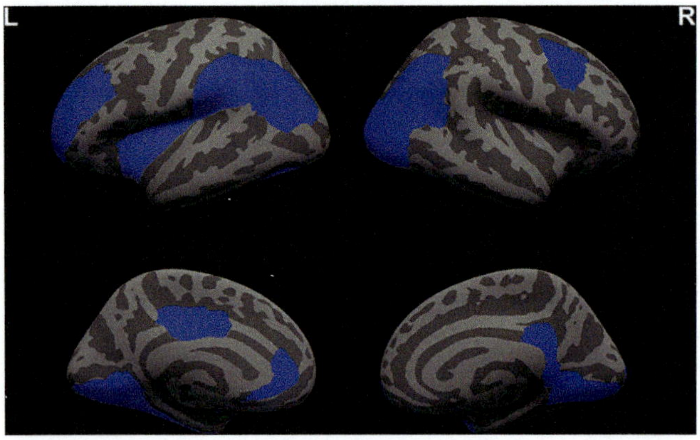

Fig. 8.5 Brain regions (labeled by blue color) contributing to diagnostic classification based on surface area or cortical thickness. *L* left hemisphere, *R* right hemisphere

Table 8.1 Brain regions contributing to discrimination between first episode schizophrenia and healthy control groups based on surface area or cortical thickness

Regions	Weight	Network
Surface area		
lh_fusiform_area	0.037163317	Visual network
lh_lingual_area	0.394043481	Visual network
lh_posterior_cingulate_area	0.373321496	Default mode network
lh_supramarginal_area	0.002481527	Language network
lh_insula_area	0.044973661	Salience network
rh_isthmus_cingulate_area	0.016799451	Default mode network
rh_lateral_occipital_area	0.256421248	Visual network
rh_lingual_area	0.076792878	Visual network
rh_frontal_pole_area	0.010835031	Default mode network
Cortical thickness		
lh_inferior_parietal_thickness	0.747446630	Default mode network
lh_rostral_anterior_cingulate_thickness	0.073074305	Salience network
lh_rostral_middle_frontal_thickness	0.123998723	Central executive network
rh_caudal_middle_frontal_thickness	0.148789386	Central executive network
rh_inferior_parietal_thickness	0.457086964	Default mode network
rh_lingual_thickness	0.065754951	Visual network
rh_temporal_pole_thickness	0.012785662	Salience network

LH left hemisphere, *RH* right hemisphere

independent dataset of patients from the multi-site research consortium (Fig. 8.6) [12]. Pooled data also displayed 3-subgroup solution and different morphological alterations (Figs. 8.6 and 8.7) [12]. Similarity of classification patterns between these two patient cohorts suggests that the 3-group typology is relatively stable across the course of illness. Cognitive functions were worse in subgroup 1 with mid-course SZ than those in subgroup 3, supporting clinical differences in the MRI-defined illness subtypes. Regardless of clinical presentation and stage of illness, anatomic MR subgrouping biomarkers can separate neurobiologically distinct subgroups of SZ patients based on brain anatomy features.

Major Depressive Disorder (MDD)

Neuroimaging models can also be used for differential diagnosis and patient subtyping. For instance, we applied Support-Vector-Machine (SVM) to distinguish patients with refractory depressive disorder (RDD) and non-refractory depressive disorder (NDD) and found different classification accuracies with gray matter (69.57%) and white matter (65.22%) (Fig. 8.8) [13]. Our results may serve as an initial step towards the use of biological markers to inform clinical treatment. Another recent study based on resting-state functional connectivity data grouped 458 depression patients into four depression biotypes that were differentially responsive

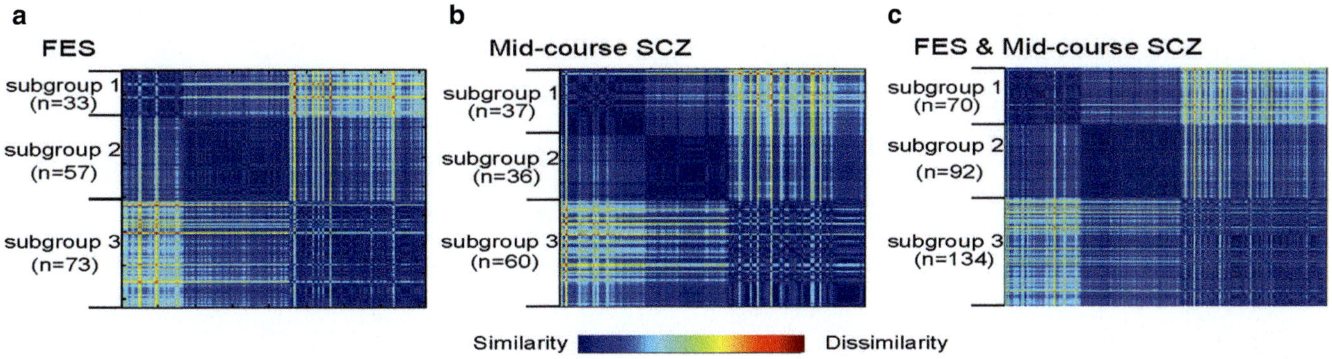

Fig. 8.6 Clustering results illustrated by dissimilarity matrices for treatment naïve first episode schizophrenia patients (FES) (**a**), mid-course schizophrenia (SCZ) patients from Bipolar and Schizophrenia Network for Intermediate Phenotypes (B-SNIP) study (**b**) and the combined sample (**c**) [12]

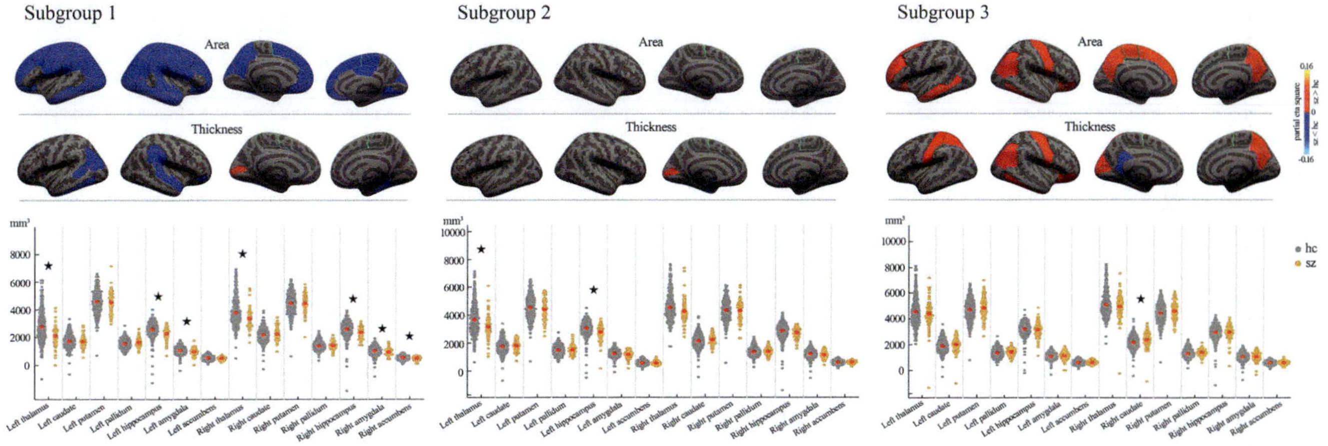

Fig. 8.7 Cortical/subcortical structural alterations in the three subgroups of pooled patients compared with healthy controls (cold color: decreased cortical measurement in patients; asterisk indicates significant alterations for group comparison on subcortical morphology)

to transcranial magnetic stimulation (Fig. 8.9) [14]. Such models provide typologies for diagnosis and treatment that complement existing typologies based on clinical symptoms.

Obsessive Compulsive Disorder (OCD)

There are many different clinical manifestations between youths and adults with obsessive-compulsive disorder, including gender distribution, comorbidity, and treatment options. However, the differences in neural correlates between these two populations remain elusive. One coordinate-based meta-analytic investigation provided neuroimaging evidence regarding this issue (Fig. 8.10) [15]. This study demonstrated that, apart from the consistent prefrontal-striatal model in OCD, abnormalities of the visual cortex might be associated with pathology in OCD youths, while deficits in the limbic-cerebellar circuit may play an important role in the pathophysiology of OCD adults. These findings suggest that OCD youths and OCD adults might belong to different clinical subtypes.

Post-Traumatic Stress Disorder (PTSD)

PTSD is a traumatic- and stressor-related disorder characterized by re-experiencing, arousal, avoidance symptoms, and negative cognitions and emotion [16]. In recent decades, neuroimaging studies have demonstrated structural and functional brain changes in PTSD that might be associated with the identification and subtyping of PTSD. Based on whole brain neuroanatomy and the support vector machine, a neuroimaging study discriminated adult PTSD patients from non-PTSD controls with 91% accuracy (Fig. 8.11) [17]. Using relevance vector regression, successful prediction of individual PCL scores has been achieved using resting-state functional MRI data in a large group of adult survivors with and without PTSD [18].

DSM-5 includes an additional subtype of PTSD: PTSD with prominent dissociative symptoms (PTSD+DS), denoting a particular class of patients that exhibit symptoms of depersonalization/derealization [16]. Imaging-based parameters could provide an objective marker for subtyping PTSD. Using Multiclass Gaussian Process

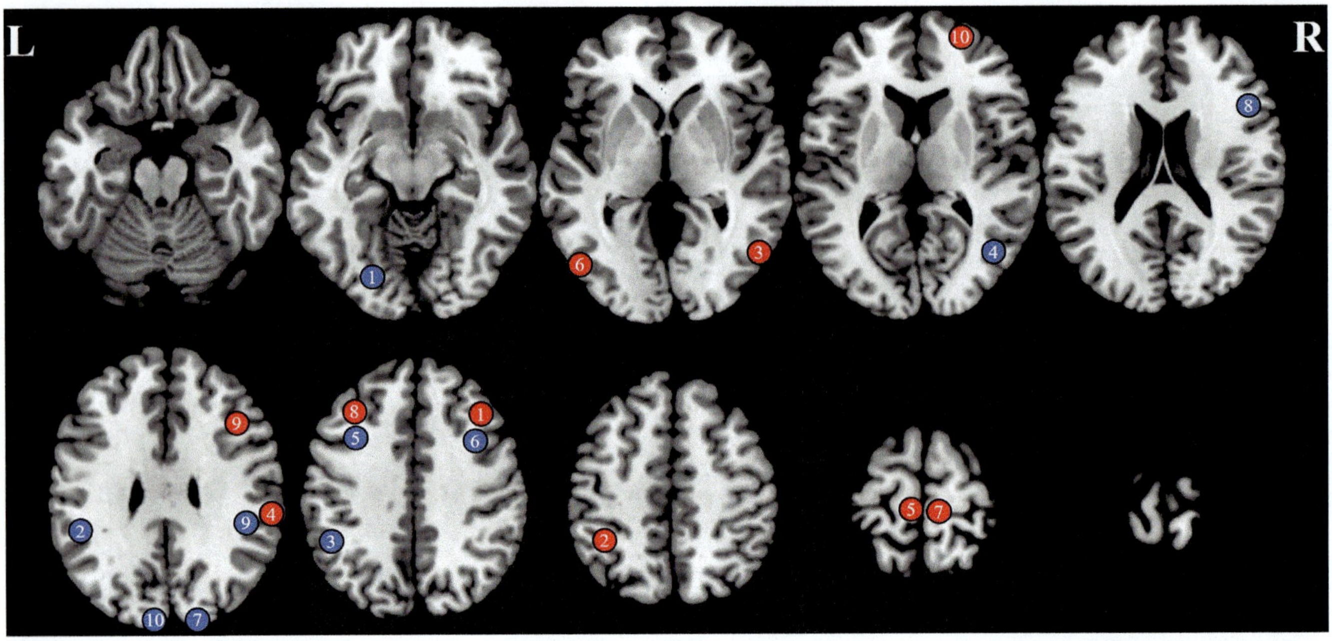

Fig. 8.8 Most important regions discriminating between RDD and NDD. Gray matter regions (red dots) which showed the highest prognostic value included right middle frontal (1), left inferior parietal (2), right middle temporal (3), right supramarginal (4), left paracentral (5), left middle temporal (6), right paracentral (7), left middle frontal (8), right superior frontal (9), and right superior frontal (10) cortex. White matter regions (blue dots) which showed the highest prognostic value included left lingual (1), left supramarginal (2), left inferior parietal (3), right middle temporal (4), left middle frontal (5), right middle frontal (6), and right superior occipital (7), right inferior frontal (8), right supramarginal (9), and left superior occipital (10) white matter. *L* left, *NDD* non-refractory depressive disorder, *R* right, *RDD* refractory depressive disorder

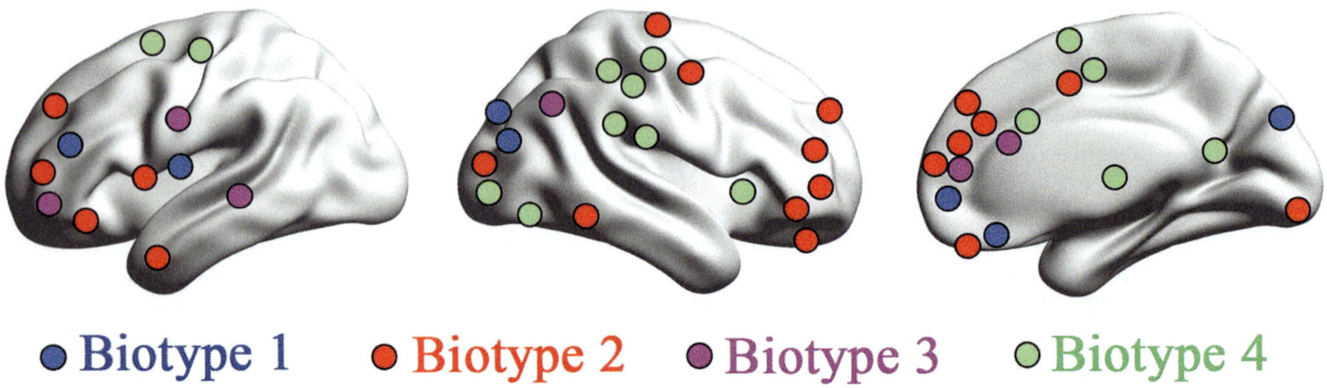

Fig. 8.9 Neuroanatomical distribution of dysfunctional connectivity features for four depression biotypes. Nodes are colored to indicate the biotype with the most abnormal connectivity features

Classification, a recent functional neuroimaging study has successfully predicted the diagnosis of PTSD, PTSD + DS, and healthy individuals using individual amygdala functional connectivity maps. The classification accuracy was 83.67% for PTSD + DS patients and 85.37% for PTSD patients (Fig. 8.12) [19].

Attention-Deficit/Hyperactivity Disorder (ADHD)

Attention-deficit/hyperactivity disorder (ADHD) is one of the most common childhood-onset neurodevelopmental disorders characterized by age-inappropriate inattention, hyperactivity, and impulsivity. The diagnosis and subtyping of ADHD are based on clinical and behavioral evaluations for a long time [20]. However, ADHD is a highly heterogeneous disorder with various symptoms and a high psychiatric comorbidity rate [21]. Therefore, the subjective clinical assessments could not discriminate patients with ADHD from typically developing controls precisely.

Imaging-based parameters could provide an objective marker for diagnosing and subtyping ADHD. A recent study

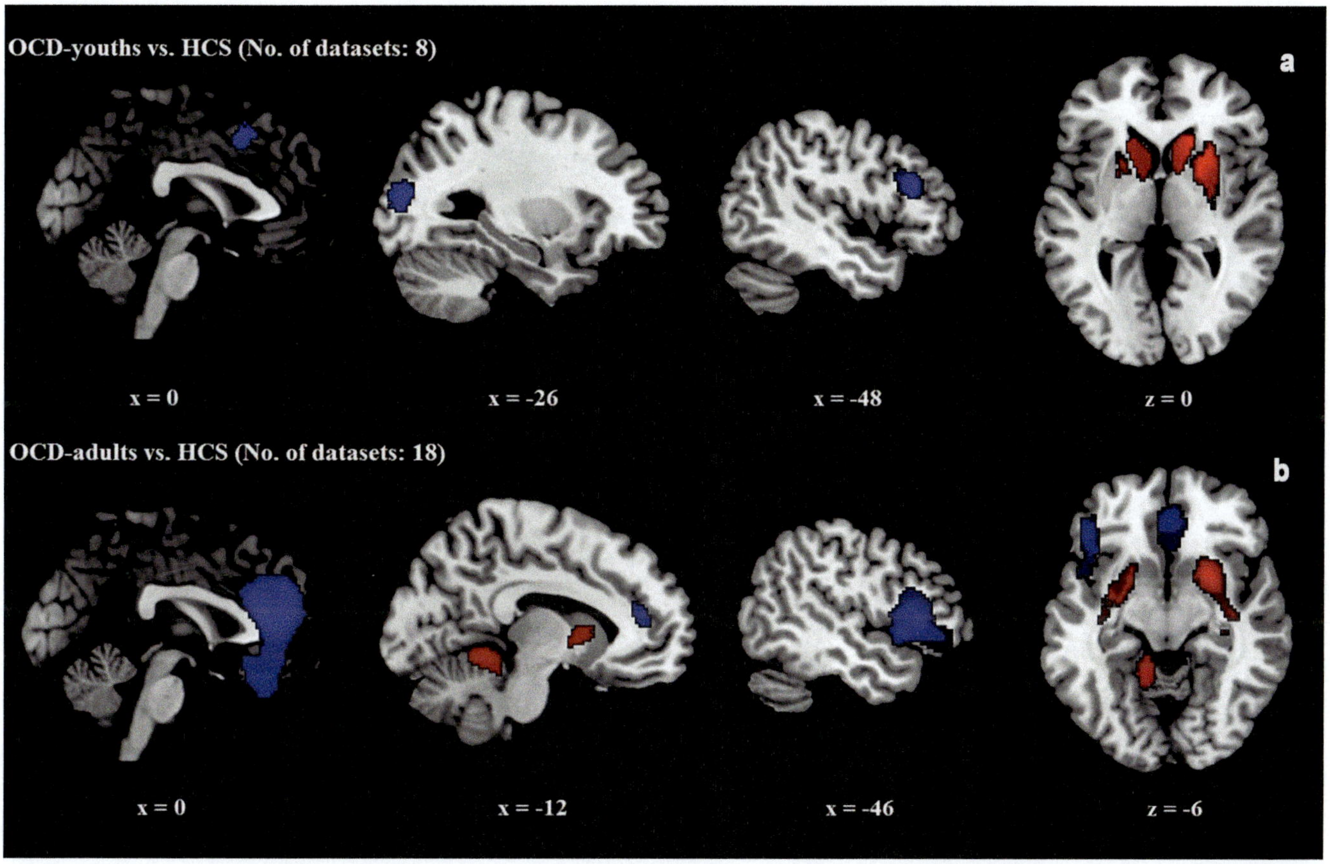

Fig. 8.10 The meta-analytic maps of gray matter (GM) changes in patients with obsessive-compulsive disorder (OCD) compared with the healthy controls (HCS). (**a**) Regions of GM alterations in OCD-youths compared to HCS. (**b**) Regions of GM alterations in OCD-adults compared to HCS

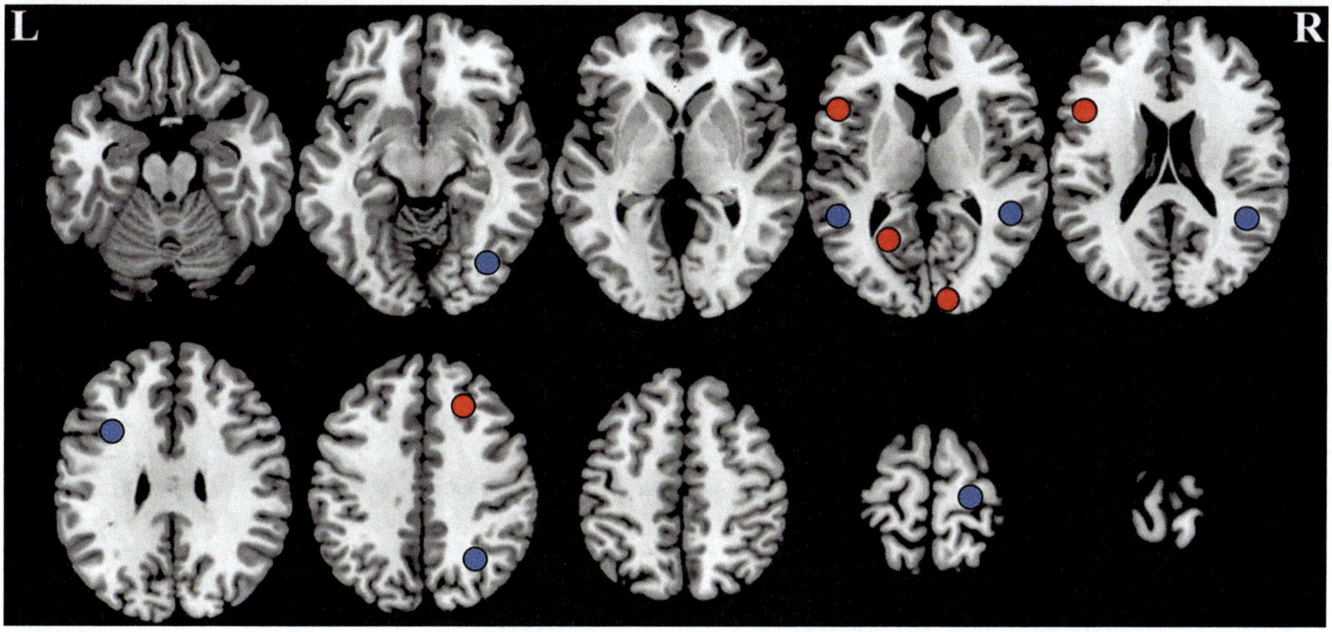

Fig. 8.11 Grey matter regions that showed the highest discriminative value for the comparison between PTSD patients and non-PTSD controls. Regions were identified by setting the threshold to the top 30% of the maximum absolute weight vector score. Red indicates higher values in the group of survivors with PTSD, while blue indicates higher values for survivors without PTSD. PTSD posttraumatic stress disorder; non-PTSD, trauma-exposed controls without PTSD

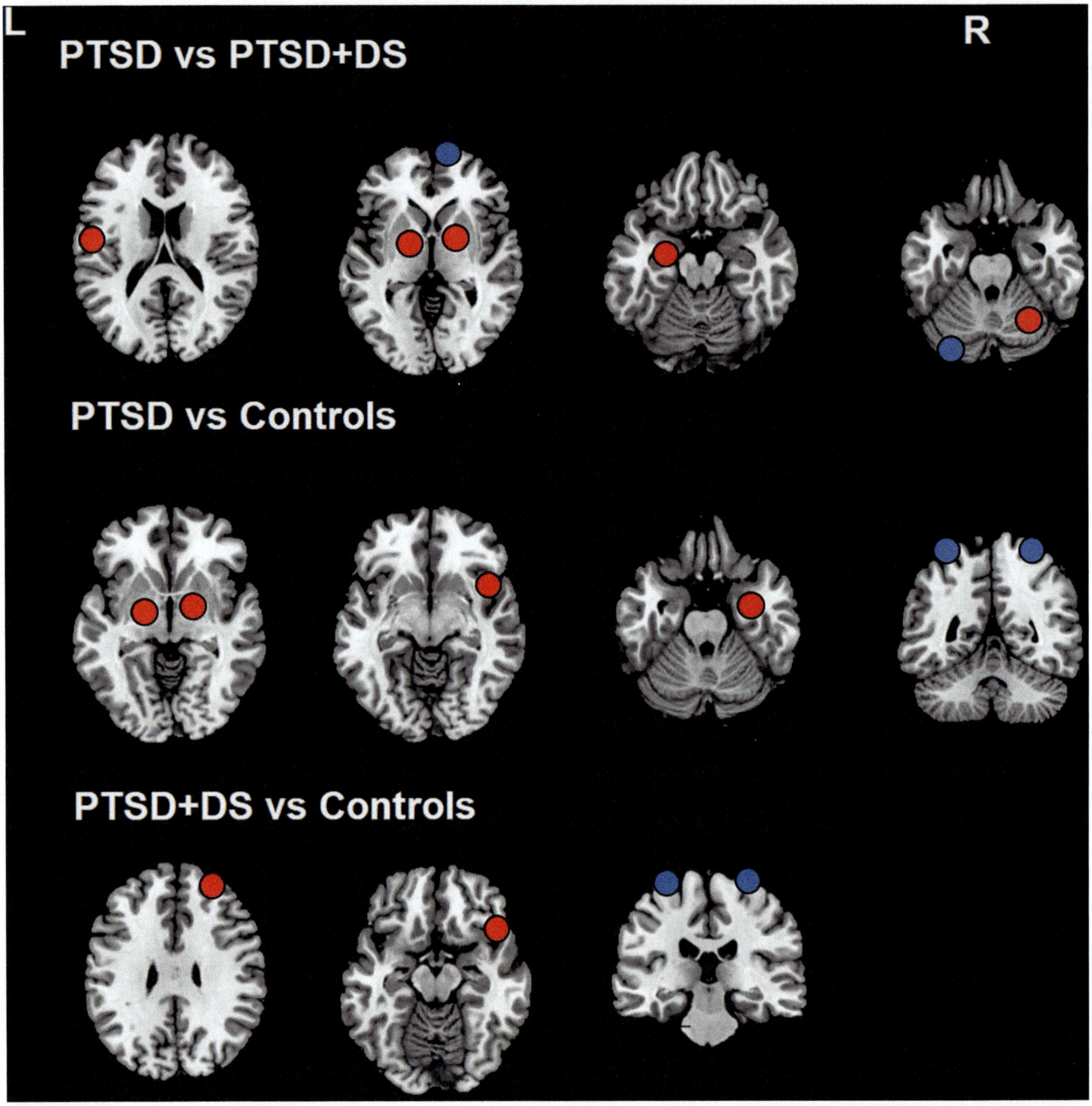

Fig. 8.12 Whole-brain corrected t test for mALFF resting-state activation, comparing PTSD patients, PTSD + DS patients, and healthy controls. Red circles represent increased mALFF, and blue circles represent decreased mALFF. *PTSD* posttraumatic stress disorder, *PTSD + DS* dissociative subtype posttraumatic stress disorder patients, *mALFF* mean amplitude of low-frequency fluctuations

used radiomics and machine learning analyses to identify imaging features (including gray matter properties and white matter properties) relevant to ADHD and constructed random forest classifiers based on these features (Table 8.2 and Fig. 8.13). The accuracies for discriminating ADHD patients from controls and ADHD inattentive patients from combined inattentive and hyperactive subtypes were 73.7% and 80.1%, respectively [22].

Table 8.2 Significant features for discriminating ADHD and TDC, ADHD-I, and ADHD-C subtypes

Hemisphere	Location	Feature type	ADHD	TDC	ADHD-I	ADHD-C
Left	Superior temporal sulcus	Convexity	−0.81 ± 0.11	−0.78 ± 0.08		
Right	Cuneus	Local thickness	2.01 ± 0.16	1.92 ± 0.17		
Left	Precentral	Mean curvature	−0.33 ± 0.43	−0.41 ± 0.51		
Left	Superior temporal	Travel depth	−0.46 ± 0.13	−0.40 ± 0.11		
Left	Cerebral peduncle	FA	−0.14 ± 0.16	−0.24 ± 0.15		
Left	Postcentral	Mean curvature	−0.26 ± 0.66	−0.48 ± 0.46		
Left	Circular sulcus	Travel depth			−19.75 ± 1.26	20.05 ± 1.12
Left	Posterior cingulate	Mean curvature			−1.13 ± 0.08	−1.17 ± 0.11
Left	Sylvian fissure	Mean curvature			−0.41 ± 0.30	−0.31 ± 0.34
Left	Pars triangularis	Mean curvature			−0.85 ± 0.16	−0.72 ± 0.16
Left	External capsule	FA			−0.13 ± 0.14	0.20 ± 0.20

ADHD attention-deficit/hyperactivity disorder, *TDC* typically developing controls, *ADHD-I* ADHD-inattentive subtype, *ADHD-C* ADHD-combined subtype, *FA* fractional anisotropy

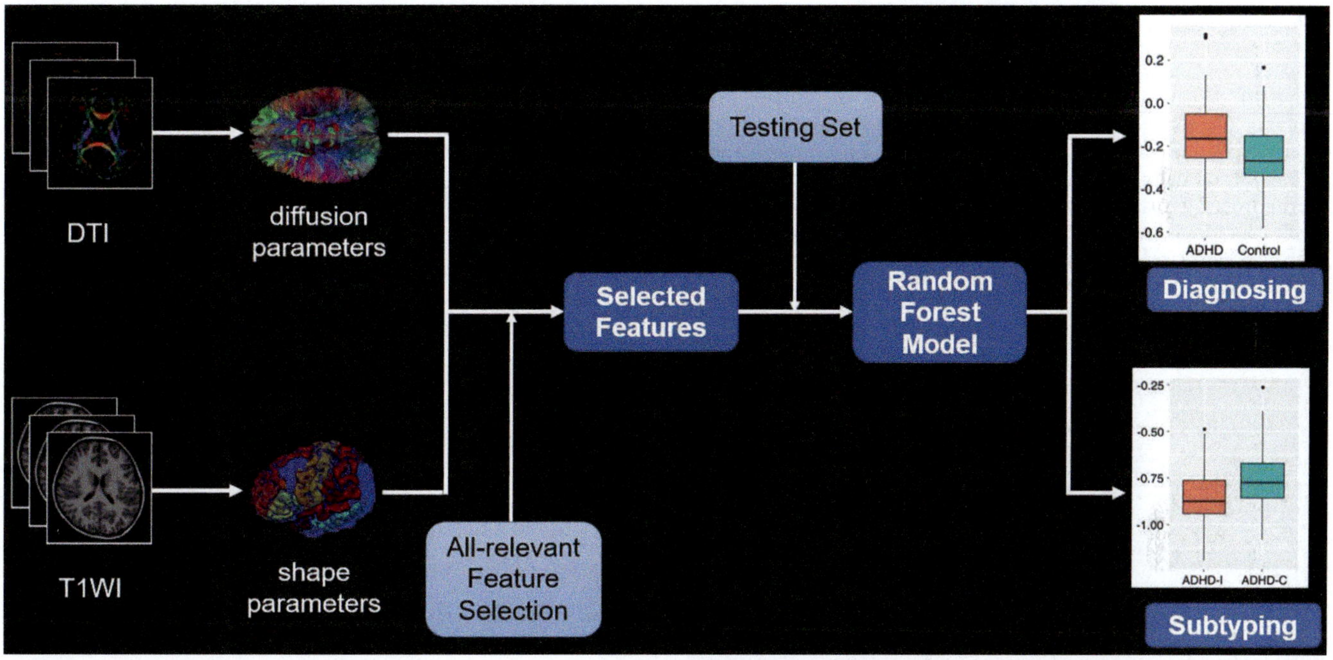

Fig. 8.13 The workflow of radiomics analysis. First, radiomics parameters were extracted from T1-weighted and diffusion-tensor images. Then, the features relevant to diagnosing ADHD were selected by using the all-relevant feature selection approach. Finally, the random forest model was constructed for group and subtype discrimination. *DTI* diffusion tensor image, *T1WI* T1-weighted image

Predicting and Monitoring

Predictions of Illness Onset, Relapse, and Long-Term Prognosis

Schizophrenia

The MRI studies suggested that SZ is associated with progressive structural and functional alternations in the prefrontal, temporal, and thalamus (Fig. 8.14), making it possible to predict and monitor brain changes over the different stages of SZ. These regions might involve alterations in the cortico-cerebellar-thalamic-cortical loop (Fig. 8.15). Selective evidence was shown below:

(a) In individuals with ultra-high risk for psychosis, structural abnormalities of the thalamocortical circuit may be a potential marker for transition to psychosis [23].
(b) In first-episode SZ, a meta-analysis [24] reviewed 11 structural studies in patients in the first 12 months of illness. Alterations in medial temporal and prefrontal cortical regions, and in the networks that connect them with subcortical areas, are potential neuroanatomical markers for poor symptomatic and functional outcomes.
(c) Another article [25] systematically reviewed resting-sate functional MRI studies and found SZ-related abnormalities in the cortico-cerebellar-thalamic-cortical networks.

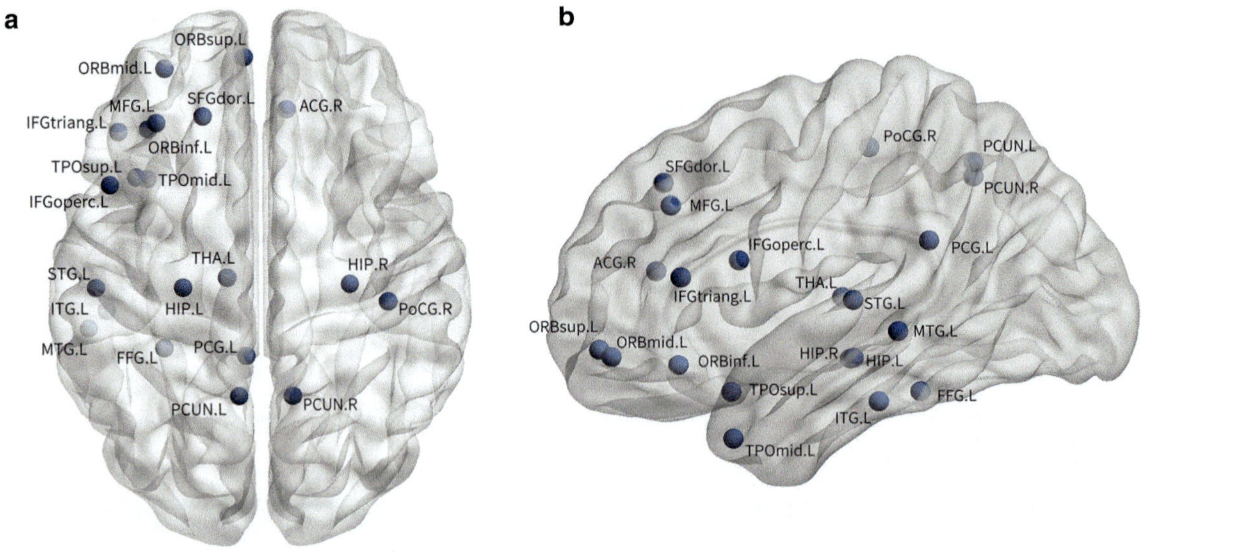

Fig. 8.14 Structural and functional alternations in schizophrenia involving in cortical and subcortical regions. (**a**) superior view and (**b**) sagittal view. *SFGdor. L* left superior frontal gyrus, dorsolateral, *ORBmid. L* orbital part of left middle frontal gyrus, *IFGoperc. L* left inferior frontal gyrus, pars opercularis, *IFGtriang. L* left inferior frontal gyrus, pars triangularis, *ORBsup. L* orbital part of left superior frontal gyrus, *ORBinf. L* orbital part of left inferior frontal gyrus, *TPOmid. L* left temporal pole, middle temporal gyrus, *TPOsup. L* left temporal pole, superior temporal gyrus, *STG. L* left superior temporal gyrus, *THA. L* left thalamus, *PCUN. L* left precuneus, *PCUN. R* right precuneus, *PCG. L* left posterior cingulate gyrus, *HIP. L* left hippocampus, *HIP. R* right hippocampus, *ITG.L* left inferior temporal gyrus, *FFG. L* left fusiform gyrus, *MFG. L* left middle frontal gyrus, *ACG. R* right anterior cingulate gyrus, *MTG. L* left middle temporal gyrus, *PoCG. R* right postcentral gyrus

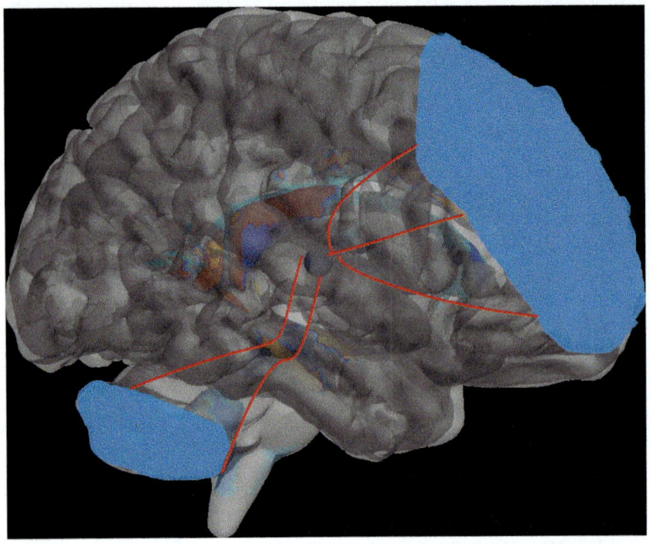

Fig. 8.15 The demonstration of Cortico-Cerebellar-Thalamic-Cortical Circuit

However, they did not observe the unique relationships between distinct cognitive domains and specific network abnormalities, suggesting that the disturbances of functional connectivity in the circuitry may contribute to a general cognitive deficit in SZ.

(d) One longitudinal MRI study [26] found the relapse duration was related to both total cerebral volume and regional (e.g., frontal volume) brain measures, while the number of relapses was uncorrelated to brain measures.
(e) Studies focusing on patients with chronic SZ showed that gray matter decreased to a greater extent in the thalamus, frontal, and temporal areas, especially in poor-outcome patients [27].

Major Depressive Disorder (MDD)

Previous MRI studies have proposed that neurobiological alterations may contribute to illness onset, relapse, and prognosis of major depressive disorder (MDD). Among the affected regions and networks, the deficits of the default mode network (DMN) have most consistently been identified in structural and functional MRI studies in medication-free depressed patients (Fig. 8.16) [28, 29]. Family risk studies have shown that the function of the DMN may be a resilience factor to MDD [30]. Earlier fMRI findings suggest a dissociation within the DMN, where abnormal functional connectivity within the anterior subnetwork of DMN may be a biomarker for relapse [31]. Spies et al. found that DMN activity changes can be successfully used to predict early treatment response [32].

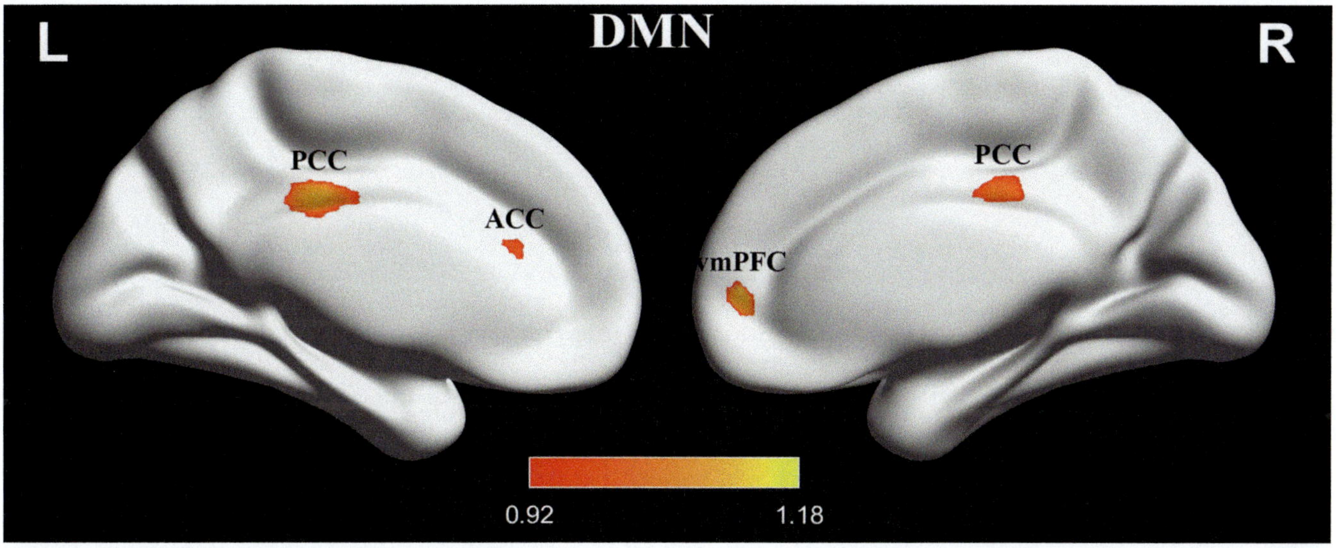

Fig. 8.16 Medication-free patients with major depressive disorder showed increased cortical thickness in default mode network (DMN) compared to healthy controls. Regions of increased cortical thickness (warm color) in medication-free patients with major depressive disorder than healthy controls. *ACC* anterior cingulate cortex, *L* left, *PCC* posterior cingulate cortex, *vmPFC* ventromedial prefrontal cortex, *R* right

Obsessive Compulsive Disorder (OCD)

Recent advances in resting-state functional magnetic resonance imaging (rs-fMRI) have proposed that the pathophysiology of obsessive-compulsive disorder (OCD) encompasses a specific cortico-striato-limbic network. However, the vast majority of these studies published so far have been based on average differences between groups. Whether functional neuroimaging could be used to inform the clinical assessment of individual OCD patients remains unclear. One study applied Support Vector Machine (SVM) to distinguish drug-naive OCD patients from healthy control subjects (HCS) based on four common rs-fMRI parameters including the amplitude of low-frequency fluctuation (ALFF), the fractional amplitude of low-frequency fluctuation (fALFF), regional homogeneity (ReHo), and functional connectivity strength (FCS) [33]. This study showed that the four common rs-fMRI parameters exhibited significant differences in predicting the diagnosis of OCD (Fig. 8.17). In particular, the ALFF showed the highest accuracy, sensitivity and specificity, suggesting its potential in clinical practice to help identify OCD at the individual level.

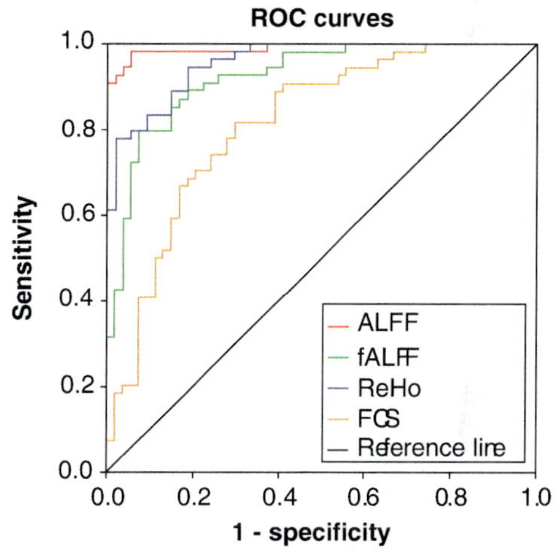

Fig. 8.17 Receiver operating characteristic (ROC) curves for the assessment of SVM performance using different resting-state functional MRI parameters to distinguish OCD patients from HCS. *ALFF* amplitude of low frequency fluctuation, *fALFF* fractional amplitude of low frequency fluctuation, *FCS* functional connectivity strength, *HCS* healthy control subjects, *MRI* magnetic resonance imaging, *OCD* obsessive-compulsive disorder, *ReHo* regional homogeneity, *SVM* support vector machine

Post-Traumatic Stress Disorder (PTSD)

The identification of posttraumatic stress disorder (PTSD) among natural disaster survivors is remarkably challenging, and there are no reliable objective features available to assist clinical diagnosis. One study used 108 brain nodes based on the Schaefer atlas (Fig. 8.18) and their connections to represent each subject's functional connectivity profile [34]. Multivariate pattern analysis with a relevance vector machine was used to distinguish PTSD patients from trauma-exposed healthy controls (TEHCs). A promising diagnostic accuracy of 89.2% in distinguishing PTSD patients from TEHCs was obtained. The most predictive connections for PTSD were between the default mode network, visual network, somatomotor network, limbic network, and dorsal attention network, which may provide potential features to facilitate clinical diagnosis.

A sizable minority of veterans who initially experience prominent symptoms of PTSD eventually experience remission [35]. However, the underlying neural correlates of remission are still unclear. One study explored the differ-

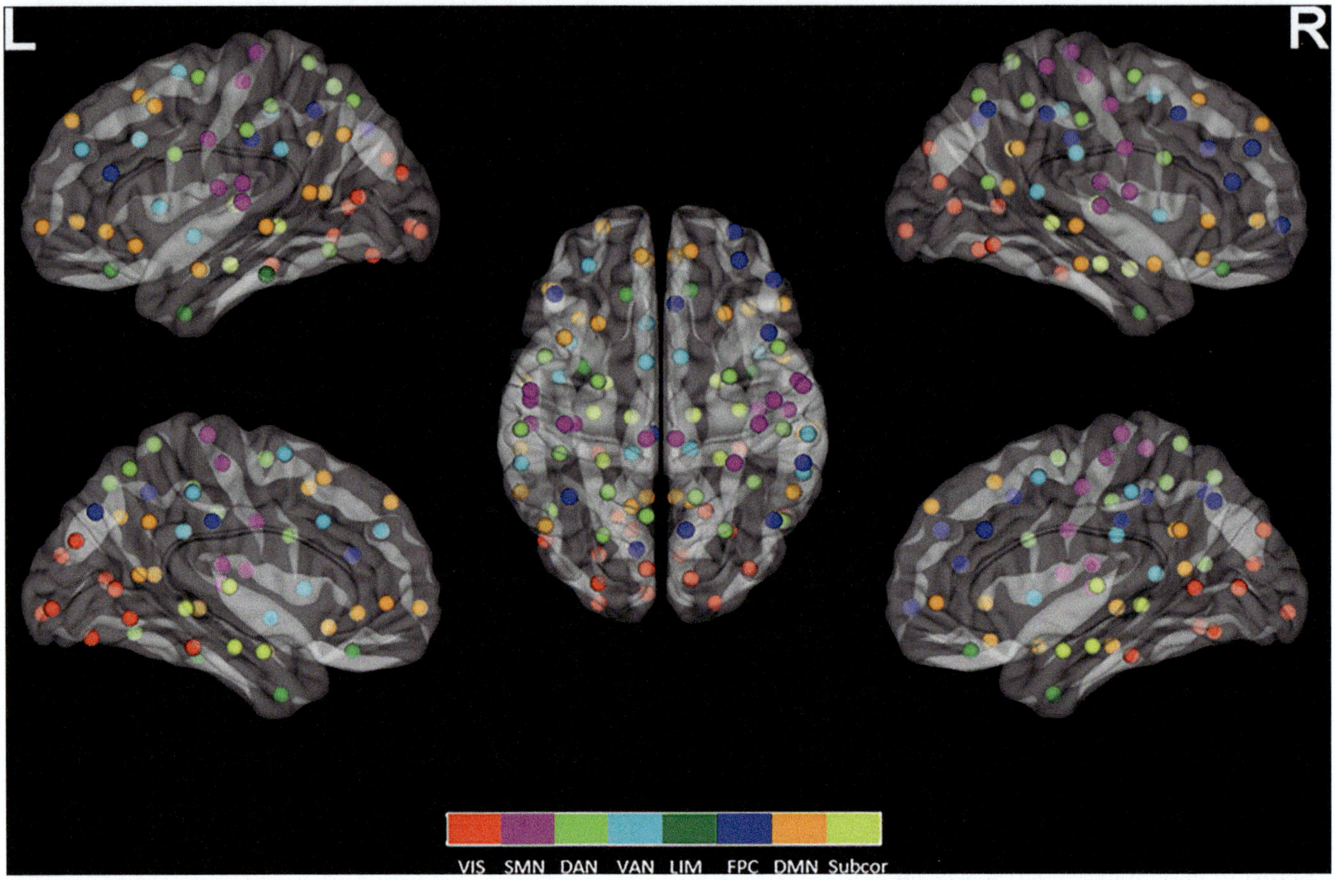

Fig. 8.18 The demonstration of 108 brain nodes associated with eight networks based on the Schaefer atlas. Each node denotes a brain region and further mapped onto the cortical surface using the BrainNet Viewer package (www.nitrc.org/projects/bnv). Associations of these nodes with specific brain networks are shown in different color. *L* left, *R* right, *VIS* visual network, *SMN* somatomotor network, *DAN* dorsal attention network, *VAN* ventral attention network, *LIM* limbic network, *FPC* frontoparietal control network, *DMN* default mode network, *Subcor* subcortical regions

ences in structural covariance networks between remitted PTSD, current PTSD, and TEHCs [36]. Cortical thickness was assessed for 148 cortical regions using the aparc.a2009s template and interregional partial correlations of cortical thickness across subjects were computed in each group. The centrality of the right subcallosal gyrus, left frontal pole, and right superior frontal sulcus may play a role in remission, current symptoms, and PTSD history, respectively.

Attention-Deficit/Hyperactivity Disorder (ADHD)

Approximately 60% of childhood ADHD patients demonstrate symptom persistence in adulthood [37], 20–30% retain full syndrome, and the rest show either partial or full remission [38, 39]. Simply relying on demographics, clinical information, and neuropsychological data cannot accurately predict the outcome of an ADHD child [40]. Therefore, recent studies sought to explore objective measures of the brain and revealed their potential predictive roles in clinical outcomes. For example, one longitudinal study investigated 205 clinically followed participants with ADHD since childhood by using functional MRI and magnetoencephalography (MEG), and found that persistent inattentive symptoms were associated with atypical connectivity within the default mode network (DMN) and between the DMN and networks pertinent to attention and cognitive control [41] (Fig. 8.19).

Predicting and Monitoring Treatment Response

Schizophrenia

The topological organization of the brain network is related to response to antipsychotic treatment in SZ. Both never-treated and antipsychotic-treated SZ patients showed altered nodal centralities in left pre–/postcentral gyri relative to controls; however, decreased nodal centralities in right amygdala/hippocampus and bilateral putamen/caudate were detected in never-treated patients relative to antipsychotic-treated patients and controls, supporting the effect of treatment (Fig. 8.20) [42]. Furthermore, different antipsychotics can act differently in structural networks. Patients treated

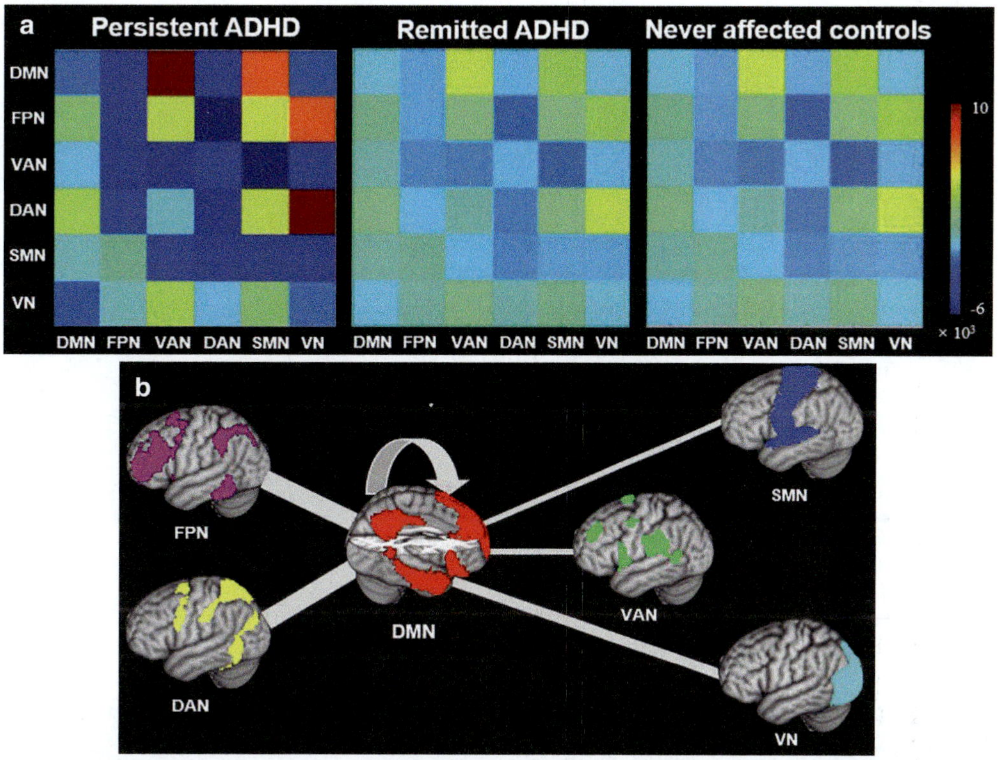

Fig. 8.19 (**a**) Group differences in the functional networks associated with inattention among the persistent, remitted ADHD and never-affected controls. The heat map shows the strength of intra- and internetwork connectivity for each group. Hotter colors indicate stronger connectivity. (**b**) Network connectivity patterns associated with inattention identified in MEG. The thickness of the lines correspond to the strength of the connectivity. *DMN* default mode network, *FPN* frontoparietal network, *DAN* dorsal attention network, *VAN* ventral attention network, *SMN* somatomotor, *VN* visual network, *ADHD* attention-deficit/hyperactivity disorder

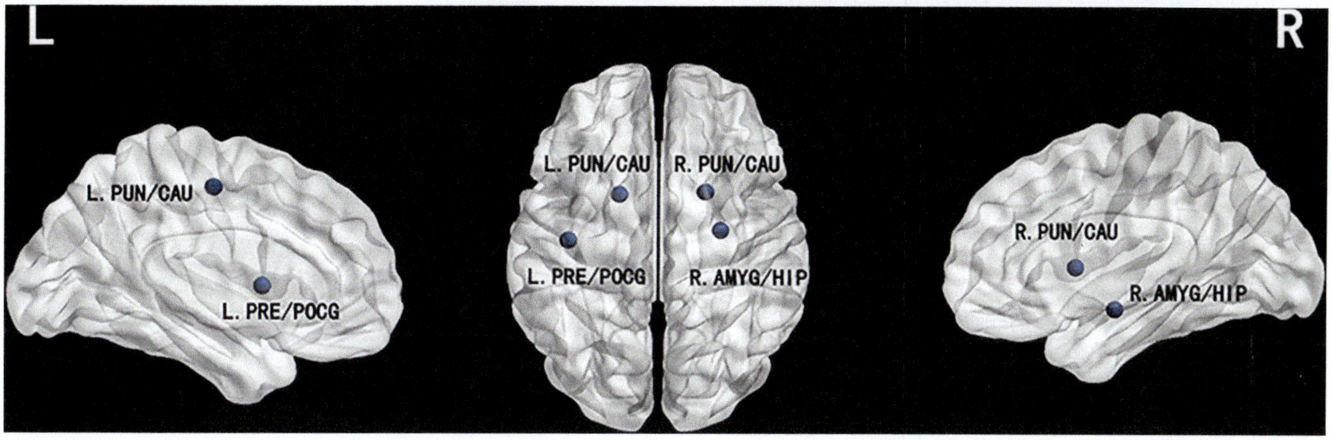

Fig. 8.20 Group differences in functional topological properties among never-treated schizophrenia patients, chronically treated schizophrenia patients, and healthy controls. Both never-treated schizophrenia patients and chronically treated schizophrenia patient groups showed lower nodal efficiency of left pre-/post-central gyri within functional network; only never-treated patients showed decreased nodal efficiency of bilateral putamen/caudate and right amygdala/hippocampus. *PUT* putamen, *CAU* caudate, *AMYG* amygdala, *HIP* hippocampus, *PRE/POCG* pre-/post-central gyri, *L* left, *R* right

with risperidone showed higher nodal degree than patients treated with clozapine in the right thalamus, cuneus, and precentral gyrus (Fig. 8.21) [43]; the decreased pattern of FA-weighted white matter network was more prominent in clozapine-treated patients, as indicated by significantly lower values than in risperidone-treated patients, which primarily involved subcortical, prefrontal, and also some occipital regions. The findings above provided a potential method for the selection of antipsychotics (Fig. 8.22) [43].

Major Depressive Disorder (MDD)

Since depression is associated with substantial morbidity, mortality, and family burden, it is particularly pressing to k for potential predictors for treatment response [44–46]. A broad array of studies have focused on neuroimaging biomarkers in MDD after first-line treatments (i.e., evidence-based psychotherapy and pharmacotherapy) and interventions reserved for highly treatment-resistant patients, such as stimulation treatments or unconventional medications [44].

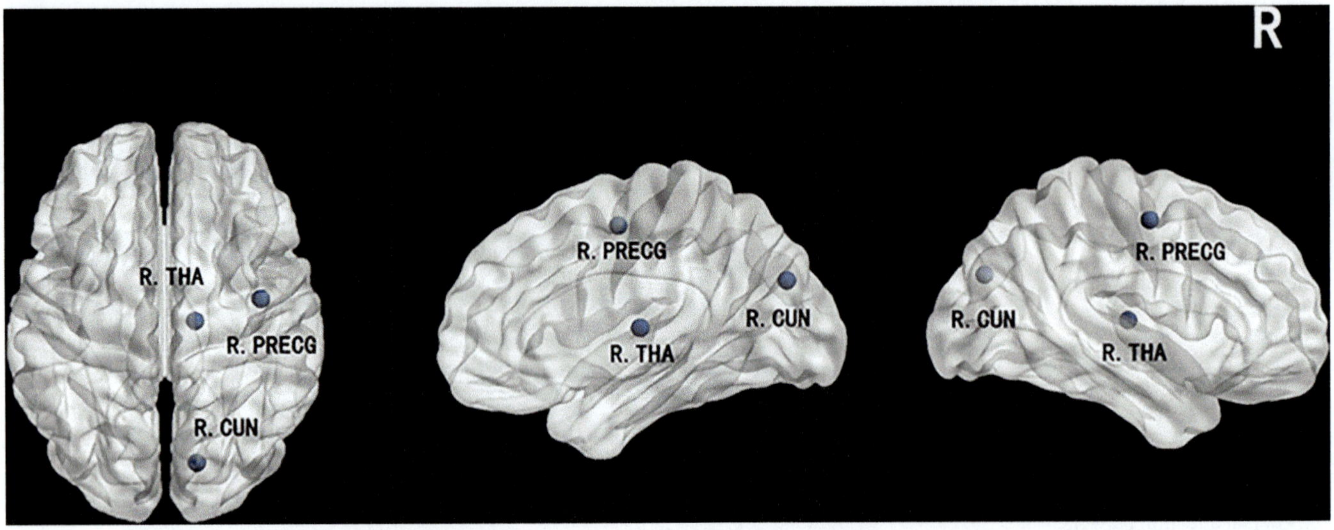

Fig. 8.21 Group differences in structural topological properties between clozapine-treated and risperidone-treated schizophrenia patients. The direct comparison between the clozapine-treated and risperidone-treated group revealed significant differences in right thalamus, right cuneus, and right precentral gyrus, with higher nodal degrees in the risperidone group. *THA* thalamus, *CUN* cuneus, *PRECG*, pre-central gyrus, *R* right

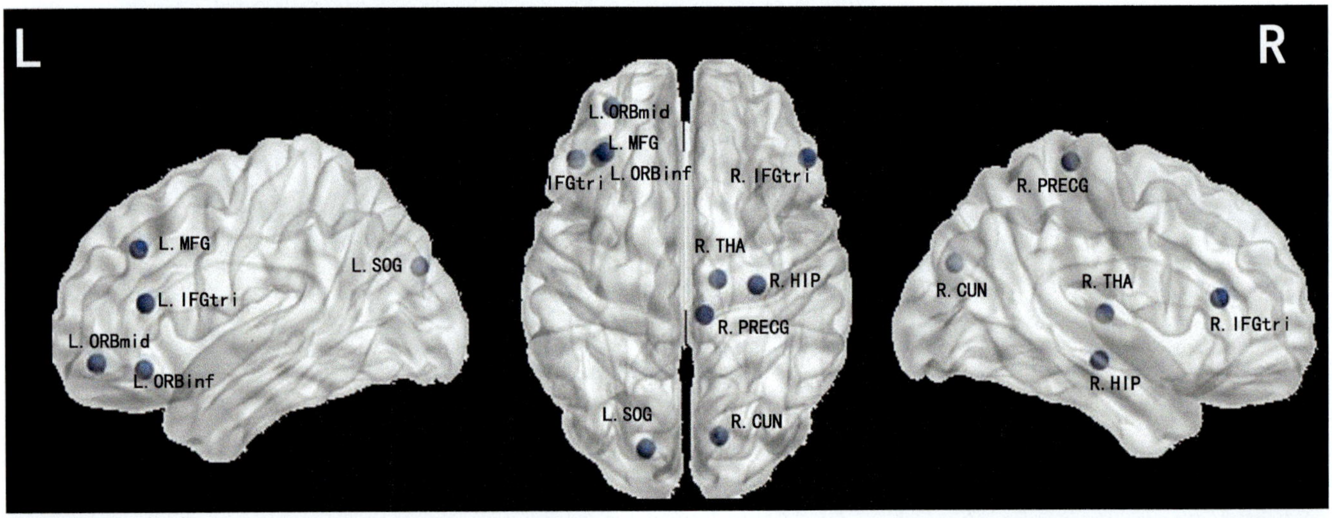

Fig. 8.22 Group differences in FA-weighted white matter network between clozapine-treated and risperidone-treated schizophrenia patients. The Post-hoc tests revealed lower values in risperidone-treated patients than clozapine-treated patients with FA-weighted white matter network, which primarily involved subcortical, prefrontal, and also some occipital regions. *L* left, *R* right, *MFG* middle frontal gyrus, *IFGtri* inferior frontal gyrus, pars triangularis, *ORBinf* orbital part of inferior frontal gyrus, *ORBmid* orbital part of middle frontal gyrus, *SOG* superior occipital gyrus, *HIP* hippocampus, *THA* thalamus, *CUN* cuneus, *PRECG* pre-central gyrus

Volumetric reductions in the hippocampus are well-replicated findings in MDD patients versus healthy controls, where studies have identified reduced volume of the hippocampus as a structural imaging predictor for poorer response to antidepressant medication [47–51] (Fig. 8.23). Treatment with antidepressant medication [47, 52] has been reported to be associated with increases in hippocampal volume. A group of studies have investigated the relations between resting-state functional-MRI and treatment response in MDD, and found the associations between treatment (ie, antidepressant medications and transcranial magnetic stimulation) response and functional connectivity regarding frontal and limbic brain regions, subcallosal cingulate cortex, visual recognition circuits, default mode network, and cognitive control network (Fig. 8.24) [53]. The prediction reached an accuracy of 75% (74% positive predictive value, 76% negative predictive value) using task-based connectivity measures between the right superior anterior temporal lobe and the subgenual cingulate cortex [54]. Studies reported consistent findings of altered DTI measures (ie, fractional anisotropy, mean diffusivity and radial diffusivity) in frontolimbic circuits in remitted MDD patients compared with non-remitters.

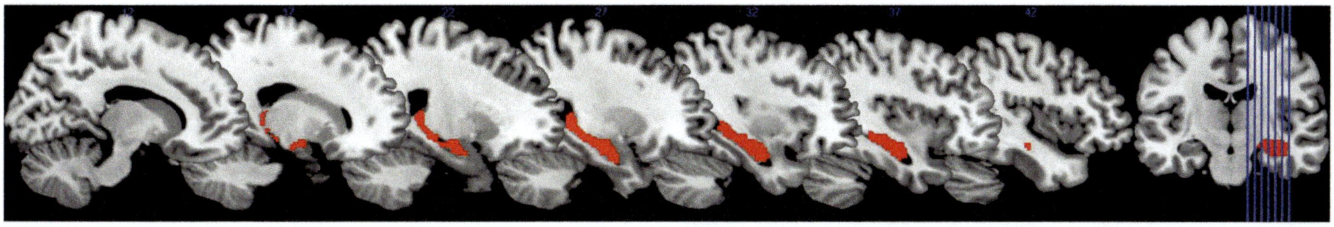

Fig. 8.23 Reduced volume of the hippocampus as predictors of poor response to antidepressant medication

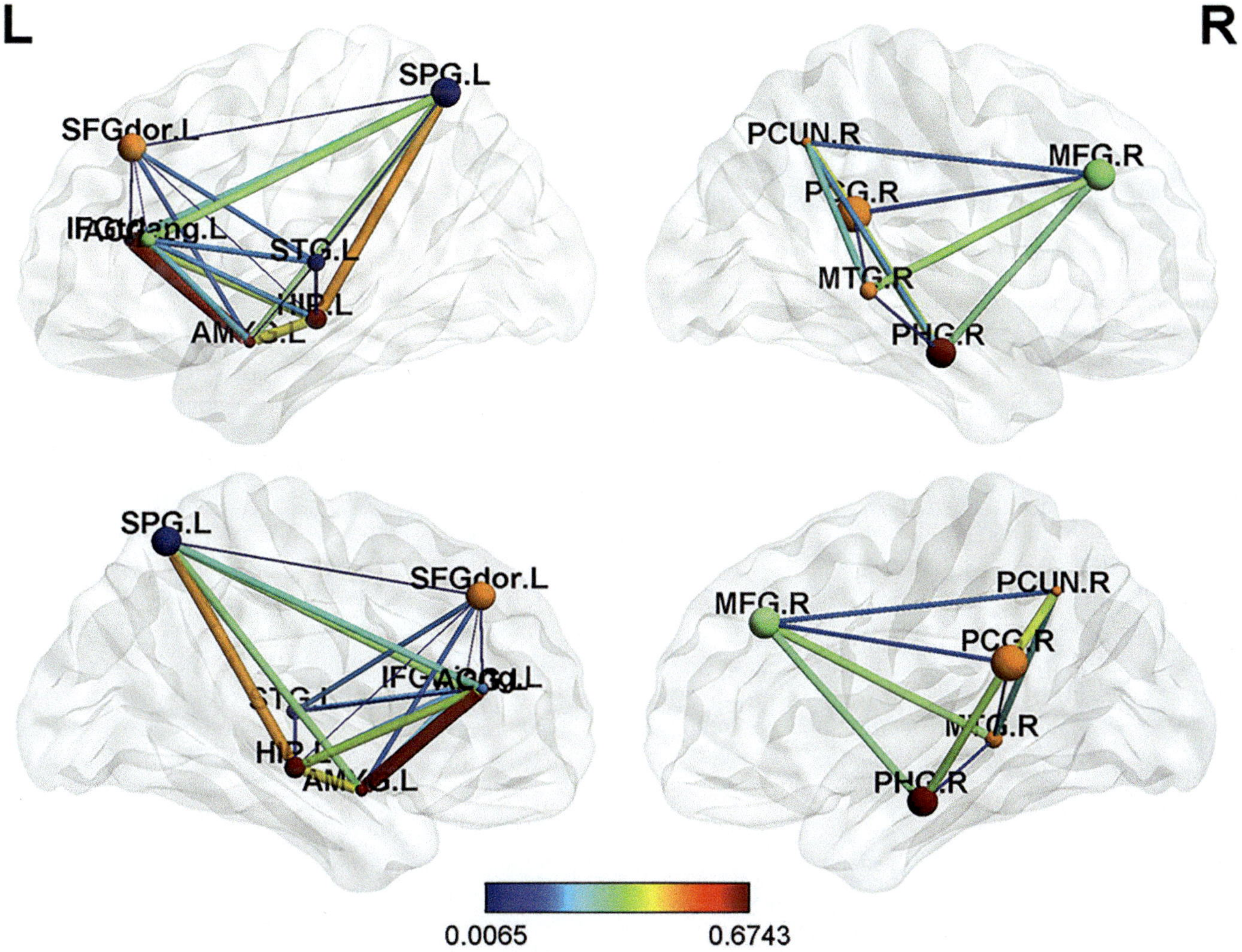

Fig. 8.24 Resting-state functional networks associated with treatment response in major depressive disorder (MDD). *MFG.R* right middle frontal gyrus, *SFGdor. L* left superior frontal gyrus, dorsolateral, *IFGtriang.L* left inferior frontal gyrus, triangular part, *ACG.L* left anterior cingulate and paracingulate gyri, *PCG.R* right posterior cingulate gyrus, *HIP.L* left hippocampus, *PHG.R* right parahippocampal gyrus, *AMYG.L* left amygdala, *SPG.L* left superior parietal gyrus, *PCUN.R* right precuneus, *STG.L* left superior temporal gyrus, *MTG.R* right middle temporal gyrus

Obsessive Compulsive Disorder (OCD)

Identifying clinically predictive biomarkers that differentiate responders from nonresponders is important for improving treatment efficacy for obsessive-compulsive disorder (OCD). Neuroimaging techniques hold the promise to predict treatment responses in OCD. One review summarized neuroimaging findings about treatment-refractory obsessive-compulsive disorder and imaging markers that predict response to neurotherapeutic interventions [55]. This review indicated that the orbitofrontal cortex (OFC) is a key region for the prediction of conventional psychiatric interventions including pharmacotherapy and psychotherapy, while the anterior cingulate cortex (ACC) is a core neuroanatomical structure to predict the response of invasive neurotherapeutic interventions such as deep brain stimulation (DBS) (Fig. 8.25).

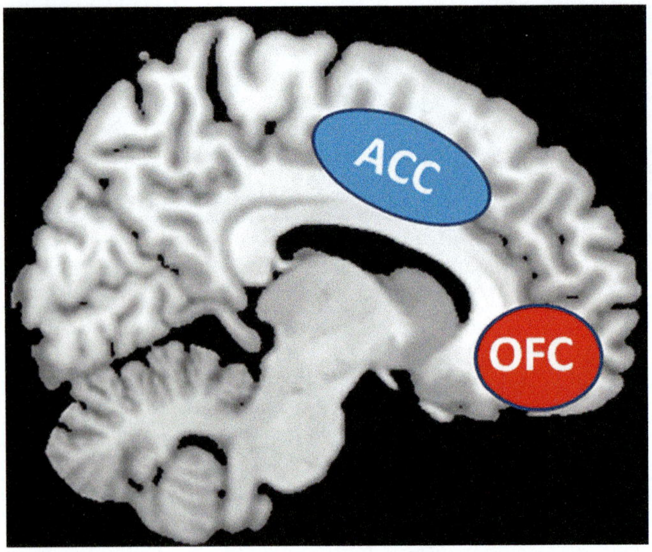

Fig. 8.25 Brain anatomical regions predicting the treatment response for conventional psychiatric interventions (red) and invasive neurotherapeutic interventions (blue) in the obsessive-compulsive disorder. *ACC* anterior cingulate cortex, *OFC* orbitofrontal cortex

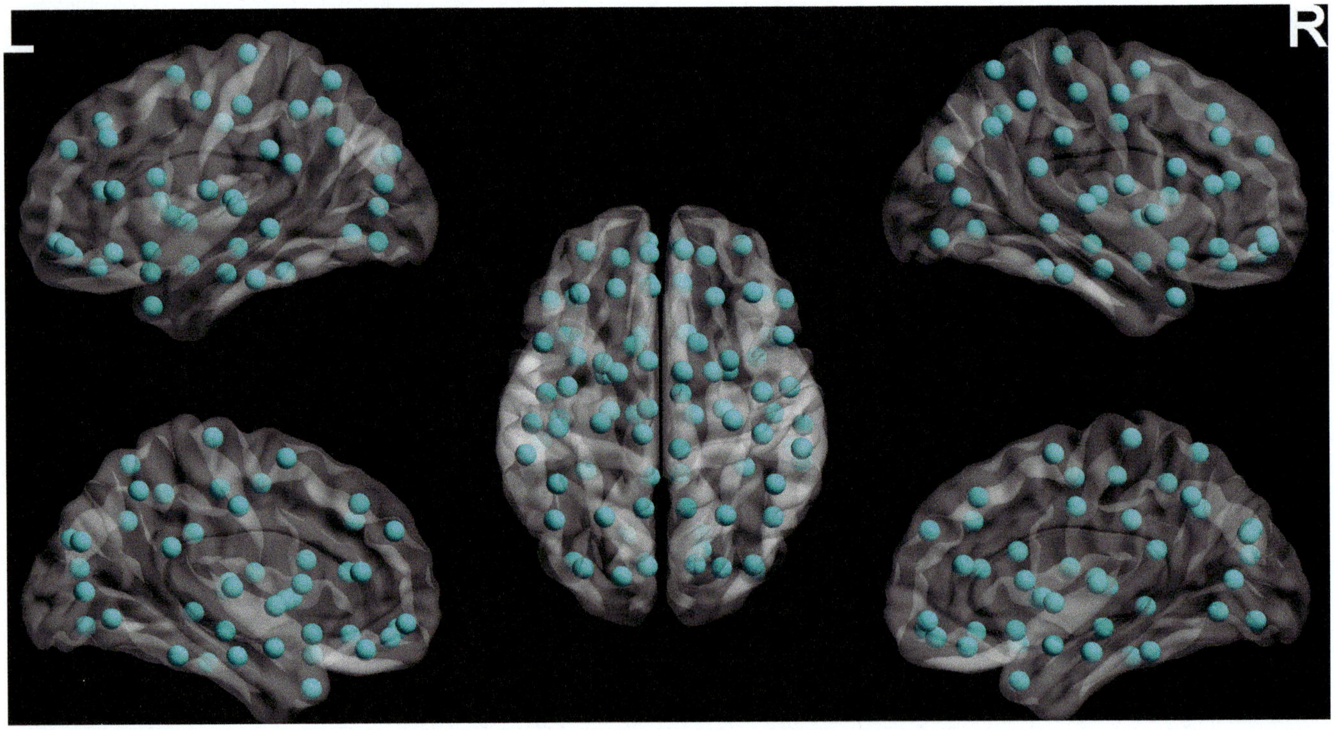

Fig. 8.26 The demonstration of 90 brain nodes based on Automated Anatomical Labeling atlas. Each node denotes a brain region and further mapped onto the cortical surface using the BrainNet Viewer package (www.nitrc.org/projects/bnv). *L* left, *R* right

Post-Traumatic Stress Disorder (PTSD)

Trauma-focused cognitive behavior therapy (TF-CBT) is a recommended treatment strategy for PTSD [56]. Despite the promise of TF-CBT, approximately one-third of patients do not respond to this approach [57]. Therefore, there is a need to examine biomarkers for identifying patients who are not responsive to TF-CBT. One study aimed to identify neural markers of treatment response to TF-CBT when participants are reappraising aversive material and to test the hypotheses regarding neural activation associated with emotional reactivity [58]. The neural circuitry of negative emotion processing (including the anterior cingulate cortex, bilateral amygdala, insula, and hippocampus) was defined using the Automated Anatomical Labeling (AAL) atlas (Fig. 8.26). Lower connectivity of the left amygdala with the anterior cingulate cortex and right insula, and of the left hippocampus with the right amygdala were associated with symptom improvement (Fig. 8.27).

Attention-Deficit/Hyperactivity Disorder (ADHD)

Psychostimulants are generally considered a first-line pharmacologic treatment for ADHD. Among them, methylphenidate (MPH) is currently the most used drug with a high response rate of approximately 70% [59]. Although stimulants are successful in reducing core symptoms of ADHD, early assessment of treatment response is also crucial, which may help check whether the currently used stimulant is effective and if an alternative treatment is needed. Previous structural MRI and PET/SPECT studies revealed psychoradiological characteristics could be potential predictive biomarkers of treatment response in ADHD [60, 61] (Table 8.3 and Fig. 8.28). Few functional MRI studies have been utilized to investigate the relationship between treatment response and brain function. One d-based functional connectivity study found that a good response to MPH was associated with lower functional connectivity between striatal subregions and frontal cortices in ADHD children [62] (Fig. 8.29).

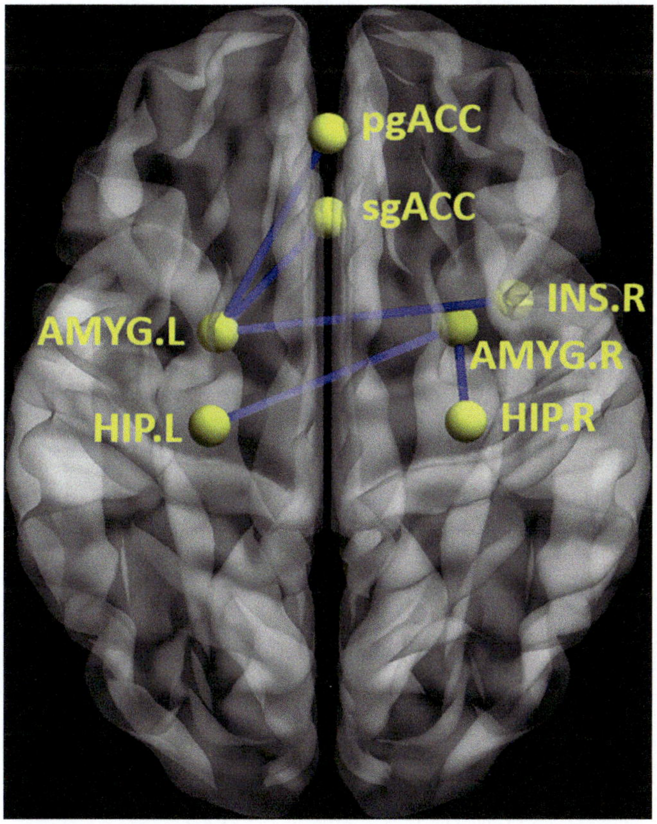

Fig. 8.27 Functional connectivity during emotion reactivity correlated with improvement in post-traumatic stress disorder (PTSD) symptoms. The brain map depicts connectivity between the negative affect networks that is significantly correlated with a change in symptom improvement. *sgACC* subgenual anterior cingulate cortex, *pgACC* pregenual anterior cingulate cortex, *AMYG* amygdala, *INS* insula, *Hip* hippocampus

Table 8.3 Predictive biomarkers of good response to MPH in ADHD

Imaging index	Psychoradiological characteristics
Structural volume	↑ volume caudate, nucleus accumbens, cerebellum, corpus callosum, prefrontal cortex in children
CBF	↓ CBF in midbrain, posterior cerebellum, middle frontal gyrus, ACC, and the claustrum in children and adults
DAT	↑ striatal DAT in adults, ↓ DAT in children

↑ indicates increase, ↓ indicates reduction, *MPH* methylphenidate, *ADHD* attention-deficit/hyperactivity disorder, *CBF* cerebral blood flow, *DAT* dopamine transporter, *ACC* anterior cingulate cortex

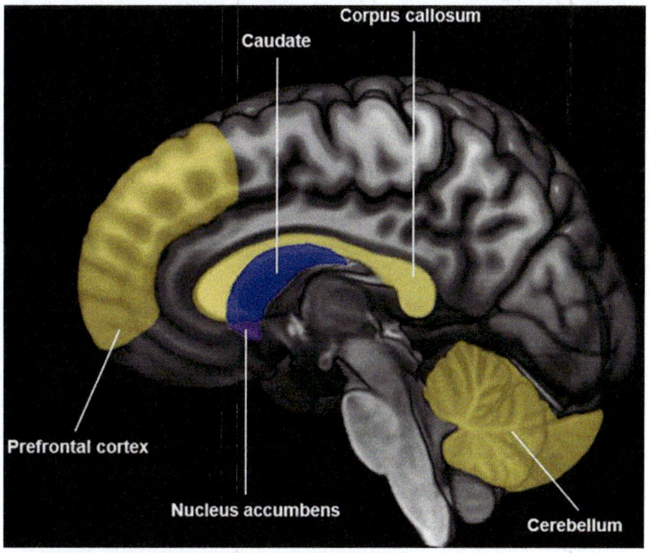

Fig. 8.28 Structural predictive biomarkers of good response to methylphenidate (MPH) in ADHD. Increase volume of caudate, nucleus accumbens, cerebellum, corpus callosum, and prefrontal cortex could predict good response to MPH in ADHD children

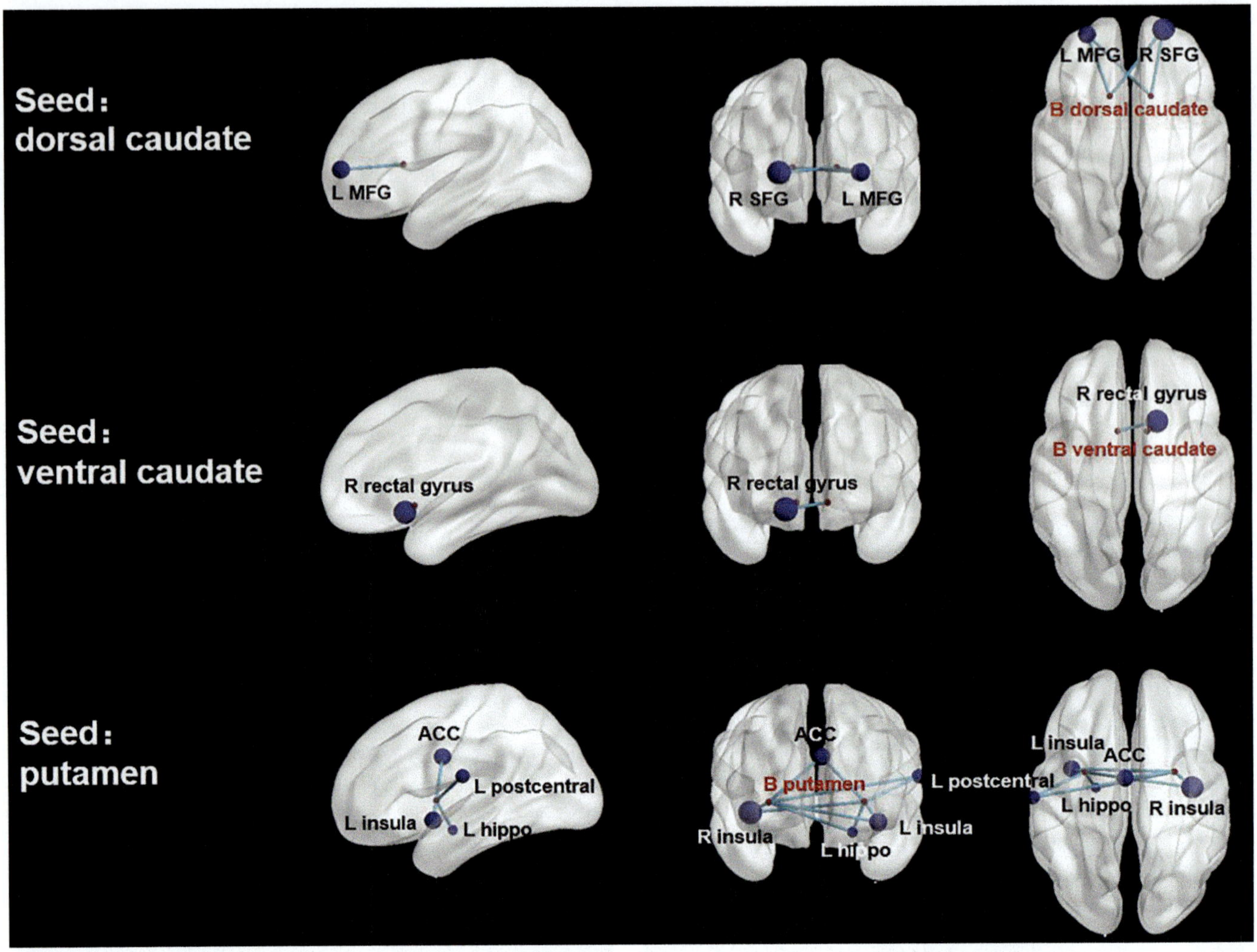

Fig. 8.29 Significantly decreased striatal functional connectivity in good responders to methylphenidate compared with poor responders of ADHD. The red spheres indicate d regions; the blue spheres indicate effect regions; the blue lines indicate functional connectivity between ds and effect regions. *MFG* middle frontal gyrus, *SFG* superior frontal gyrus, *ACC* anterior cingulate cortex, *hippo* hippocampus, *L* left, *R* right, *B* bilateral

Diagnostic Neuroimaging of ECT

For the first time, single photon emission computed tomography (SPECT) and positron emission tomography (PET) have achieved the goal of studying brain function in vivo with useful clinical information. Emission computed tomography (ECT) can observe changes in cerebral blood flow, cerebral oxygen consumption, cerebral glucose metabolism, brain protein synthesis, and brain neurotransmitters and receptors, which opens up new approaches for the study of psychiatric diseases and provides a new method for the study of neurobiology (Fig. 8.30).

^{99m}TC-ECD (99mTc-ethylcysteinate dimer) imaging of SZ patients showed hypoperfusion in frontal and temporal lobes (Fig. 8.31). One study using this method for SZ patients has found reduced regional cerebral blood flow (rCBF) perfusion in early-onset SZ group including the precentral and inferior frontal gyri, and reduced cerebral blood flow perfusion in the bilateral postcentral gyrus in late-onset SZ patients [63]. These results revealed a significant difference in brain perfusion between early-onset SZ and late-onset SZ and suggesting that the characteristic changes in regional cerebral blood flow are related to onset-age in SZ.

Dopamine (DA) receptor and transporter dysfunction play an important role in the pathophysiology of neuropsychiatric disorders including SZ. Compared with other psychiatry diseases, the function of DA in SZ is impaired in the substantia nigra striatum and the mesocortical system; the availability of DA is increased in the striatum cortex, and the availability of DA is decreased in the mesocortical pathway [64]. These results indicate various modes of neurotransmitter action in SZ.

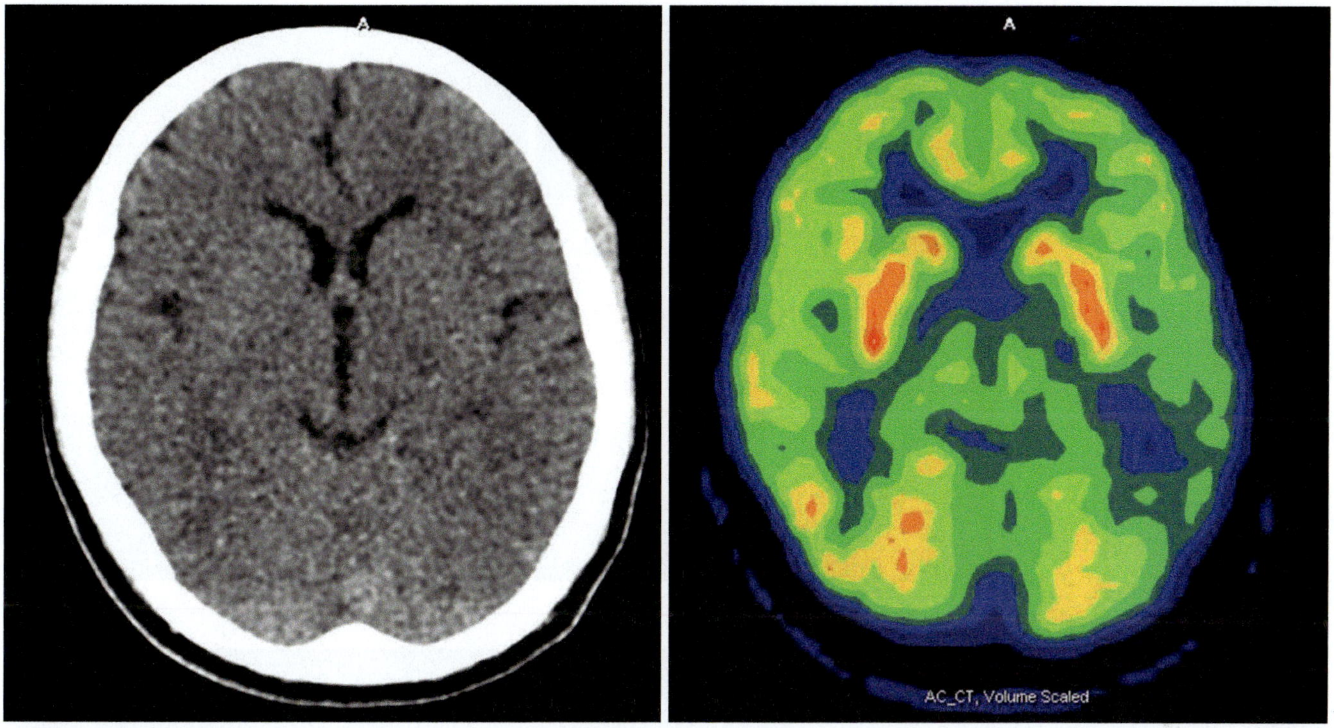

Fig. 8.30 FDG-PET/CT imaging in a healthy person. A indicates the anterior position

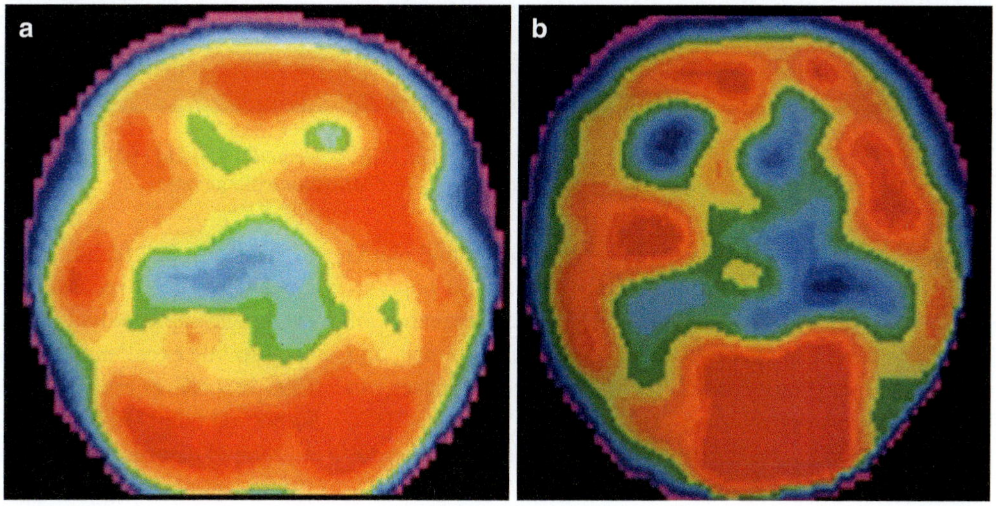

Fig. 8.31 ^{99m}TC-ECD SPECT/CT imaging in a healthy person (**a**) and a representative schizophrenia patient (**b**). Patients with schizophrenia showed increased rCBF perfusion in the right temporal lobe

The physiological or pathological condition of regional cerebral blood flow can be objectively described through real-time observation of the functional activity of the living brain by using SPECT, to the pathological basis of depression and the related brain function (Fig. 8.32). Most of the research results showed that depressed patients had abnormal blood perfusion in the frontal and temporal lobes, among which the anterior and ventral cingulate cortex of the knee of the corpus callosum were the most frequently reported [65]. Neuroreceptor imaging is also a hot topic in depression research. Studies have shown that compared with the placebo group, depressive symptoms in patients treated with Gonadotropin-releasing hormone agonist (GnRHa) are correlated with the increase of 5-HT (5-hydroxytryptamine) transporter binding in the cortical brain [66].

To sum up, SPECT and PET cerebral imaging can observe the local energy metabolism, oxygen metabolism, brain blood perfusion, and the change of various neurotransmitters and receptors using various physiological tracer, which allows brain function research from multiple levels and multiple perspectives (Fig. 8.33). Until now, SPECT and PET have been widely used in psychiatric research of SZ,

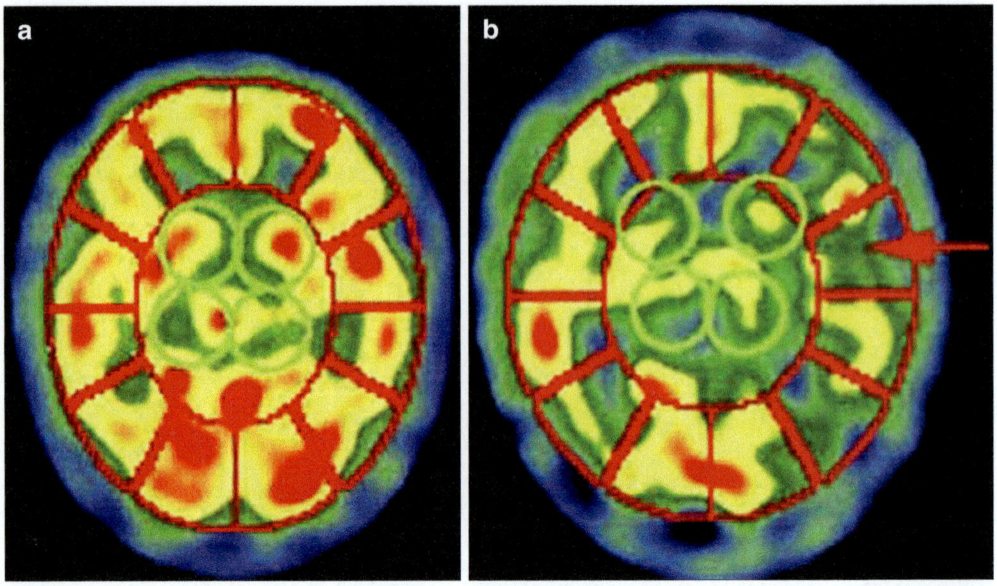

Fig. 8.32 ^{99m}TC-ECD SPECT/CT imaging in a healthy person (**a**) and a representative depression patient (**b**). Red arrow indicated reduced rCBF in the left frontal lobe in depressed patients

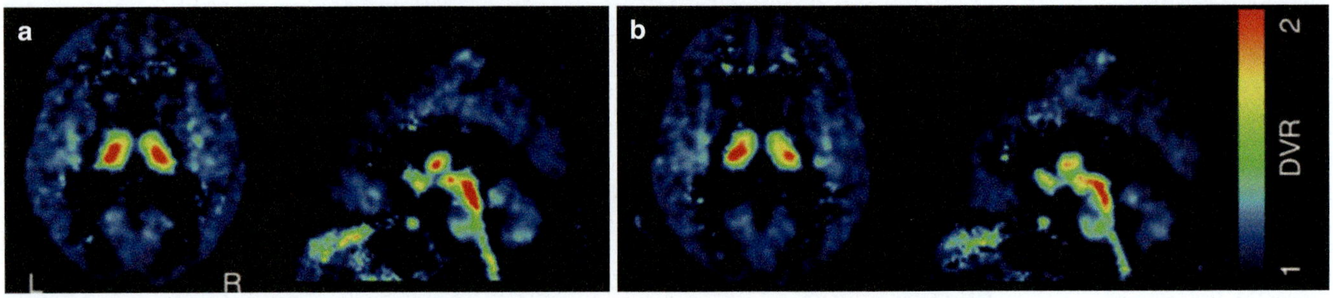

Fig. 8.33 PET imaging using the norepinephrine transporter (NET)-selective (S,S)-O-[11C] methylreboxetine in healthy controls (**a**) and attention-deficit/hyperactivity disorder (ADHD) patients (**b**). *DVR* distribution volume ratio

depression, anxiety disorder, personality disorder, and mania [67]. It is believed that with the improvement and popularization of SPECT and PET technology, the research of SPECT and PET in psychiatry will be further deepened, and the etiology and pathophysiology of psychiatric diseases can be better understood.

Diagnostic Neuroimaging of Quantitive EEG

With the advanced technology development of electrical engineering, computer, and signal processing in the 1980s, EEG and event-related brain potentials (ERPs) were becoming popular in both basic and clinical studies. EEG is a direct measurement of neuronal activity with a sampling frequency as high as dozens of kHz, resulting in extremely high temporal resolution. Compared to other neuroimaging techniques, which are used to investigate brain function (e.g., PET and fMRI), EEG is much cheaper, since the equipment is relatively cheaper and the disposable supplies required for experimenting are less. Moreover, in contrast to other electrophysiological techniques, the EEG technique is noninvasive. Thus, EEG recordings can be collected from subjects easily and repeatedly. In addition, EEG and ERP techniques can provide excellent temporal resolution. For these reasons, EEG recordings are becoming more and more popular as an important complement to PET and fMRI techniques.

Mental disorder is a syndrome characterized by clinically significant abnormalities in cognitive function, emotion regulation, and social behavior, which reflects an individual's obstacles in the development of psychological, biological, or social functions. A mass scientific epidemic survey found that there are 970 million people with mental disorders in the world. From 2010 to 2030, the cumulative loss of global economic output caused by mental illness is expected to reach US$16 trillion, equivalent to 25% of global GDP in 2010. However, the pathological mechanism of mental disorders is complex and the symptoms are diverse, which brings many difficulties to basic research and clinical practice in this field. In addition, traditional clinical diagnosis methods are also affected by the subjective factors of clinicians. It is difficult to illustrate the pathological mechanism of mental disorders only from the view of an objective evaluation of the symptoms of mental disorders. Finding objective biomarkers of mental disorders is an important way to solve these problems.

Biomarkers are objective indicators that can be repeatedly measured and reflect the medical status of patients. They can help clinicians, epidemiologists, and scientists to study various diseases and determine treatment goals by confirming the disease and tracking the course of the disease, as well as evaluating the efficacy of drugs. Currently, the most concerning mental disorder biomarkers mainly come from non-invasive neuroelectrophysiology or imaging techniques such as EEG and MRI. Researchers use the above tools to find the neural structure and functional state associated with specific mental disorders to find biologically based objective indicators or biomarkers. Compared with MRI, EEG equipment is cheaper and is easier to generalize and can sensitively and effectively evaluate the various stages of cognitive processing. The high time resolution also makes EEG widely used in cognitive neuroscience, and this type of research has accumulated considerable physiological evidence for mental disorders.

Neural Basis and Measurement of Quantitive EEG

EEG is defined as the electrical activity, which is generated by the firing of neurons within the human brain, and normally recorded at the brain scalp [68]. It is commonly recognized that the EEG originates from summed synchronized synaptic activities in populations of cortical neurons, with the main contribution from pyramidal cells. The information transmitted and processed in these neurons is realized by electrochemical signaling, via specialized connections called synapses. The relationship between the cortical processing within the brain and the electrical activity measured at the scalp is not formatted in a straightforward manner. The pyramidal neurons, which are the main composition of the cerebral cortex and close to the scalp, are highly polarized with the major orientation perpendicular to the cortical surface. Therefore, the cortical pyramidal neurons are the primary generators of the scalp EEG.

To obtain high quality EEG signals, the EEG measurement system should consist of several necessary elements, including electrodes with conductive media, amplifiers with filters, an analog-to-digital (A/D) converter, and a recording device. Specifically, the microvolt signals recorded from electrodes at the scalp were transformed by amplifiers into signals within a proper range of voltage. Then, signals were transformed by a converter from an analog format to a digital one and finally stored via the recording device. In 1958, a standard protocol for EEG electrode placement was developed by the American Electroencephalographic Society [69, 70]. It is called the International 10–20 System, which is widely used for defining electrode placement. This system contains standardized locations of 75 electrodes on the scalp (Fig. 8.34). The electrodes are placed at 10% and 20% points along lines of latitude and longitude, and this is the reason why the system is called the 10–20 system.

The recordings of the spontaneous electrical activity, called spontaneous EEG activity, exhibit certain characteristic waveforms that dominate in a wide range of frequencies and are normally applied in various clinical diagnoses. The spontaneous EEG activity is normally classified according to the frequency bands. Empirically, spontaneous EEG activity is divided into five frequency bands (Fig. 8.35): delta (δ, <4 Hz), theta (θ, 4–8 Hz), alpha (α, 8–13 Hz), beta (β, 13–30 Hz), and gamma (γ, >30 Hz). The rhythmic activity at each of these frequency bands characterizes by a certain distribution over the scalp and a certain biological significance.

When a stimulus associated with a specific sensory, cognitive, or motor event occurs, the neural responses disturb and can be extracted from the spontaneous EEG activity using a simple averaging technique. Specifically, the averaged responses are called ERPs to denote the fact that they are electrical potentials and related to the target events. Some researchers showed that ERPs appear to be an additional activity and independent of the ongoing spontaneous EEG activity [68]. In most cases, the magnitude of ERPs is often several factors smaller than the magnitude of the background EEG activity. Therefore, the identification of ERPs relies on signal processing methods for enhancing the SNR by means of the across-trial averaging in the time domain. And the averaged ERPs often comprise monophasic deflections which are characterized by their polarity, latency, amplitude, and scalp distribution.

Common Auditory and Visual ERP Components

The presentation of an auditory stimulus evokes a set of brainstem auditory evoked potentials (BAEPs), which reflects the flow of information from the cochlea through the brainstem and into the thalamus (Fig. 8.36). These auditory brainstem responses are typically labeled with Roman numerals (waves I–VI) and probably represent the activation of acoustic nerve (wave I), cochlear nuclear nuclei (wave II), superior olives (wave III), lateral lemniscus tracts and nuclei (wave IV), and inferior colliculi (wave V). Wave VI presumably arises from the medial geniculate body but is not considered clinically useful. BAEPs are highly automatic and relatively unaffected by sleep and anesthesia. Therefore, BAEPs can be used to assess the integrity of the auditory pathways, especially for newborns and infants. It is an extraordinary tool for the early identification of hearing impairment or hearing loss, aiding in early intervention.

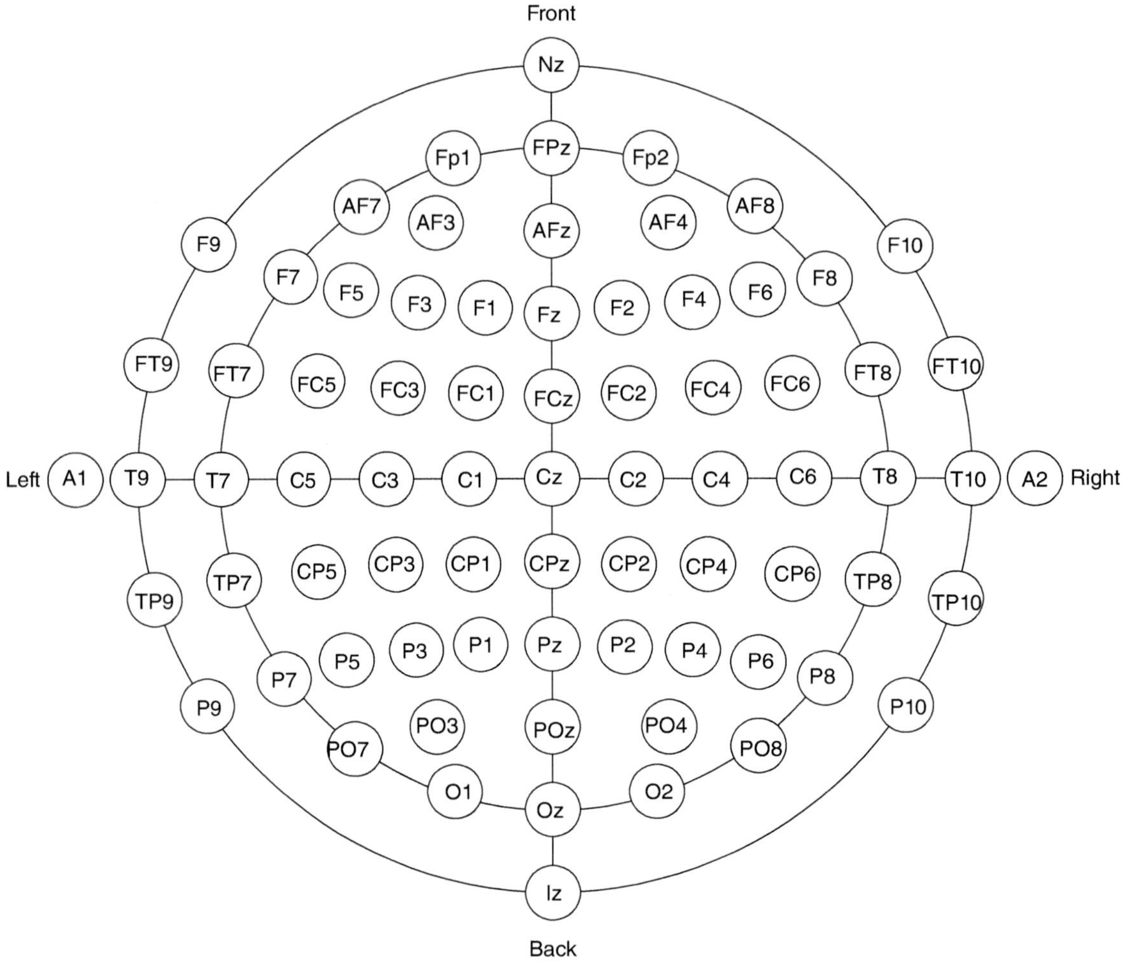

Fig. 8.34 International 10–20 System for electrode placement

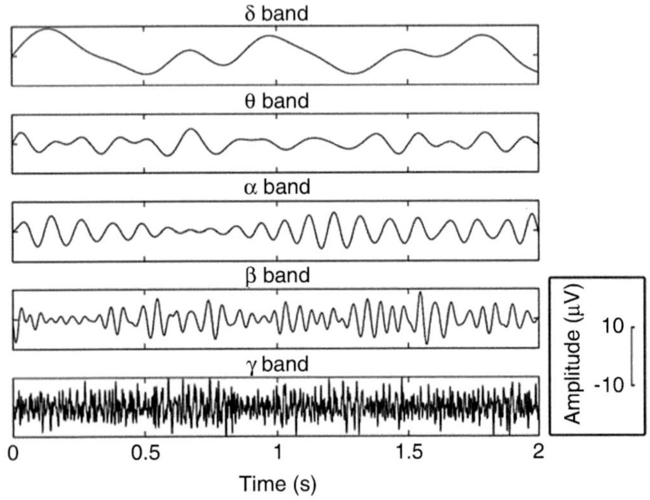

Fig. 8.35 Rhythmic EEG activity patterns. The rhythmic EEG activity is often divided into bands by frequency. Empirically, spontaneous EEG activity is divided into five frequency bands: delta (δ, < 4 Hz), theta (θ, 4–8 Hz), alpha (α, 8–13 Hz), beta (β, 13–30 Hz), and gamma (γ, > 30 Hz)

The BAEPs are followed by the mid-latency responses potentials (such as P1, N1, and P2), which probably arise at least in part from the medial geniculate nucleus and the primary auditory cortex, and the long-latency responses potentials (such as N2) [71]. The auditory N1 wave with a peak latency between 50 and 150 ms is one of the most prominent components during an auditory task. The auditory N1 is sensitive to attention. It has several distinct subcomponents that sum together to form the N1 peak, including a set of specific subcomponents that associated with the physical and temporal aspects of the stimulus and general state of the subject and a set of subcomponents. When deviant stimuli are occasionally presented within the repetitive train, a larger N2 amplitude is evoked in response to the deviants. This effect can be divided into three subcomponents—N2a, N2b, and N2c. The N2a is an automatic effect that occurs mainly for auditory mismatches, even if they are task-irrelevant, which is more commonly known as the auditory mismatch negativity (MMN). Specifically, MMN is generated by a relatively automatic response to an auditory stimulus that differs from

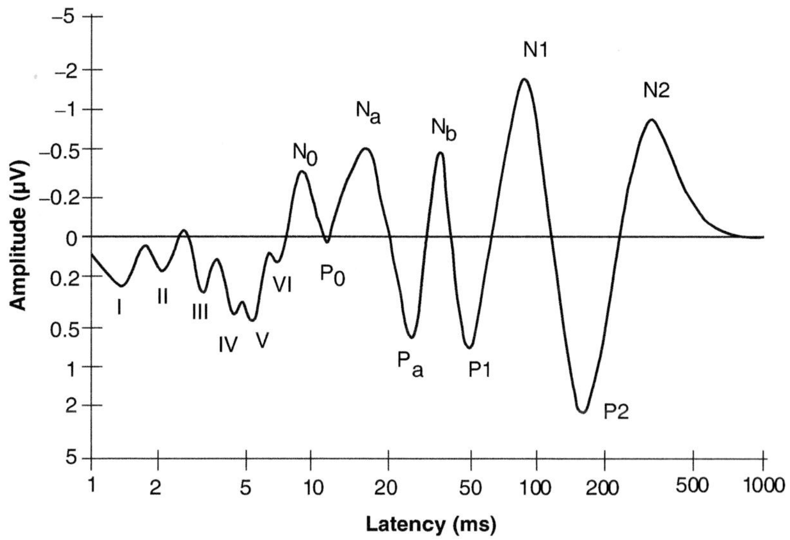

Fig. 8.36 Typical sequence of auditory evoked components. The waveform elicited by an auditory stimulus is shown over a period of time to demonstrate the auditory brainstem responses (waves I–VI), the mid-latency responses, and the long-latency responses

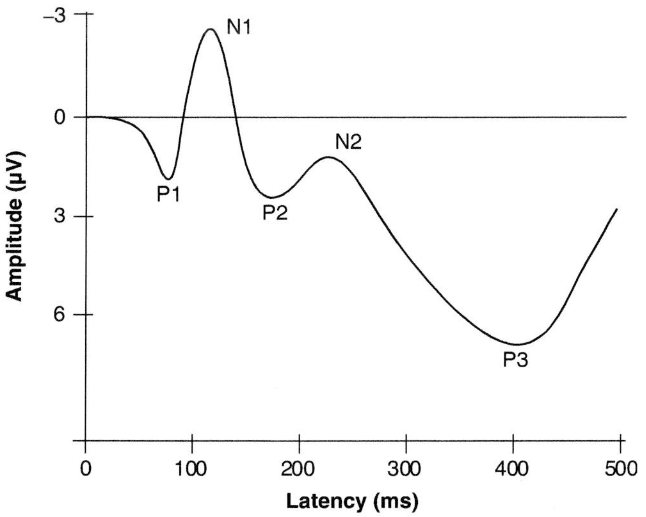

Fig. 8.37 Typical visual evoked components, including P1, N1, P2, N2, and P3 components

the preceding stimuli, that is, an infrequent change in homogeneous repetitive stimuli even in the absence of attention.

Visual evoked potentials include P1 and N1 (Fig. 8.37). Typically, the first major visual ERP component is the P1 wave. Visual P1 is maximal at lateral occipital electrode sites and onsets 60–90 ms poststimulus with a peak between 100 and 130 ms. The P1 wave is sensitive to variations in stimulus parameters and can be modulated by selective attention as well as by the individual's state of arousal [72]. It is believed that the P1 component is mainly generated in extrastriate visual areas. Following the P1 wave is the visual N1 wave, which is highly refractory. Like auditory N1, there are several visual N1 subcomponents. The earliest N1 subcomponent peaks at 100–150 ms poststimulus at anterior electrode sites, and there appear to be at least two posterior N1 components that peak at 150–200 ms poststimulus, arising from parietal cortex and lateral occipital cortex, respectively. It has shown that all three N1 subcomponents are influenced by spatial attention.

Diagnostic Performance of ERP Measures

EEG measures the electric potential generated by the synchronous firing of neurons by placing electrodes on multiple positions on the scalp. It can detect the electric potential generated by the cerebral cortex and some subcortical areas, thereby providing the brain's neural activity in milliseconds. In the EEG research of mental disorders, ERPs are mostly measured as outcome variables. ERP is calculated from the activity of EEG in some data periods and makes full use of the inherent high time resolution advantages of EEG technology. The selected data period is time-locked to some event of interest, such as an external stimulus or the subject's response, and the time-locked data period is averaged to produce a separate ERP waveform. In addition, EEG equipment is inexpensive and it is easy to operate, and its cost is much lower than that of MRI and MEG. It can analyze the electrophysiological characteristics of the brain economically and effectively. This also makes EEG expected to be widely used in the basic research of neuroscience and the clinical practice of individual medicine. In recent years, in order to more accurately assess the cognitive function characteristics of patients with mental disorders and high-risk groups, researchers have combined EEG technology and meta-analysis to carry out neuro-electrophysiological evidence-based medicine research on mental disorders. It also provides more objective and reliable biomarkers for the establishment of a new diagnostic framework for mental disorders.

The neuro-electrophysiological research of mental disorders has made considerable achievements in identifying objective biomarkers of SZ, anxiety, and obsessive-compulsive disorder. The cognitive deficits of patients and high-risk populations provide reliable empirical data. However, the existing evidence-based medicine research on mental disorders has different perspectives, and most studies only explore the components of a single type of ERP in a certain mental disorder. And the abnormal conditions in the EEG frequency band also make it difficult to form a consistent view of cognitive deficits in patients with mental disorders in theoretical construction and clinical practice. The time domain and frequency domain characteristics of EEG and the cognitive activities reflected in EEG-like research results not only help to form a systematic understanding of the cognitive impairment of specific mental disorders, but also help to compare the cognitive deficits of various mental disorders horizontally, and then establish a new mental disorder diagnostic framework and disease clustering. Recent neuro-electrophysiological research integrating evidence-based medicine has provided an important way for this and has achieved considerable research results. However, the existing research results are still controversial and difficult to reach a consensus.

The ERP Components as Potential Endophenotypes

An endophenotype is defined as an internal phenotype that is discoverable using biochemical or microscopic tests. Endophenotypes form the causal links between genetic influences and overt phenotypic expression and are therefore key in the understanding of the underlying biological mechanisms of disease risk and expression. Unlike biological markers, which may not be heritable, criteria for an endophenotype include heritability of the marker as well as a higher prevalence of the marker in non-affected family members relative to the general population. The strategy for validating endophenotypes for mental disorders first involves identifying deficits in patients, followed by exploring evidence of heritability in unaffected relatives. For example, SZ is a complex disease that involves a combination of numerous genetic and environmental factors. It has been consistently demonstrated that patients with SZ exhibit deficits in sensory and cognitive processing. Many studies have aimed to further explore these deficits using EEG to measure (ERPs. Three specific components, the P50, P300, and mismatch negativity (MMN) have been shown to reliably differ between patients with SZ and healthy controls in response to auditory stimuli (Fig. 8.38).

The P50 ERP component is a positive deflection occurring approximately 50 ms after stimulus onset and generally shows a decrease in amplitude to repeated stimuli, termed P50 suppression. Specifically, when two identical stimuli are presented successively, a decrease in P50 amplitude to the second stimulus is generally found. P50 is mostly thought to reflect a sensory gating mechanism or filtering of redundant stimuli. The P300 component is a positive deflection occurring between 250 and 500 ms after stimulus onset and is thought to reflect attentional processes. This component is often recorded using an oddball paradigm, in which the subject is presented with frequent and infrequent stimuli and asked to respond to the infrequent stimuli. An increase in amplitude to the infrequent relative to the frequent stimuli is generally found. It has been demonstrated that P300 amplitude is related to the number of attentional resources devoted to the task, whereas P300 latency indexes stimulus classification speed. The oddball paradigm also induces the MMN component that occurs in response to deviant stimuli. This response is elicited by auditory tones differing in a variety of perceptual features, such as frequency or duration. The MMN generally occurs 150–250 ms after the onset of the deviant stimulus is maximal over frontocentral scalp locations and is related to the degree of deviance. Unlike the P300, the MMN is elicited even in the absence of attention. The MMN reflects automatic auditory processing, perceptual discrimination ability, and sensory memory.

To sum up, the SZ patients showed a change of perception from early to late defects in processing, cognitive control, semantic processing, affect, and social cognition. Many studies have demonstrated robust deficits in P50 suppression, as reflected by larger P50 ratios for patients with SZ relative to healthy controls. Attention deficit/hyperactivity disorder has cognitive control defects from early to late, anxiety and obsessive-compulsive disorder have early cognitive control defects, and autism spectrum disorders have early perceptual processing and social cognitive deficits. Deficits in MMN generation are robust in patients with most of the mental disorders. In addition, the decrease in P300 amplitude and the increase in latency, which index attention allocation and processing speed, span multiple diagnostic types, indicating that this component may reflect the generality of cognitive deficits of mental disorders, and may be related to high-level cross-diagnostic factors. In the future, existing data sets and multi-center databases can be used to develop the "gold standard" of neuroelectrophysiological markers for clinical practice, and integrate machine learning and multi-modality. Imaging indicators to further enhance the reliability and effectiveness of biomarkers for mental disorders.

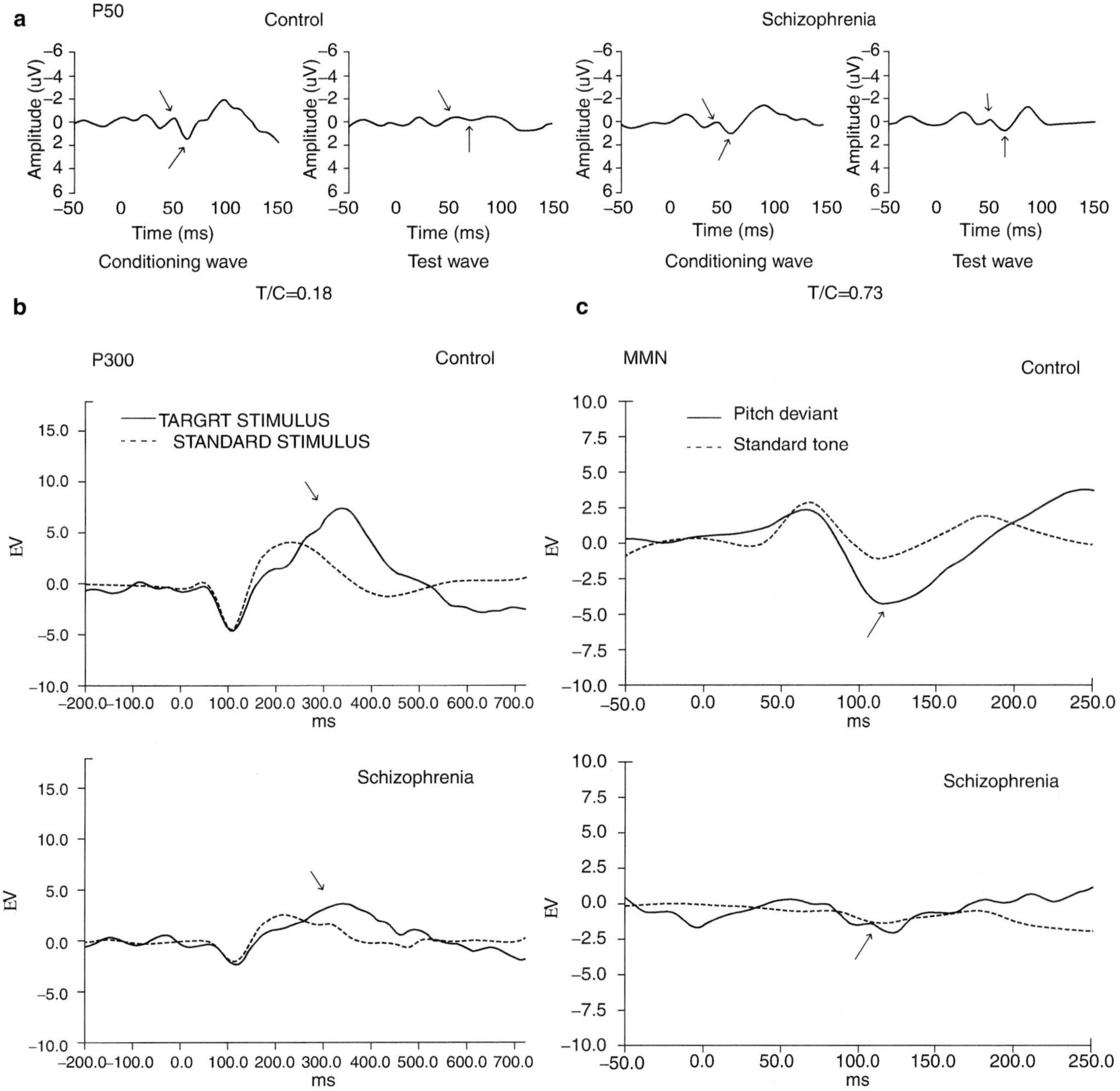

Fig. 8.38 Example component waveforms. (**a**) Example auditory-evoked response from a healthy control (left) and patient with schizophrenia (right). Arrows mark the location of the P50 wave for the conditioning stimulus and identical test stimulus. T/C indicates the test-to-conditioning ratio for each subject. The P50 response to the second stimulus is attenuated for the healthy control subject, but not for patient with schizophrenia. (**b**) Grand average waveforms for 38 healthy control subjects (top) and 52 patients with schizophrenia (bottom) in response to an infrequent auditory stimulus to which participants made a button press. As marked by arrows, patients with schizophrenia exhibit smaller P300 amplitudes than healthy controls. (**c**) Grand average mismatch negativity (MMN) response to an auditory pitchdeviant stimulus for 20 healthy control subjects (top) and 19 patients with schizophrenia (bottom). As marked by arrows, patients with schizophrenia exhibit smaller MMN amplitudes than healthy controls. (*From* Turetsky et al. [89]; *with permission*)

Diagnostic Neuroimaging of Magnetoencephalography

As a noninvasive functional imaging tool, magnetoencephalography (MEG) is featured by a fine combination of high spatial and temporal resolutions, offering a unique view in psychiatry diagnosis. Although MEG and EEG share the same origin of postsynaptic potentials, there are important differences due to the physics of detected signals (Table 8.4 for a detailed comparison between EEG and MEG). Since the magnetic fields are hardly affected by the skull or other brain tissues, MEG has better sensitivity in event-related responses and brain oscillations detection compared with EEG.

Apart from clinically detecting abnormal neuronal activities such as epilepsy, MEG has also been used in the search for biomarkers in psychiatry. It has been found that autism spectrum disorders (ASD) patients show a significantly delayed MEG auditory response around 100 ms (M100) in right-hemispheres, indicating impaired auditory processing in its early stage. Detailed MEG results also revealed a frequency-dependent latency shared by ASD patients (Fig. 8.39) [73]. As for SZ, the MEG recordings of wide-band neural oscillation provide the detection of gamma band or even high gamma band abnormalities apart from 40-Hz frequency range commonly used with EEG (Fig. 8.40) [74]. Also, by investigating the alteration of the resting-state network across brain regions and rhythms, MEG could potentially act as research tool for psychiatric patients such as Alzheimer's disease (AD) [75]. Finally, recent studies also show the possibility of combing brain stimulation such as transcranial electrical stimulation (tES) with MEG [76], providing concurrent monitoring and evaluation of the entrainment of brain oscillations.

Table 8.4 Comparison between EEG and MEG

Parameter	EEG	MEG
Spatial resolution	Centimeter range	Up to millimeter range
Temporal resolution	Millisecond range	Millisecond range
Forward model	Three-layer BEM or FEM[a]	Spherical approximation or single-layer BEM
Frequency of interest	Below 60 Hz[b]	Up to 500 Hz
Source direction	Radial and tangential	Tangential
Channels	Up to ~1000	Up to ~300
Non-invasiveness	Requires contact with electrodes and conductive gel	No physical contact required
Artifacts	Muscular, cardiac, ocular	Muscular, cardiac, ocular, environmental magnetic noise
Cost	Low	High

[a] *BEM* boundary element method, *FEM* finite element method
[b] It is widely accepted that the skull, cerebrospinal fluid and other brain tissues will act as a low-pass filter for electrical currents so that the high frequency brain oscillation signals will decay quickly before being detected by EEG

However, the research of MEG in the diagnosis of psychiatric diseases is still in its early stage with limited studies due to the high costs of commercial systems based on superconducting quantum interference devices (SQUID). Recent progress in optically-pumped magnetometers (OPM) has proposed a new generation of non-cryogenic MEG with a

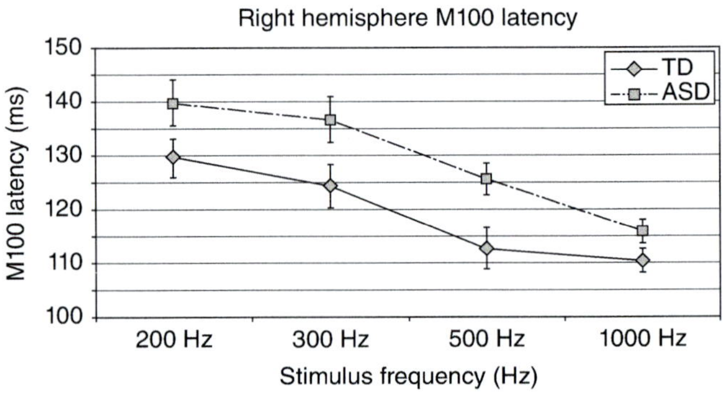

Fig. 8.39 The right hemisphere M100 response latencies in ASD patients and typical development (TD) subjects. It was found ASD patients shared a delayed of M100 response across frequencies, while the latency delay of 500 Hz was the most evident. (Error bars represent standard error of the mean, while "*" shows significant t-test result with $p < 0.05$ for Group Frequency ANOVA test.) (*From* Roberts et al. [73]; *with permission*)

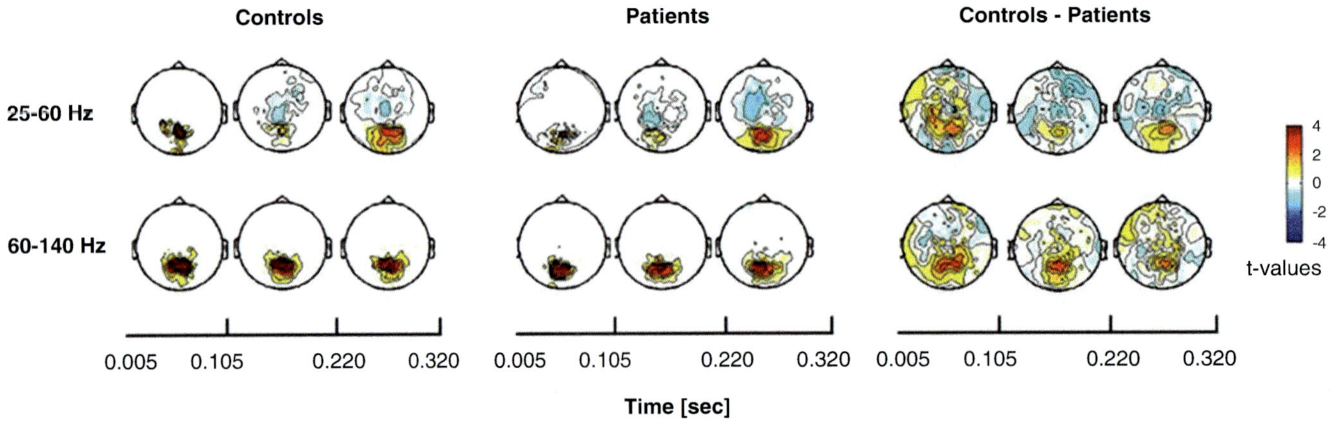

Fig. 8.40 MEG topographies of schizophrenia patients (left panels) show extent differences with controls (middle panels) in response to upright Mooney faces both in lower (25–60 Hz) and higher (60–140 Hz) gamma band. The right panels show the statistical difference where red denotes stronger activation for controls compared to patients, whereas blue represents stronger activation in patients relative to controls (FDR corrected, $q < 0.05$) (*From* Grützner et al. [74]; Creative Commons Attribution license [CC-BY])

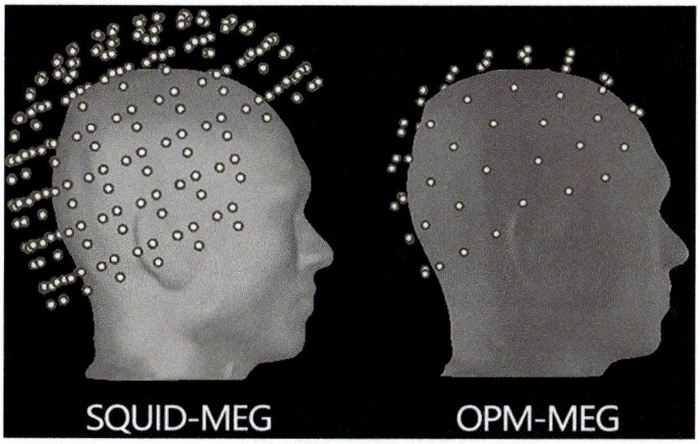

Fig. 8.41 The reconstructed SQUID (left) and OPM (right) sensor array positions relative to the head. By getting rid of the Dewar in the SQUID system, the OPM sensors can get much closer to the scalp, with the distance between sensitive point and scalp less than 1 mm. *SQUID* superconducting quantum interference devices, *OPM* superconducting quantum interference devices, *MEG* magnetoencephalography

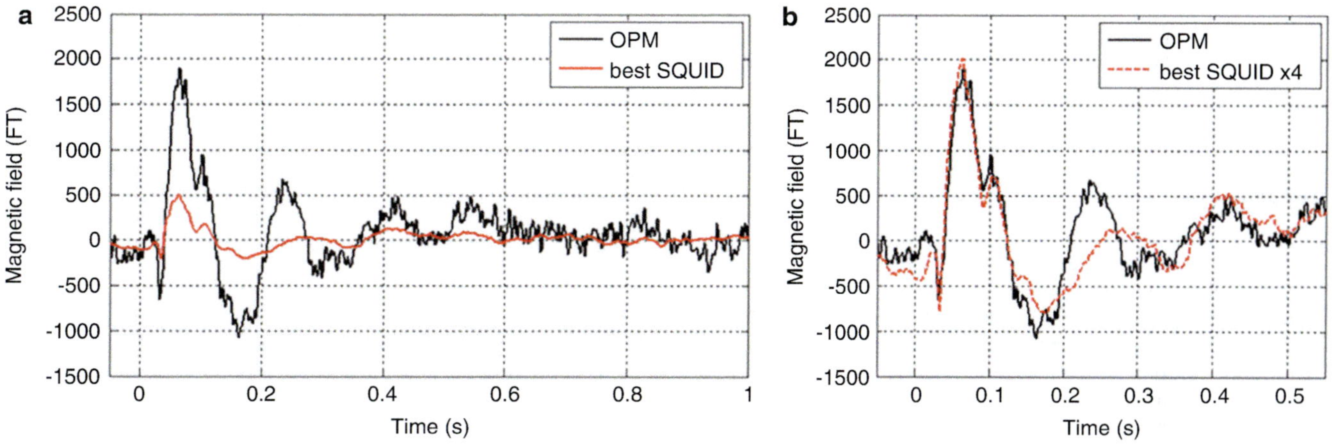

Fig. 8.42 Comparison of the magnitudes between OPM and SQUID in detecting evoked responses. (**a**) Measurements of the median nerve stimulation responses (in fT) of both OPM (black line) and SQUID (read line). (**b**) The OPM response shares the similar amplitude and profile as SQUID time course multiplied by four. *SQUID* superconducting quantum interference devices, *OPM* superconducting quantum interference devices (*From* Boto et al. [79]; Attribution 4.0 International [CC BY 4.0])

much lower price [77]. The other important advantage of OPM over SQUID is the reduced distance between sensor and scalp (Fig. 8.41), which brings several times increase in signal magnitude (Fig. 8.42) [78, 79]. The OPM–MEG could also be developed as a wearable device that offers much more flexibility for clinical diagnosis and other applications [77].

Diagnostic Laboratory Tests

Genetic testing may be useful in various clinical settings. Genome -wide association studies (GWAS) evolved as a key tool to identify genetic risk variants related to complex diseases. For example, rare or de novo copy number variants and SNPs are common in individuals with SZ, autism spectrum disorder, and other psychiatric disorders. Microdeletion 22qll.l syndrome is typically caused by a recurrent 3 MB deletion of 40 genes, including TBX1. 20 to 50% of patients with this deletion develop ASD [80], and the deletion is also found in approximately 1% of people with SZ, bipolar disorder, and idiopathic Parkinson disease [81, 82]. And approximately 2.5% of SZ patients carry one of the associated copy number variants [83]. Thus, the identification of de novo CNVs could be useful in the management of severe psychiatric disorders.

Besides genetic testing, the plasma-targeted metabonomic method has also been used for the diagnosis of mental disorders. Pan et al. simultaneously quantified the levels of 19 plasma metabolites involved in the GABAergic, catecholaminergic, and serotonergic neurotransmitter systems in 50 first-episode, antidepressant drug-naïve MDD subjects by using a GC-MS coupled with LC-MS/MS-based targeted metabolomics approach, they found a panel of four candidate plasma metabolite biomarkers (GABA, dopamine, tyramine, kynurenine) could distinguish MDD subjects from health controls with an AUC of 0.968 and 0.953 in the training and testing set, respectively [84].

The pharmacological treatment of psychiatric disorders has been severely hampered by large inter-individual variations in terms of drug response and/or side effects, often leading to painful, frustrating, and inefficient trial-and-error-based changes in treatment regimens. Such variations are to a large extent due to genetic factors, with an estimated heritability of 0.6–0.8 [85]. Thus, numerous studies attempted to detect gene variants associated with individual differences in drug responsiveness or side effect. Recent GWASs have suggested that the proportion of variance in antidepressant response explained by common genetic variation is as high as 42% [86], and pharmacogenetic (ie, evaluating a single gene) and pharmacogenomic (ie, evaluating multiple genes) testing have shown promise for informing the selection of antidepressants [87, 88]. Pharmacogenetic and pharmacogenomic testing have been developed to predict which medication may yield the best treatment response and/or the lowest risk of adverse events for a given individual.

References

1. Gong Q. Psychoradiology. New York: Elsevier Inc; Neuroimaging Clinics of North America. 2020;30:1–123.
2. Lui S, Zhou XJ, Sweeney JA, Gong Q. Psychoradiology: the frontier of neuroimaging in psychiatry. Radiology. 2016;281(2):357–72.
3. Li F, Sun H, Biswal BB, Sweeney JA, Gong Q. Artificial intelligence applications in psychoradiology. Psychoradiology. 2021;2(1):94–107. https://doi.org/10.1093/psyrad/kkab009.
4. Sun H, Lui S, Yao L, Deng W, Xiao Y, Zhang W, et al. Two patterns of white matter abnormalities in medication-naive patients with first-episode schizophrenia revealed by diffusion Tensor imaging and cluster analysis. JAMA Psychiatry. 2015;72(7):678–86.
5. Li F, Wu DS, Lui S, Gong QY, Sweeney JA. Clinical strategies and technical challenges in psychoradiology. Neuroimaging Clin N Am. 2020;30(1):1–13.
6. Glasser MF, Van Essen DC. Mapping human cortical areas in vivo based on myelin content as revealed by T1- and T2-weighted MRI. J Neurosci. 2011;31(32):11597–616.
7. Reuter M, Tisdall MD, Qureshi A, Buckner RL, van der Kouwe AJW, Fischl B. Head motion during MRI acquisition reduces gray matter volume and thickness estimates. NeuroImage. 2015;107:107–15.
8. Tisdall MD, Reuter M, Qureshi A, Buckner RL, Fischl B, Kouwe AJW. Prospective motion correction with volumetric navigators (vNavs) reduces the bias and variance in brain morphometry induced by subject motion. NeuroImage. 2016;127:11–22.
9. Xiao Y, Yan ZH, Zhao YJ, Tao B, Sun HQ, Li F, et al. Support vector machine-based classification of first episode drug-naive schizophrenia patients and healthy controls using structural MRI. Schizophr Res. 2019;214:11–7.
10. Lui S, Xiao Y, Sweeney JA, Liao W, Gong QY. Heterogeneity of brain structure alterations in patients with never-treated first episode schizophrenia. Neuropsychopharmacology. 2018;43:S486.
11. Rodriguez A, Laio A. Machine learning. Clustering by fast search and find of density peaks. Science. 2014;344(6191):1492–6.
12. Xiao Y, Liao W, Long Z, Tao B, Zhao Q, Luo C, et al. Subtyping schizophrenia patients based on patterns of structural brain alterations. Schizophr Bull. 2022;48(1):241–50.
13. Gong QY, Wu QZ, Scarpazza C, Lui S, Jia ZY, Marquand A, et al. Prognostic prediction of therapeutic response in depression using high-field MR imaging. NeuroImage. 2011;55(4):1497–503.
14. Drysdale AT, Grosenick L, Downar J, Dunlop K, Mansouri F, Meng Y, et al. Resting-state connectivity biomarkers define neurophysiological subtypes of depression (vol 23, pg 28, 2016). Nat Med. 2017;23(2):264.
15. Hu XY, Du MY, Chen LZ, Li L, Zhou M, Zhang LQ, et al. Meta-analytic investigations of common and distinct grey matter alterations in youths and adults with obsessive-compulsive disorder. Neurosci Biobehav Rev. 2017;78:91–103.
16. Association, A.P. Diagnostic and statistical manual of mental disorders. 5th ed. Arlingtion, VA: American Psychiatric Association; 2013.
17. Gong Q, Li L, Tognin S, Wu Q, Pettersson-Yeo W, Lui S, et al. Using structural neuroanatomy to identify trauma survivors with and without post-traumatic stress disorder at the individual level. Psychol Med. 2014;44(1):195–203.
18. Gong Q, Li L, Du M, Pettersson-Yeo W, Crossley N, Yang X, et al. Quantitative prediction of individual psychopathology in trauma survivors using resting-state FMRI. Neuropsychopharmacology. 2014;39(3):681–7.
19. Nicholson AA, Densmore M, McKinnon MC, Neufeld RWJ, Frewen PA, Theberge J, et al. Machine learning multivariate pattern analysis predicts classification of posttraumatic stress disorder and its dissociative subtype: a multimodal neuroimaging approach. Psychol Med. 2019;49(12):2049–59.
20. Colby JB, Rudie JD, Brown JA, Douglas PK, Cohen MS, Shehzad Z. Insights into multimodal imaging classification of ADHD. Front Syst Neurosci. 2012;6:59.
21. Posner J, Polanczyk GV, Sonuga-Barke E. Attention-deficit hyperactivity disorder. Lancet. 2020;395(10222):450–62.
22. Sun H, Chen Y, Huang Q, Lui S, Huang X, Shi Y, et al. Psychoradiologic utility of MR imaging for diagnosis of attention deficit hyperactivity disorder: a radiomics analysis. Radiology. 2018;287(2):620–30.
23. Ding Y, Ou Y, Pan P, Shan X, Chen J, Liu F, et al. Brain structural abnormalities as potential markers for detecting individuals with ultra-high risk for psychosis: a systematic review and meta-analysis. Schizophr Res. 2019;209:22–31.
24. Dazzan P, Arango C, Fleischacker W, Galderisi S, Glenthøj B, Leucht S, et al. Magnetic resonance imaging and the prediction of outcome in first-episode schizophrenia: a review of current evidence and directions for future research. Schizophr Bull. 2015;41(3):574–83.
25. Sheffield JM, Barch DM. Cognition and resting-state functional connectivity in schizophrenia. Neurosci Biobehav Rev. 2016;61:108–20.
26. Andreasen NC, Liu D, Ziebell S, Vora A, Ho BC. Relapse duration, treatment intensity, and brain tissue loss in schizophrenia: a prospective longitudinal MRI study. Am J Psychiatry. 2013;170(6):609–15.
27. Dietsche B, Kircher T, Falkenberg I. Structural brain changes in schizophrenia at different stages of the illness: a selective review of longitudinal magnetic resonance imaging studies. Aust N Z J Psychiatry. 2017;51(5):500–8.
28. Li Q, Zhao Y, Chen Z, Long J, Dai J, Huang X, et al. Meta-analysis of cortical thickness abnormalities in medication-free patients with major depressive disorder. Neuropsychopharmacology. 2020;45(4):703–12.

29. Li W, Chen Z, Wu M, Zhu H, Gu L, Zhao Y, et al. Characterization of brain blood flow and the amplitude of low-frequency fluctuations in major depressive disorder: a multimodal meta-analysis. J Affect Disord. 2017;210:303–11.
30. Figueroa CA, Cabral J, Mocking RJT, Rapuano KM, van Hartevelt TJ, Deco G, et al. Altered ability to access a clinically relevant control network in patients remitted from major depressive disorder. Hum Brain Mapp. 2019;40(9):2771–86.
31. Li B, Liu L, Friston KJ, Shen H, Wang L, Zeng LL, et al. A treatment-resistant default mode subnetwork in major depression. Biol Psychiatry. 2013;74(1):48–54.
32. Spies M, Kraus C, Geissberger N, Auer B, Klöbl M, Tik M, et al. Default mode network deactivation during emotion processing predicts early antidepressant response. Transl Psychiatry. 2017;7(1):e1008.
33. Bu X, Hu X, Zhang L, Li B, Zhou M, Lu L, et al. Investigating the predictive value of different resting-state functional MRI parameters in obsessive-compulsive disorder. Transl Psychiatry. 2019;9(1):17.
34. Zhu H, Yuan M, Qiu C, Ren Z, Li Y, Wang J, et al. Multivariate classification of earthquake survivors with post-traumatic stress disorder based on large-scale brain networks. Acta Psychiatr Scand. 2020;141(3):285–98.
35. Marmar CR, Schlenger W, Henn-Haase C, Qian M, Purchia E, Li M, et al. Course of posttraumatic stress disorder 40 years after the Vietnam war: findings from the National Vietnam Veterans Longitudinal Study. JAMA Psychiat. 2015;72(9):875–81.
36. Sun D, Davis SL, Haswell CC, Swanson CA, Mid-Atlantic MW, LaBar KS, et al. Brain structural covariance network topology in remitted posttraumatic stress disorder. Front Psych. 2018;9:90.
37. Sibley MH, Swanson JM, Arnold LE, Hechtman LT, Owens EB, Stehli A, et al. Defining ADHD symptom persistence in adulthood: optimizing sensitivity and specificity. J Child Psychol Psychiatry. 2017;58(6):655–62.
38. Faraone SV, Biederman J, Mick E. The age-dependent decline of attention deficit hyperactivity disorder: a meta-analysis of follow-up studies. Psychol Med. 2006;36(2):159–65.
39. Shaw P, Malek M, Watson B, Greenstein D, de Rossi P, Sharp W. Trajectories of cerebral cortical development in childhood and adolescence and adult attention-deficit/hyperactivity disorder. Biol Psychiatry. 2013;74(8):599–606.
40. Sudre G, Mangalmurti A, Shaw P. Growing out of attention deficit hyperactivity disorder: insights from the 'remitted' brain. Neurosci Biobehav Rev. 2018;94:198–209.
41. Sudre G, Szekely E, Sharp W, Kasparek S, Shaw P. Multimodal mapping of the brain's functional connectivity and the adult outcome of attention deficit hyperactivity disorder. Proc Natl Acad Sci U S A. 2017;114(44):11787–92.
42. Yao L, Li F, Liu JK, Liao W, Li XJ, Li ML, et al. Functional brain networks in never-treated and treated long-term Ill schizophrenia patients. Neuropsychopharmacology. 2019;44(11):1940–7.
43. Luo C, Lencer R, Hu N, Xiao Y, Zhang W, Li S, et al. Characteristics of white matter structural networks in chronic schizophrenia treated with clozapine or risperidone and those never-treated. Int J Neuropsychopharmacol. 2020;23(12):799–810.
44. Dunlop BW, Mayberg HS. Neuroimaging-based biomarkers for treatment selection in major depressive disorder. Dialogues Clin Neurosci. 2014;16(4):479–90.
45. Fonseka T, MacQueen G, Kennedy S. Neuroimaging biomarkers as predictors of treatment outcome in major depressive disorder. J Affect Disord. 2018;233:21–35.
46. Kang S, Cho S. Neuroimaging biomarkers for predicting treatment response and recurrence of major depressive disorder. Int J Mol Sci. 2020;21(6):2148.
47. Frodl T, Jäger M, Smajstrlova I, Born C, Bottlender R, Palladino T, et al. Effect of hippocampal and amygdala volumes on clinical outcomes in major depression: a 3-year prospective magnetic resonance imaging study. J Psychiatry Neurosci. 2008;33(5):423–30.
48. Fu CH, Steiner H, Costafreda SG. Predictive neural biomarkers of clinical response in depression: a meta-analysis of functional and structural neuroimaging studies of pharmacological and psychological therapies. Neurobiol Dis. 2013;52:75–83.
49. Kronmüller KT, Pantel J, Köhler S, Victor D, Giesel F, Magnotta VA, et al. Hippocampal volume and 2-year outcome in depression. Br J Psychiatry. 2008;192(6):472–3.
50. MacQueen GM, Yucel K, Taylor VH, Macdonald K, Joffe R. Posterior hippocampal volumes are associated with remission rates in patients with major depressive disorder. Biol Psychiatry. 2008;64(10):880–3.
51. Sämann PG, Höhn D, Chechko N, Kloiber S, Lucae S, Ising M, et al. Prediction of antidepressant treatment response from gray matter volume across diagnostic categories. Eur Neuropsychopharmacol. 2013;23(11):1503–15.
52. Arnone D, McKie S, Elliott R, Juhasz G, Thomas EJ, Downey D, et al. State-dependent changes in hippocampal grey matter in depression. Mol Psychiatry. 2013;18(12):1265–72.
53. Dichter G, Gibbs D, Smoski M. A systematic review of relations between resting-state functional-MRI and treatment response in major depressive disorder. J Affect Disord. 2015;172:8–17.
54. Lythe K, Moll J, Gethin J, Workman C, Green S, Lambon Ralph M, et al. Self-blame-selective hyperconnectivity between anterior temporal and Subgenual cortices and prediction of recurrent depressive episodes. JAMA Psychiat. 2015;72(11):1119–26.
55. Borairi S, Dougherty DD. The use of neuroimaging to predict treatment response for neurosurgical interventions for treatment-refractory major depression and obsessive-compulsive disorder. Harv Rev Psychiatry. 2011;19(3):155–61.
56. Medicine, I.o. Treatment of posttraumatic stress disorder: an assessment of the evidence. Washington, DC, Institute of Medicine; 2008.
57. Bradley R, Greene J, Russ E, Dutra L, Westen D. A multidimensional meta-analysis of psychotherapy for PTSD. Am J Psychiatry. 2005;162(2):214–27.
58. Bryant RA, Erlinger M, Felmingham K, Klimova A, Williams LM, Malhi G, et al. Reappraisal-related neural predictors of treatment response to cognitive behavior therapy for post-traumatic stress disorder. Psychol Med. 2020;51(14):2454–64.
59. Hanwella R, Senanayake M, de Silva V. Comparative efficacy and acceptability of methylphenidate and atomoxetine in treatment of attention deficit hyperactivity disorder in children and adolescents: a meta-analysis. BMC Psychiatry. 2011;11:176.
60. Zimmer L. Contribution of clinical neuroimaging to the understanding of the pharmacology of methylphenidate. Trends Pharmacol Sci. 2017;38(7):608–20.
61. Schrantee A, Ruhe HG, Reneman L. Psychoradiological biomarkers for psychopharmaceutical effects. Neuroimaging Clin N Am. 2020;30(1):53–63.
62. Hong SB, Harrison BJ, Fornito A, Sohn CH, Song IC, Kim JW. Functional dysconnectivity of corticostriatal circuitry and differential response to methylphenidate in youth with attention-deficit/hyperactivity disorder. J Psychiatry Neurosci. 2015;40(1):46–57.
63. Wake R, Miyaoka T, Araki T, Kawakami K, Furuya M, Limoa E, et al. Regional cerebral blood flow in late-onset schizophrenia: a SPECT study using 99mTc-ECD (vol 266, pg 3, 2016). Eur Arch Psychiatry Clin Neurosci. 2016;266(1):13.
64. Nikolaus S, Mamlins E, Hautzel H, Muller HW. Acute anxiety disorder, major depressive disorder, bipolar disorder and schizophre-

nia are related to different patterns of nigrostriatal and mesolimbic dopamine dysfunction. Rev Neurosci. 2019;30(4):381–426.
65. Charney DS, Nestler EJ. Neurobiology of mental illness, vol. xx. 3rd ed. Oxford/New York: Oxford University Press; 2009. p. 1475.
66. Frokjaer VG, Pinborg A, Holst KK, Overgaard A, Henningsson S, Heede M, et al. Role of serotonin transporter changes in depressive responses to sex-steroid hormone manipulation: a positron emission tomography study. Biol Psychiatry. 2015;78(8):534–43.
67. Frankle WG, Slifstein M, Talbot PS, Laruelle M. Neuroreceptor imaging in psychiatry: theory and applications. Neuroimaging, Pt B. 2005;67:385–440.
68. Niedermeyer E, da Silva FHL. Electroencephalography, basic principles, clinical applications, and related fields. 5th ed. Philadelphia, PA: Lippincott Williams & Wilkins; 2005. 752 p.
69. Acharya JN, Hani A, Cheek J, Thirumala P, Tsuchida TN. American Clinical Neurophysiology society guideline 2: guidelines for standard electrode position nomenclature. J Clin Neurophysiol. 2016;33(4):308–11.
70. American Clinical Neurophysiology, S. Guideline 5: Guidelines for standard electrode position nomenclature. J Clin Neurophysiol. 2006;23(2):107–10.
71. Luck SJ. An introduction to the event-related potential technique. Cognitive neuroscience, vol. xii. Cambridge, MA: MIT Press; 2005. p. 374.
72. Hillyard SA, Vogel EK, Luck SJ. Sensory gain control (amplification) as a mechanism of selective attention: electrophysiological and neuroimaging evidence. Philos Trans R Soc Lond Ser B Biol Sci. 1998;353(1373):1257–70.
73. Roberts TPL, Khan SY, Rey M, Monroe JF, Cannon K, Blaskey L, et al. MEG detection of delayed auditory evoked responses in autism Spectrum disorders: towards an imaging biomarker for autism. Autism Res. 2010;3(1):8–18.
74. Grützner C, Wibral M, Sun LM, Rivolta D, Singer W, Maurer K, et al. Deficits in high- (> 60 Hz) gamma-band oscillations during visual processing in schizophrenia. Front Hum Neurosci. 2013;7:88.
75. Engels MMA, van der Flier WM, Stam CJ, Hillebrand A, Scheltens P, van Straaten ECW. Alzheimer's disease: the state of the art in resting-state magnetoencephalography. Clin Neurophysiol. 2017;128(8):1426–37.
76. Kasten FH, Herrmann CS. Recovering brain dynamics during concurrent tACS-M/EEG: an overview of analysis approaches and their methodological and interpretational pitfalls. Brain Topogr. 2019;32(6):1013–9.
77. Boto E, Holmes N, Leggett J, Roberts G, Shah V, Meyer SS, et al. Moving magnetoencephalography towards real-world applications with a wearable system. Nature. 2018;555(7698):657.
78. Sheng JW, Wan SG, Sun YF, Dou RS, Guo YH, Wei KQ, et al. Magnetoencephalography with a Cs-based high-sensitivity compact atomic magnetometer. Rev Sci Instrum. 2017;88(9):094304.
79. Boto E, Meyer SS, Shah V, Alem O, Knappe S, Kruger P, et al. A new generation of magnetoencephalography: room temperature measurements using optically-pumped magnetometers. NeuroImage. 2017;149:404–14.
80. Vorstman JAS, Morcus MEJ, Duijff SN, Klaassen PWJ, Heineman-de Boer JA, Beemer FA, et al. The 22q11.2 deletion in children: high rate of autistic disorders and early onset of psychotic symptoms. J Am Acad Child Adolesc Psychiatry. 2006;45(9):1104–13.
81. Mok KY, Sheerin U, Simon-Sanchez J, Salaka A, Chester L, Escott-Price V, et al. Deletions at 22q11.2 in idiopathic Parkinson's disease: a combined analysis of genome-wide association data. Lancet Neurol. 2016;15(6):585–96.
82. Malhotra D, Sebat J. CNVs: harbingers of a rare variant revolution in psychiatric genetics. Cell. 2012;148(6):1223–41.
83. Brand H, Pillalamarri V, Collins RL, Eggert S, O'Dushlaine C, Braaten EB, et al. Cryptic and complex chromosomal aberrations in early-onset neuropsychiatric disorders. Am J Hum Genet. 2014;95(4):454–61.
84. Pan JX, Xia JJ, Deng FL, Liang WW, Wu J, Yin BM, et al. Diagnosis of major depressive disorder based on changes in multiple plasma neurotransmitters: a targeted metabolomics study. Transl Psychiatry. 2018;8:130.
85. Pouget JG, Shams TA, Tiwari AK, Müller DJ. Pharmacogenetics and outcome with antipsychotic drugs. Dialogues Clin Neurosci. 2014;16(4):555–66.
86. Tansey KE, Guipponi M, Hu XL, Domenici E, Lewis G, Malafosse A, et al. Contribution of common genetic variants to antidepressant response. Biol Psychiatry. 2013;73(7):679–82.
87. Perlis RH. Pharmacogenomic testing and personalized treatment of depression. Clin Chem. 2014;60(1):53–9.
88. Singh AB, Bousman CA, Ng C, Berk M. Antidepressant pharmacogenetics. Curr Opin Psychiatry. 2014;27(1):43–51.
89. Turetsky BI, Calkins ME, Light GA, Olincy A, Radant AD, Swerdlow NR. Neurophysiological endophenotypes of schizophrenia: the viability of selected candidate measures. Schizophr Bull. 2007;33:69–94.

Psychiatric Emergencies: Suicide and Violence

9

Basant K. Puri

Suicide

Introduction

A deep understanding of the etiology and management of suicidal behavior cannot simply be confined to the academic discipline of psychiatry. Rather, a multidisciplinary approach needs to be taken, with due regard being paid to areas as diverse as the economy, religious and educational upbringing, and the role of television, newspapers, magazines, and social media.

Suicidal behavior disorder constitutes a psychiatric emergency. It is included as a condition for further study in DSM-5, with the proposed criteria summarized in Table 9.1. Within these criteria, DSM-5 defines a suicide attempt as "a self-initiated sequence of behaviors by an individual who, at the time of initiation, expected that the set of actions would lead to his or her own death." The "time of initiation" is defined as "the time when a behavior took place that involved applying the method" [1].

Table 9.1 A summary of the DSM-5 proposed criteria for suicidal behavior disorder

A.	Within the last 24 months, the individual has made a suicide attempt
B.	The act does not meet criteria for nonsuicidal self-injury—That is, it does not involve self-injury directed to the surface of the body undertaken to induce relief from a negative feeling/cognitive state or to achieve a positive mood state
C.	The diagnosis is not applied to suicidal ideation or to preparatory acts
D.	The act was no initiated during a state of delirium or confusion
E.	The act was not undertaken solely for a political or religious objective
Specify if:	
	Current: Not more than 12 months since the last attempt
	In early remission: 12–24 months since the last attempt

Epidemiology

According to the World Health Organization (WHO), in the year 2016 (the last year for which data were available at the time of writing), the overall global suicide rate was just under 11 per 100,000 of the population. As can be seen from the WHO breakdown of these figures shown in Fig. 9.1, the suicide rate was almost twice as high in males as in females in 2016.

Figure 9.1 also shows a marked difference in regional variation in the suicide rate, with the Eastern Mediterranean having the lowest rates in both males and females. The WHO has also published the suicide rates by country. The countries with the highest rates in 2016 are shown in Fig. 9.2.

Suicide is a major cause of mortality in young people, as shown in the WHO 2016 data of Fig. 9.3.

Indeed, in females, it is a more common cause of death in 15- to 29-year-olds than road injury, while in males in the same age range suicide is the third leading cause of death after road injury and interpersonal violence. The corresponding WHO data for 2016 are shown in Fig. 9.4.

Economic factors also play a part. There is an association between suicide and not being employed, while worldwide most suicides take place in low- and middle-income countries (see Fig. 9.5) [2].

A seasonal effect also exists. In both the northern and southern hemispheres, the rate of suicide is lowest in the winter months but highest in late spring or summer. The winter minimum is illustrated for Victoria, Australia, in Fig. 9.6 [3].

B. K. Puri (✉)
University of Winchester, Winchester, UK
e-mail: bpuri@cantab.net

W. W. IsHak (ed.), *Atlas of Psychiatry*, https://doi.org/10.1007/978-3-031-15401-0_9

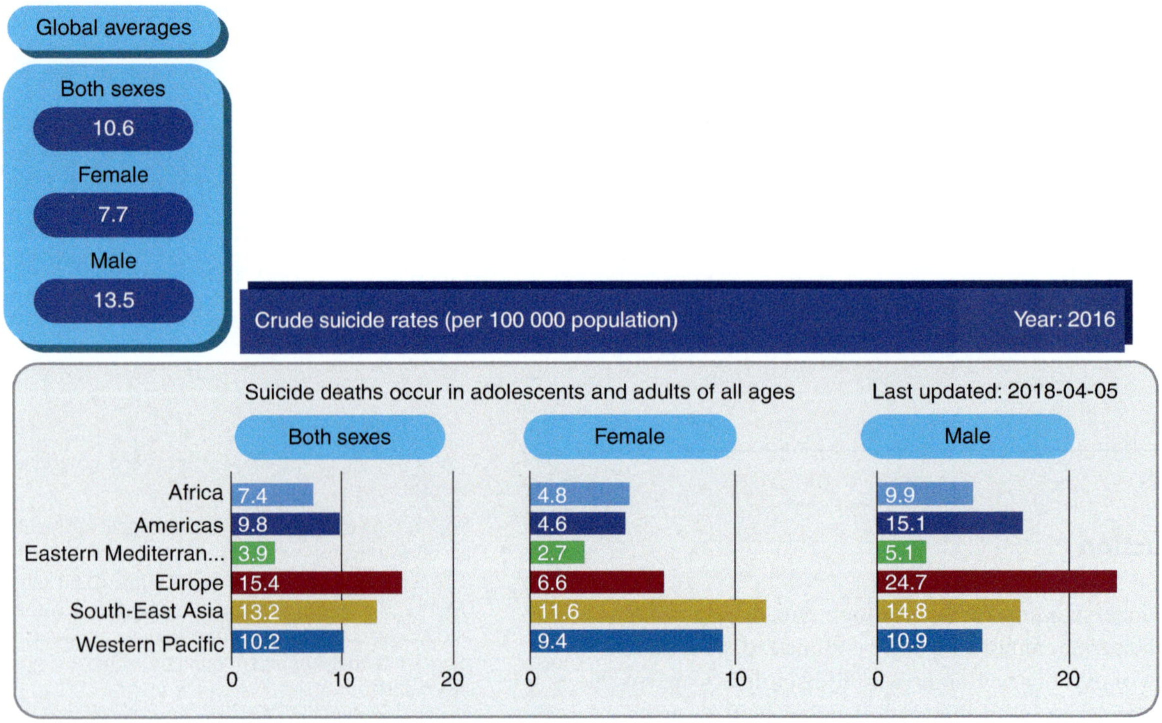

Fig. 9.1 WHO crude suicide rates (per 100,000 population) for 2016 [4]

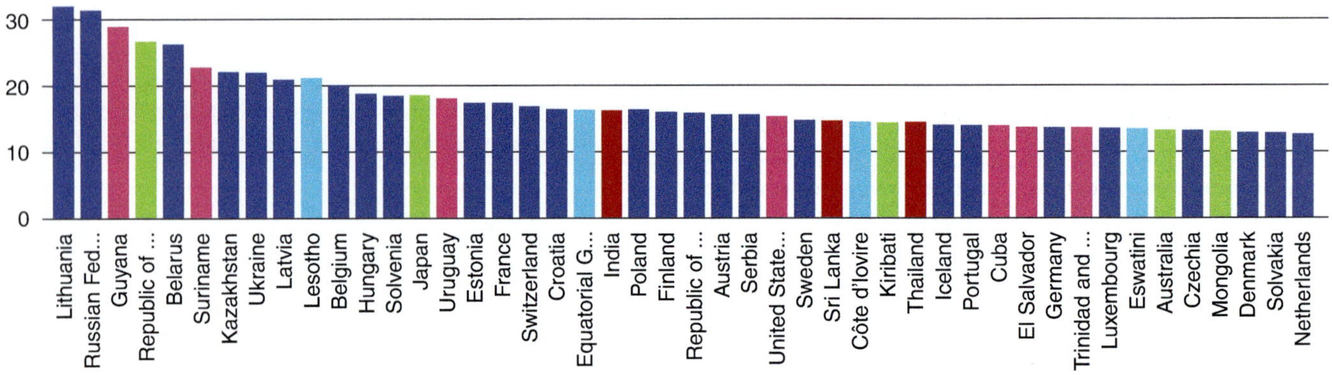

DisplayString	Africa	Americas	Eastern Mediterranean	Europe	South-East Asia	Western Pacific
Lithuania				32		
Russian Federation				31		
Guyana		29				
Republic of korea						27
Belarus				26		
Suriname		23				
Kazakhstan				23		
Ukraine				22		
Latvia				21		
Lesotho						
Belgium		21		21		
Hungary				19		
Solvenia				19		
Japan						19

Fig. 9.2 WHO crude suicide rates (per 100,000 population) for 2016 by country [4]

Fig. 9.3 WHO data on global number of suicides in 2016 in young people [4]

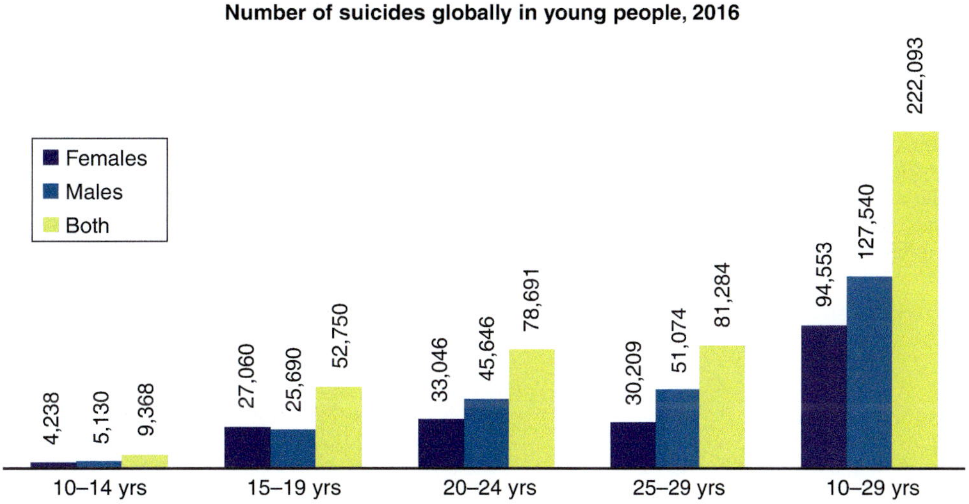

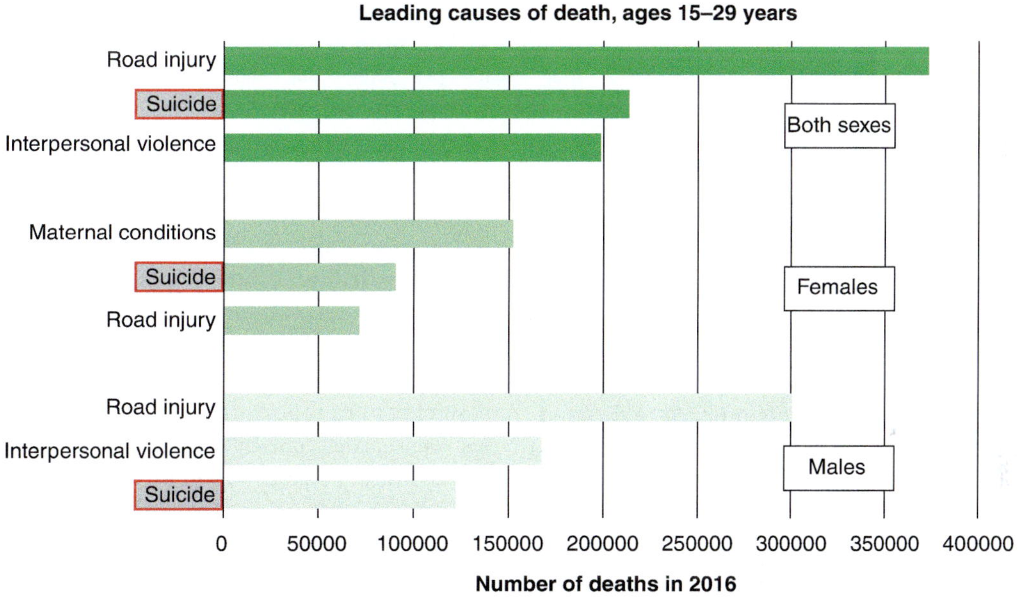

Fig. 9.4 WHO data on leading causes of death in 2016 in young people [4]

Fig. 9.5 WHO data on global suicides by age and country income level [4]

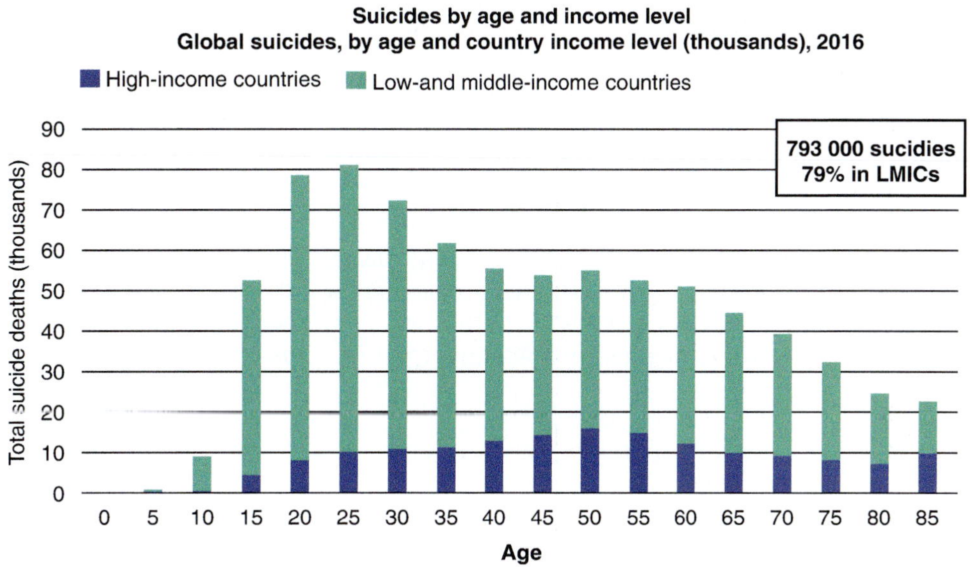

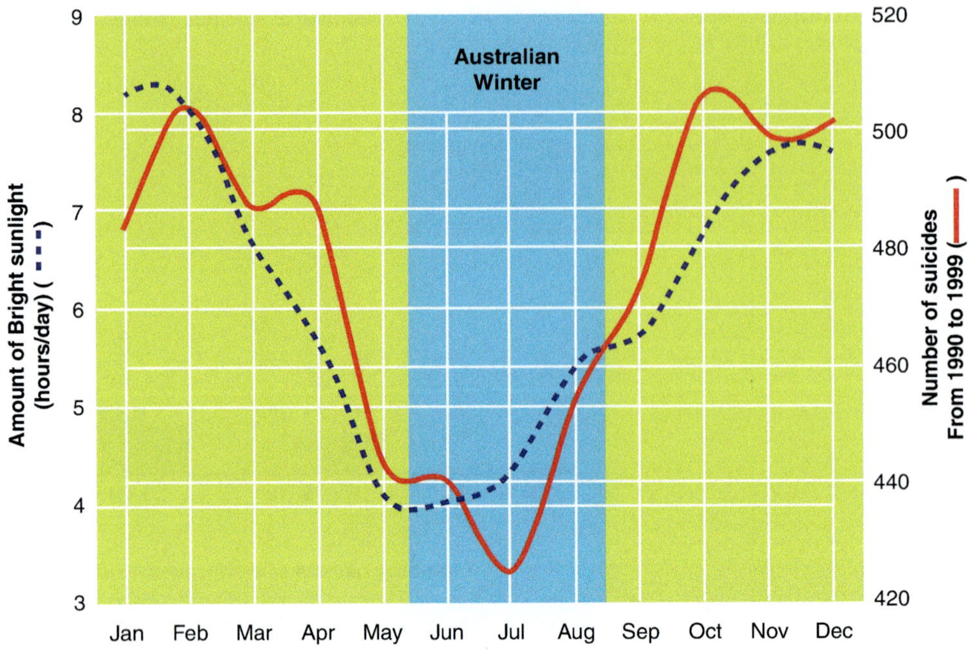

Fig. 9.6 Association between the frequency of suicide and the level of bright sunlight in Victoria, Australia, during the last decade of the twentieth century; each monthly value was calculated from the mean of the values of the previous month, the index month, and the following month [3]

Etiological Factors

A large number of putative biological factors have been implicated as risk factors for suicidal behavior. Chang and colleagues carried out a meta-analysis of longitudinal studies (through 1 January 2015) which tested the hypothesis that individual biological factors were predictive of suicidal behavior [5]. Over 2500 unique papers were initially identified. The process by which these were reduced to the studies included in the meta-analysis is shown in the Preferred Reporting Items for Systematic Reviews and Meta-analyses (PRISMA) flowchart depicted in Fig. 9.7. Table 9.2 lists the biological factors which were studied in this meta-analysis. In terms of the results of this meta-analysis, Fig. 9.8 shows a Forest plot of suicide attempt outcome cases with weighted mean odds ratios and risk factor cases, while Fig. 9.9 is a Forest plot for suicide death outcome cases, again with weighted mean odds ratios and risk factor cases. The conclusions of this large meta-analysis were as follows: "The combined effect of biological factors produced statistically significant but relatively weak prediction of suicide attempts (weighted mean odds ratio (wOR)=1.41; CI: 1.09–1.81) and suicide death (wOR=1.28; CI: 1.13–1.45). After accounting for publication bias, prediction was nonsignificant for both suicide attempts and suicide death. Only two factors remained significant after accounting for publication bias—cytokines (wOR=2.87; CI: 1.40–5.93) and low levels of fish oil nutrients (wOR=1.09; CI: 1.01–1.19). Our meta-analysis revealed that currently known biological factors are weak predictors of future suicidal behaviors." [5].

The vast majority of those who commit suicide suffer from a psychiatric disorder, including depressive disorders, bipolar disorders, substance-related and addictive disorders, personality disorders, and schizophrenia spectrum and other psychotic disorders. A systematic review and meta-analysis of suicide rates following discharge from psychiatric facilities was carried out by Chung and colleagues [6]. From 11,449 titles (1 January 1946 to 1 May 2016), they included 100 studies in their meta-analysis. Their key findings are summarized as follows: "…the postdischarge suicide rate was approximately 100 times the global suicide rate during the first 3 months after discharge and patients admitted with suicidal thoughts or behaviors had rates near 200 times the global rate. Even many years after discharge, previous psychiatric inpatients have suicide rates that are approximately 30 times higher than typical global rates." They concluded that all patients discharged from psychiatric inpatient facilities "have an enduring high suicide rate and should have ongoing access to health care resources."

Suicide is also associated with certain primarily physical disorders, such as multiple sclerosis, chronic pain, and epilepsy, and with infections such as *Toxoplasma gondii*, which is one of the commonest human parasites. Major life-stresses, such as the break-up of a relationship or financial loss, can be associated with suicide.

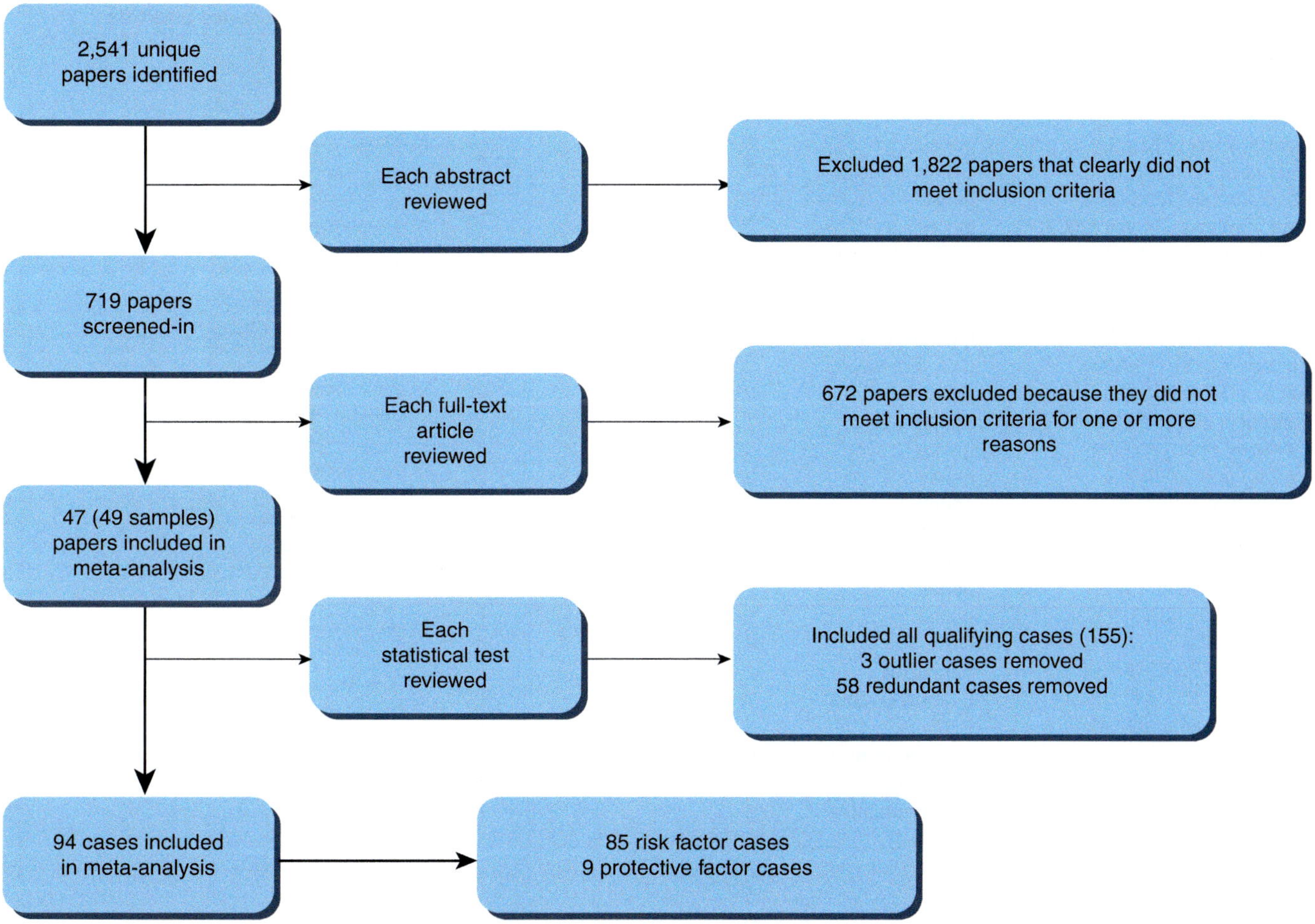

Fig. 9.7 PRISMA flowchart for the meta-analysis by Chang et al. [5]

Table 9.2 The biological factors studied in the meta-analysis by Chang et al. [5]

Blood-related factors: Glucose; cholesterol; serum tryptophan ratio; plasma oxytocin
Cerebrospinal fluid metabolite: Serotonin; dopamine; oxytocin; norepinephrine; cortisol-releasing hormone; dehydroepiandrosterone
Cytokines: Monocyte chemotactic protein-1; tumor necrosis factor-a; vascular endothelial growth factor; interleukin-10
Genes: Serotonin synthesis (tryptophan hydroxylase gene); serotonin transporter and receptor polymorphisms (5-HTT, 5-HTTLPR)
Hormone challenges/tests: Nonsuppression (or lowered suppression) on the dexamethasone suppression test; fenfluramine challenge
Molecule binding: Affinity constant of platelet serotonin [3H] paroxetine binding; maximum number of binding site (Bmax) of [3H] paroxetine
Nutrients: Serum cholesterol level; omega-3; omega-6; monosaturated fatty add; saturated fatty acid intake and serum levels
Peripheral physiology: Systolic blood pressure; forced vital capacity

Methods

The WHO report that the commonest methods of completed suicide are pesticide ingestion, hanging, and the use of firearms [7]. The first of these methods accounts for approximately one-fifth of suicides worldwide, and occurs mostly in rural parts of low- and medium-income countries [8].

In the case of hanging, unless a long drop with a thin noose leads to decapitation, which is very rare, the pathophysiological consequences shown in Table 9.3 take place [9]. Figures 9.10 and 9.11 show postmortem CT images from two men who hanged themselves.

Table 9.4 gives the commonest entrance wounds in those who commit suicide using firearms. The most common, in right-handed subjects, is the right temporal, as shown in Fig. 9.12.

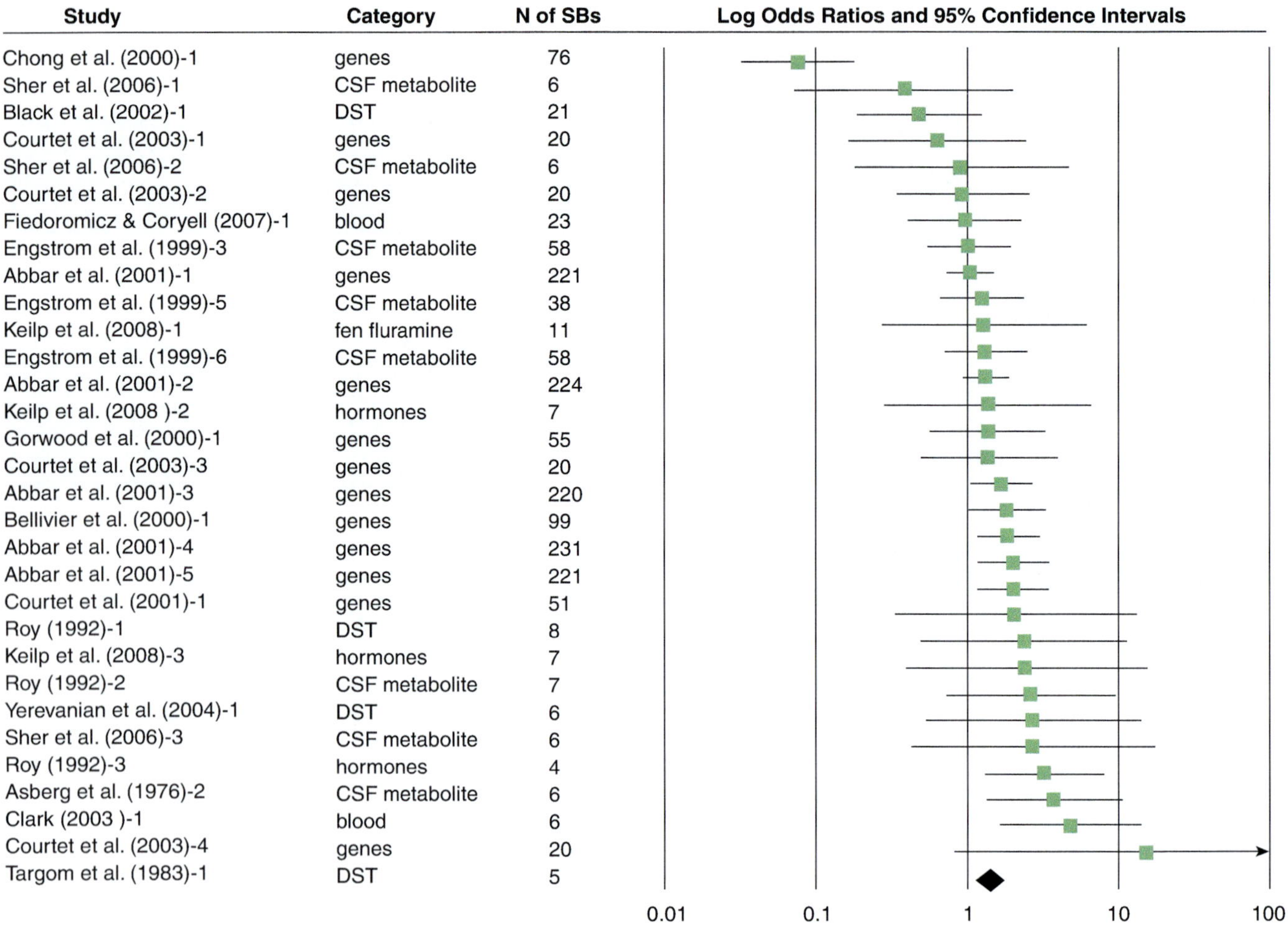

Fig. 9.8 Forest plot of suicide attempt outcome cases from the meta-analysis by Chang et al. [5]. *CSF* cerebrospinal fluid, *N of SBs* number engaging in suicide behavior

Suicide may be attempted in unusual ways in patients with schizophrenia spectrum and related psychotic disorders; this particularly applies to male patients. Figure 9.13 shows one such example of a patient who was seen by the author [10].

Assessment

The assessment of a potentially suicidal person should include a detailed exploration of any suicidal thoughts that he or she may have. Asking about these does not appear to introduce the idea of suicide to the patient. Any positive answer should be taken very seriously. Most people who commit suicide in Western countries have previously expressed suicidal thoughts and have seen their family doctor during the previous month; indeed, most psychiatric patients have seen their psychiatrist in the previous week [3]. Potential predictors of suicide risk are given in Table 9.5; information about these may need to be obtained from others, including the patient's family doctor, his or her psychiatrist (if any), relatives, and friends.

Management

The management of a person at risk of suicide may include the measures shown in Table 9.6. It should be borne in mind that patients suffering from psychomotor retardation are at particular risk of suicide when their physical symptoms improve; if their psychiatric symptoms lag, then they may

Study	Category	N of SBs
Du et al. (1999)-1	genes	24
Crawford et al. (2000)-1	genes	68
Black et al. (2002)-1	DST	21
Ingairem et al. (1999)-1	CSF metabolite	8
Engstrom et al. (1999)-2	CSF metabolite	8
Du et al. (1999)-2	genes	24
Iribarren et al (1995)-1	blood	24
Lewis et al. (2012)-1	nutrients	800
Chatrittefix et al.(2013)-1	CSF metabolite	6
Lewis et al. (2012)-2	nutrients	800
Lewis et al. (2012)-3	nutrients	800
Lewis et al. (2012)-4	nutrients	800
Engstrom et al. (1999)-4	CSF metabolite	8
Nordex m et al. (1994)-1	CSF metabolite	13
Nordex m et al. (1994)-2	CSF metabolite	14
Nordex m et al. (1994)-3	CSF metabolite	12
Nerman et al. (1990)-1	DST	13
Jekinen et al. (2007)-1	DST	36
Irung et al. (2012)-1	cytokines	7
Ceryell et al. (2006)-1	DST	13
Aaberg et al. (1976)-1	CSF metabolite	2
Irung et al. (2012)-2	cytokines	7
Jekinen et al.(2012)-1	blood	6
Jekinen et al. (2009)-1	CSF metabolite	6
Trackman et al. (1981)-1	CSF metabolite	7
Chatrittefix et al. (2013)-2	CSF metabolite	6
Ellison & Morrison (2001)-1	blood	27
Ceryell & Schlener (2007)-1	blood	8
Jekinen et al. (2012)-2	CSF metabolite	6
Yerevanian et al. (1983)-1	DST	2
Irung et al. (2012)-3	cytokines	7
Du et al. (1999)-3	genes	24
Roy et. al (1986)-1	CSF metabolite	4
Chatrittefix et al. (2013)-3	CSF metabolite	6
Jekinen et al. (2009)-2	CSF metabolite	6
Irung et al. (2012)-4	cytokines	7
Roy et. al (1986)-2	DST	4
Samuelmon et al. (2006)-1	CSF metabolite	6
Jekinen & Nordstrom (2003)-1	DST	6
Roy et. al (1986)-3	CSF metabolite	4
Yerevanian et al. (2004)-2	DST	3
Zureik et al. (1996)-3	blood	32

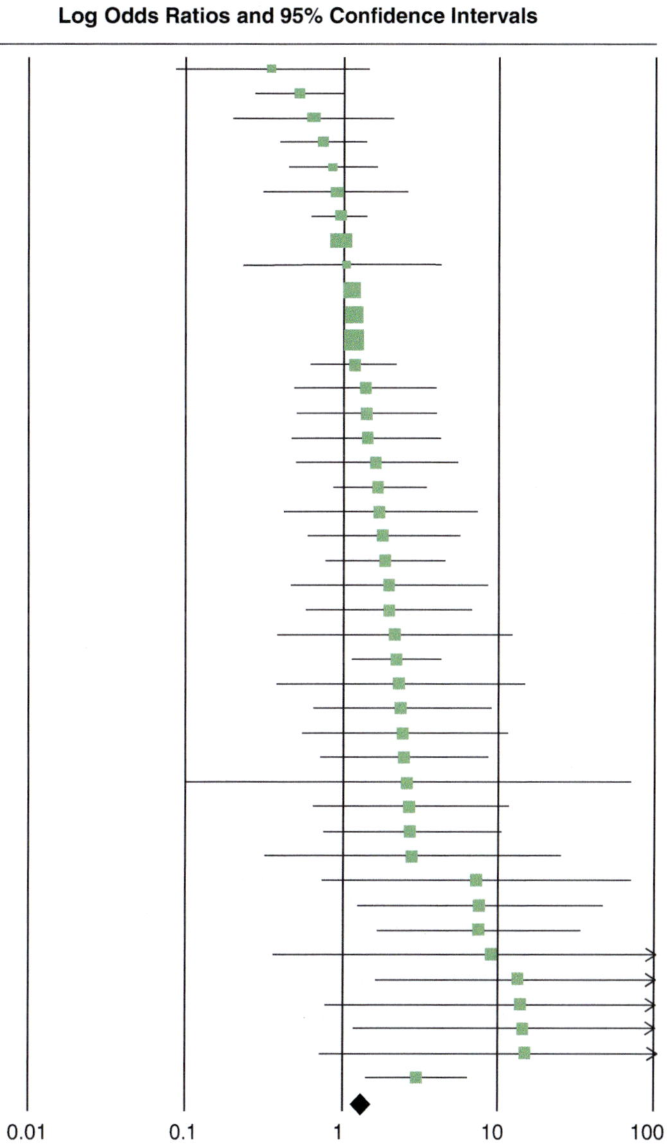

Fig. 9.9 Forest plot of suicide attempt outcome cases from the meta-analysis by Chang et al. [5]. *CSF* cerebrospinal fluid, *N of SBs* number engaging in suicide behavior

Table 9.3 Pathophysiological consequences of self-hanging, based on details in [9]

Physical cause	Consequence
Mild to moderate force of ligature on neck	Jugular vein compression • Facial & cerebral edema • Loss of consciousness
Moderate to strong force of ligature on neck	Carotid artery compression followed by vertebral artery compression • Cerebral ischemia Pressure on carotid artery nerve ganglion • Cardiac arrest
Very strong force of ligature on neck	Tracheal compression
Tongue being pushed posteriorly against posterior pharyngeal wall	Asphyxia
Ligature knot not placed anteriorly	Hyoid bone fracture Laryngeal cartilage (especially thyroid cartilage) fracture
Ligature	Muscle injury (especially the sternocleidomastoid)
Long drop (similar to a long-drop judicial hanging)	Cervical vertebral injury (especially to C2)

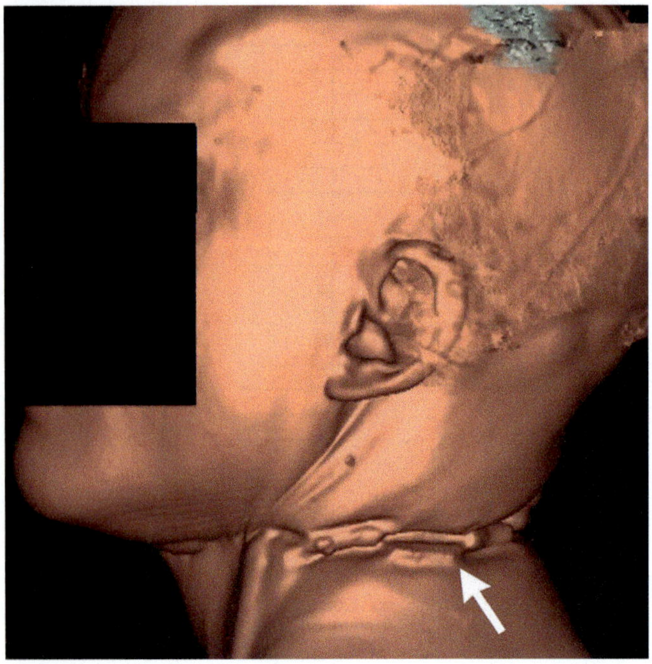

Fig. 9.10 3D volume rendered postmortem CT image from a 26-year-old man who hanged himself. The arrow points to the ligature mark on the posterior neck which resulted from an anterior position of the knot [9]

enter a phase when they are still suicidal but now have enough energy to enact a plan of suicide.

D'Anci et al. carried out a systematic qualitative review of treatment, both pharmacological and non-pharmacological, for the prevention and management of suicide [11]. They concluded that both cognitive behavioral therapy (CBT) and dialectical behavior therapy "showed modest benefit in reducing suicidal ideation" and that "CBT also reduced suicide attempts compared with [treatment as usual]" [11]. In terms of phamacological treatments, both ketamine and lithium were found to reduce the rate of suicide compared with placebo.

Table 9.4 Site of entry wound in suicides by firearms [9]

Site	Percentage
Head	75
• Right temporal	67
• Mouth	16
• Frontal	7
• Left temporal	6
• Below the chin	2
Chest	15
Abdomen	3

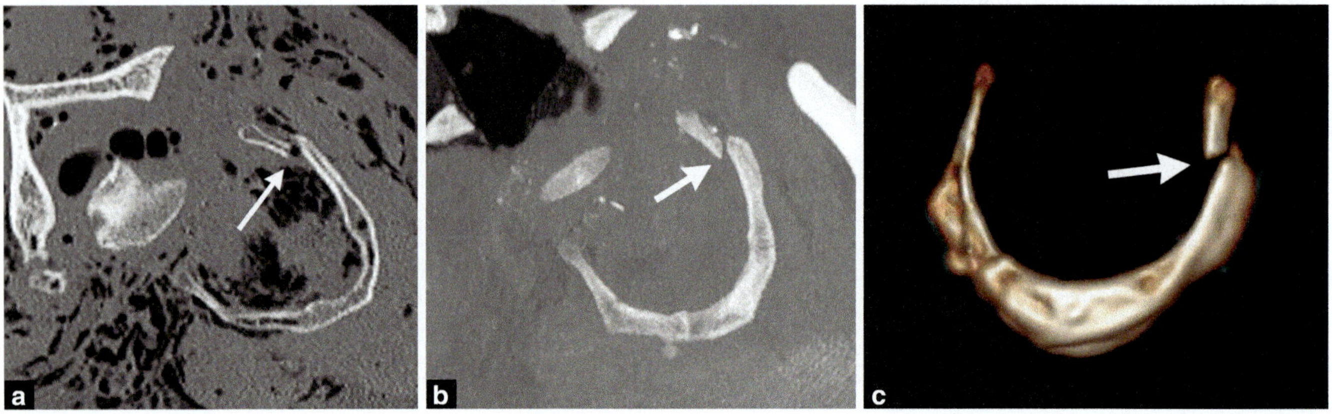

Fig. 9.11 (**a**) Multiplanar, (**b**) maximum intensity projection, and (**c**) 3D volume rendered postmortem CT images from a 39-year-old man who hanged himself, showing a fractured greater horn of the hyoid (see arrow) [9]

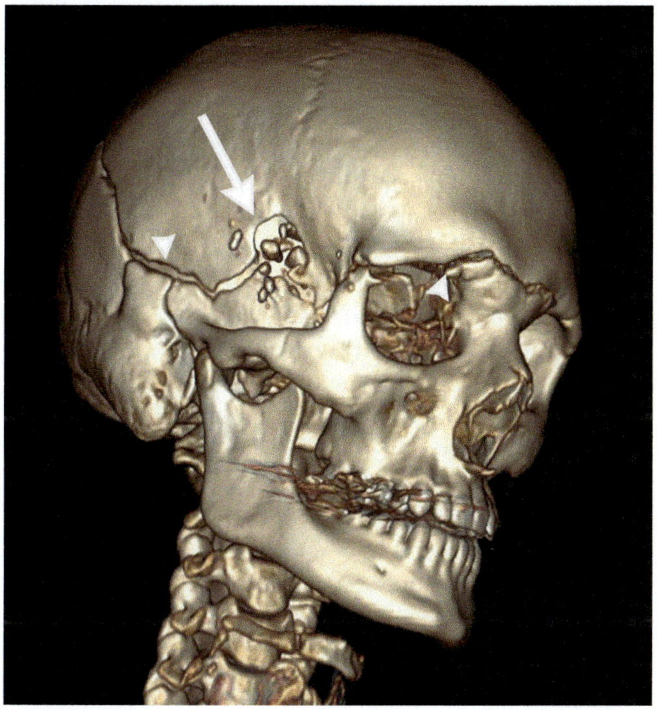

Fig. 9.12 3D volume rendered postmortem CT image of the skull of a 24-year-old man who committed suicide using a firearm; the right temporal entry wound is marked by an arrow, while arrowheads indicate associated radiating fracture lines [9]

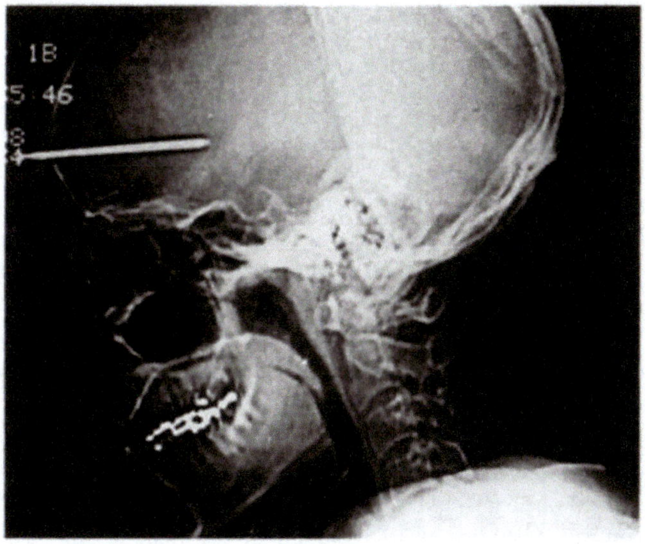

Fig. 9.13 Lateral skull radiograph of a 36-year-old male patient who, while suffering from persecutory delusions, tried to commit suicide by head-butting a three-inch masonry nail until it was fully driven into his forehead, as can be seen in the image [10]

Table 9.5 Potential predictors of suicide [3]

Potential predictor
A previous attempt to commit suicide
Expressing suicidal thoughts
Suffering from a psychiatric and/or physical disorder associated with increased suicide risk (see main text)
Major life stress
• Relationship break-up
• Financial loss
• Death of a relative or close friend
• Loss of employment
• Loss of position or status in society (e.g. following arrest for shoplifting)
Loneliness
Reduced or no social contacts

Table 9.6 Management of a person at risk of suicide [3]

Issue	Measures to be taken
High risk	Hospitalization, compulsorily if need be. Staff should establish a good rapport with the patient. Objects which can be used in a suicide attempt should be removed from the patient (e.g. belts, cords, shoelaces, sharp objects)
In-patient at very high risk	Continuous nursing observations. Patient to be accompanied at all times, even at night and to the lavatory or bathroom
Suffering from a psychiatric and/or physical disorder associated with increased suicide risk	If possible, treat the illness appropriately. In the case of severe depressive episodes, electroconvulsive therapy may need to be considered
Potential method(s) in the community	Reduce, or preferably eliminate, access to methods such as guns, medication which can be lethal in overdose, pesticides (for farmers in rural low- and medium-income countries)
Loneliness	Encourage social contact. Social work input
Recent bereavement	Bereavement counselling
Other major life stress	Counselling or other psychotherapeutic intervention

Violence

Introduction

The majority of violent acts are perpetrated by men. In their Declaration on the Elimination of Violence against Women, The United Nations defined violence against women as "any act of gender-based violence that results in, or is likely to result in, physical, sexual, or mental harm or suffering to women, including threats of such acts, coercion or arbitrary deprivation of liberty, whether occurring in public or in private life" [12].

In this section, the emphasis is on violence perpetrated by those suffering from a psychiatric disorder at the material time.

Epidemiology

The WHO estimates that, worldwide, presently one in three women has experienced physical and/or sexual violence, usually by an intimate partner [12]. The WHO also point out that one in two children aged between 2 and 17 years has suffered from violence in the previous year.

Etiology

Some potential psychiatric causes of violent behavior are given in Table 9.7.

Table 9.7 Potential psychiatric causes of violence

Previous history of violence	Including threats of violence
Schizophrenia spectrum and other psychotic disorders	Schizophrenia Delusional disorder Brief psychotic disorder Schizophreniform disorder Schizoaffective disorder Substance/medication-induced psychotic disorder Psychotic disorder due to another medical condition
Bipolar and related disorders	Bipolar I disorder Bipolar II disorder Substance/medication-induced bipolar and related disorder Bipolar and related disorder due to another medical condition
Depressive disorders	Major depressive disorder Substance/medication-induced depressive disorder
Trauma- and stress-related disorders	Posttraumatic stress disorder Acute stress disorder
Dissociative state	
Parasomnia	Rapid eye movement sleep behavior disorder
Disruptive, impulse-control, and conduct disorders	Intermittent explosive disorder Conduct disorder
Substance-related and addictive disorders	Substance intoxication and withdrawal
Neurocognitive disorders	
Personality disorders	Antisocial personality disorder Borderline personality disorder

At the present time, there is no strong association between violence and genetic polymorphisms [13]. However, there is some preliminary evidence pointing to a relatively low level in the cerebrospinal fluid (CSF) of the serotonin metabolite 5-hydroxyindolacetic acid (5-HIAA) in some violent offenders; an example is shown in Fig. 9.14 [14, 15].

In a follow-up study (carried out 6–8 years following forensic psychiatric evaluation) of 14 men who had committed violent offenses, the serum tri-iodothyronine (T3) was found to be positively correlated with measures of both detachment and irritability (Fig. 9.15), indicating a potential chronic change in the functioning of the hypothalamic-pituitary-thyroid axis in violent recidivists [15, 16].

There is evidence of structural brain changes in violent male offenders who were suffering from psychopathy or schizophrenia at the time of their offenses (Fig. 9.16) [17, 18].

Functional magnetic resonance imaging and neurospectroscopy studies have also indicated that violent schizophrenia is associated with significant cerebral activation deficits, poor phospholipid-related signal transduction, and changes in cerebral energy metabolism [19, 20].

Assessment

Table 9.8 summarizes the assessment of violence risk in psychiatric patients [21].

Management

Recommendations on behavioral and environmental approaches in the management of a violent patient are given in Table 9.9 [21].

Recommendations on the verbal approach to be used are given in Table 9.10 [21].

An important list of recommendations regarding patient-therapist relationship variables which can be helpful in the management of a violent patient is given in Table 9.11 [21].

A systematic review of pharmacotherapy for the treatment of aggressive behavior in general adult psychiatry was carried out by Goedhard et al. [22]. Thirty-five randomized controlled studies were included in the final review. The authors reported "weak evidence for anti-aggressive effects of antipsychotics, anti-depressants, anticonvulsants, and beta-adrenergic-blocking drugs". Within the group of antipsychotic medication, "Atypical antipsychotics appeared superior to typical antipsychotics." [22]

Fig. 9.14 CSF 5-HIAA concentrations in three patients who murdered or attempted to murder a child [14]

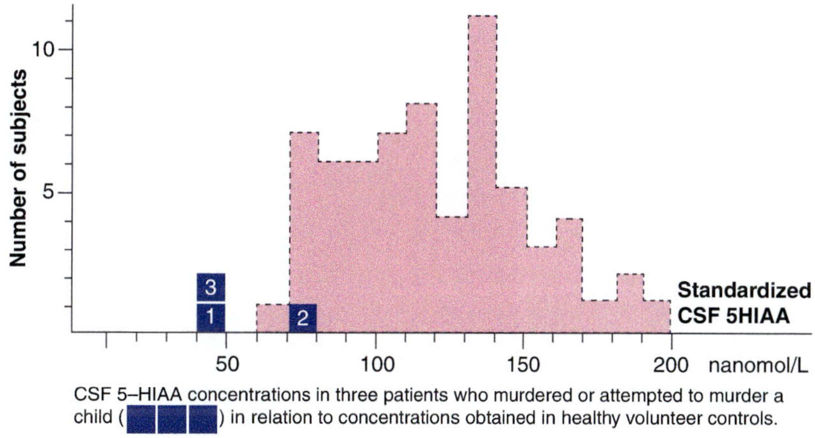

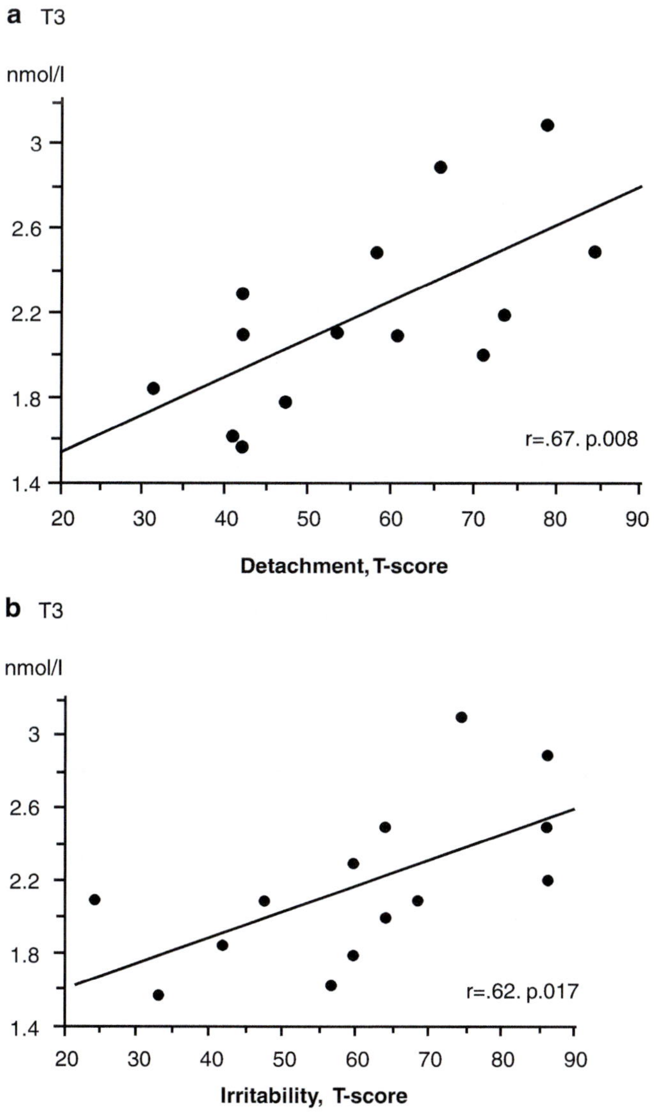

Fig. 9.15 Serum T3 concentrations versus Karolinska Scales of Personality ratings of (**a**) detachment, and (**b**) irritability, in 14 men with violent criminal recidivism [16]

Interestingly, several studies of lithium carried out on aggressive prisoners in the 1970s showed essentially positive findings. For example, Sheard et al. carried out a double-blind, placebo-controlled study of the effect of lithium on impulsive aggressive behavior in 66 male inmates of the medium security Correctional Institution, Cheshire, Connecticut [23]. The inmates were aged between 16 and 24 years, had been convicted for serious aggressive crimes, were not psychotic and were in good physical health. They received either placebo or sufficient sustained-release lithium carbonate (Priadel) to maintain a serum lithium level between 0.6 and 1.0 mM. The results are depicted in Fig. 9.17; treatment with lithium carbonate was associated with a significant reduction in aggressive behavior [23].

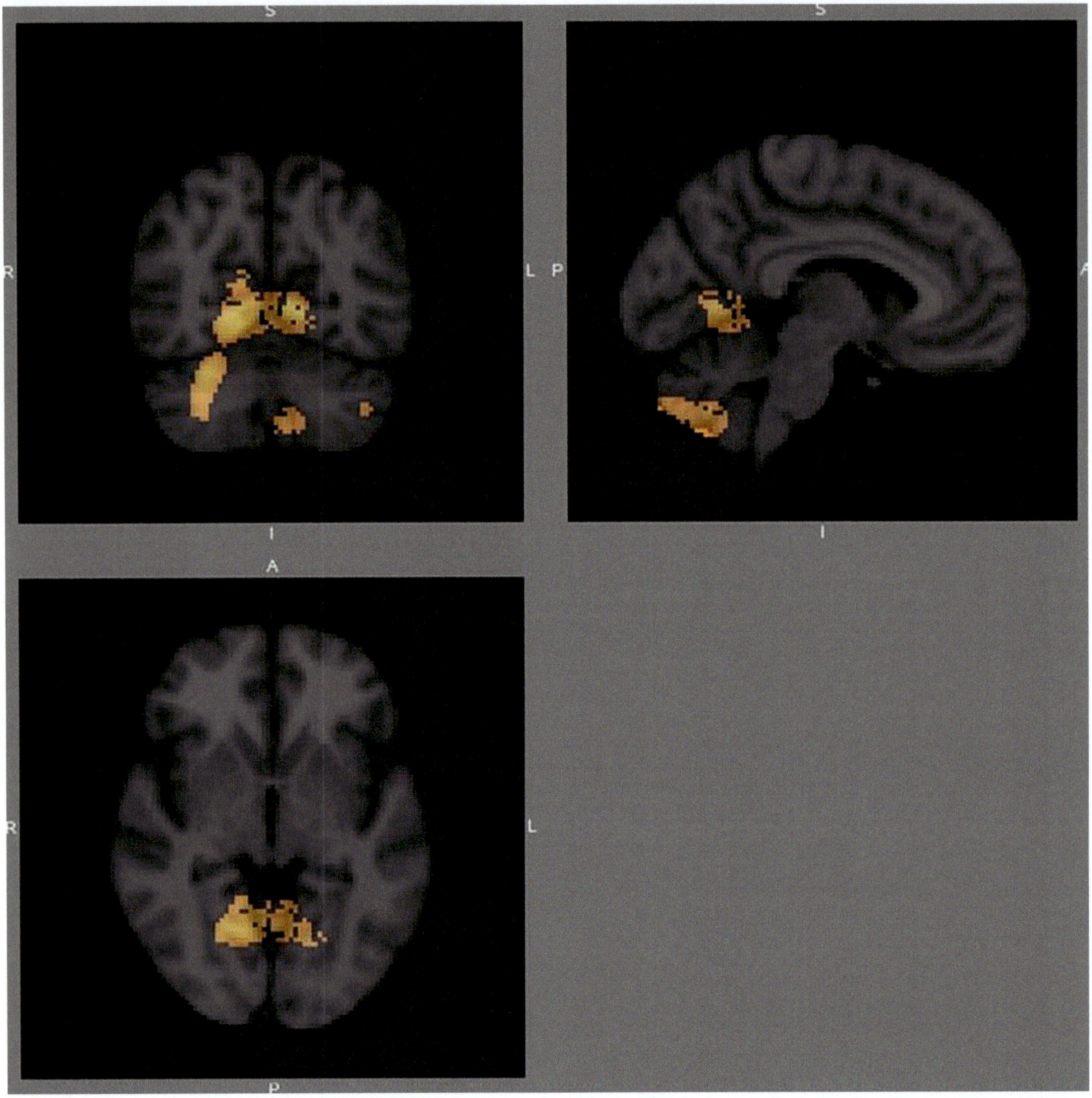

Fig. 9.16 Voxel-based morphometry study of 26 male patients with schizophrenia, half of whom had seriously and violently offended (homicide, attempted murder, or wounding with intent to cause grievous bodily harm) as a result of the schizophrenia compared with the other half who had no history of violence. The colored areas show regions with significantly reduced grey matter in the violent cohort [18]

Table 9.8 Assessment of the risk of violence in a psychiatric patient [21]

The risk of violence in psychiatric patients is associated with the following factors	
Demographic	Male Aged 15–24 years Low socioeconomic status Low educational achievement Unemployed Ethnic minority No supportive social network
Past history	Early victimization Violence Substance abuse Early onset of psychiatric disorder Poor parental model
Diagnostic	See Table 9.6
Clinical features	Command auditory hallucinations Paranoid delusions and suspiciousness Poor impulse control Poor insight Low adherence to treatment Low IQ Low global assessment of functioning score
Psychological	Low tolerance for frustration, criticism, and interpersonal closeness Low self-esteem Tendency to projection and externalization, anger, irritability Previous methods of coping with similar stressors Poor motivation and capacity to participate in the treatment process

From Rocca et al. [21]; *with permission*

Table 9.9 Recommended behavioral and environmental interventions in managing a violent patient [21]

A big room or area should be chosen	It should not be isolated, so that others can come quickly if needed
You and the patient should be positioned to allow both of you to reach the door easily	The door should be open You should be nearer the door than the patient, so that he/she cannot block your way out
The environment should be as calm as possible	Avoid intense environmental stimuli or triggers
Safe environment	There should be no potentially dangerous objects present
If a suitable room is unavailable, choose an open space	
Keep your distance	Do not be too close; the violent patient needs more room than others Never approach the patient from behind or in a rough manner
Never turn your back on the patient	
Do not be confrontational	Do not look the patient in the eyes Try to assume a neutral facial expression and tone of voice Adopt a relaxed body posture; avoid crossed arms or having your hands behind your back
Do not leave the patient alone	
If others represent a trigger for the patient's violence then ask them to leave	
Give information and support to relatives and significant others	
Debrief with the staff and if possible also with the patient	

From Rocca et al. [21]; *with permission*

Table 9.10 Recommended verbal approach in managing a violent patient [21]

Introduce yourself and explain what you are going to do
Use simple words and speak in short, clear sentences
Adopt a calm manner
Use a confidential but formal tone
Help the patient understand what is happening and reassure him/her about the diagnostic and therapeutic procedure to be undertaken
Help the patient restore orientation
At least at the start, prefer alliance-oriented questions
When possible, try to talk about the real motivations for the violence
Set limits of acceptable behavior and tell the patient that violations will not be allowed
Encourage the verbal expression of feelings, states of mind, fantasies
Discourage acting out; make clear that the patient will be held responsible for his/her actions
When you have to communicate your decisions, do so in a clear and simple way

From Rocca et al. [21]; *with permission*

Table 9.11 Recommended patient-therapist relationship factors to be adopted in the management of a violent psychiatric patient [21]

Make procedures as flexible as possible	
Prioritize the patient's requests, if possible	
Show empathy and talk about the negative aspects of the present situation	"I understand that this is not a good time for you" "It seems to me that you feel bad" "You look as if you are afraid of something"
Engage a therapeutic alliance	"In such a difficult situation, you need help" "Please allow me to help you"
Do not lie or betray the trust of the patient	
Do not challenge the patient	Do not be confrontational Do not look the patient in the eyes
Offer your help to discuss therapeutic aspects of psychiatric disorders	
Give help for problem-solving	Particularly for those who have difficulty coping, offer alternatives to violent behavior
Evaluate the presence of acute and chronic stressors	Particularly important if they act as triggers of violence and are related to past violence and victimization
Give reassurance for present or past paranoid features	
Be careful with gender issues	
If needed, give an opportunity for a time-out	Offer food and beverage If possible, allow the patient to smoke and/or to make a telephone call

From Rocca et al. [21]; *with permission*

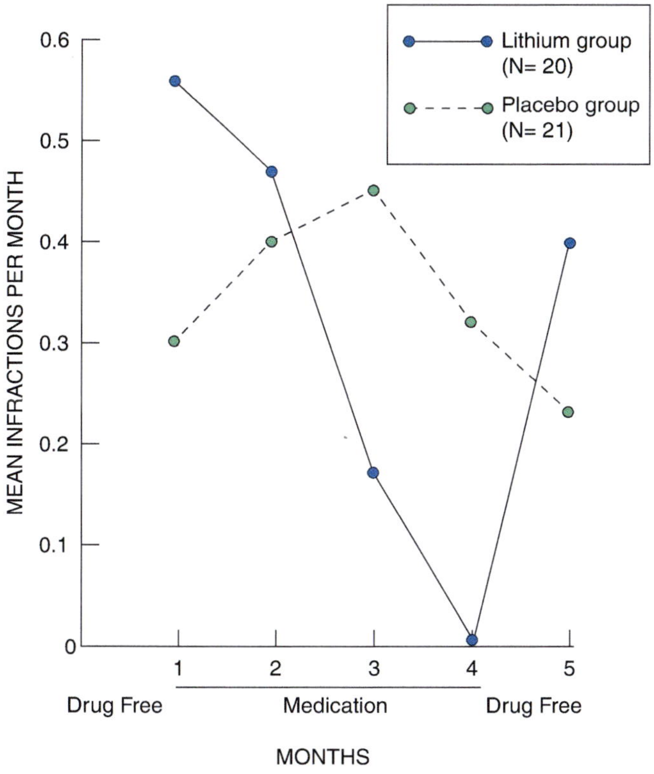

Fig. 9.17 Major infractions per month in prisoners receiving lithium compared with those receiving placebo [23]

References

1. American Psychiatric Association. Diagnostic and Statistical Manual of Mental Disorders, DSM-5. 5th ed. Washington, DC: American Psychiatric Association; 2018.
2. Puri BK, Treasaden IH. Textbook of psychiatry. 3rd ed. Edinburgh: Churchill Livingstone; 2011.
3. Lambert G, Reid C, Kaye D, Jennings G, Esler M. Increased suicide rate in the middle-aged and its association with hours of sunlight. Am J Psychiatry. 2003;160:793–5.
4. World Health Organization. World Health Statistics data visualizations dashboard. Suicide. https://apps.who.int/gho/data/node.sdg.3-4-viz-2?lang=en. Accessed 2 Dec 2022.
5. Chang BP, Franklin JC, Ribeiro JD, Fox KR, Bentley KH, Kleiman EM, Nock MK. Biological risk factors for suicidal behaviors: a meta-analysis. Transl Psychiatry. 2016;6:e887.
6. Chung DT, Ryan CJ, Hadzi-Pavlovic D, Singh SP, Stanton C, Large MM. Suicide rates after discharge from psychiatric facilities: a systematic review and meta-analysis. JAMA Psychiat. 2017;74:694–702.
7. Suicide. https://www.who.int/news-room/fact-sheets/detail/suicide. Accessed 2 Dec 2022.
8. Knipe D, Williams AJ, Hannam-Swain S, Upton S, Brown K, Bandara P, et al. Psychiatric morbidity and suicidal behaviour in low- and middle-income countries: a systematic review and meta-analysis. PLoS Med. 2019;16:e1002905.
9. Garetier M, Deloire L, Dédouit F, Dumousset E, Saccardy C, Ben SD. Postmortem computed tomography findings in suicide victims. Diagn Interv Imaging. 2017;98:101–12.
10. Puri BK, -el-Dosoky A, Barrett JS. Self-inflicted intracranial injury. Br J Psychiatry. 1994;164:841–842.
11. D'Anci KE, Uhl S, Giradi G, Martin C. Treatments for the prevention and management of suicide: a systematic review. Ann Intern Med. 2019;171:334–42.
12. Declaration on the Elimination of Violence against Women, proclaimed by General Assembly resolution 48 / 104 of 20 December 1993. 1993.
13. Puri BK. Genetics. In: Puri BK, Treasaden IH, editors. Forensic psychiatry: fundamentals of clinical practice. Boca Raton, FL: CRC Press; 2018. p. 115–21.
14. Lidberg L, Asberg M, Sundqvist-Stensman UB. 5-Hydroxyindoleacetic acid levels in attempted suicides who have killed their children. Lancet. 1984;2:928.
15. Puri BK. Endocrinological influences. In: Puri BK, Treasaden IH, editors. Forensic psychiatry: fundamentals of clinical practice. Boca Raton, FL: CRC Press; 2018. p. 15–9.
16. Stalenheim EG. Long-term validity of biological markers of psychopathy and criminal recidivism: follow-up 6-8 years after forensic psychiatric investigation. Psychiatry Res. 2004;121:281–91.
17. Puri BK. Structural neuroimaging. In: Puri BK, Treasaden IH, editors. Forensic psychiatry: fundamentals of clinical practice. Boca Raton, FL: CRC Press; 2018. p. 21–7.
18. Puri BK, Counsell SJ, Saeed N, Bustos MG, Treasaden IH, Bydder GM. Regional grey matter volumetric changes in forensic schizophrenia patients: an MRI study comparing the brain structure of patients who have seriously and violently offended with that of patients who have not. BMC Psychiatry. 2008;8(Suppl 1):S6.
19. Puri BK. Schizophrenia, psychopathy, and violent offending. In: Puri BK, Treasaden IH, editors. Forensic psychiatry: fundamentals of clinical practice. Boca Raton, FL: CRC Press; 2018. p. 29–36.
20. Puri BK. Neurospectroscopy. In: Puri BK, Treasaden IH, editors. Forensic psychiatry: fundamentals of clinical practice. Boca Raton, FL: CRC Press; 2018. p. 37–8.
21. Rocca P, Villari V, Bogetto F. Managing the aggressive and violent patient in the psychiatric emergency. Prog Neuro-Psychopharmacol Biol Psychiatry. 2006;30:586–98.
22. Goedhard LE, Stolker JJ, Heerdink ER, Nijman HLI, Olivier B, Egberts TCG. Pharmacotherapy for the treatment of aggressive behavior in general adult psychiatry: a systematic review. J Clin Psychiatry. 2006;67:1013–24.
23. Sheard MH, Marini JL, Bridges CI, Wagner E. The effect of lithium on impulsive aggressive behavior in man. Am J Psychiatry. 1976;133:1409–13.

10 Biological Treatments: Psychopharmacology, Brain Stimulation, and Innovations

Tiffany E. Schwasinger-Schmidt and Matthew Macaluso

Introduction

Psychopharmacology encompasses the diagnosis and treatment of mental illness with an emphasis on studying the effects of medications on the mind and body. A basic understanding of the principles of psychopharmacology is essential for all physicians involved in treating psychiatric conditions and must comprise a basic understanding of neuroscience including neuroanatomy, basic pharmacology including pharmacokinetics and pharmacodynamics, diagnostic criteria with the ability to formulate a broad differential diagnosis, and the treatment options available for each disorder [1].

Mental illness is estimated to affect one in five adults in the USA, which is approximately 46.6 million people, with a greater prevalence in women compared to men [2]. In 2019, approximately 23 million people received mental health services [2]. Major depression is one of the most common mental disorders that can result in severe impairments in functioning and has been estimated to occur in 7.1% of all adults in the USA, representing approximately 17.3 million people. The greatest prevalence of depression occurs in women aged 18–25 years [2]. Anxiety disorders are also common and are estimated to affect approximately 31% of adults within the USA with 23% of people with anxiety experiencing serious impairment and 34% experiencing moderate impairment in functioning [2] as assessed by the Sheehan Disability Scale. Bipolar disorder affects 4.4% of adults in the USA with 89% of patients reporting serious functional impairment, which is the highest among all mood disorders [2]. The exact prevalence of schizophrenia is difficult to determine due to the complexity of the diagnosis but is estimated at 0.25–0.64% of the population in the USA, 0.33–0.75% of the population internationally and is one of the top 15 leading causes of disability worldwide [2]. Individuals with schizophrenia have a significantly increased risk of premature mortality with an average of 29 years of lost potential life. It is estimated that 4.9% of people with Schizophrenia die by suicide with the greatest risk of death within the early stages of the disease [2]. In 2018, suicide was the tenth leading cause of death in the USA and claimed the lives of 48,000 people. Age-adjusted suicide rates have continued to increase from 17.8 per 100,000 in 1999 to 22.8 per 100,000 in 2018 [3].

The field of psychopharmacology has evolved from early studies that focused on sedation as a means to cure mental illness to the advancements in diagnostic techniques for earlier detection of disease, noninvasive targeted brain stimulation as a means of treatment, and the identification of potential biomarkers to aid in early detection, targeted drug development, and monitoring for the response to treatment. Through this long journey of the treatment of mental illness, pharmaceutical companies and researchers have worked together to advance the field and provide care to large populations of patients struggling with depression and other mental illnesses. It is through these advancements in psychiatric care that patients now have numerous options for treatment and the potential for targeted therapy using genetic and genomic information regarding drug metabolism within the body.

This chapter will focus on the history of psychopharmacology from the early investigation of plant-based therapies, through the vast growth of the pharmaceutical industry in the 1950s. Descriptions of the general principles of pharmacokinetics and pharmacodynamics will be used to provide a better understanding of what the drug does to the body and what the body does to a drug. The drug development process will be explored in detail from concept to post-marketing surveillance and will highlight timelines and the cost of developing

T. E. Schwasinger-Schmidt (✉)
Department of Internal Medicine, University of Kansas School of Medicine-Wichita, Wichita, KS, USA
e-mail: tschwasinger-schmidt@kumc.edu

M. Macaluso
Department of Psychiatry and Behavioral Neurobiology, UAB Depression and Suicide Center, Heersink School of Medicine, The University of Alabama at Birmingham, Birmingham, AL, USA
e-mail: mmacaluso@uabmc.edu

W. W. IsHak (ed.), *Atlas of Psychiatry*, https://doi.org/10.1007/978-3-031-15401-0_10

a potential compound for use in the treatment of mental disorders. Discussion of various therapies for the treatment of psychiatric illness with relevant neuroanatomy will be combined with new advancements in brain stimulation as a means for treatment. The chapter will conclude by highlighting the potential use of biomarkers as a means of early detection of mental illness and in the monitoring of treatment response.

This chapter is not meant to be a comprehensive review of all of psychopharmacology. Instead, the authors provide a high-level overview of the major topics of interest, recognizing that we have not covered every possible topic as it pertains to psychopharmacology and other biological treatments of mental disorders. Throughout this chapter, the reader will be referred to several additional textbooks and the primary medical literature for a full in-depth review of psychopharmacology. We have endeavored to cite books that are commonly used for teaching purposes at our institutions but have not listed every possible resource, textbook, or teaching tool.

Brief History of Psychopharmacology with Landmark Theories and Concepts

The history of drug development for treating psychiatric illness began as early as 1826 when French physicians began investigating the effects of natural, plant-based substances as potential treatments for mental disorders. Pierre-Alexandre Chavet has been credited with conducting initial studies in comparative psychopharmacology through the administration of opium to a variety of species in order to study the effects of this compound on animals [4]. These early experiments were followed by the work of Jacques-Joseph Moreau who was the first person to suggest a model of psychosis, which was derived from studies comparing the mental status induced using hashish to that of persons with mental illness [4, 5]. In 1859, Paolo Mantegazza was the first to introduce a comprehensive classification of psychoactive plants and plant extracts for use in the treatment of mental illness [4]. Following this pioneering work in understanding the effects of natural substances on the brain, numerous drugs were developed for the treatment of mentally ill patients with an early emphasis on achieving sedation, deep sleep, and a treatment for convulsions [5–7] (Table 10.1).

Table 10.1 Medications used in early psychopharmacology

Medication name	First use as a therapy	Indication
Morphine	1855	Sedative for excitement agitation and aggression, pain reliever, antidepressant
Potassium bromide	1857	Sedative, anticonvulsant, anxiolytic
Atropine	1860s	Drowsiness
Hyoscyamine	1860s	Drowsiness and sleep induction
Chloral hydrate	1869	Hypnotic, sleep induction,
Lithium	1870s	Gout, mania, antidepressant Bipolar disorder
Scopolamine	1880s	Drowsiness
Barbital	1912	Hypnotic, sedative, anticonvulsant, general anesthetic, insomnia
Insulin	1927	Sedation, anticonvulsant, coma, appetite stimulant, morphine withdrawal, schizophrenia
Amphetamine	1935	Antidepressant, ADHD, narcolepsy, appetite suppressant
Camphor	1937	Anticonvulsant
Iproniazid	1951	Antidepressant
Chlorpromazine	1952	Antipsychotic, mania
Reserpine	1953	Antipsychotic
Meprobamate	1955	Anxiolytic, sedative, hypnotic, muscle relaxant, anesthetic
Imipramine	1957	Antidepressant, sedative
Haloperidol	1958	Antipsychotic, sedative
Chlordiazepoxide	1960	Anxiolytic, muscle relaxant, anticonvulsant
Amitriptyline	1961	Antidepressant
Clozapine	1971	Antipsychotic

Pharmacotherapy for the treatment of mental illness progressed in three distinct phases beginning in 1808 with Dalton's atomic theory that indestructible, invisible atoms are the origin of matter in the universe. At the same time, a parallel recognition of mental illness as an organic syndrome with morphological changes observed in the brain was emerging [5]. During the late 1800s, scientists began to characterize the functional units of the brain with the most notable discoveries including the neuron as the morphological and functional unit of the nervous system by Ramon y Cajal in 1890 and the demonstration of the synapse as the functional site of neurotransmission by Sherrington in 1897 [5].

During this period in history, organic chemistry became a focus of several Swiss dye companies that formed the foundation for the growth of the pharmaceutical industry during the nineteenth century [5, 7]. One of the first medications that were widely used to treat psychiatric illness was morphine, which was initially isolated from opium in 1804, but was not used for the treatment of agitation and aggression for patients in psychiatric hospitals until the 1850s due to the invention of the hypodermic needle [4, 5, 7]. Potassium bromide, which was the second most widely used medication, initially isolated from seawater in 1826, became widely used as an antiepileptic and sedative for restlessness and anxiety in the 1850s [4, 7]. The third leading medication developed during this early phase of pharmacology was chloral hydrate which was first synthesized in 1832 but was not used until the late 1860s as a treatment for insomnia [4, 7]. The use of these medications in early psychiatry created a paradigm shift in treatment allowing for sedation to treat extremes in behavior and aggression rather than the use of physical restraints [4, 5, 7]. During this same time frame, the origins of psychiatry and understanding of the underlying changes in the brain in psychiatric illness began to emerge. By controlling extremes in behavior, early psychiatrists were able to better understand and study the phases of psychiatric illness and develop a series of classifications of mental illness based largely on observation [5].

The second phase of drug development occurred from 1900 until 1949 with a continued emphasis on behavioral control through medications that acted centrally on the brain [4, 5, 7]. Barbital, which was the first barbiturate used in clinical practice, synthesized in 1903 was used to induce sleep through hypnotic effects. By the 1950s more than 50 different barbiturates were used in clinical practice as hypnotics, sedatives, anti-epileptics, and general anesthetics [5, 7]. During this phase of drug development, insulin use became prevalent in psychiatry for the stimulation of appetite and for sedation in the 1920s, morphine withdrawal treatment in the 1930s, and as a treatment for schizophrenia in the 1940s [4, 7]. In 1935, the use of amphetamine and its derivatives became a treatment for Narcolepsy and for calming hyperactive children but was found to be of little use in treating depression. During this same timeframe, the use of nicotinic acid, penicillin, and thiamine in psychiatry led to a significant reduction in hospitalization for psychosis due to the treatment of pellagra, syphilis, and Wernicke's encephalopathy respectively [4, 5, 7]. In addition to pharmacotherapy, electroconvulsive therapy emerged as a treatment for psychosis during this timeframe [5].

The emphasis in the final phase of drug development occurring from 1951–1960 focused on psychotropic medications that were used to treat excitement, agitation, and aggression. Chlorpromazine, initially discovered through research with antihistamines, was first used in 1952 to treat delusions and hallucinations associated with psychosis [5, 8]. This was followed by reserpine in 1953 which was discovered by research into anti-hypertensive medications [7]. The antidepressants of imipramine and iproniazid were discovered in 1957 through investigations of the monoamine transport system, which was followed by the discovery of haloperidol and chlordiazepoxide as a neuroleptic and anxiolytic, respectively [5, 7, 9, 10]. The first tricyclic antidepressant, amitriptyline, was discovered in 1961 and by the 1970s there were over 64 psychotropic medications available for use in treating depression, agitation, panic disorder, anxiety, insomnia, schizophrenia, mania, and psychosis [4, 11]. The number of medications for the treatment of psychiatric conditions has continued to expand to over 700 different available therapies currently on the market.

During this final phase of drug development, a shift was made in the understanding of neurotransmission in the brain from a purely electrical-based event to a chemically mediated event [7]. By the end of 1950, six new neurotransmitters in the central nervous system were identified including acetylcholine, dopamine, gamma-aminobutyric acid, norepinephrine, serotonin, and substance P [5]. These discoveries stimulated the formation of psychopharmacology as an emerging field focused on understanding of the effects of medications on the brain and body.

General Principles in Psychopharmacology

Psychopharmacology focuses on the investigation and use of medications in treating mental disorders. This discipline requires an understanding of pharmacokinetics and pharmacodynamics in combination with knowledge of basic neuroscience and diagnostic criteria for various psychiatric conditions. Pharmacokinetics is focused on what the body does to a medication with an emphasis on understanding absorption, distribution, metabolism, and elimination [12–14] (Fig. 10.1). This information is used to determine the dose of the medication and provides insight into the behavior of the substance within the body [12].

Absorption encompasses the transportation of medication from the route of administration into general circulation [13]. Many medications used to treat psychiatric illness are administered orally with rapid and complete absorption in the small bowel and transportation to the liver through portal circulation [12]. These medications also tend to be highly lipophilic to be able to readily pass through the blood–brain barrier for effects on the central nervous system [12, 13]. Alternative methods of drug administration for psychiatric conditions are additionally available with each route having its benefits and drawbacks [12–14] (Table 10.2).

Bioavailability is the amount of medication that arrives in systemic circulation and is dependent on the method of administration [14]. This concept is especially important in orally administered medications as these substances must be processed by digestive enzymes in the stomach and small intestine before absorption by transporters into portal circulation for transport to the liver [12, 13]. Enzymes within the wall of the bowel and liver cells can metabolize a portion of the medication before reaching circulation through first-pass metabolism, which reduces the effective dose of the medication [12]. Alternatively, medications that can be administered intravenously have 100% bioavailability as the drug is directly injected or infused into the systemic circulation [13].

Distribution, or spread of medication throughout the body, is determined by the characteristics of the drug (size and binding ability) and physiology of the individual (volume status and protein concentrations) [13]. The goal of distribution is to deliver an effective amount of the drug to the target receptors to illicit the desired effect. Most medications used in psychiatry are highly protein bound and are thus affected by alterations in protein concentrations in the body

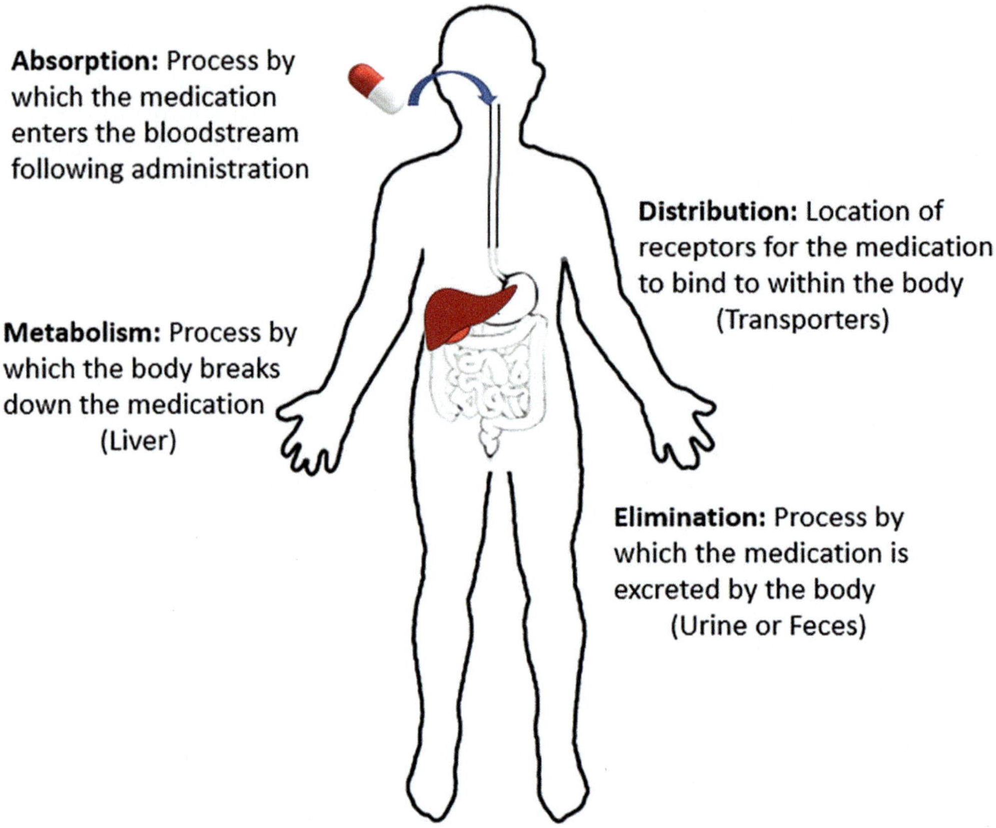

Fig. 10.1 Pharmacokinetic principles

Table 10.2 Routes of drug administration

Routes of administration	Benefits	Drawbacks
Oral	Safer, cheaper, painless, convenient for repeated and prolonged use, self-administration	Slow onset of action, unable to be used with severe vomiting and diarrhea, unable to be used in unconscious patients
Sublingual	Quick onset of action, bypasses first pass metabolism, self-administration	Unable to be used in children, bad taste
Rectal	Use in children and unconscious patients, little to no first pass metabolism, rapid onset	Inconvenient, slow absorption, irritation of mucosa
Parenteral	Rapid onset, useful in unconscious patients or patients with vomiting and diarrhea, avoids destruction in the stomach, used for irritants and drugs with high first pass metabolism	Sterile conditions, expensive, invasive techniques, not self-administered, can cause local tissue and nerve injury
Inhalation	Quick action, smaller dose, amount of drug can be regulated	Local irritation, increased respiratory secretions, bronchospasm
Intradermal	Slow absorption	Small amount of drug administered
Subcutaneous	Self-administration, can be a lipophilic substance	Volume limitations, slow absorption
Intramuscular	Rapid absorption, depot or suspensions can be used	Sterile conditions, painful, may cause injury to nerves
Intravenous	100% bioavailability, quick onset, large volume, irritant or hypertonic solutions can be used	Sterile conditions, local irritation, no self-administration, may cause tissue injury

including during malnutrition, aging, and with the use of other medications that can compete for binding sites. These factors must be considered when determining dosing of the medication [12–14].

Metabolism of most medications occurs primarily in the liver, but can also occur in the kidneys, lungs, skin, and gastrointestinal tract through enzymes that create active compounds or inactivate compounds for clearance in the urine or feces [13]. Within the liver, the majority of metabolism occurs through the cytochrome P450 enzymes, which are highly affected by other medications or substances in the body. For example, nicotine, alcohol, and anticonvulsants are all known inducers of the cytochrome enzymes resulting in increased enzymatic activity and thus lower drug concentrations; while fluoxetine, paroxetine, and antipsychotics inhibit specific cytochrome enzymes resulting in increased drug concentrations and potential toxicity [12–16]. Elimination primarily occurs in urine for many psychiatric medications as most of the medications have been converted to polar metabolites that are water soluble [12, 14].

Pharmacodynamics describes what the drug does to the body and is dependent on the effects and concentrations of enzymes, receptors, and second messengers [12]. Once the drug reaches the target receptors in sufficient quality, they activate or inactivate the receptor, which is dependent on whether the drug is an agonist (activator) or antagonist (inactivator) of the receptor. These interactions trigger a signaling cascade with resultant changes to the neuron or group of neurons producing a desired behavioral effect [12].

The half-life of a medication is the time necessary for half of the drug to be cleared from the plasma and determines the length of time for the medication to reach a steady state within the body [12]. The time for a drug to reach a steady state where the concentration of the medication has equilibrated within the various compartments of the body, including the brain, is five times the half-life of the drug [12]. Medications, like selective serotonin reuptake inhibitors that have a longer half-life will take longer to reach full effect with an average of 4–6 weeks. Knowledge of pharmacokinetics and half-lives determine the onset of action, length of action, and frequency of dosing [12]. These principles can be altered by drug-drug interactions, gender differences, and the effects of aging and disease state [12] (Fig. 10.2).

Drug Development Process

The development of new medications for use in clinical practice is a long and costly process that often begins through the identification of a biological target with a potential role in disease development or regulation [17, 18]. A review of drug development across all disciplines in medicine indicates that the process from idea to marketing of a novel therapy takes on average 12 years and costs anywhere from $1–3 billion with thousands of compounds initially tested to produce one potential therapy [17]. Central nervous system drugs, in particular, take longer to develop and have lower success rates compared to other therapeutic categories with an average approval time of 2 years compared to most other therapies at 1 year [17].

The phases of drug development can be separated into two broad categories consisting of "learn and confirm" [18] (Fig. 10.3). The "learn" phase starts with the discovery of a compound with the acquisition of information regarding pharmacokinetics, pharmacodynamics, dosage, safety, interactions, and early studies on effectiveness [17]. The "confirm" phase, however, focuses mainly on safety and efficacy in larger populations over time.

Preclinical studies and early clinical trials are smaller studies that focus on the dosing and safety of the medication [19]. Later phases of clinical trials shift to a focus on efficacy and side effects with longer enrollment times and increased study populations ranging from 300–50,000 participants [17–19] (Fig. 10.4). Phase IV studies focus on the confirma-

Changes in Pharmacokinetics in Females

Absorption and Bioavailability

- Exogenous estrogen increases absorption of many medications
- Lower acidic environment increases TCA, benzodiazepine and antipsychotic absorption
- Slower small intestine transit time delays absorption and lowers peak blood concentrations
- Protein binding is reduced in females

Changes in Pharmacokinetics with Aging and Disease

Increased Effects of Medications due to:

- Decreased Intercellular water
- Decreased protein binding
- Decreased muscle/tissue mass
- Increased total body fat

Fig. 10.2 Effects of gender and aging on pharmacokinetics

Phase 1:
Study Participants: 20-100 healthy volunteers or people with the condition
Length of Study: Several months
Purpose: Safety and dosage

70% of drugs move to the next stage

Phase 2:
Study Participants: Several 100 volunteers with the condition
Length of Study: Several months-2 years
Purpose: Efficacy and side effects

33% of drugs move to the next Stage

Phase 3:
Study Participants: 300-3,000 volunteers with the condition
Length of Study: 1-4 years
Purpose: Efficacy and monitoring of adverse reactions

25-30% of drugs move to the next stage

Phase 4:
Study Participants: Several thousand volunteers with the condition
Purpose: Safety and efficacy

Fig. 10.4 Phases of clinical trials for human subjects

Discovery → Preclinical testing → Phase 0 → Phase I → Phase II → Phase III → Phase IV*

"Learn" (Discovery through Phase II) — "Confirm" (Phase II through Phase IV)

**Approval frequently contingent upo agreement with the regulatory agency (e.g., the U.S. Food and Drug Administration [FDA] to perform specific phase IV studies to confirm findings or provide additional data on specific issues (e.g., a drug-drug interaction) or in specific populations (e.g., children and adolescents)*

Fig. 10.3 Process of drug development. (© 2011 Lippincott Williams & Wilkins. This content of this figure previously appeared in the Journal of Psychiatric Practice. The copyright in the figures, tables and illustrations in this article are owned by Dr. Sheldon Preskorn and are reproduced here with his permission) tion of initial clinical trial findings and provide additional data on drug–drug interactions and use of the medication in special populations including children and adolescents [18].

Once the developer of the medication has evidence that the drug is safe and effective for the clinical condition, the medication will be submitted to the Food and Drug Administration (FDA) for review. The initial application will include information about labeling, safety, potential drug abuse, patient information, directions for use, data from studies conducted outside of the USA and IRB compliance information [19]. If a drug receives approval from the FDA it will then be marketed and undergo post-market surveillance to continue to evaluate long-term safety.

Neuroanatomy

The pathophysiology of structural changes in the brain associated with mental illness has largely been centered in the frontal and subcortical areas of the brain including the prefrontal cortex, cingulate cortex, amygdala, hippocampus, thalamus, and basal ganglia [20]. Dysfunction within these interconnected areas of the brain has been associated with the development of mood disorders and mood regulation with related structural or functional changes that are observed in imaging studies [21] (Fig. 10.5).

Neuroimaging studies including functional MRIs and PET scans in patients with depression or bipolar disorder, for example, have shown reductions in the amount of grey matter in the left anterior cingulate cortex and the orbital and ventrolateral prefrontal cortex [21]. Additional reductions in the grey matter have been noted in the frontal anterolateral prefrontal cortex in patients with major depressive disorder and the posterior cingulate cortex and superior temporal gyrus in patients with bipolar depression [21]. Additional studies have shown reductions in the hippocampus in patients diagnosed with major depressive disorder [21]. Advancements in imaging studies have revealed differences in brain structure and function in patients with mental illness compared to normal controls, which can be used to monitor treatment response and may have a role in determining appropriate pharmacotherapy [22] (Fig. 10.6).

Antidepressants

The most recent data obtained from the Center for Disease Control (CDC) National Center for Health Statistics in 2011–2014 showed that antidepressants are one of the three most used therapeutic drug classes in the USA with approximately 13% of people over the age of 12 years on an antidepressant [23]. Females are twice as likely to be on antidepressants than males and a 5% increase was noted in antidepressant use from 1999 to 2014 in both genders [23]. While this class of medications is primarily used for the treatment of a major depressive disorder, these medications have also shown efficacy in treating generalized anxiety disorder, panic disorder, post-traumatic stress disorder, social anxiety disorder, obsessive-compulsive disorder, bulimia,

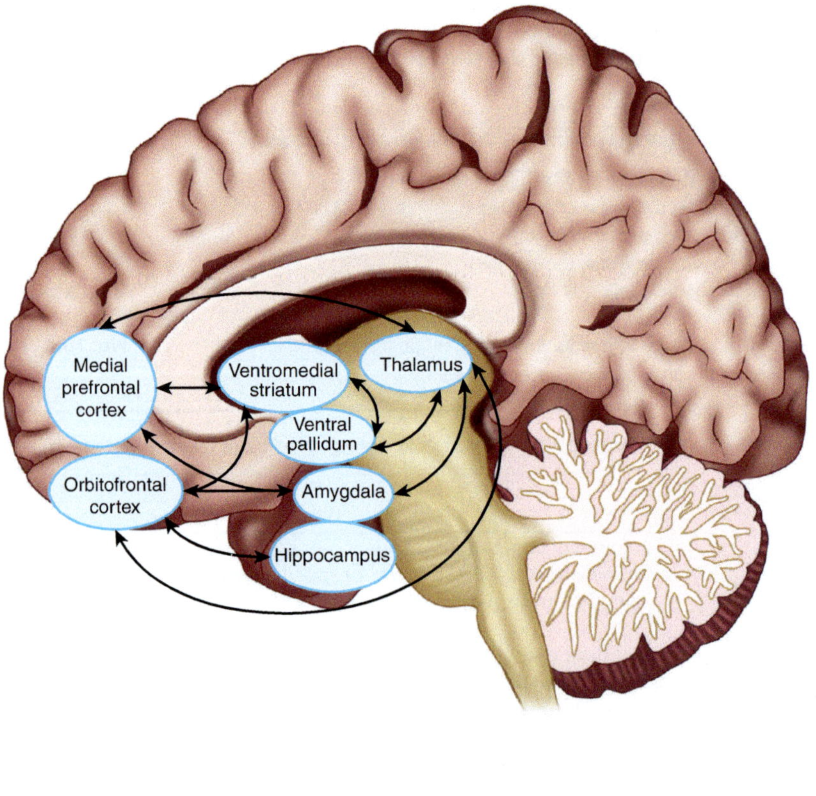

Fig. 10.5 Neuroanatomy of brain structures involved in mood disorders

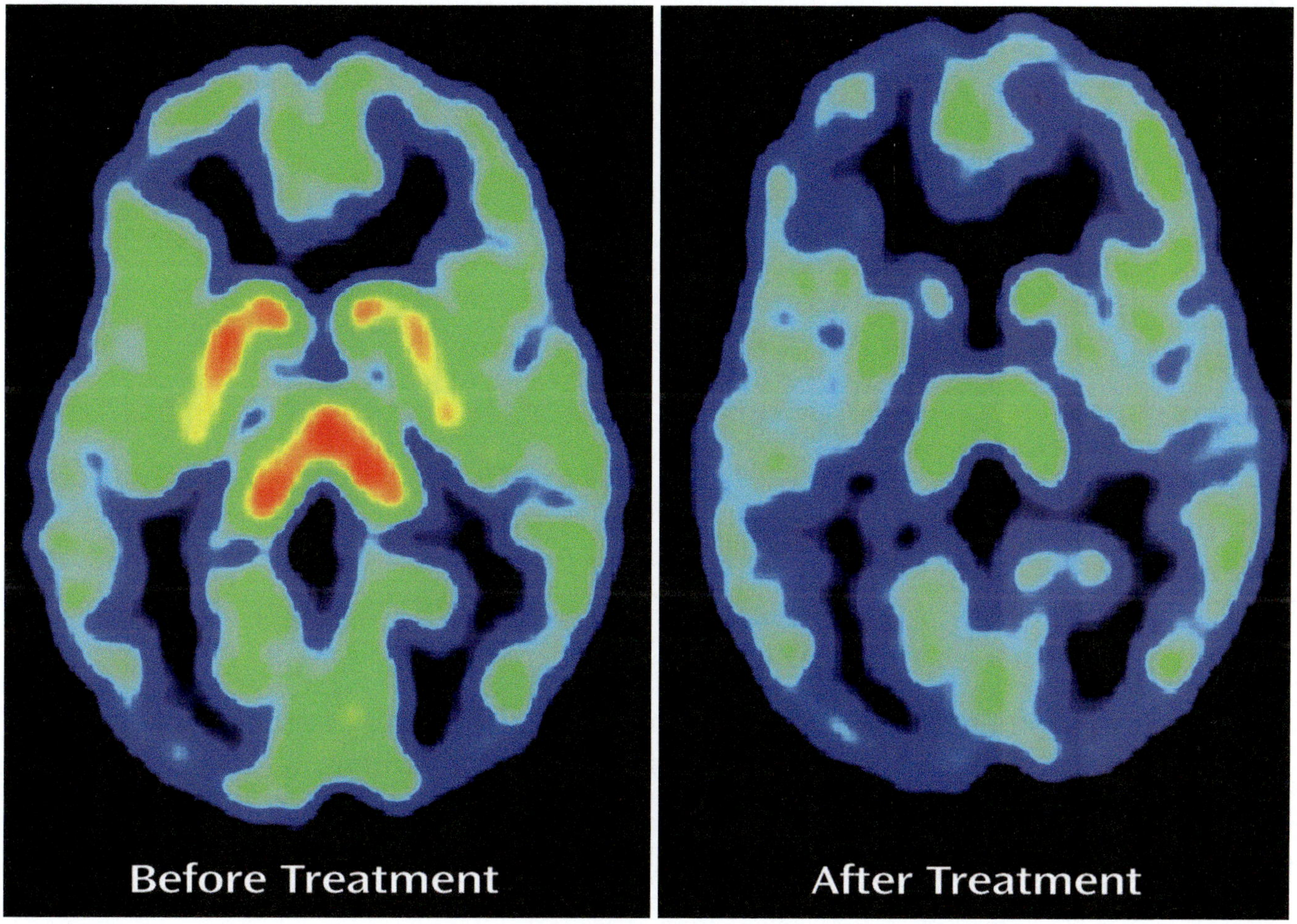

Fig. 10.6 PET scan of a depressed patient at baseline and following treatment

premenstrual dysphoric disorder, pain, fibromyalgia, smoking cessation, and enuresis [24].

One of the first medication classes used to successfully treat depression were the tricyclic antidepressants (TCAs) that were discovered through work in developing H1 antihistamines in the 1950s [25]. This class of medications was discovered in an attempt to produce an antipsychotic through modification of the structure of chlorpromazine. While the TCAs failed as antipsychotics, they treated clinical depression and allowed for the recognition of psychiatric illness as a medical condition, thus laying the groundwork for the future development of generations of antidepressants [26]. More than 20 different TCAs have been introduced into clinical practice worldwide [24–26] (Fig. 10.7) with an onset of action for the treatment of depression in 1–2 weeks with additional benefits noted at 4–6 weeks of therapy [9, 11, 27, 28] (Table 10.3).

Monoamine oxidase inhibitors (MAOIs) were pioneers in the treatment of depression and resulted in the discovery of the role of serotonin and norepinephrine in the development of depression. These medications allowed for the examination of amino acid levels in the brain during treatment which led to the recognition of neurogenesis and neuronal rescue, thus advancing depression treatment and the field of psychiatry [26]. Despite the concerns with food and drug interactions and the significant side effects, the MAOIs remain a third-line agent for treatment-resistant depression [24, 26] (Fig. 10.8) with an onset of action ranging from 1–2 weeks up to 3–6 weeks with an additional benefit in depressive symptoms noted at 4–6 weeks of therapy [29–32] (Table 10.4).

Selective serotonin reuptake inhibitors (SSRIs) were the first class of medications used for the treatment of psychiatric disease that were designed to target a specific site of action using receptor binding affinity technology [25, 33]. This was a novel approach in that prior drug discoveries were based solely on serendipity [6, 26]. SSRIs are the most commonly used drugs for the treatment of major depressive disorder worldwide due to efficacy, tolerability, and low incidence of side effects [26, 33]. These medications have proven efficacy for numerous other psychiatric conditions [24–26, 33] (Fig. 10.9) and can remain in the system for prolonged treatment duration given the longer a longer half-life of the drug. SSRIs take only 1–2 weeks to produce a clini-

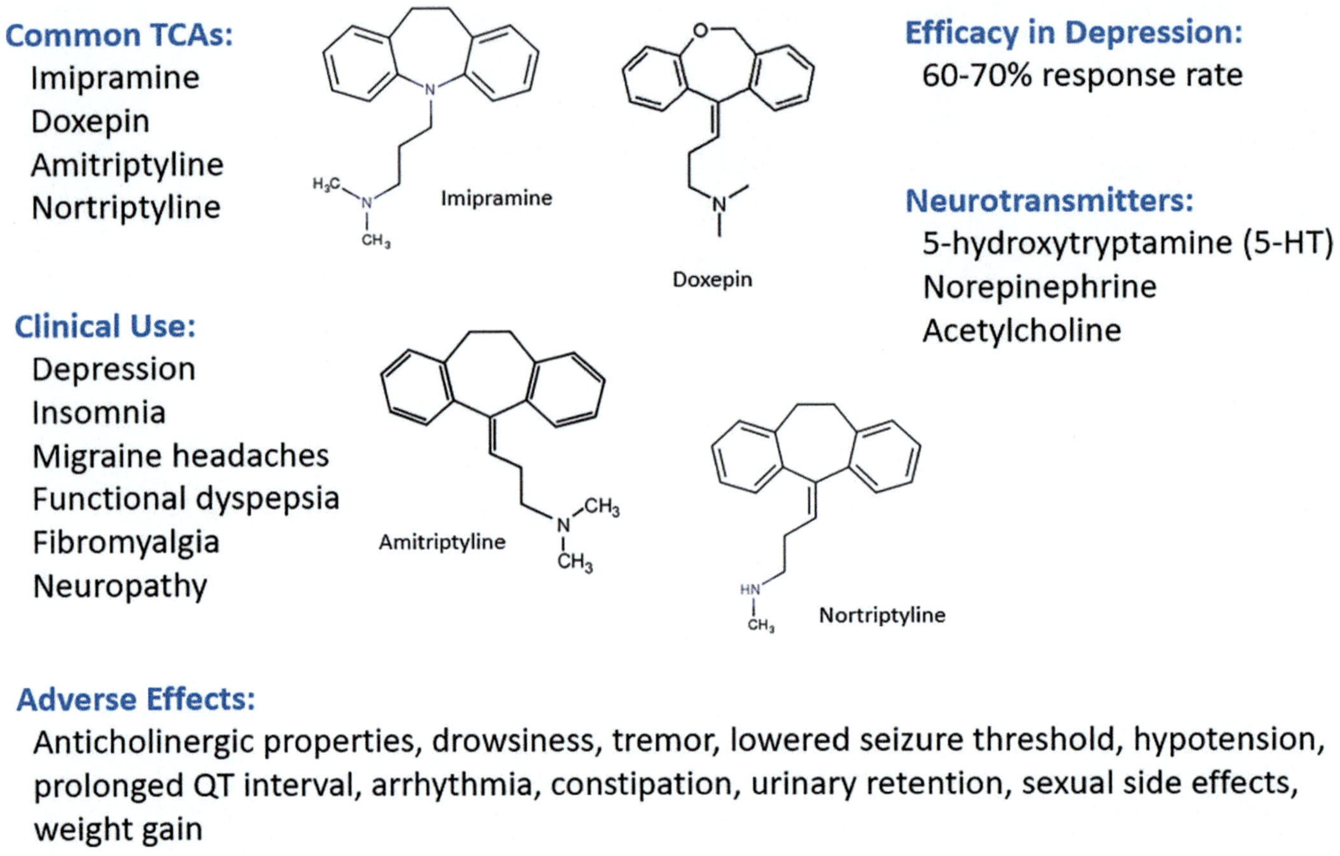

Fig. 10.7 Tricyclic antidepressants

Table 10.3 Pharmacokinetics of tricyclic antidepressants and onset of action

Medication name	Half life	Distribution	Typical dosage	Onset of action
Imipramine	16–17 h	60–96% protein bound	50–150 mg daily	1–2 weeks
Doxepin	15 h	80% protein bound	100–300 mg daily	1–2 weeks
Amitriptyline	13–36 h	>90% protein bound	100–300 mg daily	1–2 weeks
Nortriptyline	14–51 h	Extensively protein bound	75–100 mg daily	1–2 weeks

From the package inserts for each medication

cally meaningful response with full efficacy at 4–6 weeks [15, 16, 34–36] (Table 10.5).

Venlafaxine was the first selective serotonin and norepinephrine reuptake inhibitor (SNRIs) to be released for treatment of depression in the USA in 1994, and the extended-release version of this medication was the first antidepressant approved for the treatment of generalized anxiety disorder [24]. In 2004, duloxetine was approved as an antidepressant for use in patients with chronic pain and has shown efficacy in treatment-resistant depression [33]. Desvenlafaxine, which is the metabolite of venlafaxine with more potent effects on norepinephrine reuptake was approved in 2008 for the treatment of major depressive disorder [24]. Milnacipran was approved the following year for the treatment of fibromyalgia but has shown efficacy in treating depression. The SNRIs have been shown to have additional efficacy in depression and chronic pain syndromes [24, 33] (Fig. 10.10) and have dose-dependent side effects with an onset of action in 1–2 weeks with additional benefits noted at 4–6 weeks [37–41] (Table 10.6).

Additional antidepressants that do not fit into the major classifications but have an important role in the treatment of depression include bupropion, mirtazapine, trazadone, vortioxetine, vilazodone, and esketamine which target different areas of the brain [33]. Bupropion has combined effects on norepinephrine and dopamine neurotransmitters and is the only antidepressant on the market in the USA with no effect on serotonin concentrations in the brain [26, 33, 42] (Fig. 10.11). Bupropion has been shown to have similar rates of remission of depression as compared to SSRIs [33].

Mirtazapine was approved for use as an antidepressant in the USA in 1987 and works by increasing norepinephrine and serotonin release in neurons with an additional decrease in cortisol throughout the body through reduced corticotro-

Common MAOIs:
- Isocarboxazid
- Phenelzine
- Selegiline
- Tranylcypromine

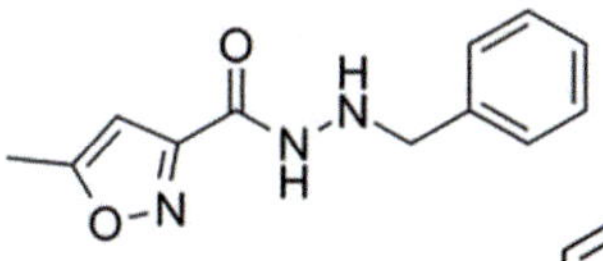

Isocarboxazid

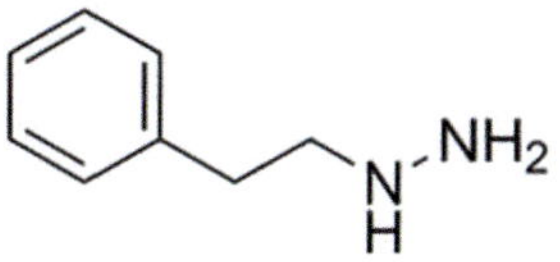

Phenelzine

Clinical Use:
- Depression
- Anxiety
- Parkinson's disease
- Social anxiety
- Panic disorder

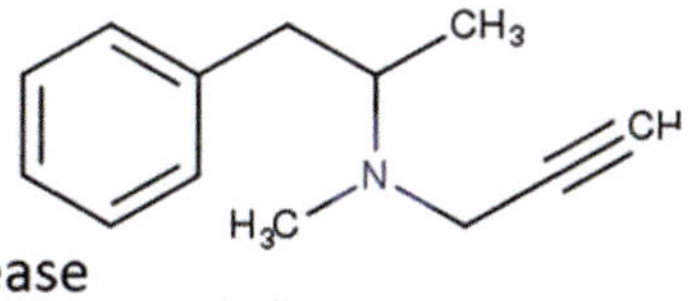

Selegiline

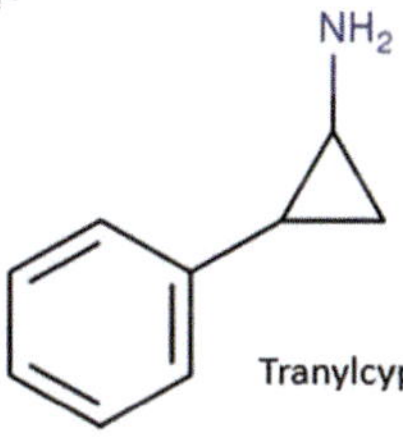

Tranylcypromine

Neurotransmitters:

MAO-A
- 5-hydroxytryptamine (5-HT)
- Norepinephrine

MAO-B
- Phenylethylamine
- Dopamine

Tyramine Containing Foods to Avoid:
- Cheese
- Red wine/Beer
- Yeast extracts
- Aged meats
- Fava or Italian green beans
- Liver

Adverse Effects:

Weight gain, hypertensive crisis, orthostatic hypotension, sexual dysfunction, dry mouth, insomnia, headache

Fig. 10.8 Monoamine oxidase inhibitors

Table 10.4 Pharmacokinetics of monoamine oxidase inhibitors and onset of action

Medication name	Half life	Typical DOSAGE	Onset of action
Isocarboxazid	1.5–4 h	20–40 mg daily	3–6 weeks
Phenelzine	11.6 h	15–45 mg daily	1–2 weeks
Selegiline	10 h	6 mg per 24 h	1–2 weeks
Tranylcypromine	2.5 h	30–60 mg daily	1–2 weeks

From the package inserts for each medication

Common SSRIs:
- Citalopram
- Escitalopram
- Fluoxetine
- Paroxetine
- Sertraline

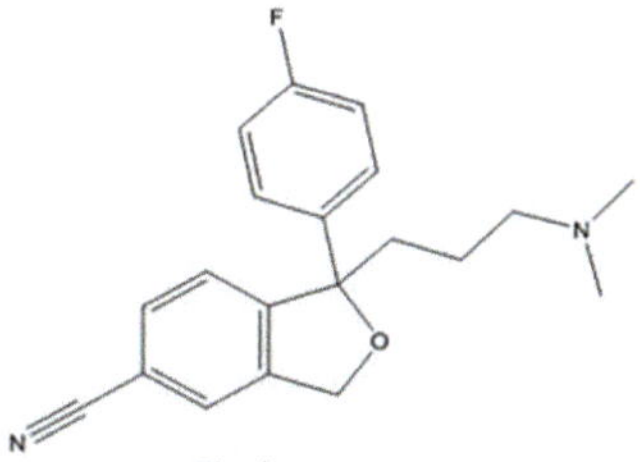

Citalopram

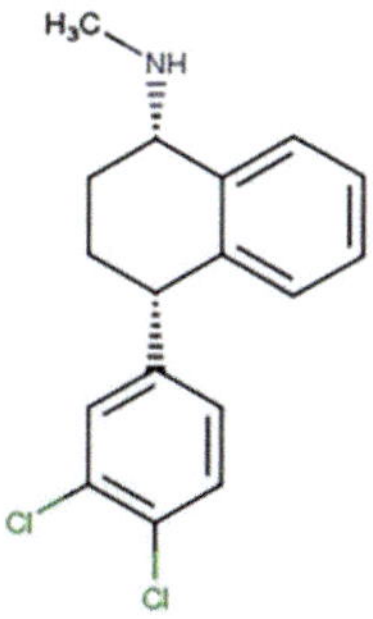

Sertraline

Efficacy in Depression:

60-80% response rate

Receptor Targets:

5-hydroxytryptamine

5-HT_{2A}, 5-HT_{2C}, $5HT_3$

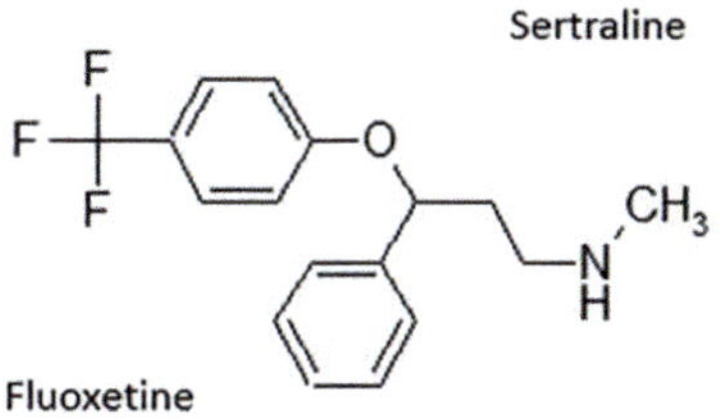

Fluoxetine

Clinical Use:
- Depression
- Panic disorder
- OCD
- Anxiety
- PTSD
- Bulimia nervosa
- Social anxiety disorder
- Premenstrual dysphoric disorder

Adverse Effects:

Nausea, diarrhea, GERD, decreased libido, delayed orgasm, headache, insomnia, dizziness, tremor, dry mouth, anxiety

Fig. 10.9 Selective serotonin reuptake inhibitors

Table 10.5 Pharmacokinetics of selective serotonin reuptake inhibitors and onset of action

Medication name	Half life	Distribution	Typical dosage	Onset of action
Citalopram	24–48 h	80% protein bound	20–40 mg daily	1–2 weeks
Escitalopram	27–32 h	56% protein bound	10–20 mg daily	1–2 weeks
Fluoxetine	1–3 days	95% protein bound	20–60 mg daily	1–2 weeks
Paroxetine	21 h	93–95% protein bound	20–40 mg daily	1–2 weeks
Sertraline	26 h	98% protein bound	50–200 mg daily	1–2 weeks

From the package inserts for each medication

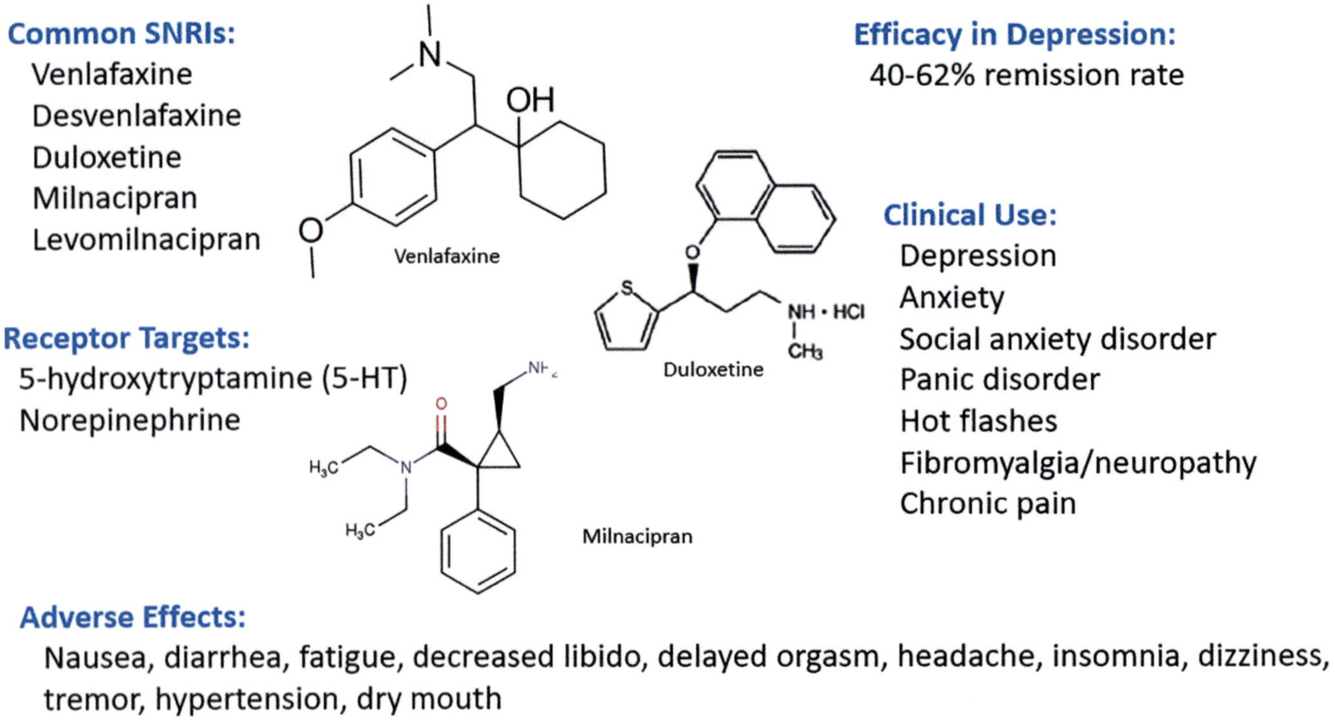

Fig. 10.10 Serotonin and norepinephrine reuptake inhibitors

Table 10.6 Pharmacokinetics of selective serotonin and norepinephrine reuptake inhibitors and onset of action

Medication name	Half life	Distribution	Typical dosage	Onset of action
Venlafaxine	5 h	27% protein bound	75–375 mg daily	1–2 weeks
Desvenlafaxine	10–11 h	30% protein bound	50–100 mg daily	1–2 weeks
Duloxetine	12 h	>90% protein bound	40–60 mg daily	1–2 weeks
Milnacipran	6–8 h	13% protein bound	100–200 mg daily	1–2 weeks
Levomilnacipran	12 h	22% protein bound	40–120 mg daily	1–2 weeks

From the package inserts for each medication

phin release [33]. Mirtazapine has been shown to have similar efficacy in depression treatment compared to TCAs, SSRIs, and SNRIs with continued response rates and lower relapse rates compared to placebo for up to 40 weeks of therapy [26, 43] (Fig. 10.12).

Trazadone was initially available in the USA in the 1980s and can be used as monotherapy or in combination with other antidepressants [33]. This medication has been used to treat numerous medical conditions but is the second most prescribed medication for the treatment of insomnia in the USA, which is an off-label use [26, 33]. Trazadone has been shown to be as effective as TCAs in the treatment of major depressive disorder with an earlier onset of action at 1 week of therapy [26, 44, 45] (Fig. 10.13).

Vortioxetine is a novel antidepressant approved in 2013 in the USA that targets the inhibition of serotonin transportation and 5-HT_{1A} receptor modulation for the treatment of depression [33]. Patients on this medication have been noted to have significant improvements in sleep, energy, and appetite within 1–2 weeks with the full effect of the medication on treatment of depression noted at 4–6 weeks [33, 46] (Fig. 10.14).

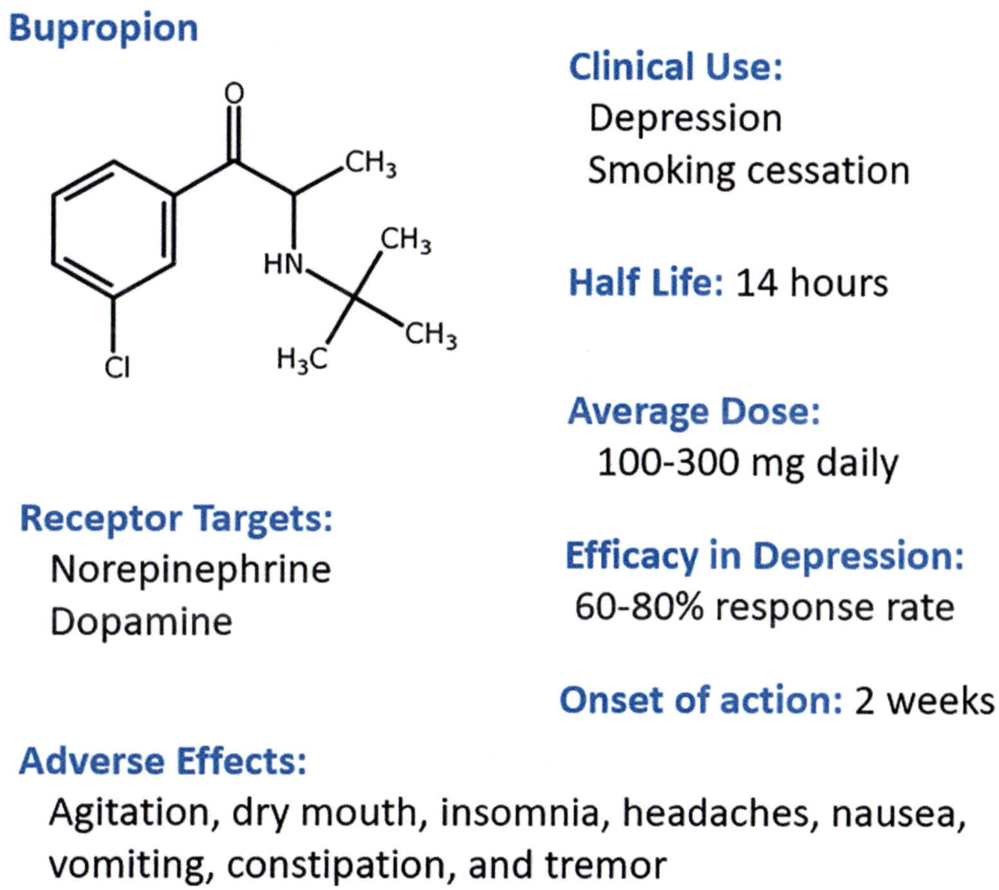

Fig. 10.11 Bupropion

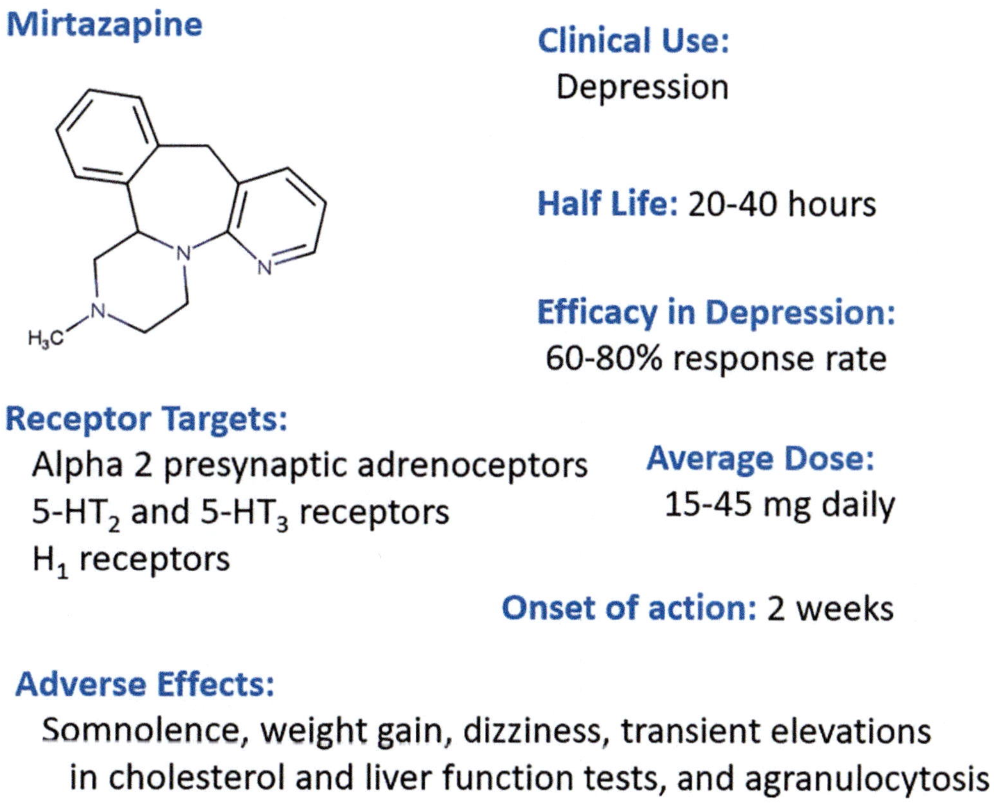

Fig. 10.12 Mirtazapine

Fig. 10.13 Trazadone

Trazadone

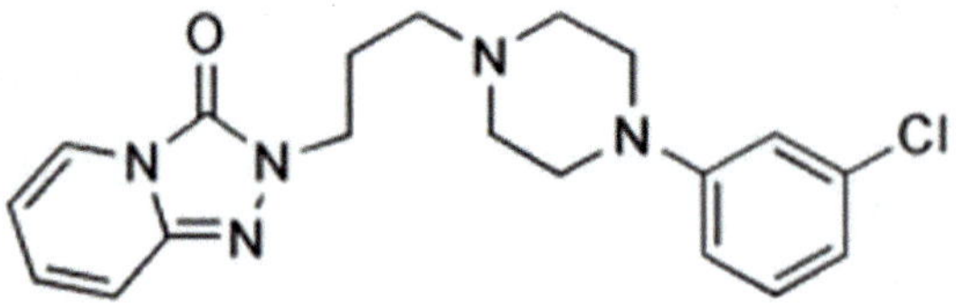

Clinical Use:
Depression
Anxiety
Insomnia
Dementia
Fibromyalgia

Receptor Targets:
Serotonin receptors
5-HT_2 receptors

Efficacy in Depression:
60-80% response rate

Average Dose:
75-150 mg daily

Half Life: 20-40 hours

Onset of action: 1 week

Adverse Effects:
Drowsiness, dizziness, dry mouth, nervousness, bradycardia, acute angle glaucoma, and hyponatremia

Fig. 10.14 Vortioxetine

Vortioxetine

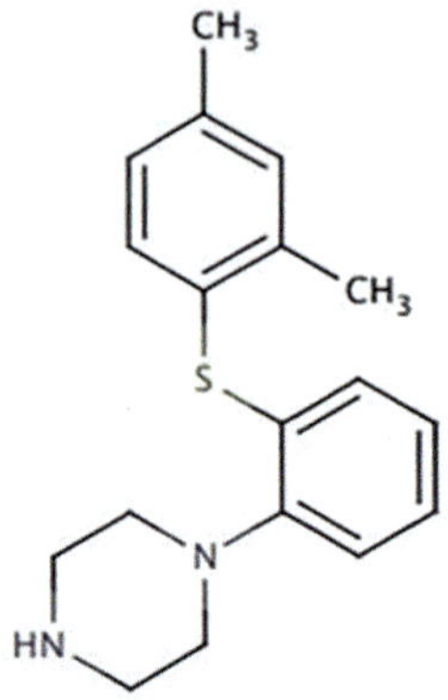

Clinical Use:
Depression

Onset of action: 1-2 weeks

Half Life: 57-66 hours

Average Dose:
10-20 mg daily

Receptor Targets:
Serotonin receptors
5-HT_3, 5-HT_{1D}, 5-HT_7,5-HT_{1A},5-HT_{1B} receptors

Adverse Effects:
Nausea, sexual dysfunction, headaches, dry mouth, dizziness, constipation, hypertensive crisis, and pancreatitis

Vilazodone was approved by the FDA in 2011 for the treatment of major depressive disorder and works by enhancing serotonergic activity in the central nervous system with no significant effects on norepinephrine or dopamine uptake [33]. This medication was noted to have similar remission rates of depression compared to citalopram at 6 weeks of therapy [33, 47] (Fig. 10.15).

Intravenous ketamine has been studied for use in treatment-resistant depression for over 20 years. Ketamine works by antagonizing the NMDA receptors, thus producing increased glutamate concentrations in the brain that activate AMPA receptors leading to the creation of new connections within the brain [48]. Additional studies suggest that ketamine has downstream effects on the opioid, aminergic, and cholinergic systems in the brain [49]. Human clinical trials have demonstrated rapid antidepressant effects of IV ketamine in patients with depression with responses 14 days after a single dose in some patients [50]. The s-enantiomer of ketamine, esketamine, was approved as a nasal spray by the FDA to be used with an oral antidepressant for treatment-resistant depression in 2019 and for suicidality associated with depression in 2020 [51] (Fig. 10.16).

Fig. 10.15 Vilazodone

Vilazodone

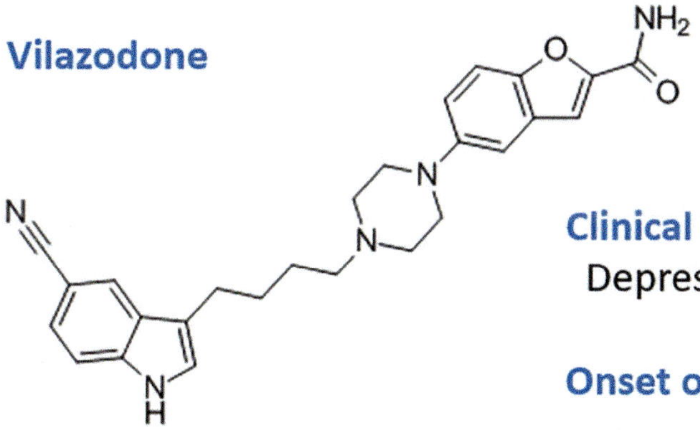

Clinical Use:
Depression

Onset of action: 1 week

Half Life: 25 hours

Receptor Targets:
Serotonin receptors
5-HT$_{1A}$ receptors

Average Dose:
20-40 mg daily

Adverse Effects:
Nausea, diarrhea, vomiting, insomnia, dizziness, dry mouth, fatigue, decreased libido, abnormal dreams, arthralgias and palpitations

Fig. 10.16 Esketamine

Esketamine

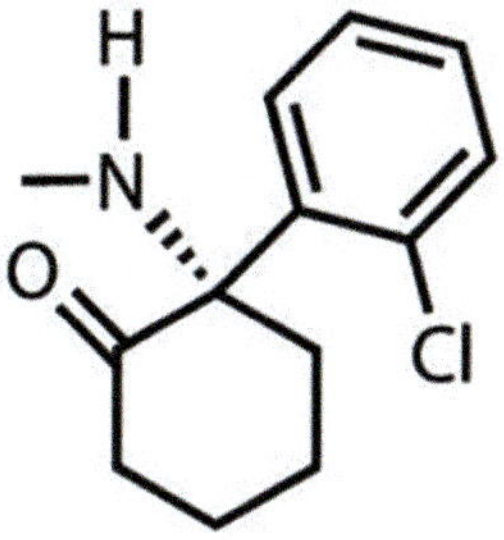

Clinical Use:
Treatment resistant depression
Suicidality in depression

Half Life: 7-12 hours

Receptor Targets:
NMDA Receptor

Adverse Effects:
Hypertension, nausea, vomiting, anxiety, depersonalization, derealization, dissociation, dizziness, headache, sedation, vertigo

The cytochrome P450 enzymes in the liver have a significant role in the metabolism of numerous drugs within the body. Multiple medications work to both enhance and inhibit these enzymes resulting in several significant drug–drug interactions that must be considered in pharmacotherapy and dosing. Figure 10.17 shows some of the inducers and inhibitors of this enzymatic system and the drugs that each enzyme metabolizes [24, 52].

Neurostimulation

Despite the numerous available pharmacotherapies for the treatment of depression, many patients are unable to obtain an adequate response with medications alone or in combination with psychotherapy. Neuromodulation as a treatment for depression uses electrical or electromagnetic energy to alter activity levels within the brain. There are only three FDA-approved modalities for neurostimulation including electroconvulsive therapy (ECT), vagal nerve stimulation (VNS), and repetitive transcranial magnetic stimulation (rTMS) [33].

ECT is one of the oldest and most effective treatments for severe depression in either acute episodes or as a form of maintenance therapy. The first therapeutic-induced seizure for the treatment of depression via ECT occurred in 1938 [12, 33]. The mechanism for benefit in depression has not yet been determined, but there are clear indications for this form of therapy with response rates of 70–90%, and remission achieved in 40–50% of patients with treatment-resistant depression [12, 33, 53] (Fig. 10.18).

Fig. 10.17 Cytochrome P450 enzyme inhibitors and inducers

Enzyme	Substrate	Inhibitor	Inducer
CYP1A2	TCAs, acetaminophen, caffeine, clozapine, duloxetine, olanzapine, diazepam	Cimetidine, fluoroquinolones, fluoxetine, fluvoxamine	Chargrilled meats, omeprazole, tobacco
CYP2C19	TCAs, citalopram, diazepam, omeprazole, warfarin	Cimetidine, fluoxetine, fluvoxamine, imipramine, sertraline, omeprazole	Rifampin
CYP2D6	TCAs, amphetamine, bupropion, clozapine, codeine, duloxetine, fluoxetine, haloperidol, nortriptyline, mirtazapine, paroxetine, oxycodone, trazodone, venlafaxine, risperidone	Bupropion, celecoxib, cimetidine, duloxetine, fluoxetine, haloperidol, paroxetine, sertraline, citalopram, fluvoxamine	Phenobarbital and rifampin
CYP3A4	TCAs, acetaminophen, alprazolam, loratadine, mirtazapine, citalopram, escitalopram	Cimetidine, fluoxetine, sertraline, fluvoxamine	Barbiturates. glucocorticoids, rifampin, St. John's wort

Fig. 10.18 Indications and relative contraindications for electroconvulsive therapy

Diagnostic Indications:

Major depressive disorder
Bipolar disorder (acute mania)
Catatonia
Schizophrenia (psychosis)
Parkinson's disease
Intractable epilepsy
Neuroleptic malignant disorder

Relative Contraindications:

Recent myocardial infarction
Unstable cardiac disease
Decompensated heart failure
Increased intercranial pressure
Increased risk of brain bleed

Clinical Indications :

Need for rapid, definitive response due to psychosis, suicide risk, severe illness or severe malnutrition
History of poor response/intolerance to pharmacotherapy
History of ECT response

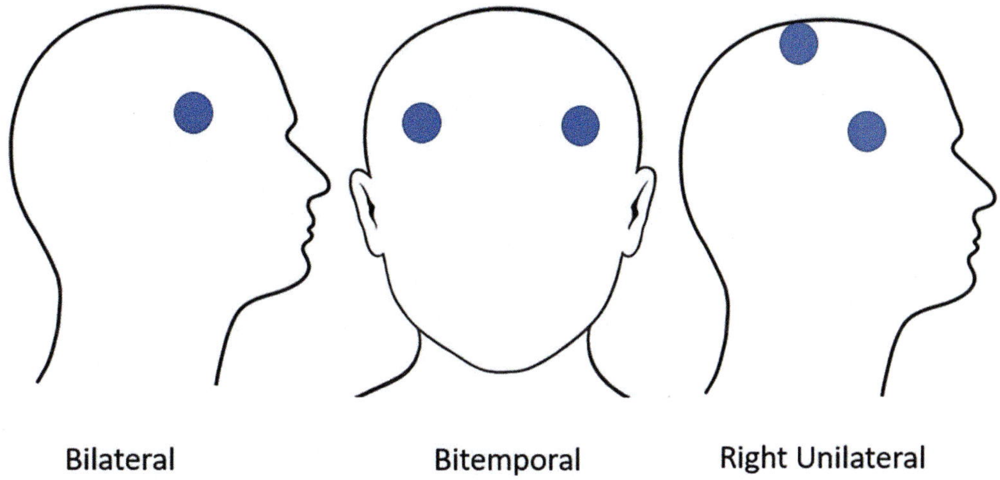

Fig. 10.19 Electroconvulsive therapy electrode placement

ECT is performed under general anesthesia with cessation of benzodiazepines, anti-epileptics, lithium, theophylline, lidocaine and reserpine prior to the procedure [33, 53]. Succinylcholine is used to prevent skeletal muscle contractions and injuries during the procedure. Three different electrode placements (Fig. 10.19) are used in ECT with bilateral placement noted to have the most predictable efficacy and speed of response in depression with the most cognitive side effects; while right unilateral placement with an electrical stimulus 500% above the seizure threshold produces similar effects with regards to symptom resolution with less cognitive dysfunction [33, 53]. Appropriate seizure monitoring during ECT, treatment course, and side effects are listed in Fig. 10.20 [12, 33].

Electroconvulsive therapy is one of the most potent forms of treatment for depression. Studies using functional MRI imaging in patients with major depressive disorder before and after treatment with ECT have shown decreased connectivity between the brain's medial cortex, left dorsolateral prefrontal cortex, and the left supermarginal gyrus, angular gyrus, and somatosensory association cortex [54] These changes have been correlated with a significant reduction in depressive symptoms in patients with treatment-resistant depression following treatment with ECT using bilateral electrode placement [54] (Fig. 10.21).

Transcranial magnetic stimulation introduces an electrical current to the brain by creating a temporary magnetic field that depolarizes neurons in the cortex through brief electromagnetic pulses [33]. This form of therapy induces long-lasting changes but is only currently FDA approved for the treatment of a major depressive disorder, mapping of the brain prior to neurosurgery, and treatment of migraine headaches with aura [33] (Fig. 10.22). The most serious adverse effect is a seizure, which can be prevented with appropriate precautions [33].

Studies have shown that repetitive TMS increases cerebral blood flow in the pre-frontal cortex, cingulate gyrus, amygdala, uncus, hippocampus, parahippocampus, thalamus, and cerebellum in patients with treatment-resistant depression [55] (Fig. 10.23). This form of therapy has been shown to improve depression symptoms in patients through changes in neuronal activity and cerebral blood flow following 10 sessions [55]. This non-invasive method of treatment has been shown to have a significant positive effect on symptoms of depression through alterations in neuroplasticity in patients that do not derive significant benefit in symptom management with medications and psychotherapy.

Optimal ECT Seizure:
20 seconds motor duration
30 seconds EEG duration

Treatment Course:
6-12 treatments 2-3 times per week
Maintenance therapy monthly or as indicated

Side Effects:
Disorientation, delirium, anterograde amnesia, retrograde amnesia, reduced autobiographical memory
Muscle soreness, jaw pain, headaches, nausea, hypotension, tachycardia, transient arrhythmias

Fig. 10.20 Electroconvulsive therapy treatment and side effects

Vagal nerve stimulation for the treatment of depression stemmed from early trials in patients with refractory epilepsy with comorbid depression that showed noted improvement in depressive symptoms following treatment [33]. This form of therapy was FDA approved in 2007 but has been limited in availability due to a lack of coverage from Medicare, Medicaid, and other insurance companies. Figure 10.24 illustrates the placement of the device and the initial settings used in therapy. Currents for the device are increased as clinically indicated and treatment lasts on average 6–12 months [33].

Additional neurostimulation techniques are under investigation for the treatment of depression. These include deep brain stimulation, magnetic seizure therapy, and trigeminal nerve stimulation [33]. Early studies using deep brain stimu-

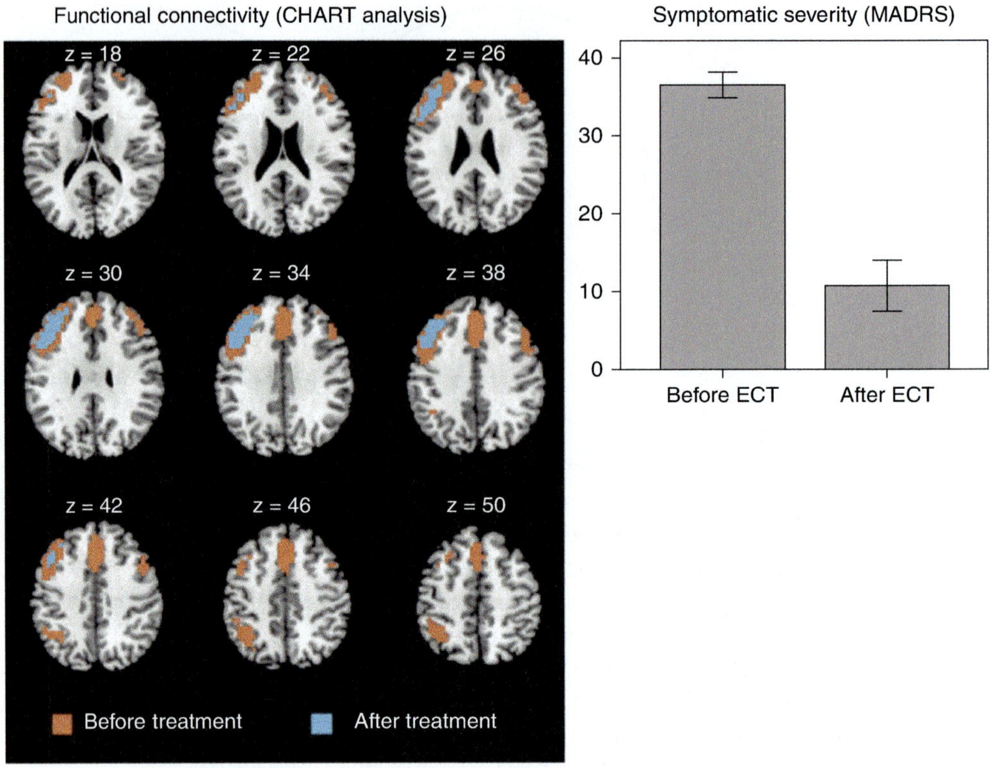

Fig. 10.21 Functional MRI scans in patients with treatment resistant depression prior to and following ECT

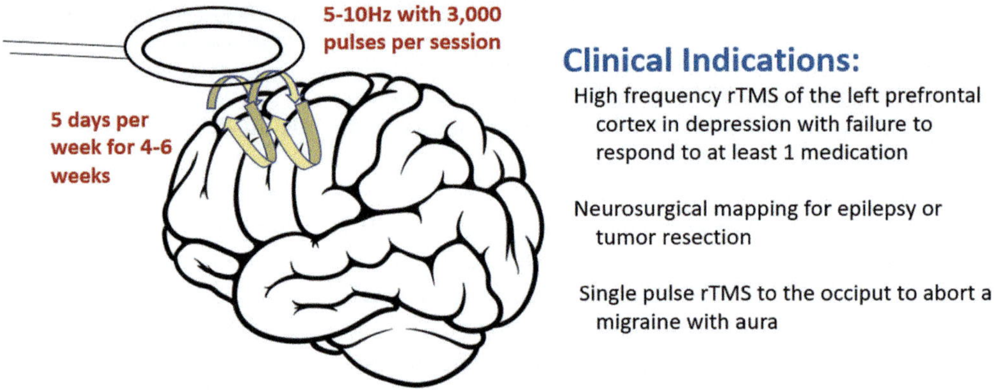

Fig. 10.22 Clinical indications for repetitive transcranial magnetic stimulation

lation in the area of the nucleus accumbens demonstrated benefits in depression treatment in the first 6 months of therapy, with approximately 50% response rates in larger, long-term studies. Similar results were achieved in studies with stimulation of the subgenual cortex with 3-year response rates up to 75% in patients with treatment-resistant depression [33]. Magnetic seizure therapy is similar to electroconvulsive therapy but uses an electromagnetic transcranial stimulation device to induce a less intense, focal seizure. This technique reduces the cognitive side effects that are observed with ECT with a variable response and remission rates in the treatment of depression [33]. Transcutaneous trigeminal nerve stimulation has shown improvements in treatment-resistant depression and quality of life measurements in early trials in patients with major depressive disorder, post-traumatic stress disorder, and epilepsy with associated mood changes [33]. Each of these modalities shows promise in the early clinical trials but will need additional testing prior to potential approval for clinical use.

Antipsychotics

Initial antipsychotic medications were developed in the 1950s following the observation that aniline dye, produced by early textile companies for its purple coloration, had a calming and sedating effect [24]. This led to the discovery of promethazine, which was initially used as an anesthetic during surgery in the early 1950s. Chlorpromazine, which was derived from promethazine, was noted to have efficacy in the treatment of psychosis with a favorable side effect profile [8, 24]. Currently, there are 11 first-generation and 14 second-

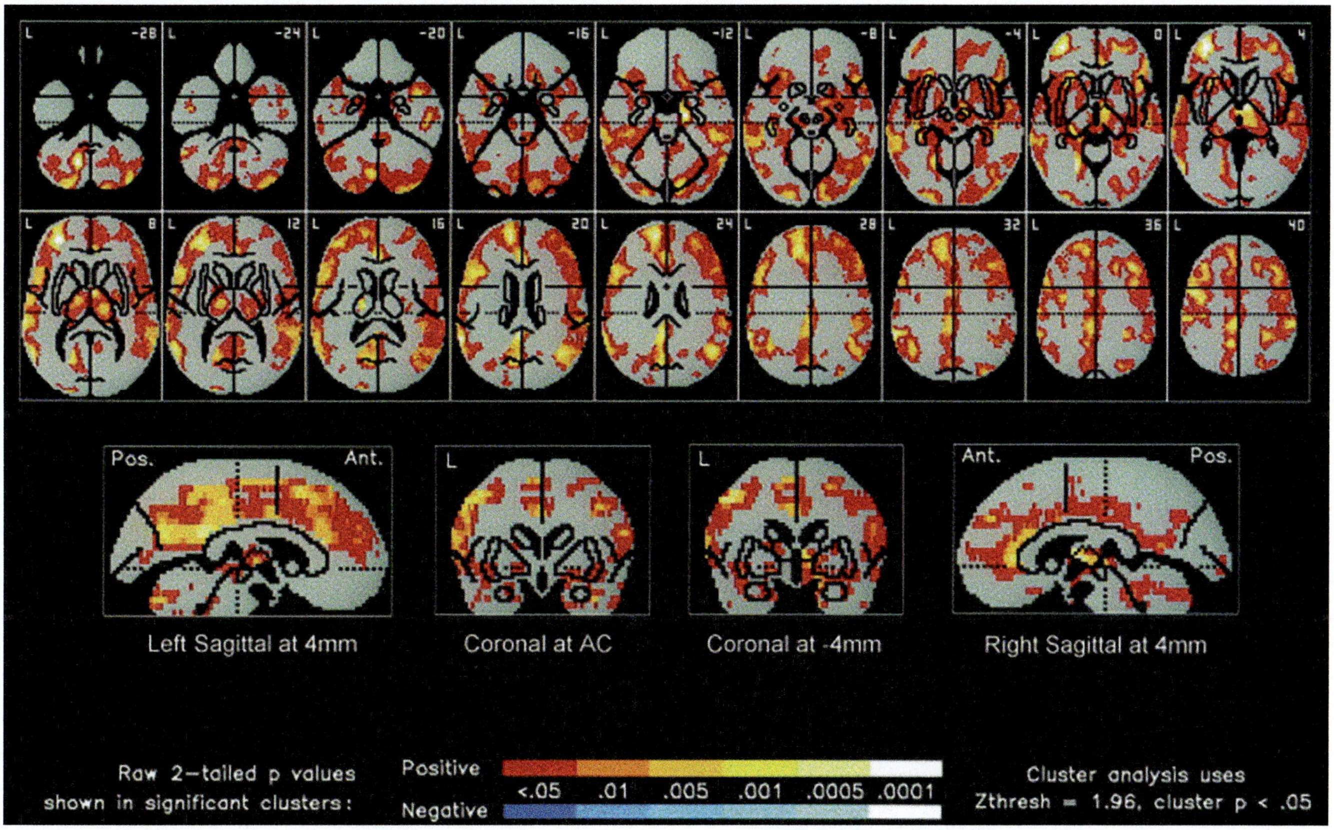

Fig. 10.23 PET scan following TMS treatment in patients with treatment resistant depression

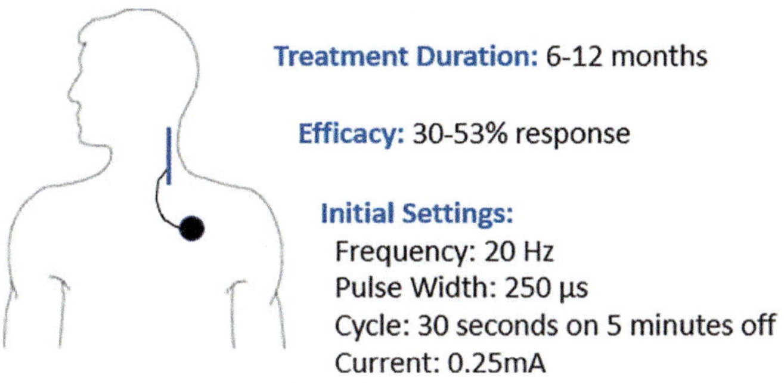

Fig. 10.24 Vagal nerve stimulation

generation antipsychotics that are FDA approved to treat schizophrenia, schizoaffective disorder, acute mania, delusional disorder, bipolar disorder, for augmentation in major depressive disorder, severe agitation, psychosis, borderline personality disorder, and Tourette's syndrome.

The first generation, or typical antipsychotics, are dopamine receptor antagonists with approximately 72% blockade of the D2 dopamine receptor in the brain [56]. These medications additionally block noradrenergic, cholinergic, and histaminergic receptors and are associated with a significant risk for extrapyramidal side effects, sedation, lowered seizure thresholds, cardiac arrythmias through QT prolongation, and blood dyscrasias [56]. Neuroleptic malignant syndrome (NMS) is a rare but fatal adverse effect that can occur with the use of these medications and is more prevalent with the first-generation typical antipsychotics, but can also be observed with the use of second-generation atypical antipsychotics. Chlorpromazine is associated with blue-grey skin discoloration and benign pigmentation of the lens and cornea [8]. Thioridazine can cause retinal pigmentation that can be permanent even after discontinuing the medication [8, 10, 24, 57] (Fig. 10.25).

Second-generation, or atypical, antipsychotics are serotonin (5-HT_{2A} receptor) and dopamine (D2 receptor) antagonists that can be administered in oral, parenteral, or sublingual forms [56]. These medications are associated with decreased extrapyramidal side effects compared to first-generation antipsychotics but are associated with weight gain and the development of metabolic syndrome in addition to an increased risk of stroke in older patients with dementia [56]. These medications are approved for the treatment of schizophrenia, mania, and bipolar depression with full benefits of the medication noted at 4 weeks to 6 months of therapy [24, 56, 58–62] (Fig. 10.26). Pimavanserin is the first antipsychotic that works on serotonin receptors instead of dopamine receptors and is FDA approved for the treatment of psychosis associated with Parkinson's disease [63]. This medication is currently being studied for additional applications in other psychiatric conditions.

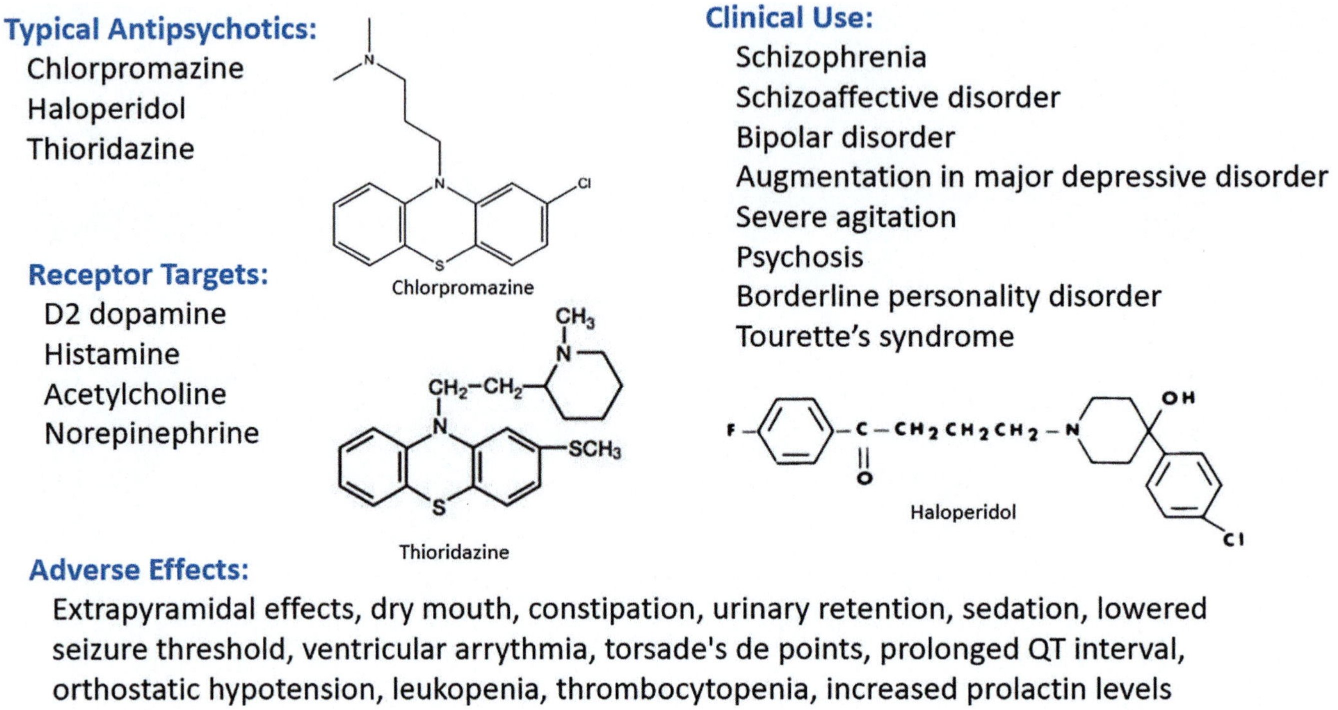

Fig. 10.25 First-generation (typical) antipsychotics)

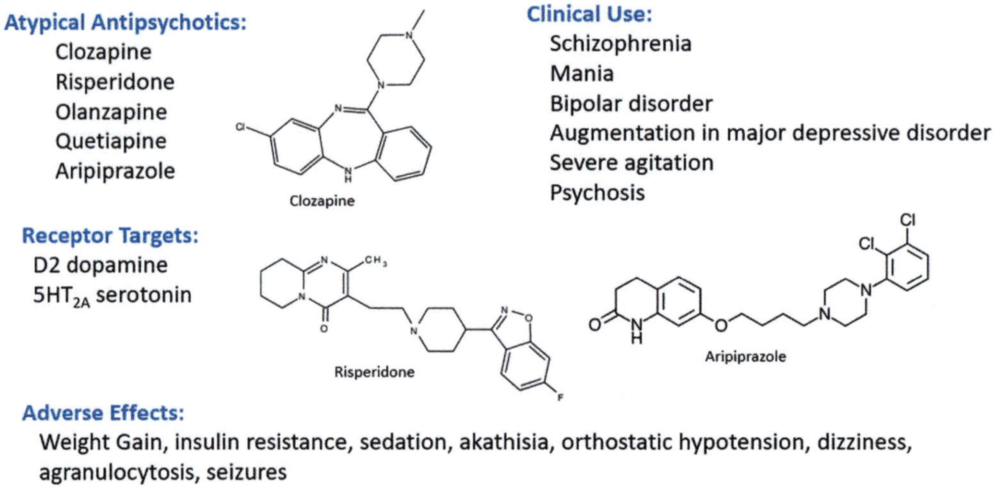

Fig. 10.26 Second-generation (atypical) antipsychotics

Both that typical and atypical antipsychotics have been extensively used in the treatment of schizophrenia. First-generation antipsychotics are more effective at treating the positive symptoms including hallucinations and delusions with a noted reduction in the incidence of repeated episodes of psychosis [56]. Second-generation antipsychotics are used to treat both the positive and negative symptoms of schizophrenia including withdrawal and ambivalence and are known to reduce relapse rates [56]. Clozapine, which is a second-generation antipsychotic has been indicated to treat treatment-resistant schizophrenia but can cause significant leukopenia and agranulocytosis requiring close monitoring of absolute neutrophil counts weekly for the first 6 months and then biweekly following this timeframe [24, 58]. Antipsychotics can be monitored for a therapeutic range 12–24 h following the last dose with Haloperidol having a therapeutic range of 2–15 ng/ml, chlorpromazine at 30–100 ng/ml, and Clozapine at plasma concentrations of 350 mg/ml or higher [8, 10, 57–67] (Table 10.7).

Mood Stabilizers

Mood stabilizers including lithium, divalproex, carbamazepine, and lamotrigine are primarily used for the treatment of bipolar disorder [24]. These medications have a relatively

Table 10.7 Pharmacokinetics of antipsychotic medications and onset of action

Medication name	Half life	Distribution	Typical Dosage	Onset of action
Chlorpromazine	2 h	92–97% protein bound	25–200 mg daily	Intramuscular 15 min Oral 30–60 min
Haloperidol	14–37 h	88–92% protein bound	2–10 mg daily	30 min
Thioridazine	5–27 h	96–99% protein bound	300–800 mg daily	Rapid
Clozapine	12 h	97% protein bound	300–400 mg daily	6–12 weeks
Risperidone	20 h	90% protein bound	4–8 mg daily	Rapid
Olanzapine	30–54 h	93% protein bound	5–10 mg daily	3–6 weeks
Quetiapine	6 h	83% protein bound	400–800 mg daily	Rapid
Aripiprazole	75–94 h	99% protein bound	10–15 mg daily	1–3 weeks
Cariprazine	2–4 days	91–97% protein bound	3–6 mg daily	3–6 h
Lurasidone	18–40 h	99% protein bound	40–80 mg daily	1–3 h
Brexpiprazole	91 h	>99% protein bound	2–4 mg daily	4 h
Paliperidone	23 h	74% protein bound	6–12 mg daily	24 h
Pimavanserin	57 h	95% protein bound	34 mg daily	6 h

From the package inserts for each medication

Table 10.8 Pharmacokinetics of mood stabilizing medications

Medication name	Half life	Distribution	Typical dosage
Lithium	18–36 h	Not protein bound	900–1800 mg daily
Divalproex	9–19 h	80–90% protein bound	1.5–2.5 g daily
Carbamazepine	25–65 h	75–90% protein bound	600–1600 mg daily
Lamotrigine	25–33 h	55% protein bound	100–400 mg daily

From the package inserts for each medication

long half-life and variability in protein binding within the body [68–71] (Table 10.8). A common mechanism of action that has been proposed for this class of medications is through the inhibition of inositol uptake resulting in alleviation of symptoms of mania and prophylaxis against the manic and depressive cycles in bipolar disorder [72].

Lithium is FDA approved for the treatment of acute mania and as maintenance, therapy to prevent recurrent episodes of bipolar disorder and has been used in psychiatry since 1949 [24, 68]. The proposed mechanism of action for lithium includes inhibition of neuronal excitation through its effects on the inositol signaling pathway, enhanced serotonin neurotransmission, modulation of norepinephrine release in both mania and depression, and alterations in dopamine regulation [24, 72]. Side effects of lithium include tremor, weight gain, nephrogenic diabetes insipidus, chronic tubulointerstitial nephritis, hypothyroidism, and cognitive alterations [24, 68, 72]. Lithium had a narrow therapeutic index and requires close monitoring of blood levels for toxicity [68] (Fig. 10.27).

Divalproex, also known as valproic acid, is FDA approved for the treatment of acute manic episodes, seizures, and migraine headache prophylaxis [72]. Divalproex enhances the inhibitory effects of GABA, which reduces neuronal firing within neural networks [24, 72]. Side effects of this medication include weight gain, nausea, vomiting, alopecia, tremor, easy bruising, hyponatremia, transaminitis, hepatotoxicity, and acute pancreatitis [69, 72]. Due to the risk of hepatotoxicity, liver enzymes must be monitored closely during the first 6 months of therapy [69] (Fig. 10.28). Despite the noted side effects, valproic acid remains one most common medications used in the USA for the treatment of bipolar disorder [24].

Carbamazepine was originally synthesized in 1957and was used in the 1960s in Europe to treat temporal lobe epilepsy [24]. It was later discovered that carbamazepine was effective for the treatment of trigeminal neuralgia, and in 1970 in Japan it was discovered to be effective for the treatment of bipolar disorder for both acute mania and mixed episodes [24, 72]. Carbamazepine downregulates the inositol transporter through inhibition of cyclic AMP resulting in its effects on mood stabilization [72]. Side effects of carbamazepine include sedation, dizziness, fatigue, nausea, vomiting, diarrhea, hyponatremia, rash, headache, diplopia, ataxia, agranulocytosis, and aplastic anemia [24, 70, 72]. Carbamazepine is traditionally regarded as a third-line treatment for bipolar disorder behind lithium and divalproex due to the high degree of pharmacokinetic interactions of the medication [70] (Fig. 10.29).

Lamotrigine received FDA approval in 2003 for the treatment of bipolar disorder following studies conducted in the early 1990s that showed improvement in mood symptoms in epileptic patients [24]. Lamotrigine reduces the frequency of excitatory postsynaptic potentials resulting in decreased glutamate release with an additional increase in the frequency and amplitude of inhibitory postsynaptic potentials that enhance GABA release [24, 72]. Additional modulation of serotonin reuptake and the blockade of dopamine uptake have further roles in the mood stabilizing properties of this medication [24]. Side effects of lamotrigine include rash, nausea, diplopia, headache, dizziness, tremor, and sedation with less associated weight gain and cognitive effects compared to other treatments for bipolar disorder [24, 71, 72].

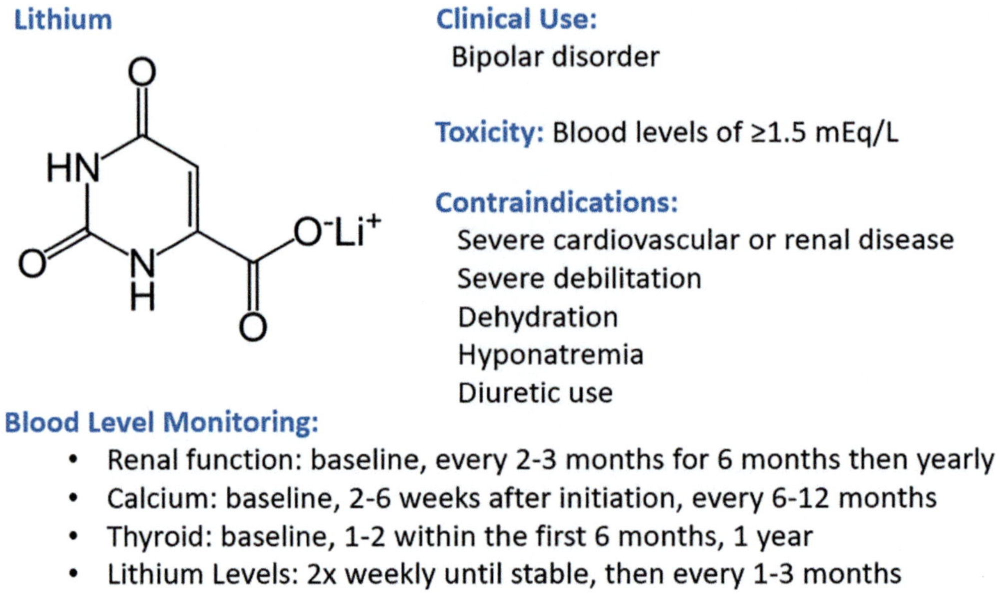

Fig. 10.27 Lithium

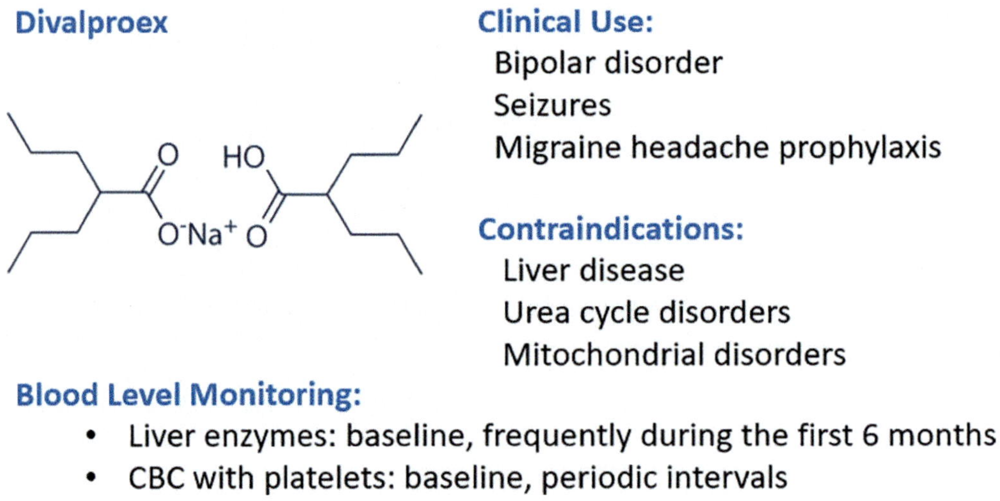

Fig. 10.28 Divalproex

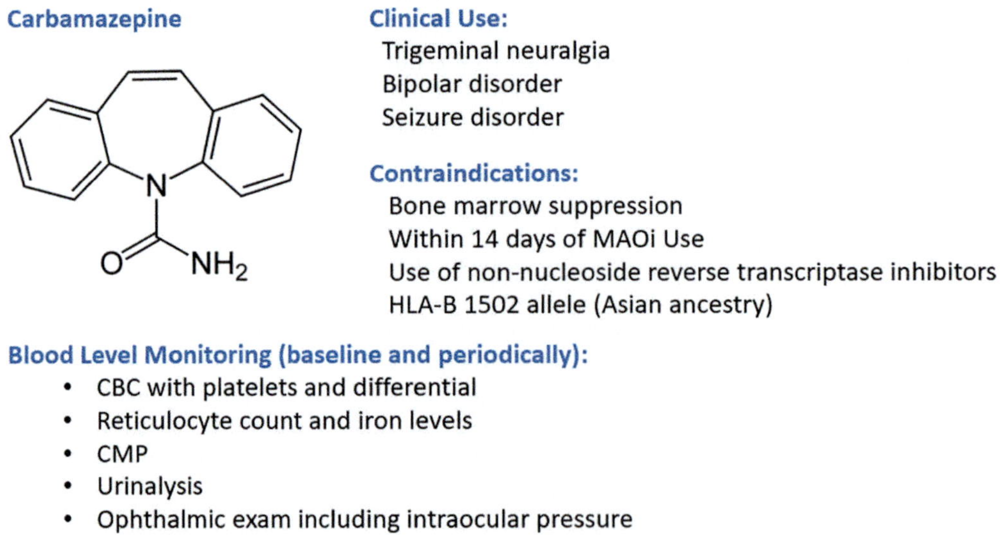

Fig. 10.29 Carbamazepine

Given the low side effect profile, lamotrigine is recommended as a second-line treatment for bipolar disorder [71] (Fig. 10.30).

Anxiolytics

Anxiety disorders are the most prevalent psychiatric condition, with a 12-month prevalence of 10.3% of the population and increased patient illness burden [73]. Medications used for the treatment of anxiety include SSRIs, SNRIs, TCAs, benzodiazepines, buspirone, and hydroxyzine [24]. A review of the effectiveness of medications used in the treatment of generalized anxiety disorder shows that benzodiazepines work the fastest to relieve symptoms, while antidepressants can take several weeks, and cognitive behavioral therapy takes 2 months or longer to alleviate symptoms [24]. Studies have shown that the combination of pharmacotherapy and psychotherapy are more effective than either therapy used in isolation [73].

Benzodiazepines were introduced in the 1960s and in the USA are used to treat 55–94% of patients with anxiety [24, 73]. These medications are FDA approved for the treatment of generalized anxiety disorder, panic disorder, insomnia, and myoclonic epilepsy and have been additionally used for the treatment of muscle tension, alcohol withdrawal, and as an anesthetic [24, 73]. Side effects of benzodiazepines include CNS depression with fatigue, dizziness, sedation, lethargy, and impaired cognitive function. These medications have a risk of dependence and withdrawal in long-term use or in patients with underlying substance use disorder [24, 73] (Fig. 10.31). Given the noted side effects and variable half-lives of these medications, benzodiazepines are often used as a second-line treatment for generalized anxiety disorder behind antidepressants, or for use in augmentation for patients already on antidepressants [74–78] (Table 10.9).

Buspirone is an anxiolytic that works as a partial $5HT_{1A}$ receptor agonist that has been shown to be effective in the treatment of generalized anxiety disorder [24, 73]. This medication is well tolerated with mild side effects and takes 2–4 weeks to reach full effect [79] (Fig. 10.32). This medication can be used as monotherapy or in augmentation with antidepressants [24, 79].

Hydroxyzine is an antihistamine that is FDA approved for the treatment of generalized itching [80]. This medication is

Table 10.9 Pharmacokinetics of benzodiazepines

Medication name	Half life	Distribution	Typical dosage
Diazepam	40 h	95–98% protein bound	5–40 mg per day
Clonazepam	17–60 h	85% protein bound	1–4 mg per day
Lorazepam	14 h	91% protein bound	1–6 mg per day
Oxazepam	9 h	96–98% protein bound	15–120 mg per day
Alprazolam	14 h	80% protein bound	1–4 mg per day

From the package inserts for each medication

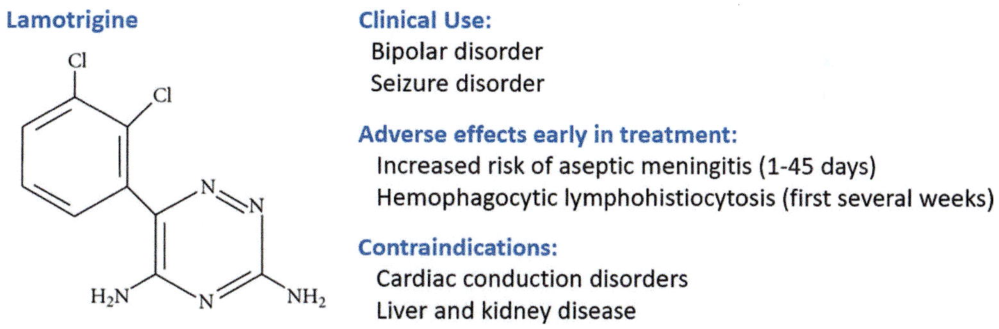

Fig. 10.30 Lamotrigine

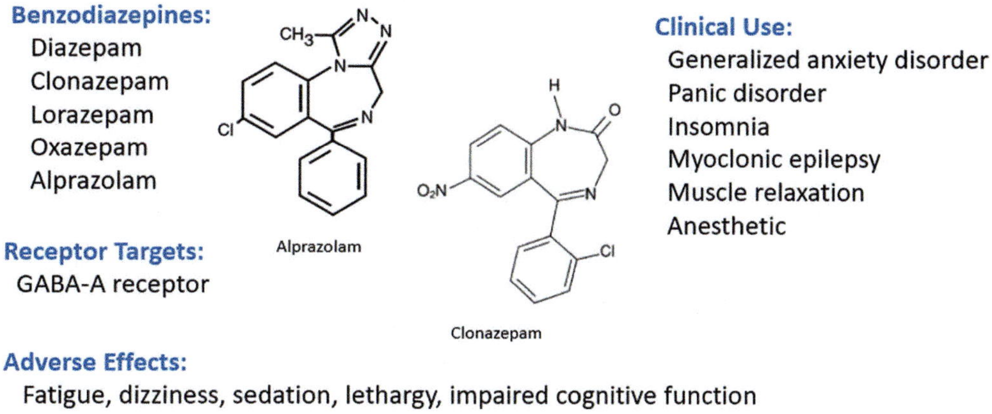

Fig. 10.31 Benzodiazepines

Buspirone

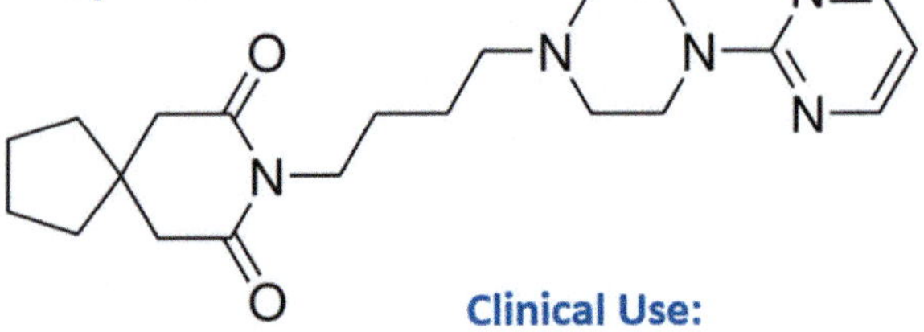

Clinical Use: Generalized anxiety disorder

Average Dose: 30-60 mg daily

Onset of action: 2-4 weeks

Adverse Effects: Headache, nausea, dizziness, and tension

Fig. 10.32 Buspirone

Hydroxyzine

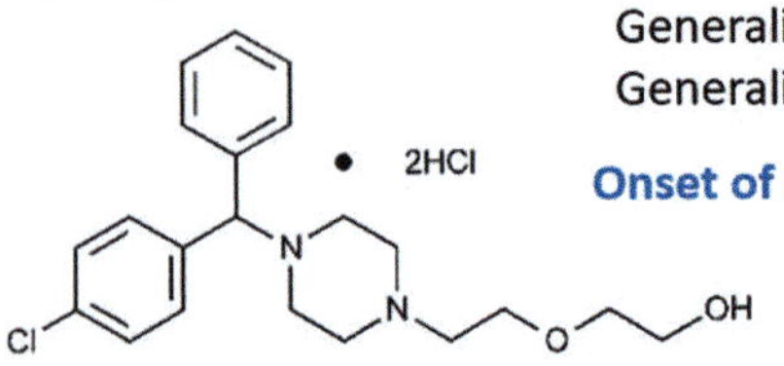

Clinical Use:
Generalized anxiety disorder
Generalized itching

Onset of action: 15-30 minutes

Average Dose: 37.5-75 mg daily

Adverse Effects: Drowsiness and dry mouth

Fig. 10.33 Hydroxyzine

often used off-label in augmentation therapy for generalized anxiety disorder and insomnia due to its sedating properties [24]. Side effects are generally well tolerated and include drowsiness and dry mouth [80] (Fig. 10.33).

Hypnotics

Sedative and hypnotic medications are largely used for the treatment of insomnia and sleep disorders associated with psychiatric conditions [24]. The medications include benzodiazepines, TCAs, non-benzodiazepine sedative-hypnotics (zolpidem, zaleplon, and eszopiclone), and diphenhydramine [81]. Barbiturates were initially used as sedative hypnotics in psychiatric disorders but are not longer used as oral therapy due to side effects and toxicities, and thus will not be discussed in detail within this chapter [24].

Non-benzodiazepine sedative-hypnotics act on the alpha 1 benzodiazepine site on the GABA-A receptor with zolpidem being among the most prescribed medications for insomnia in the USA [24]. These medications have short half-lives with relatively few side effects [24] (Fig. 10.34). These medications are becoming more limited in use due to complex sleep-related behaviors that include patients acting out dreams without awareness due to the lack of REM-based

Non-Benzodiazepine Sedative-Hypnotics:
Zolpidem
Zaleplon
Eszopiclone

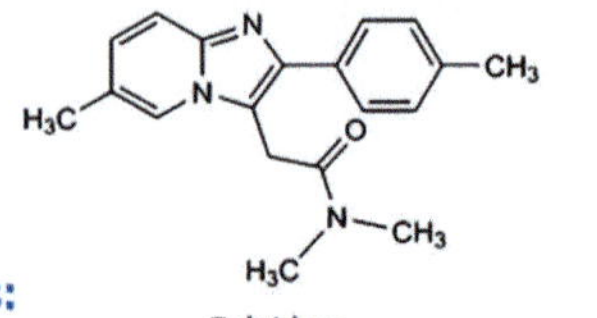

Zolpidem

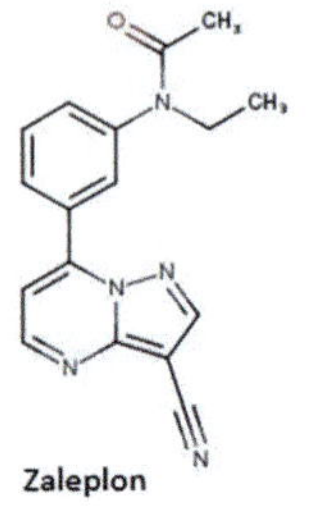

Zaleplon

Receptor Targets: GABA-A receptor

Half Lives:
Zolpidem: 2-4 hours
Zaleplon: 1-2 hours
Eszopiclone: 4-5 hours

Adverse Effects:
Drowsiness, dizziness,
Sleep related behaviors

Fig. 10.34 Non-benzodiazepine sedative hypnotics

Ramelteon

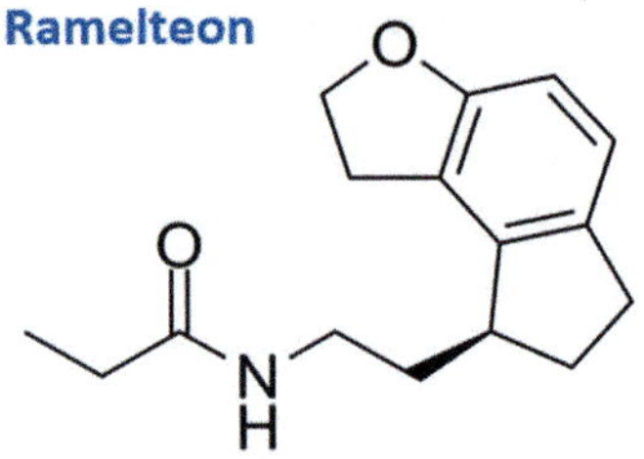

Average Dose: 8 mg daily within 30 minutes of bedtime

Adverse Effects: Headache, somnolence, fatigue, dizziness, and nausea

Fig. 10.35 Ramelteon

sleep paralysis commonly associated with normal sleep patterns [24, 81].

Ramelteon is a specific melatonin MT1 and MT2 melatonin receptor agonist that was approved for the treatment of insomnia in 2005 by the FDA. This was the first hypnotic prescription medication that was not classified as a controlled substance [24]. The use of this medication has resulted in increased total sleep time and reduced sleep latency [81]. The onset of action for sleep occurs within 30 min, however, high-fat meals delay the abruption of this medication and delay sleep onset timing. Side effects include headache, somnolence, fatigue, dizziness, and nausea [24, 81] (Fig. 10.35).

Stimulants

Stimulants have largely been used in the treatment of ADHD in psychiatry for behavioral modulation [24]. ADHD is known to affect up to 10% of children and 3% of adults in the USA and is associated with a significant degree of comorbidities including depression and long-term functional impairment [56]. Two groups of stimulates including meth-

Table 10.10 Stimulants for the treatment of ADHD

Stimulants: Names, formulations, and strengths				
Stimulant	Generic name	Brand name	Formulations and strengths	Duration of behavioral effect (h)
Amphetamines				
	d-amphetamine	Dexedrine	Tablets: 5, 10 mg	3–6
		Dexedrine Spansule	Spansules: 5, 10, 15 mg	
		ProCentra	Oral solution: 5 mg/5 mL	
	Mixed amphetamine/ dextroamphetamine	Adderall	Tablets: 5, 7.5, 10, 12.5, 15, 20, 30 mg	4–6
		Adderall XR	Capsules: 5, 10, 15, 20, 25, 30 mg	8–10
	Lisdexanofetamine dimesylate	Vyvanse	Capsules: 20, 30, 40, 50, 60, 70 mg	
	d-methamphetamine	Desoxyn	Tablet: 5 mg	
Methylphenidates				
	Methylphenidate	Ritalin	Tablets: 5, 10, 20 mg	3–4
		Methylin	Tablets, chewable: 2.5, 5, 10 mg	3–4
			Oral solution: 5 mg/5 mL, 10 mg/5 mL (500 mL)	3–4
		Ritalin sustained release	Tablet: 20 mg	5–8
		Ritalin LA	Capsules: 10, 20, 30, 40 mg	8–9
		Metadate ER	Tablets: 10, 20 mg	5–8
		Metadate CD	Capsules: 10, 20, 30 mg	8–9
		Concerta	Tablets: 18, 27, 36, 54 mg	10–12
		Daytrana	Transdermal patch: 10, 15, 20, 30 mg/9 h	9
		Quillivant XR	Oral suspension: 25 mg/5 mL	10–12
	Dexmethylphenidate	Focalin	Tablets: 2.5, 5, 10 mg	
		Focalin XR	Capsules: 5, 10, 20 mg	

From Stevens et al. [82]; Creative Commons Attribution License; https://creativecommons.org/licenses/by/4.0

ylphenidates and amphetamine are FDA-approved for the treatment of ADHD [82] (Table 10.10). The average response rate of children with ADHD treated with stimulant medications are approximately 70% and side effects are generally mild and include delayed sleep onset, headache, appetite suppression, and mood dysregulation [56].

Pharmacogenetics and Pharmacogenomics

Personalized medicine through pharmacogenetics and pharmacogenomics has long been the goal for treatment. The ability to tailor therapy based on genetic markers supersedes the standard trial and error approach allowing for earlier effectiveness of medication with the goal of quicker symptom resolution [33]. This additionally allows for the development of targeted therapies, an improved understanding of pharmacokinetics, and the ability to identify the underlying mechanisms for variability in drug responses [26]. Fig. 10.36 shows the major pharmacogenomic studies conducted to date and highlights the important findings from each study [33, 83].

The work in pharmacogenetics and pharmacogenomics to date has shed light on the effects of various genes and single nucleotide polymorphisms (SNPs) on drug metabolism in psychopharmacology, but has yet to lead to broader applications of this knowledge in clinical practice. Several pharmacogenomic tests are currently marketed as decision support tools and claim to help clinicians select safer or more effective treatments for mental disorders. This is an active area of study and controversy, where both the American Psychiatric Association and the USA FDA have advised caution in the use of these tests in clinical practice due to a lack of evidence supporting their use [84, 85]. Additional research into the effects of epigenetics and gene modifications in drug response may lead to advancements in personalized medicine and drug responsiveness, but additional work is needed before the implementation of genetic testing in clinical practice. This research does, however, show promise in drug development through targeted therapy.

Biomarkers

Biomarkers, especially markers of underlying inflammation, have been extensively used in medicine to identify early indicators of disease, including cardiovascular and rheumatologic disease, and in guiding response to therapy. Despite the noted association between depression and inflammation, the field of psychiatry has yet to identify biomarkers like

Sequenced Treatment Alternatives to Relieve Depression (STAR*D)

- Variants in serotonin receptor (HTR2A), glutamate receptor (GRIK4), and potassium channel (KCNK2) predicted improvement with citalopram
- Polymorphisms in pharmacokinetic genes was not significantly associated with improvement
- Treatment emergent suicidal ideation and sexual dysfunction were associated with glutamate receptor and immune regulatory pathway polymorphisms

Munich Antidepressant Response Signature (MARS)

- Polymorphisms in brain derived neurotrophic factor and the receptor polymorphisms are predictive of antidepressant response

Genome Based Therapeutic Drugs for Depression (GENDEP)

- Serotonin receptor (HTR2A) is associated with a response to escitalopram
- Norepinephrine transporter (SLC6A2) is associated with a response to nortriptyline

Pharmacogenomic Research Network Antidepressant Medication Pharmacogenomic Study (PGRN-AMPS)

- Single nucleotide polymorphisms in or near CYP450 (2C19) and (2D6) were associated with levels of escitalopram

Fig. 10.36 Pharmacogenomic studies on antidepressant response

Fig. 10.37 Biomarkers for treatment response

C- Reactive Protein
Marker of CNS inflammation

Escitalopram>Nortriptyline if CRP<1 mg/L
Escitalopram> Escitalopram-Bupropion if CRP<1 mg/L

Nortriptyline>Escitalopram if CRP ≥1 mg/L
Escitalopram-Bupropion>Escitalopram if CRP ≥1 mg/L

Interleukin 17
Marker of CNS inflammation

Increased IL-17 greater reduction in depression severity with Escitalopram-Bupropion

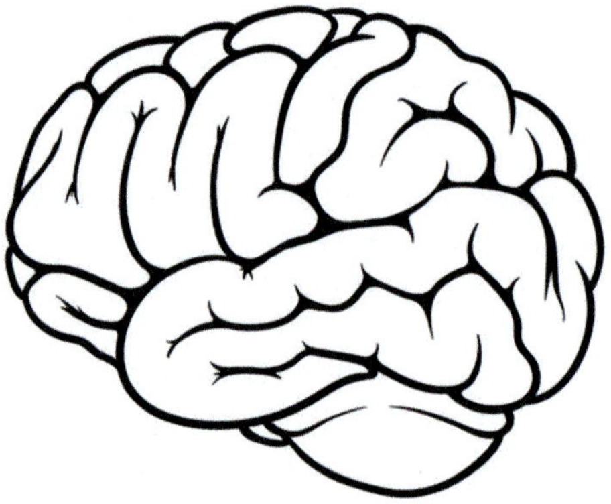

those used in medicine to aid in identifying early signs of mental illness. Two inflammatory proteins, c reactive protein (CRP) and interleukin 17(IL-17) have been identified as potential biomarkers to predict treatment response in depression [33] (Fig. 10.37).

Patients with concentrations of CRP less than 1 mg/L were found in the GENDEP study to be more responsive to escitalopram as compared to nortriptyline, and nortriptyline was found to be superior to escitalopram if CRP measurements were greater or equal to 1 mg/L [86]. In the Co-MED trial, it was shown that patients with CRP less than 1 mg/L had increased remission at 57.1% with escitalopram compared to 33.3% remission in patients on the combination of escitalopram and bupropion. In patients with CRP greater than or equal to 1 mg/L, remission rates were greater in patients on escitalopram and bupropion at 51.4% compared to escitalopram at 29.7% [87]. Elevated levels of IL-17 have been associated with increased anhedonia in males with major depressive disorder. In the CO-MED study, it was noted that elevated IL-17 levels were correlated with a greater reduction in the severity of depression in patients treated with bupropion and escitalopram with no association noted in patients treated with escitalopram as a monotherapy or in patients that received a combination of venlafaxine and mirtazapine [87].

Additional research into biomarkers with an emphasis on understanding the association between inflammation and depression will provide further insight into potential mechanisms for early diagnosis and treatment of depression and other psychiatric conditions. Currently, the diagnosis of depression occurs when patients have sufficient signs and symptoms to meet the diagnostic criteria laid forth in the

Diagnostic and Statistical Manual for Mental Disorders version 5 (DSM-5). Research suggests that these patients may be at risk for developing mental illness for months or even years prior to diagnosis and earlier intervention through the use of biomarkers may improve overall patient outcomes [88].

References

1. Janicak P, Davis J, Preskorn S, Ayd F. Principles and practice of psychopharmacology. 3nd ed. Baltimore, MD: Williams and Wilkins; 2001.
2. National Institute of Mental Health Mental Health Information Statistics. 2019. https://www.nimh.nih.gov/health/statistics/mental-illness.shtml
3. Hedegaard H, Curtin SC, Warner M. Increase in suicide mortality in the United States, 1999–2018, NCHS Data Brief, no 362. Hyattsville, MD: National Center for Health Statistics; 2020.
4. Badiani A. History of psychopharmacology. In: Stolerman I, Price L, editors. Encyclopedia of psychopharmacology. Berlin, Heidelberg: Springer; 2014.
5. Ban TA. Academic psychiatry and the pharmaceutical industry. Prog Neuro-Psychopharmacol Biol Psychiatry. 2006;30(3):429–41. https://doi.org/10.1016/j.pnpbp.2005.11.014.
6. Baumeister AA, Hawkins MF, López-Muñoz F. Toward standardized usage of the word serendipity in the historiography of psychopharmacology. J Hist Neurosci. 2010;19(3):253–70. https://doi.org/10.1080/09647040903188205.
7. Ban TA. Pharmacotherapy of mental illness—a historical analysis. Prog Neuro-Psychopharmacol Biol Psychiatry. 2001;25(4):709–27. https://doi.org/10.1016/s0278-5846(01)00160-9.
8. Chlorpromazine Prescribing Information. Sanofi-Avenits New Zealand Limited. FDA approved. 2013. https://genesight.com/wp-content/uploads/2017/05/Chlorpromazine-Thorazine-FDA-Label.pdf
9. Imipramine Pamoate Prescribing Information. Mallinckrodt Pharmaceuticals. FDA approved. 2014. https://www.accessdata.fda.gov/drugsatfda_docs/label/2014/017090s078lbl.pdf
10. Haloperidol Prescribing Information. Janssen Pharmaceuticals. FDA approved. 2011. https://www.accessdata.fda.gov/drugsatfda_docs/label/2011/018701s054lbl.pdf
11. Amitriptyline hydrochloride Prescribing Information. Sandoz Inc. FDA approved. 2014. https://www.accessdata.fda.gov/drugsatfda_docs/label/2014/085966s095,085969s084,085968s096,085971s075,085967s076,085970s072lbl.pdf
12. Janicak P, Davis J, Preskorn S, Ayd F. Principles and practice of psychopharmacology. 2nd ed. Baltimore, MD: Williams and Wilkins; 1997.
13. Currie GM. Pharmacology, part 2: introduction to pharmacokinetics. J Nucl Med Technol. 2018;46(3):221–30. https://doi.org/10.2967/jnmt.117.199638. Epub 2018 May 3
14. Grogan S, Preuss CV. Pharmacokinetics. [Updated 2020 May 17]. In: Stat Pearls [Internet]. Treasure Island, FL: Stat Pearls Publishing; 2020. https://www.ncbi.nlm.nih.gov/books/NBK557744
15. Fluoxetine Prescribing Information. Eli Lilly and Company. FDA approved. 1987. https://www.accessdata.fda.gov/drugsatfda_docs/label/2011/018936s091lbl.pdf
16. Paroxetine Prescribing Information. GlaxoSmithKline. FDA approved. 2008. https://www.accessdata.fda.gov/drugsatfda_docs/label/2008/020031s060,020936s037,020710s024lbl.pdf
17. Mohs RC, Greig NH. Drug discovery and development: Role of basic biological research. Alzheimer's Dement (N Y). 2017;3(4):651–7. Published 2017 Nov 11. https://doi.org/10.1016/j.trci.2017.10.005.
18. Macaluso M, Krams M, Preskorn S. Phase I trials: from traditional to newer approaches part II. J Psychiatr Pract. 2011;17(4):277–84.
19. United States Food and Drug Administration. The Drug Development Process. 2018. https://www.fda.gov/patients/learn-about-drug-and-device-approvals/drug-development-process.
20. Soares JC, Mann JJ. The functional neuroanatomy of mood disorders. J Psychiatric Res. 1997;31(4):393–432. ISSN 0022-3956
21. Drevets WC, Price JL, Furey ML. Brain structural and functional abnormalities in mood disorders: implications for neurocircuitry models of depression. Brain Struct Funct. 2008;213(1-2):93–118. https://doi.org/10.1007/s00429-008-0189-x. Epub 2008 Aug 13. PMID: 18704495; PMCID: PMC2522333
22. Meyer JH, Wilson AA, Ginovart N, Goulding V, Hussey D, Hood K, Houle S. Occupancy of Serotonin Transporters by Paroxetine and Citalopram during treatment of Depression. A [11C]DASB PET Imaging Study. Am J Psychiatry. 2001;158(11):1843–9.
23. Pratt LA, Brody DJ, Gu Q. Antidepressant use among persons aged 12 and over: United States, 2011–2014, NCHS data brief, no 283. Hyattsville, MD: National Center for Health Statistics; 2017.
24. Schatzberg A, Cole J, Debattista C. Manual of clinical psychopharmacology. 7th ed. Washington, DC: American Psychiatric Publishing Inc.; 2010.
25. Domino EF. History of modern psychopharmacology: a personal view with an emphasis on antidepressants. Psychosom Med. 1999;61(5):591–8.
26. Preskorn S, Feighner J, Stanga C, Ross R. Antidepressants: past, present and future. Handbook of experimental pharmacology. Switzerland: Springer; 2004.
27. Doxepin HCL Prescribing Information. Pfizer Inc. FDA approved. 2007. https://www.accessdata.fda.gov/drugsatfda_docs/label/2007/016798s054,017516s023lbl.pdf
28. Nortriptyline hydrochloride Prescribing Information. Novartis Consumer Health Inc. FDA approved. 2012. https://www.accessdata.fda.gov/drugsatfda_docs/label/2007/018012s27lbl.pdf
29. Isocarboxazid Prescribing Information. Neurocrine Biosciences Inc. FDA approved. 2017. https://www.accessdata.fda.gov/drugsatfda_docs/label/2017/209241lbl.pdf
30. Phenelzine Prescribing Information. Pfizer Inc. FDA approved. 2007. https://www.accessdata.fda.gov/drugsatfda_docs/label/2007/011909s038lbl.pdf
31. Selegiline Prescribing Information. Bristol-Myers Squibb Company. FDA approved. 2007. https://www.accessdata.fda.gov/drugsatfda_docs/label/2007/021336s002lbl.pdf
32. Tranylcypromine Prescribing Information. Concordia Pharmaceuticals Inc. FDA approved. 2015. https://www.accessdata.fda.gov/drugsatfda_docs/label/2018/012342s064lbl.pdf
33. Macaluso M, Preskorn S. Antidepressants: from biogenic amines to new mechanisms of action. Handbook of experimental pharmacology. Switzerland: Springer; 2019.
34. Citalopram Prescribing Information. Forest Pharmaceuticals Inc. FDA approved. 2009. https://www.accessdata.fda.gov/drugsatfda_docs/label/2009/020822s037,021046s015lbl.pdf
35. Escitalopram Prescribing Information. Forest Pharmaceuticals Inc. FDA approved. 2009. https://www.accessdata.fda.gov/drugsatfda_docs/label/2009/021323s032,021365s023lbl.pdf
36. Sertraline Prescribing Information. Pfizer Inc. FDA approved. 2009. https://www.accessdata.fda.gov/drugsatfda_docs/label/2009/019839s070,020990s032lbl.pdf
37. Venlafaxine Prescribing Information. Wyeth Pharmaceuticals Inc. FDA approved. 1997. https://www.accessdata.fda.gov/drugsatfda_docs/label/2017/020699s107lbl.pdf
38. Desvenlafaxine Prescribing Information. Wyeth Pharmaceuticals Inc. FDA approved. 2008. https://www.accessdata.fda.gov/drugsatfda_docs/label/2012/021992s030lbl.pdf

39. Duloxetine Prescribing Information. Eli Lilly and Company. FDA approved. 2004. https://www.accessdata.fda.gov/drugsatfda_docs/label/2010/022516lbl.pdf
40. Milnacipran Prescribing Information. Forest Pharmaceuticals Inc. FDA approved. 2009. https://www.accessdata.fda.gov/drugsatfda_docs/label/2012/022256s013lbl.pdf
41. Levomilnacipran Prescribing Information. Forest Pharmaceuticals Inc. FDA approved. 2013. https://www.accessdata.fda.gov/drugsatfda_docs/label/2013/204168s000lbl.pdf
42. Bupropion Prescribing Information. GlacoSmithKline. FDA approved. 2009. https://www.accessdata.fda.gov/drugsatfda_docs/label/2009/021515s023s024lbl.pdf
43. Mirtazapine Prescribing Information. Organon. FDA approved. 2007. https://www.accessdata.fda.gov/drugsatfda_docs/label/2007/020415s019,021208s010lbl.pdf
44. Trazodone Prescribing Information. TEVA Pharmaceuticals. FDA approved. 2014. https://www.accessdata.fda.gov/drugsatfda_docs/label/2015/071196s062lbl.pdf
45. Fagiolini A, Comandini A, Dell'Osso MC, Kasper S. Rediscovering trazadone for the treatment of major depressive disorder. CNS Drugs. 2012;26(12):1033–4.
46. Vortioxetine Prescribing Information. Takeda Pharmaceuticals America, Inc. 2013. FDA approved. https://www.accessdata.fda.gov/drugsatfda_docs/label/2013/204447s000lbl.pdf
47. Vilazadone Prescribing Information. Trovis Pharmaceutical LLC. FDA approved. 2011. https://www.accessdata.fda.gov/drugsatfda_docs/label/2011/022567s000lbl.pdf
48. Aleksandrova LR, Phillips AG, Wang YT. Antidepressant effects of ketamine and the roles of AMPA glutamate receptors and other mechanisms beyond NMDA receptor antagonism. J Psychiatry Neurosci. 2017;42(4):222–9.
49. Williams NR, Heifets BD, Blasey C, et al. Attenuation of antidepressant effects of ketamine by opioid receptor antagonism. Am J Psychiatry. 2018;175(12):1205–15.
50. Murrough JW, Perez AM, Pilemer S, et al. Rapid and longer-term antidepressant effects of repeated ketamine infusions in treatment-resistant major depression. Biol Psychiatry. 2013;74:250–6.
51. Esketamine Prescribing Information. Janssen Pharmaceutical Inc. FDA approved. 2019. https://www.accessdata.fda.gov/drugsatfda_docs/label/2019/211243lbl.pdf
52. Debattista C, Schatzberg A. Psychotropic dosing and monitoring guidelines. Primary Psychiatry. 2006;13(6):61–81.
53. Hermida AP, Glass OM, Shafi H, McDonald WM. Electroconvulsive therapy in depression: current practice and future direction. Psychiatr Clin North Am. 2018;41(3):341–53. https://doi.org/10.1016/j.psc.2018.04.001. Epub 2018 Jun 15
54. Perrin JS, Merz S, Bennett DM, Currie J, Steele DJ, Reid IC, Schwarzbauer C. ECT reduces frontal cortical connectivity. Proc Natl Acad Sci. 2012;109(14):54645468. https://doi.org/10.1073/pnas.1117206109.
55. Speer AM, Kimbrell TA, Wassermann EM, Repella JD, Willis MW, Herscovitch P, Post RM. Opposite effects of high and low frequency rTMS on regional brain activity in depressed patients. Biol Psychiatry. 2000;48(12):1133–41.
56. Chokhawala K, Stevens L. Antipsychotic Medications. [Updated 2020 May 23]. In: StatPearls [Internet]. Treasure Island, FL: StatPearls Publishing; 2020. https://www.ncbi.nlm.nih.gov/books/NBK519503/
57. Thioridazine Prescribing Information. Eli Lilly Company. FDA approved. 1987. https://www.accessdata.fda.gov/drugsatfda_docs/label/2011/018936s091lbl.pdf
58. Clozapine Prescribing Information. HLS Therapeutics INC. FDA approved. 2017. https://www.accessdata.fda.gov/drugsatfda_docs/label/2017/019758s084lbl.pdf
59. Risperidone Prescribing Information. Janssen Pharmaceuticals. FDA approved. 2009. https://www.accessdata.fda.gov/drugsatfda_docs/label/2009/020272s056,020588s044,021346s033,021444s03lbl.pdf
60. Olanzapine Prescribing Information. Eli Lilly Company. FDA approved. 2009. https://www.accessdata.fda.gov/drugsatfda_docs/label/2009/020592s051,021086s030,021253s036lbl.pdf
61. Quetiapine Prescribing Information. AstraZeneca Pharmaceuticals. FDA approved. 2003. https://www.accessdata.fda.gov/drugsatfda_docs/label/2004/20639se1-017,016_seroquel_lbl.pdf
62. Aripiprazole Prescribing Information. Otsuka Pharmaceuticals. FDA approved. 2016. https://www.accessdata.fda.gov/drugsatfda_docs/label/2016/021436s041,021713s032,021729s024,021866s026lbl.pdf
63. Pimavanserin Prescribing Information. Acadia Pharmaceuticals Inc. FDA approved. 2016. https://www.accessdata.fda.gov/drugsatfda_docs/label/2016/207318lbl.pdf
64. Cariprazine Prescribing Information. Actavis Pharma Inc. FDA approved. 2015. https://www.accessdata.fda.gov/drugsatfda_docs/label/2015/204370lbl.pdf
65. Lurasidone Prescribing Information. Sunovion Pharmaceuticals Inc. FDA approved. 2013. https://www.accessdata.fda.gov/drugsatfda_docs/label/2013/200603lbls10s11.pdf
66. Brexpiprazole Prescribing Information. Otsuka Pharmaceuticals Co. FDA approved. 2018. https://www.accessdata.fda.gov/drugsatfda_docs/label/2018/205422s003lbl.pdf
67. Paliperidone Prescribing Information. Ortho-McNeil-Janssen Pharmaceuticals Inc. FDA approved. 2010. https://www.accessdata.fda.gov/drugsatfda_docs/label/2010/021999s018lbl.pdf
68. Lithium Prescribing Information. Roxane Laboratories Inc. FDA approved. 2016. https://www.accessdata.fda.gov/drugsatfda_docs/label/2016/017812s027,018421s025,018558s021lbl.pdf
69. Divalproex Prescribing Information. Abbott Laboratories. FDA approved. 2011. https://www.accessdata.fda.gov/drugsatfda_docs/label/2011/018723s037lbl.pdf
70. Carbamazepine Prescribing Information. GlaxoSmithKline. FDA approved. 2009. https://www.accessdata.fda.gov/drugsatfda_docs/label/2009/016608s101,018281s048lbl.pdf
71. Lamotrigine Prescribing Information. GlaxoSmithKline. FDA approved. 2015. https://www.accessdata.fda.gov/drugsatfda_docs/label/2015/020241s045s051lbl.pdf
72. Nath M, Gupta V. Mood Stabilizers. [Updated 2020 Oct 5]. In: StatPearls [Internet]. Treasure Island, FL: StatPearls Publishing; 2020. https://www.ncbi.nlm.nih.gov/books/NBK556141/
73. Bandelow B, Michaelis S, Wedekind D. Treatment of anxiety disorders. Dialogues Clin Neurosci. 2017;19(2):93–107.
74. Diazepam Prescribing Information. Roche Laboratories Inc. FDA approved. 2008. https://www.accessdata.fda.gov/drugsatfda_docs/label/2008/013263s083lbl.pdf
75. Clonazepam Prescribing Information. Genetech USA Inc. FDA approved. 2013. https://www.accessdata.fda.gov/drugsatfda_docs/label/2013/017533s053,020813s009lbl.pdf
76. Lorazepam Prescribing Information. Valeant Pharmaceuticals Inc. FDA approved. 2016. https://www.accessdata.fda.gov/drugsatfda_docs/label/2016/017794s044lbl.pdf
77. Oxazepam Prescribing Information. Faulding Laboratories Inc. FDA approved. 2001. https://www.accessdata.fda.gov/drugsatfda_docs/label/2001/15539s52lbl.pdf
78. Alprazolam Prescribing Information. Pfizer Inc. FDA approved. 2011. https://www.accessdata.fda.gov/drugsatfda_docs/label/2011/018276s045lbl.pdf
79. Buspirone Prescribing Information. Bristol-Myers Squibb FDA approved. 2010. https://www.accessdata.fda.gov/drugsatfda_docs/label/2010/018731s051lbl.pdf

80. Hydroxyzine Prescribing Information. Pfizer Inc. FDA approved. 2014. https://www.accessdata.fda.gov/drugsatfda_docs/label/2014/011459s048%2C011795s025lbl.pdf
81. McMillan JM, Aitken E, Holroyd-Leduc JM. Management of insomnia and long-term use of sedative-hypnotic drugs in older patients. CMAJ. 2013;185(17):1499–505.
82. Stevens JR, Wilens TE, Stern TA. Using stimulants for attention-deficit/hyperactivity disorder: clinical approaches and challenges. Prim Care Companion CNS Disord. 2013;15(2):PCC.12f01472.
83. Laje G, Perlis RH, Rush AJ, McMahon FJ. Pharmacogenomics studies in STAR D: strengths, limitations and results. Psychiatr Serv. 2009;60:1446–57.
84. U.S. Food and Drug Administration. The FDA warns against the use of many genetic tests with unapproved claims to predict patient response to specific medications: FDA Safety Communication. October 31, 2018. https://www.fda.gov/medical-devices/safety-communications/fda-warns-against-use-many-genetic-tests-unapproved-claims-predict-patient-response-specific
85. Moran M. Task force on gene testing for antidepressant efficacy concludes tests not yet ready for widespread use. Psychiatr News July 19 2018; 2018. https://www.sandiegopsychiatricsociety.org/uncategorized/task-force-on-gene-testing-for-antidepressant-efficacy-concludes-tests-not-yet-ready-for-widespread-use
86. Uhr M, Tontsch A, Namendorf C, Ripke S, Lucae S, Ising M, Dose T, et al. Polymorphisms in the drug transporter gene ABCB1 predict antidepressant treatment response in depression. Neuron. 2008;57:203–9.
87. Mk J, Minhajuddin A, Gadad BS, Greer T, et al. Can c-reactive protein inform antidepressant medication selection in depressed outpatients? Findings from the CO-MED trial. Psychoneuroendocrinology. 2017;78:105–13.
88. Macaluso M, Preskorn SH. How biomarkers will change psychiatry: from clinical trials to practice. Part I: introduction. J Psychiatr Pract. 2012;18(2):118–21.

11 Psychosocial Treatments: Psychotherapy, Behavioral, and Cultural Interventions

Manuel Trujillo

Introduction

Psychiatry, which in the 1870s was to become the youngest of all medical disciplines, was late to incorporate prevailing information. It took its time to entertain physiological hypotheses to account for the causal chain of severe psychiatric disorders, and hesitated for far too long, to use the same conceptual framework that was being successfully applied to the rational understanding of practically all other medical disorders. Sigmund Freud, at the beginning of the twentieth century, discovered a method of scientific inquiry (psychoanalysis) from which, in addition to psychoanalysis proper, a torrent of other therapeutic applications evolved over the years under such generic names as psychoanalytic psychotherapies and psychodynamic psychotherapies. Since World War II (WWII) the growth of the discipline has been extraordinary. Numerous new effective medications have allowed patients to achieve clinical successes on par with those obtained in other areas of clinical medicine. In parallel, many other psychosocial interventions, anchored in disciplines such as systems theory, family dynamics, cultural formulations of health and illness, and many others have reached scientific recognition and therapeutic prowess. Their extraordinary diversity found an intellectual and pragmatic home under the umbrella of the biopsychosocial paradigm, first fully articulated by George Engel in a seminal paper published in 1977 [1]. Emil Kraepelin [2] and Sigmund Freud [3], at the beginning of the twentieth century, provided solid anchors for such progress. Kraepelin gave a scientific framework for clinical psychiatry and psychopathology with his classification system which still survives in our diagnostic practices. Freud discovered a method of scientific inquiry (psychoanalysis), from which, in addition to clinical psychoanalysis, and many other therapeutic applications, basic findings for a science of the mind emerge: the existence and importance of unconscious mental processes, the mechanism of defense, the structure of the mind (its id, ego, superego, and self). The value of the transference is central to contemporary science of the mind, compatible with all other biological and psychological paradigms and deeply embedded in contemporary art and culture.

Psychiatry started the twenty-first century fully equipped to produce more and better evidence-based therapies for the large and growing number of disorders that afflict contemporary societies. The reinvigoration of its scientific zeal and ambition is allowing psychiatrists to claim the neurosciences (neuroimaging, molecular neurobiology) and the rapidly evolving fields of medical genetics and epigenetics as central to its scientific and practice frameworks.

Psychosocial interventions in Psychiatry received a significant push in the turbulent cauldron of revolutionary France in the late eighteenth century, under the "Moral Treatment" philosophy developed by the legendary French physician Philippe Pinel who, myth and questioned history, have exalted as the first who liberated the mentally ill from their chains and from exclusionary labels as "deviants" or "sinners" and thus were welcomed by society as citizens, subject to the rights and privileges of all people declared equal in the radically new social order that emerged in revolutionary France (Table 11.1) [4].

Pinel has been described by many as "the father of modern psychiatry," and although Pinel always gave his colleague Pussin the credit he deserved as the actual author of the iconic act, a legend grew about Pinel single-handedly liberating the insane from their chains at Bicêtre. This legend has been immortalized in commemorated national paintings and public monuments in France, and has lived on for 200 years in history books, psychiatric textbooks and in the public imagination. In fact, it was Pussin and not Pinel, who actually removed the iron shackles from, and it was at Bicêtre, not at the Salpetriere, after Pinel had already lefBicetre for the Salpêtrière. Pinel did, indeed, remove the chains from patients at the Salpêtrière but 3 years later, when Pussin joined him there.

M. Trujillo (✉)
Department of Psychiatry, New York University School of Medicine, New York, NY, USA
e-mail: Manuel.Trujillo@nyulangone.org

W. W. IsHak (ed.), *Atlas of Psychiatry*, https://doi.org/10.1007/978-3-031-15401-0_11

Table 11.1 The moral treatment principles; an eighteenth century forerunner of the twentieth-century biopsychosocial treatment model

• Respect for patient's rights and freedom, and awareness of their dignity as citizens and the abolition of many abusive restraint practices. Maintenance of "order without violence"
• Awareness of patient's emotions and openness to consider them a focus of treatment and a causal element of the illness (the birth of the therapeutic interest and focus on the mind), together with heredity and stressed physiology
• The understanding that love could turn to grief and desperation. Sudden failures could bring about alienation. Unbridled passions (religious or political) could develop into fanaticism and overwhelm the person's reason. Pinel often traced emotions to mental states and those to physiological states
• A clinical method based on frequent physician-patient contact, careful and extensive history taking, empirical observations and on phenomenological descriptions of patient's behavior, thoughts and feelings
• And the development and maintenance of life skills through the judicious use of rehabilitative work activities, education and distractions

From such foundations, both the brand-new discipline and the status of its patients, initiated a slow but steady worldwide dissemination, with Britain and the USA being the first and most important stations in this journey.

The seeds for the final component of our current bio-psychosocial model of care, the psychosocial interventions dimension, were also enthusiastically planted in the humanistic fervor of eighteenth-century France, and it was thoroughly revitalized in the aftermath of World War II (WWII), when great numbers of US military psychiatrists returned to civilian positions at the end of the armed conflict. Back home, they applied the many clinically useful lessons learned on the battlefields of a war that had endured a high rate of psychiatric casualties. These lessons were, essentially (1) treat early, (2) treat as close as possible to the frontline, (3) maintain the soldier's connection to their units, and (4) let your treatments offer rest, emotional understanding and support, and the judicious use of the limited medical armamentarium available at the time. Since WWII the growth of the discipline has been extraordinary. Numerous new effective medications have allowed psychiatrists to achieve clinical successes on par with those obtained in other areas of clinical medicine. The domain of the mind grew exponentially as well, both in theoretical prowess and in clinical practice, first under the impetus of Sigmund Freud's psychoanalysis which, after all, presented the first scientific theory of unconscious mental function and the first comprehensive metapsychology of the mind, and then under the power of the knowledge generated by the experimental study of behavior, cognition and other mental functions not addressed in the psychoanalytic metapsychology. Thus, a very large number of therapeutic models and techniques have become available for the psychological care of patients and to facilitate the scientific study of the mind. In parallel, many other psychosocial interventions have reached scientific recognition and therapeutic prowess, anchoring themselves in disciplines such as systems theory, family dynamics, cultural formulations of health and illness, and many others. These advancements led to the development of the bio-psychosocial paradigm, first presented by George Engel in his 1977 paper referenced above [1].

The last leg of psychiatry's impressive journey is represented by the commitment of all of its contributing disciplines to submit their methods and findings, as well as their therapeutic proposals, to the rigors of the scientific method and to the standards of scientific proof. Thus, psychiatry started the twenty-first century fully equipped to produce more and better evidence-based therapies for the large and growing number of disorders that afflict the citizens of contemporary societies.

A few additional transformative steps are already visible on the horizon. The full application of neuroimaging to psychiatric clinical practice, now in development in the hands of a few pioneers, will bring psychiatry closer to Freud's long-delayed dream for our profession; to anchor his findings about the mind on the secure footing of neurobiological knowledge. As Freud wrote:

> *Biology is truly a land of unlimited possibilities. We may expect it to give us the most surprising information, and we cannot guess what answers it will return in a few dozen years. They may be of a kind which will blow away the whole of our artificial structure of hypothesis.* (Freud, *Beyond the Pleasure Principle* [1920] [5].)

For most of the last 200 years, the psychiatric care provided in the developed world had to make do with the slow expansion of the Moral Treatment philosophy championed by Pinel, and with the limited therapeutic practices flowing from such philosophy which could be implemented in the Asylums; the institutions which developed in the USA under the moral treatment principles. The Moral Treatment model found its way to a young America aided, among other forces, by the intellectual and humanitarian commitments of Benjamin Rush, and by the advocacy zeal of Dorothea Dix.

A much fuller development of such embryonic rendition of the psychosocial model did not become possible until the middle of the twentieth century, when, almost simultaneously in the USA and in other countries of the developed and developing worlds, new treatments and models of psychiatric care emerged.

A very important such model is the Community Mental Health Center Movement, a set of population-based mental health principles, clinical models, community facilities and funding mechanisms that flowed from US President John F. Kennedy's signing of the landmark Community Mental Health Act of 1963 and which represented yet another major step in the liberation of the mentally ill; this time from the restrictive, distant, therapeutically bare models of the State Psychiatric Centers which took over from the early Asylums (Fig. 11.1). The impetus this time was generated by an

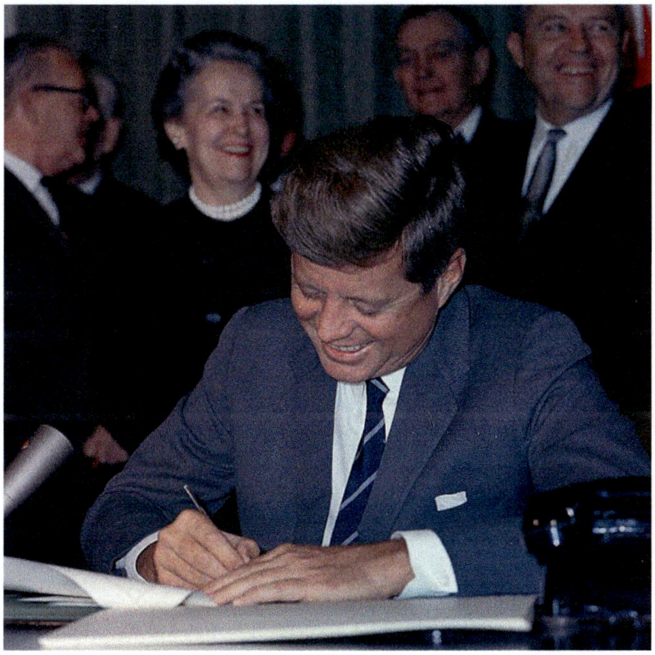

Fig. 11.1 President John F. Kennedy Signs the Community Mental Health Act

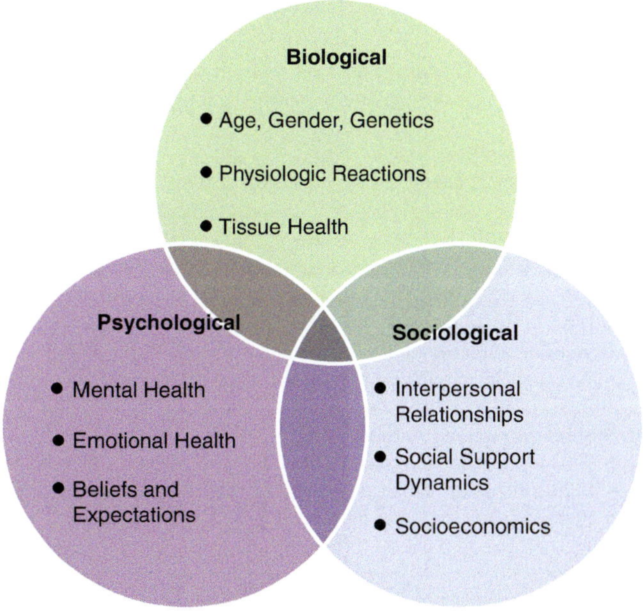

Fig. 11.2 An illustration of the biopsychosocial model comprised of biological, psychological, and sociological influences. (*From* Gliedt et al. [178]; Creative Commons Attribution 4.0 International License; http://creativecommons.org/licenses/by/4.0)

expanded bill of rights, and by Kennedy's administration philosophical passion, and political will, to integrate the psychiatric patients into their natural communities, an action which had proven singularly so helpful, on the battlefields of WWII, in restoring psychiatric casualties to health and function, and in preventing the deterioration associated with chronic institutionalization. Such views were held by many psychiatric advocates and advocacy organizations that supported progressive politicians to pass the necessary legislation.

In the 1960s, first in the USA, later in the developed countries of Europe, and then spreading worldwide, the conceptual and administrative contributions of the Community Mental Health model, assumed the monumental dual task of treating in their communities the rising number of new patients seeking counseling and care, while simultaneously trying to bring home, to their original neighborhoods, the patients being discharged in huge numbers from asylum-like state psychiatric centers. Those were the patients who were responding very positively to the new medical treatments (antipsychotic, antidepressant, and antianxiety medications) which were rolling out of pharmaceutical companies in the 1950s and 1960s. By the 1970s, the prevailing locus of care of psychiatric patients was shifting from the asylum to the community, and to psychiatric units in the general hospital where, at long last, psychiatrists and our patients, joined local communities and the mainstream of medicine.

There, in the community, the psychosocial model initial triad (respecting patients' dignity and agency, treating early and in the community, and providing robust community supports), expanded vigorously, both conceptually and functionally, generating new hope for our patients and significant excitement and optimism in the psychiatric professional community. A broad and growing array of psychosocial and psychotherapeutic interventions grew fast and furious under such a benign climate. Such developments ushered in an era of great therapeutic zeal, and a profusion of therapeutic programs and practices; practices which however slowly, came to accept the challenge of gathering supportive evidence for their efficacy and effectiveness in scientifically controlled clinical trials. Results of psychiatric treatments turned about to be comparable to the results achieved in the clinical trials conducted by the other biomedical disciplines to evaluate the treatment of their most common disorders.

Psychiatry functions now, practically worldwide, under the bio-psycho-social model of medical science; a model first promulgated by George Engel in the 1970s [1], which holds that human behavior is the product of a unique combination of interacting biological, psychological and social dimensions, and of their complex interrelations (Fig. 11.2) and presented a comprehensive critique of the biomedicine of the 1970s (Table 11.2).

Engel also described the model's applications to Psychiatry in 1980 [6]. In later years, the cultural and spiritual dimensions of human experience and behavior, have gained significant scientific and pragmatic status as legitimate foci for interventions to support health and mental health, and have been added to the bio-psycho-social model to create the more complete—if somewhat cumbersome—current formulation for the understanding and treatment of psychiatric disorders: *the bio-psychosocial-cultural-spiritual model of human behavior and behavioral disorders*. This is

Table 11.2 Engel's critique of biomedicine

1. Illness
• A biochemical alteration does not translate directly into an illness
• The appearance of illness results from the interaction of diverse causal factors, including those at the molecular, individual, and social levels And the converse
• Psychological alterations may manifest as illnesses or health problems, including, at times, biochemical correlates
• Adopting a sick role is not necessarily associated with the presence of a biological derangement
2. Biology
• The presence of a biological derangement does not shed full light on the meaning of the symptoms to the patient, nor does it necessarily infer the clinical attitude and process needed to process it well
• The success of the most biological of treatments is influenced by psychosocial factors, for example, the so-called placebo effect
3. Psychosocial factors
• Psychosocial variables are more important determinants of susceptibility, severity, and course of illness than had been previously appreciated by those who maintain a biomedical view of illness
4. Patient–physician relationship
• The patient–clinician relationship influences medical outcomes, even if only because of its influence on adherence to a chosen treatment
• Unlike inanimate subjects of scientific scrutiny, patients are profoundly influenced by the way in which they are studied, and the scientists engaged in the study are influenced by their subjects

the, more or less, explicit intellectual template from which Psychosocial interventions and treatments derive their ethos. Limits to the biopsychosocial model have been pointed out over the last few years [7], with new alternatives being presented offering more scientifically sophisticated descriptions of the causal pathways that link biological, psychological, and social domains appearing recently [8].

The cultural dimension of the model is built upon many sources: case-based epidemiological knowledge, accumulated through the years by clinicians and investigators as to the risks and protective factors, that accrue from people's cultural beliefs, intercultural conflict, mass displacements, migration, and other sociodemographic variables, which can color and influence the presentation, prognosis or outcome of classical disorders. The imprint of the academic psychiatrist Emile Kraepelin whose towering influence shaped the first thorough attempt to construct a diagnostic classification system based on scientific psychopathology, is also, to no one's surprise, found at the foundation of cultural psychopathology. Indeed, in the early 1900s he made the initial descriptions of the distinct (culture-bound) syndromes found in patients' native to the islands of Fiji. He also reported a higher incidence of manic-depressive patients displaying episodes of pure mania only (and no depression) over the course of the disorder in Fiji; a rarity in western countries where depression dominates mania over the course of the illness. Be that as it may, following this initial taxonomic interest, cultural psychiatry has experienced significant growth supported by psychiatrists and anthropologists such as Edward Taylor, Gregory Bateson, Margaret Mead, and many others [9].

As the principles and practices of Community Psychiatry took hold in the USA, UK, and worldwide, it became progressively obvious that the classical definitions and classification criteria for psychiatric disorders, promoted by the DSM system were woefully inadequate to capture the broad clinical dimensions, and the subjective experiences, of the large number of new users of care. Furthermore, the linguistic and cultural "translation" capacities of most physicians, clinicians, and psychiatric support staff who participated in the care of poor excluded, and marginalized minorities, were drastically insufficient to treat such patients across the language and cultural barriers. Thanks in part to the tireless activism of many such physicians and clinicians supported by the fact that study after study documented the shortcomings of culturally blind psychiatric practice, the American Psychiatric Association (APA), approved the publication and use of the Outline for Cultural Formulation (OCF) in DSM-IV in 1994, finally acknowledging the importance of culture in psychiatry [10]. In 2013, after nearly 20 years of experience in the field, the revision of the Cultural Formulation followed in the DSM-5. This revision included field-tested semi-structured interviews, to facilitate and normalize the process of collecting information for the OCF [11]. This set of interviews is known collectively as the Cultural Formulation Interview (CFI) and consists of a core 16-item questionnaire and 12 modules for further inquiry, as well as versions for other informants such as caregivers (Table 11.3) [12, 13].

A parallel process of science-based activism moved many other mental health stakeholders to advance, expand and test various models of cultural competence. Thus grew the whole field of health disparities; a field that tracks the differences in health, access to healthcare, outcomes of care, and healthcare attributable longevity that culture, ethnic, and class status makes, and investigates mechanisms to address and reduce such disparities.

Table 11.3 The cultural formulation interview

CFI question	Relevant OCF domain
1. What problems or concerns bring you to the clinic?	Cultural explanations of the individual's illness
2. What troubles you most about your problem?	Cultural explanations of the individual's illness
3. People often understand their problems in their own way, which may be similar or different from how doctors explain the problem. How would you describe your problem to someone else?	Cultural explanations of the individual's illness
3a. Sometimes people use particular words or phrases to talk about their problems. Is there a specific term or expression that describes your problem? 3b. What is it?	Cultural explanations of the individual's illness
4. Why do you think this is happening to you? What do you think are the particular causes of your problem?	Cultural explanations of the individual's illness
5. What, if anything, makes your problem worse, or makes it harder to cope with?	Cultural factors related to psychosocial environment and levels of functioning
5a. What have your family, friends, and other people in your life done that may have made your problem worse?	Cultural factors related to psychosocial environment and levels of functioning
6. What, if anything, makes your problem better, or helps you cope with it more easily?	Cultural factors related to psychosocial environment and levels of functioning
6a. What have your family, friends, and other people in your life done that may have made your problem better?	Cultural factors related to psychosocial environment and levels of functioning
7. Is there anything about your background for example your culture, race, ethnicity, religion or geographical origin that is causing problems for you in your current life situation? In what way?	Cultural identity of the individual
8. On the other hand, is there anything about your background that helps you to cope with your current life situation? In what way?	Cultural identity of the individual
9. Sometimes people consider various ways of making themselves feel better. What have you done on your own to cope with your problem?	Cultural explanations of the individual's illness
10. Often, people also look for help from other individuals, groups, or institutions to help them feel better. In the past, what kind of treatment or help from other sources have you sought for your problem?	Cultural explanations of the individual's illness
10a. What type of help or treatment was most useful? Why?/How?	Cultural explanations of the individual's illness
10b. What type of help or treatment was not useful? Why?/How?	Cultural explanations of the individual's illness
11. Has anything prevented you from getting the help you need—for example, cost or lack of insurance coverage, getting time off work or family responsibilities, concern about stigma or discrimination, or lack of services that understand your language or culture? What got in the way?	Cultural factors related to psychosocial environment and levels of functioning
12. Now let's talk about the help you would be getting here. Is there anything about my own background that might make it difficult for me to understand or help you with your problem? 12a. In what way?/Why not?	Cultural elements of the relationship between the individual and the clinician
13. How can I and others at our clinic be most helpful for you?	Cultural elements of the relationship between the individual and the clinician
14. What kind of help would you like from us now, as specialists in mental health?	Cultural elements of the relationship between the individual and the clinician

Abbreviations: *CFI* cultural formulation interview, *OCF—DSM-IV* outline for cultural formulation
From Aggarwal et al. [177]; *with permission*

Culture

The iconic image of the Bison of Altamira (Spain) (Fig. 11.3) depicts, better than the proverbial one thousand words, how the use of symbols represents Homo Sapiens' passage, and grounding, to the world of culture, and behavioral modernity. Behavioral modernity refers to the suite of behavioral and cognitive traits that distinguishes current homo sapiens from other modern humans and advanced primates. Such cognitive capacities include abstract thinking, planning depth, facial recognition, sophisticated "theories of mind", the use of art, ornamentation, music, and dancing, to modulate relationships and signal rank. It includes kin recognition and rules of cooperation (and opposition) to kin and not-kin. Above all, it includes new forms of learning by observation and emulation, and key to human communities is the construction of symbolic values and meanings that bind groups.

The ability to operate with symbols codifies our understanding of the world in which we live, thus serving as the referent upon which we make judgments and create value-based narratives which can transmit identity and destiny to successors. These narratives are the community's "constitutive rhetoric," defined by James Boyd White as "a discourse that creates collective identity," and demands action to rein-

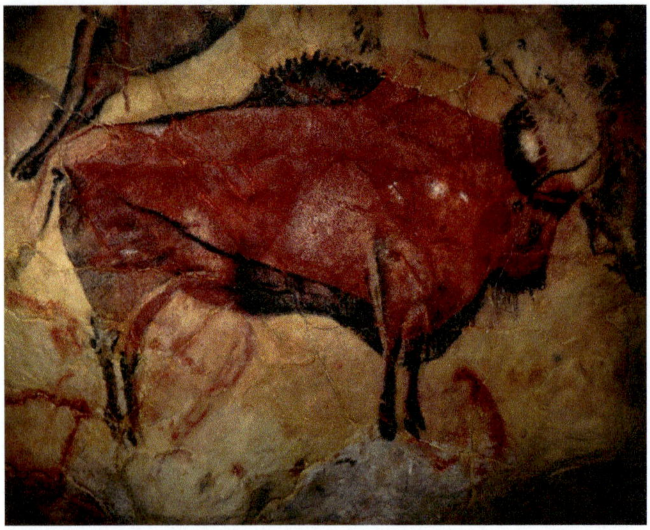

Fig. 11.3 The Bison of Altamira

force identity and the beliefs supporting identity." For White, constitutive rhetoric denotes "the art of constituting character, community and culture in language" [14].

Definition of Culture

For Cultural Psychiatry, culture can be defined as a *learned* symbolic whole that provides each individual with a unique view of the world and with language narratives that allows individuals to order such world. These narratives, include creation stories and religious beliefs often, encompassing themes of life and death and the role of ancestors (Trujillo, 2000) [15]. They provide views of our selves (identity); values and meanings to label experience and to pursue goals. It provides behavioral standards including morals, laws, norms, traditions, etiquette, and customs to relate to kin and not-kin. It often provides guidance for eating, sexual and mating behaviors, as well as complex codes to deal with deviant behaviors and practices. For clinical purposes, the APA defined Culture as: "The meanings, values and behavioral norms that are learned and transmitted in the dominant culture, influencing cognitions, feelings and self-concept and the diagnostic process and treatment decisions."

Culture Influences Psychopathology

Culture influences psychopathology through numerous direct and indirect pathways: (1) through the direct pathogenic effects of anxiety-provoking culturally prescribed roles and duties when they are at odds with healthy drives for affirmation or self-realization, (2) through the culture-specific "idioms of distress." The "ataque de nervios" which appears in certain Hispanic populations when confronted with conflicts with family authority figures often defuses a situation that might be perceived as an "offensive" challenge to a cultural prescription of deference to parents or other community authorities. (3) Through a "pathoplastic effect: culture coloring and shaping the content of symptoms such as delusions (religious content shape the ideas and delusions of religious communities, spy and secret agencies such as the C.I.A or K.G.B shape the delusions in more secular societies, auditory hallucinations may come through, animals or vegetation in some societies and through technology such as Television equipment in others). (4) Through labeling as pathological social behaviors considered unacceptable by the dominant powers: homosexuality was considered a psychiatric illness in the US until the 1970s, dissent is classified as "personality disorder" in certain societies, etc.

Cultural Competence Facilitates Diagnosis and Treatment Across the Cultural Barrier

Cultural competence: a term first defined by Cross in 1989, refers to the acquisition of a set of attitudes, skills and knowledge that makes it possible for the culturally competent professional to provide quality and effective care through the language and cultural barriers [16]. Necessary skills include understanding cultural differences between people and appreciating their impact on health beliefs and practices, an attitude of cultural humility which facilitates trust, specific knowledge about the prevalence of illness, differential clinical presentations, response to medications, treatment expectations and preferences between people [17].

Measuring Cultural Competence

To the degree that cultural competence includes phenomena and ideas that rest on cognitive concepts and insights [18], it is, in principle, a measurable parameter containing measurable dimensions and variables. Indeed, research over the last few decades has provided analytic frameworks that can measure the degree to which an individual shares with others similar views about particular cultures including their own. The medical anthropologist William Dressler has developed an analytic framework "Cultural Consensus Analysis," which uses factor analytic methods to estimate similarities and differences between respondents, and then can estimate the impact of cultural congruence, or dissonance, on the health status of respondents [19]. The philosophical and human ground from which all cultural competence models develop is situated at the boundary between anthropology and sociology, and has been well explored by Kleinman [21, 22]. The concept of Cultural Humility articulated in the concept of Cultural Humility proposed by Tervalon and Garcia in 1998

Cultural Humility: Definition

- "It is a process that requires humility [each has something of great value to learn from the other] as individuals continually engage in self-reflection and self-critique as lifelong learners and reflective practitioners... to redress power imbalances to develop mutually beneficial non-paternalistic partnerships in care"

Fig. 11.4 Cultural humility [20]

(Fig. 11.4) [20] is probably the best framer of the optimal attitude for the clinician working at the cultural barrier.

Clinical Cultural Competence: DSM-5 Cultural Formulation Interview

The development of the Cultural Formulation Interview(CFI), provides psychiatrists and psychiatric clinicians who participate in the assessment of patients, with a semi-structured sophisticated instrument and method which was developed by the DSM-5 Committee Cross-Cultural Issues subgroup (DCCIS) led by Lewis-Fernandez et al. in 2014 [13], after a complex process of evaluation of the assets and limitations of the initial DSM-IV's Outline for a Cultural Formulation (OCF).

An instrument was finally developed and extensively field tested. It consists of 16 core interview items and 12 additional supplementary modules (to cover the clinical problems of special clinical or demographic populations, or to expand the assessment obtained by the original core items).

The CFI aimed to be based on a "mini-ethnography," that explored and included in the clinical formulation, the patient's own interpretation of illness experience.

Key themes of the OCF and CFI include (1) an assessment of the cultural identity of the individual (including the complexities of multiple identities and their impact on the clinical presentation), (2) the patient's cultural explanations of their illness, including clinical features and treatment expectations, and the possible presence of a designated culture-bound syndrome. Treatment expectations are essential to ultimately provide these patients with treatment pathways syntonic with cultural narratives of illness course, ways of coping with setbacks, pain, and suffering, and syntonic procedures for conflict resolutions. (3) Cultural factors related to the specific psychosocial environment (migration status if relevant, social access and support to employment, education, and other key resources), (4) cultural aspects that may affect the relationship between clinician and patient [19–22].

Although it can be legitimately argued that the cultural formulation is potentially relevant and useful for any patient belonging to any cultural group the DSM-5 DCCIS identified five main situations when the assessment of cultural factors may be especially relevant for patient care: (1) diagnostic uncertainty, the presence of unusual symptoms or atypical expression of symptoms, (2) Clinician difficulties in assessing the severity of illness or of impairment, (3) and limited patient engagement or adherence to recommended treatment. The CFI includes an exploration of the existence of Culture-bound Syndromes (now labeled cultural idioms of distress or cultural syndromes) (Table 11.4) [23].

Since the publication of the CFI as part of DSM-5 in 2013, the literature on its use in training and clinical work has grown. The instrument is widely available and relatively easy to use. Most investigators report favorable evaluations of its clinical utility, feasibility, and acceptability to patients and clinicians alike. Training is straightforward, and even 1 h of training conveys measurable benefits to students. The time required for its completion shrinks to about 20 min after one administration. However, studies on the effectiveness of the CFI to improve clinical outcomes are lacking, and this paucity of data points to an urgent research priority [24].

Best Practices in Cultural Competence: The Cultural Consultation Model

In 1999, cultural researcher Dr. Laurence J. Kirmayer and his team undertook to develop and evaluate a specialized cultural consultation service (CCS) in mental health for the Montreal region [25, 26]. The CCS, based at Sir Mortimer B Davis—Jewish General Hospital, used a consultation-liaison conceptual model to build the cultural consultation concept and emphasized integrating medical anthropology perspectives with conventional psychiatric, cognitive-behavioral, and family systems perspectives. The Core CCS personnel included two part-time psychiatrists, as well as psychologists, social workers, psychiatric nurses, medical anthropologists, and trainees from these disciplines and from family medicine. A full-time clinical psychologist acted as a clinical coordinator and triaged all referred cases.

The consultation process was guided by a prepared protocol: consultants were asked to use an expanded version of the "Outline for Cultural Formulation" in DSM-IV"; that emphasized issues related to migration, ethnic identity, family systems, and developmental issues. The report of the first 100 cases is a treasure-trove of insights into the joys and complexity of the practice of cultural psychiatry. The cases evaluated rep-

Table 11.4 Culture bound syndromes

Name (geographical/cultural location)	Presentation
Amok (Malaysia, Indonesia, Philippines, Brunei, Singapore)	Dissociative episode—violent and homicidal behaviour, usually preceded by brooding over real or imagined insults
Ataque de nervios (nervous attack) (Latin-America)	Brief, intense release of emotion believed to be caused by family conflict or anger
Bilis (Rage)	Outburst of anger
Boufée deliriante (West Africa and Haiti)	Outburst of agitated, aggressive behaviour, marked confusion, psychomotor excitement, often with visual and auditory hallucinations or paranoid ideation
Brain fag or brain fog (West Africa)	Usually among high school or university students. Symptoms: difficulties in concentrating, remembering, and thinking
Dhat syndrome (Indian subcontinent)	Sexual/general weakness due to loss of semen through urine or feces
Falling out/blacking out (Southern USA, Caribbean)	Episodes of sudden collapse and fainting, often with hysterical blindness
Ghost sickness American Indian (Novajo)	A syndrome, associated with dead or dying, attributed to ghosts (chindi) or witchcraft. Symptoms are general weakness, loss of appetite, feeling of suffocation, recurring nightmares and a pervasive feeling of terror
Hwa-byung (Anger sickness) (Korea)	Epigastric pain, usually female, shortness of breath, flushing, indigestion, palpitations, vomiting, cold hands, dysphoria from an imagined abdominal mass, thought to be caused by suppressed or unresolved anger, disappointment or grudges
Koro (China, Malaysia, India, SEA)	Acute fear- genitalia will retract into the body (also breast into the chest in female), causing death
Latah (Malaysia, Indonesia)	Hypersensitivity to sudden fright, often with echopraxia, echolalia, command obedience, and dissociative or trancelike behaviour
Locura (Latinos in USA/Latin America)	Chronic psychosis with incoherence, agitation, auditory and visual hallucinations, inability to follow rules of social interaction, and possible violence- attributed to an inherited vulnerability or life adversities
Mal-de-ojo (Evil eye) (Mediterranean, Hispanic)	A common idiom of disease, attributed to any misfortune, and social disruption
Nervios (Latinos in USA/Latin America)	Refers to a general state of vulnerability to stressful life experiences and difficult life circumstances. A wide range of symptoms: emotional distress, somatic disturbance, and inability to function. Common symptoms: headaches, brain aches, irritability, stomach disturbances, sleep diffi- culties, nervousness, easy tearfulness, inability to concentrate, trembling, tingling sensations, and mareos (dizziness with occasional vertigo-like exacerbation)
Pibloktoq (Arctic hysteria) (Arctic circle, Inuhuit Eskimos)	Symptoms: hysterical (screaming, uncontrolled wild behavior), depression, coprophagia, echolalia, insensivity to extreme cold. Common in winter and among women
Gi-gong (Psychotic reaction) (China)	An acute, time-limited episode characterized by dissociative, paranoid, or other psychotic or nonpsychotic symptoms that occur after participating in the Chinese folk health-enhancing practice of qi-gong
Rootwork (African American, Caribbean, White population in Southern USA)	Cultural interpretations that explain illness as the result of hexing, witchcraft, voodoo, or the influence of an evil person
Sangue dormido (Portuguese in Cape Verde)	Literally "sleeping blood" with symptoms of pain, numbness, tremor, paralysis, convulsions, stroke, blindness, heart attack, infection, and miscarriage
Shenjang shuairuo (Neurasthenia) (India, China)	Mental and physical fatigue, poor concentration and memory, headache, dizziness, changes in sleep, appetite, and sexual function
Shen kui (China)	Anxiety, panic and sexual complaints with no physical findings, attributed to loss of semen or 'vital essence'
Shin-byung (Korea)	A syndrome characterized by anxiety and somatic complaints like general weakness, dizziness, fear, loss of appetite, insomnia, and gastrointestinal problems, followed by dissociation and possession by ancestral spirits
Spell (African American, White population in Southern USA)	A trance state in which individuals "communicate" with deceased relatives or with spirits
Susto (Latinos in USA, Mexico, Central America, South America)	Attributed to an illness precipitated after a frightening event that causes the soul to leave the body, leading to symptoms of unhappiness and sickness
Taijin Kyofusho (Social phobia) (Japan)	Guilt about embarrassing others- an intense fear that one's body, body parts, or bodily functions are displeasing, embarrassing, or offensive to other people
Zar (Ethiopia, Somalia, Egypt, Sudan, Iran, and Middle East)	Experience of spirit possession-presented with dissociative episodes with laughing, shouting, hitting the head against a wall, singing, or weeping

resented enormous cultural diversity, with 42 countries of origin, 28 languages, over 50 ethnocultural groups, six major religious traditions, and numerous distinct sects. This demanded a wide range of consultants, interpreters, and culture brokers.

The most common recommendations emerging from the cultural consultation involved reassessing or changing treatment (70%) or using an additional treatment (for example, medication or psychotherapy) (48%). A change in diagnosis was recommended in 23% of cases. In 9 cases, it was suggested that treatment be reorganized to enable ethnic match at the level of the clinician, service, or specific type of treatment intervention. The authors conclude by making many recommendations drawn from lessons learned while setting up the service. Recommendations for health policy, service development and training are made which, if followed, could promote significant changes in the practice of culturally competent mental health.

Outcome of Culturally Competent Interventions

Ultimately the value of culturally competent interventions (like any medical or psychiatric intervention) will be determined by the demonstration of effective inadequately focused and powered randomized clinical trials in well-selected patient populations, using valid measuring instruments and trained therapists who can practice with adequate fidelity to the designed intervention. Unfortunately, such studies, however promising, are still far from the goal.

Anderson et al., in 2003, reviewed five interventions to improve cultural competence in healthcare systems: (1) programs to recruit and retain staff members who reflect the cultural diversity of the community served, (2) use of interpreter services or bilingual providers for clients with limited English proficiency, (3) cultural competency training for healthcare providers, (4) use of linguistically and culturally appropriate health education materials, and culturally specific healthcare settings [27].

Beach et al. in 2011, in a review, that sought to synthesize studies evaluating training in cultural competence, found "Cultural competence training shows promise as a strategy for improving the knowledge, attitudes, and skills of health professionals. However, he concluded, that evidence that cultural competence improves patient adherence to therapy, health outcomes, and equity of services across racial and ethnic groups is lacking. Future research should focus on these outcomes and should determine which teaching methods and content are most effective" (Fig. 11.5) [28].

Holvart et al. in a 2014 Cochrane review of studies comparing treatment outcomes of psychiatric patients treated by culturally trained vs, non-trained professionals, including five RCTs involving 337 healthcare professionals and 8400 patients, concluded "cultural competence continues to be developed as a major strategy to address health inequities." Five studies assessed the effects of cultural competence education for health professionals on patient-related outcomes. They found positive, albeit low-quality evidence, showing outcomes improvements in the culturally and linguistically diverse patients involved in the study. "The quality of evidence is insufficient to draw generalizable conclusions, largely due to heterogeneity of the interventions in content, scope, design, duration, implementation and outcomes

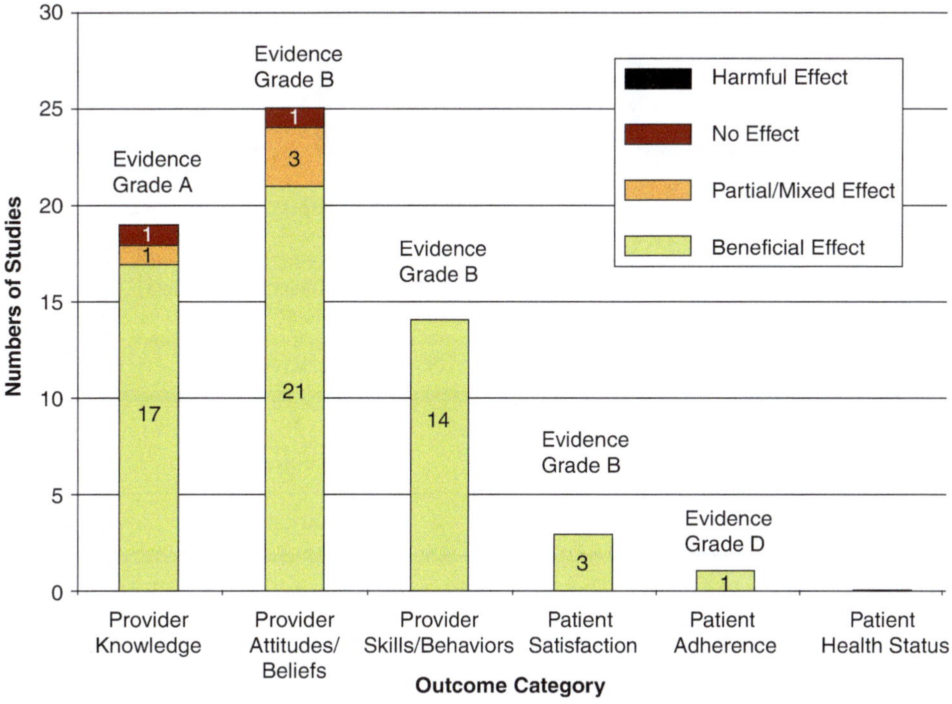

Fig. 11.5 Number of studies showing beneficial, partial/mixed, harmful, or no effect reported by outcome. (*From* Beach et al. [28]; *with permission*)

selected" [29]. Further research is required to establish greater methodological rigor and uniformity on core components of education interventions, including how they are described and evaluated.

Implementing Cultural Competence in Systems

Studies of organizational cultural competence are scarce. Investigators such as Siegel et al. since 2000 and Stork et al. in 2001 tend to support the notion that there is a relationship between the cultural competence of clinicians in a particular system, and the cultural competence of organizations [30–32]. Such relationship is visible in various indicators such as leadership selection (recruiting culturally competent leaders) and organizational planning which may include cultural competence goals that may help the system towards Cross' comprehensive definition both for clinical practitioners and for organizations: "a set of congruent behaviors, attitudes, and policies that come together in a system, agency or among professionals, and which enables that system, agency or those professionals to work effectively in cross cultural situations" [16]. At the operational level, the pathway towards that goal requires the progressive integration of evidence supported into specific standards, policies, practices, and attitudes, which are used to improve the quality of health care [33], and ultimately may produce better outcomes [34]. Table 11.5 lists some of the strategies that can be used to move organizations forward along the cultural competence Axis [35], and Fig. 11.6 provides a map of potential intervention techniques [36].

Table 11.5 System strategies to enhance cultural competence

1. Provide executive level support and accountability
2. Foster patient, community and stakeholder participation and partnerships
3. Conduct organizational cultural competence assessments
4. Develop incremental and realistic cultural competence action plans
5. Ensure linguistic competence
6. Diversify, develop, and retain a culturally competent workforce
7. Develop a system strategy for managing staff and patient grievances

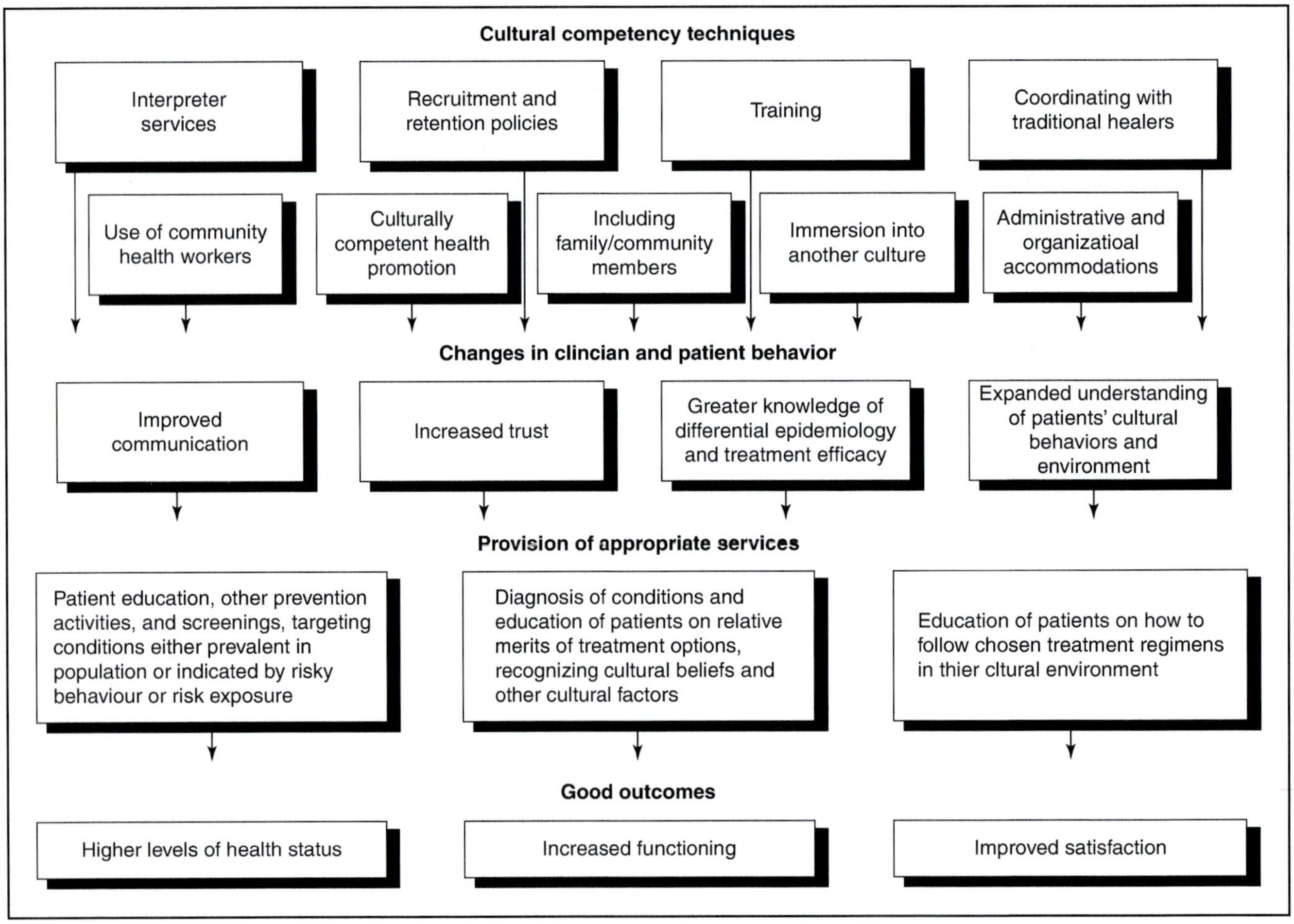

Fig. 11.6 Cultural competency techniques

Table 11.6 Sample textbooks relevant to cultural competence

Intended for psychiatry audience
Alarcon, R. D. and Wise, T. N. (2013). *Cultural Psychiatry (Advances in Psychosomatic Medicine, Vol. 33), first Edition.* S. Karger. Basel, Switzerland
Bhattacharya, R., Cross, S., and Bhugra, D. (2010). *Clinical Topics in Cultural Psychiatry.* RCPsych Publications. London, UK
Bhugra, D. and Bhui, K. (2011). *Textbook of Cultural Psychiatry.* Cambridge University Press. Cambridge, UK
Committee on Cultural Psychiatry of the Group for the Advancement of Psychiatry. (2002). *Cultural Assessment in Clinical Psychiatry.* American Psychiatric Association Publishing, Washington, DC
Kirmayer, L. J., Lemelson, R., and Cummings, C.A. (2015). *Re-Visioning Psychiatry: Cultural Phenomenology, Critical Neuroscience, and Global Mental Health.*Cambridge University Press. New York, NY
Lim, R. F. (2014). *Clinical Manual of Cultural Psychiatry: Second Edition.* American Psychiatric Publishing, Inc. Washington, DC
Tseng, W. (2003). *Clinicians Guide to Cultural Psychiatry.* Academic Press. San Diego, CA
Tseng, W. and Streltzer, J. (2004). *Cultural Competence in Clinical Psychiatry.* American Psychiatric Publishing, Inc. Washington, DC
Intended for other mental health fields
Hayes, P.A. (2016). *Addressing Cultural Complexities in Practice: Assessment, Diagnosis, and Therapy*, Third Edition. American Psychological Association, Washington, DC
Heine, S.J. (2015). *Cultural Psychology, Third Edition.* W. W. Norton & Company, New York, NY
Kitayama, S. (2010). *Handbook of Cultural Psychology.* The Guilford Press, New York, NY
Tseng, W. and Streltzer, J. (2008). *Cultural Competence in Health Care.* Springer, New York, NY

From Corral et al. [38]; *with permission*

Training for Cultural Competence

The development of culturally competent health stakeholders (clinicians, administrators, investigators and staff and community agents in general), requires significant ongoing, educational and training resources. Table 11.6 lists some of the many training and educational resources in cultural competence at all levels [37].

Psychosocial Interventions

Psychosocial interventions grew out of the principles promulgated by the humanitarian philosophers of the French revolution (remember the slogan "Liberty, Fraternity, Equality"), which generated an aspirational climate of respect and equality for the newly liberated psychiatric patients, and all other citizens alike. This climate highlighted human dignity and enhanced the value of the individual as the architect of his or her life. When transferred from the public square to the bedside, such values resulted in clinical practices such as a focus and inquiry on the patient's psychological inner experiences (the mind), and aimed to help them understand the triumphs and the sorrows of their lives. It also encouraged patient's participation in structured work and recreational activities as a way to develop or restore functional capabilities. This original triad: (1) respect for patient's autonomy rights, (2) promotion of insight, and (3) skill development and maintenance, constitute the core from which all psychosocial treatments and rehabilitation initiatives have developed. They are supported by three intellectual traditions: (1) a philosophy of human nature; an ethos, which determines for each historical era which rights belong to individuals and entitles them to the beneficial support of society, (2) theories of mental function and dysfunction which provide the scientific underpinnings for psychotherapeutic interventions, and (3) the social sciences which support social interventions.

Definition of Psychosocial Interventions

As defined by the Institute of Medicine's Committee on Developing Evidence-Standards for Psychosocial Interventions for Mental Disorders, "*Psychosocial interventions for mental health and substance use disorders are interpersonal or informational activities, techniques, or strategies that target biological, behavioral, cognitive, emotional, interpersonal, social, or environmental factors, with the aim of improving the health, functioning and well-being of the recipients*" (Fig. 11.7) [38].

Scope of the Field

The second half of the twentieth century saw dramatic socio-political changes as well as the growth of key sciences such as health and mental health epidemiology which allowed governments and International Aid Organizations to focus on global population epidemiology on health problems, among other reasons, to make possible the growth of interventions and programs based on known needs of populations and epidemiological risks. Through those instruments, we soon learned that health and mental health morbidities are vast

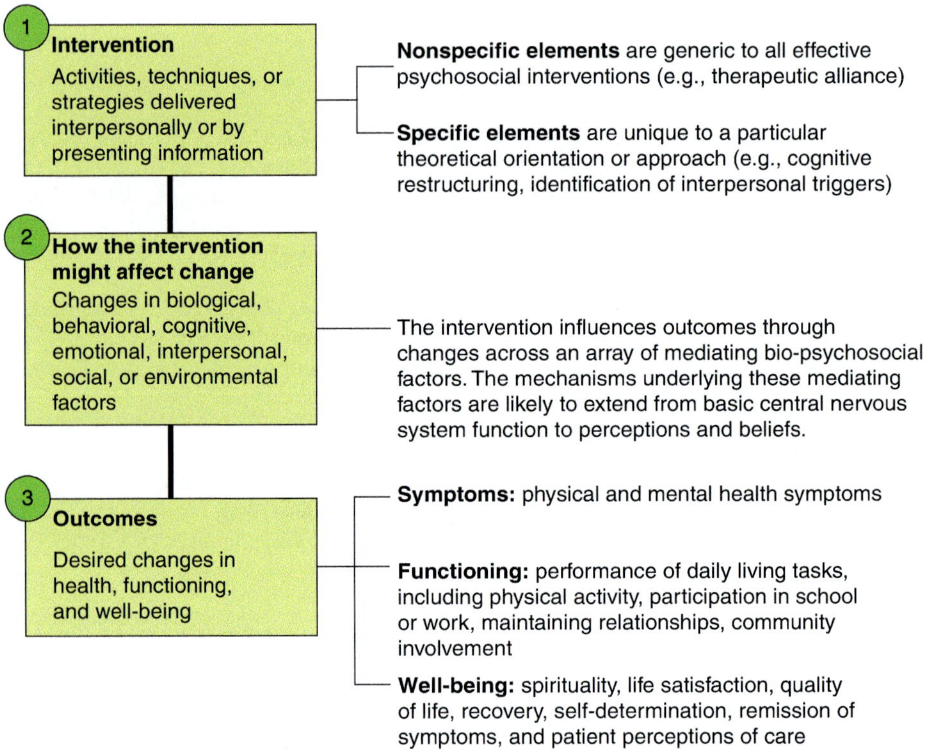

Fig. 11.7 Illustration of the three main concepts in the Institute of Medicine's Committee's definition of psychosocial interventions

and growing, and their incidence is tied to population's characteristics such as poverty, the impact of mass displacement, and other adversities which increase the morbidity of basic disorders and the special traumas of war violence, extreme exploitation, and childhood maltreatment.

Unfortunately, we also learned that most psychiatric disorders detected in populations through solid epidemiological screenings are untreated and remain untreated in the community and that comprehensive state-of-the-art psychiatric treatment reaches a small minority of the people who need it. The barriers to mental health care access are well depicted in the table below using the Healthcare Access Barriers for Vulnerable Population (HABVP) Model (see Table 11.7) [39].

Settings of Interventions

The broad range of settings in which psychosocial interventions are delivered includes all known medical, social, rehabilitation, and correctional facilities, outpatient clinics, solo provider offices, primary care clinics, schools, client homes, hospitals and other facilities (including inpatient and partial hospital care), and community settings such as senior services, religious services facilities and others [40]. Some interventions use a combination of office-based and naturalistic sites delivery, and, increasingly many psychosocial interventions are delivered in the streets. Such is the case of those directed to help homeless subjects, who are evaluated and followed up in the streets by Assertive Community Treatment (ACT) Teams until patients are willing and able to accept referrals to shelters, housing organizations, or other medical or social service organizations. The internet and other components of cyberspace are growing and promising delivery systems for the delivery of psychosocial interventions.

Table 11.7 Themes and subthemes from the Healthcare Access Barriers for Vulnerable Population (HABVP) Model

Theme	Subthemes
Financial barriers	1. Health insurance 2. Employment status 3. Affordability 4. Bribery 5. Competing priorities
Structural barriers	1. Service availability 2. Accessibility 3. Waiting times 4. Adults versus children
Cognitive barriers	1. Healthcare professional attitude and mentality 2. Language and communication 3. Vulnerable population discrimination 4. Cultural discrimination 5. Health literacy
Psychological barriers	1. Mistrust 2. Hopelessness 3. Fear 4. Anxiety

From George et al. [40];

Delivery

While historically, most psychosocial interventions have been delivered in an interpersonal format with face-to-face contact between provider and client, recent real-time alternative delivery formats in use include delivery by telephone, through digital devices, and video conferencing. Other delivery formats such as self-guiding books (bibliotherapy) and computer/Internet or video conference, with minimal face-to-face contact between provider and client, are growing in parallel with the development of new social media technologies. Many interventions combine one or more of these options. There is also a growing library of Mental Health applications (Apps) for disorders such as Anxiety and Depression, and to help stressed people achieve peace of mind, relaxation, and adequate sleep, or to facilitate the development of skills such as mindfulness, concentration, and focus. Other applications are used to enhance memory and monitor basic health parameters such as pulse, blood pressure, sleep duration, and other physiological indicators.

Formats for psychosocial interventions also vary between individual, group, family, or milieu formats, with varying intensity (length of sessions), frequency (how often in a specified time), and duration (length of treatment episode) depending on the availability of providers and the needs of the recipients.

Providers

Psychosocial interventions are delivered by many providers, including psychologists, psychiatrists, social workers, counselors/therapists, primary care and other non-psychiatric physicians, nurses, physical and occupational therapists, religious leaders, lay and peer providers, paraprofessionals, and family or voluntary caregivers. Of late, more of the care is delivered remotely (telehealth) and/or by automated providers (e.g., Internet/audio/video-delivered interventions). Combinations of provider options are often used. Slowly professional organizations and governmental licensing bodies are promulgating guidelines for training requirements, credentialing, and training standards for the various disciplines which train, license, and credential psychosocial intervention providers. A growing trend incorporates former patients as providers of care as "peer counsellors." The value and efficacy of services provided by peers are supported by a significant body of research. Self-help is a vast component of the publishing industry and it is a fascinating—if poorly studied—resource for human help human resources for mental health vary worldwide [41].

Target Population Diversity and Cultural Competence

The populations targeted by psychosocial interventions are also extremely varied, ranging from individuals at risk for, or experiencing prodromal symptoms of an illness such as schizophrenia or bipolar disorders; to individuals experiencing acute disorders; individuals who are in the remission, maintenance, or recovery phases of their disorders; and individuals who are not ill, but are challenged by daily functioning, relationship problems, adverse life events, or effortful psychological adjustment. It also includes individuals referred by social service or educational, judicial, or correctional organizations. Children and adolescents who are sexually, physically, or mentally abused, and those who are victims of severe maltreatment or abandonment are a special population for whom many science-based effective interventions have been developed [42].

Caregivers of people with severe chronic illnesses such as dementias, severe psychiatric disorders such as schizophrenias, and severe medical disorders, are also a frequent focus of targeted psychosocial interventions to alleviate the demonstrated burden of such caregiving functions [43].

Finally, asylum seekers and refugees; whether they are affected by major natural, or man-made disasters or are seeking protection from dangerous political situations in their home countries, have endured severe stress and are often recipient of psychosocial interventions in concert with other social services, giving rise to significant service research in disaster mental health. The greatest source of diversity in all these populations is probably represented not by clinical variation but by the cultural diversity of all groups mentioned in the preceding paragraph. Humans build their symbolic cultural lives between the double pull of universality ("each person is a lot like other person") and uniqueness ("each person is like no other person") [44, 45]. Each culture builds on the human universal dimensions to construct belief systems about its origin and its destination while living on earth, its religious beliefs and rituals, the nature of power and love relations between people and shapes and gives meaning to the rules that govern culturally appropriate behavior. Each culture also defines behavior in crisis, proposes what is and is not normal behavior, defines explanations for ill behaviors, and sanctions practices and practitioners to heal ill behaviors.

The disciplines of anthropology and sociology have helped shape the specially of Psychiatry (Cultural Psychiatry) that provides the scientific foundation for a culturally competent understanding and treatment of psychiatric disorders and psychological suffering.

Specific Psychosocial Interventions

As we have seen earlier, there are three conceptual human science domains generating templates from which psychosocial interventions may develop: (1) the rights and dignity of the person who suffers an emotional disorder, and their longing to exercise agency and control over their lives, (2) the discovery and cultivation of an inner personal and emotional life: the mind, (3) the personal physical and emotional capacities (skills) and expectations (roles) that bind people to their families and communities. The science of human capacities under girthing these areas of performance has been growing since the middle of the eighteenth century, and exponentially through the twentieth century. Patient Rights have evolved through the twentieth century in particular; from the protection of essential liberties, the right to refuse hospitalization and treatments, all the way to the development of the patient-generated recovery model, which supports patients directing their own treatment (and in many cases their own facilities), and which encourage all to keep a strong voice, and much autonomy, through the treatment process.

The inner space of the mind, a subject of fascination and wonder through the centuries, became an object of intense study during the nineteenth and twentieth centuries [46]. A valued scientific instrument for such study (psychoanalysis) has spawned innumerable treatments which have endured, and survived the challenges presented over the years by many other treatment models such as psychopharmacology, and other alternative therapies. Many psychoanalytically derived therapies are now meeting the new standards of scientific evaluation and are generating rigorously controlled clinical trials which demonstrate robust efficacy and effectiveness in treating many psychiatric disorders in children, adults, and geriatric populations.

In parallel to the psychoanalytic therapies, which developed with a focus on their patient's unconscious emotional, and instinctual conflicts, the cognitive component of the mind, became the core from which cognitive, and cognitive-behavioral therapies evolved, thanks in large part to the seminal insights of Aaron Beck, his long commitment to teaching and his responsiveness to efficacy research demands (Fig. 11.8) [47, 48].

These therapies (the cognitive or cognitive-behavioral therapies) have abundantly demonstrated significant efficacy and effectiveness as a primary treatment for anxiety and depressive disorders, and as effective adjuncts in the treatment of many other emotional disorders including psychosis. The domain of therapies focused on the acquisition of personal skills has undergone considerable expansion as well

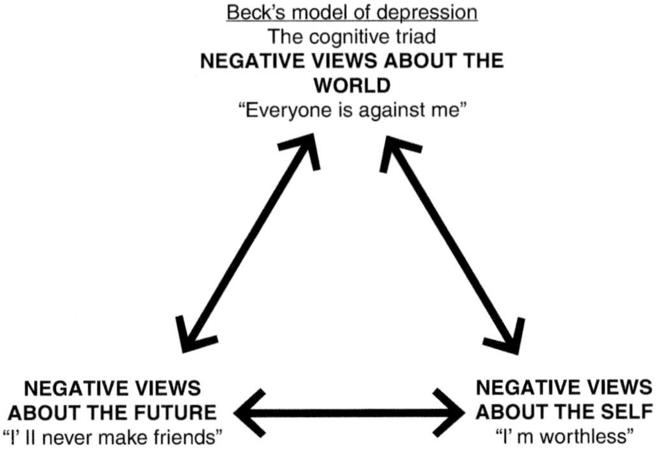

Fig. 11.8 Aaron Beck's cognitive triad. (*From* Lawrence et al. [49]; *with permission*)

and, as we will see later in the chapter, numerous models of habilitation and rehabilitation are successfully employed today to correct developmental problems, and to overcome the skills deficits that may have been caused by the primary illness, or by co-morbid psychiatric or medical disorders. An exhaustive list of psychotherapies is available on Wikipedia (https://en.wikipedia.org/wiki/List_of_psychotherapies).

The following list—by no means exhaustive—in Fig. 11.9, includes the most common interventions which have been studied in clinical trials and present adequate evidence of efficacy and effectiveness and will be discussed in detail now.

Classical psychotherapy interventions will be discussed in the following section of this chapter (see Fig. 11.10).

Psychotherapies are detailed in Fig. 11.11.

Basic Psychosocial Intervention

Counseling

Supportive counseling is commonly defined as any professional supportive, relatively unstructured therapeutic relationship where personal regard and interest in the subject's life and inner experiences, mixed with relatively unspecific basic psychological, and relational techniques common to all approaches, such as facilitating the expression of painful emotions, and experiences while providing empathic validation and support. Counseling is not aimed at necessarily seeking specific solutions or at acquiring new skills. It is based on the common idea that relief from personal problems may be achieved through reflective discussion with others. Practical knowledge about resources may be given but the patients themselves may discover new avenues and solutions as a result of the support provided [50].

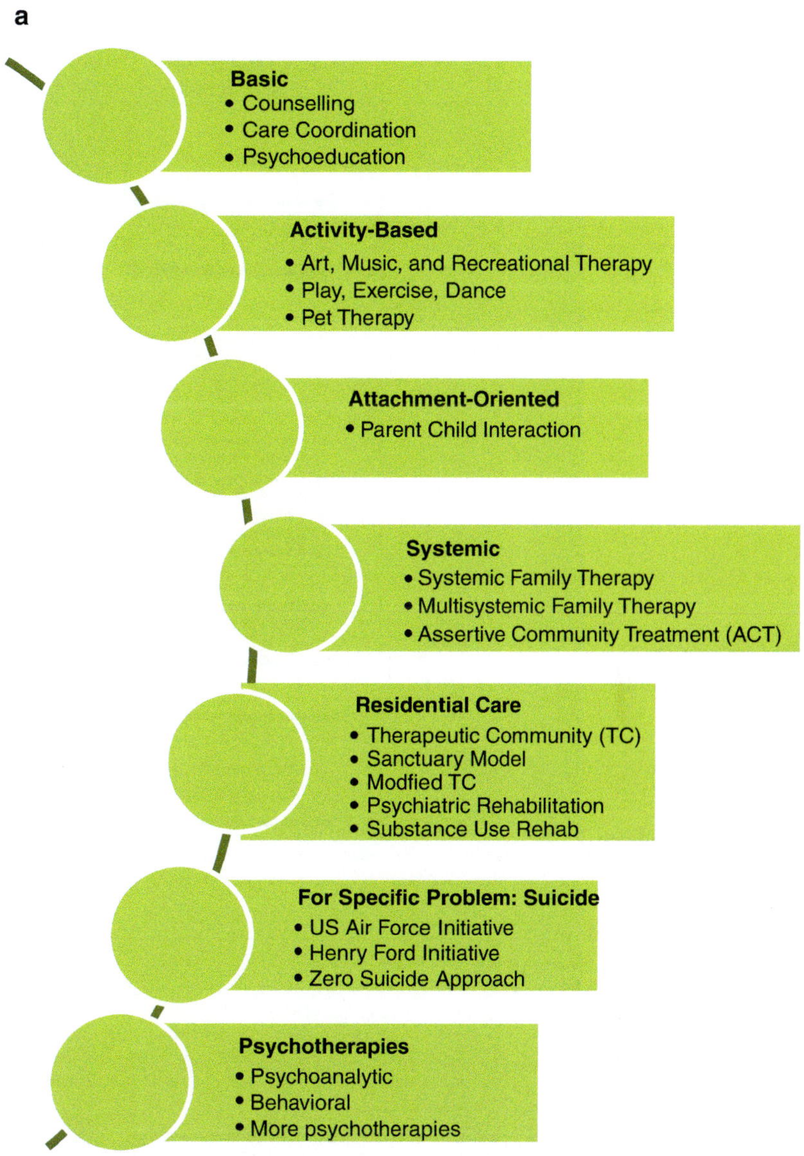

Fig. 11.9 (**a**) List of psychosocial interventions. (**b**) List of individual psychotherapies

Care Coordination

Coordinated care refers to interventions designed to provide a single point of entry to multiple services, facilitating a seamless system of service delivery. It has much in common with initiatives designed to improve interagency working. The intervention is designed to address some of the weaknesses that are inherent to situations where subjects are receiving multiple services from diverse medical, social, and legal services; a situation that is often plagued by errors and confusion, often leading to patients "falling between the cracks" of poorly coordinated planning.

Psychoeducation

As defined by by many human services agencies, at the heart of psychoeducational interventions is the view that helping people understand how their problems have arisen and how they are maintained, is an important first step in empowering them to address those problems. Information or education is therefore at the heart of psychoeducational interventions. It may include information about available needed resources, direct instruction on coping, or change strategies. The educational component is often combined with other activities designed to support change.

Psychoeducational interventions are often run-in group formats, to enable the modeling of acceptable behavior, help modify inappropriate behavior, and facilitate the acquisition of social competencies. Psychoeducation principles have been developed for specific psychiatric disorders. Several such interventions for the treatment of schizophrenia developed in the late 1980s and early 1990s for single families and for multiple families, with documented evidence of efficacy, as demonstrated by drastically reduced relapse rates post-intervention. These family-based, psychoeducational, and multi-family group approaches to treating schizophrenia

Fig. 11.9 (continued)

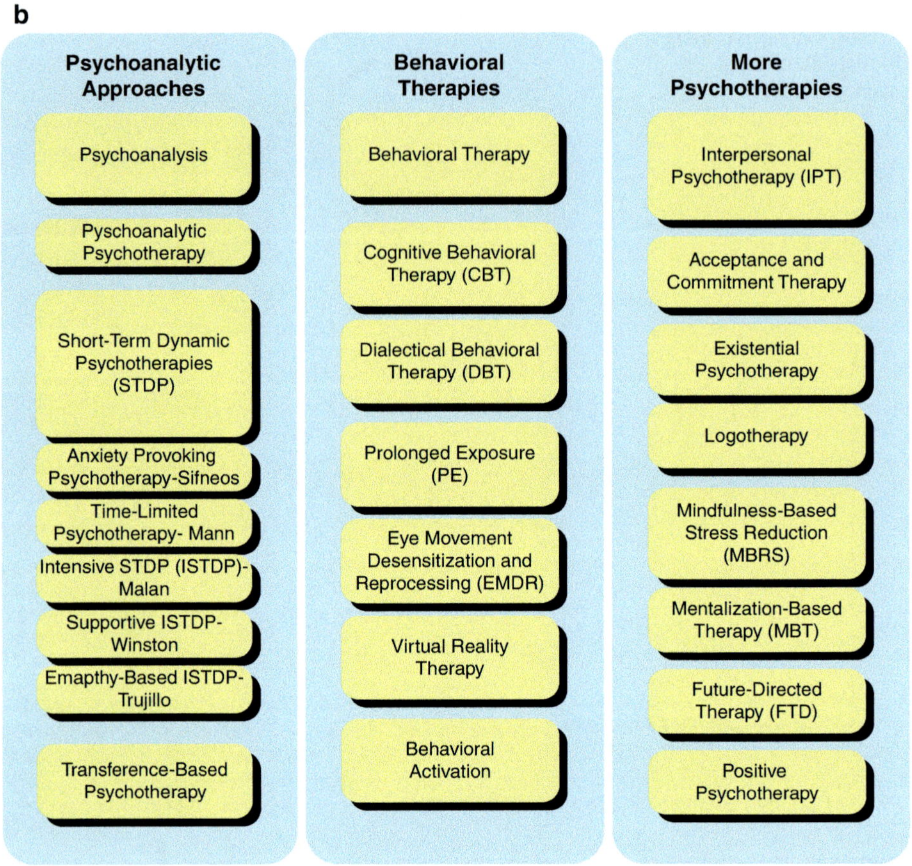

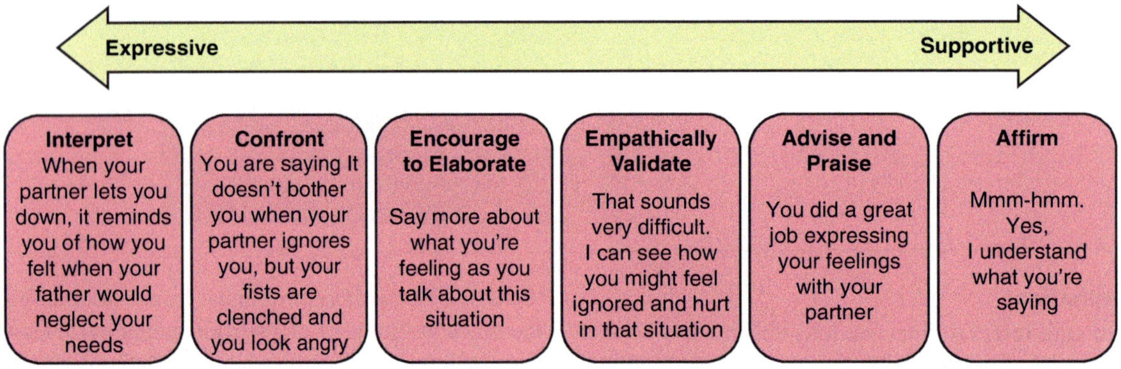

Fig. 11.10 The expressive–supportive continuum

were developed using a common strategy: influencing clinical outcomes by providing families with the information, coping, and interaction skills, and social supports that appear to be lacking in most cases.

Family psychoeducation (FPE) for psychotic disorders has been established as one of the most effective psychosocial treatments ever developed [51–53].

Overall, the relapse rate for patients provided FPE has hovered around 15% per year, across many studies in different countries (USA, China, Italy, and the Scandinavian Countries), compared to a consistent 30–40% for controls of individual therapy and medication, or medication alone [54].

Activity-Based Interventions

Art Therapy

Art Therapy is a therapeutic modality very helpful in situations that for cultural, educational, traumatic, linguistic barriers, and other reasons limit the ability of patients to engage in verbal therapies. Psychotic patients, young children, and children who have been maltreated can find it difficult to verbalize their experiences and may feel intimidated by the verbal therapeutic environment and overwhelmed by sharing publicly their intimate thoughts and/or abuse experiences. Using a variety of media—such as paint, clay, photos, poems,

The most commonly used psychoeducation model today is an amalgam of Family Psychoeducation (FPE), Behavioral family therapy and Multifamily group therapy (MFG).

- William McFarlane developed a multifamily group psychoeducational model that, beyond the specific therapeutic help provided to patients and their families, often accrues the added benefit of creating a natural social supportive network among participant families. This observation of the added value of the multifamily groups,was made early in the development of the investigatior's family model.
- At the time of designing a research protocol for single families, while also working clinically with multiple family groups with such positive results that the group felt encouraged to develop a research protocol for multifamily group (MFG) as well. When MFG model tested against the single-family model, it demonstrated significant superiority over the single family model, which was itself superior to treatment as usual. Such is the wonderful power of serendipity when it finds open minded receptive people.

Psychoeducation in schizophrenia studies in real-world settings showed results comparable to those in experimental settings.

- In keeping with these conclusions, the U.S. Department of Health and Human Services' Substance Abuse and Mental Health Services Administration includes McFarlane et al.'s multiple-family group model as an evidence-based partice and has released a "tool kit" developed by U.S. leaders in the field to promote its widespread implementation (U.S. Department of Health and Human Services).

Psychoeducation interventions for Biopolar Disorder

- The interventions provide patients with information about bipolar disorder, its triggers, and its treatment. A primary goal is to improve adherence to pharmacological treament by enhancing patient's understanding of the biological roots of the disorder, and the rationale for pharmacological treatments. Patients are also taught the early warning signs for possible future episodes, and common triggers for symptoms, as well as strategies to prevent initial symptoms form developing into a full-blown psychotic crisis.
- Psychoeducation interventions are typically-but not always-held in group format. The best tested approach for psychoeducation of bipolar disorder patients consists of 21 group sessions. Bauer has developed a successful goal-oriented group psychotherapy for Bipolar Disorder.

Fig. 11.11 Psychoeducation

storytelling, or music—arts-based therapies are thought to help facilitate the non-verbal and verbal expression of thoughts, feelings, and life narratives. In this way, arts can provide a non-verbal medium for therapeutic communication and cognitive processing, for adults and for whom verbal forms of therapy are not possible. Art Therapy is used to improve cognitive and sensory-motor functions, foster self-esteem, and self-awareness cultivate emotional resilience, promote insight, enhance social skills, reduce and resolve conflicts, modulate distress, and advance societal and ecological change. It can help to bridge the gap between the internal world and the limitations of verbal language, particularly in latency-age children and provide a mode of communication for children who are unwilling or unable to talk about what has happened to them [55].

Music Therapy

Music therapy has been utilized as a treatment for medical and psychiatric conditions. Music interventions have been shown to be correlated with changes in biomarkers of stress [56]. Music therapy incorporates patient-selected and/or therapist-selected music to treat symptoms of anxiety and depression [57].

Play/Activity Interventions

Play or activity interventions, depending on the age of the target population, are based on the premise that play and activity are vital for healthy development in general and cognitive development in particular. Play therapy views play as a 'natural medium in which children express themselves'. It, therefore, provides a way to communicate complex painful experiences and ideas which would be otherwise difficult, to communicate and integrate just through verbal means. Play facilitates engagement thus helping children make sense of their internal and external worlds [58]. Furthermore, deficits in imaginative play have been observed in children who have experienced maltreatment. Such imaginative deficits have been negatively associated with the capacity to for joy, the drive and ability to relate to peers, and the ease of problem-solving.

A study of 45 children (ages 8–12), showed that, 8 months after a play intervention, the imagination play group significantly increased performance on multiple test scores from baseline to follow. Results indicate that play skills can be improved, and cognitive play skills may have a stronger impact on affective processes than anticipated [59].

Activity-based interventions, such as sports or game-based therapies, view activity as an appropriate medium for adolescent's self-expression; among other things because a game is more enjoyable and invigorating than one-to-one office-based therapy/activity in organized games or sports also requires social skills and thus tends to facilitate learning and enhancing the patient's relations with peers. These interventions do have physiological benefits as well through physical exercise and make possible the practice of key cognitive skills, such as impulse inhibition and planning.

Physical Activity and Exercise

A meta-analysis of 122 studies by Dauwan et al. to examine the efficacy and safety of add-on exercise in depression, schizophrenia, Alzheimer's disease, Huntington's disease, multiple sclerosis, and Parkinson's disease, showed large effect size on mood, medium effect size on quality of life, and small significant effect size on cognitive functions with no complications in the 69% of studies which reported safety data [60, 61].

Dance Movement Therapy (DMT)

DMT includes individual sessions with patients using the six components shown in Fig. 11.12 below with the goal of promoting self-awareness, self-care, and coping with serious illness [62].

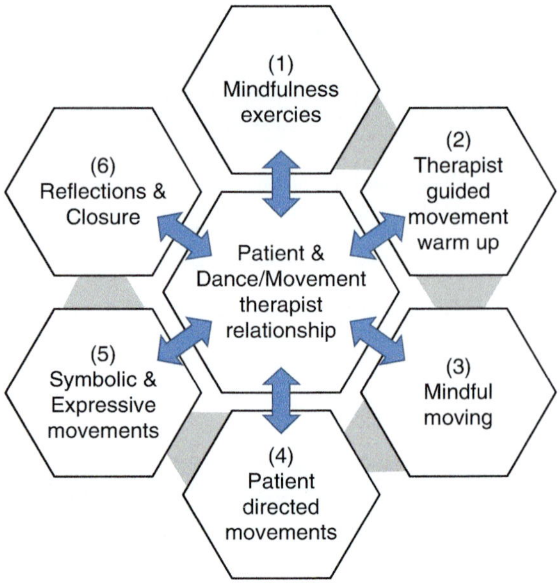

Fig. 11.12 The six components of a model for individual dance/movement therapy sessions

Pet Therapy

Pet therapy (animal therapy or animal-assisted therapy) uses animals as part of the therapeutic process in increasingly broader areas of emotional distress. Animals (from dogs to horses) are used to assist with the therapeutic process, and to support other treatment strategies. They are thought to aid the therapeutic process through the provision of warmth, tolerance and acceptance, empathy, and unconditional regard. The therapeutic use of pet therapy is supported by research that has found that the presence of animals, has improved the communication skills of therapy participants, lowered their anxiety while undergoing therapy, and enhanced their motivation for therapy [63]. A systematic review incorporating dogs into the treatment of adolescents (10–19 years old), suffering from various mental disorders, demonstrated a broad impact on symptoms of general anxiety and post-traumatic anxiety, reduced irritability, anger, and disruptive behaviors, and facilitated engagement retention and increased prosocial behaviors of treatment participants [64]. Therapy dogs were also used for children with special needs [65]. Pet therapy can be integrated with other therapies including dynamic therapies [66], as there is a robust, and growing, corpus of theory and practice which guides its application to developmental disorders (autism), traumatic stress, complex mental disorders, and other conditions [67].

Relationship-Based Interventions Attachment-Oriented Interventions

Attachment bonds between people, especially between parents and dependent children, are essential for the survival of children, as they are essential for the survival of all evolved organisms who require significant time, and learning, for the full development of their adult skills and capacities. Such prolonged survival requires that infants be protected, a considerable investment of time, effort, and commitment by the protector. The parent-infant bond, a complex neurobiological system that maintains the subject's proximity to their caregivers and alerts and stresses caregivers when the young subject strays away, is one of nature's means to secure the needed protection. Attachment can be described as an infant's strong drive to seek proximity and contact with a specific figure and to do so especially in certain situations, notably when frightened, tired, or ill, as described by John Bowlby (Fig. 11.13) [68].

Fig. 11.13 The attachment model [68]

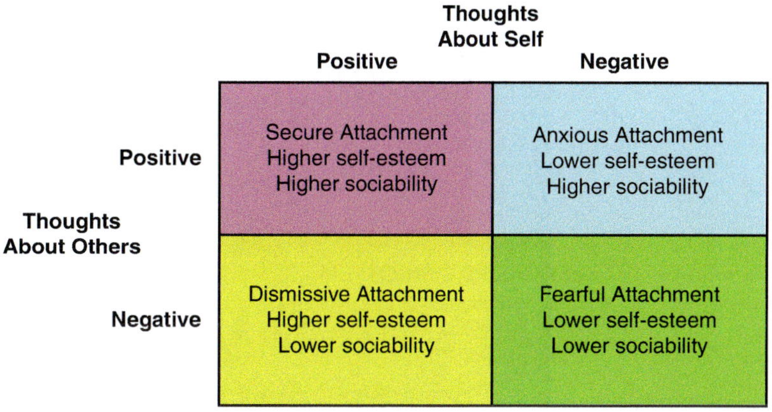

Attachment is a complex system, a product of human evolution, that involves neuroendocrine regulation, fine-tunes the reward system capacities of the developing child, and enhances the development of satisfactory loving and trusting bonds, within the basic genetic endowment of the child. Failures of this attachment process are catastrophic for emotional regulation, the development of trust, and for the development of the capacity to love; their caregivers first, of course, but also other key people in their living environments. For most infants, the relationship with the mother (or equivalent maternal person) is their first intimate relationship, and it is from the quality of that relationship that they derive (or not it is impaired) a sense of identity, self-value, and the corresponding sense of what they can expect from others (healthy entitlement). For many human populations (refugee families, abused children, children who have experienced abandonment or who are at risk of abandonment), the healing of frayed or broken human attachment bonds is an essential target of psychosocial treatments. The stress response system of humans is very sensitive to disruptions of attachment bonds and—depending upon the genetic endowment of the child he or she may have difficulties modulating stress.

The stress response involves the sympathetic and parasympathetic systems and the hypothalamic-pituitary-adrenal (HPA) axis. This system can be assessed (via morning cortisol, for example) to evaluate the baseline state of attachment stress in children and toddlers at risk and to measure a positive normalizing response following successful attachment interventions [69].

Emotional and physical neglect or abuse, loss, and exposure to violence can result in insecure, disorganized, or severely disrupted attachments: If unresolved, such disruptions will contribute to a wide range of problems: poor socio-emotional development, self-regulation difficulties, the display of maladaptive behaviors, sleep disturbances, language delays, poor peer relationships, school underachievement, and overt psychopathology and delinquency in later life. Insecure attachments have also been associated with a disturbed hypothalamic–pituitary–adrenal axis, which is key for self-regulation and stress management (Fig. 11.14) [70].

Disorganized attachment styles develop when children are emotionally and physically dependent on someone who is also a source of fear, anxiety, and/or who represents an actual threat. Disorganized attachment styles are prevalent among children living in families in which there is child maltreatment, parental depression, parental history of loss or trauma, parental dissociation, parental frightening behavior, with or without mental illness, violence or marital discord. The cascade of negative outcomes associated with a disturbed attachment has been referred to as 'toxic stress'.

There is sizable literature focused on evolving interventions that are designed to promote parental and maternal sensitivity and responsiveness [71]. Attachment interventions generally involve caregiver–infant sessions and aim to enhance parental sensitivity to emotional and behavioral cues, to improve a child's attachment security. Achieving these aims may require teaching parents, and other caregivers, child development parenting skills and coping strategies. They also may need help developing social support networks and enhancing their capacity to provide safety (Table 11.8) [72–75].

Parent-Child Interaction Therapy (PCIT)

PCIT is an evidence-based behavioral treatment program designed and tested by Dr. Sheila Eyberg, for the treatment of 3–6 years old experiencing acting out problems (externalizing Disorders) [77]. Based on a philosophical approach that blends operant conditioning behavior therapy, child development, and parenting styles concept, PCIT aims to teach parents with behavior disorders children (usually angry, despairing and feeling helpless to deal with the behavior of their children) to develop more effective parenting by promoting a balancing approach that blends authoritative limit-setting with nurturing (Table 11.9) [78].

Outcome studies have shown significant clinical and behavioral improvement at termination and at 2-year follow-up. Adaptations to internet delivery [79], as well as exten-

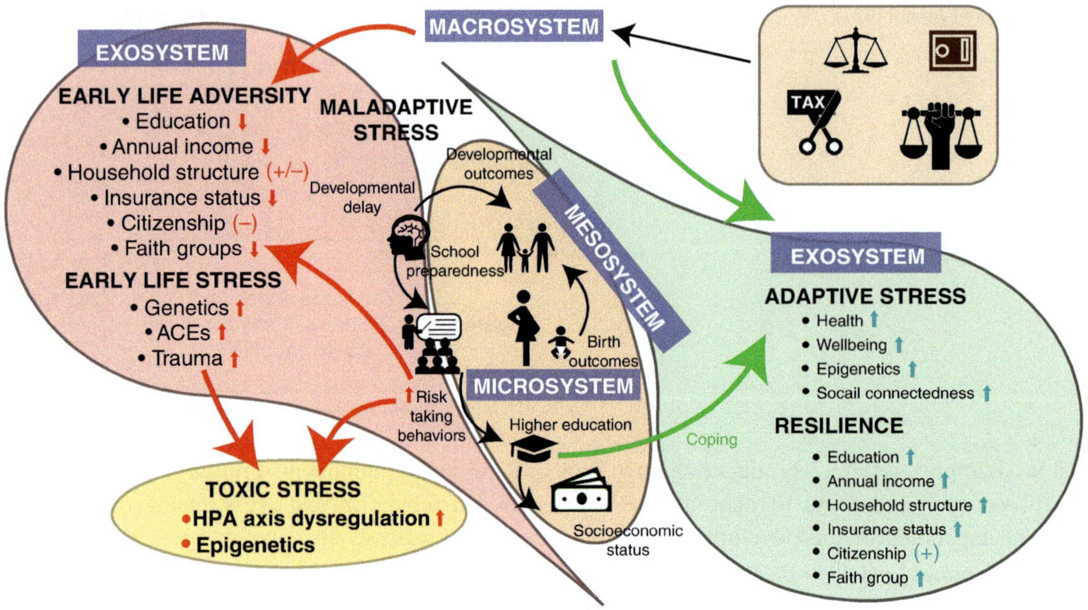

Fig. 11.14 Adverse and protective factors in a child's life are organized by Bronfenbrenner's ecological systems model. Governmental, socioeconomic, and cultural factors in the macrosystem may steer the child's exosystem either towards adversity or adaptation. ELA (red box/arrows) and adaptation (green box/arrows) may work in tandem to build a child's resilience, support education, income adequacy, health equity, and access to basic social services. The mesosystem forms an interface between the exosystem and the family unit with variable effects on the child's milieu. In the microsystem, children are exposed to ELA or prosocial affiliations that affect their developmental, cognitive, behavioral, and health outcomes. (*From* Lopez et al. [70]; *with permission*)

Table 11.8 Attachment interventions

	Child–parent psychotherapy (CPP)	Psychoeducational parenting intervention (PPI)	Promoting first relationships	Attachment and biobehavioral catch-up
Type	Attachment-based, nondirective	Psychoeducation-based, directive	Psychoeducation-based, directive	Directed psychoeducation
Description	Encourages sensitive interactions between caregivers and their children	Home-based education program	Increases caregiver's awareness, confidence, and competence	Designed to help caregivers provide nurturance when they do not spontaneously give it
Goal	To help parents form positive self-infant representations	Teaching about infant physical and mental development and about parenting		Reduces parental frightening behavior
Procedure	Therapist and mother jointly observe the infant. Offers developmental guidance if needed	Encourages mother's seeking education, employment and social support. Can be supplemented by cognitive, behavioral and skills-based therapies	Through video-feedback of parent–child interaction	When children do not signal their need helps develop self-regulation behavior
Evidence	RCT by Lieberman et al. in 2005 shows Positive effect vs Community standard [72]	Model developed by Selma Freiberg in 1975 [73]. Research by David Olds, 1990–2010 [74]	RCT by Spieker et al., in 2012 showed positive impact on toddlers on child welfare [75]	Dozier et al. research in the Infant-Caregiver Lab [76]

Table 11.9 Parent–child intervention therapy

Parent–child interaction therapy (PCIT) By Sheila Eyberg, 2001 [78]	Designed to increase prosocial behaviors reduce undesirable behaviors and establish nurturing relationships. Therapy involves coaching on the spot as parents interact with children through the one-way mirror
Attachment theory, learning theory, and parenting styles. Two components: 1. Child Directed Teaching (CDI) 2. Parent Directed Teaching (PDI)	Parents are taught behavior management skills and practice **through one-way mirror and are encouraged** to practice at home, receiving feedback
Child directed teaching	Parents learn traditional play therapy skills: praising, reflecting, expressing enthusiasm. Imitating and paying attention
Parent directed teaching	Parents learn limit setting by learning to issue commands, praise responsiveness, and use technique for control such as time-outs

sions to the treatment of children suffering from internalizing disorders [80], and ADHD have been developed.

Systemic Interventions

Systems theory posits that individuals are embedded in, and influenced by, a number of interacting systems, including—most importantly—the family. Within systems theory, the problems affecting an individual are conceptualized as a function of the relationships, and patterns of interaction, that surround him or her, opening up avenues for helping each individual through interventions aimed at modifying system parameters.

Systemic Family Therapy

There are many forms of Family Therapy (FT). Many of them are informed primarily by structural family systems theory by Salvador Minuchin in 1974 [81], but also draw from a wide range of techniques from other interventions, such as CBT. This can make assessing its effectiveness quite challenging, as some forms of therapy are essentially systems-focused cognitive–behavioral interventions. Results of a major meta-analysis confirm that for child- and adult-focused mental health problems and relationship difficulties, family therapy is effective.

The average treated case fares better than 70% of untreated control cases [82]. In cases of childhood abuse or neglect, a system approach facilitates the evaluation of the nexus of relationships that link the identified patient with the nuclear family, the extended family, the school, and the broader social system network in search of the most effective point of intervention that will ensure the end of abuse and the development of more nurturing effective family structures. A research review of family systems and multimodal interventions shows that such interventions are broadly supported by evidence in the treatment of a wide array of child and family problems beyond child maltreatment cases [83]. Oppositional behavior problems, and attention deficit disorders, have proven responsive to family member's behavioral skills training which allows children and parents to break out of dysfunctional patterns of behavior, and parents to manage the household emotional atmosphere by increasing their ability to establish, and hold, behavioral rules that promote a supportive structure where rewards and behavioral control can be balanced (Fig. 11.15) [84].

Multisystemic Family Therapy

Multisystemic therapy (MST) is a short-term, multifaceted intervention for children and young people with serious psychosocial and behavioral problems. It differs from FT in that it includes a combination of multiple systems in the treatment focus, such as family, peers, school, neighborhood, or community. Consistent with social-ecological theories of

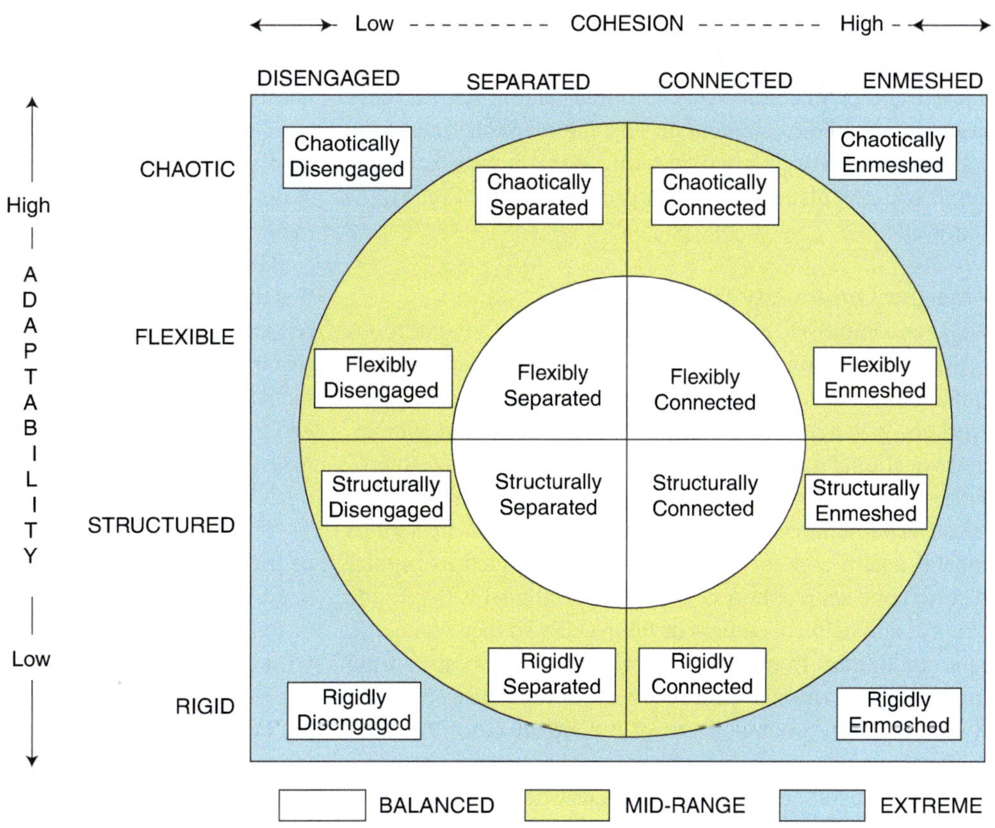

Fig. 11.15 Model of marital and family systems. Structural rules and boundaries in open vs. closed systems affect family cohesion or emotional bonding and family *adaptability* or flexibility in response to change. (*From* Olson et al. [179]; *with permission*)

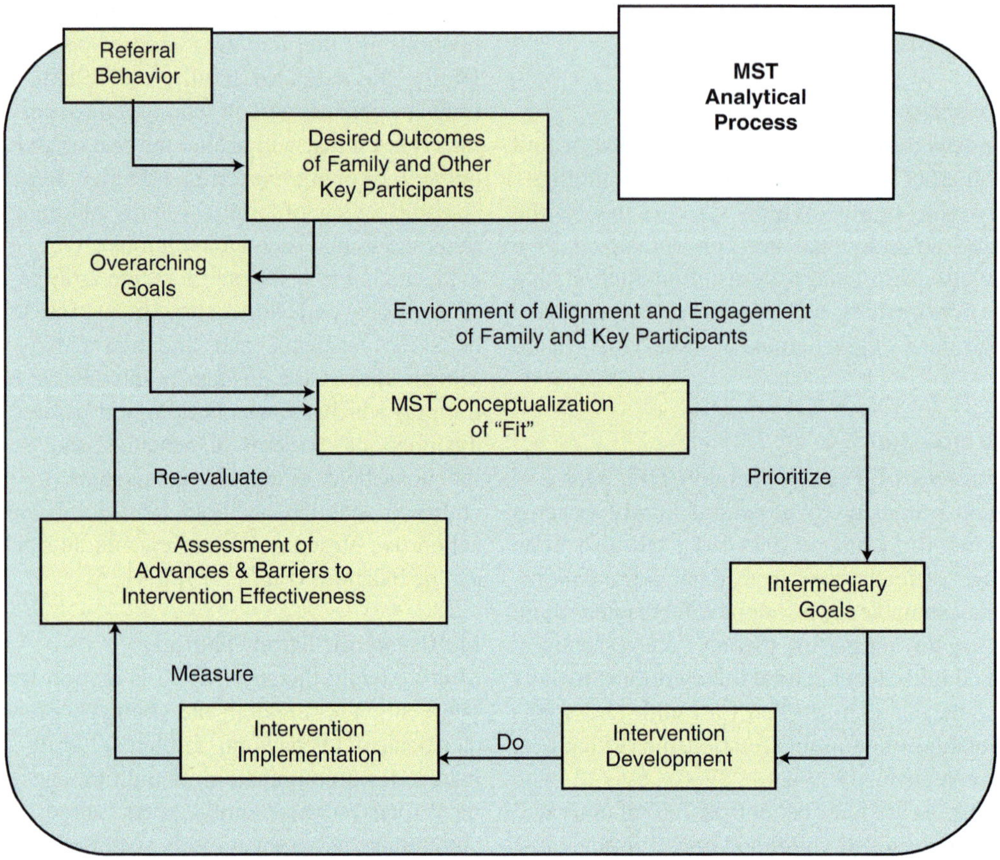

Fig. 11.16 Multisystemic therapy (MST) analytic process (aka "Do-Loop")

human development, this broader focus is based on the view of the program developers, that children's difficulties are caused and/or maintained by multiple factors within these systems and their interaction. The intervention, therefore, focuses on identifying and targeting these factors to reduce symptoms and distress as well as promote health (Fig. 11.16) [85, 86].

Assertive Community Treatment (ACT)

ACT encompasses an array of services and interventions provided by a community-based, multidisciplinary, mobile treatment team, consisting of case managers, peer support workers, psychiatrists, social workers, psychologists, nurses, and vocational specialists. The approach is designed to provide comprehensive, community-based psychiatric treatment, rehabilitation, and support, to persons with serious mental health and substance use disorders, such as bipolar disorder and schizophrenia. A fundamental goal is to provide support and help consumers develop skills so they can maintain community living, avoid hospitalization, improve their quality of life, and strive for recovery. Core features of assertive community treatment are an individualization of treatment plans and flexibility of services based on a patient's specific recovery goals. Key characteristics of these interventions are small caseloads; assertive outreach, ongoing treatment, and support including medications and 24-h availability with crisis readiness. A range of other psychosocial interventions, such as family psychoeducation, supported employment, dual-disorder substance abuse treatment, and skills development. and motivational interviewing can be made available if needed (Fig. 11.17) [87].

The original Stein and Test 1980 study of ACT, showed that the use of the community program for 14 months, greatly reduced the need to hospitalize patients and enhanced the community tenure and adjustment of patients in the experimental arm. When the special programming was discontinued, many of the gains were lost, and the use of the hospital rose sharply, clearly suggesting that community programming should be comprehensive and ongoing [88].

Yet despite the time-tested efficacy and the effectiveness of this intervention, there is still a large (over 40%) unmet need for ACT Teams. A recent study found that only 13% of the 12,826 surveyed US facilities reported offering ACT, with significant variability among states [89]. Of the facilities offering ACT, only 19.2% reported offering all core ACT services. Few facilities offered peer support, employment, and housing services. Facilities with ACT programs offering these comprehensive services were more likely

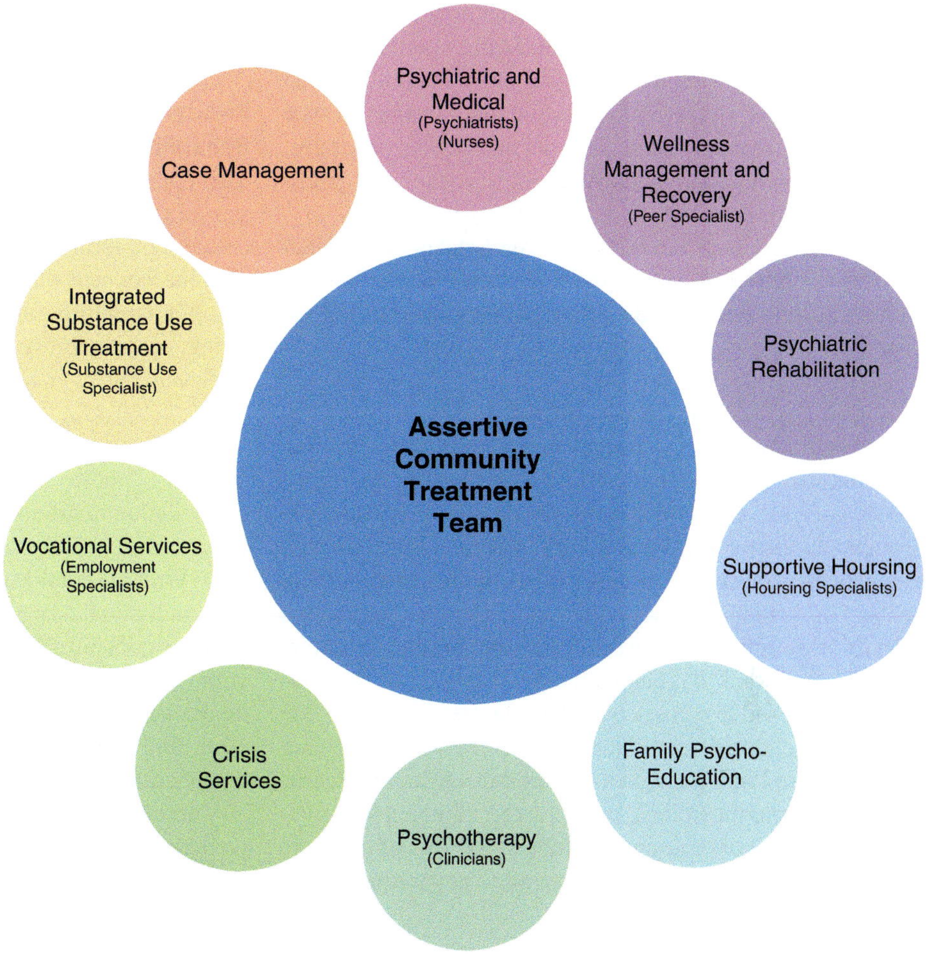

Fig. 11.17 Assertiveness community treatment team

publicly sponsored end received direct federal funding or grant funding. investigators also found a significant decrease in the proportion of facilities offering ACT from 2010 to 2016.

Residential Care

Therapeutic Communities: Maxwell Jones

It was Maxwell Jones (1907–1990) who most enthusiastically developed the concepts of the therapeutic community both in Britain and in the USA and attempted to spread those concepts to institutions outside of the formal psychiatric system [90]. Just like other army psychiatrists who had developed community treatments to apply the community lessons of WWII, Jones first developed a program during the war to treat soldiers suffering from "effort syndrome," a psychosomatic disorder that was related to combat fatigue a forerunner of today's Posttraumatic Stress Disorders (Table 11.10) [90].

The patients of Jones' communities had mixed diagnoses, were usually unemployed when admitted, and came to the Hospital demoralized, depressed, isolated, and with profound feelings of failure. Dr. Jones reported good outcomes after 2–6 months of therapy, including a 50% employment rate of formally unemployed participants. In addition to hospital-based therapeutic communities (TCs), a parallel system of. TCs evolved; an evidence-based, self-help approach, that developed outside the mainstream of psychiatry, psychology, and medicine facilities and which serves diverse populations, especially patients suffering from substance use disorders. The TC's basic approach is to treat the whole person through the use of peer communities employing community-imposed sanctions and penalties as well as earned advancement of status and privileges as part of the recovery and growth process.

Table 11.10 Maxwell Jones therapeutic community concept

1. A philosophical stance embracing an **egalitarian ethos** that flattened the traditional rigid hierarchies of doctors, nurses, aides, and patients, then prevailing in most hospitals
2. Making the promotion of **human bonding through group** activities the central clinical paradigm
3. The use of **drama as an effective tool of social therapy**. Under its tenets, each patient would reimagine, write, and enact their life narrative story with the support of other patients with the aim to achieve an intense and therapeutic emotional experience

In the late 1960s within the US correctional system, the Asklepion Foundation initiated therapeutic communities in the Marion Federal Penitentiary, and other institutions that included clinical interventions based upon Transactional Analysis, the Synanon Game, internal twelve-step programs, and similar therapeutic modalities. Some of these programs lasted into the mid-1980s.

Other correctional facilities in several states in the USA currently continue to use a modified form of therapeutic communities to treat dual diagnosis patients and report good results [91].

Modified Therapeutic Communities

The therapeutic ideas, principles, and practices flowing from the various therapeutic community models described above, got a second wind through the revolutionary changes brought about by the Community Mental Health Act of 1963. In the optimistic mindset of the community mental health movement, therapeutic communities expanded broadly through the many administrative and political changes, turf wars that accompanied change, and the constraints imposed by cost-control initiatives, distorted the natural development of such initiatives. Managed care companies and the many cost-cutting initiatives of governments and insurance plans, often forced clinician administrators to make cost management the key driver of program organization, however unsupported by any clinical evidence such strategy was.

The Sanctuary Model

At its heart, much as was the case with Pinel's moral treatment philosophy, The Sanctuary Model represents an organizational, value-based system committed to the following seven principles: nonviolence, promotion of emotional intelligence, social learning, democracy, open communication, growth and change, and social responsibility.

The Sanctuary Model is not a clinical intervention; rather, it is a method for creating an organizational culture that can more effectively provide a cohesive context within which healing from biological, psychological, and socially derived forms of traumatic experience can be addressed. Chapters are organized around the seven Sanctuary commitments, providing step-by-step, realistic guidance to creating and sustaining fundamental change. "Restoring Sanctuary" an idea that flows from the same philosophy of community healing, is a roadmap to recovery that has been promoted for the resolution of the structural problems said to plague our nation's systems of care. It explores the notion that organizations are living systems themselves, and as such they manifest various degrees of health and dysfunction, analogous to those of individuals. Becoming a truly trauma-informed system, therefore, requires a process of reconstitution within helping organizations, top to bottom. A system cannot be truly trauma-informed unless the system can create and sustain a process of understanding itself and healing itself [92].

Residential Psychiatric and Substance Use Rehabilitation

The common elements of residential treatments are their shared philosophical conviction of the therapeutic value of certain community environments ("milieus"), which generated the concept of milieu therapy and emphasizes a well-thought structure to promote relatively egalitarian group living, accountability (Fig. 11.18).

Seven basic assumptions in Milieu therapy evoke the deeply felt healing power of community (Fig. 11.19).

Following the concept of "community as (clinical) method," these therapeutic communities use active participation in group living and activities to drive individual change and to support the attainment of therapeutic goals [93]. With an emphasis on social learning and mutual self-help, individual participants, as part of their recovery, take on some responsibility for their peers' recovery. This aid to others is seen as an important part of changing oneself. The theory supporting the model, the methods and interventions used, and the effectiveness of both have been abundantly documented by De Leon [94].

Therapeutic communities (TCs) for Substance use patients have a *recovery* orientation (NIDA 2020), focusing on the whole person and overall lifestyle changes, not simply

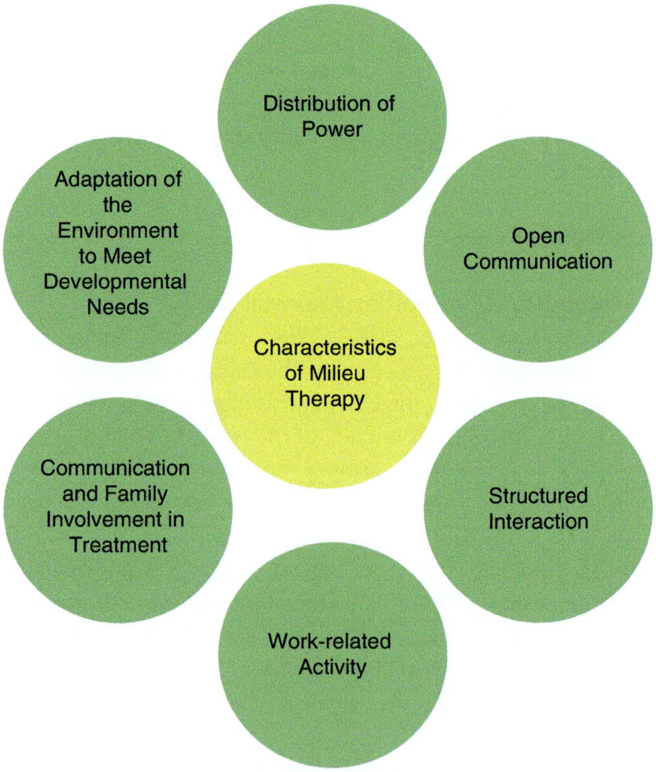

Fig. 11.18 Components of milieu therapy

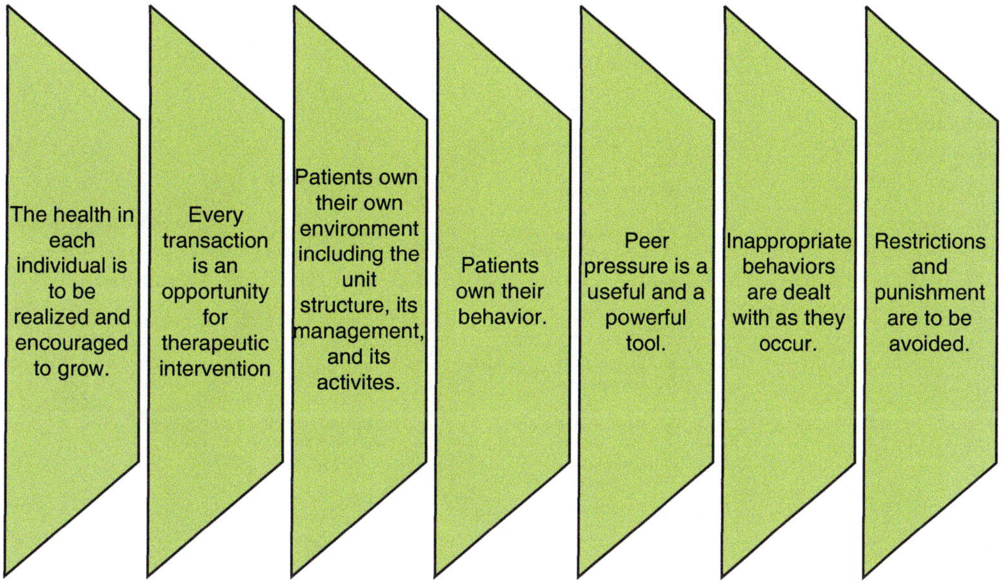

Fig. 11.19 A matrix of accountability from the seven basic assumptions in milieu therapy

abstinence from drug use. This orientation acknowledges the chronic, relapsing nature of substance use disorders (SUDs) and holds the view that relapses are learning opportunities. Recovery is seen as a gradual ongoing process of cognitive, emotional and skills change, achieved through clinical interventions, and it is expected that it will take time for program participants to advance through the stages of treatment, setting personal objectives along the way. Overall, studies find that TC participants show improvements in substance use, criminal behavior, and mental health symptoms; this is especially true of participants who enter treatment with the most severe problems [95, 96]. The largest long-term outcome study of addiction treatment interventions to date was the NIDA-sponsored Drug Abuse Treatment Outcome Studies (DATOS), which examined the effectiveness of several types of drug abuse treatment programs in the USA including TCs, methadone maintenance, outpatient drug-free treatment, and short-term inpatient programs. DATOS found TCs to be effective [97]. Participants who showed improved behavior after 1 year continued to do so after 5 years, which was also true for the other modalities studied [98]. Table 11.11 summarizes the therapeutic philosophy and the core clinical model of substance abuse therapeutic communities.

Table 11.11 Core clinical model of therapeutic communities

Therapeutic model:	Recovery abstinence plus lifestyle-changes
Clinical objectives:	Change cognition. Develop prosocial behaviors
Clinical model:	Group driven. "Community as Method" Social learning. All assume responsibility for others
Community structure	Highly structured, with community jobs, performance expectations in a context of interwoven rewards behavioral rewards (praise and status)
Learning focus	Skills, attitudes and values related performance, accountability, self-efficacy, social responsibility
Treatment stages	1. Immersion into the community 2. Evidenced-based therapies are part of the second stage (CBT: strategic psychotherapy) 3. Preparation for community reintegration Job seeking, community educational resources 4. Community treatment support

Residential Care in the Context of a Full Continuum of Care

Many experts in healthcare delivery have come to agree that what is needed now, is a new beginning that creates a robust system, which provides sufficient, criteria driven. levels of care in an integrated continuum. A system that is supported by evidence, organized around practical goals, such as the achievement of robust clinical outcomes, increased staff satisfaction, and increased leadership competence, and which develops technology for creating and sustaining healthier systems for healthier patients. Such changes can empower our mental health and social service systems to make a more effective contribution to the overall health of the nation. After a careful analysis, a 2017 document developed jointly by the National Association of State Mental Health Directors and the Advocacy Treatment Center [99], makes recommendations to guide the development of a full continuum of care which includes (1) involvement of all significant stakeholders, including, families and nontraditional partners in planning (2) create a comprehensive continuum of programs, technology friendly, integrated, evidence-based and outcome-focused, (3) be alert and aware of systems gaps and provide for robust "hands-off protocols."

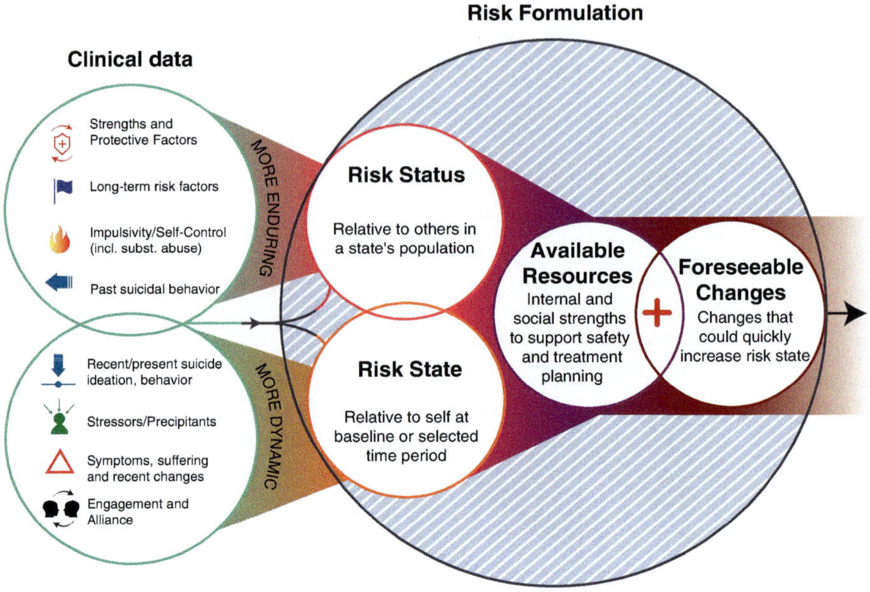

Fig. 11.20 Suicide risk stratification graphic. (*From* Pisani et al. [103]; Creative Commons Attribution 4.0 International License; https://creativecommons.org/licenses/by/4.0/)

Psychosocial Interventions for Specific Problems

Suicide

Suicide rates have been rising steadily in the USA in the last decades of the twentieth century and the first decades of the twenty-first despite considerable investments in mental health science and services, the extension of insurance coverage for psychiatric disorders, and the new therapies and medications developed during those years. There have been, however, a few landmark population-based initiatives that have achieved considerable reductions in rates of suicide in the populations covered by specific interventions. The US Airforce Initiative (1990–2002) which encompassed 11 interventions across 15 functional areas was associated with a 33% reduction in suicide deaths in the target population [100]. The Henry Ford Health System Initiative (HFHFI) through a comprehensive approach to depression care, emphasizing strong leadership on patient safety and continuous quality improvement, achieved a 75% reduction in suicide among patients receiving psychiatric care (from 96 per 100,000 in 2001 to 24 per 100,000 in 2010) [101].

Zero Suicide Toolkit uses research findings, clinical screening and other tools, and educational materials including videos, to walk implementers through putting the Zero Suicide framework into practice. Institutional leadership and monitored execution are key components of any suicide prevention initiative, together with a tight identification of risk among patients through all the levels of care, the use of clinical care pathways supported by evidence, collaborative safety planning including reducing access to means, management of transitions of care (discharges after emergency care, inpatient to outpatient transitions for example), and continuous improvement of care through data-driven feedback and identification of gaps (Fig. 11.20) [101, 102].

Psychotherapy

Merriam-Webster's Dictionary defines *psychotherapy* as "a procedure for the treatment of the mental or emotional disorder, or of related bodily ills, by psychological means." Psychotherapy professionals view psychotherapy as "the informed and intentional application of clinical methods, and interpersonal stances, derived from established psychological principles to assist people to modify their behaviors, cognitions, emotions, and/or other personal characteristics in directions that the participants deem desirable" as defined by Norcross [104].

Psychotherapy is also colloquially called "talk therapy," following the early naming of psychoanalysis as "the talking cure," reflecting the link between "the word" and healing. Of course, the spoken word is the angular stone for the building of human culture and thus is probably responsible for human's ecological singularity. The Bible says, "In the beginning was the word" (John 1:1) (Fig. 11.21).

"Word" originates from the Greek *Logos*, a word with multiple meanings such as "ground," "plea," "opinion," "expectation," "word," "speech," "account," "reason," "proportion," and "discourse." Heraclitus is said to be the first to use it in a philosophical context with the meaning of "a principle of order and knowledge." All meanings signal that logos is the gift that has allowed humans to provide order to

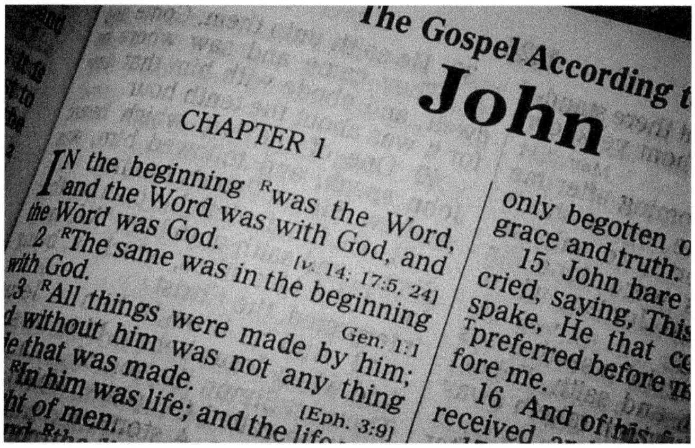

Fig. 11.21 "In the beginning was the word" (John 1:1)

their inner worlds and to build the complex systems of symbols, signs, and communication that constitute human culture. Through words, humans have influenced the behavior of others for thousands of years. Words have been used to soothe and calm, to woo, seduce, or inspire, console, threaten, and elicit obedient behavior, and guide, exclude, and support or oppose the infinite number of actions that constitute human culture. Through the ages, consummate users (orators) had probably been guided in constructing their speech, by the codes of behavior inscribed by nature through evolution in the neurobiology of humans. As people evolved, the scientific method discovered ways to use such a wonderful resource to help others to understand themselves, regulate their emotions, and constructively overcome and resolve conflict. Freud is legitimately credited with the development of modern psychotherapy at the beginning of the twentieth century, thus opening a door to a scientific inquiry into the nature of the mind (Fig. 11.22).

There are many schools of psychotherapy active in health and academia today. At their core, they all contain the four fundamental conceptual elements that already in the eighteenth century defined Pinel's moral treatment: (1) they originate in general philosophy of human life and human nature, (2) they construct a theory of behavior, of their causes, and motivations (both healthy and pathological), and—when possible—of the pathophysiology that explains syndromes or disorders, (3) they identify the "basic fault" which generates pathological behavior, and (4) design interventions and treatments aimed to promote healing.

Such healing behavior, deeply inscribed in the ethos of medical practice is best summarized by the often-quoted adage: "To cure sometimes, to relieve often, to comfort always."

Such wonderfully poetic description of the actions of physicians and healers has been attributed over the years to Hippocrates, Sir William Osler, Edward Trudeau, and other eminent physicians without arriving at a definitive ascertainment of ownership.

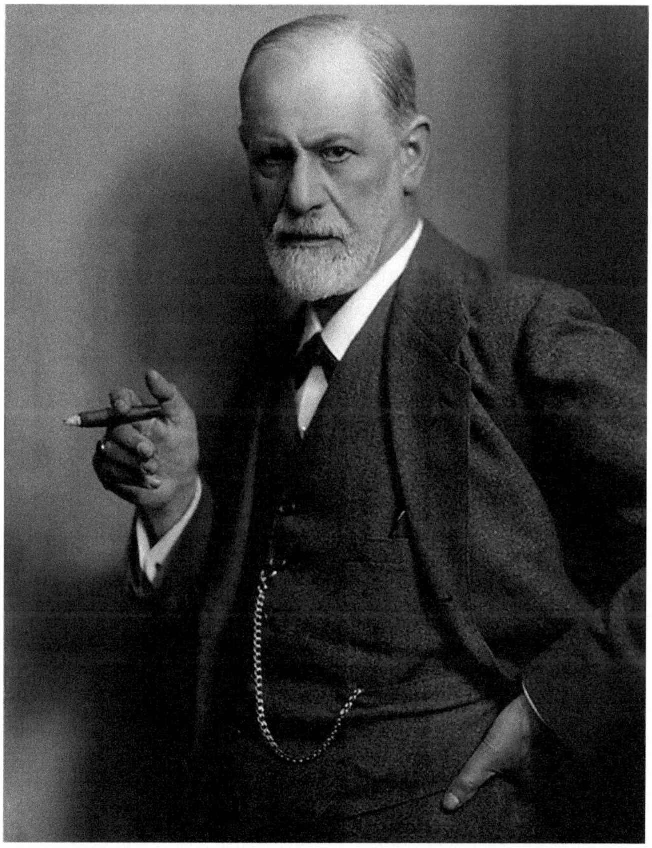

Fig. 11.22 Sigmund Freud and the development of modern psychotherapy

Psychoanalysis

Historically, therapeutic interventions have originated from various theories of human behavior.

Freud, at the end of the nineteenth and the beginning of the twentieth centuries, adopted the philosophical position that neuroses, and other illnesses of the mind, must be considered natural processes which follow natural laws and that could be understood with methods similar, if not identical to, to those used to investigate the natural sciences. He applied rigorous observations to the products of the minds of his neurotic patients as seen in Fig. 11.23.

This core process theory, when adapted by other psychoanalysts to different patients living in different circumstances spawned many psychoanalytically based therapies, as followers of Freud ideas added new elements in accordance with new observations, and with a new hypothesis about the human mind, the causes of its disorders and the techniques necessary to treat them.

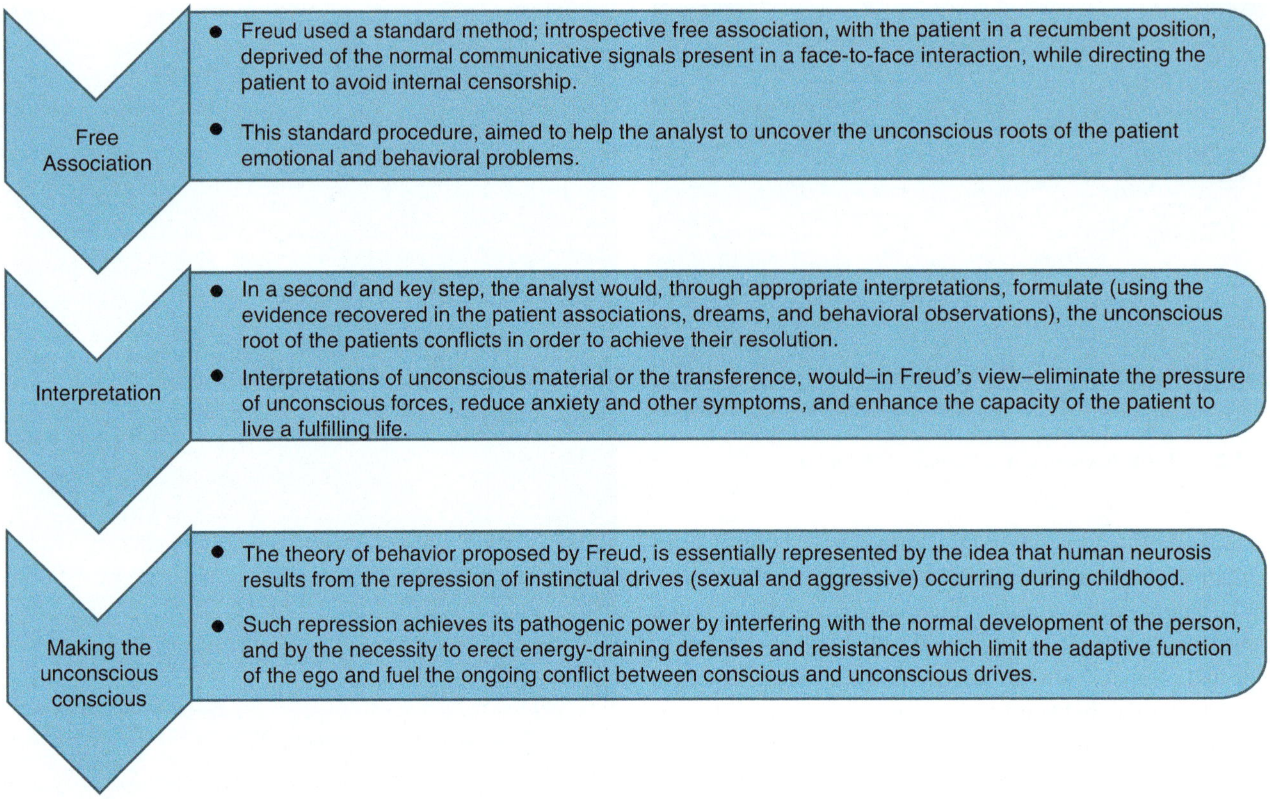

Fig. 11.23 The method of psychoanalysis

Psychoanalytic Psychotherapies

Freud's original theory of the unconscious, and its technical application in the treatment of neurosis (the triad of free-association, transference development, and well-timed interpretation of impulses and feelings), has undergone a century of fruitful evolution. Beyond psychoanalysis proper, it has spawned a broad spectrum of psychoanalytically based psychotherapies which have demonstrated, in multiple well-controlled clinical trials, efficacy and effectiveness on par with state-of-the-art psychopharmacology and alternative psychosocial empirically validated models such as cognitive therapy (Table 11.12).

All psychoanalytically based psychotherapies share a core of the classical view of the therapeutic process; a process in which unconscious conflicts are recovered from memory (through free associations, dreams, and other means), and are verbally expressed, re-experienced in the transference, reconstructed by the analyst through well-timed interpretations, and ultimately resolved through the special form of understanding called "insight." Freud referred to those processes as "recollection, repetition, and working through."

Along the way, the psychoanalytic enterprise itself has evolved beyond an instinctual focus, to include and expand Heinz Kohut's (Fig. 11.24) ideas about the development of the self, its disorders and its treatments, and Otto Kernberg's contributions to the definition and treatment of borderline personality disorders (transference-based psychotherapy), and to incorporate many other modifications of the theory and process of treatment (Fig. 11.25).

Table 11.12 Conceptual matrix common to all therapies

A philosophy of human nature
A theory of behavior in health and illness
A presumed psychophysiology to explain syndromes or disorders
A set of interventions to correct, alleviate, or compensate for disorders

In addition, clinicians can now count on a very broad spectrum of psychoanalytically derived, effective short-term techniques to treat classical neurotic patients, (now diagnosed using DSM rules as suffering largely from anxiety and depressive disorders, interpersonal, work and personality problems). These therapies range from Supportive [105], to Anxiety Provoking Psychotherapy [106], the Time-Limited Psychotherapy of James Mann [107], to Intensive Dynamic Psychotherapy by David Malan [108].

For patients with added character pathology, clinicians can depend on models and techniques proposed by Habib Davanloo [109], and first tested through randomized clinical trials by Winston, Trujillo (principal investigators), and others. For a patient with significant pathogenic narcissistic traits or disorders, Manuel Trujillo has developed a model of

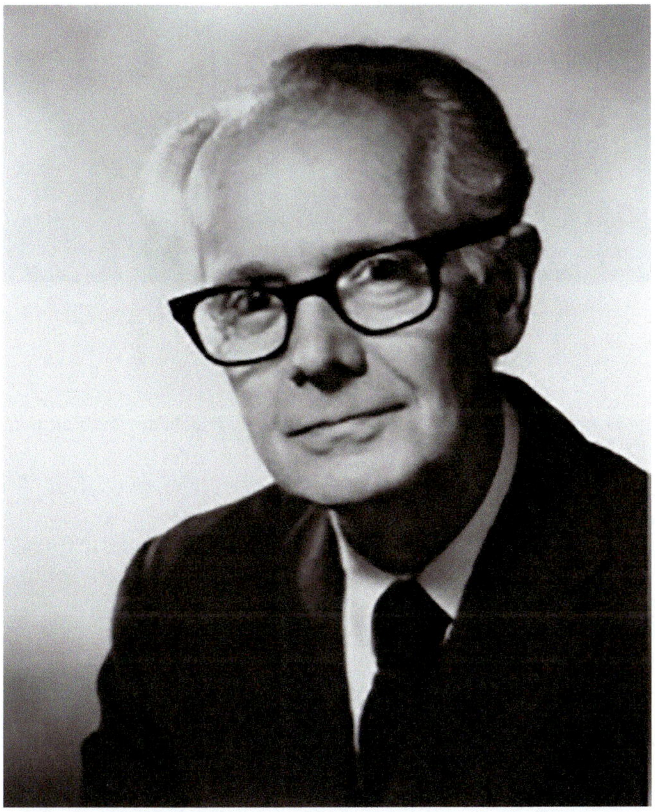

Fig. 11.24 Heinz Kohut

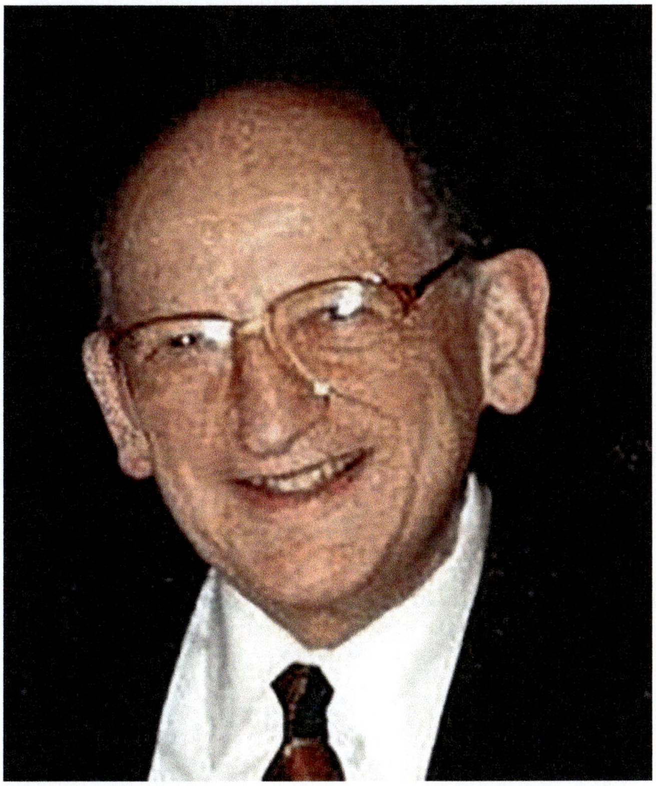

Fig. 11.25 Otto Kernberg

treatment which is based on active utilization of transference and empathy: empathy-based psychotherapy [110–112]. All of these therapeutic developments retain a core of classical psychoanalytic thinking on which they build technique-specific structures [112] (Fig. 11.26).

Table 11.13 summarizes the spectrum of psychoanalytically derived therapies that evolved from the classical model, and which are practiced today [113].

Short-Term Dynamic Psychotherapies

The modern era of short-term psychotherapy can be dated to the 1940s and linked to Franz Alexander who, by then a prominent psychoanalytic leader in Chicago, focused his efforts on pioneering research projects aimed at making psychoanalytic treatment more effective, to specify the core techniques (process variables) necessary to achieve such a goal, and to shorten the duration of the average course of treatment. More than 600 patients were included in his studies, the findings of which were reported in 1946 in the book Psychoanalytic Therapy coauthored with Thomas French [114].

Alexander emphasized, that among the "process variables" that led to success, the therapist increased activity and the maintenance of the therapeutic focus on the patient's emotional experience—thus his emphasis on what he called the "corrective emotional experience," an experience that he considered essential to any successful therapy. Such corrective emotional experience allows the patient to relive, in the safe and supportive presence of the therapist, the original childhood traumatic experiences at the root of the patient's neurotic symptoms and maladaptive defenses.

Alexander reported therapeutic results comparable to those of long-term psychotherapy, and emphasized the fact that, besides symptomatic improvement, short-term therapies did also promote significant character changes [114]. The ideas of Franz Alexander received significant opposition from the psychoanalytic community and did not become part of the academic mainstream, which at the time was significantly dominated by Academic Chairs from orthodox Psychoanalytic Institutes.

Short-Term Anxiety Provoking Psychotherapy: Peter Sifneos

In the 1960s, another Boston psychoanalyst, Dr. Peter Sifneos, responding to the request of a patient who sought treatment with him, but could only stay in Boston for a few months, acceded to treat him and modified his usual therapeutic stance to accommodate the patient's time-frame. He became more active, developed a therapeutic focus with his patient, and conducted the treatment by making use of positive transference and using classical interpretations of

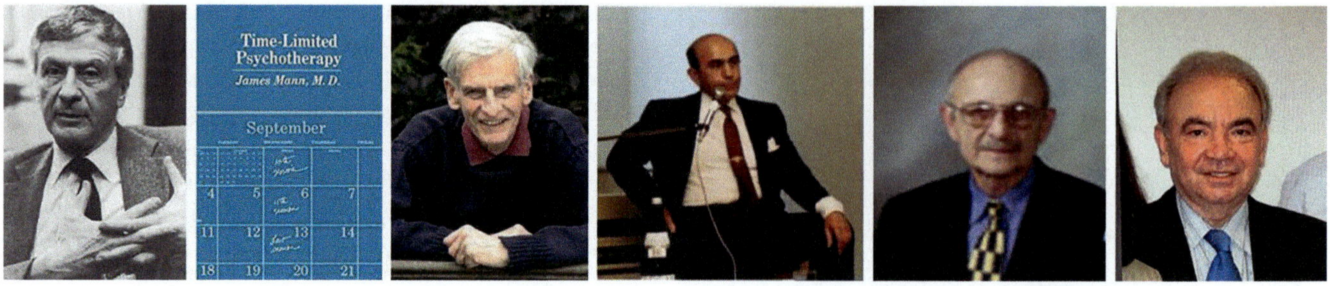

Fig. 11.26 Contributors to short-term dynamic psychotherapy

Table 11.13 Spectrum of psychoanalytic psychodynamic therapies. Adapted from Kaplan and Sadock's Synopsis of Psychiatry 12th edition. Baltimore: Wolters Kluwer; 2021, p.745

Features	"Classic" analytic	Expressive mode (exploratory)	Supportive mode
Target patient population	Neuroses; mild character psychopathology	Neuroses; mild to moderate character psychopathology, especially narcissistic and borderline disorders	Severe character disorders, latent or manifest psychoses, acute crises, physical illness, actual life stresses
Selection criteria	High motivation, psychological mindedness, good previous object relationships, ability to maintain transference neuroses, good frustration tolerance	High, moderate motivation and psychological-mindedness, ability to form therapeutic alliance, some frustration tolerance	Some degree of motivation and ability to form therapeutic alliance
Basic goals	Structural reorganization of personality; resolution of unconscious conflicts leading to reduced guilt. Enhanced ego flexibility; insight into intrapsychic events Symptom relief an indirect result	Partial reorganization of personality and defenses; resolution of Preconscious derivatives of conflicts; insight into interpersonal events; improved object relations; symptom relief a goal or prelude to further exploration	Reintegration of self, ability to cope; restoration of pre-existing equilibrium; strengthening of defenses; acceptance of pathology; symptom relief and environmental restructuring as primary goals
Major techniques	Free association method predominates; full dynamic interpretation (including confrontation, clarification, and working through), with emphasis on genetic reconstruction	Limited free association, confrontation, clarification, and partial interpretation predominate, with emphasis on here-and- now interpretation, and limited genetic interpretation	Free association method contraindicated; suggestion (advice) predominates; abreaction useful; confrontation, clarification, and interpretation in the here-and-now are secondary; genetic interpretation is not indicated
Therapeutic blueprint	Primary focus on analyst and intrasession events Systematic analysis of all positive and negative transference and resistance Transference neurosis facilitated; regression encouraged	Partial analysis of dynamics and defenses; focus on current interpersonal events and transference to others outside of sessions; analysis of negative transference; positive transference left unexplored unless it impedes progress; limited regression encouraged	Formation of therapeutic alliance and real object relationship; analysis of transference not indicated with rare exceptions; focus on conscious external events; regression discouraged. Reality testing promoted. Resilience enhanced
Therapist role	Absolute neutrality; frustration of patient; reflector/mirror role	Modified neutrality; implicit gratification of patient by greater activity of therapist	Neutrality suspended; limited explicit gratification, direction, and disclosure
Frequency of sessions	Regular 4–5 times/wk.; "50-min hour"	Regular 1–3 times/wk.; $^{1}/2$ to full hour	Flexible 1 time/wk. or less; or as needed$^{1}/2$ to full hour
Setting	Patient primarily on couch with analyst out of view	Patient and therapist face to face; occasional use of the couch	Patient and therapist face-to-face; couch not indicated
Duration	Long term; usually 3–5+ years; maybe considerably longer	Short or long term; several sessions to months or years	Short or intermittent long term; single session to lifetime
Change agent	Insight predominates within relatively deprived environment Emotional insight of transference useful and healing.	Insight within more empathic environment; identification with benevolent object	Auxiliary or surrogate ego as a temporary substitute. Holding environment; insight to the degree possible
Adjuncts treatments	Primarily avoided; if applied, all negative and positive meanings and implications thoroughly analyzed more recently, medication adjunct	May be necessary, e.g., psychotropic drugs as temporary measure. If applied, negative implications are explored and resolved.	Often necessary, e.g., psychotropic drugs, family rehabilitative therapy, or hospitalization; if applied, positive implications are emphasized

impulses. To his surprise, he was able to terminate the treatment (the patient suffered from moderate anxiety and phobic behavior) in about nine sessions and obtained a good outcome which was confirmed at follow-up a year later. That experience inspired Dr. Sifneos to launch a vast clinical research project which generated a major contribution to short-term psychoanalytically based therapy which Sifneos called Short-Term Anxiety Provoking Psychotherapy (STAPP) [106].

Short-Term Dynamic Psychotherapy: David Malan

Simultaneously, but independent from each other, other clinical investigators such as David Malan at the Tavistock clinic in London, and others, generated models of psychoanalytically based psychodynamic psychotherapies applicable to increasingly broader, and more impaired, patient populations (Short-Term Dynamic Psychotherapy or STDP) [108]. With significant boldness for the time, these clinician investigators provided transcripts, audio recordings, or videotapes of treatment sessions, thus facilitating the training of new therapists. These authors used the evidence produced by these means to define in very specific terms their treatment techniques and to evaluate the outcomes of their treatments.

The basic map that moves these therapies forward from the initial evaluation, can be conceptualized using two triangles: the triangle of conflict (Menninger) and the triangle of the person (Malan) (Fig. 11.27). Additional short-term models were developed by Mann, Horowitz, Luborski, Strupp, Wolberg, and the members of the New York Beth Israel group (Winston, Trujillo, Pollack, Been, Flaggenheimer, Laikin, McCullough) [105, 125].

Intensive Short-Term Dynamic Psychotherapy: Habib Davanloo

Habib Davanloo in Montreal's McGill University, starting in the 1960s has revolutionized the domain of Short Term Dynamic Psychotherapies, through the development of Intensive Short Term Dynamic Psychotherapy (ISTDP); a psychotherapy characterized by a setof powerful techniques designed to breakthrough the rigid defenses protecting the very vulnerable core of character disordered patients. Such patients had often suffered significant past traumas, held multiple foci of conflict and loss, and were dealing with primitive, poorly organized, difficult-to-manage rage that required substantial defenses to suppress [109]. These patients had been very difficult to reach and help with psychodynamic techniques, had poor outcomes with most treatments, and the accumulated despair of many episodes of failed treatments, enhanced their resistances.

For Davanloo the key therapeutic intervention necessary to treat these patients involves the mobilization of a powerful therapeutic alliance through a highly specialized form of interviews, designed to deal with the patient's overwhelming resistance. The delineation of such resistances and the ways to breakthrough them is one of Davvanloo's major contributions. A second major area of scientific inquiry for Davanloo concerns his views on the centrality of the process of attachment for human development, and the importance of its disruptions to psychopathology. For Davanloo, it is the severe traumatization of core attachment bonds during development that causes psychic traumas through the accumulation of the pathogenic forces of the pain of trauma, the mobilization of primitive rage and murderous impulses, and the guilt, grief, and character distortions that make their way to the character structure of these complicated psychoneurotic patients (Fig. 11.28) [115].

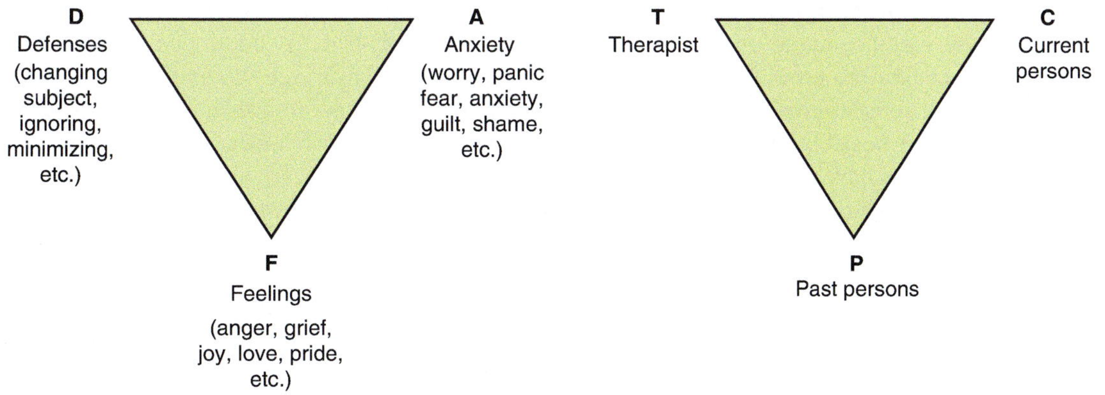

Fig. 11.27 The triangle of conflict (Left) and the triangle of the person (Right)

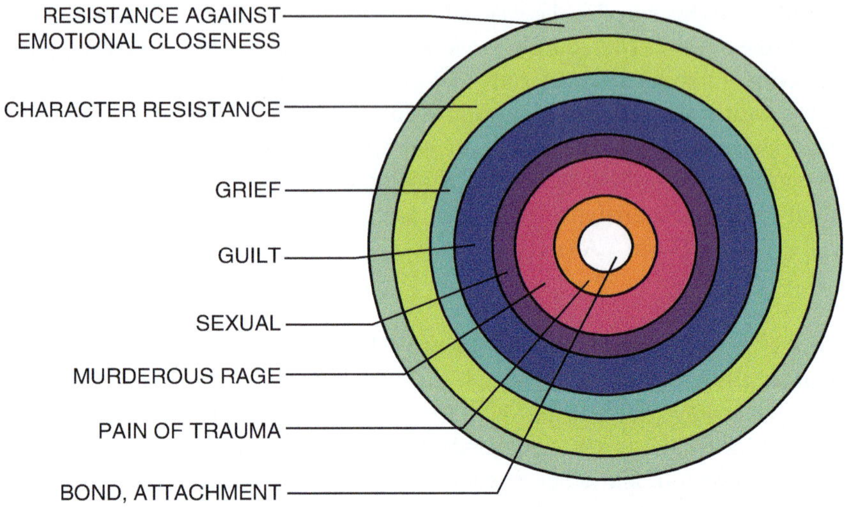

Fig. 11.28 Davanloo's concentric circles

Table 11.14 shows the essential dimensions, goals, and treatment techniques for the following therapies: Short Term Dynamic Psychotherapy techniques STAPP [106], STDP (Malan) [108, 118, 119], ISTDP (Davanloo) [109, 121, 122], The therapeutic process in these three therapies share many common features: they are all based on a psychoanalytic view of psychopathology, with pathogenic unconscious impulses and feelings eliciting rigid maladaptive defenses and pathological behavior, and rigid, break down under internal or external pressures and facilitate the appearance of symptoms.

All these techniques value the early identification and use of the transference relationship and transference interpretations as essential to the success of the therapy. Sifneos and Malan rely on positive transference to move the treatment forward, Malan works with the fear of loss of the therapists midway through his therapies to treat the more characterologically impaired patients whose psychopathology often involves a focus of loss. Davanloo works (via complex challenges to the patient's initial resistances) with the transference resistance from the very beginning of the evaluation. Such a challenge often evokes the arousal of very intense rage towards the therapist, intense grief, or a sequence of rage and grief, that makes it possible to reach the nuclear deep despair that these patients have repeatedly experienced through their childhood and which they have held, barely repressed through impenetrable defenses, over the years. Such dynamic forces have sculpted, through many disheartening experiences, the complex character pathology that they often exhibit at their clinical presentations. After the defenses' breakdown, torrents of dramatic feelings often emerge, providing—for the patient as well—a very clear and serene view of the roots of their suffering.

Figure 11.28 portrays how severe disruptions to the attachment bonds are severely traumatic to humans, produce deep pain, and profoundly destructive rage, and layer upon layer of defenses to avoid such pain, and limit the discharge of almost uncontainable aggression. Coming to terms with profound rage and painful guilt promotes the resolution of guilt-induced self-destructive attitudes and behaviors, a substantial softening of character defenses, and the freeing up of serene, joyful living.

Barth (1998) [116] provided a comprehensive assessment of change in patients treated with STDP.

The Beth Israel group and other investigators such as Abbass, Town, and Johanson [122–124] have contributed seminal outcome research studies demonstrating the efficacy and effectiveness of STDP and ISTDP, as well as its broad applicability to the treatment of patients suffering from severe acute, and often recurrent and chronic anxiety, depression. Personality disorders, and somatic disorders..

Empathy-Based Short-Term Dynamic Psychotherapy: Manuel Trujillo

Little did the cultural historian Christopher Lasch know when he published his book *The Culture of Narcissism: American Life in an Age of Diminishing Expectations*, that the term narcissism, until then living an obscure life within limited psychological circles, would undergo a "viral" entry into daily life, culture, art, and politics, and it would become the most often used term to describe the behavior, and the persona, of many people in the public space such as celebrities, masters of the universe captains of industry, and notably, our last White House occupant. Lasch asserted that post-WWII America produced a personality type closely parallel to the clinical prototype of narcissistic personality disorders. Also, in the 1970s the psychoanalyst, Heinz Kohut, building on careful observations gathered during analytic work with his patients and described in his book "The Analysis of the Self, developed and presented a comprehen-

Table 11.14 Spectrum of short-term psychodynamic psychotherapies

Key figure	Peter Sifneos STAPP	David Malan STDP	Habib Davanloo ISTDP
Frequency	Standard: 1 time/wk.; 50-min hour but flexible alternatives allowed	Standard: 1 time/wk.; to full hour	Standard: 1 time/wk. for 1 h. Double-triple sessions as needed for initial evaluation
Duration	Up to 15–20 1-h sessions	Up to 20–30 1-h sessions	Up to 40 1-h sessions
Setting	Patient and therapist face-to-face	Patient and therapist face-to-face	Patient and therapist face-to-face
Target patient population	Neuroses; mild character psychopathology. Moderate anxiety, depression, interpersonal difficulties, developmental crisis	Neuroses; character psychopathology, anxiety, depression, severe interpersonal and work problems, emotional dependency and separation fears	Severe character disorders, with recurrent acute crises, situations physical illness. Protracted anxiety disorders and severe recurrent depression. Personality disorders
Patient selection criteria	High motivation, psychological mindedness, at least one good previous object relationships, ability to interact with the evaluator, good frustration tolerance	High or moderate motivation and psychological-mindedness, ability to form therapeutic alliance, tolerate painful affects	Minimal motivation BUT ability to respond to "trial therapy" evaluation achieving a breakthrough of painful feelings related to deep core pathology
Analyst/therapist role	Basic neutrality maintained except for activity in support of selected focus, awareness of instinctual conflicts, and interpretation of its roots in the past. Outside of that activity "reflector/mirror role maintained." "The therapist encourages a therapeutic alliance in a learning atmosphere"	Basic neutrality maintained except for greater activity of therapist to develop foci for therapy and empathic response to feelings of separation and loss to avoid regression. "Selective interpretation, selective attention and selective neglect"	Basic neutrality maintained except for greater activity of therapist to develop foci. Confrontation of defenses through multiple channels, challenges of resistance as required by patient's complexity. At times dramatic, prolonged challenges as in the "head on collision"
Therapeutic blueprint	Maintenance and exploration of selected focus or foci, awareness but not interpretation of all positive and negative transference. Avoid entanglement with resistances and push through them. Active interpretation of primary conflict (usually oedipal). Regression avoided	Active exploration of pathogenic foci (impulse and loss) and their consequences on current interpersonal life. Make active interpretations of transference(I), past(P) and to relevant others (C) (TRIANGLE OF CONFLICT AND TRIANGLE OF PERSON) analysis of negative transference related to loss at termination; positive transference left unexplored unless it impedes progress; avoid regression	Active exploration of deep instinctual conflict, primitive murderous rage, sadness, loss and deep grief which increases therapeutic alliance. Active challenges of defenses and resistances particularly transference resistance (distancing for example.) regression discouraged
Basic goals	Obtain resolution of unconscious conflicts related to selected focus or foci; achieve insight into pathogenic dynamics linking instinctual problems with behavior and intrapsychic events; symptom relief	Partial reorganization of personality and defenses; resolution of preconscious and conscious derivatives of instinctual conflicts and fear of loss; insight into current interpersonal events (particularly dependence and its roots); improved object relations and symptom relief particularly of depression	Significant restructuring of personality through resolution of self-destructive activities related to primitive guilt. Experience and resolve deep, well repressed murderous impulses and deep grief. Liberation of loving and creative impulses formerly frozen by guilt and self-punishment
Major techniques	Free association method limited around the selected foci, activity of the therapy to point out evasive avoidant responses. Mild challenges to defenses are required; full dynamic interpretation (including confrontation, clarification, working through). Emphasis on genetic reconstruction within the selected foci	Free association method limited to selected foci. Activity of the therapist required to maintain focus of therapy. Transference interpreted to limit regression. Key is the transference-Past- Interpretation (TCP Link) which Malan has demonstrated as key to better results. Emphasis on links between here- and-now interpretation, and as full as possible genetic interpretation	Free association method limited by patient's characterological defenses and resistances. Mayor techniques include difficult challenges of defenses, at times of long duration, to achieve a **breakthrough** of impulses (murderous rage), deep feelings of grief, deep transferential feelings. Exploration and linkages of the many pathogenic foci that these patients sometimes hold. A well-defined challenge sequence labelled by Davanloo "the head on collision"
Perceived change agents	Insight (cognitive an emotional). Behavioral change in relation to selected foci (i.e., phobias), generate momentum for further change	Insight, reduced symptoms and pathological affects promote more mature relationships. Work through of dependence results in search for better object relations	Deep emotional awareness and resolution of primitive rage and the self-punitive guilt ridden corollary. Corrective emotional transference experiences promote liberation of frozen capacities

(continued)

Table 11.14 (continued)

Key figure	Peter Sifneos STAPP	David Malan STDP	Habib Davanloo ISTDP
Dynamic results	Resolution of unconscious conflicts related to the selected therapeutic foci; insight; symptom relief	Partial reorganization of interpersonal defenses; resolution of unconscious conflicts related to impulses (sexual and aggressive). and feelings of loss and unresolved grief; insight into current interpersonal events; improved relations with others, symptom relief and improved function	Significant reorganization of interpersonal defenses and dysfunctional personality traits. Resolution of primitive aggressive impulses and derived conflicts. Significant shifts in self-regard and reductions of guilt and masochistic, self- destructive actions
Adjunct treatments	If clinically indicated medications and other biological therapies to primary pathology and co-morbidities. Transferential responses should be thoroughly analyzed if they become a source of resistance	For many of these patients' medications maybe absolutely necessary. When used implications (for views of patient of self and transference) are explored	Like for STDP patients, for many of these patients' medications may be necessary. When used implications (for views of patient of self and transference) are explored
Research	**Sifneos P et al., (1980)** **RCT STAAP Vs. Wait List. 14/**22 STAPP pts. achieved remission vs 0/8 wait list [106] **Barth et al (1988)-**44 eligible for STAPP STDP were assessed ten patients were ascribed to STAPP, 22 Malan's BT and 12 Eclectic brief therapy [116]. 78% of the patients completed with good results for all three therapies. Improvement was sustained throughout the 2-year follow-up period **Svartberg M**, Seltzer MH, Stiles TC (1998) RCT to STAPP or a "common factor" control condition. Patients improved greatly. The therapeutic alliance was a strong predictor of symptom improvement [117]	**Two studies (Malan D 63,76)** generated many seminal therapeutic insights. Findings confirmed that neither severity of symptoms nor chronicity predicted outcome at termination, Motivation for insight was highly predictive of success. Use of transference and transference–past-present (T-C-P) links was highly predictive of positive outcome [117, 118] **Husby R. (1985)-39** out-patients neurotic personality structure, treated with short-term dynamic psychotherapy. 33 patients were followed up 2 years. At f.u 24 (67%) had symptom relief and 11(31%) substantial dynamic change [120]. **Barth et al (1988)-**44 eligible for STAPP STDP were assessed ten patients were ascribed to STAPP, 22 Malan's BT,12 eclectic form of brief therapy. 78% of the patients completed with good results for therapies. Improvement was sustained throughout the 2-year follow-up period [116]	**Davanloo H (1978)** Report of 475 pt's evaluated and 115 treated successfully in ISTDP [121] **The Beth Israel (NY) group** (Winston **A, Trujillo M PI's**) conducted the first study of STDP vs, supportive dynamic psychotherapy with Cluster C Personality Disorder Patients. They showed superiority of STDP v. waiting list conditions. Equal to supportive in most, superior in some outcomes [105] **Town, JM (2020).** STDP in treatment resistant depression (TRD) found moderate to large effect sizes (Cohen d 0.64–0.70) for the 30 STDP pt.'s vs the 30 controls, sustained at 6 and 18 months, proving long- term [122] efficacy and cost-value **Abbass A,Town J, Driesen E(2012)** in meta-analysis of 13 controlled studies of anxiety,depression, personality and somatic disorders found significant effects and superiority over controlled conditions (Cohen d bet 0.84–1.51) maintained at follow-up. ISTDP is a short, affordable treatment that may be effective for, and applicable to a broad range of patients. Abbass et al. have found adequate efficacy in pain, somatic problems, medically unexplained symptoms [123] **Johansson R, Town J, Abass A (2014)** An ISTDP study of 402 patients showed large effect sizes (>0.80). Unlocking the unconscious was associated with significantly larger treatment outcome [124]

sive metapsychology of patients suffering from narcissistic vulnerabilities (self-disorders), and discussed the necessary modifications of the classical psychoanalytic technique required to mobilize narcissistically derived transferences (grandiose, idealizing, mirror) needed to successfully treat these patients who until Kohut demonstrated otherwise, were viewed as unanalyzable as a function of their incapacity to form transferences. At the root of self-disorders, lie deeply distorted images, perceptions, and emotions related to the Self (and its many dimensions: body, attitudes and dispositions, intelligence, virtuosity, human special capacities) and to others; more specifically toward the subject's perception of Others and their impact on his or her self-representation. The core element in the area of Self-experience is identity, and the central unconscious question is, who am I, am I worthy of love and admiration? This domain of human experience represents one step deeper than the attachment bond, but it is inevitably related to attachment bonds. Normal development proceeds in a never-ending dialectic between Identity (self) and Attachment. Attachment objects normally facilitate the discovery and affirmation of Self (with no more than the reality imposed necessary limits). Unfortunately, often enough in self-disordered development, the person's core identity is deeply injured, and the bonds with others are severely disrupted. The core pain effect here is a shame, and the defenses and resistances include emotional distancing from others, and severe dissociation from core aspects of self-experience to avoid such pain and to limit the discharge of almost uncontainable rage. Maintaining a steady therapy focus is facilitated by using the triangle of the self as a guide to the process (Fig. 11.29).

Experiencing, and coming to terms with such profound rage and painful guilt during the therapeutic process—a challenging occurrence for both the patient and the therapist—promotes the resolution of guilt-induced self-destructive attitudes and behaviors, and result in a substantial softening of character defenses and the freeing up of the patient's "true self" and capacity joyful living. Trujillo (Fig. 11.30) has built on Kohut's metapsychology and added theoretical and technical recommendations that make the short-term treatment of many self-disordered patients possible [126].

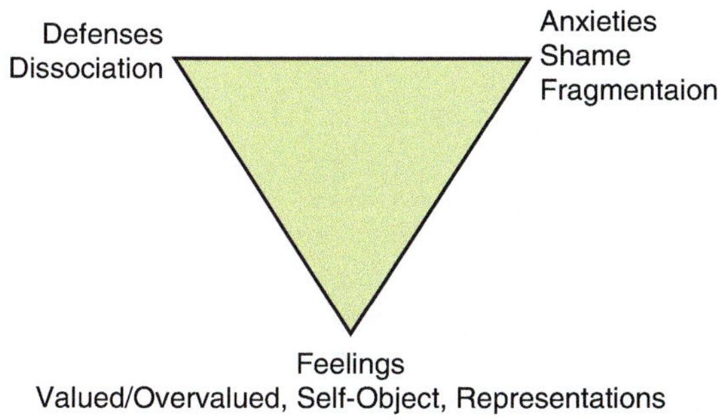

Fig. 11.29 Triangle of the self

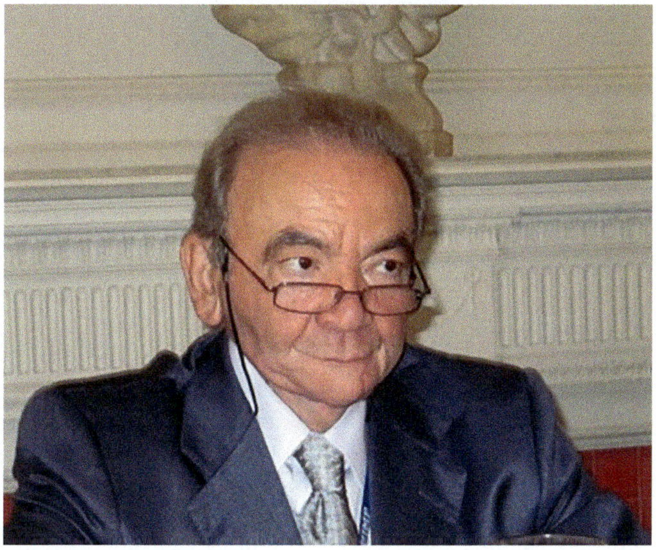

Fig. 11.30 Manuel Trujillo

The triangle of the Self guides the therapeutic work necessary to heal narcissistic psychopathology. It helps the therapist focus, as appropriate, from challenging the defenses (including dissociation), to dealing with the anxiety and shame evoked and then to the vital work of correcting the Self and Object distortions that lie at the root of this pathology.

For Trujillo, when this preliminary work is done using Davanloo's techniques to challenge defenses and open up primal rage, guilt, and grief stemming from the patient's very painful past abuses and corresponding traumas, a state of very intense transferences and positive therapeutic alliance develops and both make possible the necessary reconstruction of the patient's damaged self, the reactivation of the patient's healthy self-images and experiences; work that can proceed fast enough to fit into a time-limited therapeutic framework [126]. Empathy can be said to drive this process, as the heightened empathically supported detection of the and—at times light acknowledgment—of the patient's true capacities and real self affects such as joy and love and ideals, facilitates for the patient an often radical shift in self-experience and basic attitudes to others. (see Fig. 11.31).

Transference-Based Psychotherapies for Borderline Personality Disorders: Otto Kernberg

Psychoanalysis and the psychiatric community in general, owe much credit to Dr. Otto Kernberg, whose long career has spawned many contributions to the theory and practice of classical psychoanalysis, and has developed psychoanalytic applications to many areas outside of the clinical domain, such as medical administration, human organizations, and the nature of leadership. His contributions to the understanding of narcissism, and borderline personality disorder (BPD), are especially relevant given the pervasive growth of such pathologies in our current societies, (the prevalence of BPD is estimated to be 1–2.5% in the general population and 10–50% in psychiatric outpatient and inpatient settings), the significant morbidity they carry (suicide rates over 10%), and the dearth of evidenced-based, effective psychosocial treatments available for such patients. For Borderline Personality, its essential psychopathology, and possible treatments, Kernberg's theoretical contributions are transformative. Based upon this theoretical understanding, Kernberg has also developed, applied, and ultimately thoroughly researched, the technical modifications to the classical techniques necessary for the successful treatment of patients suffering from such devastating disorders. He has named this therapy Transference Based Psychotherapy: TFP [127, 128].

Central to TFP is a negotiated treatment contract between patient and therapist, which creates the treatment

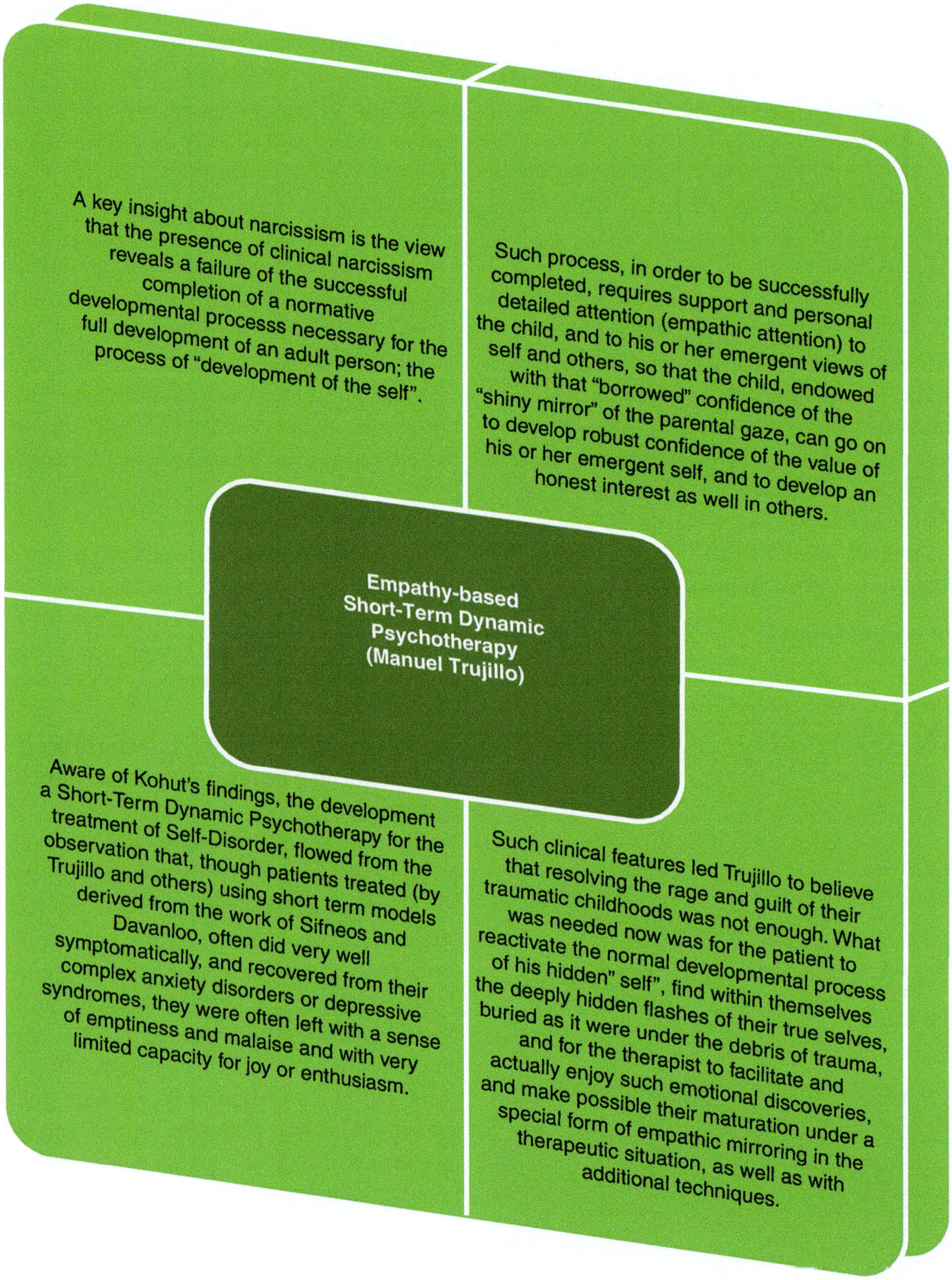

Fig. 11.31 Empathy-based short-term dynamic psychotherapy [126]

frame. Change is achieved through analyzing and interpreting the transference relationship, focusing on the here-and-now context to avoid severe regression. Other prominent techniques are exploration, confrontation, and interpretation. Recovery in TFP is reached when formerly split and separate good and bad representations of self (and of others) are integrated, and when fixed primitive internalized object relations based on those self-others distortions are resolved.

Table 11.15 provides a summary of both Transference-Focused Psychotherapy for Borderline conditions (discussed above TFP) and Empathy-Based Short-Term Psychotherapy of Narcissistic and other Self-Disorders (ESTDP) [126–128].

Supportive Psychotherapy

Supportive psychotherapy is one of the most commonly provided psychotherapies. Figure 11.32 shows the working framework to structure the therapeutic relationship [132].

Table 11.15 Psychoanalytic dynamic therapies for borderline and narcissistic personality disorders

Type of therapy author	Transference-focused psychotherapy Otto Kernberg	Empathy-based short-term psychotherapy Manuel Trujillo
Frequency	Regular 2 times/wk.; 50-min	Regular 1–2 times/wk.; 50′ to full hour. Flexible alternative blocks
Duration	Long term; usually at 1-year positive results. May last longer	Usually, 40–50 sessions show significant results
Setting	Face to face	Patient and therapist face to face
Patient population	In Kernberg studies, pts. had a BPD disorder diagnosis and exclusion of major comorbidities (Bipolar disorder, severe addiction, antisocial personality)	In clinical practice patient had a Dx of NPD with severe anxiety, depression, serious work interpersonal problems, no psychotic or active serious addictive disorders
Selection criteria	Acceptance of therapeutic contract to create a reality frame for therapy	Acceptance of the usual psychotherapy frame (non-censorship, attendance to sessions, payment)
Core theoretical and clinical concepts	Key dynamic for Kernberg is "identity diffusion" which creates broad dysfunctions (self, others, goals ideals and morals). Split good-bad Self (and object), drives destructive, self-destructive affects and behaviors	Key dynamic for Trujillo is multilevel dissociation of self. Immature and dissociated forms of self-identity (grandiose, devalued) drive relationships, work, intimacy, and interpersonal relationships
Basic goals	To achieve significant stable clinical improvement and quality of life gains, as reflected in BPD Scale scores below the threshold of "patient." Evidence of reduced good bad split, maturation of object relationships	Significant, stable clinical improvement and quality of life as reflected in reduced symptoms (below clinical significance), reduced dissociation of self, and maturation of child-like grandiosity or self-devaluation. Realistic self-other views. Enhanced joy and creativity
Major techniques	Gold standard technique is transference interpretation in the here and now. Other interventions, (clarification and confrontation) identify, and interpret split off Self- Object dyads which drive pathology. Promote integration of split off self(good-bad) and Object	Gold standard technique is the empathic identification and interpretation of narcissistic transference (idealized, twin and mirror) as they appear in the transference and—as derivatives—in dreams and fantasies. The focus is held on the repeated identification, exploration and working through of those transferences. The use of "imaginary reconstruction" helps patients to experience their craving for "perfect" parental figures and to grieve and let go of perfection needs flowing from those
Therapist role	Maintain the frame created by the therapeutic contract and confront and interpret the patient's avoidance of it. Identify and interpret the transference in the here and now. Identify, confront and work-through split self-objects leading to integration	Maintain the focus on the dynamic template of the initial dynamic formulation: (core-genetic-developmental pathology which drive unconscious dynamics which generate conscious symptoms and functional problems). Promote reintegration of split off whole self-images (grandiose or devalued) via empathic focus. Facilitation of their emotional experience and their gradual integration into the mature ego
Change agents	Repeated identification of self-object distortions promotes development of reflective function on self-object experiences. This helps the resolution of core identity diffusion, reduces affect arousal and dysregulation	Empathy based, and transference fueled feelings; full experiences of past healthy self-images and gradual linking with self- objects free of distortions, rage and guilt
Adjunct treatment	Many (50% in research studies) are on medications (antidepressants, antipsychotic, anxiolytics, mood regulators). Some are able to reduce the use of medications as their therapy progresses. Use of medications, and its transference implications are analyzed	May be necessary a temporary or long term for symptomatic or co-morbid mood dysregulation, depression and anxiety. Use of medications, and its transference implications are analyzed
Research outcomes	A study of TFP vs Schema Cognitive therapy (88) patients, showed that TFP provedtobeeffective in reducing borderline personality disorder–specific and general psychopathologic dysfunction and measures of TFP concepts and in improving quality of life. (Giesen-Bloo et al., 2006) [129]. TFP has been shown to be an effective treatment for (BPD) in one uncontrolled study (Clarkin et al., 2001) and two randomized controlled trials (Clarkin, Levy, Lenzenweger, & Kernberg, 2007) [130], Doering et al., 2010) [131]	A 54-patient RCT of patient with BPD by Reneses and Trujillo (Co-PI's) in 2013, showed that Psychic Representation focused Psychotherapy (PRFP), a manualized psychodynamic psychotherapy based on self-representations, achieved significantly better outcomes in all the main variables measured, and in most of the secondary ones. PRFP may represent an important contribution for the treatment of BPD patients [132]

(continued)

Table 11.15 (continued)

Type of therapy author	Transference-focused psychotherapy Otto Kernberg	Empathy-based short-term psychotherapy Manuel Trujillo
As the great theoretician of psychoanalysis Otto Fenichel, referring to the explanatory power of psychoanalytic constructs, wrote, "There are many ways to treat neuroses, but there is only one way to understand them." Since the 1970's the evolving analytic enterprise has gradually incorporated the findings produced by the direct clinical study of narcissistic and borderline personality disorders. Both disorders (examples of a broader class of Self-Disorders), present, in addition to the instinctually derived problems posited by the classical psychoanalytic theory of neurosis, with additional specific disturbances of the self. The self was described by Kohut as a supraordinate agency of the mind which relates to the classical Freudian mental agencies, the id, the ego and the superego, modulates their function, and is in turn influenced by feedback from the actions of such agencies. The self maintains, for each person, a continuous evolving representation of the person's perception of their own lived value as a person, (an intimate "ranking" as it were), and of the value of their physical, emotional or intellectual assets and capacities. The self also manages, and denotes, the vicissitudes of emotional bonds with others. For the self, the fundamental and ongoing questions are: who am I, am I worthy of love, am I loved? and while the "other" (objects) are in the person's horizon, the questions are, can I love? is he or she worthy of my love? Thus, both instinctually based normative experiences such as sexuality, aggression, assertion, and their conflicts on the one hand, and disturbances of self (problems of self-esteem or of modulating ambition on the other), constitute the therapeutic domain for a wide range of psychoanalytically based psychotherapies; both open ended and short-term		

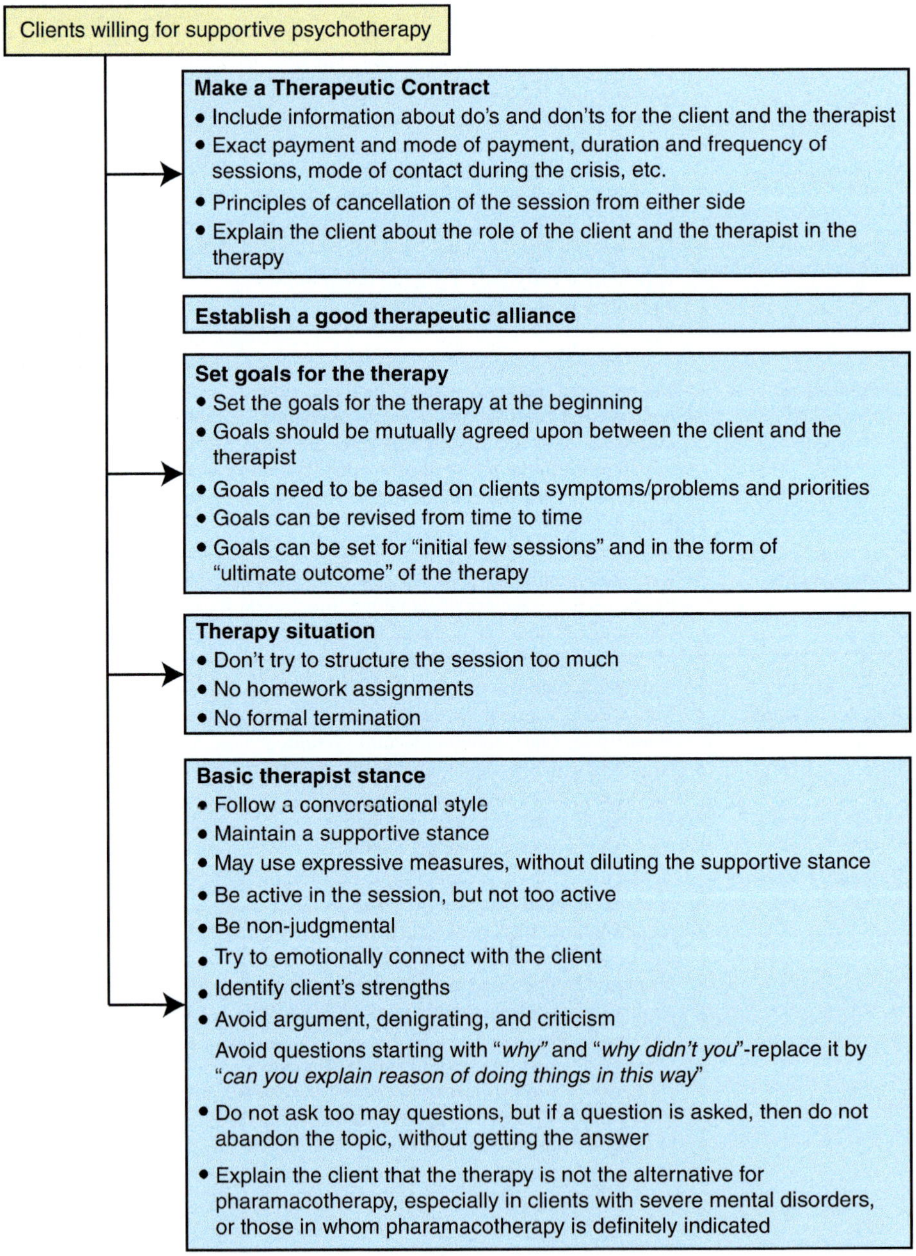

Fig. 11.32 General principles of supportive psychotherapy (*From* Grover et al. [133]; Creative Commons Attribution 4.0 International License; https://creativecommons.org/licenses/by/4.0/)

Behavioral and Cognitive Therapies

Other clinicians inside and outside the psychoanalytic tradition, have developed alternative explanations for the development of normal and abnormal behavior, and crafted procedures and techniques for the treatment of such abnormal behaviors congruent with their theoretical orientations. Early in the century, behaviorism appeared as new scientific psychology based partly on the works of Ivan Pavlov, who applied the rigorous scientific methods of physiology to study the phenomenon he called conditioned reflexes. Watson introduced behaviorism in 1913 with a somewhat radical manifesto: "Psychology, as the behaviorist views it, is a purely objective experimental branch of natural science. Its theoretical goal is the prediction and control of behavior. Introspection forms no essential part of its methods, nor is the scientific value of its data dependent upon the readiness with which they lend themselves to interpretation in terms of consciousness."

B. F. Skinner, in the late 1930s, introduced the notion of operant conditioning, enriching the limited therapeutic possibilities of Pavlov's classical conditioning for therapeutic application.

Behavior Therapy

Behavior therapy (BT), a term originated by Arnold Lazarus, refers now to many different therapies that treat many common mental health disorders. Behavior therapy's key scientific assumption is that behavior associated with psychological problems develops through the same processes of learning that affect the development of all other behaviors; a development that is rooted in classical conditioning and its experimental principles (Table 11.16). Ivan Pavlov's classical conditioning, as well as counterconditioning, are the basis for much of clinical behavior therapy, which now also includes other techniques, such as operant conditioning, contingency management, and modeling. A frequently noted behavior therapy is systematic desensitization, which was first demonstrated by Joseph Wolpe and Arnold Lazarus [134].

Lazarus, who originated the term behavior therapy, wrote the first text in Cognitive Behavior Therapy ("Behavior Therapy and Beyond") and also devised Multi-Modal Therapy (MMT), after acknowledging the importance of certain personality dimensions (variables among people) to the success of behavior and cognitive therapies. MMT involves those relevant dimensions from the seven that form the complete matrix: behavior, affect, bodily sensations, imagery, cognition, interpersonal relationships, and drugs when used. Other therapies associated with classical conditioning are aversion therapy, systematic desensitization, and flooding. Systematic desensitization is a treatment for phobias in which the patient is trained to relax while being exposed to anxiety-provoking stimuli (e.g., angry words), in a progressive sequence from the lower to the higher intensity, while reducing the anxiety response of the patient to tolerable limits via various relaxation techniques. Aversion therapy is a type of behavior therapy designed to make patients cease an undesirable habit by associating the habit with a strong unpleasant unconditioned stimulus. For example, a medication might be used to associate the taste of alcohol with stomach upset. It is said that behaviorism has expanded wildly over the years, as it developed new therapeutic applications and re-considered its foundational radical manifesto and its commitment to purely objective definitions of behavior and behavioral interventions [135].

Table 11.16 The basics of behavior therapy

Underlying philosophy of human nature	Psychology, as the behaviorist views it, is a purely objective experimental branch of natural science (Watson 1913)
Theory of behavior in health and illness	Behavior (healthy and pathological) are learned and maintained through Pavlovian conditioning mechanism and their derivatives (classical, operant, counterconditioning)
A presumed psychophysiology to explain syndromes or disorders	Faulty learning derails simple and complex conditional processes
A set of interventions to correct, alleviate or compensate for disorders	Procedures derived from classical and operant conditioning (rewards or punishment to enhance or extinguish adverse behaviors). Contingency management and modeling
Other interventions	Aversion therapy, systematic desensitization, exposure therapies, functional behavioral analysis

Today behaviorism encompasses schools as diverse as the Radical Behaviorism of Skinner, Moore, and others; the contextualist behaviorism of Hayes and Hayes (and the derived Acceptance and Commitment therapies), Rachlin's experimental analysis of behavior and Staddon's theoretical behaviorism with its cognitive, and learning theory, derivatives. Functional behavioral analysis is yet another derivative of behavior therapy. The assets and liabilities of these diverse branches of behaviorism are reviewed in Arabia in 2020 [135]. A 2013 Cochrane Review by Shinohara et al., concludes: "*We found low- to moderate- quality evidence that behavioral* therapies and other psychological therapies are equally effective. The current evidence base is very weak. This limits our confidence in both the size of the effect and its precision. Studies recruiting larger samples with improved reporting of therapy design and fidelity to treatment would improve the quality of evidence in this review" [136].

Cognitive Behavioral Therapy

Though the 1950s and 1960s saw the emergence of a few psychotherapy brands that anchored their theory and techniques on cognition, it is to the credit of Aaron Beck (Fig. 11.33) that he systematically unfolded a long-lasting program of clinical practice, defined the application of CBT to many clinical disorders, and has conducted numerous research studies which have established the efficacy and effectiveness of these techniques on broad populations of patients and disorders, making Cognitive behavior therapy (CBT) one of the most (if not the most) practiced psychotherapy worldwide. CBT's philosophical roots are deep: they go back to the Greek Stoic philosophers (who get their names from the great philosopher Zeno of Citium, the founder of the Stoic's school who is said to have done his teaching at the public colonnade or porch (stoa).

The stoic line of thinking arrives at Beck through Adler and Ellis. As Beck himself proclaims: *"These assumptions converge on a relatively new approach to emotional disorders. The philosophical underpinnings go back thousands of years, certainly to the time of the Stoics who considered man's conceptions (or misconceptions of events, rather than the events themselves) as the key to emotional upsets"* [137].

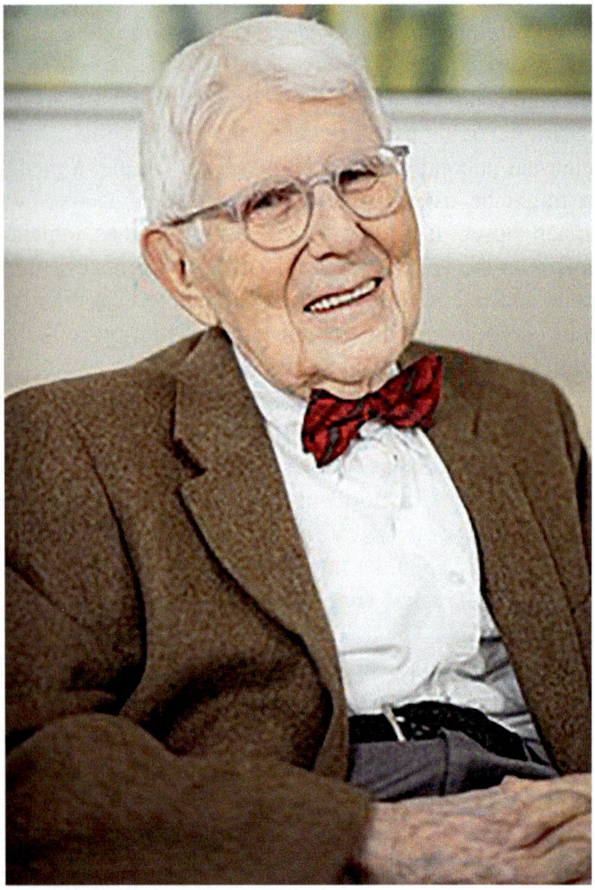

Fig. 11.33 Aaron Beck in 2016

The other significant experience contributing to Beck's development of cognitive therapy came from his observations of patients' thoughts while they underwent classical psychoanalytic treatment for depression. Some of these patients, in addition to the conventional psychoanalytic free-associative discourse, entertained a parallel and separate flow of "casual" thoughts, unrelated to the main content of the analysis, but which influenced their moods in and out of the session deeply. One of such patients admitted to feeling sad during and after each psychoanalytic session; not so much because of the content discussed but because of the "idle chatter "going on in parallel to the conventional discourse consisting of thoughts like "I hate myself; I think he is bored with me" … "he must hate me… How could he not… we are not making progress and he resents it ..."

A cascade of additional self-directed negative thoughts would ensue, ending up in the reported sadness and depression. Upon inquiry, one such patient told Beck that, not only was she having these thoughts during the session but all day long and in most contexts. From such observations, Beck built a theory of how thought distortions (in this case "I am boring him" for example, however unfounded) affected the patient's mood and behavior. He then devised techniques for the systematic more realistic evaluation of the thoughts and the correction of thought's distortions [137].

Today, cognitive-behavioral therapy is used for a wide array of mental health and substance use disorders. It combines behavioral techniques with cognitive psychology—the scientific study of mental processes, such as perception, memory, reasoning, decision making, and problem-solving. The goal is to replace maladaptive behavior and faulty cognitions with thoughts and self-statements that promote adaptive behavior [47]. One example is to replace a defeatist expectation, such as "I can't do anything right," with a positive expectation, such as "I can do this (specific task) right."

Figure 11.34 portrays the web of relationships between thoughts, feelings, and behavior. Streams if automatic thoughts, most adaptive, some pathogenic) flow from the person's development and associated experiences. Such thoughts frame deeply held views of Self, Others (and the World at large), and the future. Thoughts in turn mobilize feelings: fear and anxiety if thoughts predict threats, and sadness and depression if they anticipate failure or loss. Thoughts are aggregated into beliefs schemas that automate this process and may make it quite pervasive.

CBT focuses primarily on the "here and now" and imparts a directive or guiding role to the therapist, as well as the main responsibility for the structuring of the psychotherapy sessions. Some additional elements of cognitive-behavioral

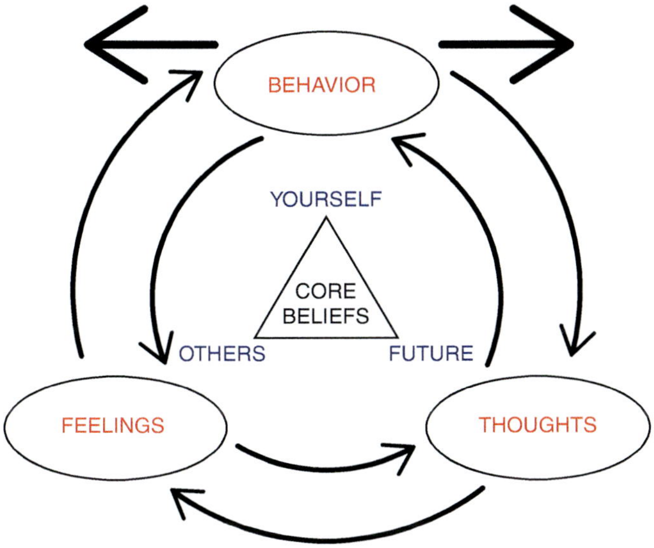

Fig. 11.34 Cognitive behavioral therapy (CBT). The diagram depicts how feelings, thoughts, and behaviors all influence each other. The triangle in the middle represents CBT's tenet that all humans' core beliefs can be summed up in three categories: self, others, future

therapy include cognitive restructuring, exposure techniques, behavioral activation, relaxation training, self-monitoring, and relapse prevention. CBT has a dense portfolio of high-quality research supporting its efficacy in the treatment of anxiety and depressive disorders, as an adjunct in the psychiatric rehabilitation of schizophrenia and bipolar disorders, and borderline personality disorders [138]. It has established efficacy for the treatment of women with alcohol or eating behavior problems. It has established presumed efficacy for specific phobias, antisocial and avoidant personalities, and anxiety disorders and depression in children and adolescents (Table 11.17) [139, 140].

Table 11.17 Cognitive behavior therapy

A philosophy of human nature	The philosophical underpinnings go back the Stoics who considered man's conceptions, rather than the events themselves) as the key to emotional upsets" [137]
A theory of behavior in health and illness	The anchor science is cognitive psychology: the scientific study of broad mental processes such as cognition, perception, reasoning, decision making
A presumed psychophysiology to explain syndromes or disorders	People form triads linking their views (beliefs) about self, others and the world. Such schemas influence physiology and behavior for health or disease
A set of interventions to correct, alleviate or compensate for disorders	Basic interventions include: (1) challenging unhelpful distortions of thinking or unsupported beliefs, (2) improving emotion regulation, (3) promoting coping skills
Research	CBT has demonstrated broad efficacy and effectiveness in the treatment of depression, anxiety, personality, body dysmorphic, eating disorders in adults, children, and adolescent It has also proven effective as a primary or adjunct therapy for the treatment of OCD and PTSD, psychosis including schizophrenia and many other Axis I and Somatic conditions

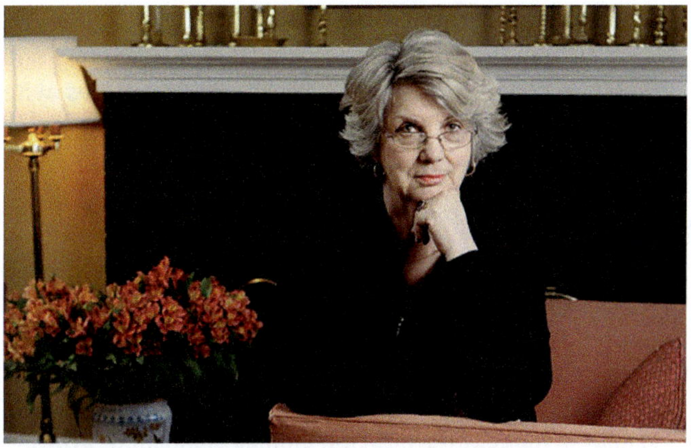

Fig. 11.35 Dr. Marsha Linehan

Dialectical Behavior Therapy (DBT)

Dialectical Behavior therapy evolved from the efforts of Dr. Marsha Linehan to find effective treatments for suicidal, young women with multiple life problems beyond their diagnostic labels. She found that classical CBT interventions were often misunderstood and rejected by these patients (Fig. 11.35) [141].

Linehan discovered the potential application of the dialectical philosophical framework to the, often contradictory emotions which fuel psychological and psychiatric problems; The dialectical framework makes it possible to address the impossible challenge of integrating the many opposing dichotomies experienced by these patients and their therapists. Challenges such as balancing needs for acceptance vs, needs for change, dependence vs independence, and many others. Maintaining a dialog between opposing, intensely experienced emotions is facilitated by the idea of dialectical integration. In the classic definition of dialectics by the German philosopher Fichte, dialectics is a process of addressing opposing ideas by a methodical examination of an idea or proposition (thesis), and its opposite, (antithesis), to arrive at a reasoned integrated synthesis (Fig. 11.36) [141].

DBT therapy originally targeted a subset of patients who experienced emotions far more intensely than others, and who have limited ability to modulate the emotions or the behaviors which flow from such emotional storms. In order to regulate their heightened emotions, these patients often

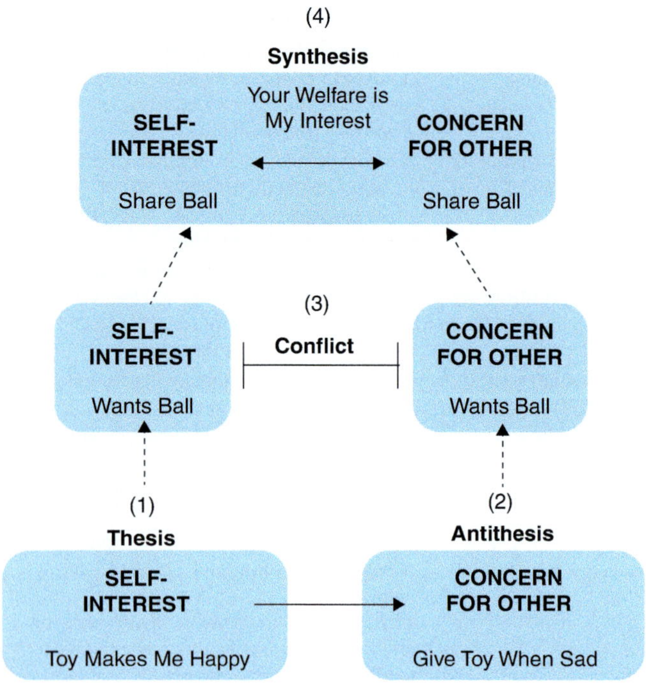

Fig. 11.36 The dialectical development of moral identity. (*From* Marginean et al. [180]; *with permission*)

reacted in an extreme and impulsive manner (e.g., self-harm, suicide attempts). It is thought that a lack of awareness and acceptance of these emotional experiences interferes with developing effective coping strategies to manage distress. Dialectical behavior therapy teaches clients behavioral skills such as mindfulness, distress tolerance, interpersonal effectiveness, and emotion regulation (Table 11.18).

The therapy is structured in individual and group sessions, and a therapist consultation team, which provides much-needed support and perspective for therapists who must deal with the intense, demanding emotions of their patients (Fig. 11.36) [141].

There is plethora of research studies stablishing efficacy of DBT in borderline personality disorders with suicidal risk [142] and with severely dysfunctional patients with substance abuse [143, 144].

DBT can be considered a "bridge therapy "between classical CBT and the so-called "third wave" therapies such as Mindfulness and Acceptance and Commitment therapies. DBT is rich in the promotion of skills; What skills (observe, describe, experience), How skills, action skills (doing what works and doing it well). More generally, a skill focus is applied to learning mindfulness, distress tolerance, and effective interpersonal and functional skills.

A list of DBT Skills is available at a DBT self-help website: https://www.dbtselfhelp.com. The Linehan Institute Training Company (www.behavioraltech.com) has large

Table 11.18 Dialectical behavior therapy—DBT

Underlying philosophy	A dialectical philosophical framework aims for the integrated resolution of these patients, often extremes emotional dichotomies
Pathophysiology results from vulnerability to emotional dysregulation, often coupled by an environment of invalidation	Often the invalidating environment and the emotional vulnerability get locked in a vicious circle of ever-growing, intense, variable and often conflicting emotions ("emotional dysregulation") which rules the lives of these patients and drives behavioral dysregulation and destructiveness
Therapeutic methods	Therapy is a composite of (1) strong structure, (2) methods to facilitate acceptance of emotions and mindfulness, (3) skills development in areas such as mindfulness, distress tolerance and effective interpersonal and functional skills
Therapy structure	1. Individual therapy (1 week outpatient) 1 a day (inpatient). Focuses on destructive behaviors through behavior analytics 2. Group therapy to develop skills 3. Consultation team to support therapists' efforts and to keep balance of therapeutic techniques
Research Linehan (2006) a RCT (101 females Dx of BPD w suicide attempts [142]	DBT achieved better outcomes, in the intent-to- treat analysis than community treatment by experts in most target areas during the 2-year treatment and follow-up period. DBT subjects were half as likely to make a suicide attempt ($P = 0.005$), required less hospitalization for suicide ideation ($P = 0.004$), and had lower medical risk ($P = 0.04$) across all suicide attempts and self-injurious acts combined. DBT subjects were less likely to drop out of treatment ($P < 0.001$) and had fewer psychiatric hospitalizations ($P = 0.007$) and psychiatric emergency visits ($P = 0.04$).Study showed DBT appears to be uniquely effective in reducing suicide attempts [142]
Linehan (1999) [143]	DBT has shown to be more effective than treatment-as-usual in treating drug abuse in this study, providing more support for DBT as an effective treatment for severely dysfunctional BPD patients across a range of presenting problems [143]
Linehan (2015) [144]	Single blind RTC, 2 years follow-up of 89 females with BPD with 2 suicide attempts or non-suicidal self-injury (NSSI). To evaluate the impact of the skills training component of BPD DBT interventions with therapists trained in the DBT suicide risk assessment and management protocol are effective for reducing suicide attempts and NSSI episodes. Interventions that include DBT skills training are more effective than DBT without skills training [144]

catalogs of clinical, training, and research information about DBT end professional and patient informational guides and papers which are updated often.

Research has shown efficacy and effectiveness for the treatment of many aspects of Borderline Personality Disorder and its risks, including suicide. DBT has also been applied successfully to patients with BPD plus substance abuse. More research is needed to ascertain, which components of the DBT therapeutic arsenal are preferentially effective for what conditions and under what circumstances. Such challenges are shared with many, if not most, effective psychosocial treatments [141].

Prolonged Exposure (PE)

Prolonged Exposure is based on imagined as well as real prolonged and repeated exposure to trauma in a safe supportive environment in psychotherapy in order to enable extinction of avoidance and fear responses to traumatic stimuli. PE was introduced by Edna Foa and has been shown to be effective in PTSD [145]. PE is delivered in 8–15 weekly 90-min sessions covering the key components in the figure below (see Fig. 11.37) [146].

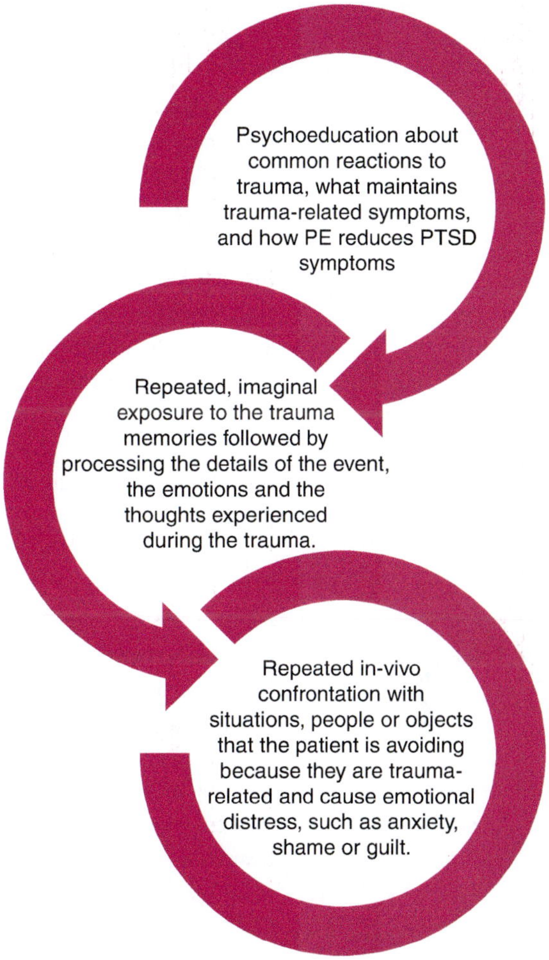

Fig. 11.37 Prolonged exposure (PE) key components

Eye Movement Desensitization and Reprocessing (EMDR)

EMDR, an empirically validated psychotherapy, is based on identifying and processing target memories using bilateral sensory stimulation. Depending on the patient's comfort level, this stimulation could involve following the clinician's finger or tapping among other visual and auditory stimuli. EMDR was introduced by Francine Shapiro and is delivered in 6–12 weekly or biweekly 60–90-min sessions covering the key components in Fig. 11.38 [147].

Virtual Reality Therapy (VR)

VR is becoming a treatment modality for a variety of medical and psychological conditions such as chronic pain, fear of heights (acrophobia), PTSD, and OCD. A new specialty in medicine is evolving called virtual therapeutics as outlined by Spiegel in 2020 [148], where technology shown in the figure below as an example, includes the successful use of a smartphone-based virtual reality exposure for acrophobia showing significant improvements in subjective fear and avoidance behaviors with cost and accessibility advantages for professional and self-help uses [149].

Behavioral Activation (BA)

BA is an evidence-based patient-centered psychotherapy that emphasizes engagement in enjoyable and valued personalized activities selected by the patient. BA has been shown to be effective in depression in more than 25 randomized clinical trials with effects comparable to CBT and with less intensive and costly training [150].

Example activities for BA include calling a friend, coloring, cooking, drawing, gardening, hiking, swimming, going to a museum, looking at old photos, playing games, reading a book, singing, spend time with a friend, take a walk, watch a movie, watch the sunset, and write in your journal.

Phase	Purpose	Procedures
History taking	Obtain background information. Identify suitability for EMDR treatment Identify processing targets from events in client's life according to standardized three-pronged protocol	Standard history-taking questionnaires and diagnostic psychometrics Review of selection criteria Questions and techniques (e.g., Floatback) to identify (1) past events that have laid the groundwork for the pathology, (2) current triggers, and (3) future needs
Preparation	Prepare appropriate clients for EMDR processing of targets	Education regarding the symptom picture Metaphors and techniques that foster stabilization and a sense of personal control (e.g., Safe Place)
Assessment	Access the target for EMDR processing by stimulating primary aspects of the memory	Elicit the image, negative belief currently held, desired positive belief, current emotion, and physical sensation and baseline measures
Desensitization	Process experiences toward an adaptive resolution (no distress)	Standardized protocols incorporating eye movements (taps or tones) that allow the spontaneous emergence of insights, emotions, physical sensations, and other memories
Installation	Increase connections to positive cognitive networks	Enhance the validity of the desired positive belief and fully integrate within the memory network
Body scan	Complete processing of any residual disturbance associated with the target	Concentration on and processing of any residual physical sensations
Closure	Ensure client stability at the completion of an EMDR therapy session and between sessions	Use of self-control techniques if needed Briefing regarding expectations and behavioral reports between sessions
Reassessment	Ensure maintenance of therapeutic outcomes and stability of client	Evaluation of treatment effects Evaluation of integration within larger social system

Fig. 11.38 Overview of eight-phase Eye Movement Desensitization and Reprocessing (EMDR) therapy treatment. Source: https://link.springer.com/chapter/10.1007/978-3-319-46138-0_13#Tab1. Permission needed Table 13.1 from [147]

Other Psychotherapies

Interpersonal Psychotherapy (IPT)

IPT which was introduced by Gerald Klerman and Myrna Weissman is an evidence-based psychotherapy, based on the close relationship between depression and interpersonal disruptions such as a struggle with a significant other (*role dispute*), the beginning or end of a marriage or other relationship, or becoming physically ill (*a role transition*), or the death of a loved one (*complicated bereavement*) [151]. IPT is administered weekly for 12–16 weeks with three phases: a beginning, middle, and end as detailed below.

The first phase of IPT is an assessment phase in which an area of focus is selected among the following options: interpersonal role dispute, interpersonal role transition, grief, and interpersonal sensitivity and the therapeutic task is to link the depressive feelings with one or two of these themes. The second phase aims to alleviate the symptoms of depression, by recognizing and expressing of depressive and associated effects, and by active engagement in developing or reactivating the patient's interpersonal network. The third phase is focused on the transition to ending therapy, the expression of feelings associated with the loss, and the review and support of learned strategies to prevent relapses [152, 153].

Acceptance and Commitment Therapy (ACT)

ACT, developed by Stephens C. Hayes in 1982, has philosophical roots in the philosophy of functional contextualism, an approach which focuses on the behavior of individuals within their historical and situational contexts. ACT seeks to predict and influence events using empirically based concepts and rules [154]. ACT draws on a comprehensive theory of language, relational frame theory (RFT), which accounts for the influence of culturally shaped language processes on learning and human behavior.

Taking a step beyond CBT, ACT's focus is on freeing up energy for committed action by changing the function of psychological events such as cognitions and promoting psychological flexibility. Psychological flexibility is established through six core ACT processes: cognitive diffusion, acceptance, being present, values, committed action, and self as context. Through techniques such as acceptance, mindfulness, and cognitive diffusion, clients learn to accept into awareness, and reconceptualize avoided or feared thoughts, feelings, memories, and physical sensations in an adaptive manner. Acceptance and commitment therapy is achieving significant recognition and is supported by a growing body of research that demonstrates its efficacy with a wide variety of problems and suggests that it works by its theorized mechanism of change, an important fact that is unfortunately very necessary but not that common in psychotherapy research. ACT is being tested in controlled trials with encouraging, though not yet clearly superior results [155, 156]. Research has established efficacy in a wide range of problems: Depression, Anxiety Disorders, Posttraumatic Stress Disorders, OCD spectrum, Borderline Personality Disorder. It has been studied also for medical problems such as multiple sclerosis, substance use disorder (tobacco) chronic pain (Table 11.19).

Table 11.19 The structure of acceptance and commitment therapy

A philosophy of human nature	The underlying philosophy is functional contextualism. Situational context help predict behavioral events
A theory of behavior in health and illness	For ACT psychological suffering is usually caused by the interface between human language and cognition, and the control of human behavior by direct experience. Psychological inflexibility is argued to emerge from experiential avoidance, cognitive entanglement, attachment of a conceptualized self, loss of contact with the present, and the resulting failure to take needed behavioral steps in accord with core values
A presumed pathogenic pathway	A core process that can lead to pathology is cognitive fusion, which refers to the domination of behavior regulatory functions, by relational networks, based in particular on the failure to distinguish the process and products of relational responding. Psychological flexibility is established through six core ACT processes: cognitive diffusion, acceptance, being present, values, committed action, self as context
A set of interventions to correct, alleviate or compensate for disorders	Cognitive diffusion, which aims develop a non-judgmental and mindful perspective of self and environment, facilitating a commitment to pursue life goals. Other techniques include being present, accepting the experience of negative emotions, sensations and thoughts. Mindful meditation to reduce distress
Supporting research: 1. Powers MB (2009) 18 RTC, 917 Pts [155]	Acceptance and commitment therapy was more effective than control conditions across several disorders, but there was no evidence that it was more effective than established treatments
2. A-Tjak, JG (2015) 39 RTC,1827 Pts [156]	Findings indicate that ACT is more effective than treatment as usual or placebo and that ACT may be as effective in treating anxiety disorders, depression, addiction, and somatic health problems as established psychological interventions

Existential Psychotherapy

Existential Psychotherapy, is a therapeutic intervention derived from the philosophy espoused by leading European intellectuals after WWII: existentialism, which flowed from the disillusioned climate about the human condition

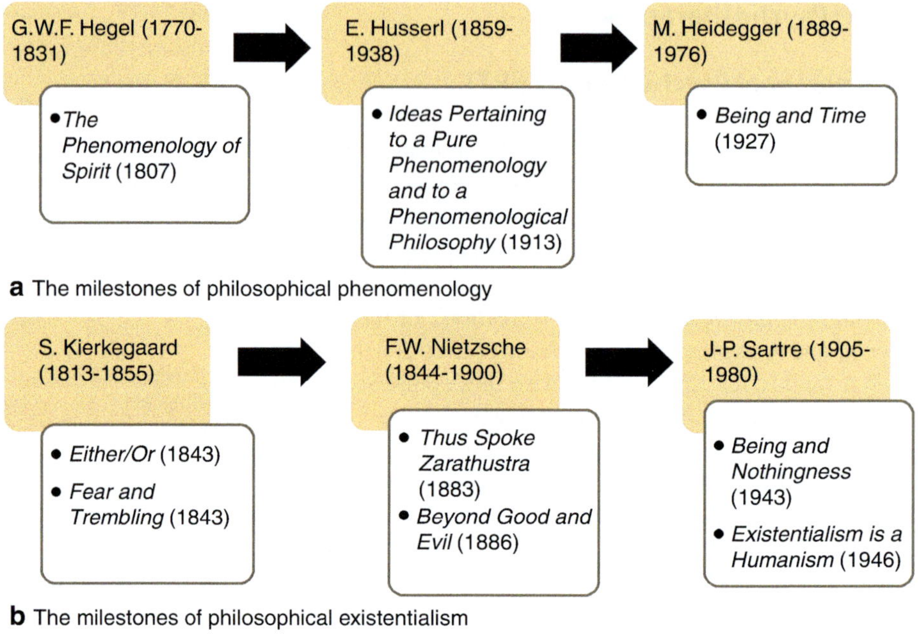

Fig. 11.39 Milestones of philosophical existentialism. (*From* Balogh et al. [157]; Creative Commons Attribution 4.0 International License; https://creativecommons.org/licenses/by/4.0/)

which followed the contemplation of the atrocities which presumed enlightened people, from a Christian background, were capable of committing. Existential philosophies gave rise to numerous therapeutic approaches. The existential philosophy (greatly influenced by Nietzsche and Kierkegaard) posits the central importance of a lived, experienced life, starting from the position of the individual and its radical aloneness.

The person must see him/herself as separate and independent from any inherited values or external sources of meaning. To feel whole the individual must embrace that radical solitude and its attendant feelings of loneliness and dread before joining external sources of meaning. Only after struggling with the deep feelings of anxiety, isolation, and the dread of existing in a meaningless world, that such a radical individualism brings about, can the person begin to find what is alive and authentic within themselves. The cultivation and expansion of such roots will allow the person to create enduring values and to give meaning to their lives (Fig. 11.39) [157].

A good number of therapists, Irwin Yalom and Rollo May in the US, R.D. Laing, Cooper, Medar Boss L Bingswanger, and Victor Frankl in Europe, attempted to create therapies sensitive to common "life crises" springing from the essential bleakness of the human self-awareness of post-war societies, making available to many the existential approach to life, previously accessible only through the complex writings of existential philosophers (Fig. 11.40).

Patients who often seek, and benefit from such therapy tend to be in an existential crisis themselves: they may be loners or feel empathically drawn to the pain of others, or feel confused, and lost in a world that feels gray and dreadful. They tend to be introspective and feel no visceral bonds with people or causes.

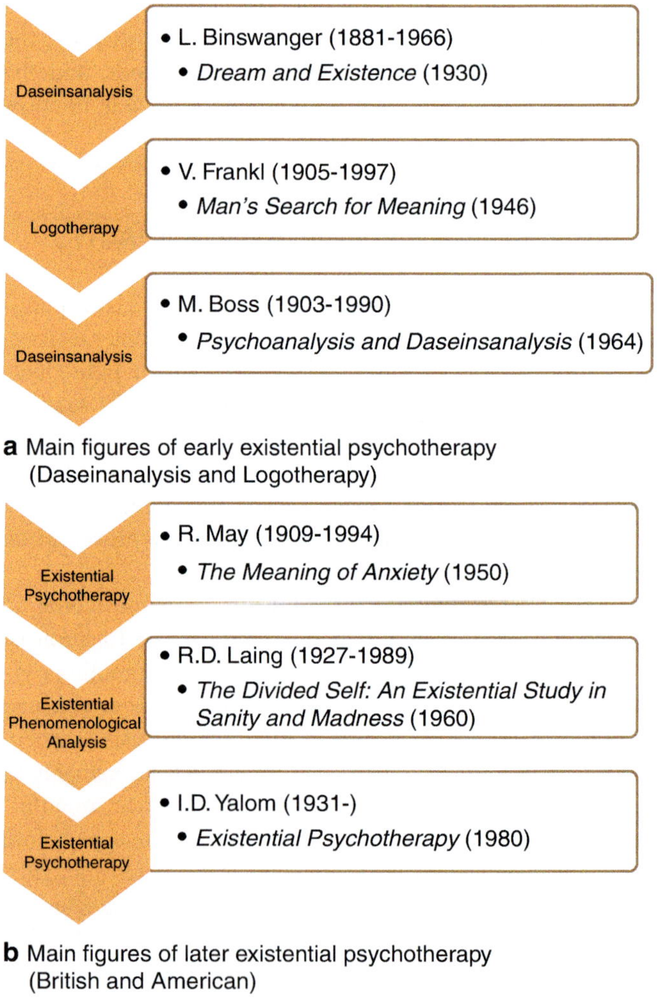

Fig. 11.40 Milestones of philosophical existentialism. (*From* Balogh et al. [157]; Creative Commons Attribution 4.0 International License; https://creativecommons.org/licenses/by/4.0/)

Logotherapy

Logotherapy, an existential humanistic therapy based on people's search for meaning, is the work of Viktor Frankl (Fig. 11.41) [158].

As an inmate in a WWII concentration camp, where he lost most of his family, Dr. Frankl was able to endure the catastrophic experience and survive with some sense of wholeness and integrity, sustained by the conviction that life matters, and that it can be lived with integrity by finding within yourself what constitutes your own unique mission in life: Nietzsche's why.

He who has a why to live for can bear with almost any how.
Friedrich Nietzsche.

Logotherapy's basic philosophy asserts that humans have the freedom to take their stance toward internal (psychological) and external (biological and social) conditions and that the search for meaning is seen as the primary motivation of humans.

The therapy assists clients in finding and pursuing deeply personal and meaningful goals for their lives. However, they are not offered specific meanings; they are encouraged instead to realize some of the "meaning possibilities" they have detected within themselves. Frankl identified three pathways to realizing meaning in life: (1) through "creative values that flow with our actions, our work and our other creations { creative values }. (2) through experiencing truth and beauty, art, nature, the universe, or encountering love: "experiential values" (3) "through the adoption of a courageous and exemplary attitude in situations of great and unavoidable suffering: "attitudinal values" [158].

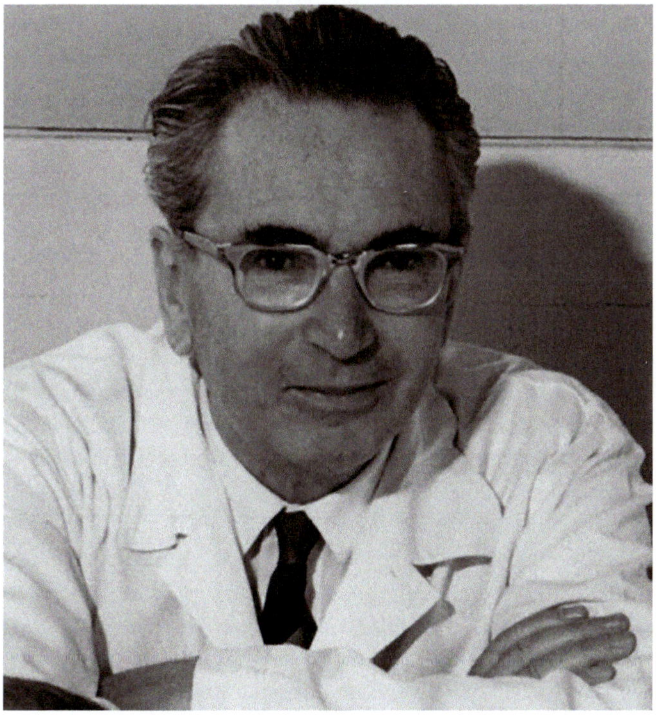

Fig. 11.41 Viktor Frankl

Employing specific techniques, such as self-distancing (learning to distance the self from the immediacy of the psychological pain, relativizing it through humor for example), Socratic dialogue (interviewing designed to elicit the patient's own wisdom and to elicit attitudes that deepen the patients suffering: nihilism, radical pessimism, skepticism), and de-reflection (redirecting attention from the self towards other people or meaningful goals), logotherapy promotes the adoption of a radically optimistic view of human potential (Frankl's tragic optimism) and the ability to transcend the self through the pursuit of meaning that is specific to one's own life. For Frankl, one can "find meaning in a deed, in a work, or in love" or in the attitude that one adopts in the face of a predicament that cannot be changed as detailed by Frankl in 1988 [158].

Mindfulness-Based Stress Reduction (MBSR)

MBSR is an evidence-based therapy that is based on. MBSR was introduced by Jon Kabat-Zinn and consists of 8 weekly 2–2.5-h sessions. MBSR has shown effectiveness in the treatment of a variety of psychological and medical problems (Table 11.20). Explains MBSR on a week-by-week basis [159].

Mentalization-Based Therapy (MBT)

MBT is an evidence-based psychotherapy, based on establishing an enduring attachment relationship and stimulating a

Table 11.20 The 8-week Mindfulness-based Stress Reduction (MBSR). Adapted from Kabat- Zinn J. *Full catastrophe living.* New York: Random House; 2013

Week	Topic	Details
Week 1	Simple awareness	Raisin meditation and the body scan
Week 2	Attention and the brain	Introduction to sitting meditation
Week 3	Dealing with thoughts	Introduction to yoga
Week 4	Stress: responding vs. reacting	STOP: The 1-min breathing space
Week 5	Dealing with difficult emotions or physical pain	Turning toward
Week 6	Mindfulness and communication	Lake and mountain meditations
Week 7	Mindfulness and compassion	Lovingkindness meditation
Week 8	Conclusion	Developing a practice of your own

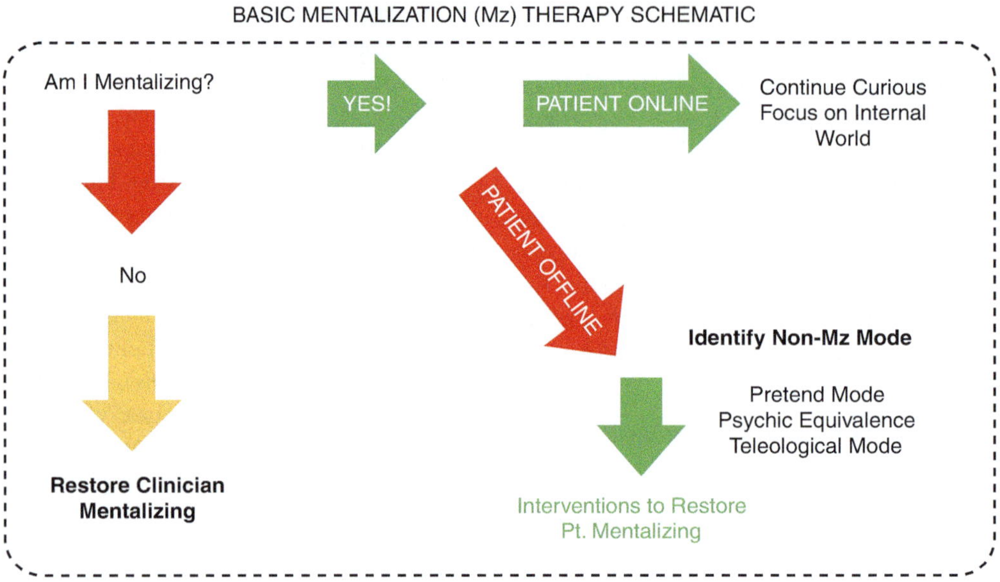

Fig. 11.42 Basic mentalization. (*From* MacMillian [161]; *with permission*)

mentalizing process in the patient which involves the ability to reflect upon, to understand one's own and others state of mind and to have insight how and why one and others are feeling (Fig. 11.42) [160]. MBT was introduced by Peter Fonagy and Anthony Bateman for the treatment of borderline personality disorder and is administered weekly for 18 months starting with assessment and introductory sessions and followed by weekly individual and group therapy [161, 162].

Future-Directed Therapy (FTD)

FTD is an evidence-based psychotherapy, based on three primary concepts: (1) the desire to thrive is the primary drive of all human beings because it promotes the evolutionary process; (2) thought and behavior are limited resources that humans utilize to promote their thriving, and (3) preparing for the future is essential to thriving and much of human functioning has evolved to create such future [163]. FTD was introduced by Jennice Vilhauer and is administered weekly for 10 weeks.

Positive Psychotherapy (PPT)

PPT is an evidence-based psychotherapy, based on positive emotion, engagement, and meaning rather than directly targeting depressive symptoms. PPT was introduced as a self-help intervention in the 1980s by Pesechkian, and then as a manualized psychotherapy with robust research studies by Seligman and Tayyeb, and is administered weekly for 12 weeks (see Table 11.21) [164].

Group Psychotherapy

Group psychotherapy involves composing and organizing a group of patients to work together to achieve their individual goals with the help of a group leader. Group psychotherapy orientations include supportive, psychodynamic, self-help, or cognitive-behavioral, with the use of mutual support. Other significant therapeutic factors to effect change in group psychotherapy include abreaction, acceptance, altruism, catharsis, cohesion, and consensual validation. Contagion, corrective emotional experience, empathy, identification, imitation, inspiration, insight, interpretation, reality testing, and validation.

The Future of Psychotherapy and Psychosocial Interventions

Is Psychotherapy Effective?

Controversy has plagued psychotherapy since the beginning of the modern era: is Psychotherapy effective? The first challenge to the effectiveness of Psychotherapy was presented by Hanks Eysenck's assertion that psychotherapies are not effective in the treatment of mental disorders [113]. This first salvo in the war over the effectiveness of psychotherapy generated many fireworks but not much light. It took the work of Mary Lee Smith and Gene Glass to show, after conducting a comprehensive meta-analysis of controlled studies of psychotherapy, that psychotherapy was indeed effective, with a standardized mean difference (SMD) between treated and untreated patients of approximately 0.70, a relatively large effect [165, 166]. Munde et al., in 2019

Table 11.21 Outline of PPT sessions based on Pesechkian, Seligman, and Tayyeb

Session and topic	Description
Orientation to PPT; current positive resources	Psychological distress is discussed as a lack of positive resources, such as positive emotions, relationships, meaning, and accomplishment To explore this, the therapist might use an exercise that encourages the individual to write a one-page, real-life story that calls for the best in them and has a positive ending
Individual character strengths	In this session, individual character strengths are explored, and the concept of engagement and flow is introduced To begin exploring individual character strengths, the individual may be asked to identify what they believe are their signature strengths both in the session and through an online self-report They may also ask two other close persons to rate their signature strengths
Signature strengths and positive emotions	Following on from the last session, signature strengths are discussed in more detail As an exercise, the therapist may ask the individual to compile a signature strengths profile, which could include setting SMART (specific, measurable, achievable, realistic, and timely) goals
Good vs. bad Experiences, symptoms or memories	The concept of how negative experiences and symptoms can be perpetuated is discussed in alignment with positive experiences The therapist might use an exercise that asks the individual to explore a memory or experience that elicited feelings of anger, bitterness, or resentment and how these feelings further perpetuated the negative experience
Forgiveness	Forgiveness is explored as a resource to reframe negative symptoms and feelings into more positive emotions. The therapist might use a **letter-writing exercise** that asks the participant to remember a negative experience and to write out a letter of forgiveness towards the perceived transgressor/s of the scenario—themselves included
Gratitude	Alongside forgiveness, gratitude is explored as a resource for generating better balance, and to view individual circumstances more positively The role of positive and negative memories, feelings, and symptoms are discussed with an emphasis on gratitude for all the lessons both of these states have allowed for. The therapist might use gratitude journaling as an exercise to help build more focus and awareness of all the things for which the individual is grateful
Mid-therapy check	At this point, the therapist may follow up on any at-home tasks related to the forgiveness and gratitude sessions, and to revisit any of the previous sessions that may feel unresolved This is also the opportunity for the individual to discuss their perceived gains or hurdles they might be experiencing so far as an outcome of the sessions As an exercise, the therapist may seek to explore different ways the individual can overcome any of the hurdles, utilizing their signature strengths uncovered previously
Satisficing vs. maximizing	The therapist may now introduce the two concepts of satisficing (mainly, being 'good enough') and maximizing The individual may be asked to explore the different ways in life they have not felt 'good enough' and to tell the story of one experience where they did feel good enough, and one where they did not Again, these can be explored regarding the individual's signature strengths
Hope and optimism	The additional concepts of optimism and hope are explored
Positive	As an exercise, the therapist may ask the individual to think about a time when they may have felt they lost out on something, only to discover it opened up new opportunities
Communication	Various interventions that involve developing positive communication, such as active-constructive, are explored and referenced in association to the individual's signature strengths
Signature strengths of others	The importance of recognizing, acknowledging, and associating with the signature strengths of the key people the individual has close relationships with is explored As an exercise, the therapist may ask the individual to draw up a 'Family Strengths Tree' where the individual asks their significant relationships to complete an online self-report strengths test and identify their signature strengths These can then be discussed in the session
Savoring	The concept of **savoring** is explored, as well as some of the techniques and strategies that can be used to prevent adaptation, along with techniques and strategies to safeguard against adaptation
Gift of time and positive legacy	The benefits of kindness, sharing, and helping others are explored and discussed in alignment with therapeutic outcomes As an exercise, the therapist might ask the individual to make plans for how they might give the gift of their time utilizing their signature strengths
The full life	In the final session, 'The Full Life' is discussed in terms of what the individual feels they have that leads to this Therapeutic gains are discussed, focusing on positive emotions, engagement, and meaning How to keep this momentum going is also discussed, and ways of doing this are devised with the individual taking the lead and considering their signature strengths to achieve this

From Mead [176]; Creative Commons Attribution 4.0 International License; http://creativecommons.org/licenses/by/4.0/

once again, revisited the controversy and after significant reanalysis of the data provided by both camps, concluded: "The SMD for all interventions and for psychotherapy compared to Wait List controls was approximately 0.70, a value consistent with past estimates of the effectiveness of psychotherapy. Psychotherapy was also found to be more effective than care-as-usual (SMD = 0.31) and then other control conditions (SMD = 0.43)" [167]. Many other investigators have found effect sizes (ES) of 0.78 at termination to 1.31 at 1-year follow-up in a large sample of subjects in many studies [168–171]. In general ES for symptomatic improvement tends to be larger (ES ranging from 1.03 at termination to 1.67 at 1 year follow-up) than ES for personality changes 0.52–1.31).

Of interest, the conclusions of these studies include that supportive mechanism were present in all therapies including psychoanalysis and accounted for more of the achieved outcomes and structural changes than anticipated [172].

Visualizing the Effects of Psychotherapy USING Neuroimaging Brain Imaging Before and After Psychotherapy

Sankar et al. conducted a systematic review and meta-analysis of fMRI, PET, SPECT, and MRS studies, and showed increased activation of the left rostral anterior cingulate in depressed patients during affective visual processing tasks after psychotherapy. Their findings suggest that psychological therapy may increase emotional responsivity and regulation in patients with major depressive disorder (Fig. 11.43) [173].

Neuroimaging and the Effects of Psychotherapy on Borderline Personality Disorder

Neuroimaging showed that structural brain abnormalities in borderline personality disorder correlate with clinical severity and predict psychotherapy response (Fig. 11.44) [174].

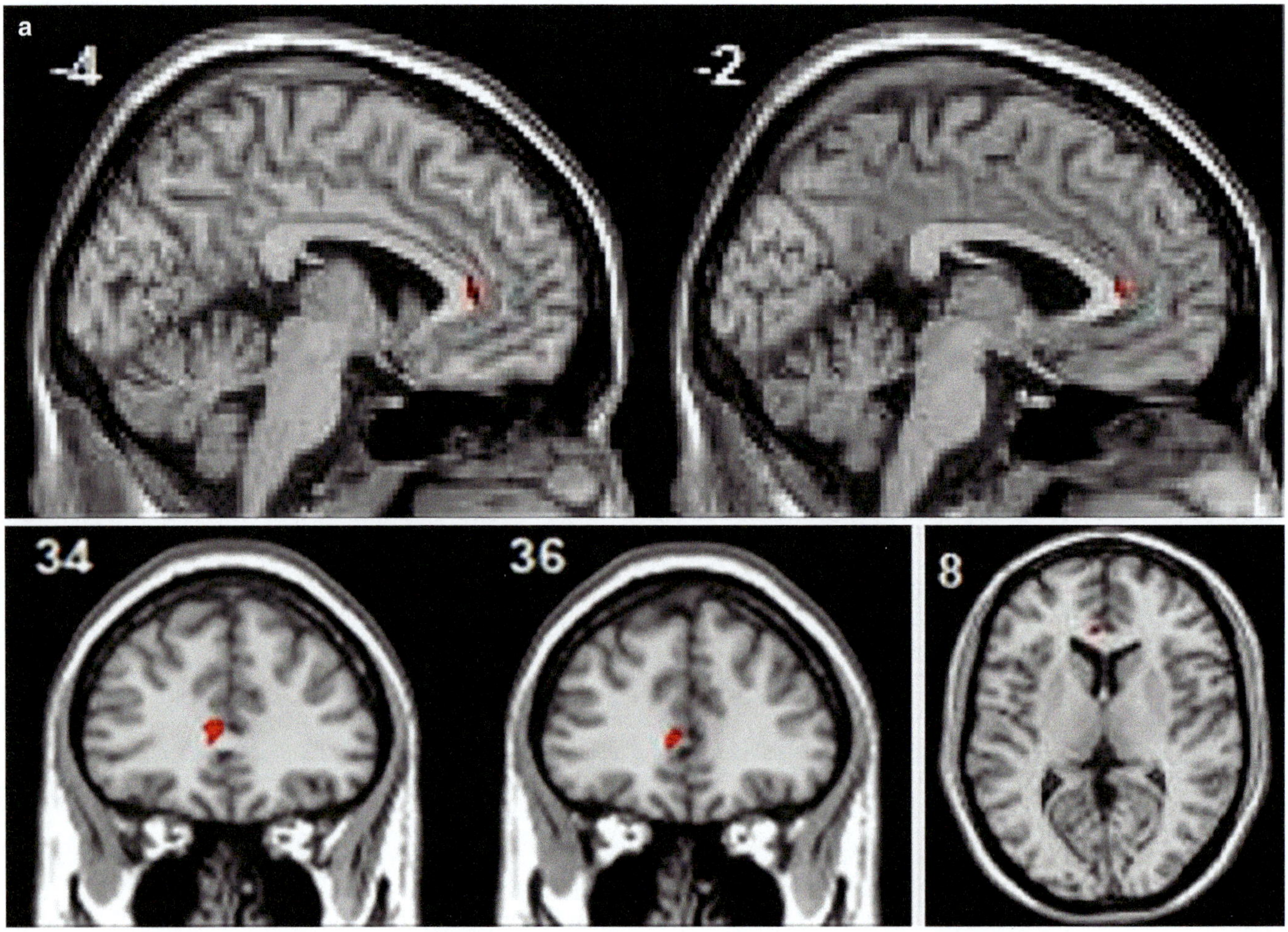

Fig. 11.43 Imaging showing findings indicative of improvements in emotion responsivity that may be achieved following psychotherapy, in a systematic review and meta-analysis of psychotherapy treatment studies measuring neural function and metabolism using fMRI, PET, SPECT and MRS. (**a**) Group by time interaction effects of psychological therapies. There was a significant group by time interaction in the left rostral anterior cingulate cortex, in which participants with major depression showed increased activity following psychological therapy while healthy participants showed a reduction in activity at the follow up scan. (**b**) Longitudinal changes following psychological therapies. There was a main effect of in the left precentral gyrus, which showed decreased activity following psychological therapy in major depression. (*From* Sankar et al. [173]; *with permission*)

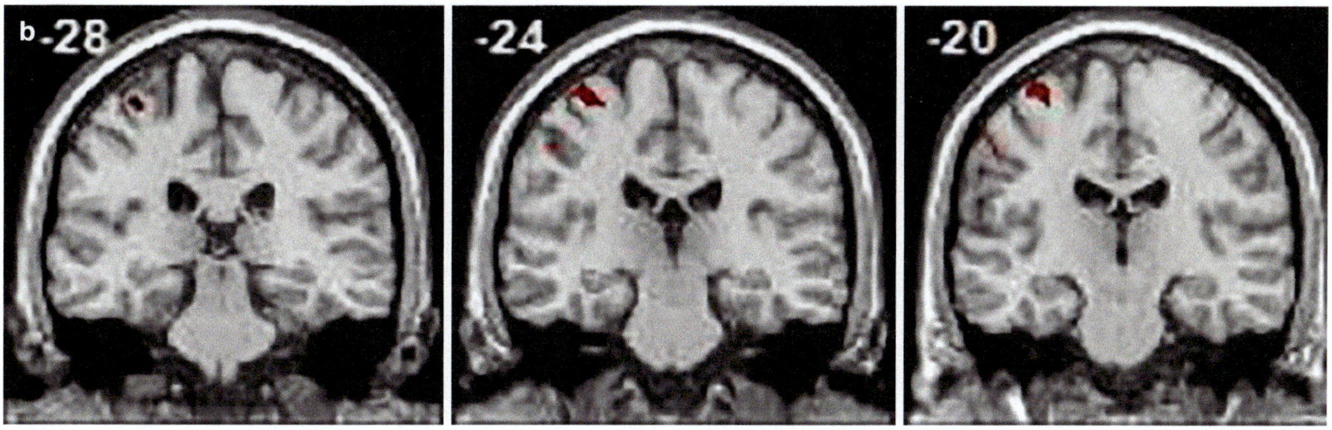

Fig. 11.43 (continued)

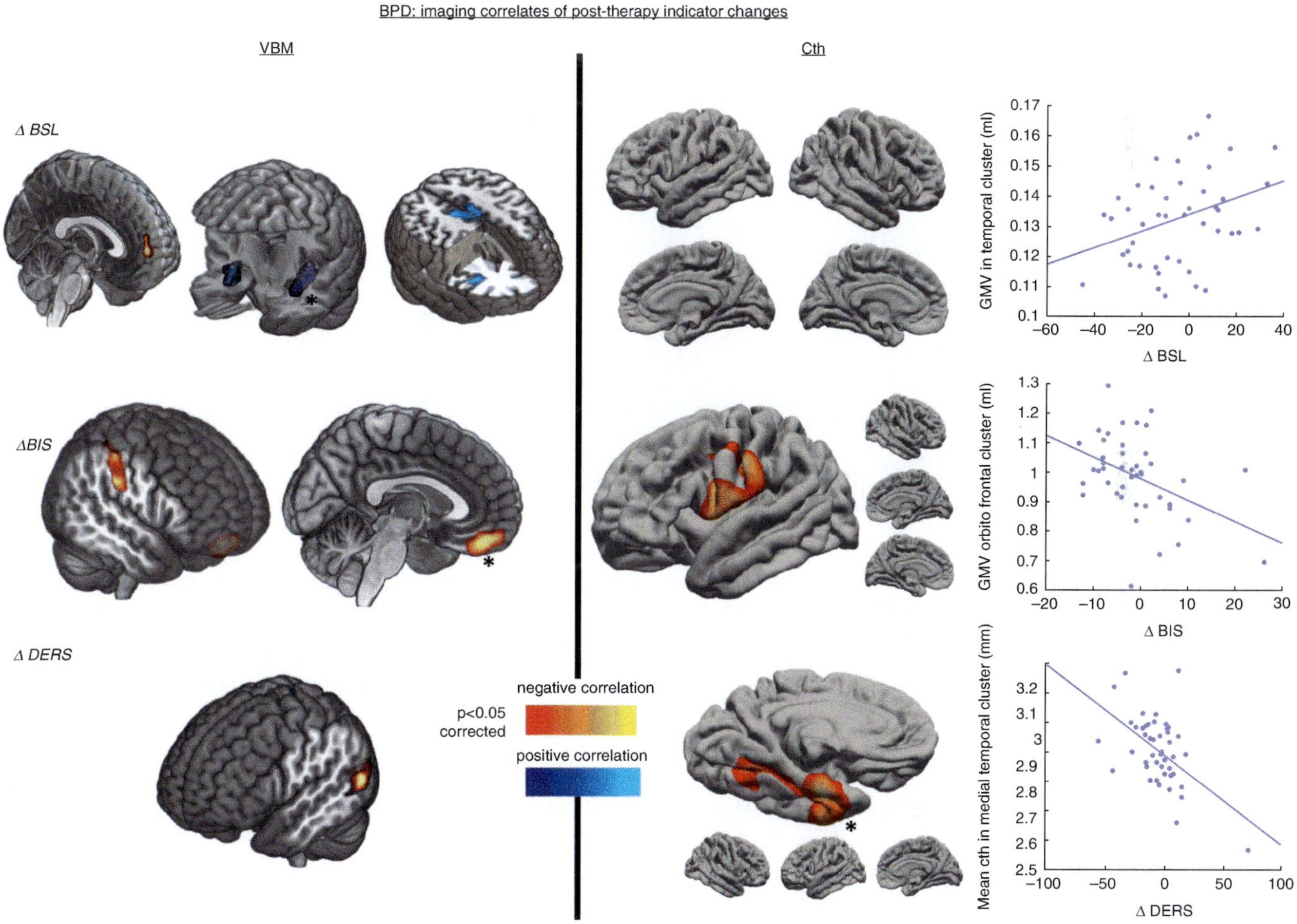

Fig. 11.44 Correlates of post-therapeutic changes in clinical indicators with baseline imaging in Borderline Personality Disorder. V oxel-based morphometry (VBM) and cortical thickness (Cth) correlates of post-therapeutic c hanges in clinical indicators with baseline imaging in the BPD group, controlling for age, sex, and educational level ($p < 0.05$ corrected). Scatter plots illustrate the direction of the correlations by showing the direct relationship between the changes in clinical indicators (post—pre) and the VBM/Cth values at the clusters marked with an asterisk. (*From* Sampedro et al. [174]; *with permission*)

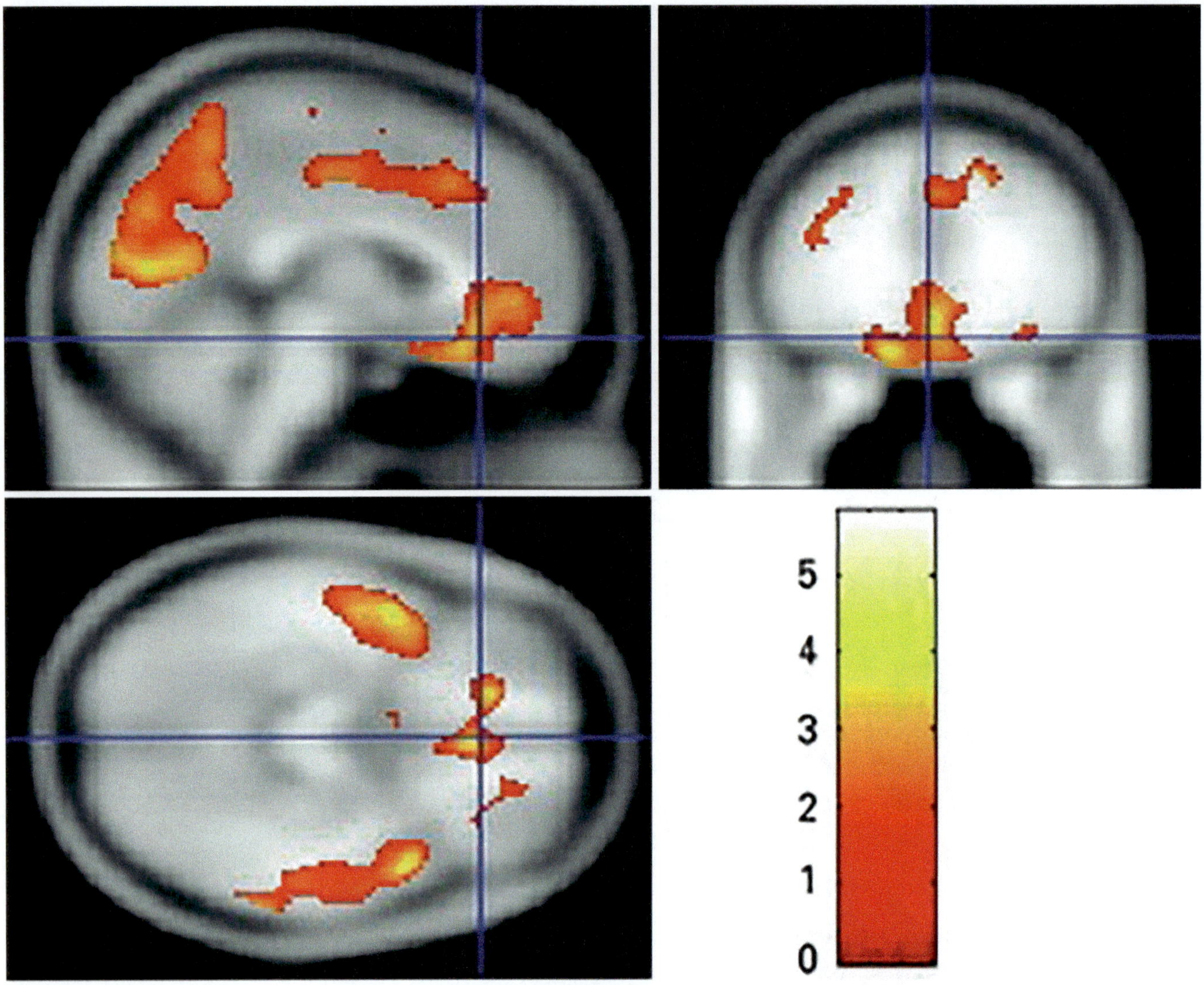

Fig. 11.45 Significant increase in frontal, parietal, and temporal cortex 5-HT1A density in the Short Term Dynamic Psychotherapy group as compared with the fluoxetine group. Visualization of the results from the SPM analysis. The analysis of parametric [carbonyl-^{11}C]WAY-100635 binding potential (BPND) maps at the voxel level showed two large clusters [*k* E = 9515, *T* max = 5.82 at (−26, 0, −38) and *k* *E* = 18,231 voxels, *T* max = 4.10 at (−46, −20, 42)] located mainly in frontal, temporal and parietal cortex. These clusters represent significantly increased BPND in the psychotherapy group as compared with the fluoxetine group. The results are visualized on a T1-weighted MRI template in stereotactic standard space; the color bar represents the *T* statistic at voxel level. (*From* Karlsson et al. [175]; *with permission*)

Neuroimaging and the Effects of Short-Term Dynamic Psychotherapy

Karlsson et al. demonstrated a significant increase in frontal, parietal, and temporal cortex 5- HT1A density following Short Term Dynamic Psychotherapy group compared with fluoxetine (see Fig. 11.45) [175].

The Future of Psychosocial Interventions in Psychiatry

Anyone reviewing the progress of Psychosocial Interventions in the last few decades must recognize that the improvements made in that period were nothing short of impressive. New therapies have been developed by the hundreds. A large percentage of them have already shown efficacy and effectiveness in controlled studies, and a therapist today, can count on a significant array of best practices to serve the needs of a growing population with complex problems; many made worse by trauma. Even better standards are on the horizon. The Institute of Medicine's Committee on Developing Standards for Psychosocial Interventions for Mental Disorders 2015, has developed a set of comprehensive recommendations aimed at further improving the quality of the evidence supporting future psychosocial intervention studies. A significant sample of their recommendations includes expanding the evidence base, standardizing interventions, and identifying the main drivers of the therapeutic effect to differentiate from specific effects: the large unresolved conceptual problem of all therapies [38].

Beyond the improvements that can be achieved through this framework, there are existing initiatives that could potentially expand the availability and efficacy of psychosocial interventions. Among them Make use of technology to facilitate delivery. One such valid initiative is SAMSHA's My Mental Health Crisis Apps, available from Apple App Store and Google Play.

All such innovations open optimistic vistas for our patients as they will reinforce with solid science the supporting columns of the bio-psycho-social framework; a framework which has undergirded incredible progress over the past 200 years.

References

1. Engel GL. The need for a new medical model: a challenge for biomedicine. Science. 1977;196(4286):129–36. https://doi.org/10.1126/science.
2. Kraepelin E. Lectures on clinical psychiatry. New York: William Wood & Co.; 1904. https://doi.org/10.1037/10789-000.
3. Freud S. An outline of psychoanalysis. London: Hogarth Press; 1949.
4. Weiner DB. Philippe Pinel's "Memoir on Madness" of December 11, 1794: a fundamental text of modern psychiatry. Am J Psychiatry. 1992;149(6):725–32. https://doi.org/10.1176/ajp.149.6.725.
5. Freud S. Beyond the pleasure principle. New York, NY: Dover Publications; 2015. - original text 1920
6. Engel GL. The clinical application of the biopsychosocial model. Am J Psychiatry. 1980;137(5):535–44. https://doi.org/10.1176/ajp.137.5.535.
7. Borrell-Carrió F, Suchman AL, Epstein RM. The biopsychosocial model 25 years later: principles, practice, and scientific inquiry. Ann Fam Med. 2004;2(6):576–82. https://doi.org/10.1370/afm.245.
8. Karunamuni N, Imayama I, Goonetilleke D. Pathways to well-being: Untangling the causal relationships among biopsychosocial variables. Soc Sci Med. 2021;272:112846. https://doi.org/10.1016/j.socscimed.2020.112846.
9. Forrester J, Cameron L. Discipline formation – psychology, english, philosophy. In Freud in Cambridge. Cambridge: Cambridge University Press; 2017. p. 203–362. https://doi.org/10.1017/9781139020862.006.
10. American Psychiatric Association. Diagnostic and statistical manual of mental disorders. 4th ed. Arlington, VA: American Psychiatric Publishing, Inc.; 1994.
11. American Psychiatric Association. Diagnostic and statistical manual of mental disorders. 5th ed. Arlington, VA: American Psychiatric Publishing, Inc.; 2013.
12. Lewis-Fernández R, Aggarwal NK, Bäärnhielm S, Rohlof H, Kirmayer LJ, Weiss MG, Jadhav S, Hinton L, Alarcón RD, Bhugra D, Groen S, van Dijk R, Qureshi A, Collazos F, Rousseau C, Caballero L, Ramos M, Lu F. Culture and psychiatric evaluation: operationalizing cultural formulation for DSM-5. Psychiatry. 2014;77(2):130–54. https://doi.org/10.1521/psyc.2014.77.2.130.
13. Lewis-Fernández R, Aggarwal NK, Hinton L, Hinton DE, Kirmayer LJ, editors. DSM-5® handbook on the cultural formulation interview. Arlington, VA: American Psychiatric Publishing, Inc.; 2016.
14. White JB. Law as rhetoric, rhetoric as law: the arts of cultural and communal life. Univ Chic Law Rev. 1985;52(3):Article 4. https://chicagounbound.uchicago.edu/uclrev/vol52/iss3/4. Accessed 1 May 2021
15. Trujillo M. Cultural psychiatry. In: Sadock BJ, Sadock VA, editors. Kaplan & Sadock's comprehensive textbook of psychiatry. 7th ed. Baltimore, MD: Williams & Wilkins Publishers; 2000.
16. Cross T, Bazron B, Dennis K, Isaacs M. Towards a culturally competent system of care (Vol. 1). Washington, DC: Georgetown University Child Development Center, CASSP Technical Assistance Center; 1989.
17. Betancourt JR, Green AR, Carrillo JE, Park ER. Cultural competence and health care disparities: key perspectives and trends. Health Aff. 2005;24(2):499–505. https://doi.org/10.1377/hlthaff.24.2.499.
18. Office of the Surgeon General (US); Center for Mental Health Services (US); National Institute of Mental Health (US). Mental health: culture, race, and ethnicity: a supplement to mental health: a report of the surgeon general. Rockville, MD: Substance Abuse and Mental Health Services Administration (US); 2001.
19. Dressler WW. Cultural consensus and cultural consonance: advancing a cognitive theory of culture. Field Methods. 2020;32(4):383–98. https://doi.org/10.1177/1525822X20935599.
20. Tervalon M, Murray-García J. Cultural humility versus cultural competence: a critical distinction in defining physician training outcomes in multicultural education. J Health Care Poor Underserved. 1998;9(2):117–25. https://doi.org/10.1353/hpu.2010.0233.
21. Kleinman AM. Depression, somatization and the "new cross-cultural psychiatry". Soc Sci Med. 1977;11(1):3–10. https://doi.org/10.1016/0037-7856(77)90138-x.
22. Kleinman A. Patients and healers in the context of culture an exploration of the borderland between anthropology, medicine, and psychiatry. Berkeley, CA: University of California Press; 1980. https://doi.org/10.1525/9780520340848.
23. Trujillo M. Culture-bound syndromes. In: Sadock BJ, Sadock VA, editors. Kaplan and Sadock's comprehensive textbook of psychiatry. 8th ed. Baltimore, MD: Williams & Wilkins Publishers; 2004.
24. Jarvis GE, Kirmayer LJ, Gómez-Carrillo A, Aggarwal NK, Lewis-Fernández R. Update on the cultural formulation interview. Focus (Am Psychiatr Publ). 2020;18(1):40–6. https://doi.org/10.1176/appi.focus.20190037.
25. Kirmayer LJ, Groleau D, Guzder J, Blake C, Jarvis E. Cultural consultation: a model of mental health service for multicultural societies. Can J Psychiatry. 2003;48(3):145–53. https://doi.org/10.1177/070674370304800302.

26. Kirmayer LJ, Groleau D, Rousseau C. Development and Evaluation of the Cultural Consultation Service. In: Kirmayer L, Guzder J, Rousseau C, editors. Cultural consultation. International and Cultural Psychology. New York, NY: Springer; 2014. https://doi.org/10.1007/978-1-4614-7615-3_2.
27. Anderson LM, Scrimshaw SC, Fullilove MT, Fielding JE, Normand J, Task Force on Community Preventive Services. Culturally competent healthcare systems. A systematic review. Am J Prev Med. 2003;24(3 Suppl):68–79. https://doi.org/10.1016/s0749-3797(02)00657-8.
28. Beach MC, Price EG, Gary TL, Robinson KA, Gozu A, Palacio A, Smarth C, Jenckes MW, Feuerstein C, Bass EB, Powe NR, Cooper LA. Cultural competence: a systematic review of health care provider educational interventions. Med Care. 2005;43(4):356–73. https://doi.org/10.1097/01.mlr.0000156861.58905.96.
29. Horvat L, Horey D, Romios P, Kis-Rigo J. Cultural competence education for health professionals. Cochrane Database Syst Rev. 2014;(5):CD009405. https://doi.org/10.1002/14651858.CD009405.pub2.
30. Siegel C, Davis-Chambers E, Haugland G, Bank R, Aponte C, McCombs H. Performance measures of cultural competency in mental health organizations. Adm Policy Ment Health. 2000;28(2):91–106. https://doi.org/10.1023/a:1026603406481.
31. Siegel C, Haugland G, Chambers ED. Performance measures and their benchmarks for assessing organizational cultural competency in behavioral health care service delivery. Adm Policy Ment Health. 2003;31(2):141–70. https://doi.org/10.1023/b:apih.0000003019.97009.15.
32. Stork E, Scholle S, Greeno C, Copeland VC, Kelleher K. Monitoring and enforcing cultural competence in Medicaid managed behavioral health care. Ment Health Serv Res. 2001;3(3):169–77. https://doi.org/10.1023/a:1011575632212.
33. Trujillo M. Culture and the organization of psychiatric care. In Cultural Psychiatry: International Perspectives, Mezzich J, and Fabrega H (Eds). Psychiatr Clin North Am. 2001;24(3):539–52. https://doi.org/10.1016/S0193-953X(05)70246-X.
34. Davis JH. The what and the whether of the U: cultural implications of understanding development in graphic symbolization. Hum Dev. 1997;40:145–54. https://doi.org/10.1159/000278717.
35. Delphin-Rittmon ME, Andres-Hyman R, Flanagan EH, Davidson L. Seven essential strategies for promoting and sustaining systemic cultural competence. Psychiatry Q. 2013;84(1):53–64. https://doi.org/10.1007/s11126-012-9226-2.
36. Brach C, Fraserirector I. Can cultural competency reduce racial and ethnic health disparities? A review and conceptual model. Med Care Res Rev. 2000;57(1_suppl):181–217. https://doi.org/10.1177/1077558700057001S09.
37. Corral I, Johnson TL, Shelton PG, et al. Psychiatry resident training in cultural competence: an educator's toolkit. Psychiatry Q. 2017;88:295–306. https://doi.org/10.1007/s11126-016-9472-9.
38. Institute of Medicine. Psychosocial interventions for mental and substance use disorders: a framework for establishing evidence-based standards. Washington, DC: The National Academies Press (US); 2015. https://doi.org/10.17226/19013.
39. George S, Daniels K, Fioratou E. A qualitative study into the perceived barriers of accessing healthcare among a vulnerable population involved with a community centre in Romania. Int J Equity Health. 2018;17:41. https://doi.org/10.1186/s12939-018-0753-9.
40. Kopelovich SL, Monroe-DeVita M, Buck BE, et al. Community mental health care delivery during the COVID-19 pandemic: practical strategies for improving care for people with serious mental illness. Community Ment Health J. 2021;57:405–15. https://doi.org/10.1007/s10597-020-00662-z.
41. Saxena S, Thornicroft G, Knapp M, Whiteford H. Resources for mental health: scarcity, inequity, and inefficiency. Lancet. 2007;370(9590):878–89. https://doi.org/10.1016/S0140-6736(07)61239-2.
42. Kadir A, Shenoda S, Goldhagen J, Pitterman S. The effects of armed conflict on children. Pediatrics. 2018;142(6):e20182586. https://doi.org/10.1542/peds.2018-2586. https://pediatrics.aappublications.org/content/142/6/e20182586
43. Ayalew M, Workicho A, Tesfaye E, et al. Burden among caregivers of people with mental illness at Jimma University Medical Center, Southwest Ethiopia: a cross-sectional study. Ann Gen Psychiatry. 2019;18:10. https://doi.org/10.1186/s12991-019-0233-7.
44. Hofstede G, Hofstede GJ. Cultures and organizations: software of the mind. New York: McGraw-Hill; 2005.
45. Nazir A, Enz S, Lim MY, et al. Culture–personality based affective model. AI Soc. 2009;24:281–93. https://doi.org/10.1007/s00146-009-0217-2.
46. Freud S. The Ego and the Id. London: The Hogarth Press Ltd.; 1949. (original text in 1923)
47. Campbell J, Pile S. Telepathy and its vicissitudes: Freud, thought transference and the hidden lives of the (repressed and non-repressed) unconscious. Subjectivity. 2010;3:403–25. https://doi.org/10.1057/sub.2010.22.
48. Beck AT, Rush A, Shaw B, Emery G. Cognitive therapy of depression. New York, NY: The Guilford Press; 1979.
49. Lawrence HR, Buffie ML, Schwartz-Mette RA, Nangle DW. Cognitive behavioral therapy with depressed youth. In: Friedberg R, Nakamura B, editors. Cognitive behavioral therapy in youth: tradition and innovation, Neuromethods, vol. 156. New York, NY: Humana; 2020. https://doi.org/10.1007/978-1-0716-0700-8_2.
50. Prout T, Wadkins M. Chapter 1: introduction to counseling and interviewing in essential interviewing and counseling skills an integrated approach to practice. New York, NY: Springe; 2014.
51. McFarlane WR, Lukens E, Link B, Dushay R, Deakins SA, Newmark M, Dunne EJ, Horen B, Toran J. Multiple-family groups and psychoeducation in the treatment of schizophrenia. Arch Gen Psychiatry. 1995;52(8):679–87. https://doi.org/10.1001/archpsyc.1995.03950200069016.
52. McFarlane WR. Family interventions for schizophrenia and the psychoses: a review. Fam Process. 2016;55(3):460–82. https://doi.org/10.1111/famp.12235.
53. Colom F, Vieta E, Scott J. Psychoeducation manual for bipolar disorder. Cambridge: Cambridge University Press; 2006. https://doi.org/10.1017/CBO9780511543685.
54. Bauer MS, McBride L. Structured group psychotherapy for bipolar disorder: the life goals program. 2nd ed. New York, NY: Springer; 2003.
55. Brillantes-Evangelista G. An evaluation of visual arts and poetry as therapeutic interventions with abused adolescents. Arts Psychother. 2013;40(1):71–84. https://doi.org/10.1016/j.aip.2012.11.005.
56. Ishak M, Herrera N, Martin C, Jeffrey J. Music therapy for depression in adolescents: a systematic review of randomized controlled trials. Int J Psychiatr Res. 2021;4(1):1–5.
57. Leubner D, Hinterberger T. Reviewing the effectiveness of music interventions in treating depression. Front Psychol. 2017;8:1109. https://doi.org/10.3389/fpsyg.2017.01109.
58. Quiñones G, Ridgway A, Li L. Holding hands: Toddlers' imaginary peer play. In: Ridgway A, Quiñones G, Li L, editors. Peer play and relationships in early childhood, International Perspectives on Early Childhood Education and Development, vol. 30. Cham: Springer; 2020. https://doi.org/10.1007/978-3-030-42331-5_6.
59. Moore AL, Carpenter DM 2nd, Miller TM, Ledbetter C. Clinician-delivered cognitive training for children with attention problems: effects on cognition and behavior from the ThinkRx randomized

controlled trial. Neuropsychiatr Dis Treat. 2018;14:1671–83. https://doi.org/10.2147/NDT.S165418.
60. Dauwan M, Begemann MJH, Slot MIE, Lee EHM, Scheltens P, Sommer IEC. Physical exercise improves quality of life, depressive symptoms, and cognition across chronic brain disorders: a transdiagnostic systematic review and meta-analysis of randomized controlled trials. J Neurol. 2021;268(4):1222–46. https://doi.org/10.1007/s00415-019-09493-9.
61. Sutherland ME. Physical activity and depression. Nat Hum Behav. 2019;3:320. https://doi.org/10.1038/s41562-019-0559-9.
62. Millrod E. Medical dance/movement therapy in the infusion room: a model for individual sessions with adults in active treatment. Am J Dance Ther. 2020;42:61–89. https://doi.org/10.1007/s10465-020-09323-w.
63. Dietz TJ, Davis D, Pennings J. Evaluating animal-assisted therapy in group treatment for child sexual abuse. J Child Sex Abus. 2012;21(6):665–83. https://doi.org/10.1080/10538712.2012.726700.
64. Jones MG, Rice SM, Cotton SM. Incorporating animal-assisted therapy in mental health treatments for adolescents: a systematic review of canine assisted psychotherapy. PLoS One. 2019;14(1):e0210761. https://doi.org/10.1371/journal.pone.0210761.
65. Renck Jalongo M, Petro J. Promoting children's well-being: therapy dogs. In: Renck JM, editor. Children, dogs and education. Cham: Springer; 2018. https://doi.org/10.1007/978-3-319-77845-7_9.
66. Parish-Plass N. Animal-assisted therapy with children suffering from insecure attachment due to abuse and neglect: a method to lower the risk of intergenerational transmission of abuse? Clin Child Psychol Psychiatry. 2008;13(1):7–30. https://doi.org/10.1177/1359104507086338.
67. Fine AH. Handbook on animal assisted psychotherapy. 5th ed. London: Elsevier Academic Press; 2019.
68. Bowlby J. Attachment and loss. New York, NY: Basic Books; 1969.
69. Nelson EM, Spieker SJ. Intervention Effects on morning and stimulated cortisol responses among toddlers in foster care. Infant Ment Health J. 2013;34(3) https://doi.org/10.1002/imhj.21382.
70. Lopez M, Ruiz MO, Rovnaghi CR, et al. The social ecology of childhood and early life adversity. Pediatr Res. 2021;89:353–67. https://doi.org/10.1038/s41390-020-01264-x.
71. van Ijzendoorn MH, Schuengel C, Bakermans-Kranenburg MJ. Disorganized attachment in early childhood: meta-analysis of precursors, concomitants, and sequelae. Dev Psychopathol. 1999;11(2):225–49. https://doi.org/10.1017/s0954579499002035.
72. Lieberman AF, Van Horn P, Ozer EJ. Preschooler witnesses of marital violence: predictors and mediators of child behavior problems. Dev Psychopathol. 2005;17(2):385–96. https://doi.org/10.1017/s0954579405050182.
73. Fraiberg S, Adelson E, Shapiro V. Ghosts in the nursery. A psychoanalytic approach to the problems of impaired infant-mother relationships. J Am Acad Child Adolesc Psychiatry. 1975;14(3):387–421.
74. Olds D. The nurse-family partnership: from trials to practice. In: Reynolds A, Rolnick A, Englund M, Temple J, editors. Childhood programs and practices in the first decade of life: a human capital integration. Cambridge: Cambridge University Press; 2010. p. 49–75. https://doi.org/10.1017/CBO9780511762666.004.
75. Spieker SJ, Oxford ML, Kelly JF, Nelson EM, Fleming CB. Promoting first relationships: randomized trial of a relationship-based intervention for toddlers in child welfare. Child Maltreat. 2012;17(4):271–86. https://doi.org/10.1177/1077559512458176.
76. Dozier M, Lindhiem O. This is my child: differences among foster parents in commitment to their young children. Child Maltreat. 2006;11(4):338–45. https://doi.org/10.1177/1077559506291263.
77. Eyberg SM, Funderburk BW, Hembree-Kigin TL, CB MN, Querido JG, Hood KK. Parent- child interaction therapy with behavior problem children: one and two year maintenance of treatment effects in the family. Child Fam Behav Ther. 2001;23:1–20. https://doi.org/10.1300/J019v23n04_01.
78. Eyberg SM, Funderburk BW. Parent-child interaction therapy protocol. Gainesville, FL: PCIT International; 2011.
79. Comer JS, Myers K. Future directions in the use of telemental health to improve the accessibility and quality of children's mental health services. J Child Adolesc Psychopharmacol. 2016;26(3):296–300. https://doi.org/10.1089/cap.2015.0079.
80. Carpenter AL, Puliafico AC, Kurtz SM, Pincus DB, Comer JS. Extending parent-child interaction therapy for early childhood internalizing problems: new advances for an overlooked population. Clin Child Fam Psychol Rev. 2014;17(4):340–56. https://doi.org/10.1007/s10567-014-0172-4.
81. Minuchin S. Families and family therapy. Cambridge, MA: Harvard University Press; 1974. https://doi.org/10.2307/j.ctvjz83h8.
82. Shadish WR, Montgomery LM, Wilson P, Wilson MR, Bright I, Okwumabua T. Effects of family and marital psychotherapies: a meta-analysis. J Consult Clin Psychol. 1993;61(6):992–1002. https://doi.org/10.1037//0022-006x.61.6.992.
83. Carr A. Evidence-based practice in family therapy and systemic consultation. J Family Therapy. 2000;22:29–60. https://doi.org/10.1111/1467-6427.00137.
84. Fromme DK. Family systems and couples approaches. In: Systems of psychotherapy. New York, NY: Springer; 2011. https://doi.org/10.1007/978-1-4419-7308-5_12.
85. Schoenwald SK. The Multisystemic Therapy® Quality Assurance/Quality Improvement System. In: O'Donohue W, Maragakis A, editors. Quality improvement in behavioral health. Cham: Springer; 2016. https://doi.org/10.1007/978-3-319-26209-3_12.
86. Pilling S, Fonagy P, Allison E, Barnett P, Campbell C, Constantinou M, et al. Long-term outcomes of psychological interventions on children and young people's mental health: a systematic review and meta-analysis. PLoS One. 2020;15(11):e0236525. https://doi.org/10.1371/journal.pone.0236525.
87. Bond GR, Drake RE, Mueser KT, et al. Assertive community treatment for people with severe mental illness. Dis Manage Health Outcomes. 2001;9:141–59. https://doi.org/10.2165/00115677-200109030-00003.
88. Stein LI, Test MA. Alternative to mental hospital treatment. I. Conceptual model, treatment program, and clinical evaluation. Arch Gen Psychiatry. 1980;37(4):392–7. https://doi.org/10.1001/archpsyc.1980.01780170034003.
89. Spivak S, Cullen BA, Green C, Firth T, Sater H, Mojtabai R. Availability of assertive community treatment in the United States: 2010 to 2016. Psychiatr Serv. 2019;70:948–51.
90. Jones M. The therapeutic community; a new treatment method in psychiatry. New York, NY: Basic Books; 1953.
91. Perry AE, Neilson M, Martyn-St James M, Glanville JM, Woodhouse R, Godfrey C, Hewitt C. Pharmacological interventions for drug-using offenders. Cochrane Database Syst Rev. 2015;6:CD010862. https://doi.org/10.1002/14651858.CD010862.pub2.
92. BloomSL. The sanctuary model. 2011. Retrieved May 18, 2021 from. http://www.sanctuaryweb.com/trauma-informedsystems.php
93. Dye MH, Ducharme LJ, Johnson JA, Knudsen HK, Roman PM. Modified therapeutic communities and adherence to tra-

ditional elements. J Psychoactive Drugs. 2009;41(3):275–83. https://doi.org/10.1080/02791072.2009.10400538.
94. De Leon G. The therapeutic community: theory, model, and method. New York, NY: Springer; 2000.
95. De Leon G. Is the therapeutic community an evidence based treatment? What the evidence says. Int J Therap Commun. 2010;31(2):104–28.
96. Vanderplasschen W, Colpaert K, Autrique M, Rapp RC, Pearce S, Broekaert E, Vandevelde S. Therapeutic communities for addictions: a review of their effectiveness from a recovery- oriented perspective. Sci World J. 2013;2013:Article ID 427817. https://doi.org/10.1155/2013/427817.
97. National Institute Drug Abuse. Are therapeutic communities effective? National Institute on Drug Abuse website; 2013. https://www.drugabuse.gov/publications/research-reports/therapeutic-communities/are-therapeutic-communities-effective. Accessed 1 May 2021.
98. Hubbard RL, Craddock SG, Anderson J. Overview of 5-year followup outcomes in the drug abuse treatment outcome studies (DATOS). J Subst Abuse Treat. 2003;25(3):125–34. https://doi.org/10.1016/s0740-5472(03)00130-2.
99. Pinals DA, Fuller DA. Beyond beds: the vital role of a full continuum of psychiatric care. Alexandria, VA: National Association of State Mental Health Program Directors; 2017. https://www.treatmentadvocacycenter.org/beyond-beds/ Accessed 1 May 2021
100. Knox KL, Litts DA, Talcott GW, Feig JC, Caine ED. Risk of suicide and related adverse outcomes after exposure to a suicide prevention programme in the US Air Force: cohort study. BMJ. 2003;327(7428):1376. https://doi.org/10.1136/bmj.327.7428.1376.
101. Coffey MJ, Coffey CE, Ahmedani BK. Suicide in a health maintenance organization population. JAMA Psychiat. 2015;72(3):294–6. https://doi.org/10.1001/jamapsychiatry.2014.2440.
102. Labouliere CD, Vasan P, Kramer A, Brown G, Green K, Rahman M, Kammer J, Finnerty M, Stanley B. "Zero Suicide" - A model for reducing suicide in United States behavioral healthcare. Suicidologi. 2018;23(1):22–30.
103. Pisani AR, Murrie DC, Silverman MM. Reformulating suicide risk formulation: from prediction to prevention. Acad Psychiatry. 2016;40(4):623–9. https://doi.org/10.1007/s40596-015-0434-6.
104. Norcross JC. An eclectic definition of psychotherapy. In: Zeig JK, Munion WM, editors. What is psychotherapy? Contemporary perspectives. San Francisco, CA: Jossey-Bass; 1990. p. 218–20.
105. Winston A, Pollack J, McCullough L, Flegenheimer W, Kestenbaum R, Trujillo M. Brief psychotherapy of personality disorders. J Nerv Ment Dis. 1991;179(4):188–93. https://doi.org/10.1097/00005053-199104000-00002.
106. Sifneos PE. Short-term anxiety-provoking psychotherapy: a treatment manual. New York, NY: Plenum; 1992.
107. Mann J. Time-limited psychotherapy. Cambridge, MA: Harvard University Press; 1980.
108. Malan D. Towards the validation of dynamic psychotherapy. New York: Plenum Press; 1976.
109. Davanloo H. Intensive short-term dynamic psychotherapy. Chichester: Wiley; 2000.
110. Trujillo M. Short-term dynamic psychotherapy of narcissistic disorders. In: Comprehensive handbook of psychotherapy: psychodynamic/object relations. New York, NY: John Wiley & Sons, Inc.; 2002. p. 345–64.
111. Trujillo M. Intensive dynamic psychotherapy of anxiety and depression. Primary Psychiatry. 2006;13(5):77–86.
112. Trujillo M. Treating pathological narcissism with short-term dynamic psychotherapy. In: Ogrodniczuk JS, editor. Understanding and treating pathological narcissism. Washington, DC: American Psychological Association; 2013. https://doi.org/10.1037/14041-000.
113. Kaplan and Sadock's Synopsis of Psychiatry. 12th edition. Baltimore, MD: Wolters Kluwer; 2021. p. 755–757.
114. Alexander F, French TM. Psychoanalytic therapy: principles and application. New York: Ronald Press; 1946.
115. Hickey C. Davanloo's technique of total removal of resistance and optimum mobilization of the transference component of the resistance. Psychodyn Psychiatry. 2015;43(4):601–21.
116. Barth K, Nielsen G, Haver B, Havik OE, Mølstad E, Rogge H, Skåtun M. Comprehensive assessment of change in patients treated with short-term dynamic psychotherapy: an overview. A 2-year follow-up study of 34 cases. Psychother Psychosom. 1988;50(3):141–50. https://doi.org/10.1159/000288112.
117. Svartberg M, Seltzer MH, Stiles TC. The effects of common and specific factors in short-term anxiety-provoking psychotherapy: a pilot process-outcome study. J Nerv Ment Dis. 1998;186(11):691–6. https://doi.org/10.1097/00005053-199811000-00005.
118. Malan DH. Beyond interpretation: initial evaluation and technique in short-term dynamic psychotherapy. Part I. Int J Short-Term Psychother. 1986;1:59–82.
119. Malan DH. Beyond interpretation: initial evaluation and technique in short-term dynamic psychotherapy. Part II. Int J Intensive Short-Term Dyn Psychother. 1986;1:83–106.
120. Husby R, Dahl AA, Dahl CI, Heiberg AN, Olafsen OM, Weisaeth L. Short-term dynamic psychotherapy. II. Prognostic value of characteristics of patients studied by a 2-year follow-up of 39 neurotic patients. Psychother Psychosom. 1985;43(1):8–16. https://doi.org/10.1159/000287851.
121. Davanloo H. Short-term dynamic psychotherapy. New York, NY: Jason Aronson; 1980.
122. Town JM, Abbass A, Stride C, Nunes A, Bernier D, Berrigan P. Efficacy and cost- effectiveness of intensive short-term dynamic psychotherapy for treatment resistant depression: 18-Month follow-up of the Halifax depression trial. J Affect Disord. 2020;273:194–202. https://doi.org/10.1016/j.jad.2020.04.035.
123. Abbass A, Town J, Driessen E. Intensive short-term dynamic psychotherapy: a systematic review and meta-analysis of outcome research. Harv Rev Psychiatry. 2012;20(2):97–108. https://doi.org/10.3109/10673229.2012.677347.
124. Johansson R, Town JM, Abbass A. Davanloo's intensive short-term dynamic psychotherapy in a tertiary psychotherapy service: overall effectiveness and association between unlocking the unconscious and outcome. PeerJ. 2014;2:e548. https://doi.org/10.7717/peerj.548.
125. Eppel A. The emergence of short-term psychodynamic psychotherapy. In: Short-term psychodynamic psychotherapy. Cham: Springer; 2018. https://doi.org/10.1007/978-3-319-74995-2_1.
126. Trujillo M. Intensive short-term dynamic psychotherapies. In: Sadock BJ, Sadock VA, Ruiz P, editors. Kaplan & Sadock's comprehensive textbook of psychiatry. 10th ed. Philadelphia, PA: Wolters Kluwer; 2017. p. 2796–815.
127. Kernberg O. Borderline conditions and pathological narcissism. New York: Jason Aronson; 1975.
128. Foelsch PA, Kernberg OF. Transference-focused psychotherapy for borderline personality disorders. Psychother Pract. 1998;4(2):67–90. https://doi.org/10.1002/(SICI)1520-6572(199822)4:2<67::AID-SESS5>3.0.CO;2-5.
129. Giesen-Bloo J, van Dyck R, Spinhoven P, van Tilburg W, Dirksen C, van Asselt T, Kremers I, Nadort M, Arntz A. Outpatient psychotherapy for borderline personality disorder: randomized trial of schema-focused therapy vs transference-focused psychotherapy. Arch Gen Psychiatry. 2006;63(6):649–58. https://doi.org/10.1001/archpsyc.63.6.649.

130. Clarkin JF, Levy KN, Lenzenweger MF, Kernberg OF. Evaluating three treatments for borderline personality disorder: a multiwave study. Am J Psychiatry. 2007;164(6):922–8. https://doi.org/10.1176/ajp.2007.164.6.922.
131. Doering S, Hörz S, Rentrop M, Fischer-Kern M, Schuster P, Benecke C, Buchheim A, Martius P, Buchheim P. Transference-focused psychotherapy v. treatment by community psychotherapists for borderline personality disorder: randomised controlled trial. Br J Psychiatry. 2010;196(5):389–95. https://doi.org/10.1192/bjp.bp.109.070177.
132. Reneses B, Galián M, Serrano R, Figuera D, Fernandez Del Moral A, López-Ibor JJ, Fuentes M, Trujillo M. A new time limited psychotherapy for BPD: preliminary results of a randomized and controlled trial. Actas Esp Psiquiatr. 2013;41(3):139–48.
133. Grover S, Avasthi A, Jagiwala M. Clinical practice guidelines for practice of supportive psychotherapy. Indian J Psychiatry. 2020;62(Suppl 2):S173–82. https://doi.org/10.4103/psychiatry.IndianJPsychiatry_768_19.
134. Wolpe J, Lazarus A. Behavior therapy techniques. A Guide to the Treatment of Neuroses. Oxford: Pergamon Press; 1966.
135. Araiba S. Current diversification of behaviorism. Perspect Behav Sci. 2019;43(1):157–75. https://doi.org/10.1007/s40614-019-00207-0.
136. Shinohara K, Honyashiki M, Imai H, Hunot V, Caldwell DM, Davies P, Moore TH, Furukawa TA, Churchill R. Behavioural therapies versus other psychological therapies for depression. Cochrane Database Syst Rev. 2013;2013(10):CD008696. https://doi.org/10.1002/14651858.CD008696.pub2.
137. Beck AT. Cognitive therapy and the emotional disorders. New York: Meridian; 1976.
138. INSERM Collective Expertise Centre. INSERM Collective Expert Reports [Internet]. Paris: Institut national de la santé et de la recherche médicale; 2000–. Psychotherapy: Three approaches evaluated. 2004. https://pubmed.ncbi.nlm.nih.gov/21348158/. Accessed 1 May 2021.
139. Pompoli A, Furukawa TA, Imai H, Tajika A, Efthimiou O, Salanti G. Psychological therapies for panic disorder with or without agoraphobia in adults: a network meta-analysis. Cochrane Database Syst Rev. 2016;4(4):CD011004. https://doi.org/10.1002/14651858.CD011004.pub2.
140. Wampold BE, Minami T, Baskin TW, Callen TS. A meta-(re) analysis of the effects of cognitive therapy versus 'other therapies' for depression. J Affect Disord. 2002;68(2-3):159–65. https://doi.org/10.1016/s0165-0327(00)00287-1.
141. Linehan M. Cognitive-behavioral treatment of borderline personality disorder. New York, NY: Guilford Press; 1993.
142. Linehan MM, Comtois KA, Murray AM, Brown MZ, Gallop RJ, Heard HL, Korslund KE, Tutek DA, Reynolds SK, Lindenboim N. Two-year randomized controlled trial and follow-up of dialectical behavior therapy vs therapy by experts for suicidal behaviors and borderline personality disorder. Arch Gen Psychiatry. 2006;63:757–66. https://doi.org/10.1001/Archpsyc.63.7.757.
143. Linehan MM, Schmidt H, Dimeff LA, Craft JC, Kanter J, Comtois KA. Dialectical behavior therapy for patients with borderline personality disorder and drug-dependence. Am J Addict. 1999;8:279–92. https://doi.org/10.1080/105504999305686.
144. Linehan MM, Korslund KE, Harned MS, Gallop RJ, Lungu A, Neacsiu AD, McDavid J, Comtois KA, Murray-Gregory AM. Dialectical behavior therapy for high suicide risk in individuals with borderline personality disorder: a randomized clinical trial and component analysis. JAMA Psychiat. 2015;72(5):475–82. https://doi.org/10.1001/jamapsychiatry.2014.3039.
145. Foa EB, McLean CP, Brown LA, et al. The effects of a prolonged exposure workshop with and without consultation on provider and patient outcomes: a randomized implementation trial. Implement Sci. 2020;15:59. https://doi.org/10.1186/s13012-020-01014-x.
146. McSweeney L, Rauch S, Norman S, Hamblen J. Prolonged Exposure for PTSD. US Department of Veterans Affairs National Center for PTSD. https://www.ptsd.va.gov/professional/treat/txessentials/prolonged_exposure_pro.asp. Accessed 1 May 2021.
147. Shapiro F, Wesselmann D, Mevissen L. Eye movement desensitization and reprocessing therapy (EMDR). In: Landolt M, Cloitre M, Schnyder U, editors. Evidence-based treatments for trauma related disorders in children and adolescents. Cham: Springer; 2017. https://doi.org/10.1007/978-3-319-46138-0_13.
148. Spiegel B. VRx: how virtual therapeutics will revolutionize medicine. New York, NY: Basic Books; 2020.
149. Bentz D, Wang N, Ibach MK, et al. Effectiveness of a stand-alone, smartphone-based virtual reality exposure app to reduce fear of heights in real-life: a randomized trial. npj Digit Med. 2021;4:16. https://doi.org/10.1038/s41746-021-00387-7.
150. Richards DA, Ekers D, McMillan D, Taylor RS, Byford S, Warren FC, Barrett B, Farrand PA, Gilbody S, Kuyken W, O'Mahen H, Watkins ER, Wright KA, Hollon SD, Reed N, Rhodes S, Fletcher E, Finning K. Cost and outcome of behavioural activation versus cognitive behavioural therapy for depression (COBRA): a randomised, controlled, non-inferiority trial. Lancet. 2016;388(10047):871–80. https://doi.org/10.1016/S0140-6736(16)31140-0.
151. Markowitz JC, Weissman MM. Interpersonal psychotherapy: principles and applications. World Psychiatry. 2004;3(3):136–9.
152. Brakemeier EL, Frase L. Interpersonal psychotherapy (IPT) in major depressive disorder. Eur Arch Psychiatry Clin Neurosci. 2012;262:117–21. https://doi.org/10.1007/s00406-012-0357-0.
153. Law R. Interpersonal psychotherapy for depression. Adv Psychiatric Treat. 2011;17(1):23–31. https://doi.org/10.1192/apt.bp.109.007641.
154. Hayes SC, Strosahl KD, Wilson KG. Acceptance and commitment therapy: the process and practice of mindful change. 2nd ed. New York: Guilford Press; 2012.
155. Powers MB, Vording ZVS, MB, Emmelkamp PM. Acceptance and commitment therapy: a meta-analytic review. Psychother Psychosom. 2009;78(2):73–80. https://doi.org/10.1159/000190790.
156. A-Tjak JG, Davis ML, Morina N, Powers MB, Smits JA, Emmelkamp PM. A meta-analysis of the efficacy of acceptance and commitment therapy for clinically relevant mental and physical health problems. Psychother Psychosom. 2015;84(1):30–6. https://doi.org/10.1159/000365764.
157. Balogh L, Tanaka M, Török N, Vécsei L, Taguchi S. Crosstalk between existential phenomenological psychotherapy and neurological sciences in mood and anxiety disorders. Biomedicine. 2021;9(4):340. Published 2021 Mar 27. https://doi.org/10.3390/biomedicines9040340.
158. Frankl VE. The will to meaning: foundations and applications of logotherapy. New York, NY: Penguin; 1988.
159. Kabat-Zinn J. Full catastrophe living. New York: Random House; 2013.
160. Fonagy P, Bateman A. Mechanisms of change in mentalization based therapy of borderline personality disorder. J Clinic Psych. 2006;62:411–30.
161. Bateman A, Fonagy P. Mentalization-based treatment. Psychoanal Inq. 2013;33(6):595–613. https://doi.org/10.1080/07351690.2013.835170.
162. MacMillan C. Mentalization-based treatment plays well with others. In: Williams L, Muir O, editors. Adolescent suicide and self-injury. Cham: Springer; 2020. https://doi.org/10.1007/978-3-030-42875-4_7.

163. Vilhauer JS, Young S, Kealoha C, et al. Treating major depression by creating positive expectations for the future: a pilot study for the effectiveness of future-directed therapy (FDT) on symptom severity and quality of life. CNS Neurosci Ther. 2012;18(2):102–9. https://doi.org/10.1111/j.1755-5949.2011.00235.
164. Seligman MEP, Rashid T, Parks AC. Positive psychotherapy. Am Psychol. 2006;61(8):774–88. https://doi.org/10.1037/0003-066X.61.8.774.
165. Eysenck HJ. The effects of psychotherapy: an evaluation. J Consult Psychol. 1952;16:319–24.
166. Smith ML, Glass GV. Meta-analysis of psychotherapy outcome studies. Am Psychol. 1977;32(9):752–60.
167. Smith ML, Glass GV, Miller TI. The benefits of psychotherapy. Baltimore, MD: The Johns Hopkins University Press; 1980.
168. Munder T, Flückiger C, Leichsenring F, Abbass AA, Hilsenroth MJ, Luyten P, Rabung S, Steinert C, Wampold BE. Is psychotherapy effective? A re-analysis of treatments for depression. Epidemiol Psychiatr Sci. 2019;28(3):268–74. https://doi.org/10.1017/S2045796018000355.
169. Fonagy P. The effectiveness of psychodynamic psychotherapies: an update. World Psychiatry. 2015;14(2):137–50. https://doi.org/10.1002/wps.20235. PMID: 26043322; PMCID: PMC4471961
170. de Maat S, de Jonghe F, Schoevers R, Dekker J. The effectiveness of long-term psychoanalytic therapy: a systematic review of empirical studies. Harv Rev Psychiatry. 2009;17(1):1–23. https://doi.org/10.1080/10673220902742476.
171. de Maat S, de Jonghe F, de Kraker R, Leichsenring F, Abbass A, Luyten P, Barber JP, Van R, Dekker J. The current state of the empirical evidence for psychoanalysis: a meta-analytic approach. Harv Rev Psychiatry. 2013;21(3):107–37. https://doi.org/10.1097/HRP.0b013e318294f5fd.
172. WallersteinRS.Thepsychotherapyresearchprojectofthemenninger foundation: an overview. J Consult Clin Psychol. 1989;57(2):195–205. https://doi.org/10.1037/0022-006X.57.2.195.
173. Sankar A, Melin A, Lorenzetti V, Horton P, Costafreda SG, Fu CHY. A systematic review and meta-analysis of the neural correlates of psychological therapies in major depression. Psychiatry Res Neuroimaging. 2018;279:31–9. https://doi.org/10.1016/j.pscychresns.2018.07.002.
174. Sampedro F, Farrés CCI, Soler J, et al. Structural brain abnormalities in borderline personality disorder correlate with clinical severity and predict psychotherapy response. Brain Imaging Behav. 2021;15(5):2502–12. https://doi.org/10.1007/s11682-021-00451-6.
175. Karlsson H, Hirvonen J, Kajander J, Markkula J, Rasi-Hakala H, Salminen JK, Någren K, Aalto S, Hietala J. Research letter: Psychotherapy increases brain serotonin 5-HT1A receptors in patients with major depressive disorder. Psychol Med. 2010;40(3):523–8. https://doi.org/10.1017/S0033291709991607.
176. Mead E. What is positive psychotherapy? Positivepsychology.com. https://positivepsychology.com/positive-psychotherapy-research-effects-treatment/.
177. Aggarwal NK, Nicasio AV, DeSilva R, et al. Barriers to implementing the DSM-5 cultural formulation interview: a qualitative study. Cult Med Psychiatry. 2013;37:505–33. https://doi.org/10.1007/s11013-013-9325-z.
178. Gliedt JA, Schneider MJ, Evans MW, et al. The biopsychosocial model and chiropractic: a commentary with recommendations for the chiropractic profession. Chiropr Man Therap. 2017;25:16. https://doi.org/10.1186/s12998-017-0147-x.
179. Olson DH, Russell C, Sprenkle DH. Circumplex model of marital and family systems: VI: theoretical update. Fam Process. 1983;22:69–83.
180. Marginean D, Derian SL, LaTorre J, et al. Constructing intercultural selves: bridging cultural conflict through dialectical engagement. Psychol Stud. 2019;64:365–75. https://doi.org/10.1007/s12646-019-00528-9.

Neurodevelopmental, Disruptive, Impulse-Control, and Conduct Disorders

12

Elizabeth Dohrmann and Benjamin Schneider

Introduction

Understanding development is the key to understanding human possibility, human pathology, and each person's unique constellation of strengths and vulnerabilities. Regardless of a patient's age, a thoughtful developmental history is essential to accurate diagnosis and treatment (Fig. 12.1). Timely and specialized assessment of neurodevelopment is required to identify disorders such as intellectual disability and autism spectrum disorder, where early diagnosis and intervention are essential to improving the life-long trajectory. Other neurodevelopmental disorders, such as attention-deficit/hyperactivity disorder and specific learning disorder, may declare themselves in early or late

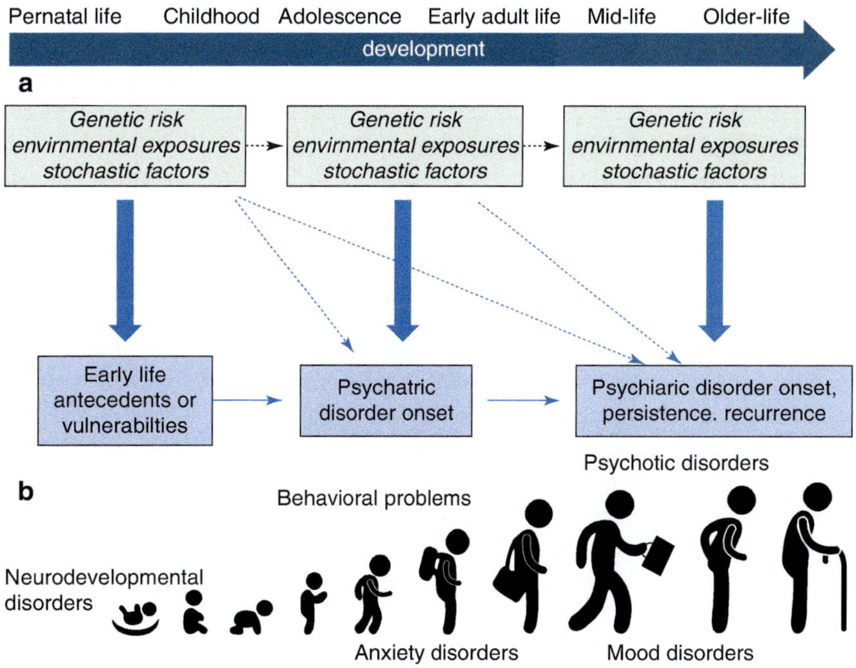

Fig. 12.1 (**a**) A developmental view of psychiatric disorders. (**b**) Typical ages of onset for different classes of psychiatric disorders. (*From* Thapar and Riglin [188]; Creative Commons Attribution 4.0 International License; http://creativecommons.org/licenses/by/4.0/)

E. Dohrmann (✉)
Los Angeles County Department of Mental Health, Los Angeles, CA, USA
e-mail: edohrmann@dmh.lacounty.gov

B. Schneider
David Geffen School of Medicine, University of California at Los Angeles, Los Angeles, CA, USA
e-mail: BSchneider@mednet.ucla.edu

W. W. IsHak (ed.), *Atlas of Psychiatry*, https://doi.org/10.1007/978-3-031-15401-0_12

school-age, requiring vigilant observation by teachers, caretakers, and mental health professionals in order to diagnose and treat problems that have significant downstream academic and social effects. Developmental processes, including environmental disruptions, are also essential to understanding how some children develop disruptive, impulse-control, and conduct disorders, which are among the most widely diagnosed, and widely pathologized, disorders of childhood and adolescence. Both a child's underlying neural substrate and the environmental pressures experienced at critical times in development select for the behaviors classified under these disorders.

Many of the diagnoses described below can present comorbid with one another. It is not uncommon, for example, for a child with autism spectrum disorder to also have intellectual disability, attention-deficit/hyperactivity disorder, and a tic disorder. Similarly, a child with attention-deficit/hyperactivity disorder should in most cases be assessed for underlying specific learning disorders that may be contributing to present academic difficulties. In children with oppositional defiant disorder or conduct disorder, it is possible that they will also have underlying mood or impulse-control disorders, although these may or may not be diagnosed. In all cases, investigation of a thorough developmental differential is the best way to understand each patient's strengths and proactively mitigate their vulnerabilities.

Intellectual Disability and Global Developmental Delay

Introduction

Intellectual disability (ID) involves impairments in three domains of adaptive reasoning: *conceptual* (i.e., language, reading, writing, math, memory), *social* (interpersonal communication, development of reciprocal relationships, social judgment), and *practical* (self-care, using transportation, cooking, finance management, employment). The American Association on Intellectual and Developmental Disabilities (AAIDD) has led the field in defining ID, with current DSM criteria overlapping substantially. For a diagnosis of ID, an individual must demonstrate deficits in the above areas of adaptive reasoning before the age of 18, and these deficits must be measurable by clinical assessment and standardized testing, such as the use of validated IQ scales and adaptive functioning measures (Table 12.1). The severity of ID, as defined by DSM, is based on the degree of deficit and level of support required for self-care. Although IQ scores are frequently used in order to determine eligibility for services—with a Full Scale IQ (FSIQ) score of 70 generally being the required cut-off—it is important to evaluate adaptive skills when making a diagnosis of ID (Fig. 12.2).

Table 12.1 Quick reference: Intellectual disability

Core features: Impairments in general mental abilities that affect adaptive behavior functioning in conceptual, social, and practical domains. Specified as mild, moderate, severe or profound
Age: No specific age requirement, but deficits must present in the developmental period
Diagnosis: Requires comprehensive clinical assessment, including clinical exam, IQ testing, and adaptive functioning measures

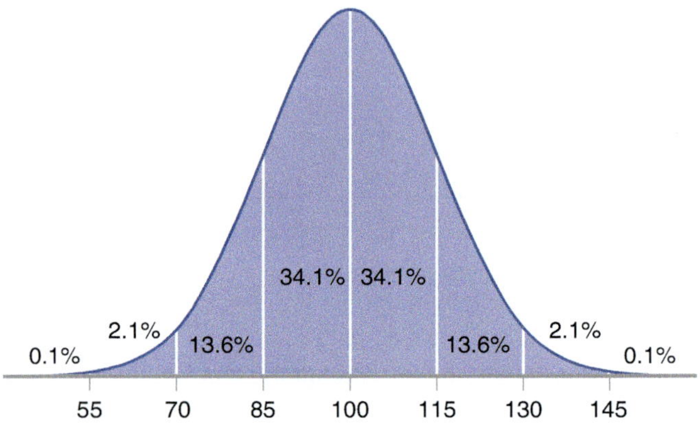

Fig. 12.2 A standardized bell curve, including standard deviations and population percentages under the curve. The mean standardized IQ score is 100; two standard deviations below the mean is 70, the typical cut-off for a diagnosis of ID

Intellectual disability is diagnosed through a comprehensive assessment of the individual's cognition and adaptive skills. In very young children, targeted psychometric testing can confirm the presence of developmental delays in gross and fine motor skills, speech and language, cognition, social skills, and practical adaptive skills through normative comparison. Due to developmental constraints, tests at very young ages may only yield an estimate of IQ. The goal at these ages is to assess for delays, provide access to early intervention services, and monitor progress.

If a child under age 5 is found to have a significant delay in two or more developmental areas, he or she may be diagnosed with global developmental delay (GDD) (Table 12.2). The more severe and global the delays, the more likely the child will meet the criteria for intellectual disability when he or she completes appropriate IQ testing. In cases of severe or profound impairments, the diagnosis of ID may be made earlier.

Table 12.2 Quick reference: Global developmental delay

Core features: Scores at least two SD below age-appropriate means in at least two of the following areas: • Gross or fine motor • Speech/language • Cognition • Social/personal • Activities of daily living
Age: Under 5 years only
Diagnosis: Direct observation/developmental testing/caregiver report

It is important to note that IQ testing was originally developed by French psychologist Alfred Binet in the early 1900s in order to assess intellectual strengths and weaknesses with the aim of providing targeted educational assistance. This was in response to an increase in undereducated and impoverished youth entering schools post-Industrial Revolution, with the intent of assessing their intellectual needs. However, in the context of the American eugenics movement, such testing was coopted in an attempt to "prove" innate intellectual disparities between races and classes and demonstrate the superiority of white people [1]. This weaponization of standardized testing into "scientific racism" has wrought significant damage that is ongoing [2].

With this acknowledgment, standardized testing remains helpful when used to evaluate specific areas of functioning and to develop educational supports. However, when reviewing data from standardized tests, it is important to understand the test's reliability and validity, what preparation is or is not required to master the tasks being tested, and what access the child has to such preparation. In the case of ID, a child will not only score in low ranges globally over a consistent period of time, but they will also have clear adaptive behavior deficits as described above.

Epidemiology

The prevalence estimate for intellectual disability across a global meta-analysis is approximately 1%, with somewhat higher prevalence rates in low- and middle-income countries and among males [3]. Among those with intellectual disability, 85% of cases are estimated to be "mild," 10% of cases are "moderate," 5% are "severe," and "profound" ID is found in <1% of cases (Fig. 12.3) [4].

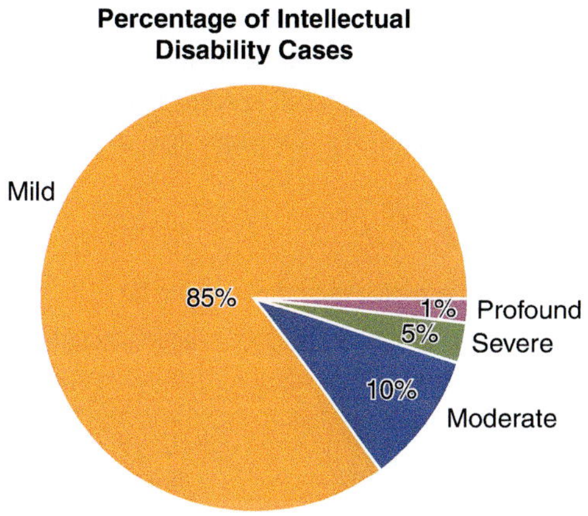

Fig. 12.3 Percentage of cases of ID based on severity

Etiology

In approximately 50% of reported cases of intellectual disability, the causative factors are unknown [3]. For the remaining cases, identifiable causes include *antenatal* (e.g., genetic syndromes), *perinatal* (e.g., intrauterine growth restriction, substance exposure, prematurity, birth trauma, or asphyxia), and *postnatal factors* (e.g., infections, traumatic brain injury). The increased prevalence rates seen in low- and middle-income countries, almost twice the rate of high-income countries, may be at least partially attributable to reduced antenatal screening, increased maternal morbidity, or nutritional deficiencies [3].

ID is associated with a wide range of genetic mutations, ranging from aneuploidies to patterns of recessive, dominant, or X-linked inheritance, to spontaneous de novo copy number variants (CNVs) [5]. Trisomy 21 is the most commonly known genetic cause of ID. Other syndromes commonly associated include fetal alcohol spectrum disorder, Fragile X syndrome (FMR1 gene), Rett syndrome (MECP2 gene), Prader–Willi syndrome (15q11.13 chromosome), Angelman syndrome (15q11.13 chromosome), Williams syndrome (7q11.23 chromosome), velocardiofacial or DiGeorge syndrome (22q11.2 chromosome), 16p11.2 Deletion Syndrome, and various disorders of inborn errors of metabolism (IEM), including phenylketonuria (PAH gene), Lesch–Nyhan syndrome (HPRT1 gene), and glycogen and lysosomal storage diseases (Table 12.3). Because of these strong genetic correlates and the treatment implications for identifying an underlying genetic disorder that may affect multiple organ systems, genetic testing is recommended for youth and adults with ID. Options for testing include a karyotype, array comparative genomic hybridization (aCGH, or "chromosomal microarray"), fluorescence in situ hybridization (FISH), whole-exome sequencing (WES), and whole-genome sequencing (WGS) (Figs. 12.4, 12.5, and 12.6). If

Table 12.3 Known genetic syndromes causing ID

Name	Genetic problem	Clinical features
Down syndrome	Chromosome 21	Dysmorphia, hypotonia, medical complications
Fragile X	FMR1 gene	Physical anomalies, social/behavioral problems
Rett syndrome	MECP2 gene	Rapid loss of speech and motor skills
Prader–Willi syndrome	Chromosome 15q11.13	Overeating, OCD, behavioral problems
Angelman syndrome	Chromosome 15q11.13	Speech impairment, persistent social smile
Williams syndrome	Chromosome 7q11.23	Facial anomalies, sociable, verbal strengths
DiGeorge syndrome	Chromosome 22q11.2	Range of physical medical problems
16p11.2	Deletion syndrome	Language and social delays, ASD
Phenylketonuria	PAH gene	If untreated, ID, hyperactivity, behavior problems
Lesch–Nyhan syndrome	HPRT1 gene, X-linked	Kidney/bladder stones, dystonia, self-injurious behavior

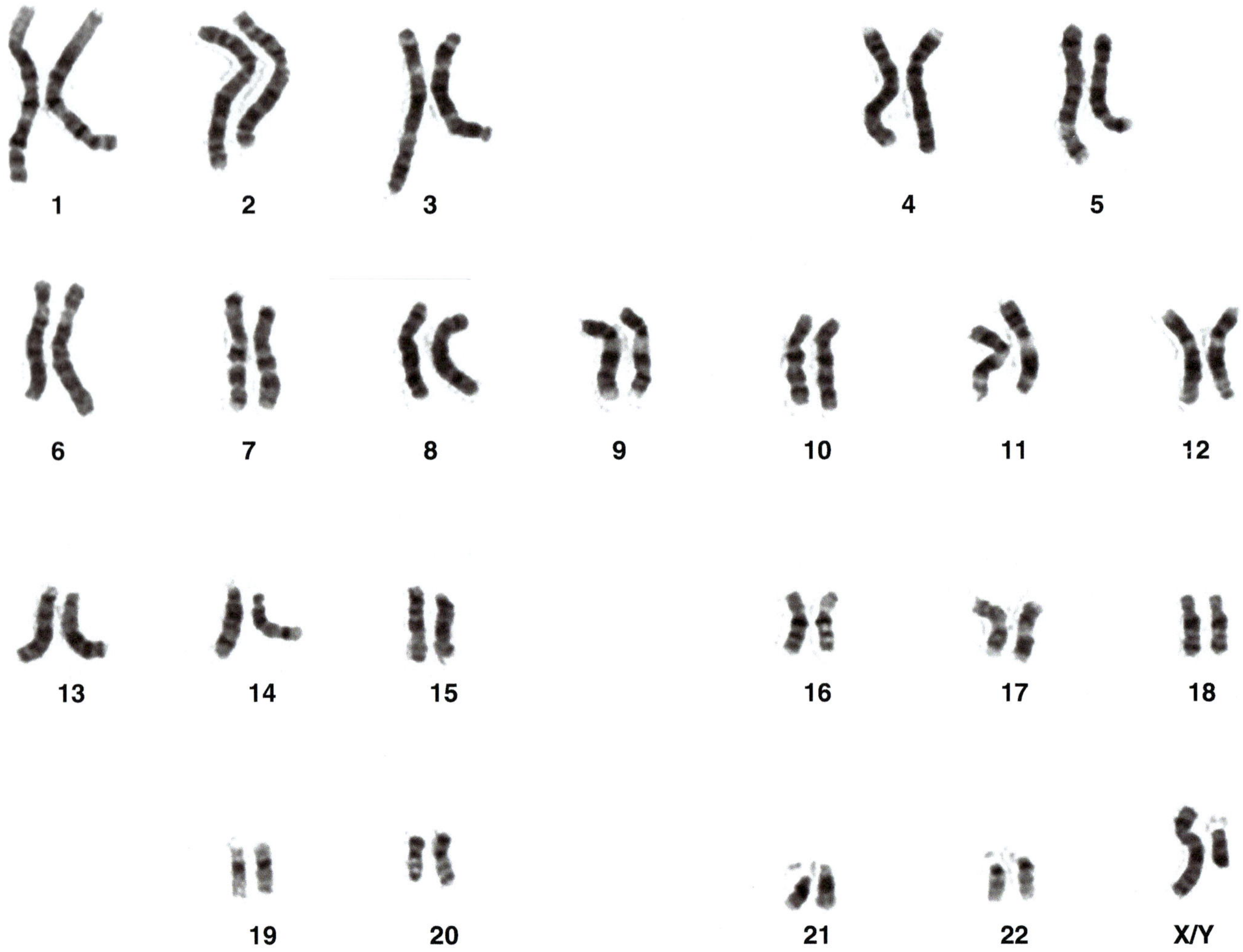

Fig. 12.4 Normal human male karyotype

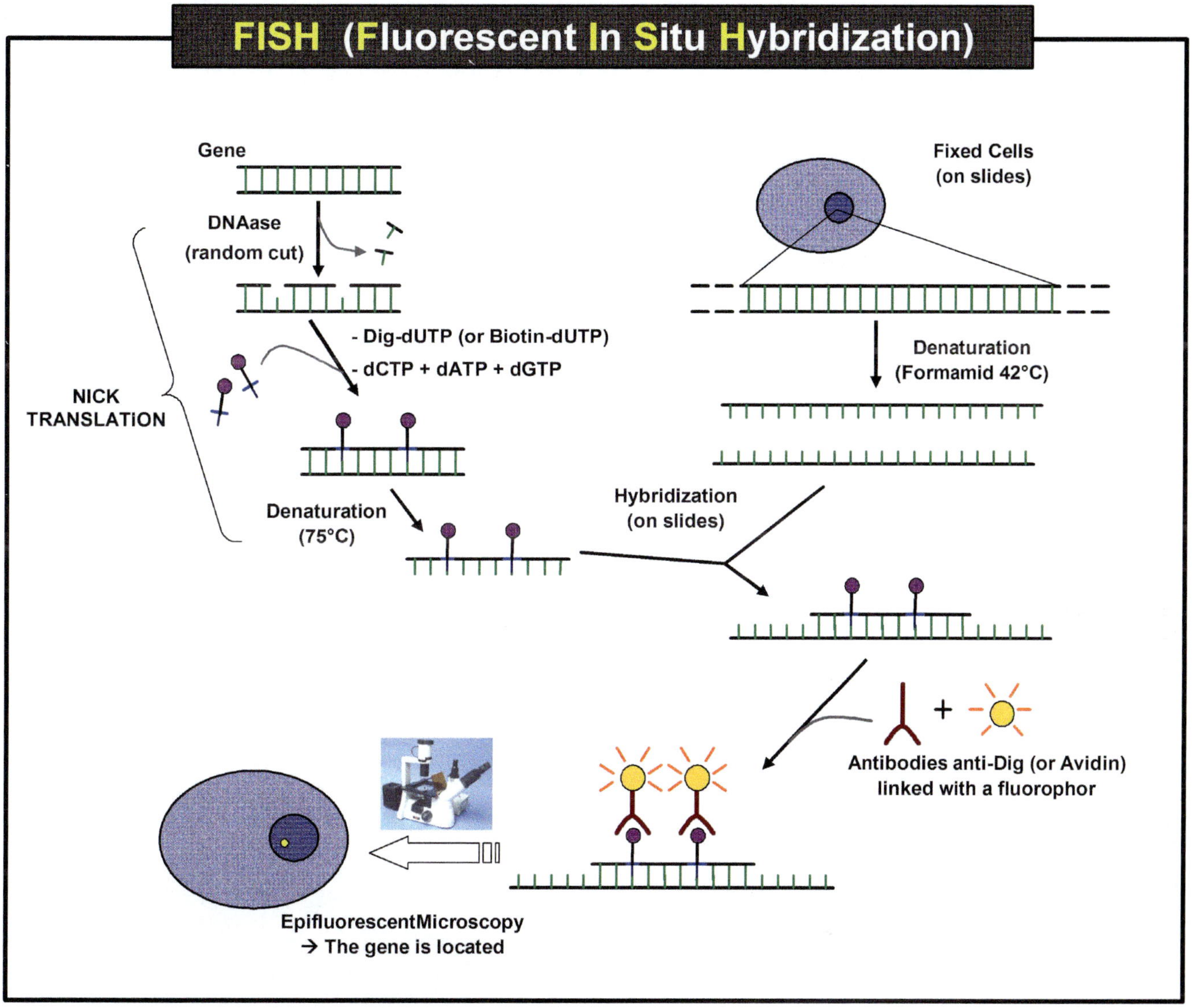

Fig. 12.5 Fluorescence in situ hybridization (FISH): process used to locate a specific DNA sequence on a chromosome by exposing the DNA sample to the target DNA sequence that has a fluorescent molecule attached to it. Used in the diagnoses of Prader–Willie syndrome (after PCR), Angelman syndrome (after PCR), Williams syndrome, and DiGeorge syndrome. (Creative Commons Attribution-Share Alike 3.0 Unported; https://creativecommons.org/licenses/by-sa/3.0; https://commons.wikimedia.org/wiki/File:FISH_(Fluorescent_In_Situ_Hybridization).jpg)

Fragile X syndrome is suspected, testing involves polymerase chain reaction (PCR) and Southern blot analysis. Updated guidelines from the American Academy of Child and Adolescent Psychiatry (AACAP) provide an algorithm for conducting genetic testing in youth with intellectual and developmental disabilities (Fig. 12.7) [6].

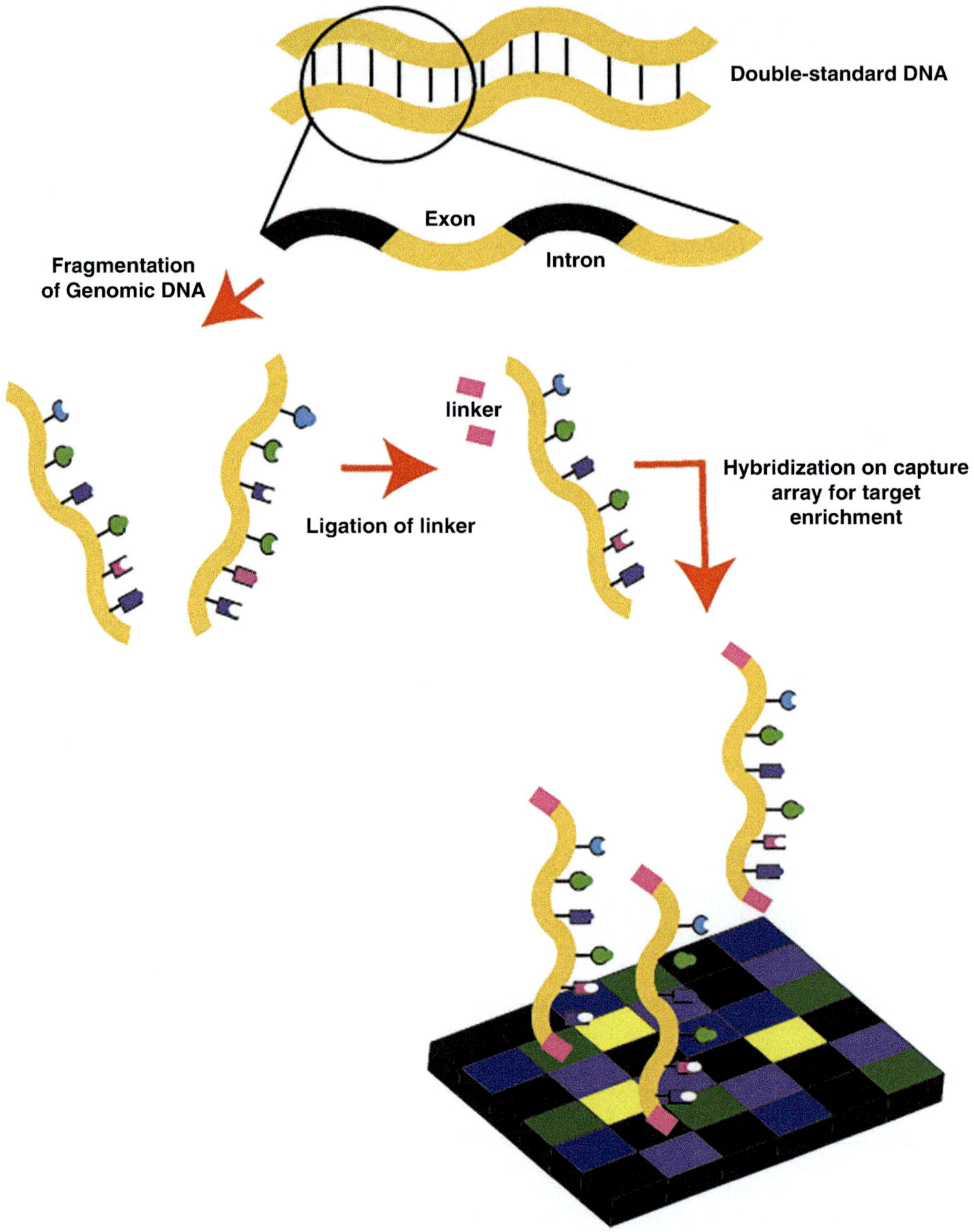

Fig. 12.6 Whole exome sequencing: exons make up 1% of the human genome and include all protein-coding regions. They are the source of most known disease mutations, and analysis of the exome is more cost effective than analysis of the entire genome. Exome sequencing may find aberrations that other genetic studies miss and are also useful in research. Shown here: double-stranded genomic DNA is fragmented by sonication. Linkers are then attached to the DNA fragments, which are then hybridized to a capture microarray designed to target only the exons. (Creative Commons Attribution-Share Alike 3.0 Unported; https://creativecommons.org/licenses/by-sa/3.0; https://commons.wikimedia.org/wiki/File:Exome_Sequencing_Workflow_1a.png)

Pathophysiology

Intellectual disability is a lifelong disorder stemming from one or more primary insults, genetic or peri-postnatal, and leading to substantive differences in brain development and function over the lifespan. Due to shared signaling by many developmental pathways, deficits in adaptive reasoning may also coincide with increased rates of metabolic problems, motor problems, specific physical characteristics/dysmorphia, or psychiatric illness. In the latter category, the prevalence of psychiatric disorders in children with ID ranges from 30% to 50%, with rates of behavioral problems three to seven times higher than in typically developing children [7]. Importantly, accurate and timely diagnosis of both co-occurring psychiatric disorders and medical disorders is often precluded by "diagnostic overshadowing" in clinicians, whereby signs and symptoms of sometimes life-threatening medical disease may be attributed to underlying intellectual

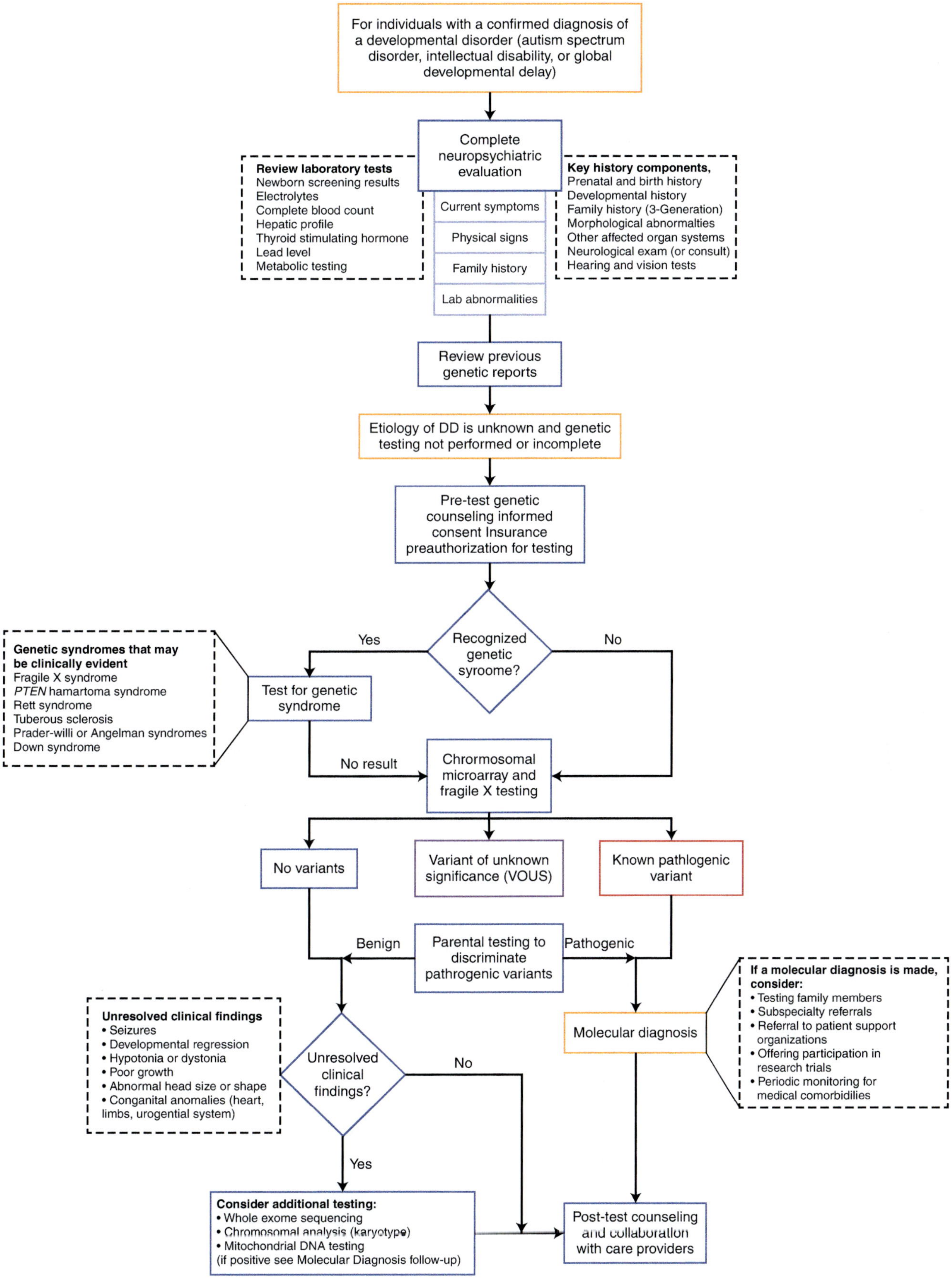

Fig. 12.7 Diagnostic testing algorithm for youth with neurodevelopmental disorders. Guidelines compiled from the American College of Medical Genetics, the American Academy of Child and Adolescent Psychiatry, the American Academy of Neurology, and the American Academy of Pediatrics. (*From* Muhle et al. [191]; *with permission*)

disability instead of adequately diagnosing co-occurring physical problems, for example, in a nonverbal adult who is crying without clear cause but is suffering from a bowel obstruction [8, 9].

Phenomenology

Individuals living with intellectual disability present in various ways. Some may be nonverbal, and some may have noticeable dysmorphic features or gross or fine motor abnormalities. It is common for affected individuals to have repetitive or stereotyped behaviors, such as rocking their body back and forth, pacing, or flapping their arms or hands. These behaviors can be seen in individuals with ID only or with both autism spectrum disorders and ID. For verbal individuals with ID, thought content is likely to be concrete, with limited ability to follow abstract or complex thought processes. They may have difficulty in concealing truths due to younger developmental age; this may translate into difficulty understanding when others are not telling the truth or have different intentions from what is explicitly stated. Depending on developmental level, some may be able to use language to identify emotional states and comprehend cause and effect related to their behaviors. Those more severely affected may not be able to label emotions or sources of physical discomfort, such as pain and hunger. In these cases, distress may be expressed through behaviors, including self-injury or aggression, rather than language, requiring a thorough examination of all possible contributing factors—medical, emotional, and behavioral—in order to understand the root cause of the behavior.

Treatment

Because intellectual disability is a lifelong disorder, the most effective treatment attempts at prevention. Routine prenatal care, screening for genetic disease, avoiding exposure to intrauterine substances, and folic acid supplementation may all help to decrease the incidence of ID. Similarly, appropriate medical treatment, such as in the cases of inborn errors of metabolism, may prevent or reduce cognitive delays. In all cases, early identification of delayed milestones and early intervention are essential and may improve the child's developmental trajectory.

Under the age of 3 years, children in the United States are eligible for services through their local public early intervention system, which assesses the child and creates an individualized family service plan (IFSP). These systems are federally mandated to provide services to children from birth to 2 years, 11 months under the Individuals with Disabilities Education Act (IDEA). After the child reaches 3 years old, he or she is guaranteed special education and related services through the local public school system and associated agencies until the age of 21 years. In most states, individuals with intellectual disability are eligible for publicly funded support throughout their lifespan (Table 12.4).

The behavioral principles underlying applied behavior analysis (ABA) have a strong evidence base in intellectual disability and are the first line for examining problem behaviors by identifying the antecedent and the function of the behavior (Table 12.5). Support and assistance in communication, whether by gestures or visual symbols, may significantly reduce frustration and corresponding challenging behavior. Educationally, individuals with ID require personalized educational approaches that identify specific strengths and weaknesses and make use of increased visual and hands-on activities rather than exclusively verbal instruction. All children with ID should have an individualized education program (IEP) developed collaboratively with their school, therapeutic staff, and caregivers. Additionally, community supports in the form of in-home behavioral teams, respite services, and crisis intervention services are all important in supporting children with ID and their families. In order to generalize skill development across settings, consistency between teachers, caregivers, and aides is vital.

Personal safety is a particular worry for individuals with ID. Due to difficulty understanding social situations, impairments in judgment, developmental levels differing from sexual maturation level, and reduced ability to identify or report

Table 12.4 Federally protected services for youth with NDDs

Age	Legal provision	Institution	Services
0–2 years 11 months	IDEA Medicaid	Early intervention programs (varies by state)	Speech and language (SLP), physical therapy (PT), occupational therapy (OT), applied behavior analysis (ABA), etc.
3–21 years	IDEA Medicaid	Public schools	SLP, PT, OT, individualized education program (IEP)
21+	IDEA Medicaid Social security (18+)	Federal government and Medicaid-accepting state programs	Medicaid, Medicaid waiver, supplemental security income (SSI), social security disability insurance (SSDI), job assistance, caregiver support, etc.

Table 12.5 Functional behavior assessment example

	Antecedent	Behavior	Consequence	Possible function of behavior
Example 1	Mark is hungry	He yells and hits his brother	Mark gets food	To get something
Example 2	Mom tells Mark to do homework	Mark hits mother	Mom takes away homework	To get away from something

abuse, individuals with ID are at increased risk of victimization and trauma exposure. It follows that individuals with mild or moderate ID may benefit from social skills supports to practice basic skills for developing friendships and staying safe when interacting with new people [10]. Other psychotherapeutic modalities have also shown promise with adapted content that is developmentally accessible and appropriate. Individual psychotherapy using Cognitive Behavior Therapy (CBT), for example, has shown benefits in studies of adults with ID [11].

It is important to take developmental age into account in assessing individuals with intellectual disability. Behaviors that may seem inappropriate for an individual's chronological age may actually be appropriate for his or her developmental age. For example, an adult with ID who believes he will become a famous actor may be misdiagnosed as having psychosis if his mental age is not adequately assessed. On the other hand, individuals with ID have higher rates of comorbid depression, anxiety, and psychosis than the baseline population, with attentional and executive functioning deficits being particularly common. Careful assessment is key.

It is estimated that more than a third of individuals with ID are prescribed psychotropic medication, with the most common agents being stimulants, antipsychotics, antidepressants, and anticonvulsants, often to manage disruptive symptoms without a clear diagnostic correlate [12]. Clinical trials of these medications in the ID population are limited, as ID is often an exclusionary criterion for drug trials. However, both of the atypical antipsychotics risperidone and aripiprazole are approved for the treatment of irritability, aggression, and self-injury in children with autism spectrum disorders, many of whom have comorbid ID. When looking specifically at RTCs involving individuals with ID, risperidone and methylphenidate show the most robust evidence of benefit [6]. Individuals with ID are more likely to have adverse or paradoxical reactions to medications and therefore require thoughtful selection and slow titration of select agents for specific, targeted symptoms. Movement side effects such as akathisia and parkinsonism, for example, have been found to be more common in adults with ID taking antipsychotic medications than in adults without ID on these drugs [13].

Specific Learning Disorders

Introduction

A "learning disorder" can mean different things in different contexts. In terms of the DSM-5, this category encompasses three specific learning disorders (SLDs)—reading, written expression, and mathematics—as well as six communication disorders and two motor disorders (Table 12.6). In the field of education, specific learning disabilities are defined somewhat differently, with the core areas of reading, writing, and mathematics broken down further to include basic reading skills, reading fluency skills, reading comprehension, written expression, mathematics calculation, and mathematics problem solving (see http://idea.ed.gov). Children with SLDs are the largest group of students served under the Individuals with Disabilities Education Act (IDEA), representing 33% of served students in the 2018–2019 school year (Fig. 12.8) [14].

Table 12.6 Quick reference: Specific learning disorders

Core features: • Difficulty with one of the following: – Reading or understanding the meaning of written content – Spelling or written expression – Number concepts or mathematical reasoning • Academic skills in the above area(s) are substantially below age expectations and cause problems • Difficulties are not due to ID, vision or hearing problems, a neurologic condition, lack of fluency in teaching language, or economic/environmental disadvantage
Age: Difficulties start during school age
Diagnosis: Comprehensive clinical assessment through school reports, observation, interviews, history, and neuropsychological testing

Children are often assessed for learning disorders in the context of a recognized skill deficit leading to functional impairment, which is not responsive to basic interventions and leads to the youth performing below grade level. By definition, a learning disability is not diagnosed if the skill deficits are due to visual, hearing, motor, or intellectual disabilities, or the use of a nonprimary language in assessing the child. Multiple neuropsychological and psychoeducational tests have been developed to assess for learning disabilities; however, some domains are more straightforward to assess than others. The specific skill deficits are important, as treatment approaches vary substantially depending on which learning process is affected. Notably, the same learning skill deficit may affect multiple areas of learning, leading to an overlap of underlying deficits in a number of cases. In fact, a recent study found that comorbid learning disorders occurred as frequently as isolated learning disorders in all three DSM-5 domains [15].

Epidemiology

According to the DSM-5, prevalence rates are estimated to be between 4% and 9% for reading deficits and 3% and 7% for deficits in mathematics [4]. The estimated prevalence of deficits in writing skills, including spelling, handwriting, and written expression, ranges from 1% to 4% [16]. Recent research has found that more girls than boys meet the criteria

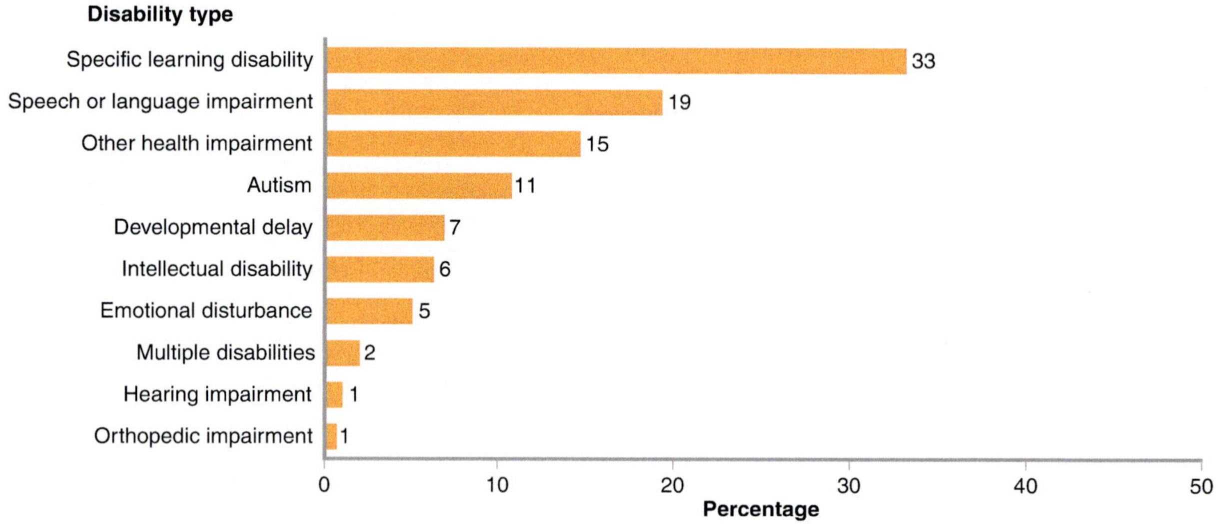

Fig. 12.8 Percentage distribution of students aged 3–12 receiving services under IDEA, according to disability, during the 2018–2019 school year. Not all disability categories are included

for mathematics disorder, while more boys have problems with spelling [17]. Some research teams have found that gender ratios do not substantially differ for reading problems, and others have found that reading disorders, such as dyslexia, are more common in males. More boys than girls are identified with combined literary deficits (such as reading and spelling problems) [17].

Etiology

While it is widely accepted that learning disorders have a degree of heritability, genetic studies are limited. Like intellectual disability, learning disorders are found in a variety of genetic syndromes, including X-linked disorders (affecting primarily males), deletions, and de novo mutations [18]. Some studies have indicated that certain cognitive processes appear to underlie learning disorders, such as processing speed, temporal processing, and working memory [15]. Notably, these processes are also impaired in attention-deficit/hyperactivity disorder, another neurodevelopmental disorder with a high comorbidity with learning disabilities.

Genetic heritability has been established for mathematics disorders through twin studies, with rates of concordance among monozygotic twins approaching 60%; however, specific candidate genes have yet to be identified [19]. There have been significant efforts to delineate the genetic etiology of dyslexia, which has not been adopted as a DSM-5 diagnosis but can be tentatively mapped onto specific learning disorder with impairment in reading. Like other SLDs, the etiology of dyslexia is thought to involve impairments in multiple processing pathways, and depending on the phenotypic definition used and the population assessed, twin studies have yielded heritability estimates of approximately 60% [20]. However, due to a lack of universally accepted criteria to define dyslexia and the resulting phenotypic variability, it has been challenging to isolate particular candidate genes, although over 14 have been described [21].

Pathophysiology

Within the broad category of learning disabilities, several areas can be broken down into specific affected skills. For instance, basic reading skills are dependent on the processes of *phonological awareness* (i.e., breaking down letters into sounds), *rapid naming* (i.e., naming letters and digits), *phonological memory* (i.e., working memory retention of sounds and words), *word recognition*, and *spelling*. Reading fluency is based on the speed of reading connected text and can be easily measured. Reading comprehension involves a variety of processes, including working memory, attention, processing speed, and the ability to self-monitor. Evidence suggests that these skills are orchestrated by three broadly defined left hemisphere brain regions: the visual word form area (VWFA) in the left occipitotemporal/fusiform region; the left temporoparietal region with the inferior parietal lobule and Wernicke's area; and the left inferior frontal gyrus (IFG), including Broca's area [22].

Mathematics involves number sense, memorization of arithmetic facts, accurate calculation, and accurate math reasoning. It requires the use of language, working and long-term memory, phonological decoding, attention, sight word recognition, and other basic skills in problem-solving and concept formation. Because of all the processes required, an interruption at any one of these steps may lead to difficulties in mathematics and other skills. Despite these complexities, repeated studies indicate that the parietal lobe is responsible for most basic number processing skills [23]. The left angular gyrus in the parietal lobe may be a localized area of dysfunction in children with comorbid math and reading disabilities, impacting verbal working memory, semantic memory, and quantitative reasoning (Fig. 12.9) [24].

Written expression takes longer to develop, with deficits often not noted until fourth or fifth grades. Writing requires the integration of multiple skills—motor, memory, language, self-organization, spelling, punctuation, syntax, and concept formation. It is often self-evident when motor processing is impaired, with the result of very poor handwriting, i.e., dysgraphia. This may occur in isolation or in the context of other difficulties with written expression. Reflecting the complexity of the writing process, a broad span of brain areas has been implicated in the process of writing, including areas in all lobes and the cerebellum [25].

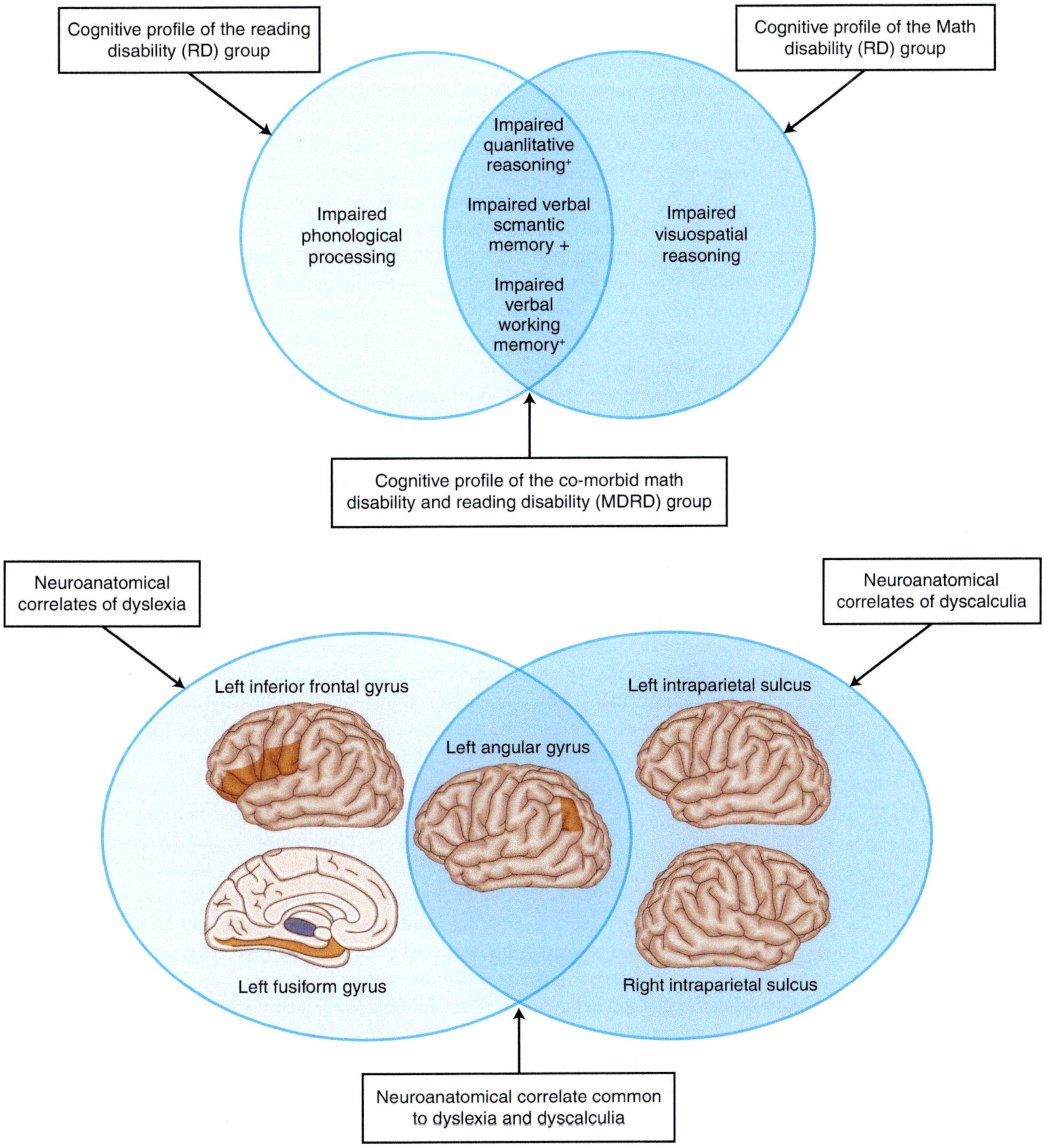

Fig. 12.9 A hypothetical neurologic model of dyslexia-dyscalculia comorbidity, demonstrating identified neuroanatomical correlates of both disorders and possible shared neuroanatomic area

Recent data suggest that across all specific learning disabilities, particular deficits are seen in working memory and processing speed [26]. This implies that both of these domains are of great importance in the development of academic skills across reading, mathematics, and writing domains.

Phenomenology

Learning disorders present in various ways. Some skills, such as number sense (the ability to discriminate numbers and perform simple arithmetic), develop early, before 5 years of age. Other skills, such as written expression, require many more processes and develop later. For these reasons, children should be monitored throughout their development to identify difficulties, as the affected processes may have significant downstream effects over time.

In some children, behavioral problems in school and declining school performance may be the first indication that something is amiss. In children with depressive, anxiety, or externalizing symptoms, an underlying driver may be difficulties with school performance. Children with ADHD should be evaluated for specific learning disabilities, as they are often co-occurring. Without adequate supports, children with learning disabilities are at elevated risk for underachievement, school drop-out, substance use, criminal-legal involvement, and underemployment [27–30]. In some cases, highly involved parents may compensate for their child's deficits by assisting in schoolwork; however, this may ultimately reduce the child's confidence, motivation, and sense of self-efficacy. In children who have significant strengths in other cognitive areas, teachers and parents may not immediately notice relative areas of weakness. In these cases, it is helpful to evaluate for avoided areas of schoolwork, which may provide clues as to areas of relative difficulty. In all children, and particularly those with significant weaknesses, identification of cognitive strengths is invaluable for bolstering self-esteem and designing access points to the school curriculum.

Treatment

Because multiple basic skills can underlie each learning difficulty, thorough neuropsychological and psychoeducational assessments are important for identifying the specific deficits and developing a treatment plan. As described earlier, under the age of three, children in the United States are eligible for services through their local public early intervention system, which assesses the child and creates an individualized family service plan (IFSP), and after the age of 3 years old, they are guaranteed special education and related services through their local public school system and associated agencies until the age of 21 years. Caretakers of children with a suspected SLD should be empowered to request an assessment for an individualized education program (IEP), which provides federally funded supports for specialized instruction to the child in order for them to access the curriculum in the least restrictive setting, under the protection of the Individuals with Disabilities Education Act (IDEA). If the child is not found to meet the criteria for an IEP (i.e., a covered disability requiring specialized instruction), the family should request an evaluation for a 504 Plan (named for Section 504 of the Rehabilitation Act of 1973), which does not provide specialized instruction, but has broader definitions of disability and incorporates basic accommodations in order for the child to have equal access to the curriculum (Fig. 12.10). Both IEPs and 504 Plans should be updated annually to evaluate measurable growth and update goals and interventions.

In young children, if language development has been delayed, early intervention services should include speech and language intervention, which can serve to both actively encourage speech production while assessing specific areas of skill deficit that may affect later skill development, such as phonological awareness or word recognition. For older children with difficulty in reading, interventions for reading fluency may involve repeated use of words and phrases with a speech and language therapist, exercises supporting executive functioning and working memory skills, and support for reading comprehension (i.e., use of semantics, phonology (sound of the word), and orthography (spelling of word) (Fig. 12.11). Multiple phonics methods are available, with studies demonstrating that "systematic phonics" (i.e., learning letter–sound relationships by a specific sequence) may be the most effective phonics method [31].

For children with mathematics difficulties, intervention targets include phonological coding of number names, orthographic coding of symbols, oral naming of codes, writing codes, using working memory, fact retrieval, learning concepts, and executive functioning skills. A review of mathematics interventions found that the use of peer tutoring, explicit and direct instruction, and periodic performance updates to the child and caregivers all led to benefits regardless of intervention [32].

For children with writing difficulties showing signs of dysgraphia, a fine motor assessment with possible occupational therapy is warranted. Whether writing on the computer or with a pencil, written expression requires a complex pro-

Fig. 12.10 Comparison between IEP and 504 Plans

IEP vs 504	Individualized Education Plan (IEP)	Section 504 Plan
Law	Special Education - Individuals with Disabilities Act (IDEA)	Civil Rights - Rehabilitation Act of 1973
Department	Department of Education	Office of Civil Rights
Requirements for eligibility	Has a disability that: a) meets criteria under IDEA, b) significantly impacts educational performance, and c) requires specialized services	Has a disability that significantly impacts a major life function
What is typically included?	Specialized education services, accommodations, related services	Accommodations, modifications, and related services
Age limits	IEP offered through 12th grade or until age 21 when required	No age limits with a 504 plan
Where is the plan used?	Educationally, through the 12th grade Does not transfer to college	School, work, and college Eligibility and plan creation occurs at each institution
Discipline	A Manifestation Determination meeting must be held to determine if the offense is a manifestation of the disability by the 10th day of suspension Services are required during long-term suspension	A Manifestation Determination meeting must be held to determine if the offense is a manifestation of the disability by the 10th day of suspension May require reevaluation

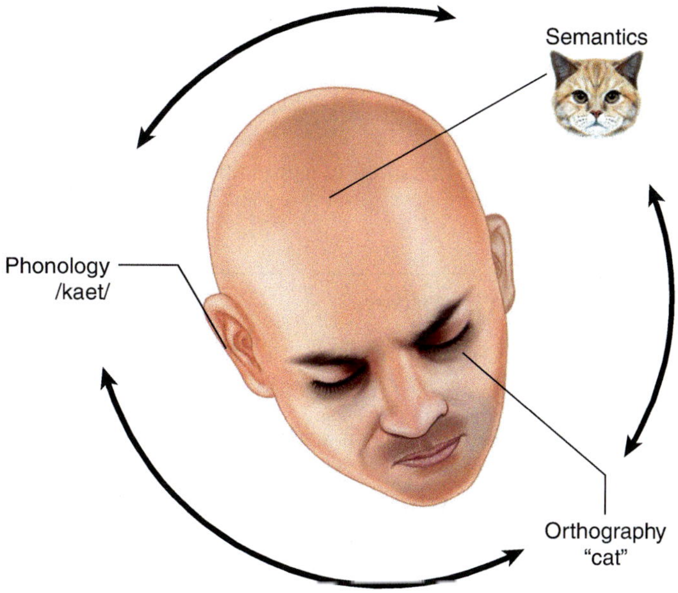

Fig. 12.11 Illustration of the reading process

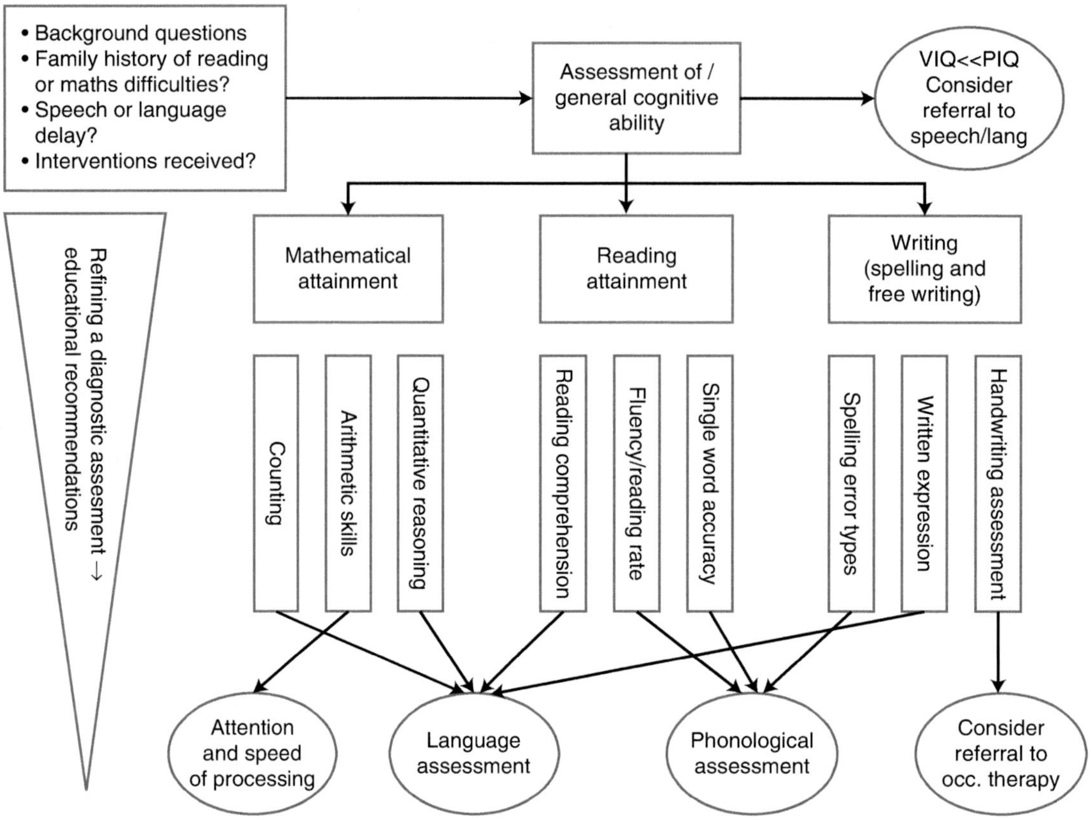

Fig. 12.12 Comprehensive assessment for SLD

cess of thought organization and optimization of attention. A recent meta-analysis of writing interventions identified that the most successful modalities involved strategy instruction (i.e., executive planning reminders), the use of dictation through recording devices, goal-setting for the specific assignment, and "process writing," involving the use of a step-to-step guide [33]. In all cases of specific learning disabilities, thoughtful assessment and educational modifications can lead to improved academic performance, increased self-confidence, and maximization of autonomous achievement (Fig. 12.12).

Autism Spectrum Disorder

Introduction

Autism spectrum disorder (ASD) is a classification used to describe individuals who have a specific combination of developmental impairments in social communication, repetitive behaviors, and restricted interests starting early in life. It is a highly heritable disorder with a high global incidence and is a diagnosis shared by individuals with a wide range of cognitive abilities. The core features of autism spectrum disorder have been described for hundreds of years, moving from case descriptions such as the "Wild Boy of Aveyron" in 1790 to, over a century later, Eugene Bleuer coining the concept of "autistic" (self-based) thinking in his early construct of schizophrenia [34]. In the 1940s, within 1 year of each other, both Leo Kanner and Hans Asperger described children and adults with "autistic" psychopathology. Initially, etiological theories related to environmental causes were dominant, including Bruno Bettelheim's blaming of "refrigerator mothers" in the 1940s [35]. By the late 1960s, the field began to acknowledge ASD as a neurodevelopmental disorder requiring targeted therapies, and the first twin study examining genetic underpinnings took place in the 1970s. Around this time, researchers also began noting the wide heterogeneity between individuals with ASD, who shared the core deficits but differed in deficit severity and intellectual profiles. This heterogeneity has contributed to the ongoing challenges in the reliability of diagnosis among clinicians with various training backgrounds due to the specialized training required to diagnose ASD accurately. As a result of these difficulties, diagnostic criteria have evolved over time to more specifically capture the primary deficits and streamline diagnostic groupings, resulting in the DSM-5 work group removing the catch-all category of Pervasive Developmental Disorder (PDD) and, more controversially, the designation of Asperger disorder, in preference of a sin-

Table 12.7 Quick reference: Autism Spectrum disorder

Core features: 1. Persistent deficits in social communication and social interaction across multiple contexts (e.g., social-emotional reciprocity, nonverbal communication, developing and understanding relationships) 2. Restricted, repetitive patterns of behavior, interests, or activities (i.e., at least two of the following: Stereotyped motor movements, routine inflexibility, restricted interests, and sensory hypersensitivity)
Age: Symptoms must start in the early developmental period, although some youth may be able to compensate for deficits, delaying diagnosis
Diagnosis: Screening (e.g., M-CHAT, SCQ, SRS-2), cognitive testing, adaptive skill testing, an autism-specific clinical interview with child and parents (gold standards: ADOS-2 and ADI-R)

gle Autism Spectrum Disorder diagnosis with three levels of severity (Table 12.7).

The diagnostic process for ASD includes screening, autism-specific diagnostic instruments, cognitive assessments, and adaptive functioning assessments. Earlier diagnosis, when coupled with early intervention, can lead to sustained improved outcomes [36]. Children with ASD who also have GDD or ID are generally identified earlier, although the average age of diagnosis remains 4 years, and is often much later for girls, children of color, and children from lower-income backgrounds [37, 38]. While universal screening for ASD at 18 and 24 months was recommended by the American Academy of Pediatrics in 2007, the US Preventive Services Task Force concluded in 2016 that there was insufficient evidence for this recommendation due to a lack of data on universal screening [39, 40]. In response, the Children's Hospital of Philadelphia Pediatric Network screened approximately 26,000 children and followed them from 4 to 8 years of age [41]. In achieving nearly universal screening (91%) with the M-CHAT (see description of screener below), the group found an ASD prevalence of 2.2%, a sensitivity of 38.8%, and a positive predictive value (PPV) of 14.6%. Notably, sensitivity was higher in older toddlers with repeated screenings, PPV was lower in girls, and both PPV and specificity were lower in children of color and those from lower-income backgrounds. These results highlight the continued need for improved screening methods and implementation in order to detect ASD, particularly in girls and in children from historically underrepresented groups.

Despite the limitations described above, the Modified Checklist for Autism in Toddlers—Revised with Follow-Up (M-CHAT-R/F) is the preferred screening instrument for young children at this time. It is standardized for children with 16–30 months of age and assesses for early validated markers of ASD, including deficits in pointing, language development, and joint attention. The Social Communication Questionnaire (SCQ) and Social Responsiveness Scale—Second Version (SRS-2) are additional valuable screening tools, particularly for older children. Following a positive screen and/or clinical concern, the child should receive specialized, autism-specific testing performed by trained clinicians. The gold standard instruments are the Autism Diagnostic Observation Schedule—2 (ADOS-2), a semi-structured play-based assessment, and the Autism Diagnostic Interview—Revised (ADI-R), which is a standardized developmental history interview completed with the primary caretaker(s) [42, 43].

An essential component of any ASD evaluation is an assessment of cognitive and adaptive functioning. While past estimates of concurrent ID in ASD hovered at more than 75%, updated estimates accounting for the increased sensitivity in detecting ASD-specific deficits in the absence of gross cognitive delays indicate a lower rate of 30–40% [44]. Cognitive assessments such as the Mullen Scales of Early Learning and the Wechsler Intelligence Scale for Children provide essential information about cognitive strengths and weaknesses and may reveal trends that are relatively ASD-specific, such as stronger nonverbal skills relative to verbal skills [45]. A comprehensive understanding of a child's global functioning also requires an assessment of adaptive functioning, often by using the Vineland Adaptive Behavior Scales [46]. Through understanding a child's cognitive and adaptive profile in the context of ASD-specific deficits, clinicians and families are better able to implement interventions and prognosticate for the future.

Epidemiology

Prevalence estimates of ASD vary based on the source study; however, the 2010 Global Burden of Disease study estimated that 52 million people had autism globally, yielding a prevalence of 1 in 132 individuals [47]. In the United States, the Centers for Disease Control (CDC) estimates a higher estimated prevalence of 1 in 54 children and a trend of increasing prevalence annually (Fig. 12.13) [48]. Accounting for a likely underdiagnosis of females, a recent study indicated an incidence rate of 3:1 in affected males versus females [49]. Although there has been a widespread concern for the rates of ASD increasing over time, when methodological variations between studies are accounted for, there appears to be no clear evidence of change in the prevalence of autism between 1990 and 2010 [47]. Intuitively, however, one may attribute increased prevalence to improvements in earlier diagnosis, changes in diagnostic criteria encompassing a broader range of cognitive profiles, and/or educational use of ASD diagnosis for increased access to service interventions. For now, consensus on prevalence shifts and potential underlying causes remains elusive.

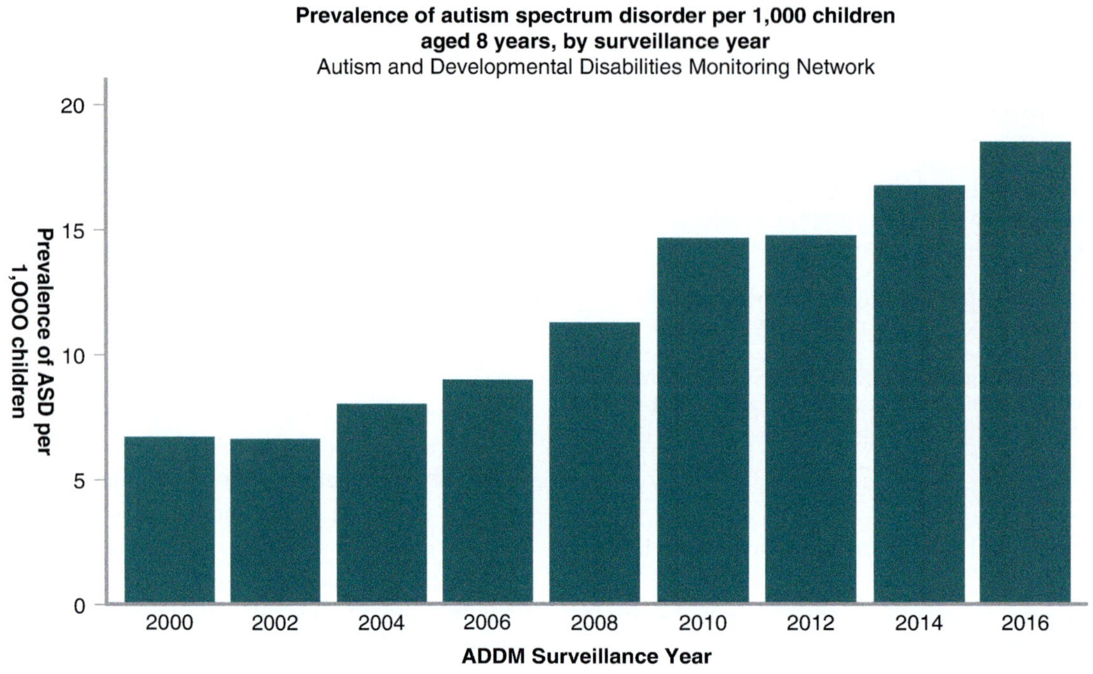

Fig. 12.13 Estimated prevalence rates of ASD in the United States based on data from the 2016 ADDM Network Surveillance Summary Supplemental Slides, https://www.cdc.gov/ncbddd/autism/data.html. Of note, 18.5/1000 children equal a rate of 1/54 children

Etiology

With the heritability of ASD estimated to be high, genetic research has boomed. Multiple baby sibling studies have prospectively assessed development in younger siblings of youth diagnosed with ASD. Based on these studies, twin studies, and larger family studies, twin heritability has been estimated to be over 50%, and siblings of a child with ASD have a risk of at least 10% of also having ASD [50, 51]. There appears to be no single genetic explanation for autism. Instead, researchers have identified numerous candidate genes, including over 100 single-gene, germline loss-of-function point mutations, and many rare de novo mutations in common genes [52]. Most of these genes individually have small effect sizes. This supports the position that although heritability is high, there may be many different neurobiological subgroups within individuals diagnosed with ASD.

Currently, it is conservatively estimated that at least 11% of individuals with ASD have a de novo rare point mutation or CNV that is contributing to their disorder [53]. This probability increases if the individual has intellectual disability, is female, has multiple unaffected siblings, or has a seizure disorder. The more of these characteristics a child has, the more likely it is to discover a genetic contribution.

Most identified autism risk genes have multiple downstream effects on the developing brain through various types of gene and protein expression. This makes it challenging to determine the impact of a particular gene or genetic region on the expression of an individual's specific ASD phenotype. A potential key for further elucidation involves the examination of clearly defined neurodevelopmental syndromes where individuals sometimes present with an ASD phenotype. These disorders include fragile X, tuberous sclerosis, Angelman, and Rett syndromes, which are all monogenic in cause. Identifying where autism risk genes converge to share pathological mechanisms in these disorders may propel efforts to elucidate ASD's molecular pathophysiology. In the meantime, the current standard of care supported by the American Academy of Pediatrics and the American College of Medical Genetics involves chromosomal microarray testing and fragile X testing for all individuals with ASD [54].

A number of environmental risk factors may contribute to the development of ASD, although the strength of these data is variable. Notable positive associations include older parental age, hypoxia at birth, maternal obesity, maternal valproic acid use, and gestational diabetes [55]. Notable negative associations, where there appears to be no contributory relationship, include assisted reproductive technologies, prolonged labor, and, importantly, vaccinations [56].

Pathophysiology

Animal models, neuroimaging, and post-mortem studies of ASD have demonstrated macro- and micro-level changes in neural structures and other organ systems. Neurologically, some individuals with ASD demonstrate accelerated brain growth in early development, although these findings are confounded by biased norm comparisons, making implications unclear [57]. Compellingly, however, a high-resolution magnetic resonance imaging (MRI) study of infants with high familial risk for ASD who met ASD criteria (HR-ASD) showed a significantly increased surface area growth rate from 6 to 12 months of age compared to both the HR-negative and low familial risk for ASD (LR) groups, linking the timing of brain overgrowth with the emergence and severity of ASD social deficits and diagnosis (Fig. 12.14) [58].

There is also increasing evidence of focal cortical dysplasias in ASD due to abnormal neuronal migration, resulting in smaller pyramidal neurons in the frontal lobe; these findings may contribute to the high rate of seizure disorders and sensory differences seen in people with ASD [59]. Increased rates of both seizure disorders and sleep disorders are seen in ASD and appear to have some reciprocal adverse effects [60].

Additionally, individuals with ASD have a high prevalence of gastrointestinal dysfunction that appears unrelated to diet or medication status, with the most common problems being chronic constipation and gastroesophageal reflux [61]. Also frequently observable are fine and gross motor impairments, which may affect hand–eye coordination, imitation, gait, posture, balance, and speed of movement [62]. Data from the Autism Treatment Network (ATN), a multisite clinical research group that has collected medical registry data for almost 7000 youth with ASD since 2005, tracks these and other medical and psychiatric comorbidities, demonstrating the heavy medical burden families with an ASD child face (Fig. 12.15) [63].

Phenomenology

Dr. Stephen Shore, an Autism Advocate who is also on the spectrum, has famously said: "If you've met one person with autism, you've met one person with autism." This quote reflects the diversity of the autism spectrum—within one diagnosis exists individuals who are verbal and nonverbal, with varying degrees of social motivation and compensatory skills. Although there is a wide range of functional independence among people who share an ASD diagnosis, all people on the spectrum have differences in social communication and repetitive behaviors that lead to developmental challenges.

Through the years, more individuals have described firsthand their experience living with ASD. Notable examples include the memoirs *Thinking in Pictures: My Life with Autism* by Temple Grandin and *The Reason I Jump: The Inner Voice of a Thirteen-Year-Old Boy with Autism* by Naoki Higashida. Common themes from first-person accounts include difficulty understanding nonverbal social communication, difficulty understanding the psychological states of other people, difficulty with idiomatic or figurative use of

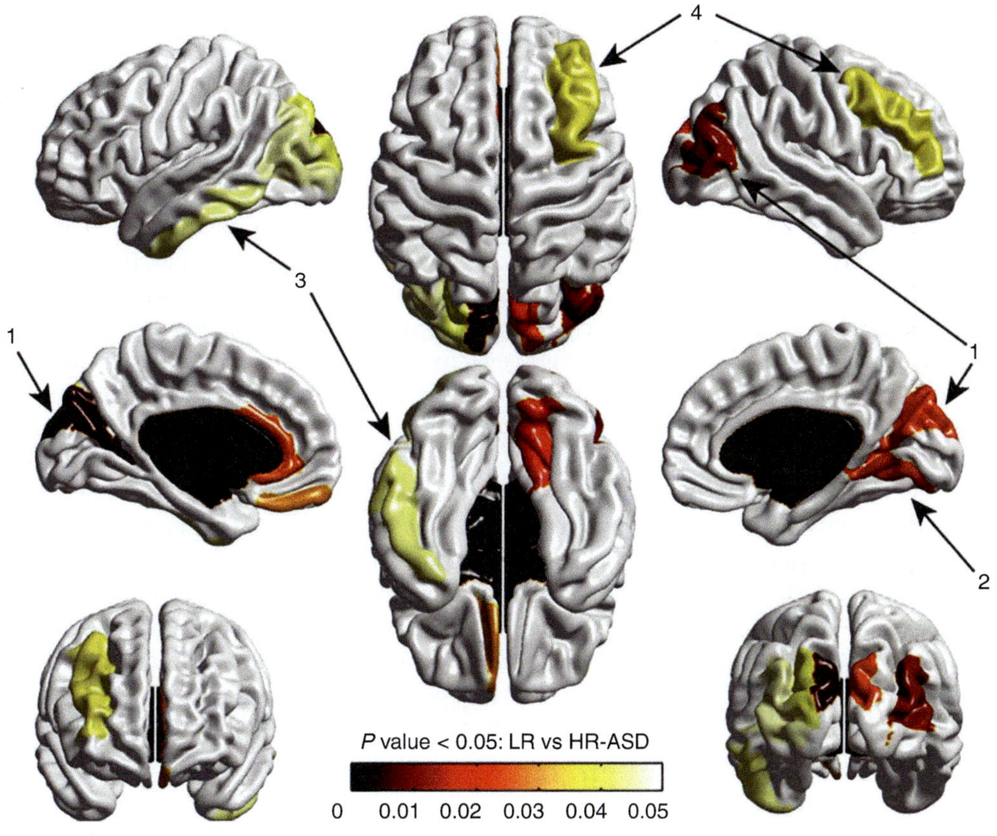

Fig. 12.14 A map of significant group differences in surface area from 6 to 12 months. The colored areas show the group effect for the HR-ASD versus LR subjects. Compared to the LR group, the HR-ASD group had significant expansion in the cortical surface area in the left/right middle occipital gyrus and right cuneus (1), right lingual gyrus (2), and to a lesser extent in the left inferior temporal gyrus (3), and middle frontal gyrus (4) (HR-ASD, $n = 34$; LR, $n = 84$). (*From* Hazlett et al. [58]; *with permission*)

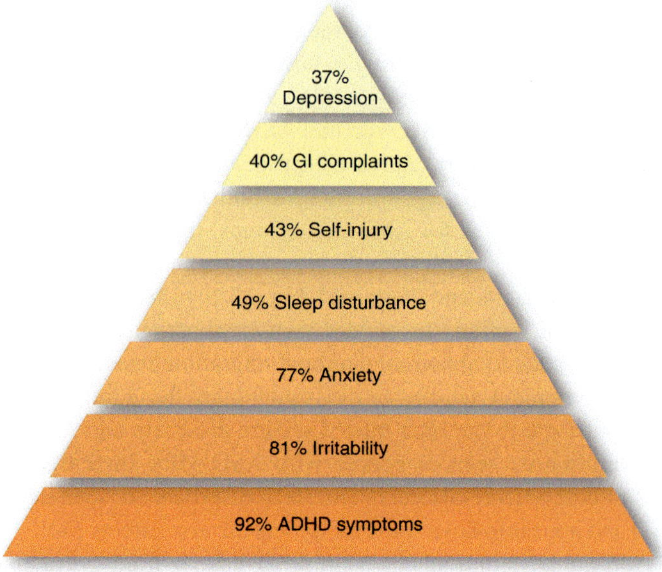

Fig. 12.15 Percentage of caregivers of youth with ASD reporting co-occurring medical problems in a sample of 500 registrants to the Autism Learning Health Network (ALHN). Data adapted from the Autism Treatment Network and Autism Intervention Research Network on Physical Health Annual Report 2019 https://www.autismspeaks.org/sites/default/files/ATN_2019_Annual_Report.pdf

language, sensory sensitivities or the urge to seek out certain sensory sensations, and the general experience of feeling different from other people. Although secure primary relationships are important for all individuals, people on the spectrum vary in respect to their interest in fostering various interpersonal relationships, including friendships and romantic relationships. For those motivated to connect socially with others, resulting difficulties can be a source of significant distress, making social skill interventions, such as those described below, a primary treatment modality.

Treatment

Given the pervasive social communication difficulties in children with ASD that affect all downstream learning and behavior, early intervention is the strongest recommendation. The earlier the interventions, the higher the child's neuroplasticity and the greater the chances of narrowing gaps in development. At the same time, it is never too late to bolster the skills of a person with autism, and individuals should receive services at whatever time problems are identified.

Access to early intervention services can vary based on the individual's community and resources. Early intervention modalities vary in length (weeks to years), intensity (hours per week), and delivery (therapist vs. parent). However, the National Research Council recommends a minimum of 25 h of intervention a week, 5 days a week, 12 months a year [64]. As described in previous sections, children younger than 3 years in the United States are eligible for services through their local public early intervention system, which assesses the child and creates an individualized family service plan (IFSP). After the child reaches 3 years old, he or she is guaranteed special education and related services through their local public school system and associated agencies until the age of 21 years. It is important that families are made aware of their right to access services through these systems and are supported in obtaining them.

Behavioral therapies modeled on applied behavior analysis (ABA) have the strongest evidence base in ASD, using principles of operant conditioning to reinforce appropriate social communication and problem-solving. Discrete trial training (DTT) is the best-known behavioral therapy modeled on ABA principles, but a number of more naturalistic ABA applications are empirically validated. Examples of these modalities, known collectively as Naturalistic Developmental Behavioral Interventions (NDBI), include pivotal response training (PRT), which incorporates the child's preferences to increase the motivation to learn; the Early Start Denver Model (ESDM); and Joint Attention Symbolic Play Engagement and Regulation (JASPER) [65].

Continued interventions—including ABA, speech and language, and occupational therapies—are recommended throughout school-age, adolescence, and adulthood, with the targeted skills and behaviors evolving over time. Evidence is building for structured, ecologically-valid social skills training, such as the UCLA PEERS Program [66]. Improved skills in social communication can lead to significant improvements in relationship development and overall quality of life, particularly for teens and young adults with ASD who struggle with social isolation. For children and adults with limited verbal language, the development of a viable communication method significantly improves the quality of life and may involve the use of augmentative communication strategies such as the Picture Exchange Communication Program (PECS), a program for facilitating nonverbal symbolic communication using ABA principles.

There are relatively few treatment studies examining adults with ASDs; however, treatment during this life stage often emphasizes the development of social and work skills, increasing adaptive behavior skills, and adequately managing co-occurring mental disorders. Because individuals with ASD have high rates of comorbidity of ADHD, anxiety, OCD, and disruptive behavior, among others, treatment at any stage may focus on providing training to parents on behavioral management, adapted individual psychotherapy, or medication management when appropriate. Importantly, medications do not treat ASD itself but rather select associated symptoms, such as irritability and agitation, poor attention and focus, impulsivity, and obsessiveness (Fig. 12.16). Both of the atypical antipsychotics risperidone and aripiprazole are FDA approved for the treatment of irritability, aggression, and self-injury in children with autism spectrum disorders. Treatment of ADHD symptoms and sleep disturbances are also primary psychopharmacologic targets. Medication treatment can be very helpful but should be chosen with close attention to risks of side effects and paradoxical responses, which are both more common in youth with developmental disabilities.

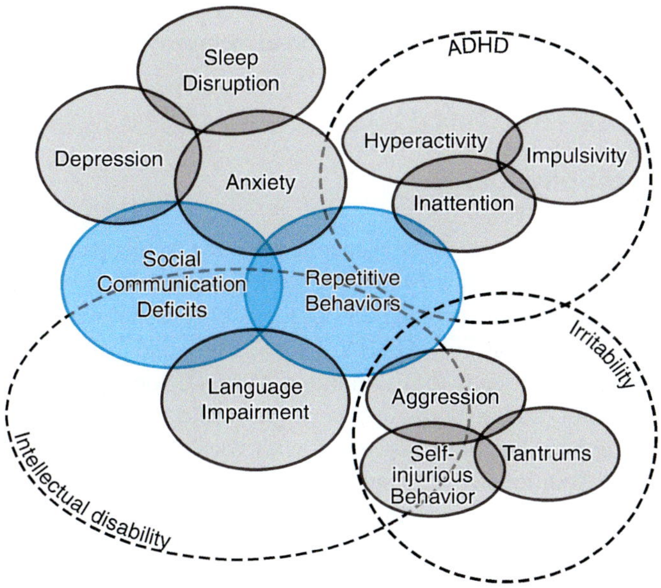

Fig. 12.16 Overlapping clusters of psychiatric symptoms commonly present in ASD. In blue are core ASD deficits. In gray are frequent co-occurring symptoms. In the dotted lines are overlapping symptom clusters consistent with ID, ADHD, and general irritability. While core ASD deficits have not been found responsive to medication management, other symptom clusters such as sleep disruption, depression, anxiety, ADHD symptoms, and irritability symptoms do have effective psychotropic correlates [192]

Tic Disorders

Introductory Text

Tic disorders have been described for over 200 years. In 1885, French neurologist George Gilles de la Tourette reviewed nine cases of individuals with motor and vocal tics, a combination of problems that became an eponymous syndrome. Motor tics are sudden, brief, repetitive, stereotyped movements occurring in voluntary muscles. They often appear in the facial voluntary muscles first (e.g., eye blinking, nose twitching) before progressing to other muscle groups in the neck, shoulders, trunk, back, arms, and legs. Vocal tics, if present, often manifest later than motor tics and may range from sounds such as throat clearing, sniffing, and barking, to more complex vocalizations such as stuttering, blurting out words, or, in fewer than 10% of cases, obscene language (i.e., coprolalia). Tics involving relatively few muscles or sounds are called "simple tics," while tics that involve multiple muscle groups or sounds are called "complex tics." In any individual, certain tics may wax and wane at various times of life, but the peak incidence of tic disorders is between ages 4 and 7 years, with symptoms often worse in late childhood and early adolescence [67]. Tics generally improve by early adulthood, although some individuals may continue to have severe symptoms.

Tics are not voluntary, but they are influenced by the environment and context. Many individuals, particularly older children or adults, are aware of a "premonitory urge"—a strong need to release the tic, after which tension and anxiety briefly subside. Depending on the severity, some individuals may be able to suppress tics to a degree for a limited amount of time. It is common for individuals with tics to have increased tics while discussing their symptoms, and tics may mimic others' movements or words (i.e., echopraxia or echolalia). Tics generally fluctuate through the day, occur in groupings separated by time, and are not present in sleep. They are known to be aggravated by stress. In addition to the clinical interview, self-report measures such as the Yale Global Tic Severity Scale (YGTSS) can be useful [68]. In the DSM-5, tic disorders include (1) provisional tic disorder (tics less than 1 year), (2) persistent motor or vocal tic disorder (tics of either type persistent for more than 1 year), and (3) Tourette's syndrome (TS; a combination of motor and vocal tics persisting for more than 1 year) (Table 12.8).

Tic disorders are highly comorbid with ADHD, OCD, anxiety disorders, and major depressive disorder. ADHD is estimated to be present in 21–90% of individuals with TD; up to 80% may have OCD, an estimated 30% have comorbid anxiety disorders, and up to 75% may have major depressive disorder [69]. Individuals with autism spectrum disorders also have higher rates of tic disorders than other youth, which present differently from stereotypies (i.e., self-soothing,

Table 12.8 Quick reference: Tic disorders

Core features: • Sudden, rapid, recurrent, nonrhythmic motor movements or vocalizations that have been present (a) less than 1 year, (b) more than 1 year but only motor or only vocal, not mixed, or (c) more than 1 year with both motor and vocal *Age:* Onset before 18 years *Diagnosis:* Comprehensive clinical assessment, rating scales

intentional complex body movements) [70]. The above comorbidities affect the choice of the treatment plan for tics and may present challenges. For example, in children with both ADHD and a tic disorder, attentional deficits may limit the child's therapeutic engagement in behavioral tic treatments, but treating their ADHD with stimulants may in turn transiently exacerbate tics (further discussion below).

Epidemiology

A 2012 meta-analysis of tic disorders estimates a prevalence rate of 0.77% for TS, with a higher rate in boys (1.06%) than in girls (0.25%) [67]. Transient motor tics alone are more common than the combined motor and vocal tics. Accordingly, provisional tic disorder is the most common tic disorder diagnosis, affecting 2.99% of children studied. Comparatively, the prevalence rate of TS in adults was estimated to be 0.05%, likely due to significant remission of symptoms by adulthood (Fig. 12.17).

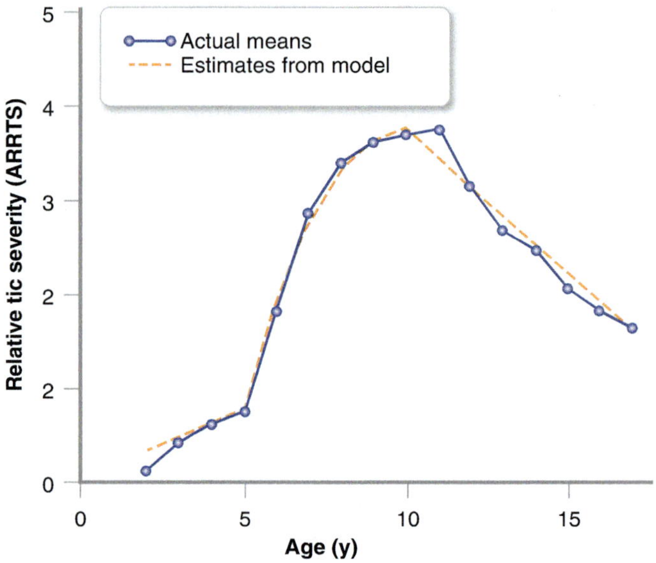

Fig. 12.17 Plot of mean tic severity from ages 2 to 18 years using the Annual Rating of Relative Tic Severity Scores (ARRTS), with inflection points noted at the age of tic onset and age of worst-ever tic severity. The dashed line shows a mathematical model designed to best fit clinical data. (*From* Bloch and Leckman [193]; *with permission*)

Etiology

TS is currently understood to have a complex etiology involving multiple genes interacting with environmental factors. Although an example of monogenic TS exists, linkage studies from large multigenerational pedigrees have not found reproducible genetic inheritance patterns [71]. Twin concordance rates for TD have been found to be 53–56% in monozygotic pairs and 8% for dizygotic pairs. To date, multiple candidate genes, chromosomal aberrations, copy number variants, and signals from genome-wide association studies are being investigated for possible etiological pathways.

Environmentally, maternal smoking and low birth weight may be risk factors [72]. Infection with group A beta-hemolytic streptococci (GABHS) may also contribute to a small number of cases with acute-onset tics and OCD symptoms. The proposed mechanism involves an autoimmune response that results in autoantibodies that attack the basal ganglia, causing tic behaviors or chorea. When the infection triggering the symptoms is found to be GABHS, the syndrome is referred to as pediatric autoimmune neuropsychiatric disorders associated with streptococcal infections (PANDAS). When the inciting etiology is unknown, it is referred to as pediatric acute-onset neuropsychiatric syndrome (PANS) [73].

Pathophysiology

Tics are thought to be generated by the same pathways involved in voluntary motor control, including the cortico-striatal-thalamo-cortical (CSTC) loops [74]. In animal models, disruption of GABA, dopamine, and glutamate transmission leads to disinhibition of CSTC loops resulting in motor tics, and disruption of the same in the nucleus accumbens has been associated with vocal tics (Fig. 12.18) [75]. Additionally, reduced cholinergic interneurons in the dorsal striatum and disrupted histamine synthesis are both potential pathways. The insular cortex appears to be associated with the experience of premonitory urges, and voluntary tic inhibition is associated with control stemming from the prefrontal cortex [74].

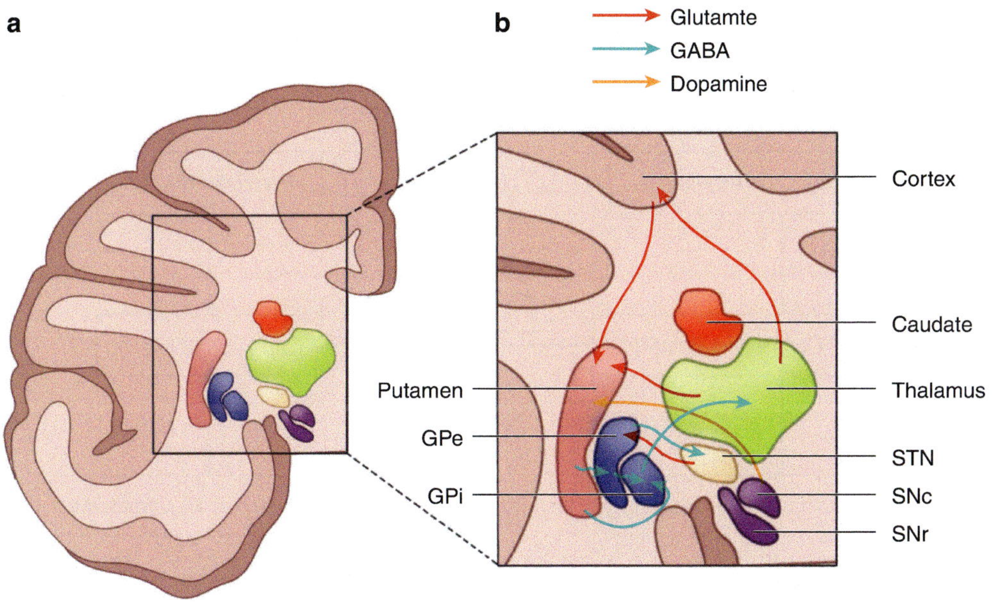

Fig. 12.18 Structure and compartments of the CSTC circuit. (**a**) Representation of a left side of the human brain coronal section showing the basal ganglia and cerebral cortex. (**b**) Schematic illustration of the CSTC internal network within the circuit showing the glutamatergic (red arrow), GABAergic (blue arrow), and dopaminergic connection (yellow arrow). Abbreviations: *GPe* globus pallidus pars externa, *GPi* globus pallidus pars interna, *STN* nucleus subthalamicus, *SNc* substantia nigra pars compact, *SNr* substantia nigra pars reticulata (From *Nespoli* et al. [75]; Creative Commons Attribution License 4.0; https://creativecommons.org/licenses/by/4.0/)

Phenomenology

Individuals with tics consistently describe 1) premonitory urges, defined by a physical sensation or thought that leads to the urge to complete the tic, and 2) obsessions and/or compulsions, for example, distressing aggressive or sexual thoughts or the need for symmetry or repetition. In assessing premonitory urges, Leckman and team conducted interviews with patients, one of whom described, "A need to tic is an intense feeling that unless I tic or twitch I feel as if I'm going to burst. Unless I can physically tic, all of my mental thoughts center on ticking until I am able to let it out" [76]. The need to suppress tics in certain situations often contributes to increased anxiety, low mood, decreased self-esteem, and social embarrassment. The cumulative effects can be deleterious in youth and young adults. Severe tics can affect the pursuit of friendships, employment, and romantic relationships, which may lead to a cycle of shame, avoidance, and isolation.

Treatment

Recommended treatment for tic disorders varies based on the severity of the tics and the motivation of the patient. In many cases, psychotherapeutic treatment, specifically habit reversal therapy (HRT), is recommended. This therapy involves tracking and observing tic behaviors, facilitating the patient's recognition of any premonitory urges, and then developing a "competing response": a motor action that is done at the same time as the tic that restricts the patient's ability to proceed with the tic and is minimally noticeable to observers (Fig. 12.19) [77]. For motivated patients, treatment using HRT may involve eight to ten sessions of treatment and lead to lasting improvements.

Dopamine antagonists—such as haloperidol, risperidone, aripiprazole, ziprasidone, and pimozide—are the most studied pharmacologic treatments for tics and have demonstrated notable rates of symptom reduction. Alpha-2 adrenergic agonists, such as clonidine and guanfacine, also have demonstrated utility in tic reduction, although with less rigorous evidence. In particularly intractable cases with high tic severity and a lack of response to three different medication trials, deep brain stimulation (DBS) may be considered, although consensus on DBS targets remains unclear [74].

Of note, while tics can increase transiently in patients with both tics and ADHD who take stimulants, stimulants remain the first-line agents for treating ADHD symptoms in this population. Longitudinal studies have demonstrated that tics do not substantially increase with stimulant treatment

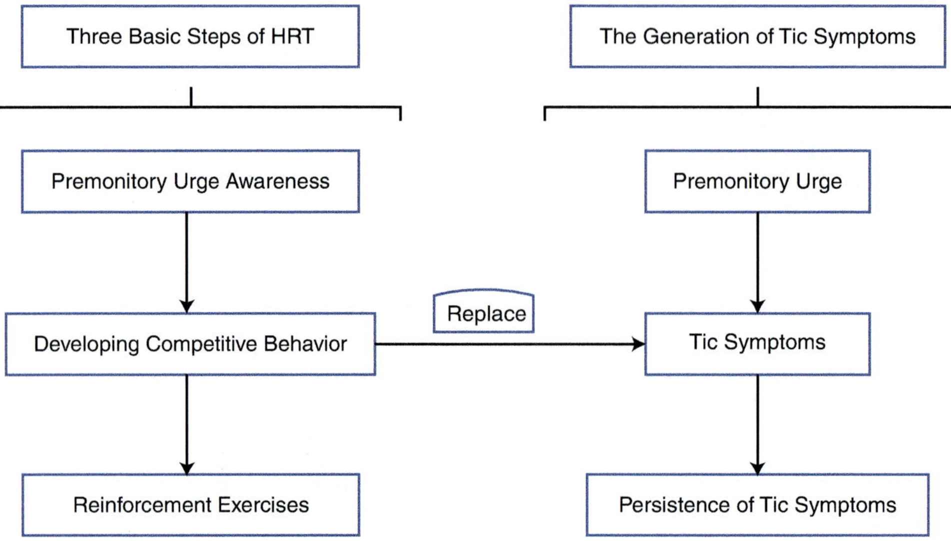

Fig. 12.19 Simplified steps of habit reversal therapy (HRT). (*From* Liu et al. [194]; *with permission*)

and may even decrease; however, it is common to see a 25% worsening in tics when any new medication is given [78]. For individuals with ADHD and tic disorders who cannot tolerate stimulants or alpha agonists, data supports the use of atomoxetine as an alternative. In cases of cooccurring OCD, the strongest evidence supports the use of cognitive behavioral therapy with consideration of a serotonin reuptake inhibitor (SRI), with or without a dopamine antagonist for augmentation as indicated [79].

Attention-Deficit/Hyperactivity Disorder

Introduction

In the early 1900s, clinicians began writing about hyperactive youth, labeling their condition a "hyperkinetic syndrome." It wasn't until the 1970s that researchers identified the executive dysfunction (i.e., inattention) that often accompanies excessive hyperactivity and impulsivity, leading to our modern understanding of Attention-Deficit/Hyperactivity Disorder (ADHD) [80]. In addition to these core symptoms, children with ADHD often present with significant comorbidities, including motor delays, learning disabilities, or autism spectrum disorder. ADHD also has high rates of comorbidity with anxiety disorders (up to 33%), major depressive disorder (up to 11%), and chronic emotional dysregulation that may be categorized as disruptive mood dysregulation disorder (DMDD, up to 50%) [81, 82]. The cooccurrence of ADHD with oppositional defiant disorder (ODD) and conduct disorder (CD) has been extensively studied; please see corresponding sections for further discussion.

Table 12.9 Quick reference: Attention-deficit/hyperactivity disorder

Core features:
Persistent pattern of inattention and/or hyperactivity-impulsivity lasting >6 months characterized by
1. Six or more inattention symptoms
2. Six or more hyperactivity-impulsivity symptoms

Age: Onset before 12 years
Diagnosis: Comprehensive clinical assessment including caregiver/teacher questionnaires (e.g., SNAP-IV, Vanderbilt, Connors 3). Symptoms must be present in 2 or more settings

ADHD is generally recognized earliest in children who are hyperactive and impulsive, often to a disruptive degree. These children move about their classrooms restlessly, shifting from one activity or topic to another, and may be impulsively intrusive both verbally and physically. Teachers and parents usually notice these differences as compared to peers in preschool or elementary school years. In addition to academic problems resulting from difficulty following directions and completing tasks, over time peers of these children become less tolerant of their activity level and social difficulties increase. Children with hyperactivity and impulsivity typically also demonstrate symptoms of inattention.

Children who are inattentive but not significantly hyperactive or disruptive tend to be identified later. These children generally have fewer social difficulties but become increasingly aware that they struggle more than their friends in focusing in class, completing schoolwork, and staying on a task outside the classroom. Without proper support, children with inattention may begin to think of themselves as less capable and may reduce their efforts in school due to the assumption that they will not achieve the level expected.

The diagnosis of ADHD remains clinical. There is no single test to identify the disorder, although there are a number of useful tools. In addition to clinical interviews with the family and child, information from teachers, after-school staff, and other adults is both helpful and necessary to establish the diagnosis. Symptoms must be chronic, present in more than two settings, and begin prior to the age of 12 years (Table 12.9). When assessing symptom history from these sources, it is helpful to use standardized self-report questionnaires that can be objectively compared across time and settings, such as the Swanson, Nolan, and Pelham Questionnaire (SNAP), Vanderbilt Assessment Scales, or Conners' 3 scales [83–85].

Importantly, a child's behavior in a one-on-one session with the clinician alone is not sufficient for a diagnosis; structured and brief sessions may not yield significant symptoms unless the child's presentation is severe, and even then, symptoms in more than one setting are necessary for diagnosis. Importantly, individuals with ADHD generally do not report difficulty in sustaining attention in preferred activities, for example video games or sports. Symptoms of inattention manifest in attending to activities of lower salience and enjoyment, such as school, homework, or chores.

Neuropsychological testing is not required for diagnosis, may not be financially feasible for many families, and has not been shown to be a reliable diagnostic tool on its own. However, such testing can be useful in evaluating areas of known deficit in ADHD, such as spatial working memory, planning ability, stop-task response suppression, and naming speed. Continuous performance tasks that evaluate sustained attention, such as the Test of Variables of Attention (TOVA) and the Connors' Continuous Performance Test (CPT), may also yield deficits. Children with ADHD may also demonstrate differential responses to reward and delay aversion, i.e., being unable to wait for an anticipated reward or showing a lack of responsiveness to a reward [86]. These findings help explain why children with ADHD may not respond as expected to routine behavioral parenting methods.

As children with ADHD age, hyperactivity symptoms may subside. The motor-driven behavior from the preschool years often recedes into mild restlessness as youth approach young adulthood [87]. Conversely, symptoms of inattention and executive dysfunction tend to persist into adulthood and beyond and are the primary concerns of older youth and adults seeking treatment for ADHD (Fig. 12.20) [88]. Based on results from the Multimodal Treatment Assessment (MTA) study of 1999 and subsequent follow-up studies, approximately one-third of children continued to exhibit significant ADHD symptoms in their teenage years with resulting worsened academic performance and a higher number of police contacts, arrests, and substance use [89–91]. One can better understand this when considering that when untreated, ADHD symptoms can lead to lower achievement in school, increased conflict with teachers and/or peers, corresponding reduced school engagement and more unscheduled time, dif-

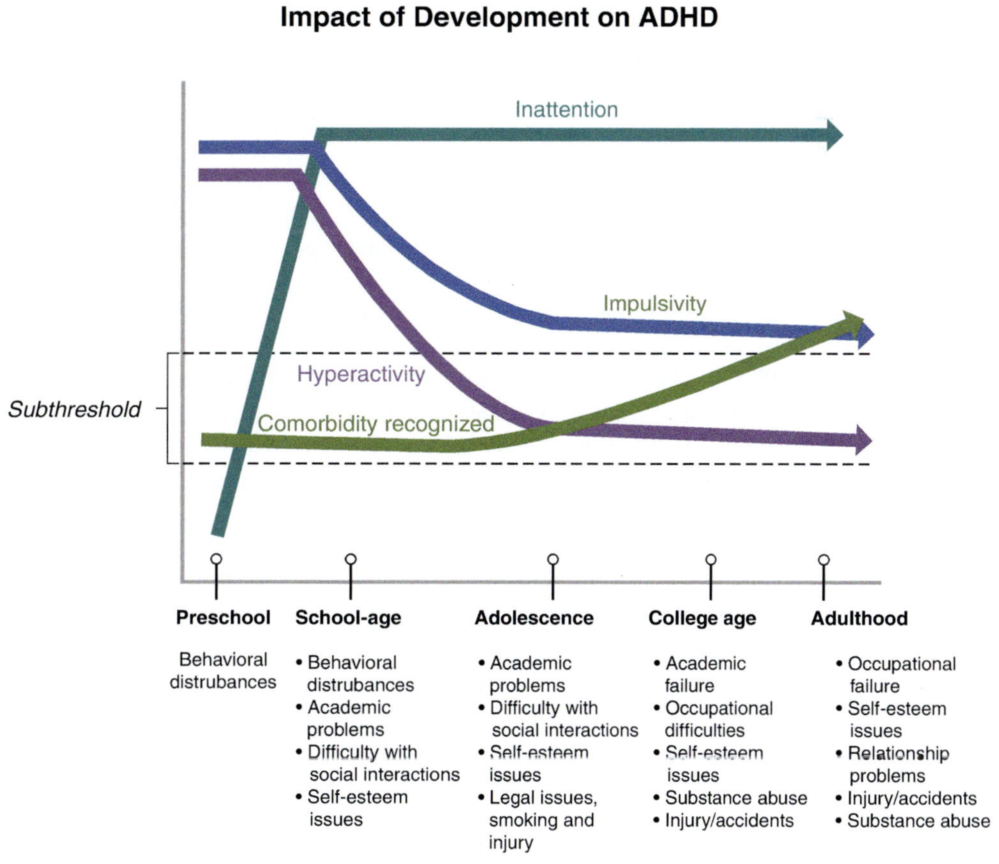

Fig. 12.20 Trajectory of ADHD symptoms over the lifespan. Hyperactivity and impulsivity tend to improve as youth age into adolescence. Inattentiveness remains persistent and results in common presenting symptoms of adult ADHD, including disorganization and difficulties with keeping a schedule, managing money, or attentiveness in relationships. Psychiatric comorbidities, such as SLD or anxiety disorders, are increasingly recognized during the lifespan [195]

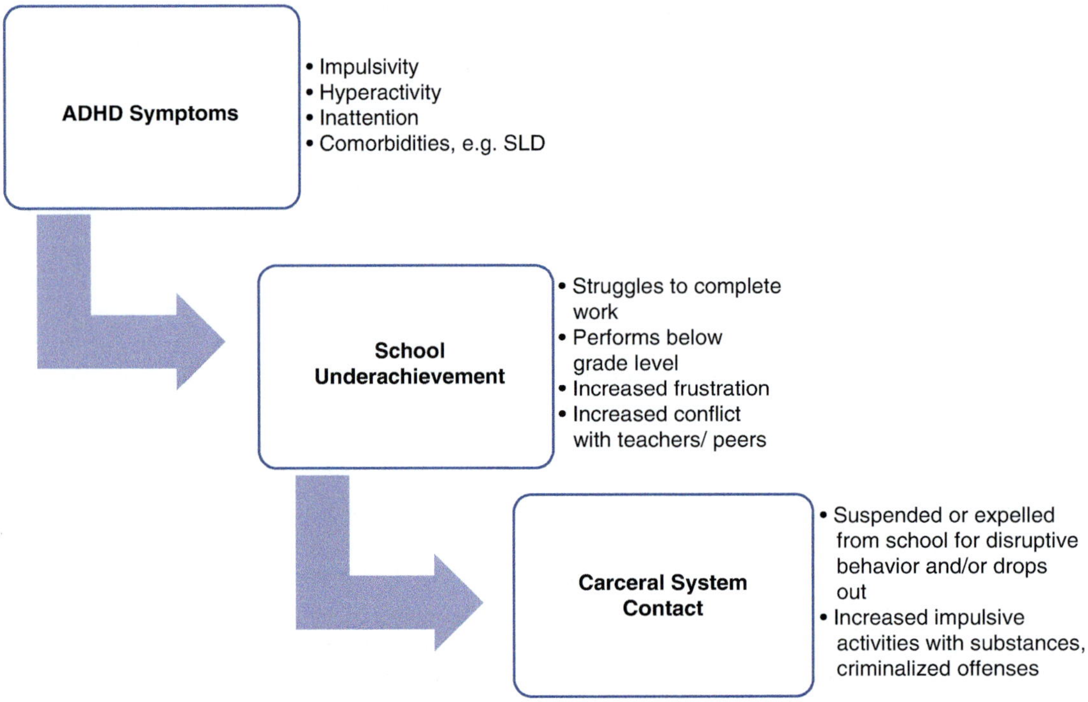

Fig. 12.21 Common trajectory for youth with severe undertreated ADHD symptoms and contribution psychosocial factors

ficulties with self-directed planning, and increased impulsive risk-taking behavior with other youth who are often experiencing similar difficulties (Fig. 12.21).

Epidemiology

ADHD is among the most common childhood disorders, with an estimated worldwide prevalence rate of 5.3% [92]. This number was higher in a national survey within the United States, with 11% of parents of children aged 4–17 years indicating that their child had been given an ADHD diagnosis in the past and 6.1% reporting that their child was prescribed medication for ADHD [93]. As in autism spectrum disorder and other neurodevelopmental syndromes, males are more frequently diagnosed than females, although this may be due to underdiagnosis. Females appear to show more inattentive symptoms than hyperactive symptoms, often leading to later diagnosis. Children and especially females with predominantly inattentive symptoms appear more likely to demonstrate internalizing symptoms, such as anxiety or depression, and may be bullied more often than other children [94].

Etiology

ADHD appears highly heritable and familial, with inherited variance rates of up to 90%; however, no single or group of genes has shown true genome-wide significance [95, 96]. Despite this, linkage and association studies in several ADHD subtypes have demonstrated inherited dysfunction in the dopamine transport gene (DAT1) on chromosome 5, the dopamine receptor D4 gene, and the dopamine receptor D5 gene, located on chromosomes 11 and 4, respectively [97]. Dysfunction of these receptors supports the prevailing monoamine hypothesis of ADHD, which suggests that symptoms are caused by a deficiency of dopamine and norepinephrine in prime cortical areas.

As with most psychiatric disorders, expression of ADHD appears to involve genetic predispositions and environmental contributions, with the latter including maternal smoking, lead exposure, and traumatic brain injury [95, 98]. Notably, the immediate family environment does not appear to significantly contribute to the development of the disorder, indicating a larger role for genetic inheritance and perinatal factors [97].

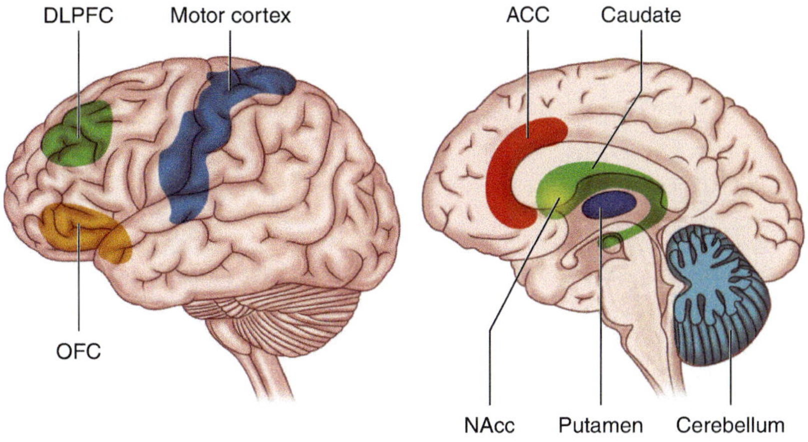

Fig. 12.22 Cortico-striatal network regions implicated in ADHD. Abbreviations: *ACC* anterior cingulate cortex, *DLPFC* dorsolateral prefrontal cortex, *NAcc* nucleus accumbens, *OFC* orbitofrontal cortex

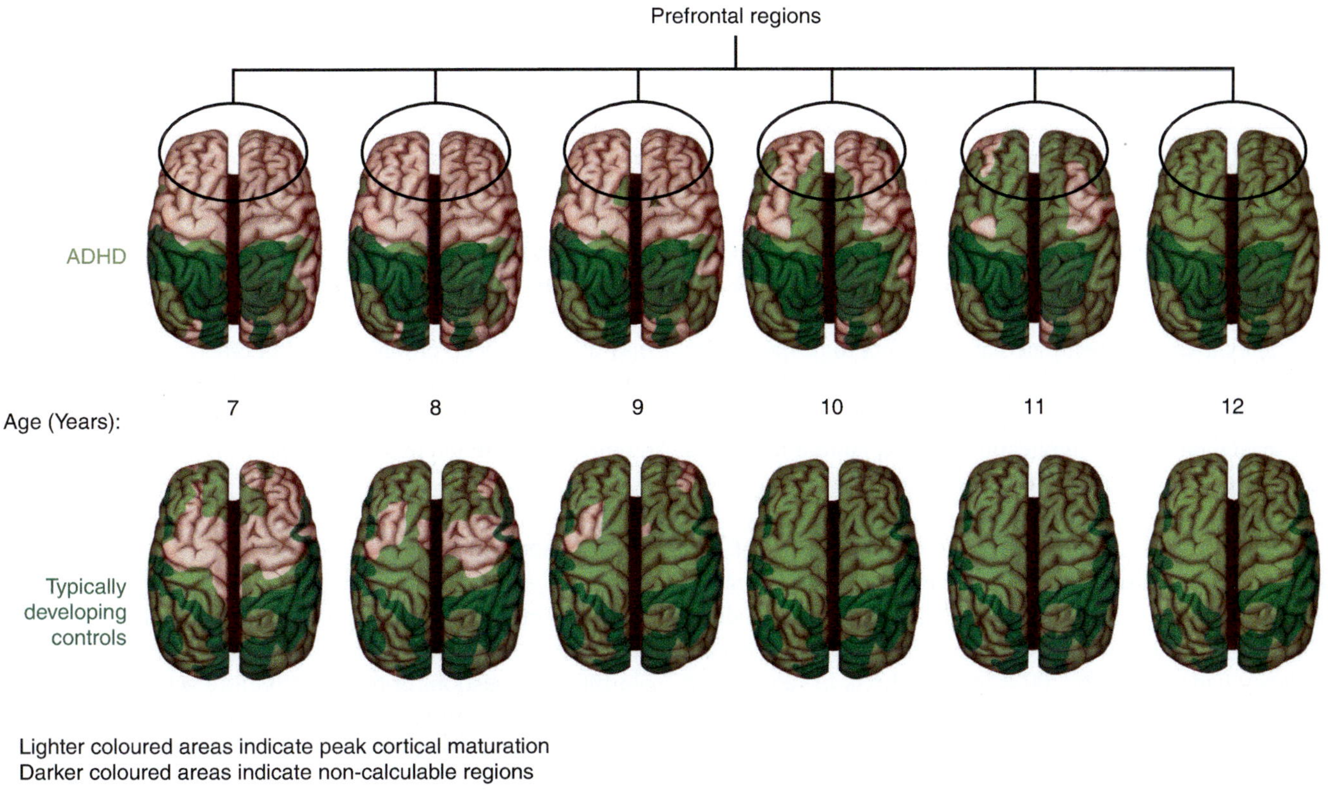

Fig. 12.23 Cortical maturation in patients with and without ADHD. In youth with ADHD compared to comparative controls, prefrontal regions are slower to mature and develop peak cortical thickness. Light blue and purple show peak cortical maturation, and darker colored areas indicate noncalculable regions. (*From* Shaw et al. [101]; *with permission*)

Pathophysiology

Researchers have identified several brain regions and circuits that play important roles in ADHD, all of which are innervated by dopaminergic and norepinephrinergic neurons. These regions include the dorsolateral prefrontal cortex (DLPFC), the orbitofrontal cortex (OFC), the anterior cingulate cortex (ACC), and the primary motor cortices, which work together with the striatum to provide working memory, response-inhibition, reward processing, and coordination of motor movements (Fig. 12.22) [99, 100]. In terms of neuroanatomy, MRI studies have consistently demonstrated reduced brain volumes, delayed cortical maturation, less cortical surface area, and thinner cortical thickness in individuals with ADHD when compared to controls (Figs. 12.23 and 12.24) [101]. Evidence also suggests that the default mode network (DMN), a brain circuit active dur-

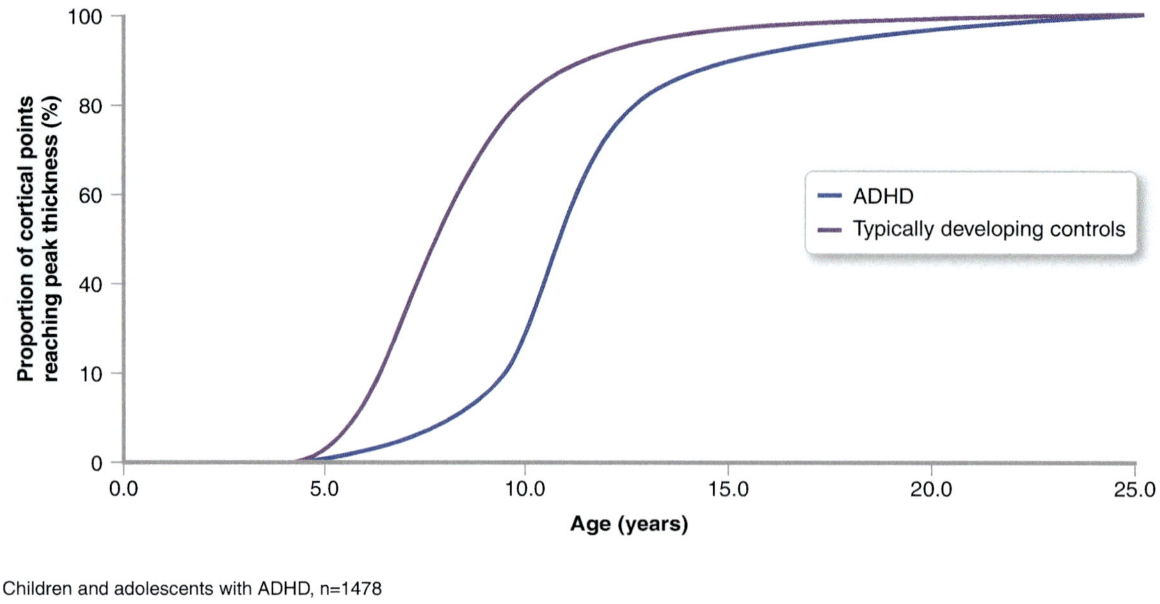

Fig. 12.24 Rate of cortical maturation as measured by peak cortical thickness in patients with and without ADHD. (*From* Shaw et al. [101]; *with permission*)

ing nonattentive states and suppressed when attention circuits are activated, may not be adequately suppressed in people with ADHD [102]. Differential responses to reward and delay aversion, mentioned above, seem to be caused by reduced ventral striatal activation, making normal rewards less motivating [103]. This hypo-responsiveness of the ventral striatal circuit has implications for explaining increased reward-seeking behavior (e.g., substance use) and mood dysregulation.

Individuals with ADHD have a higher incidence of seizures and sleep disorders than other children. In both cases, the relationship appears bidirectional. In a longitudinal cohort of over 900,000 children in Denmark, children with epilepsy had a 150% to 200% increased risk of developing ADHD, and children with a history of febrile seizures had a 20%–35% increased risk [104]. Similarly, children with a history of an ADHD diagnosis are 2.5–3.5-fold more likely than controls to have an unprovoked seizure, suggesting a common antecedent for both disorders [105].

Parent report indicates a high frequency of sleep problems in these children, most commonly involving sleep-onset delay with or without bedtime resistance. Primary sleep disorders, such as obstructive sleep apnea or restless leg syndrome, also occur regularly. Results from polysomnography have been mixed; there is some evidence for higher periodic limb movements in sleep in youth with ADHD than in controls [106]. In some cases, treating ADHD symptoms may alleviate sleep problems, and in other cases treating the primary sleep disorder may reduce ADHD symptoms. In most cases, the two appear to exacerbate each other and require an integrated treatment approach.

Phenomenology

Common manifestations of ADHD symptoms include distractedness, frequently asking for something to be repeated, blurting out questions or responses before waiting for others, restless movement that may be hard to redirect, and frequent complaints of boredom when asked to stay working on one task. People with ADHD may also present with apparent thought disorders, moving tangentially from one subject to another, not completing a thought before following another one, in what has been called "multiple tracks of thought" [107]. This occurs in the context of other ADHD symptoms and in the absence of other psychotic symptoms. Individuals often subjectively report improvement in thought cohesion with stimulant treatment [107].

In a 2008 qualitative study involving interviews with young adults reflecting on their challenges with ADHD symptoms, prominent themes included: difficulty getting along with parents due to trouble following through on tasks; feeling different from peers and "missing a lot" at school; and feeling "misunderstood" in friendships due to interpersonal difficulties, e.g., interrupting, offending others, and inattentiveness to conversation [108]. These challenges directly map onto core symptoms and are correlated with long-term adverse outcomes associated with an ADHD diagnosis, such as not completing high school, increased unemployment, increased substance use, increased comorbid psychiatric conditions, and increased rates of legal detainment or incarceration [109].

Treatment

ADHD is best treated by a combination of medication management, implementation of school supports, and behavioral treatment. Longitudinal data from the MTA study and a recent meta-analysis indicate that behavioral treatment on its own may not significantly reduce ADHD symptoms [110]. The response rates to stimulants, however, are the highest of any psychiatric medications. An estimated 65–75% of youth will respond to either methylphenidate or amphetamine, increasing to 85% if both types of stimulants are trialed [111]. Both methylphenidates and amphetamines increase reuptake inhibition of dopamine and are effective in all ages, albeit with somewhat reduced efficacy in preschool-age children [111]. Stimulants often cause mild increases in heart rate and blood pressure, but in the absence of a cardiac history, no association between stimulant use in youth and sudden cardiac events has been found [112]. Similarly, despite the addictive potential of stimulants, they have not been associated with an increased risk of developing a substance use disorder [113]. In fact, evidence suggests that appropriate treatment with stimulants may actually decrease the risk of substance use in adults with ADHD [114].

The most prominent side effects of stimulants are appetite suppression and insomnia, but they may also worsen anxiety or unmask or transiently worsen tics. For youth whose tics do not improve with decreasing the dose or changing the stimulant, alternate medications are available. Alpha-2 adrenergic agonists, for example, may be used as both an addition or alternative to stimulant treatment. Although they do not address core ADHD symptoms as effectively as stimulants, they can improve insomnia, tics, and residual hyperactivity or aggression. When stimulants are not tolerated due to side effects, atomoxetine may be used as an alternative, although with much lower response rates. Side effects to atomoxetine are common, but benefits include anxiolytic properties, no abuse potential (due to primary action on norepinephrine rather than dopamine), and a lower rate of tics. In all cases, a comprehensive assessment of comorbid psychiatric symptoms is important to guide the selection of psychopharmacologic agents in ADHD. A child with severe anxiety or depressive symptoms, for example, may do best with atomoxetine, bupropion (which has some limited evidence of benefit for ADHD symptoms), or treatment with an SSRI prior to initiation of a stimulant trial (Fig. 12.25).

In addition to medications, children with ADHD require school supports or accommodations in order to achieve their maximum potential. This may be achieved through an IEP or 504 Plan, as described above, and through after-school assistance, such as tutoring or organizational skills training.

While not efficacious at reducing core ADHD symptoms directly, behavioral parent training (described in more detail below) can help caregivers by providing instruction on how to use consistent routines and rewards, clear consequences and rules, and simple directions [110]. These strategies are particularly important in children with ADHD due to their challenges in responding to behavioral reinforcement.

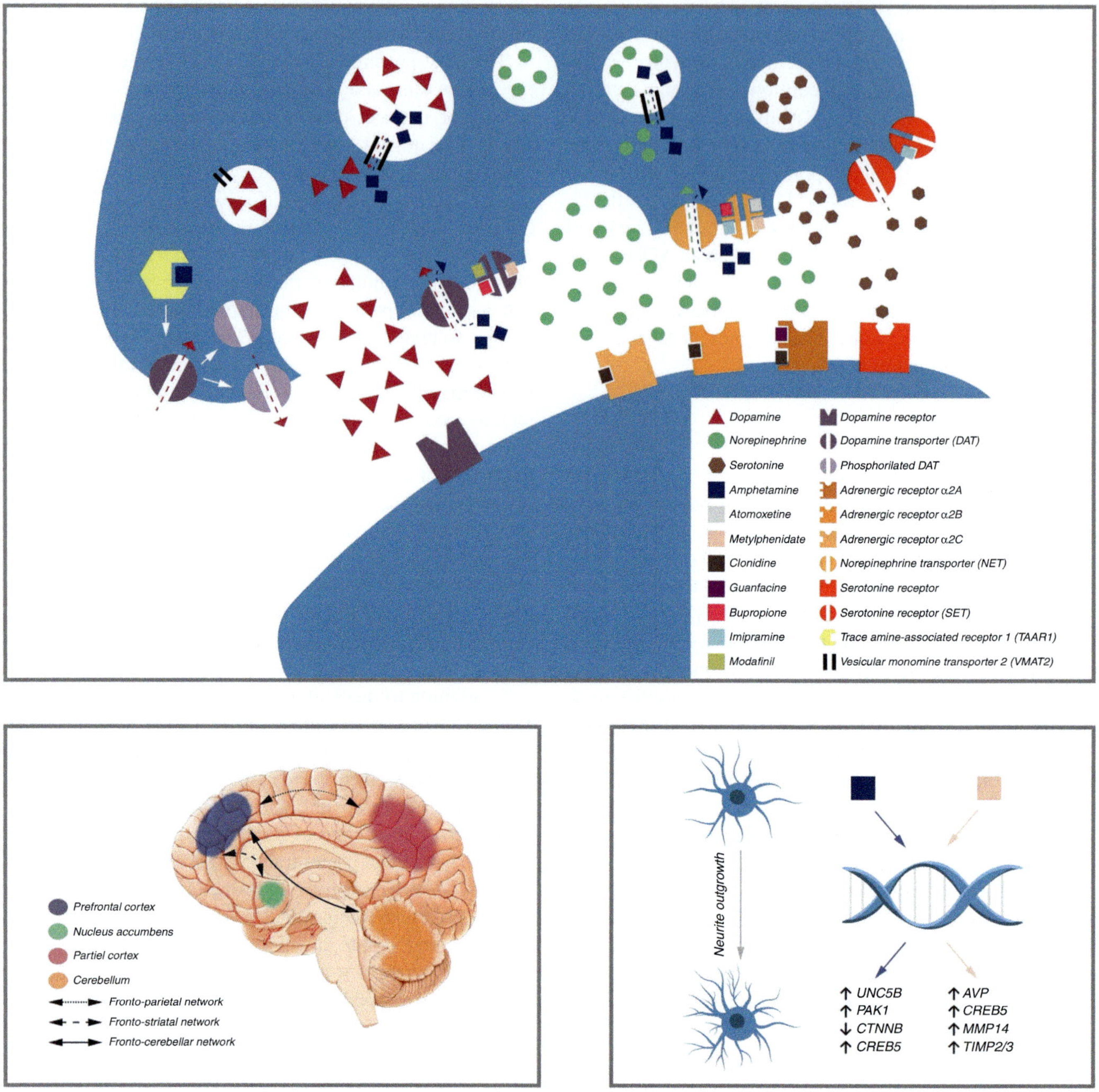

Fig. 12.25 Proposed mechanisms of action for the medications commonly used to treat ADHD. *Pharmacodynamics (superior panel)*: **Amphetamines** have at least three mechanisms of action: (1) they are transported by the monoamine transporters DAT and NET, thus competing with those neurotransmitters and decreasing their reuptake in the synapse; (2) they also cause trace amine-associated receptor 1 (TAAR1) to phosphorylate DAT, and the phosphorylated DAT is either internalized into the presynaptic neuron and ceases transport or inverses the efflux of dopamine; (3) they enter the presynaptic monoamine vesicle and cause efflux of neurotransmitters off the vesicle, which in turn augments the efflux toward the synapse. These mechanisms are more studied and established for dopamine neurotransmission but are thought to occur similarly for norepinephrine. **Atomoxetine** binds to NET, inhibiting the reuptake of norepinephrine. In the prefrontal cortex, where there is much less expression of DAT, dopamine reuptake by NET is also inhibited by the action of atomoxetine. **Methylphenidate** binds to NET and DAT, inhibiting the reuptake of norepinephrine and dopamine. **Clonidine** binds to and activates alpha-2 adrenergic receptors. **Guanfacine** binds to and activates specifically alpha-2A adrenergic receptors. **Bupropion** inhibits DAT and NET weakly. **Imipramine** inhibits NET and SET. **Modafinil** inhibits DAT to a weaker extent than other psychostimulants. *Brain network activation (left inferior panel)*: Pharmacological treatment acutely enhances activation and normalizes brain networks involved in attention, cognitive control, and working memory in children with ADHD. *Neurodevelopmental signal (right inferior panel)*: ADHD medications regulate the expression of genes involved in neurite outgrowth. In the panel, for illustration, we provide mechanisms for methylphenidate and amphetamines. (*From* Caye et al. [189]; *with permission*)

Regarding Racial Bias, ADHD, and Disruptive Disorders

In most of medicine, objective parameters such as vital signs, lab values, radiography, or genetic testing can confirm a diagnosis. In psychiatry, a diagnosis relies exclusively on clinician assessment using qualitative tools, few of which are standardized, and even fewer of which are standardized in demographically diverse populations. As a result, psychiatric diagnoses are more vulnerable to racial, ethnic, and cultural biases than other medical diagnoses. Persistent misdiagnoses can have damaging effects and may lead to inaccurate prognosis, increased stigma, and inappropriate or even unsafe treatments.

Repeated national surveys indicate that African American and Latinx youth with ADHD symptoms are less likely to receive an ADHD diagnosis than white youth and are more likely to receive a disruptive behavior disorder diagnosis, such as oppositional defiant disorder (ODD) or conduct disorder (CD) [115–117]. As a result, these minoritized youth are also less likely to receive ADHD-specific treatments, including medication management [115, 116, 118]. ADHD is a highly heritable disorder with relatively conserved prevalence rates across populations. Therefore, measured prevalence rates between racial or ethnic groups, which are social and not biologic constructs, should theoretically not differ. However, when Getahun and colleagues derived prevalence estimates from over 800,000 youth between 2001 and 2010, they found an ADHD prevalence of 5.6% in white youth, 4.1% in Black youth, and 2.5% in Latinx youth [119]. These disparities appear driven by minoritized youth not receiving an ADHD diagnosis when indicated and not by white children being over-diagnosed [118]. Additionally, youth from families with higher incomes are more likely to receive an ADHD diagnosis than youth using public insurance programs, who are five times more likely to be given disruptive behavior diagnoses [116].

Various factors may contribute to these diagnostic patterns. Clinician implicit bias plays a role and may lead practitioners to interpret underlying anxiety, mood, and post-traumatic symptoms as "oppositional" behaviors [120]. In white youth, the same behaviors are more likely to yield diagnoses of mood, anxiety, or adjustment disorder diagnoses [121]. While ADHD is understood to be strongly genetic, ODD and CD diagnoses are behavioral diagnoses more often associated with family and environmental factors and are therefore more stigmatized. This may help explain why the latter diagnoses are given more often to children living in challenging family circumstances with fewer resources.

Youth who enter the juvenile carceral system in the United States are disproportionately Black and Brown and are particularly affected by these diagnostic trends. Frequently these children carry an ODD or CD diagnosis, but when closely evaluated, they have high rates of ADHD, learning disorders, trauma disorders, and affective or anxiety disorders that have not been adequately diagnosed or treated. For example, in evaluating over 500 detained male youth with diagnoses of CD, Drerup and colleagues found that 92% met the criteria for MDD, GAD, or PTSD, but had not been diagnosed with any of these disorders [122]. Similarly, 30% of carcerally involved youth and 26% of carcerally involved adults have a diagnosis of ADHD, and these numbers are likely underestimates. Improved accuracy of diagnosis and access to treatment has the potential to shift these trends. As it stands, a familiar trajectory to detention involves youth with attention and/or learning problems, with insufficient school supports, reduced access to and/or engagement with mental health care, increased rates of trauma exposure when compared to the general population, increased reactive aggression as a byproduct to such traumas, compounded problems in the classroom with ensuing suspensions or expulsions, limited supervision outside of school, and engagement in substance use and other impulsive activity [123–125].

In cases where ODD or CD are on the differential, best practice involves evaluating for ADHD, underlying learning or intellectual disabilities, mood and anxiety disorders, and post-traumatic stress symptoms, any of which may be driving the problematic behaviors (Fig. 12.26). As diagnoses, CD and ODD capture clusters of behaviors, but these behaviors are driven by other primary factors that require further investigation.

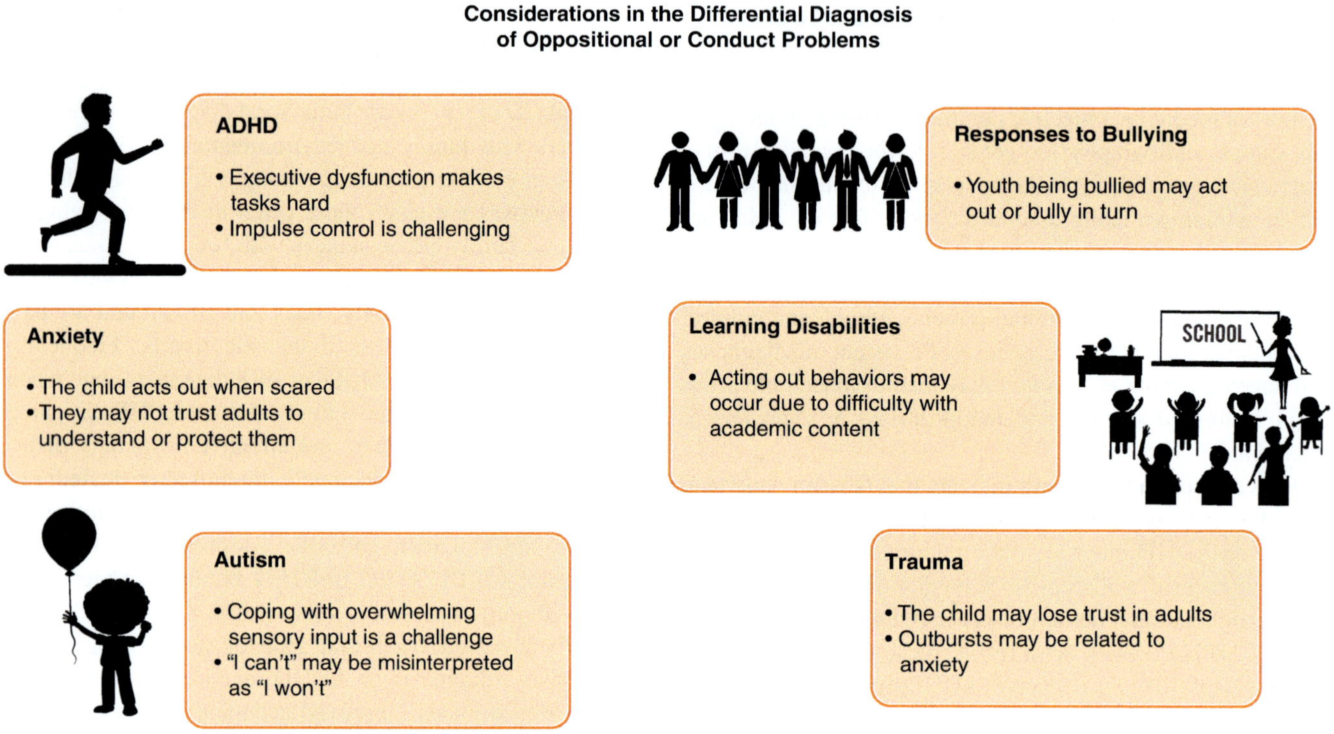

Fig. 12.26 Important diagnostic and etiologic considerations when evaluating oppositional or conduct problems

Oppositional Defiant Disorder

Introduction

Most children engage in oppositional behavior beginning in toddlerhood without long-term impairment. But for some, chronically irritable moods, repeated arguing with authority figures, and periodic vindictiveness can become impairing, affecting their ability to engage with their families, peers, and teachers as they enter school-age years. In these cases, a diagnosis of oppositional defiant disorder (ODD) may be appropriate (Table 12.10). Children meeting the criteria for ODD commonly have comorbid ADHD, requiring true oppositional symptoms to be differentiated from those driven by inattention and poor working memory—for example, is a child not following her parents' instructions because she got distracted or because she actively decided to do the opposite? [126].

Children with ODD are also more likely than other children to have concurrent anxiety or mood disorders, such as major depressive disorder (MDD) or disruptive mood dysregulation disorder (DMDD) [127]. In these cases, depressive symptoms may manifest as pronounced irritability, and anxiety may lead to severe tantrums or rigid resistance to authority figures. Additionally, children diagnosed with ODD are more likely to misinterpret certain social cues as threats and react with aggression, leading to increased interpersonal conflict [128]. A large subset of children with disruptive behavior also have academic underachievement due to learning disorders, which may lead to frustration and acting out behaviors that may be punished through suspension or expulsion [129]. Diagnosis should therefore involve a thorough assessment of mood symptoms, anxiety symptoms, neurodevelopmental profile, and other psychiatric areas. Rating scales such as the Child Behavior Checklist (CBC) are helpful in the differential diagnosis of ODD by comparing the degree of oppositional behaviors to developmental norms [130].

Table 12.10 Quick reference: oppositional defiant disorder

Core features: Pattern of angry/irritable mood, argumentative/defiant behavior, or vindictiveness lasting >6 months and including 4 of 8 defined behaviors *Age:* Under 5 years, behaviors should occur on most days; over 5 years, behaviors should occur at least once per week *Diagnosis:* Comprehensive clinical assessment, parent and teacher rating scales

ODD has commonly been thought of as a precursor to conduct disorder (CD), and there is some diagnostic overlap, particularly in cases of child-onset CD [131]. In prior editions of the Diagnostic and Statistical Manual of Mental Disorders (DSM), a diagnosis of ODD was precluded when the child also met the criteria for CD. However, current data indicate that these are different behavior clusters, and not all youth with ODD go on to develop CD [80]. Similarly, older youth with CD often did not meet the criteria for an ODD diagnosis in childhood. Additionally, unlike in CD, a diagnosis of ODD is associated with and predicts depressive and anxiety disorders, both in childhood and in early adulthood [132]. For these reasons, if a child meets the criteria for both ODD and CD, she or he may be at a higher risk for an underlying affective disorder than the child who has CD alone [80]. Due to these findings, the diagnosis of CD does not preclude the diagnosis of ODD in the current DSM-5.

Epidemiology

Prevalence estimates for ODD vary from 1% to 11% [133]. However, a recent estimate for lifetime prevalence in American youth was 10.2%, with 92.4% of these individuals meeting the criteria for at least one other lifetime psychiatric disorder, including ADHD or CD (68.2%), anxiety disorders (62.3%), mood disorders (45.8%), and substance use disorders (47.2%) [134]. Rates are consistently higher in youth from minoritized and lower-income families. Rates among males and females are equivalent among teenagers, with slightly higher rates in males during grade-school years [135].

Etiology

Several studies suggest that youth with ODD may share genetic comorbidities with ADHD and, to a lesser extent, CD; however, the etiology of ODD is largely viewed as polygenic and multifactorial [136, 137]. Most studies examining disruptive behaviors group ODD, CD, and ADHD together, complicating attempts to identify etiological factors for ODD alone. Liu and colleagues, however, found that a pattern of single nucleotide polymorphisms (SNPs) in the norepinephrine transporter gene (NET1) was more common in youth with ADHD and ODD than in youth with only ADHD [138]. Further studies in this area may better clarify genetic subtypes in these disorders.

Pathophysiology

As in genetic studies, research into the neurobiological underpinnings of ODD has been complicated by the comorbidity of ADHD and the frequent collapsing of ODD and CD into a single diagnostic entity. Temperament and attachment theories are often used to explain trajectories to behavior problems, but current evidence best supports a model based on neurobiologic responses to environmental factors. Increased family stress, poor cohesion, domestic violence, child abuse or neglect, parental substance or personality disorder, parental incarceration, community violence, and experiencing racism have all been correlated with higher rates of oppositional behaviors [139]. Van Goozen and colleagues found that when compared to controls and children with only ADHD, children with ODD had elevated levels of dehydroepiandrosterone sulfate (DHEAS), indicating a change in ACTH functioning in the hypothalamic-pituitary-adrenal (HPA) axis leading to decreased cortisol reactivity, likely due to genetic factors and/or early stressors, such as those above [140].

Developmental theory supports the idea that caregiver response to normally occurring oppositional behavior predicts whether the child will develop adaptive coping skills or become more behaviorally entrenched. Indeed, parental strategies that are punishment-based, inconsistent, or frankly abusive are associated with increased oppositional behavior in children [141]. There may also, however, be biological differences that contribute to a child's response to parent limit-setting. Some parents may find that strategies that work with other children do not work for the child with ODD; youth with ODD have shown reduced responsiveness to warnings of impending consequences when compared to other children [142]. These differences in consequence processing appear to be accompanied by differences in reward processing (i.e., hyposensitivity to reward with decreased dopaminergic functioning) and cognitive control (i.e., impaired reward- and punishment-related decision-making) [143]. Such differences are driven by alternations in the functioning of the autonomic nervous system, HPA axis, amygdala, serotonin and dopamine neurotransmitters, and the cerebral cortex.

Some researchers suggest teasing apart the symptoms of ODD into a behavioral cluster (e.g., arguing, blaming others) and an irritability cluster (e.g., tantrums, easy annoyance, resentment), with the former mapping onto the development of CD and the latter associated with the development of comorbid anxiety or mood disorders [144]. The question remains as to whether these proposed domains are substantiated by reproducible differences in neural system functioning [143, 145].

Phenomenology

Children with ODD often dominate the agenda in their families. In some cases, this may be due to intergenerational exposures to traumatic events that make it difficult for parents to create a reliable and safe environment with structure, limits, and supervision within the home. This may result in inconsistent caregiving that inadvertently cedes control to the child. In other cases, the child may perceive that their parents yield to their demands when they employ predictable oppositional behaviors, which reinforces this pattern. In any case, interrupting the child's control over the family takes consistency and perseverance and often involves an "extinction burst," whereby the child ups the ante of oppositional behavior until the caregiver demonstrates reliable and consistent limits that are clear and predictable.

Treatment

A number of early supports may help reduce the chance that a child will struggle with ODD. Foremost among these are increased access to early preschool programs, for example, Head Start, which use functional assessments to determine the underlying drivers of disruptive behaviors and support the development of self-regulatory and parenting skills [146]. Early identification of neurodevelopmental, learning, and regulatory problems with the initiation of corresponding interventions can make a significant downstream impact.

Depending on the age of the child with problematic oppositional symptoms, behavioral interventions, including parent–child interaction training (PCIT) and parent management training (PMT), have a strong evidence base for improving parenting skills for challenging behaviors, with the result of reducing disruptive behavior and increasing positive interactions between children and their parents [147, 148]. For caregivers for whom in-person training may not be possible, parent training media have also been shown to contribute to long-term improvements [149]. The common components of effective parent training involve an emphasis on positive reinforcement, limited and predictable use of appropriate consequences, practice in making effective commands, ignoring unwanted behaviors, and using behavioral reward systems (Fig. 12.27).

There are no psychopharmacologic interventions that are FDA-approved specifically for targeting ODD symptoms, although medications may be useful for treating underlying comorbidities, such as ADHD, anxiety disorders, or depressive disorders. Accurate identification and treatment of comorbid disorders often lessen the frequency and intensity of disruptive behaviors. When ADHD is present, stimulants and/or alpha agonists may both improve ADHD symptoms and reduce ODD behaviors [150].

The past 20 years have seen an increase in the frequency of atypical antipsychotic and mood stabilizer treatment in children with disruptive behaviors. In fact, an estimated 38% of all antipsychotic prescriptions are written for youth diagnosed with disruptive behavior disorders [151]. Youth covered by Medicaid are four times more likely to be prescribed an antipsychotic than privately-insured youth, and youth in foster care are even more likely than other Medicaid-covered youth to receive such a prescription [151, 152]. Such youth

Understanding children's behaviors:

Behaviors are learned and serve to fulfill a need

Behaviors are preceded by an antecedent and followed by a consequence

Our responses to a behavior (the consequences) can serve to increase or decrease that behavior

Behaviors you like and want to see more of:	**Behaviors you don't like and want to see less of:**	**Unsafe Behaviors**
Parent response: Praise and positive attending	**Parent response:** Planned ignoring	**Parent response:** limit setting and consequences

Fig. 12.27 Example of caregiver worksheet introducing concepts of behavioral parent training

are exceptionally vulnerable and often have a higher burden of psychiatric symptoms due to high trauma loads. For these youth, evidence-based intensive behavioral supports should be implemented first and every effort should be made to accurately diagnose the underlying problems prior to initiation of psychiatric medication.

In cases where behavioral supports have been maximized and acutely dangerous behaviors remain problematic, antipsychotic medications may have a role, although the evidence for their improving aggression in children without a cooccurring neurodevelopmental disorder is limited [153]. Among the mood stabilizers, lithium and valproic acid have demonstrated some short-term benefits in improving disruptive behaviors, most likely by treating underlying mood symptoms [154, 155]. These medications are off-label options for children with severe behavioral symptoms and should be prescribed with care given their limited data, significant side-effect profiles, and the ongoing racial and socioeconomic inequities in prescribing practices.

Conduct Disorder

Introduction

As classified by the DSM-5, conduct disorder (CD) is a diagnosis of persistent behavioral patterns within four specific areas: aggression to people or animals, destruction of property, deceitfulness or theft, or serious violations of rules (Table 12.11). Because of the large number of specific behavior combinations that may meet the criteria for CD, significant heterogeneity and prognosis within the diagnosis exist. In attempts to predict trajectories to ongoing antisocial behaviors or antisocial personality disorder, researchers have defined two subtypes of CD: childhood-onset type, where some diagnostic criteria are met before the age of 10 years, and adolescent-onset type, with symptoms starting after 10 years. Youth with childhood-onset are at greater risk for long-term disruptive and antisocial behaviors than those with symptoms beginning in adolescence [131].

Table 12.11 Quick reference: conduct disorder

Core features: Pattern of violating others' rights or societal norms meeting 3 of 15 specified criteria during the past 12 months in areas of • Aggression to people or animals • Destruction of Property • Deceit/theft • Serious rule violations *Age:* "Childhood-onset" if at least one symptom prior to age 10 years; "adolescent-onset" if symptoms first occur after age 10 years *Diagnosis:* Comprehensive clinical assessment with information from caregiver and teachers

DSM-5 criteria include a further specifier of limited prosocial emotions, with criteria including a lack of remorse or guilt, a callous lack of empathy, a lack of concern about performance, or shallow or deficient affect. These "callous-unemotional" traits have been used to predict later psychopathy; however, outcomes have been mixed, and only about one-third of youth with these traits also meet the criteria for CD, demonstrating the complexity of these associations [132, 156]. Additionally, viewed within a trauma-informed model, criteria such as a lack of concern about performance or deficient affect may be viewed as developmental adaptations to environments where it is not safe to show vulnerability or emotion, for example, or where academic achievement is undermined by learning or behavioral difficulties that lead the child to believe that it is better not to try since failure seems certain regardless of effort [157]. Therefore, it is important to thoughtfully assess these traits in the context of each child's full developmental profile in an effort to identify the underlying causes of the associated problematic behaviors.

This is particularly relevant given that CD is frequently comorbid with ADHD, and impulse problems often precede conduct problems [158]. Not surprisingly, children with childhood-onset CD frequently have higher rates of ADHD, lower IQ scores, and an increased rate of other psychiatric and neurodevelopmental disorders when compared to youth with adolescent-onset CD [135]. Substance use is also frequently associated with a diagnosis of CD, possibly driven by both higher rates of impulsivity and social factors selecting for the adoption of these behaviors. Anxiety disorders frequently co-occur with CD; the combination of anxiety symptoms, impulsivity, and attention deficits appear to be prominent risk factors. Depressive symptoms have been found to precede CD behaviors in some cases, with documented improvement in such behaviors when these symptoms abate [158].

Youth with CD typically progress from minor problematic behaviors to more frequent and serious behaviors, with 45–90% of youth continuing to meet criteria three or 4 years after diagnosis [159]. Continued problems in adulthood may be compounded by continued maladaptive behaviors, psychiatric comorbidities, and consequences of the former (e.g., underemployment or incarceration).

Epidemiology

Prevalence rates of CD range from 2% to 10%, with an average rate of 5%; however, lifetime prevalence has been estimated at 9.5% in the United States, with a 12% rate for males and 7.1% rate for females [158, 160]. Research reflects a steady increase of prevalence rates in males as they age as compared to females, where rates are highest in the teen years [161].

Behaviors included under the diagnosis of CD vary in frequency as a function of age, with physical fighting more common in childhood, for instance, and higher lethality assaults increasing in adolescence and adulthood. As discussed, CD is more commonly diagnosed in minoritized youth, youth living in communities with higher crime and violence rates, and youth from families of lower socioeconomic status [139]. These findings indicate a need for a deeper understanding of developmental and societal factors promoting the emergence of CD behaviors and deeper reflection on how these behaviors are best diagnostically classified and treated.

Etiology

Although multiple biological, psychological, and sociological factors likely contribute to the development of CD, it is widely accepted that CD is a heterogeneous syndrome driven largely by adverse environmental impacts on critical developmental periods. Underlying ADHD appears to increase the risk of developing CD behaviors [162]. Early toxic exposures, such as to maternal smoking, lead, and opioids, have also been correlated with the development of CD, although causality remains unclear [163–165].

Conduct problems are generally correlated with executive functioning deficits and other ADHD symptoms, impaired verbal ability, intellectual disability, and poor social skills [166, 167]. Physical abuse, neglect, domestic violence, parental substance use or mental illness, community violence and disorganization, and affiliation with youth gangs all increase the odds of CD behaviors [139, 168] (Fig. 12.28). Notably, children who are sexually abused have been found to be 12 times more likely than other youth to develop CD [169].

Pathophysiology

Central to understanding the pathophysiology of CD behaviors is the examination of the biological effects of developmental trauma. For instance, males with a variant gene for low monoamine oxidase A (MAO-A) activity were found to be twice as likely to develop CD when compared to controls,

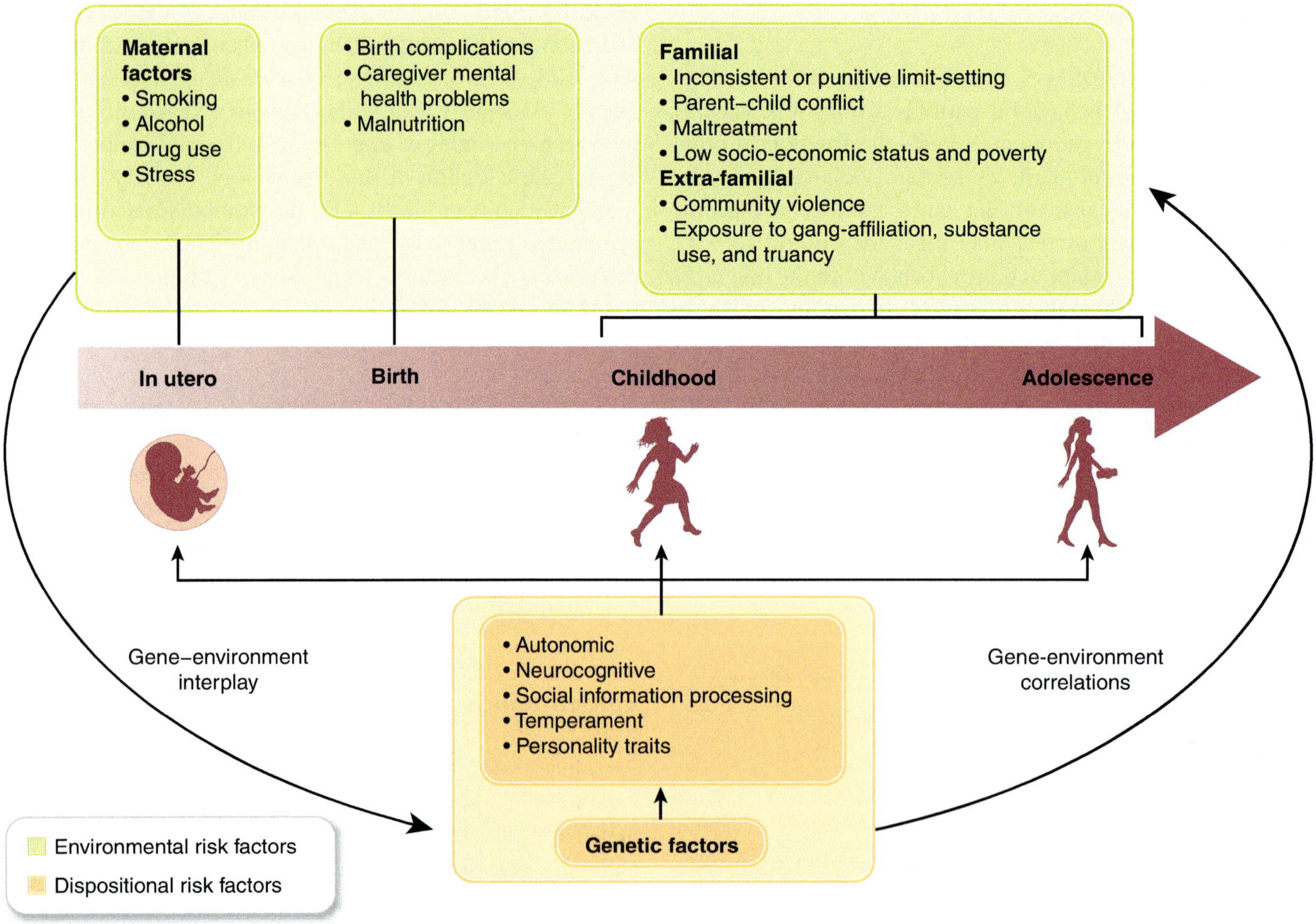

Fig. 12.28 Risk factors for conduct problems at different developmental phases. (*From* Fairchild et al. [190]; *with permission*)

but only if they had a history of childhood abuse [170]. In reviewing three genetic variants including MAO-A, Cicchetti and colleagues similarly found no difference in antisocial behavior in youth with genetic variants who had not experienced maltreatment, while in children experiencing early and/or recurrent abuse, polymorphisms of MAO-A, the short allele of the serotonin transporter gene promoter region (5HTTLPR), and polymorphisms of tryptophan hydroxylase 1 (TPH1) were all associated with increased antisocial behaviors [171].

Additional findings reflect physiologic changes likely driven by traumatic adaptations, although not all reports are consistent. For example, cerebral spinal fluid levels of serotonin metabolite 5-HIAA have been found to be low in youth with CD, although high peripheral serotonin blood levels seem correlated to childhood-onset CD [172, 173]. Low resting heart rate, low skin conductance to intense stimuli, and low salivary cortisol have all been correlated with CD and antisocial behaviors and are linked to neurobiological trauma adaptations [174–176].

Functional neuroimaging studies have highlighted several neural circuits implicated in CD that affect regulation. Rubia and colleagues, for instance, found that youth with CD showed reduced amygdala and ventral prefrontal cortex activation when compared with youth with only ADHD, inferring that orbitofrontal-paralimbic abnormalities appear specific to CD (Fig. 12.29) [177]. Supporting this theory is the work by Sterzer and colleagues, which demonstrated decreased bilateral medial amygdala and anterior insula gray matter volumes that correlated to reduced empathy scores and increased aggressive behavior (Fig. 12.30) [178]. Further investigation may yield biologic insights into the theoretical distinctions between reactive aggression (i.e., aggression in response to a real or perceived provocation, often linked to prior traumatic exposures) and proactive or planned aggression, with possible implications for treatment response and prognosis [143].

Phenomenology

Most individuals with CD have other developmental, behavioral, or psychiatric disorders that affect their presentation. Most children engage in some degree of aggressive behavior through preschool, but children with CD, by definition, develop a consistent pattern of either overt or covert conduct problems after preschool due to difficulties regulating aggression. Covert conduct problems may include truancy or stealing without violence. Overt conduct problems involve either reactive aggression—such as impulsively threatening others or initiating physical fights in response to a perceived threat or provocation—or proactive aggression, such as bullying others, initiating fights, or engaging in unprovoked physical cruelty toward people or animals. Reactive aggression is more common in children who have been abused or bullied, while proactive aggression is thought to be learned through modeling by authority figures and positive reinforcement [179]. Both forms of aggression can develop by multiple pathways (Fig. 12.31).

Problem behaviors associated with CD vary by age, with fighting, bullying, and telling falsehoods being most common in school-age boys and stealing and truancy emerging in early adolescence [180]. As discussed above, youth with childhood-onset CD have a higher prevalence of other neurodevelopmental disorders, lower IQ, and more additional psychiatric disorders than youth who first show problem behaviors in adolescence. They also have a more guarded prognosis, given the complex nature of their underlying developmental problems and the common additional impact of traumatic experiences. Youth who develop CD behaviors in adolescence frequently transition away from these behaviors as they enter adulthood, although complications such as substance use disorders, gang involvement, and incarceration may impede their progress. Caregivers of youth with CD, particularly those with chronic issues themselves, may struggle to engage in treatment and effectively set limits. Interventions supporting these families are of primary importance in the treatment of CD.

Treatment

Psychosocial treatments are the first line in CD, often with a longer timeframe and with more entities involved than for youth with ODD. Effective intervention requires the engagement of all relevant social agencies involved in the youth's care, which may include school, mental health, the juvenile carceral system, and child protection programs. Interventions involving the youth's family in behavioral-skills training are the most effective and include Parent Management Training (PMT, best for less severe cases), Functional Family Therapy (FFT), and Multisystemic Therapy (MST). FFT involves all family members and focuses on improving family communication, while MST is an intensive, home-based program interfacing with all systems in which the child is involved and has been shown to be similar in efficacy to residential programs [181, 182].

In addition to these interventions, each youth should be assessed for comorbid developmental and psychiatric conditions and treated for them. In the school setting, this includes requesting an assessment for an Individualized Education Program (IEP) and a Functional Behavioral Assessment (FBA) to thoroughly assess the antecedents to problem behavior.

Psychiatric medications have a limited role in treating CD and are best employed in treating underlying disorders, such

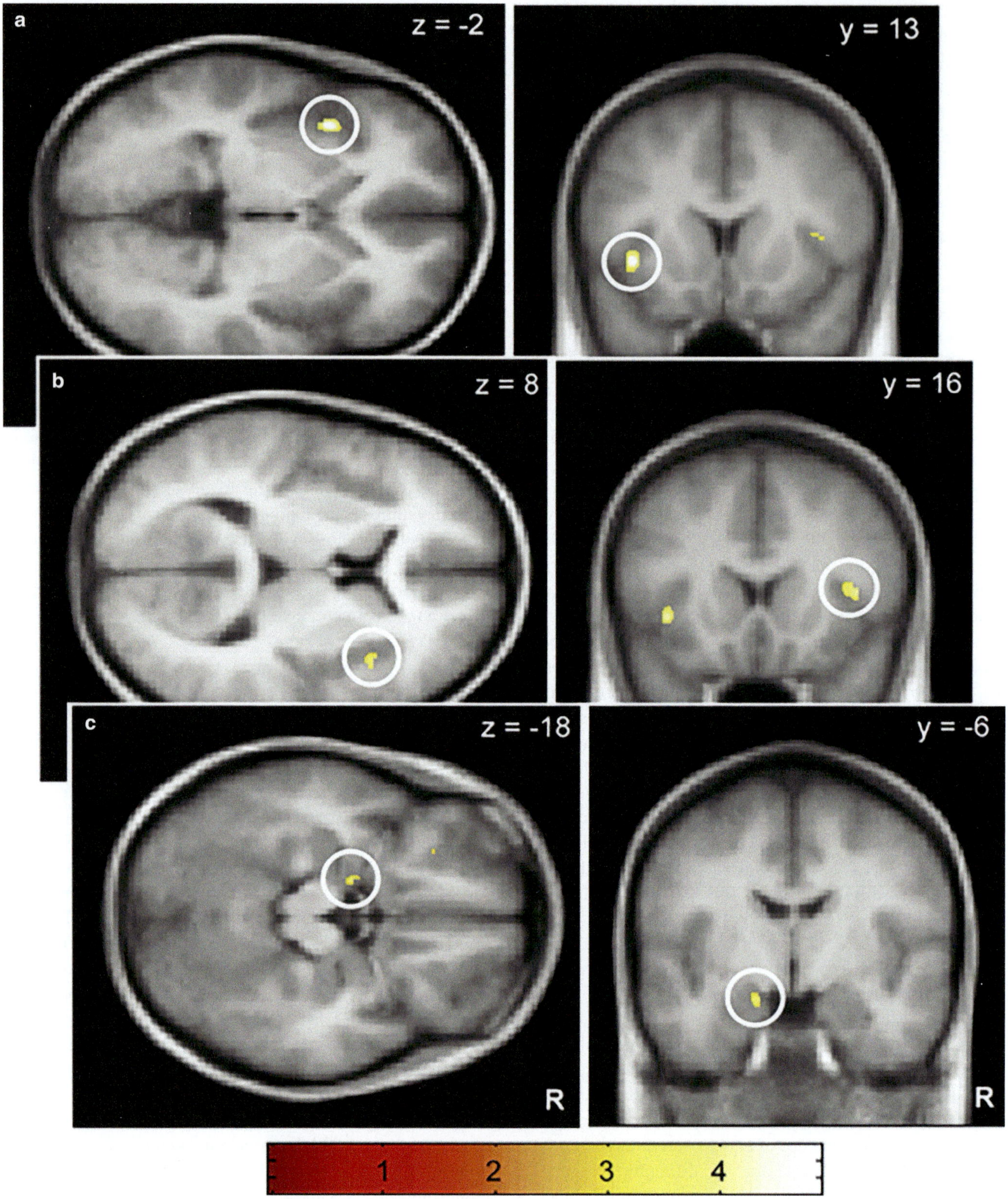

Fig. 12.29 Areas of reduced gray matter volume in adolescents with conduct disorder compared with age- and IQ-matched controls ($n = 12$, respectively) are rendered onto transversal and coronal sections of the mean structural scan of all participants. The scale represents t scores. Significant differences were observed in the left (**a**) and right (**b**) anterior insula and in the left amygdala (**c**). (*From* Sterzer et al. [178]; *with permission*)

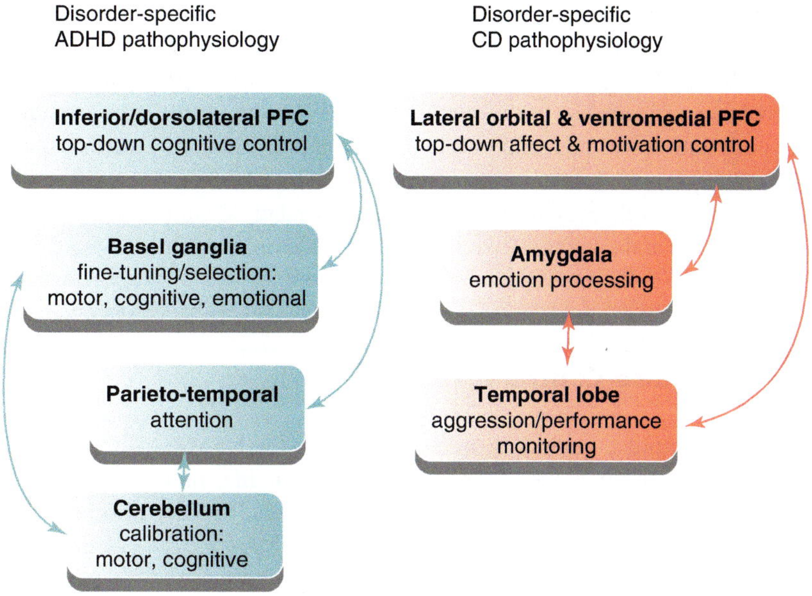

Fig. 12.30 Schematic representation of fMRI evidence for disorder-specific structural and functional brain abnormalities in children with ADHD when compared to children with CD. *ADHD* attention-deficit/hyperactivity disorder, *CD* conduct disorder, *PFC* prefrontal cortex. (*From* Rubia [177]; *with permission*)

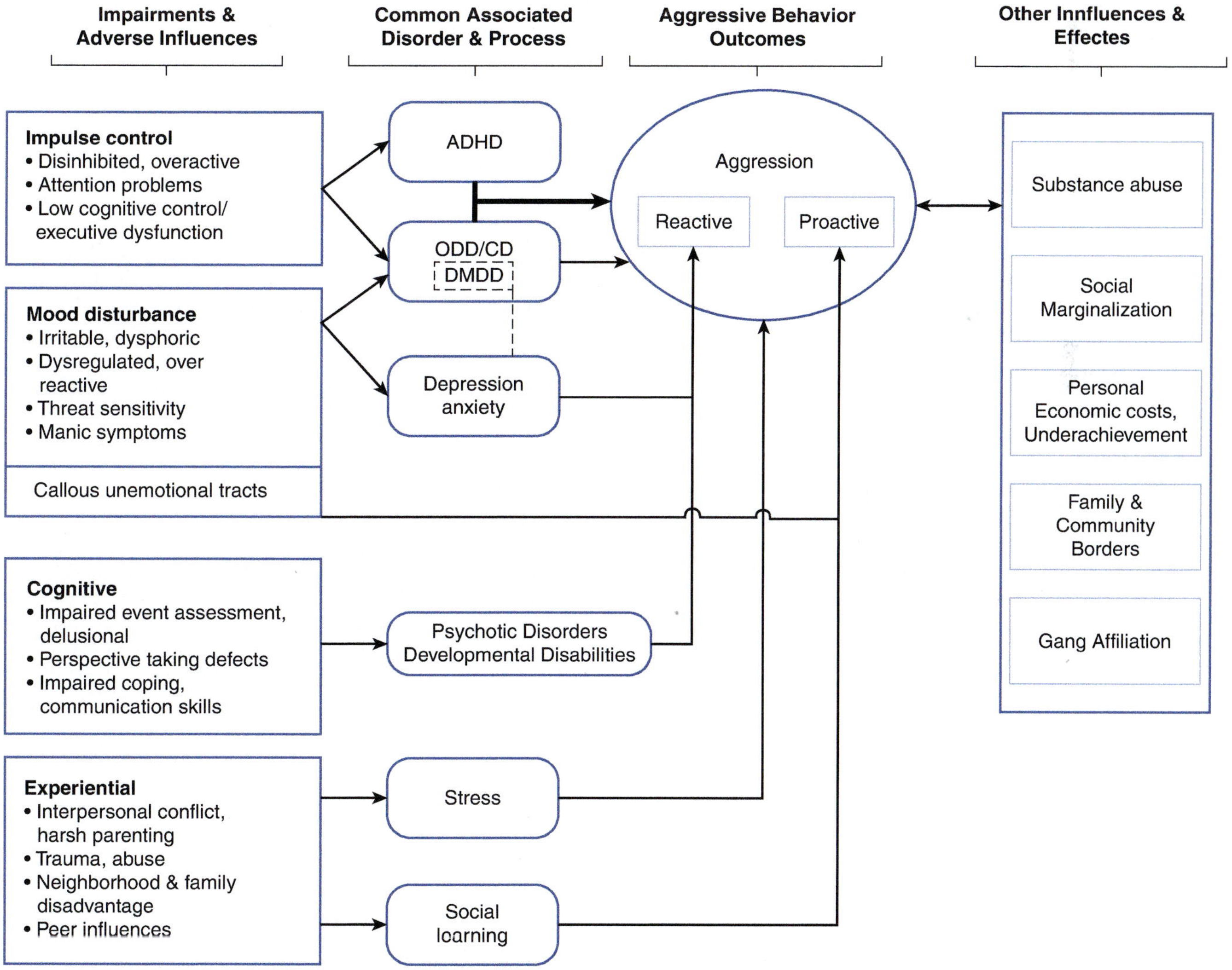

Fig. 12.31 Schematic of influences on the development of aggressive behavior. *ADHD* attention-deficit/hyperactivity disorder, *ODD* oppositional defiant disorder, *CD* conduct disorder, *DMDD* disruptive mood dysregulation disorder. (*From* Blader and Jensen [195]; *with permission*)

as ADHD, anxiety, or depressive symptoms. Appropriate treatment of ADHD symptoms with stimulants can reduce impulsive and aggressive behaviors. In cases of extreme aggression, efficacy has been found in the use of risperidone in youth with lower IQs, and to a lesser extent with lithium, clonidine, propranolol, and anticonvulsants [183, 184]. As in ODD, pharmacotherapy for CD is entirely off-label, should be thoughtful and symptom-specific, and is best employed in the context of fully maximized behavioral supports.

Other Impulse-Control Disorders

Additional impulse-control disorders included in the DSM-5 are intermittent explosive disorder (IED), pyromania, and kleptomania, all of which are behavioral diagnoses. IED is characterized by recurrent behavioral outbursts with aggressive impulses that are out of proportion to the provocation, manifested by verbal or physical aggression toward property, animals, or other people, with or without resulting damage or physical injury (Table 12.12). This aggression is notably impulsive rather than premeditated, and some patients with these symptoms may be best understood through the lens of any co-occurring and predisposing neurodevelopmental disorders, such as ASD or ADHD.

Pyromania and kleptomania are older terms that have a long history in the field, albeit with limited dedicated research (Tables 12.13 and 12.14). They refer to impulsive urges to set fires or steal, respectively, and involve a sense of tension before the act with gratification after the act. Essential to both diagnoses is that these acts are not performed for external gain, response to a delusion or hallucination, in the context of a manic episode, or in attempts to enact vengeance or other anger. As in all diagnoses, ascertainment of the patient's development level is essential in order to determine the reasons for the behavior. For instance, in children, fire-setting is commonly associated with ADHD and may develop in the context of family stress, trauma, or even boredom and can be associated with shame and suicidality [185, 186] (Fig. 12.32).

Kleptomania is also associated with multiple comorbid psychiatric diagnoses, including ADHD, eating disorders, depressive and anxiety disorders, gambling disorder, hoarding disorder, and obsessive-compulsive disorder (OCD). In fact, a validated screener for kleptomania is an adaption of the Yale–Brown Obsessive Compulsive Scale (YBOCS), known as the K-YBOCS (YBOCS, Modified for Kleptomania) [187]. Psychotherapy and behavioral treatments are often used for all three of these disorders. Research on psychotropic medication specifically used for these symptoms is limited; however, the opioid antagonist naltrexone has shown some benefit in treating kleptomania [187]. Otherwise, given the high degree of psychiatric comorbidity, prescribers may choose to use medications to target underlying symptoms of impulsivity, obsessive thoughts, or aggression in order to globally reduce symptoms that may worsen these behaviors.

Table 12.12 Quick reference: intermittent explosive disorder

Core features: Recurrent behavioral outbursts involving aggression toward property, animals, or people, occurring on average twice weekly for 3 months, or resulting in 3 instances of damage or injury within the last 12 months. Outbursts are disproportionate to the precipitating event and are not used as a means to achieve an end
Age: Age must be greater than 6 years
Diagnosis: Requires rule out of aggressive behavior related to adjustment disorders.

Table 12.13 Quick reference: pyromania

Core features: Deliberate setting of more than one fire with tension or arousal before act, fascination with fire or paraphernalia, pleasure or gratification when fire set, and no other external motive for fire-setting
Age: No age stipulation
Diagnosis: Do not diagnose if better explained by manic symptoms, conduct disorder, or antisocial personality disorder

Table 12.14 Quick reference: kleptomania

Core features: Recurrent failure to steal objects not needed for personal use or monetary value, associated with tension before theft and gratification afterward, and not associated with motivations related to anger, delusions, or hallucinations
Age: No age stipulation
Diagnosis: Do not diagnose if better explained by manic symptoms, conduct disorder, or antisocial personality disorder

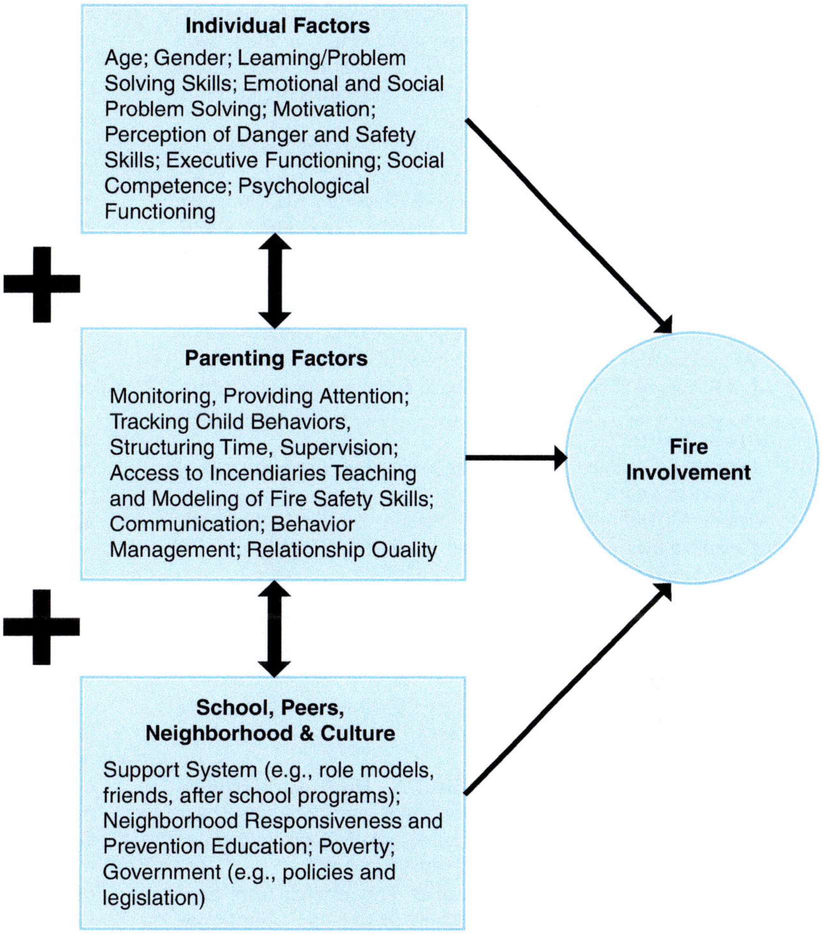

Fig. 12.32 Possible contributing factors to nonpyromania fire-setting in youth. (*From* Barreto et al. [196]; *with permission*)

Conclusion

Through the thoughtful assessment of neurodevelopment, clinicians can make sense of the complex constellation of problems with which children and their families present. A strong foundation in this developmental perspective opens the door for a more comprehensive understanding of patients of all ages. Accurate assessment and treatment of neurodevelopmental, disruptive, impulse-control, and conduct disorders require a team, repeated observation, and awareness of structural forces that have led to racial and other inequities in diagnosis and treatment. Attempting to uncover the root sources of the problem behaviors is key, and comorbidity is the rule rather than the exception. By honing these skills, clinicians are better positioned to provide accurate, effective, compassionate, and strength-based care.

References

1. Winston AS, Winston AS. Scientific Racism and North American psychology. In: Oxford research encyclopedia of psychology; 2020.
2. Hudson JB. Scientific racism: the politics of tests, race and genetics. Black Scholar. 1995;25(1):3–10.
3. Maulik PK, Mascarenhas MN, Mathers CD, Dua T, Saxena S. Prevalence of intellectual disability: a meta-analysis of population-based studies. Res Dev Disabil. 2011;32(2):419–36.
4. American Psychiatric Association. American Psychiatric Association: diagnostic and statistical manual of mental disorders 5th Edition. 2013.
5. Moeschler JB. Neurodevelopmental disabilities. 7th ed. Philadelphia, PA: Elsevier Inc.; 2018.
6. Siegel M, et al. Practice parameter for the assessment and treatment of psychiatric disorders in children and adolescents with intellectual disability (intellectual developmental disorder). J Am Acad Child Adolesc Psychiatry. 2020;59(4):468–96.
7. Dykens EM. Annotation: psychopathology in children with intellectual disability. J Child Psychol Psychiatry Allied Discip. 2000;41(4):407–17.
8. Reiss S, Szyszko J. Diagnostic overshadowing and professional experience with mentally retarded persons. Am J Ment Defic. 1983;87(4):396–402.
9. Ali A, Hassiotis A. Illness in people with intellectual disabilities. BMJ. 2008;336(7644):570–1. https://doi.org/10.1136/bmj.39490.543137.80.
10. O'Handley RD, Ford WB, Radley KC, Helbig KA, Wimberly JK. Social skills training for adolescents with intellectual disabilities: a school-based evaluation. Behav Modif. 2016;40(4). https://doi.org/10.1177/0145445516629.
11. Vereenooghe L, Langdon PE. Psychological therapies for people with intellectual disabilities: a systematic review and meta-analysis. Res Dev Disabil. 2013;34(11):4085–102.
12. Shireman TI, Reichard A, Rigler SK. Medicaid youths with disabilities. J Child Adolesc Psychopharmacol. 2005;15(1):107–15.

13. Sheehan R, Horsfall L, Strydom A, Osborn D, Walters K, Hassiotis A. Movement side effects of antipsychotic drugs in adults with and without intellectual disability: UK population-based cohort study. BMJ Open. 2017;7(8):e017406. https://doi.org/10.1136/bmjopen-2017-017406.
14. Snyder T.D, de Brey C, Dillow SA. Digest of education statistics 2018 (NCES 2020–009). 2019.
15. Moll K, Göbel SM, Gooch D, Landerl K, Snowling MJ. Cognitive risk factors for specific learning disorder: processing speed, temporal processing, and working memory. J Learn Disabil. 2014;49(3):272–81.
16. Berninger VW, Hart TM. A developmental neuropsychological perspective for Reading and writing acquisition. Educ Psychol. 1992. https://doi.org/10.1207/S15326985EP2704_2.
17. Moll K, Kunze S, Neuhoff N, Bruder J, Schulte-Körne G. Specific learning disorder: Prevalence and gender differences. PLoS One. 2014;9(7):e103537.
18. Muir WJ. Genetics advances and learning disability. Br J Psychiatry. 2000;176:12–9.
19. Alarcón M, DeFries JC, Light JG, Pennington BF. A twin study of mathematics disability. J Learn Disabil. 1997;30(6):617–23. https://doi.org/10.1177/002221949703000605.
20. Paracchini S, Diaz R, Stein J. Advances in dyslexia genetics—new insights into the role of brain asymmetries, Adv Genet. 2016;96:53–97. https://doi.org/10.1016/bs.adgen.2016.08.003. Epub 2016 Oct 5.
21. Carrion-Castillo A, Franke B, Fisher SE. Molecular genetics of dyslexia: an overview. Dyslexia. 2013;19(4):214–40. https://doi.org/10.1002/dys.1464.
22. Ashkenazi S, Black JM, Abrams DA, Hoeft F, Menon V. Neurobiological underpinnings of math and Reading learning disabilities. J Learn Disabil. 2013;46(6):549–69. https://doi.org/10.1177/0022219413483174. Epub 2013 Apr 9.
23. Butterworth B, Varma S, Laurillard D. Dyscalculia: from brain to education. Science. 2011;332(6033):1049–53. https://doi.org/10.1126/science.1201536.
24. Grant JG, Siegel LS, D'Angiulli A. From schools to scans: a neuroeducational approach to comorbid math and reading disabilities. Front Public Heal. 2020;8:469. https://doi.org/10.3389/fpubh.2020.00469.
25. Richards TL, Berninger VW, Stock P, Altemeier L, Trivedi P, Maravilla K. Functional magnetic resonance imaging sequential-finger movement activation differentiating good and poor writers. J Clin Exp Neuropsychol. 2009;31(8):967–83. https://doi.org/10.1080/13803390902780201. Epub 2009 Apr 8.
26. Toffalini E, Giofrè D, Cornoldi C. Strengths and weaknesses in the intellectual profile of different subtypes of specific learning disorder: a study on 1,049 diagnosed children. Clin Psychol Sci. 2017;5(2):402–9.
27. McNamara JK, Willoughby T. A longitudinal study of risk-taking behavior in adolescents with learning disabilities. Learn Disabil Res Pract. 2010;25(1):11–24.
28. Cortiella, Candace and Horowitz, Sheldon H. The State of Learning Disabilities: Facts, Trends and Emerging Issues. New York: National Center for Learning Disabilities, 2014.
29. Korhonen J, Linnanmäki K, Aunio P. Learning difficulties, academic Well-being and educational dropout: a person-centred approach. Learn Individ Differ. 2014;31:1–10.
30. George GB, Kathleen MM, Maureen AM. Self-concept of students with learning disabilities: A Meta-analysis, school psychology Review, 2002;31(3)405–27. https://doi.org/10.1080/02796015.2002.12086165.
31. Torgerson CJ, Brooks G, Hall J. A systematic review of the research literature on the use of phonics in the teaching of Reading and spelling. Nottingham DfES Publ. 2006. http://www.dcsf.gov.uk/research/data/uploadfiles/RR711_.pdf.
32. Baker S, Gersten R, Lee DS. A synthesis of empirical research on teaching mathematics to low-achieving students. Elem Sch J. 2002;103:1. https://doi.org/10.1086/499715.
33. Gillespie A, Graham S. A meta-analysis of writing interventions for students with learning disabilities. Except Child. 2014;80(4). https://doi.org/10.1177/00144029145272.
34. Wing L. The history of ideas on autism - legends, myths and reality. Autism. 1997;1(1). https://doi.org/10.1177/136236139701100.
35. Bettelheim B. The autistic anlage. In: The empty fortress: infantile autism and the birth of the self; 1967. The Free Press, 866 Third Avenue, New York, New York.
36. Zwaigenbaum L, et al. Early intervention for children with autism spectrum disorder under 3 years of age: recommendations for practice and research. Pediatrics. 2015;136(1):S60–81. https://doi.org/10.1542/peds.2014-3667E.
37. Mandell DS, Morales KH, Xie M, Lawer LJ, Stahmer AC, Marcus SC. Age of diagnosis among medicaid-enrolled children with autism, 2001-2004. Psychiatr Serv. 2010;61(8):822–9. https://doi.org/10.1176/ps.2010.61.8.822.
38. Mandell DS, Listerud J, Levy SE, Pinto-Martin JA. Race differences in the age at diagnosis among medicaid-eligible children with autism. J Am Acad Child Adolesc Psychiatry. 2002;J Am Acad Child Adolesc Psychiatry. 2002;41(12):1447–53. https://doi.org/10.1097/00004583-200212000-00016.
39. Myers SM, Johnson CP, Council on Children With Disabilities. Management of children with autism spectrum disorders the council on children with disabilities. Pediatrics. 2007;120(5):1162–82. https://doi.org/10.1542/peds.2007-2362.
40. A. L. Siu, "Screening for autism spectrum disorder in young children US preventive services task force recommendation statement," JAMA - J Am Med Assoc, 2016.
41. Guthrie W, et al. Accuracy of autism screening in a large pediatric network. Pediatrics. 2019;144(4):e20183963. https://doi.org/10.1542/peds.2018-3963.
42. Lord C, Rutter M, DiLavore P, Risi S, Gotham K, Bishop S. Autism diagnostic observation schedule, (ADOS-2) Modules 1–4. 2012. WPS Publishers, Torrance, CA.
43. Lord C, Rutter M, Le Couteur A. Autism diagnostic interview-revised: a revised version of a diagnostic interview for caregivers of individuals with possible pervasive developmental disorders. J Autism Dev Disord. 1994;24(5):659–85. https://doi.org/10.1007/BF02172145.
44. Christensen DL, et al. Prevalence and characteristics of autism spectrum disorder among children aged 8 years - autism and developmental disabilities monitoring network, 11 sites, United States, 2012. MMWR Surveill Summ; 2016.
45. Ankenman K, Elgin J, Sullivan K, Vincent L, Bernier R. Nonverbal and verbal cognitive discrepancy profiles in autism spectrum disorders: influence of age and gender. Am J Intellect Dev Disabil. 2014;119(1):84–99. https://doi.org/10.1352/1944-7558-119.1.84.
46. Sparrow SS, Cicchetti DV, Balla DA. Vineland adaptive behavior scales (2nd ed.). Circle Pines, MN: American Guidance Service. 2005.
47. Baxter AJ, Brugha TS, Erskine HE, Scheurer RW, Vos T, Scott JG. The epidemiology and global burden of autism spectrum disorders. Psychol Med. 2015;45(3):601–13.
48. Maenner MJ, et al. Prevalence of autism spectrum disorder among children aged 8 years-autism and developmental disabilities monitoring network, 11 sites, United States, 2016. MMWR Surveill Summ; 2020.
49. Loomes R, Hull L, Mandy WPL. What is the male-to-female ratio in autism Spectrum disorder? A systematic review and meta-analysis. J Am Acad Child Adolesc Psychiatry. 2017;56(6):466–74.
50. Tick B, Bolton P, Happé F, Rutter M, Rijsdijk F. Heritability of autism spectrum disorders: a meta-analysis of twin studies. J Child Psychol Psychiatry Allied Discip. 2016;57(5):585–95. https://doi.org/10.1111/jcpp.12499.

51. Risch N, Hoffmann TJ, Anderson M, Croen LA, Grether JK, Windham GC. Familial recurrence of autism spectrum disorder: evaluating genetic and environmental contributions. Am J Psychiatry. 2014;171(11):1206–13. https://doi.org/10.1176/appi.ajp.2014.13101359.
52. Lord C, et al. Autism spectrum disorder. Nat Rev Dis Prim. 2020;6(1):1–23.
53. Sanders SJ, et al. Insights into autism Spectrum disorder genomic architecture and biology from 71 risk loci. Neuron. 2015;87(6):1215–33.
54. Shen Y, et al. Clinical genetic testing for patients with autism spectrum disorders. Pediatrics. 2010;125(4):e727–35. https://doi.org/10.1542/peds.2009-1684.
55. Modabbernia A, Velthorst E, Reichenberg A. Environmental risk factors for autism: an evidence-based review of systematic reviews and meta-analyses. Mol Autism. 2017;8(1):1–16.
56. Taylor LE, Swerdfeger AL, Eslick GD. Vaccines are not associated with autism: an evidence-based meta-analysis of case-control and cohort studies. Vaccine. 2014;32(29):3623–9.
57. Raznahan A, et al. Compared to what? Early brain overgrowth in autism and the perils of population norms. Biol Psychiatry. 2013;74(8):563–75. https://doi.org/10.1016/j.biopsych.2013.03.022.
58. Hazlett HC, et al. Early brain development in infants at high risk for autism spectrum disorder. Nature. 2017;542(7641):348–51. https://doi.org/10.1038/nature21369.
59. Casanova MF, et al. Focal cortical dysplasias in autism spectrum disorders. Acta Neuropathol Commun. 2014;1:67. https://doi.org/10.1186/2051-5960-1-67.
60. Malow BA. Sleep disorders, epilepsy, and autism. Ment Retard Dev Disabil Res Rev. 2004;10(2):122–5. https://doi.org/10.1002/mrdd.20023.
61. Gorrindo P, Williams KC, Lee EB, Walker LS, McGrew SG, Levitt P. Gastrointestinal dysfunction in autism: parental report, clinical evaluation, and associated factors. Autism Res. 2012;5(2):101–8. https://doi.org/10.1002/aur.237.
62. Lloyd M, MacDonald M, Lord C. Motor skills of toddlers with autism spectrum disorders. Autism. 2013;17(2):133–46. https://doi.org/10.1177/1362361311402230.
63. Coury D, Jones NE, Klatka K, Winklosky B, Perrin JM. Healthcare for children with autism: the autism treatment network. Curr Opin Pediatr. 2009;21(6):828–32. https://doi.org/10.1097/MOP.0b013e328331eaaa.
64. Educating Children with Autism 2001. National Academy of Sciences - National Research Council, Washington, DC.; National Academy of Sciences - National Research Council, Washington, DC. Commission on Behavioral and Social Sciences and Education. National Academy Press, Washington, DC.
65. Schreibman L, et al. Naturalistic developmental behavioral interventions: empirically validated treatments for autism Spectrum disorder. J Autism Dev Disord. 2015;45(8):2411–28. https://doi.org/10.1007/s10803-015-2407-8.
66. Laugeson EA, Frankel F, Gantman A, Dillon AR, Mogil C. Evidence-based social skills training for adolescents with autism spectrum disorders: the UCLA PEERS program. J Autism Dev Disord. 2012;42(6):1025–36. https://doi.org/10.1007/s10803-011-1339-1.
67. Knight T, Steeves T, Day L, Lowerison M, Jette N, Pringsheim T. Prevalence of tic disorders: a systematic review and meta-analysis. Pediatr Neurol. 2012;47(2):77–90. https://doi.org/10.1016/j.pediatrneurol.2012.05.002.
68. Leckman JF, Riddle MA, Hardin MT, et al. J Am Acad Child Adolesc Psychiatry. 1989;28(4):566–73. https://doi.org/10.1097/00004583-198907000-00015.
69. Robertson MM. Attention deficit hyperactivity disorder, tics and Tourette's syndrome: the relationship and treatment implications. A commentary. Eur Child Adolesc Psychiatry. 2006;15(1):1–11. https://doi.org/10.1007/s00787-006-0505-z.
70. Simonoff E, Pickles A, Charman T, Chandler S, Loucas T, Baird G. Psychiatric disorders in children with autism spectrum disorders: prevalence, comorbidity, and associated factors in a population-derived sample. J Am Acad Child Adolesc Psychiatry. 2008;47(8):921–9. https://doi.org/10.1097/CHI.0b013e318179964f.
71. State MW. The genetics of Tourette disorder. Curr Opin Genet Dev. 2011;Curr Opin Genet Dev. 2011;21(3):302–9. https://doi.org/10.1016/j.gde.2011.01.007.
72. Leckman JF, Fernandez TV. The origins of Tourette syndrome: prenatal risk factors and the promise of birth cohort studies. J Am Acad Child Adolesc Psychiatry. 2016;55(9):751–3. https://doi.org/10.1016/j.jaac.2016.06.009.
73. Swedo SE. From research subgroup to clinical syndrome: modifying the PANDAS criteria to describe PANS (pediatric acute-onset neuropsychiatric syndrome). Pediatr Ther. 2012;2(2):1–8.
74. Ganos C. Tics and Tourette's: update on pathophysiology and tic control. Curr Opin Neurol. 2016;29(4):513–8. https://doi.org/10.1097/WCO.0000000000000356.
75. Nespoli E, Rizzo F, Boeckers TM, Hengerer B, Ludolph AG. Addressing the complexity of Tourette's syndrome through the use of animal models. Front Neurosci. 2016;10:133. https://doi.org/10.3389/fnins.2016.00133.
76. Leckman JF, Walker DE, Cohen DJ. Premonitory urges in Tourette's syndrome. Am J Psychiatry. 1993;150(1):98–102. https://doi.org/10.1176/ajp.150.1.98.
77. Piacentini J, et al. Behavior therapy for children with Tourette disorder. JAMA. 2010;303(19):1929–37. https://doi.org/10.1001/jama.2010.607.
78. Kurlan R, et al. Treatment of ADHD in children with tics: a randomized controlled trial. Neurology. 2002;58(4):527–36. https://doi.org/10.1212/wnl.58.4.527.
79. Goodman WK, Storch EA, Geffken GR, Murphy TK. Obsessive-compulsive disorder in Tourette syndrome. J Child Neurol. 2006;21(8):704–14. https://doi.org/10.1177/08830738060210081201.
80. Frick PJ, Nigg JT. Current issues in the diagnosis of attention deficit hyperactivity disorder, oppositional defiant disorder, and conduct disorder. Annu Rev Clin Psychol. 2012;8:77–107. https://doi.org/10.1146/annurev-clinpsy-032511-143150.
81. Swanson J, et al. Evidence, interpretation, and qualification from multiple reports of long-term outcomes in the multimodal treatment study of children with ADHD (MTA): part II: supporting details. J Atten Disord. 2008;12(1):4–14. https://doi.org/10.1177/1087054708319345.
82. Shaw P, Stringaris A, Nigg J, Leibenluft E. Emotion dysregulation in attention deficit hyperactivity disorder. Am J Psychiatr. 2014;171(3):276–93. https://doi.org/10.1176/appi.ajp.2013.13070966.
83. Swanson JM, et al. Categorical and dimensional definitions and evaluations of symptoms of ADHD: history of the SNAP and the SWAN rating scales. Int J Educ Psychol Assess. 2012;10(1):51–70.
84. Wolraich ML, Lambert W, Doffing MA, Bickman L, Simmons T, Worley K. Psychometric properties of the Vanderbilt ADHD diagnostic parent rating scale in a referred population. J Pediatr Psychol. 2003;28(8):559–67. https://doi.org/10.1093/jpepsy/jsg046.
85. Conners CK. Conners 3rd edition (Conners 3). 2008. WPS Publishers: Torrance, CA.
86. Sonuga-Barke EJS, Sergeant JA, Nigg J, Willcutt E. Executive dysfunction and delay aversion in attention deficit hyperactivity disorder: nosologic and diagnostic implications. Child Adolesc Psychiatr Clin N Am. 2008;17(2):367–84, ix. https://doi.org/10.1016/j.chc.2007.11.008.

87. Adler L, Cohen J. Diagnosis and evaluation of adults with attention-deficit/hyperactivity disorder. Psychiatr Clin N Am. 2004;27(2):187–201. https://doi.org/10.1016/j.psc.2003.12.003.
88. Adler LA, Faraone SV, Spencer TJ, Berglund P, Alperin S, Kessler RC. The structure of adult ADHD. Int J Methods Psychiatr Res. 2017;26(1):e1555. https://doi.org/10.1002/mpr.1555.
89. Jensen PS. A 14-month randomized clinical trial of treatment strategies for attention-deficit/hyperactivity disorder. Arch Gen Psychiatry. 1999;56(12):1073–86. https://doi.org/10.1001/archpsyc.56.12.1073.
90. Molina BSG, et al. The MTA at 8 years: prospective follow-up of children treated for combined-type ADHD in a multisite study. J Am Acad Child Adolesc Psychiatry. 2009;48(5):484–500. https://doi.org/10.1097/CHI.0b013e31819c23d0.
91. Molina BSG, et al. Adolescent substance use in the multimodal treatment study of attention-deficit/hyperactivity disorder (ADHD) (MTA) as a function of childhood ADHD, random assignment to childhood treatments, and subsequent medication. J Am Acad Child Adolesc Psychiatry. 2013;52(3):250–63. https://doi.org/10.1016/j.jaac.2012.12.014.
92. Polanczyk G, De Lima MS, Horta BL, Biederman J, Rohde LA. The worldwide prevalence of ADHD: a systematic review and metaregression analysis. Am J Psychiatry. 2007;164(6):942–8. https://doi.org/10.1176/ajp.2007.164.6.942.
93. Visser SN, et al. Treatment of attention deficit/hyperactivity disorder among children with special health care needs. J Pediatr. 2015;166(6):1423–30.e2.
94. Elkins IJ, Malone S, Keyes M, Iacono WG, Mcgue M. The impact of attention-deficit/hyperactivity disorder on preadolescent adjustment may be greater for girls than for boys. J Clin Child Adolesc Psychol. 2011;40(4):532–45. https://doi.org/10.1080/15374416.2011.581621.
95. Thapar A, Cooper M, Eyre O, Langley K. What have we learnt about the causes of ADHD? J Child Psychol Psychiatry. 2013;54(1):3–16.
96. Neale BM, et al. Meta-analysis of genome-wide association studies of attention-deficit/ hyperactivity disorder. J Am Acad Child Adolesc Psychiatry. 2010;49(9):884–97. https://doi.org/10.1016/j.jaac.2010.06.008.
97. Sharp SI, McQuillin A, Gurling HMD. Genetics of attention-deficit hyperactivity disorder (ADHD). Neuropharmacology. 2009;57(7–8):590–600. https://doi.org/10.1016/j.neuropharm.2009.08.011.
98. Nigg JT, Nikolas M, Mark Knottnerus G, Cavanagh K, Friderici K. Confirmation and extension of association of blood lead with attention-deficit/hyperactivity disorder (ADHD) and ADHD symptom domains at population-typical exposure levels. J Child Psychol Psychiatry Allied Discip. 2010;51(1):58–65. https://doi.org/10.1111/j.1469-7610.2009.02135.x.
99. Arnsten AFT. Catecholamine influences on dorsolateral prefrontal cortical networks. Biol Psychiatry. 2011;69(12):e89–99. https://doi.org/10.1016/j.biopsych.2011.01.027.
100. Oldehinkel M, Beckmann CF, Pruim RH, van Oort ES, Franke B, Hartman CA, Hoekstra PJ, Oosterlaan J, Heslenfeld D, Buitelaar JK, Mennes M. Attention-Deficit/Hyperactivity Disorder symptoms coincide with altered striatal connectivity. Biol Psychiatry Cogn Neurosci Neuroimaging. 2016;1(4):353–63. https://doi.org/10.1016/j.bpsc.2016.03.008. Epub 2016 Apr 13. PMID: 27812554; PMCID: PMC5087803.
101. Shaw P, Malek M, Watson B, Sharp W, Evans A, Greenstein D. Development of cortical surface area and gyrification in attention-deficit/hyperactivity disorder. Biol Psychiatry. 2012;72(3):191–7. https://doi.org/10.1016/j.biopsych.2012.01.031.
102. Sripada C, Kessler D, Fang Y, Welsh RC, Prem Kumar K, Angstadt M. Disrupted network architecture of the resting brain in attention-deficit/hyperactivity disorder. Hum Brain Mapp. 2014;35(9):4693–705. https://doi.org/10.1002/hbm.22504.
103. Plichta MM, Scheres A. Ventral-striatal responsiveness during reward anticipation in ADHD and its relation to trait impulsivity in the healthy population: a meta-analytic review of the fMRI literature. Neurosci Biobehav Rev. 2014;38:125–34. https://doi.org/10.1016/j.neubiorev.2013.07.012.
104. Bertelsen EN, Larsen JT, Petersen L, Christensen J, Dalsgaard S. Childhood epilepsy, febrile seizures, and subsequent risk of ADHD. Pediatrics. 2016;138(2):e20154654. https://doi.org/10.1542/peds.2015-4654.
105. Hesdorffer DC, Ludvigsson P, Olafsson E, Gudmundsson G, Kjartansson O, Hauser WA. ADHD as a risk factor for incident unprovoked seizures and epilepsy in children. Arch Gen Psychiatry. 2004;61(7):731–6. https://doi.org/10.1001/archpsyc.61.7.731.
106. Sadeh A, Pergamin L, Bar-Haim Y. Sleep in children with attention-deficit hyperactivity disorder: a meta-analysis of polysomnographic studies. Sleep Med Rev. 2006;10(6):381–98. https://doi.org/10.1016/j.smrv.2006.03.004.
107. Jerome L. Some observations on the phenomenology of thought disorder; a neglected sign in attention-deficit hyperperactivity disorder. Can Child Adolesc Psychiatr Rev. 2003;12(3):92–93.
108. Shattell MM, Bartlett R, Rowe T. 'I have always felt different': the experience of attention-deficit/hyperactivity disorder in childhood. J Pediatr Nurs. 2008;23(1):49–57. https://doi.org/10.1016/j.pedn.2007.07.010.
109. Erskine HE, et al. Long-term outcomes of attention-deficit/hyperactivity disorder and conduct disorder: a systematic review and meta-analysis. J Am Acad Child Adolesc Psychiatry. 2016;55(10):841–50.
110. Goode AP, et al. Nonpharmacologic treatments for attention-deficit/hyperactivity disorder: a systematic review. Pediatrics. 2018;141(6):e20180094. https://doi.org/10.1542/peds.2018-0094.
111. Arnold LE. Methylphenidate vs. amphetamine: comparative review. J Atten Disord. 2000;3:200–11.
112. Winterstein AG, et al. Cardiovascular safety of central nervous system stimulants in children and adolescents: population based cohort study. BMJ. 2012;345:e4627. https://doi.org/10.1136/bmj.e4627.
113. Humphreys KL, Eng T, Lee SS. Stimulant medication and substance use outcomes ameta-analysis. JAMA, Psychiatry. 2013;70(7):740–9. https://doi.org/10.1001/jamapsychiatry.2013.1273.
114. P. Lichtenstein et al., "Medication for Attention Deficit–Hyperactivity Disorder and Criminality," N Engl J Med, 2012. 367:2006–2014.
115. Stevens J, Harman JS, Kelleher KJ. Race/ethnicity and insurance status as factors associated with ADHD treatment patterns. J Child Adolesc Psychopharmacol. 2005;15(1):88–96. https://doi.org/10.1089/cap.2005.15.88.
116. Pastor PN, Reuben CA. Recent trends in childhood attention-deficit/hyperactivity disorder. Public Health Rep. 2005;167(3):282–8. https://doi.org/10.1001/2013.jamapediatrics.401.
117. Flores G, Lin H. Trends in racial/ethnic disparities in medical and oral health, access to care, and use of services in US children: has anything changed over the years? Int J Equity Health. 2013;12:10. https://doi.org/10.1186/1475-9276-12-10.
118. Coker TR, et al. Racial and ethnic disparities in ADHD diagnosis and treatment. Pediatrics. 2016;138(3):e20160407. https://doi.org/10.1542/peds.2016-0407.
119. Getahun D, Jacobsen SJ, Fassett MJ, Chen W, Demissie K, Rhoads GG. Recent trends in childhood attention-deficit/hyperactivity disorder. JAMA Pediatr. 2013;167(3):282–8. https://doi.org/10.1001/2013.jamapediatrics.401.
120. Fadus MC, et al. Unconscious bias and the diagnosis of disruptive behavior disorders and ADHD in African American and Hispanic youth. Acad Psychiatry. 2020;44(1):95–102. https://doi.org/10.1007/s40596-019-01127-6.

121. Feisthamel K, Schwartz R. Differences in mental health counselors' diagnoses based on client race: an investigation of adjustment, childhood, and substance-related disorders. J Ment Heal Couns. 2009;31:47–59.
122. Drerup LC, Croysdale A, Hoffmann NG. Patterns of behavioral health conditions among adolescents in a juvenile justice system. Prof Psychol Res Pract. 2008;39:122–8.
123. Crouch JL, Hanson RF, Saunders BE, Kilpatrick DG, Resnick HS. Income, race/ethnicity, and exposure to violence in youth: results from the national survey of adolescents. J Community Psychol. 2000;28(6):625–41.
124. Nyborg VM, Curry JF. The impact of perceived racism: psychological symptoms among African American boys. J Clin Child Adolesc Psychol. 2003;32(2):258–66. https://doi.org/10.1207/S15374424JCCP3202_11.
125. Suh S, Suh J. Risk factors and levels of risk for high school dropouts. Prof Sch Couns. 2007;10(3):297–306.
126. Lahey B.B, Miller TL, Gordon RA, Riley AW. Developmental epidemiology of the disruptive behavior disorders. In Handbook of disruptive behavior disorders; 1999.
127. Rowe R, Maughan B, Moran P, Ford T, Briskman J, Goodman R. The role of callous and unemotional traits in the diagnosis of conduct disorder. J Child Psychol Psychiatry Allied Discip. 2010;51(6):688–95. https://doi.org/10.1111/j.1469-7610.2009.02199.x.
128. Coy K, Speltz ML, DeKlyen M, Jones K. Social-cognitive processes in preschool boys with and without oppositional defiant disorder. J Abnorm Child Psychol. 2001;29(2):107–19. https://doi.org/10.1023/a:1005279828676.
129. Dodge KA, Pettit GS. A biopsychosocial model of the development of chronic conduct problems in adolescence. Dev Psychol. 2003;39(2):349–71.
130. Achenbach TM, Ruffle TM. The child behavior checklist and related forms for assessing behavioral/emotional problems and competencies. Pediatr Rev. 2000;21(8):265–71. https://doi.org/10.1542/pir.21-8-265.
131. Burke JD, Waldman I, Lahey BB. Predictive validity of childhood oppositional defiant disorder and conduct disorder: implications for the DSM-V. J Abnorm Psychol. 2010;119(4):739–51. https://doi.org/10.1037/a0019708.
132. Rowe R, Costello EJ, Angold A, Copeland WE, Maughan B. Developmental pathways in oppositional defiant disorder and conduct disorder. J Abnorm Psychol. 2010;119(4):726–38. https://doi.org/10.1037/a0020798.
133. Canino G, Polanczyk G, Bauermeister JJ, Rohde LA, Frick PJ. Does the prevalence of CD and ODD vary across cultures? Soc Psychiatry Psychiatr Epidemiol. 2010;45(7):695–704.
134. Nock MK, Kazdin AE, Hiripi E, Kessler RC. Lifetime prevalence, correlates, and persistence of oppositional defiant disorder: Results from the National Comorbidity Survey Replication. J Child Psychol Psychiatry Allied Discip. 2007;48(7):703–13. https://doi.org/10.1111/j.1469-7610.2007.01733.x.
135. Loeber R, Burke JD, Lahey BB, Winters A, Zera M. Oppositional defiant and conduct disorder: a review of the past 10 years, part I. J Am Acad Child Adolesc Psychiatry. 2000;39(12):1468–84. https://doi.org/10.1097/00004583-200012000-00007.
136. Nadder TS, Rutter M, Silberg JL, Maes HH, Eaves LJ. Genetic effects on the variation and covariation of attention deficit-hyperactivity disorder (ADHD) and oppositional-defiant disorder/conduct disorder (ODD/CD) symptomatologies across informant and occasion of measurement. Psychol Med. 2002;32(1):39–53. https://doi.org/10.1017/s0033291701004792.
137. Comings DE, et al. Multivariate analysis of associations of 42 genes in ADHD, ODD and conduct disorder. Clin Genet. 2000;58(1):31–40. https://doi.org/10.1034/j.1399-0004.2000.580106.x.
138. Liu L, Cheng J, Li H, Yang L, Qian Q, Wang Y. The possible involvement of genetic variants of NET1 in the etiology of attention-deficit/hyperactivity disorder comorbid with oppositional defiant disorder. J Child Psychol Psychiatry Allied Discip. 2015;56(1):58–66. https://doi.org/10.1111/jcpp.12278.
139. Burke JD, Loeber R, Birmaher B. Oppositional defiant disorder and conduct disorder: a review of the past 10 years, part II. J Am Acad Child Adolesc Psychiatry. 2002;41(11):1275–93. https://doi.org/10.1097/00004583-200211000-00009.
140. Van Goozen SHM, Van Den Ban E, Matthys W, Cohen-Kettenis PT, Thijssen JHH, Van Engeland H. Increased adrenal androgen functioning in children with oppositional defiant disorder: a comparison with psychiatric and normal controls. J Am Acad Child Adolesc Psychiatry. 2000;39(11):1446–51. https://doi.org/10.1097/00004583-200011000-00020.
141. Gold J, Sullivan MW, Lewis M. The relation between abuse and violent delinquency: the conversion of shame to blame in juvenile offenders. Child Abuse Negl. 2011;35(7):459–67. https://doi.org/10.1016/j.chiabu.2011.02.007. Epub 2011 Jul 23. PMID: 21783253; PMCID: PMC3763505.
142. van Goozen SHM, Cohen-Kettenis PT, Snoek H, Matthys W, Swaab-Barneveld H, van Engeland H. Executive functioning in children: a comparison of hospitalised ODD and ODD/ADHD children and normal controls. J Child Psychol Psychiatry Allied Discip. 2004;45(2):284–92. https://doi.org/10.1111/j.1469-7610.2004.00220.x.
143. Matthys W, Vanderschuren LJMJ, Schutter DJLG. The neurobiology of oppositional defiant disorder and conduct disorder: altered functioning in three mental domains. Dev Psychopathol. 2013;25(1):193–207. https://doi.org/10.1017/S0954579412000272.
144. Stringaris A, Goodman R. Longitudinal outcome of youth oppositionality: irritable, headstrong, and hurtful behaviors have distinctive predictions. J Am Acad Child Adolesc Psychiatry. 2009;48(4):404–12. https://doi.org/10.1097/CHI.0b013e3181984f30.
145. Nelson RJ, Trainor BC. Neural mechanisms of aggression. Nat Rev Neurosci. 2007;8(7):536–46. https://doi.org/10.1038/nrn2174.
146. Dufrene BA, Doggett RA, Henington C, Watson TS. Functional assessment and intervention for disruptive classroom behaviors in preschool and head start classrooms. J Behav Educ. 2007;16(4) p368–88.
147. Herschell AD, Calzada EJ, Eyberg SM, McNeil CB. Parent-child interaction therapy: new directions in research. Cogn Behav Pract. 2002;9:9–16.
148. Kazdin AE. Problem-solving skills training and parent management training for oppositional defiant disorder and conduct disorder. In Evidence-based psychotherapies for children and adolescents; 2012. Guilford Press, NY: NY.
149. Montgomery P, Bjornstad GJ, Dennis JA. Media-based behavioural treatments for behavioural problems in children. Cochrane Database Syst Rev. 2006;2006(1):CD002206.
150. Connor DF, Barkley RA, Davis HT. A pilot study of methylphenidate, clonidine, or the combination in ADHD comorbid with aggressive oppositional defiant or conduct disorder. Clin Pediatr (Phila). 2000;39(1):15–25. https://doi.org/10.1177/000992280003900102.
151. Crystal S, Olfson M, Huang C, Pincus H, Gerhard T. Broadened use of atypical antipsychotics: safety, effectiveness, and policy challenges. Health Aff. 2009;28(5):w770–81. https://doi.org/10.1377/hlthaff.28.5.w770.
152. DosReis S, Yoon Y, Rubin DM, Riddle MA, Noll E, Rothbard A. Antipsychotic treatment among youth in foster care. Pediatrics. 2011;128(6):e1459–e1466

153. Loy JH, Merry SN, Hetrick SE, Stasiak K. Atypical antipsychotics for disruptive behaviour disorders in children and youths. Cochrane Database Syst Rev. 2017;8(8):CD008559.
154. Ipser J, Stein DJ. Systematic review of pharmacotherapy of disruptive behavior disorders in children and adolescents. Psychopharmacology. 2007;191(1):127–40.
155. Donovan SJ, et al. Divalproex treatment for youth with explosive temper and mood lability: a double-blind, placebo-controlled crossover design. Am J Psychiatry. 2000;157(5):818–20. https://doi.org/10.1176/appi.ajp.157.5.818.
156. Lahey BB. What we need to know about callous-unemotional traits: comment on frick, ray, Thornton, and kahn (2014). Psychol Bull. 2014;140(1):58–63. https://doi.org/10.1037/a0033387.
157. Dvir Y, Ford JD, Hill M, Frazier JA. Childhood maltreatment, emotional dysregulation, and psychiatric comorbidities. Harv Rev Psychiatry. 2014;22(3):149–61. https://doi.org/10.1097/HRP.0000000000000014.
158. Nock MK, Kazdin AE, Hiripi E, Kessler RC. Prevalence, subtypes, and correlates of DSM-IV conduct disorder in the National Comorbidity Survey Replication. Psychol Med. 2006;36(5):699–710. https://doi.org/10.1017/S0033291706007082.
159. Loeber R, Burke JD, Pardini DA. Development and etiology of disruptive and delinquent behavior. Annu Rev Clin Psychol. 2009;5:291–310. https://doi.org/10.1146/annurev.clinpsy.032408.153631.
160. Costello EJ, Egger H, Angold A. 10-year research update review: the epidemiology of child and adolescent psychiatric disorders: I. methods and public health burden. J Am Acad Child Adolesc Psychiatry. 2005;44(10):972–86. https://doi.org/10.1097/01.chi.0000172552.41596.6f.
161. Maughan B, Rowe R, Messer J, Goodman R, Meltzer H. Conduct disorder and oppositional defiant disorder in a national sample: developmental epidemiology. J Child Psychol Psychiatry Allied Discip. 2004;45(3):609–21. https://doi.org/10.1111/j.1469-7610.2004.00250.x.
162. Thapar A, Langley K, Asherson P, Gill M. Gene-environment interplay in attention-deficit hyperactivity disorder and the importance of a developmental perspective. Br J Psychiatry. 2007;190:1–3. https://doi.org/10.1192/bjp.bp.106.027003.
163. Wakschlag LS, Pickett KE, Kasza KE, Loeber R. Is prenatal smoking associated with a developmental pattern of conduct problems in young boys? J Am Acad Child Adolesc Psychiatry. 2006;45(4):461–7. https://doi.org/10.1097/01.chi.0000198597.53572.3e.
164. Needleman HL, Riess JA, Tobin MJ, Biesecker GE, Greenhouse JB. Bone lead levels and delinquent behavior. J Am Med Assoc. 1996;275(5):363–9.
165. de Cubas MM, Field T. Children of methadone-dependent women: developmental outcomes. Am J Orthopsychiatry. 1993;63(2):266–76. https://doi.org/10.1037/h0079429.
166. Simonoff E, Elander J, Holmshaw J, Pickles A, Murray R, Rutter M. Predictors of antisocial personality: continuities from childhood to adult life. Br J Psychiatry. 2004;184:118–27. https://doi.org/10.1192/bjp.184.2.118.
167. Lahey BB, et al. Four-year longitudinal study of conduct disorder in boys: patterns and predictors of persistence. J Abnorm Psychol. 1995;104(1):83–93.
168. Thomas CR, Holzer CE, Wall JA. Serious delinquency and gang membership. Adolesc Psychiatry (Hilversum). 2003;27:61–81.
169. Trickett PK, Putnam FW. Developmental consequences of child sexual abuse. In: Violence against children in the family and the community; 2004. American Psychological Association: Washington, D.C.
170. Caspi A, et al. Role of genotype in the cycle of violence in maltreated children. Science. 2002;297(5582):851–4. https://doi.org/10.1126/science.1072290.
171. Cicchetti D, Rogosch FA, Thibodeau EL. The effects of child maltreatment on early signs of antisocial behavior: genetic moderation by tryptophan hydroxylase, serotonin transporter, and monoamine oxidase a genes. Dev Psychopathol. 2012;24(3):907–28. https://doi.org/10.1017/S0954579412000442.
172. Soderstrom H, Blennow K, Sjodin AK, Forsman A. New evidence for an association between the CSF HVA:5-HIAA ratio and psychopathic traits. J Neurol Neurosurg Psychiatry. 2003;74(7):918–21. https://doi.org/10.1136/jnnp.74.7.918.
173. Unis AS, et al. Platelet serotonin measures in adolescents with conduct disorder. Biol Psychiatry. 1997;42(7):553–9. https://doi.org/10.1016/S0006-3223(96)00465-9.
174. Ortiz J, Raine A. Heart rate level and antisocial behavior in children and adolescents: A meta-analysis. Journal of the American Academy of Child & Adolescent Psychiatry. 2004;43:154–162.
175. Herpertz SC, Wenning B, Mueller B, Qunaibi M, Sass H, Herpertz-Dahlmann B. Psychophysiological responses in ADHD boys with and without conduct disorder: implications for adult antisocial behavior. J Am Acad Child Adolesc Psychiatry. 2001;40(10):1222–30. https://doi.org/10.1097/00004583-200110000-00017.
176. Vanyukov MM, Moss HB, Plail JA, Blackson T, Mezzich AC, Tarter RE. Antisocial symptoms in preadolescent boys and in their parents: associations with cortisol. Psychiatry Res. 1993;46(1):9–17. https://doi.org/10.1016/0165-1781(93)90003-y.
177. Rubia K. 'Cool' inferior frontostriatal dysfunction in attention-deficit/hyperactivity disorder versus 'hot' ventromedial orbitofrontal-limbic dysfunction in conduct disorder: a review. Biol Psychiatry. 2011;69(12):e69–87. https://doi.org/10.1016/j.biopsych.2010.09.023.
178. Sterzer P, Stadler C, Poustka F, Kleinschmidt A. A structural neural deficit in adolescents with conduct disorder and its association with lack of empathy. NeuroImage. 2007;37(1):335–42.
179. Hubbard JA, McAuliffe MD, Morrow MT, Romano LJ. Reactive and proactive aggression in childhood and adolescence: precursors, outcomes, processes, experiences, and measurement. J Pers. 2010;78(1):95–118.
180. Simonoff E, Elander J, Holmshaw J, Pickles A, Murray R, Rutter M. Predictors of antisocial personality. Continuities from childhood to adult life. Br J Psychiatry. 2004;184:118–27. https://doi.org/10.1192/bjp.184.2.118. PMID: 14754823.
181. Alexander, J.F., and Parsons, B.V. 1973. Short-term family intervention: A therapy outcome study. Journal of Consulting and Clinical Psychology 2:195–201.
182. Henggeler SW, Schaeffer CM. Multisystemic Therapy(®): clinical overview, outcomes, and implementation research. Fam Process. 2016;55(3):514–28.
183. LeBlanc JC, et al. Risperidone reduces aggression in boys with a disruptive behaviour disorder and below average intelligence quotient: analysis of two placebo-controlled randomized trials. Int Clin Psychopharmacol. 2005;20(5):275–83.
184. Pappadopulos E, Woolston S, Chait A, Perkins M, Connor DF, Jensen PS. Pharmacotherapy of aggression in children and adolescents: efficacy and effect size. J Can Acad Child Adolesc Psychiatry. 2006;15(1):27–39.
185. Lambie I, Ioane J, Randell I, Seymour F. Offending behaviours of child and adolescent firesetters over a 10-year follow-up. J Child Psychol Psychiatry Allied Discip. 2013;54(12):1295–307.
186. Root C, MacKay S, Henderson J, Del Bove G, Warling D. The link between maltreatment and juvenile firesetting: correlates and underlying mechanisms. Child Abus. Negl. 2008;32(2):161–76.
187. Grant JE, Kim SW, Odlaug BL. A double-blind, placebo-controlled study of the opiate antagonist, naltrexone, in the treatment of kleptomania. Biol Psychiatry. 2009;65(7):600–6.

188. Thapar A, Riglin L. The importance of a developmental perspective in psychiatry: what do recent genetic-epidemiological findings show? Mol Psychiatry. 2020;25:1631–9. https://doi.org/10.1038/s41380-020-0648-1.
189. Caye A, Swanson JM, Coghill D, et al. Treatment strategies for ADHD: an evidence-based guide to select optimal treatment. Mol Psychiatry. 2019;24:390–408. https://doi.org/10.1038/s41380-018-0116-3.
190. Fairchild G, Hawes DJ, Frick PJ, et al. Conduct disorder. Nat Rev Dis Primers. 2019;5:43. https://doi.org/10.1038/s41572-019-0095-y.
191. Muhle RA, Reed HE, Vo LC, et al. Clinical diagnostic genetic testing for individuals with developmental disorders. J Am Acad Child Adolesc Psychiatry. 2017;56:910–3.
192. McCraken JT, Gandal M. Psychopharmacology of autism spectrum disorder. In: McDougle C, editor. Autism Spectrum disorder. Oxford: Oxford University Press; 2015. https://oxfordmedicine.com/view/10.1093/med/9780199349722.001.0001/med-9780199349722-chapter-16.
193. Bloch MH, Leckman JF. Tic disorders. In: Martin A, Volkmar FR, Bloch WH, editors. Lewis's child and adolescent psychiatry: a comprehensive textbook. 4th ed. Philadelphia, PA: Wolters Kluwer/Lippincott Williams & Wilkins; 2017.
194. Liu S, Li Y, Cui Y. Review of habit reversal training for tic disorders. Pediatr Invest. 2020;4:127–32. https://doi.org/10.1002/ped4.12190.
195. Stahl SM. Attention deficit hyperactivity disorder and its treatment. Stahl's essential psychopharmacology. 5th ed. Cambridge: Cambridge University Press; 2014.
196. Barreto SJ, Zeff KR, Boekamp JR, Paccione-Dyszlewski M. Fire behavior in children and adolescents. In: Martin A, Volkmar FR, Bloch WH, editors. Lewis's child and adolescent psychiatry: a comprehensive textbook. 4th ed. Philadelphia, PA: Wolters Kluwer/Lippincott Williams & Wilkins; 2017.

Neurocognitive Disorders

13

Jothi Ramalingam, Adith Mohan,
and Perminder S. Sachdev

Introduction

Neurocognitive disorders (NCDs) are characterized by the presence of cognitive impairment as the prominent and defining feature of the disorder. NCDs capture all conditions generally referred to as dementias and mild cognitive impairment (MCI), and in this chapter, we will be using the terms major and mild NCD for these conditions, respectively, in line with DSM-5 [1]. The term dementia, while not favored, is used parenthetically for major NCD in DSM-5, although there are some differences in how major NCD is defined and the traditional definition of dementia used in DSM-IV [2] and some other classifications. The number of people with dementia in the world is growing with an increasing and aging population. This growth is particularly striking in low- and middle-income countries, while there are some encouraging positive trends of reducing the incidence of dementia in high-income countries in recent cohorts. Our knowledge of the diseases causing dementia is expanding rapidly, but the promise of disease-modifying treatments has not yet been realized. Patients with NCDs are likely to be seen in a variety of settings. It is important for clinicians to have a good understanding of NCDs to improve the recognition and management of these disorders.

In this chapter, we will outline the general approach to NCDs and describe the salient features of the most common etiological subtypes given the brevity of the chapter. Readers are encouraged to read the articles in the reference list when seeking more information.

J. Ramalingam (✉) · P. S. Sachdev
Department of Psychiatry, Northern Beaches Hospital, Frenchs Forest, NSW, Australia
e-mail: p.sachdev@unsw.edu.au

A. Mohan
Department of Psychiatry, Northern Beaches Hospital, Frenchs Forest, NSW, Australia
e-mail: a.mohan@unsw.edu.au

Classification

Major and mild NCDs represent categorical diagnoses on the spectrum of severity of cognitive deficits and associated functional impairment. The cognitive impairment should represent a change from a previously attained level of functioning, thereby distinguishing NCDs from neurodevelopmental disorders. Cognitive deficits are also present in other psychiatric disorders in which they are not the defining feature. NCDs are divided into delirium, major and mild NCDs, each with a range of etiologies.

For a diagnosis of major NCD, a significant decline in cognition must be demonstrated, which leads to an impairment of independent functioning at a minimum in instrumental activities of daily living. A modest decline in cognition that does not interfere with independent functioning, with or without the use of compensatory behaviors or increased effort, would meet the criteria for the diagnosis of mild NCD. A significant number of people with mild NCD progress to a major NCD, with a meta-analysis estimating a 6.7% adjusted annual progression rate from 41 cohorts and a 38.2% progression rate from six studies in which patients were followed up for over 5 years [3]; others either remain stable or return to normal cognitive function over time.

DSM-5 also describes criteria for various etiological subtypes, and these are further categorized as possible and probable diagnoses depending on the level of certainty. There are other organizations and interest groups that have developed similar diagnostic criteria. In this chapter, we will mostly adhere to DSM-5 criteria. As a testament to our improving knowledge of biomarkers in NCDs, DSM-5 and others have incorporated biomarkers in their criteria in some of the etiological subtypes. Boxes 13.1 and 13.2 list the DSM-5 criteria for major and mild NCDs.

W. W. IsHak (ed.), *Atlas of Psychiatry*, https://doi.org/10.1007/978-3-031-15401-0_13

Box 13.1 DSM-5 Diagnostic Criteria for Major Neurocognitive Disorder

Evidence of significant cognitive decline from a previous level of performance in one or more cognitive domains (complex attention, executive function, learning and memory, language, perceptual-motor, or social cognition) based on

1. Concern of the individual, a knowledgeable informant, or the clinician that there has been a significant decline in cognitive function; and
2. A substantial impairment in cognitive performance, preferably documented by standardized neuropsychological testing or, in its absence, another quantified clinical assessment.

The cognitive deficits interfere with independence in everyday activities (i.e., at a minimum, requiring assistance with complex instrumental activities of daily living such as paying bills or managing medications).

The cognitive deficits do not occur exclusively in the context of a delirium.

The cognitive deficits are not better explained by another mental disorder (e.g., major depressive disorder, schizophrenia).

Box 13.2 DSM-5 Diagnostic Criteria for Mild Neurocognitive Disorder

Evidence of modest cognitive decline from a previous level of performance in one or more cognitive domains (complex attention, executive function, learning and memory, language, perceptual-motor, or social cognition) based on

1. Concern of the individual, a knowledgeable informant, or the clinician that there has been a mild decline in cognitive function; and
2. A modest impairment in cognitive performance, preferably documented by standardized neuropsychological testing or, in its absence, another quantified clinical assessment.

The cognitive deficits do not interfere with the capacity for independence in everyday activities (i.e., complex instrumental activities of daily living such as paying bills or managing medications are preserved, but greater effort, compensatory strategies, or accommodation may be required).

The cognitive deficits do not occur exclusively in the context of a delirium.

The cognitive deficits are not better explained by another mental disorder (e.g., major depressive disorder, schizophrenia).

Clinical Approach

In evaluating a person with a cognitive complaint, which could be a concern from the individual, an informant or clinician, it is essential to understand the nature, severity, and course of cognitive symptoms. DSM-5 recognizes six domains of cognition, viz. complex attention, executive function, learning and memory, language, perceptual-motor, and social cognition. Figure 13.1 shows the various subdomains within each domain [4]. Examples of symptoms of cognitive decline and assessments pertaining to various cognitive domains from DSM-5 are presented in Table 13.1.

Box 13.3 Examples of Age-Related Cognitive Change

- Sometimes forgetting names or appointments but remembering them later
- Occasionally needing help to use the settings on a microwave or record a television show
- Getting confused about the day of the week but figuring it out later
- Vision changes related to cataracts, glaucoma, or age-related macular degeneration
- Sometimes having trouble finding the right word
- Misplacing things from time to time and retracing steps to find them
- Making a bad decision once in a while
- Sometimes feeling weary of work, family, and social obligations
- Developing very specific ways of doing things and becoming irritable when a routine is disrupted [6]

Figure 13.2 outlines a stepwise approach to clinical evaluation. More careful evaluation is required to delineate age-related cognitive change from minor NCD, particularly in older adults. Box 13.3 contains some examples of age-related cognitive changes. A neuropsychological evaluation is generally required to evaluate cognitive function and should typically be in the 3rd–16th percentile range or 1–2 SD below reference values based on age-, sex-, and education-matched normative data for a diagnosis of mild NCD.

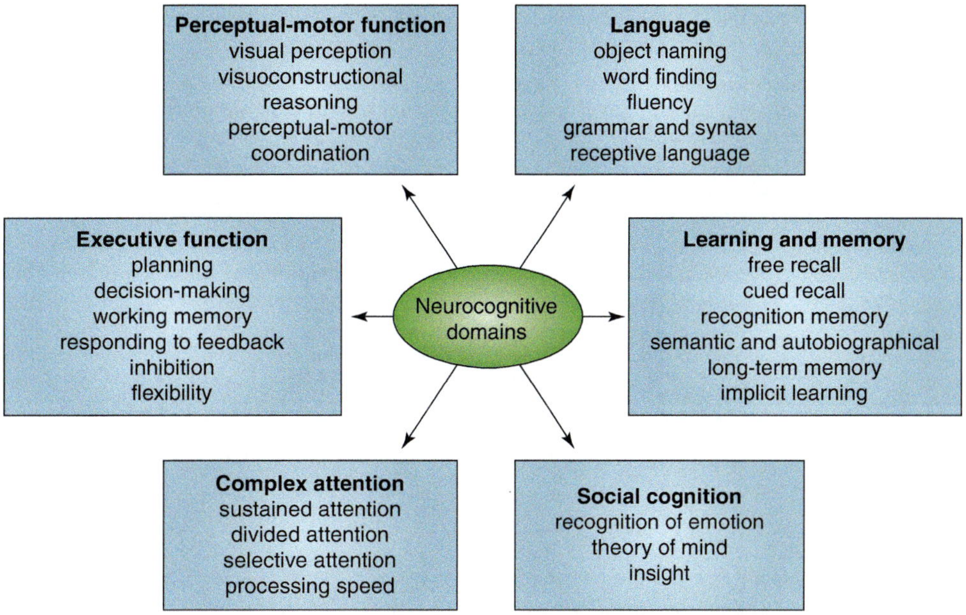

Fig. 13.1 Domains of cognitive impairment. (*From* Sachdev et al. [4]; *with permission*)

Table 13.1 Neurocognitive domains from DSM-5

Cognitive domain	Examples of symptoms or observations	Examples of assessments
Complex attention (sustained attention, divided attention, selective attention, processing speed)	Major: Has increased difficulty in environments with multiple stimuli (TV, radio, conversation); is easily distracted by competing events in the environment. Is unable to attend unless input is restricted and simplified. Has difficulty holding new information in mind, such as recalling phone numbers or addresses just given, or reporting what was just said. Is unable to perform mental calculations. All thinking takes longer than usual, and components to be processed must be simplified to one or a few. Mild: Normal tasks take longer than previously. Begins to find errors in routine tasks; finds work needs more double-checking than previously. Thinking is easier when not competing with other things (radio, TV, other conversations, cell phone, driving)	Sustained attention: Maintenance of attention over time (e.g., pressing a button every time a tone is heard, and over a period of time). Selective attention: Maintenance of attention despite competing stimuli and/or distractors: hearing numbers and letters read and asked to count only letters. Divided attention: Attending to two tasks within the same time period: rapidly tapping while learning a story being read. Processing speed can be quantified on any task by timing it (e.g., time to put together a design of blocks; time to match symbols with numbers; speed in responding, such as counting speed or serial 3 speed)
Executive function (planning, decision-making, working memory, responding to feedback/ error correction, overriding habits/ inhibition, mental flexibility)	Major: Abandons complex projects. Needs to focus on one task at a time. Needs to rely on others to plan instrumental activities of daily living or make decisions. Mild: Increased effort required to complete multistage projects. Has increased difficulty multitasking or difficulty resuming a task interrupted by a visitor or phone call. May complain of increased fatigue from the extra effort required to organize, plan, and make decisions. May report that large social gatherings are more taxing or less enjoyable because of the increased effort required to follow shifting conversations	Planning: Ability to find the exit to a maze; interpret a sequential picture or object arrangement. Decision-making: Performance of tasks that assess the process of deciding in the face of competing alternatives (e.g., simulated gambling). Working memory: Ability to hold information for a brief period and to manipulate it (e.g., adding up a list of numbers or repeating a series of numbers or words backward). Feedback/error utilization: Ability to benefit from feedback to infer the rules for solving a problem. Overriding habits/inhibition: Ability to choose a more complex and effortful solution to be correct (e.g., looking away from the direction indicated by an arrow; naming the color of a word's font rather than naming the word). Mental/cognitive flexibility: Ability to shift between two concepts, tasks, or response rules (e.g., from number to letter, from verbal to key-press response, from adding numbers to ordering numbers, from ordering objects by size to ordering by color)

(continued)

Table 13.1 (continued)

Cognitive domain	Examples of symptoms or observations	Examples of assessments
Learning and memory (immediate memory, recent memory [including free recall, cued recall, and recognition memory], very-long-term memory [semantic; autobiographical], implicit learning)	Major: Repeats self in conversation, often within the same conversation. Cannot keep track of a short list of items when shopping or of plans for the day. Requires frequent reminders to orient to the task at hand. Mild: Has difficulty recalling recent events and relies increasingly on list making or calendar. Needs occasional reminders or re-reading to keep track of characters in a movie or novel. Occasionally may repeat self over a few weeks to the same person. Loses track of whether bills have already been paid. **Note:** Except in severe forms of major neurocognitive disorder, semantic, autobiographical, and implicit memory are relatively preserved, compared with recent memory	Immediate memory span: Ability to repeat a list of words or digits. **Note:** Immediate memory sometimes subsumed under "working memory" (see "Executive Function"). Recent memory: Assesses the process of encoding new information (e.g., word lists, a short story, or diagrams). The aspects of recent memory that can be tested include 1) free recall (the person is asked to recall as many words, diagrams, or elements of a story as possible); 2) cued recall (examiner aids recall by providing semantic cues such as "List all the food items on the list" or "Name all of the children from the story"); and 3) recognition memory (examiner asks about specific items—e.g., "Was 'apple' on the list?" or "Did you see this diagram or figure?"). Other aspects of memory that can be assessed include semantic memory (memory for facts), autobiographical memory (memory for personal events or people), and implicit (procedural) learning (unconscious learning of skills)
Language (expressive language [including naming, word finding, fluency, grammar, and syntax] and receptive language)	Major: Has significant difficulties with expressive or receptive language. Often uses general-use phrases such as "that thing" and "you know what I mean," and prefers general pronouns rather than names. With severe impairment, may not even recall names of closer friends and family. Idiosyncratic word usage, grammatical errors, and spontaneity of output and economy of utterances occur. Stereotypy of speech occurs; echolalia and automatic speech typically precede mutism. Mild: Has noticeable word-finding difficulty. May substitute general for specific terms. May avoid the use of specific names of acquaintances. Grammatical errors involve subtle omission or incorrect use of articles, prepositions, auxiliary verbs, etc.	Expressive language: Confrontational naming (identification of objects or pictures); fluency (e.g., name as many items as possible in a semantic [e.g., animals] or phonemic [e.g., words starting with "f"] category in 1 min). Grammar and syntax (e.g., omission or incorrect use of articles, prepositions, auxiliary verbs): Errors observed during naming and fluency tests are compared with norms to assess frequency of errors and compare with normal slips of the tongue. Receptive language: Comprehension (word definition and object-pointing tasks involving animate and inanimate stimuli): performance of actions/activities according to verbal command
Perceptual-motor (includes abilities subsumed under the terms visual perception, visuoconstructional, perceptual-motor, praxis, and gnosis)	Major: Has significant difficulties with previously familiar activities (using tools, driving motor vehicle), navigating in familiar environments; is often more confused at dusk, when shadows and lowering levels of light change perceptions. Mild: May need to rely more on maps or others for directions. Uses notes and follows others to get to a new place. May find self-lost or turned around when not concentrating on task. Is less precise in parking. Needs to expend greater effort for spatial tasks such as carpentry, assembly, sewing, or knitting	Visual perception: Line bisection tasks can be used to detect basic visual defects or attentional neglect. Motor-free perceptual tasks (including facial recognition) require the identification and/or matching of figures—best when tasks cannot be verbally mediated (e.g., figures are not objects); some require the decision of whether a figure can be "real" or not based on dimensionality. Visuoconstructional: Assembly of items requiring hand–eye coordination, such as drawing, copying, and block assembly. Perceptual-motor: Integrating perception with purposeful movement (e.g., inserting blocks into a form board without visual cues; rapidly inserting pegs into a slotted board). Praxis: Integrity of learned movements, such as ability to imitate gestures (wave goodbye) or pantomime use of objects to command ("Show me how you would use a hammer"). Gnosis: Perceptual integrity of awareness and recognition, such as recognition of faces and colors

Table 13.1 (continued)

Cognitive domain	Examples of symptoms or observations	Examples of assessments
Social cognition (recognition of emotions, theory of mind)	Major: Behavior clearly out of acceptable social range; shows insensitivity to social standards of modesty in dress or of political, religious, or sexual topics of conversation. Focuses excessively on a topic despite group's disinterest or direct feedback. Behavioral intention without regard to family or friends. Makes decisions without regard to safety (e.g., inappropriate clothing for weather or social setting). Typically, has little insight into these changes. Mild: Has subtle changes in behavior or attitude, often described as a change in personality, such as less ability to recognize social cues or read facial expressions, decreased empathy, increased extraversion or introversion, decreased inhibition, or subtle or episodic apathy or restlessness	Recognition of emotions: Identification of emotion in images of faces representing a variety of both positive and negative emotions. Theory of mind: Ability to consider another person's mental state (thoughts, desires, intentions) or experience—story cards with questions to elicit information about the mental state of the individuals portrayed, such as "Where will the girl look for the lost bag?" or "Why is the boy sad?"

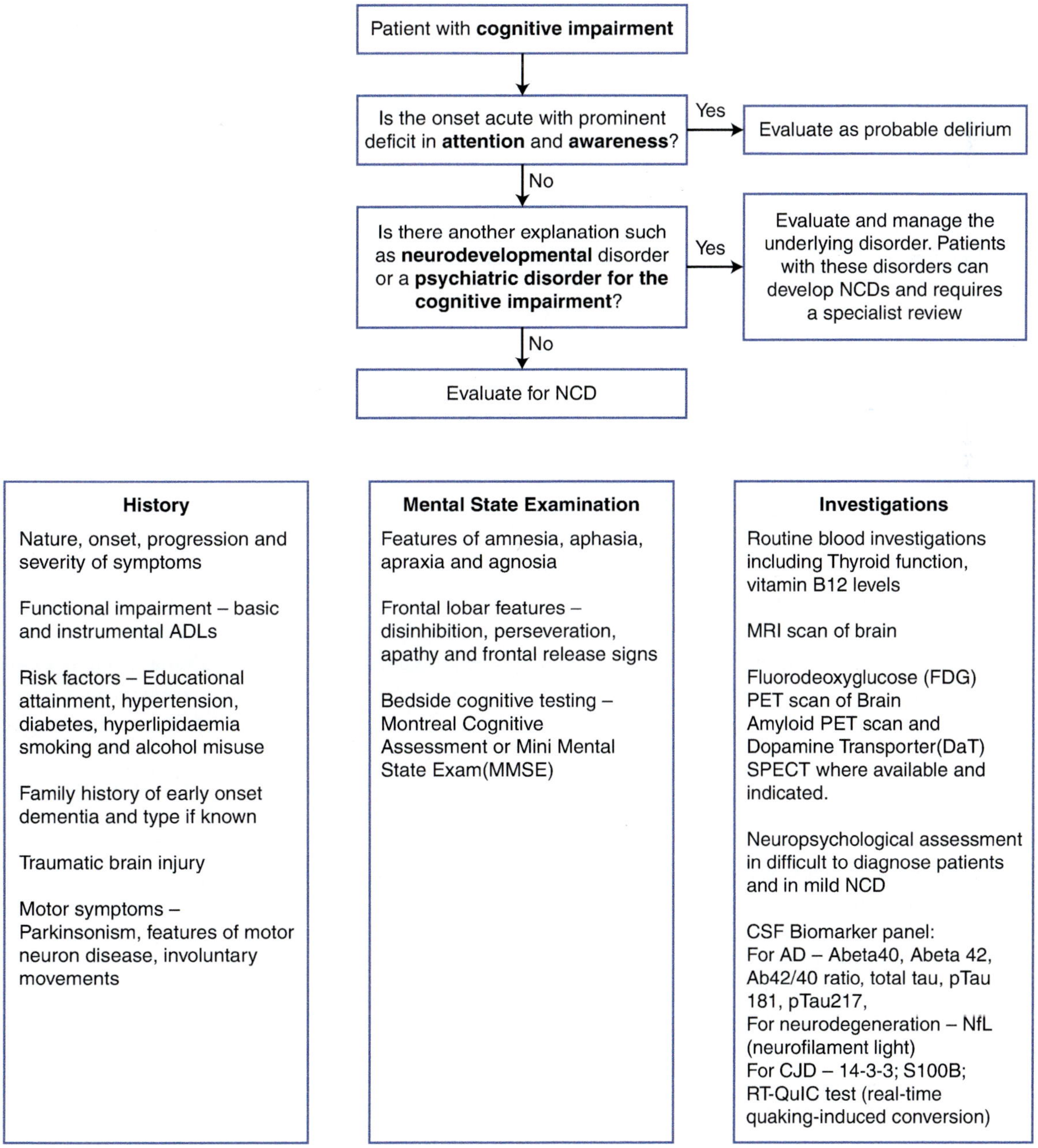

Fig. 13.2 Clinical approach to a patient with cognitive impairment

Once a diagnosis of major or mild NCD is made, etiological subtyping should be pursued. Since various etiologies (Box 13.4) account for NCDs, a good understanding of their clinical features, risk factors, and biomarkers is essential, and the next section will focus on the four common etiological types: Alzheimer's disease (AD), Lewy body disease or dementia with Lewy bodies (DLB), frontotemporal lobar degeneration (FTLD), and vascular neurocognitive disorder. Other etiologies will not be discussed in this chapter.

Box 13.4 List of Etiologies of Neurocognitive Disorders with Criteria in DSM-5

Alzheimer's disease
Frontotemporal lobar degeneration
Lewy body disease
Vascular disease
Traumatic brain injury
Substance/medication use
HIV infection
Prion disease
Parkinson's disease
Huntington's disease
Another medical condition
Multiple etiologies
Unspecified

Alzheimer's Disease

The first case of Alzheimer's disease was described in 1906 by Alois Alzheimer, who described characteristic neuropathological features of amyloid plaques and neurofibrillary tangles in that patient. However, it was in the 1960s that Alzheimer's disease was recognized as a common disease with the same neuropathological changes described by Alzheimer. Since then, there has been a great deal of research done in understanding the pathological mechanisms, and we might be indeed at the verge of having disease-modifying therapies.

Epidemiology

In 2015, 46.8 million people were estimated to be living with dementia in the world, and this was expected to reach 74.7 million in 2030 and double every 20 years [5]. In the United States alone, 5.8 million people were estimated to be living with dementia in 2019 [6]. Alzheimer disease accounts for more than 50% of dementias in those over 65 s (see Fig. 13.3), but concomitant pathology of AD exists with vascular dementia and DLB in more than two-thirds of patients [7].

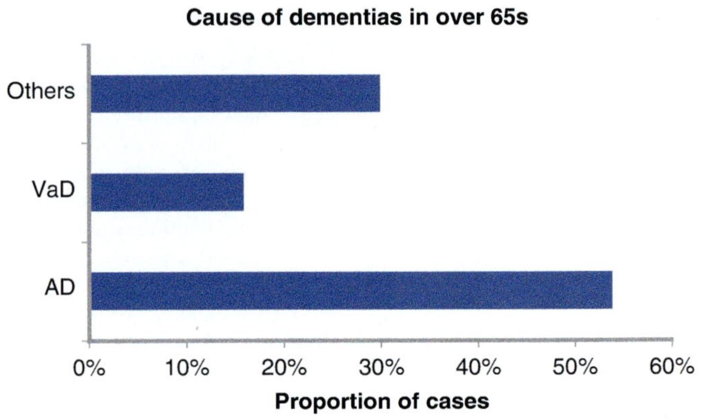

Fig. 13.3 Causes of dementia in those over 65 s. (*From* Barker et al. [7]; *with permission*)

Clinical Presentation

The onset is insidious, with symptoms developing over months to a few years, usually in the eighth and ninth decades of life, with a mean survival of 10 years following diagnosis. The most common presenting complaint in AD is impairment of recent episodic memory demonstrated by a diminished ability to learn new information. When patients are in the mild NCD stage, they tend to compensate for these deficits by using diaries, reminders, strict adherence to routines in a number of settings, and employing visual cues. Other deficits emerge over time in executive functioning, word finding, and visuo-constructional domains. At this point, a diagnosis of major NCD is usually made. Social cognition tends to be preserved until later. Box 13.5 lists the DSM-5 criteria for AD. Probable diagnosis of AD for mild NCD requires evidence of a genetic mutation from either genetic testing or family history, and probable AD for major NCD requires evidence of genetic mutation or robust clinical evidence.

Box 13.5 DSM-5 Diagnostic Criteria for Major or Mild Neurocognitive Disorder Due to Alzheimer's Disease

1. The criteria are met for major or mild neurocognitive disorder.
2. There is insidious onset and gradual progression of impairment in one or more cognitive domains (for major neurocognitive disorder, at least two domains must be impaired).
3. Criteria are met for either probable or possible Alzheimer's disease as follows:

   For major neurocognitive disorder:

   Probable Alzheimer's disease is diagnosed if either of the following is present; otherwise, possible Alzheimer's disease should be diagnosed.

(a) Evidence of a causative Alzheimer's disease genetic mutation from family history or genetic testing.
(b) All three of the following are present:
(i) Clear evidence of a decline in memory and learning and at least one other cognitive domain (based on detailed history or serial neuropsychological testing).
(ii) Steadily progressive, gradual decline in cognition, without extended plateaus.
(iii) No evidence of mixed etiology (i.e., absence of other neurodegenerative or cerebrovascular disease, or another neurological, mental, or systemic disease or condition likely contributing to cognitive decline).

For mild neurocognitive disorder:

Probable Alzheimer's disease is diagnosed if there is evidence of a causative Alzheimer's disease genetic mutation from either genetic testing or family history.

Possible Alzheimer's disease is diagnosed if there is no evidence of a causative Alzheimer's disease genetic mutation from either genetic testing or family history, and all three of the following are present:
(a) Clear evidence of a decline in memory and learning.
(b) Steadily progressive, gradual decline in cognition, without extended plateaus.
(c) No evidence of mixed etiology (i.e., absence of other neurodegenerative or cerebrovascular diseases, or another neurological or systemic disease or condition likely contributing to cognitive decline).

4. The disturbance is not better explained by cerebrovascular disease, another neurodegenerative disease, the effects of a substance, or another mental, neurological, or systemic disorder.

Many patients manifest behavioral and psychological features in the form of apathy and depression in the early stages and psychosis and agitation in the later stages. In the late stages, swallowing difficulties, sleep–wake cycle disturbances, and reduced mobility occur, and patients can become bedbound.

Not all patients with AD have the above typical presentation and variants associated with AD pathology have been described, in particular posterior cortical atrophy (PCA) [8] and logopenic variant of primary progressive aphasia. Key features of these variants are presented in Boxes 13.6 and 13.7. Figure 13.4 shows the typical visuospatial impairment and the MRI, fluorodeoxyglucose–positron emission tomography (FDG-PET), and amyloid PET scan findings in a patient with PCA.

Box 13.6 Posterior Cortical Atrophy

- Onset mid-50s to early 60s.
- Neuropsychological deficits: Visuospatial and visuo-perceptual impairments, alexia, and features of Bálint's syndrome (simultanagnosia, oculomotor apraxia, optic ataxia, environmental agnosia) and Gerstmann's syndrome (acalculia, agraphia, finger agnosia, left–right disorientation). Anterograde memory, executive dysfunction, and language are preserved early but deteriorate in some patients.
- Phenomenology: Prolonged after images, perception of the movement of static stimuli, visual disorientation, reverse size phenomena, visual crowding, dyspraxia, dyscalculia, and problems with spelling.
- Neuroimaging: Voxel-based morphometry in patients with PCA compared to healthy individuals shows reductions in occipital, parietal, and temporal lobes. When compared to patients with AD, patients with PCA have greater right parietal and less left temporal and hippocampal atrophy.

Box 13.7 Logopenic Variant of Primary Progressive Aphasia

- Spontaneous speech is halting with incomplete words and word-finding pauses.
- Grammatical processing and motor function of speech are preserved.
- Repetition of complex and long sentences is impaired and is key to the diagnosis.
- Single polysyllabic word repetition is preserved, unlike in nonfluent variants.
- Patients with phonological paraphasias are found to be associated with amyloid-positive PET scans, aligning closely with AD pathology.

Genetics in Early-Onset Familial AD and APOE Polymorphism

Three genes have been identified from mendelian families of AD with autosomal dominant inheritance patterns in which there is an early onset of the disease. These genes cause excessive amyloid deposition by affecting the cleavage of amyloid precursor protein (APP) or aggregation or generat-

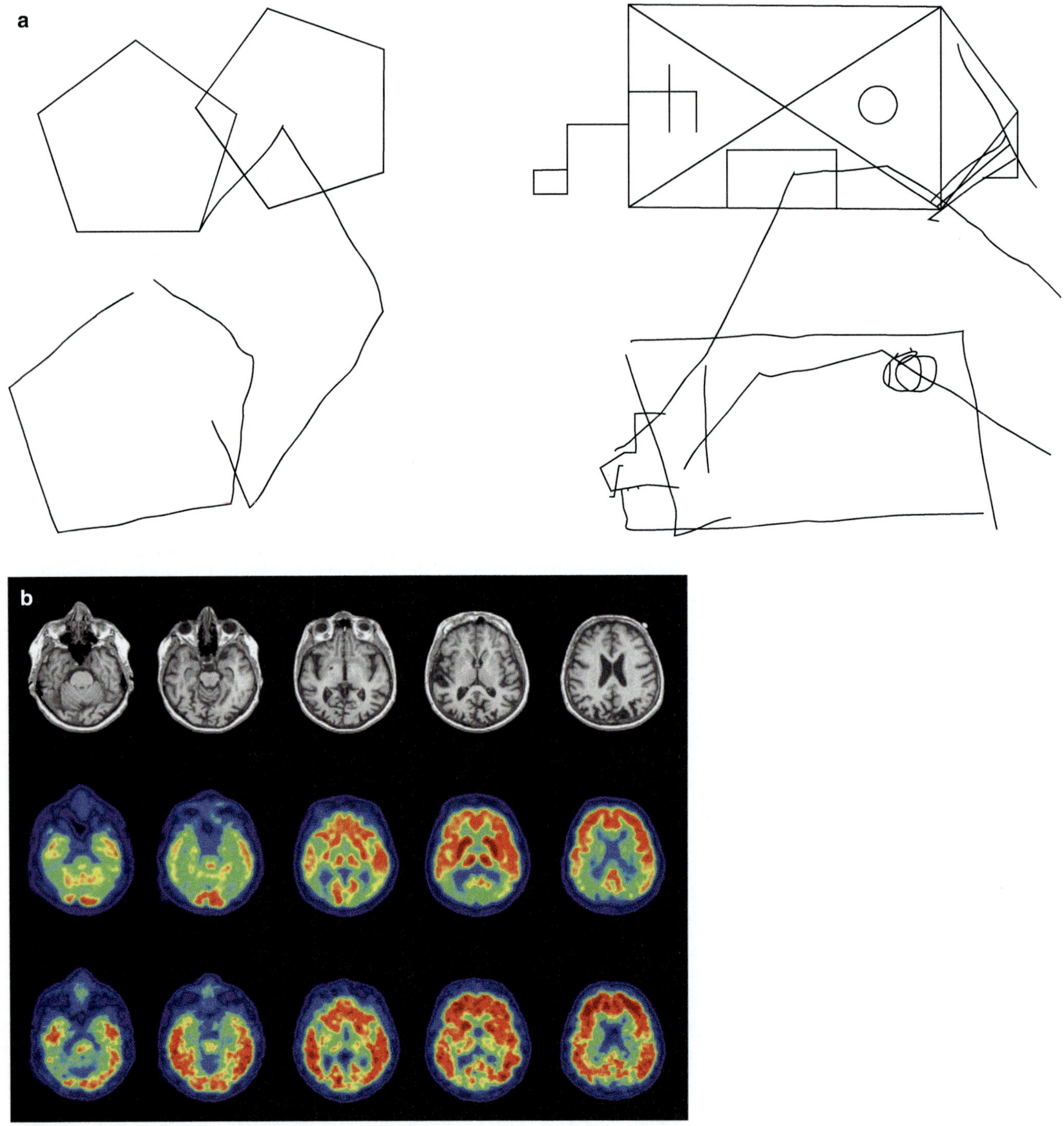

Fig. 13.4 (**a**) Demonstrates severe impairment when copying intersecting pentagons and the Benson figure in a patient with a posterior cortical variant of AD. (**b**) Brain MRI in this patient showed striking atrophy in bilateral parietal, posterior temporal, and lateral occipital cortex (upper row), and fluorodeoxyglucose (FDG)-PET (middle row) showed hypometabolism in the same regions, left worse than right. Frontal cortex, medial temporal cortex, and hippocampus were spared. Pittsburgh compound (PiB)-PET showed diffuse cortical uptake throughout posterior and anterior cortical regions alike (lower row), consistent with underlying amyloid-β plaques. (*From* Crutch et al. [8]; *Creative Commons*; https://creativecommons.org/licenses/by/3.0/)

ing hydrophobic forms. In sporadic cases, the inheritance is polygenic, with over 50 loci associated with an increased risk of AD and apolipoprotein E (APOE). A polygenic risk score predicts AD with 90% accuracy [9]. Apolipoprotein E polymorphism was the first and to date the strongest risk factor for late-onset AD. Apolipoprotein E is thought to play a role in clearing Aβ and possibly other processes and the increased risk is thought to be mediated through a conformational change that affects the ability of apolipoprotein E to bind with these ligands, thereby reducing the clearance. The ε4 allele confers an increased risk of AD while ε2 allele is somewhat protective. Table 13.2 has the salient points on genetic aspects of AD.

Risk Factors

A number of risk factors have been associated with AD, which are listed in Table 13.3. A number of modifiable risk factors are targets for intervention.

Table 13.2 Genetics of Alzheimer's disease

Familial onset AD	Sporadic cases
• Usually onset before the age of 65 • Genes with mutations • Presenilin 1 on chromosome 14 accounts for 60% of mendelian families • Presenilin 2 in chromosome 1 is the least common cause • Amyloid Protein Precursor gene (APP in chromosome 21) accounts for 15%	• More than 50 genes are associated with AD • Apolipoprotein E (APOE) has the strongest association with AD • APOE alleles—ε2, ε3, and ε4 • ε2 offers some protective effect while ε 4 increases risk • Compared with the common ε3/ε3 genotype, ε2/ε2 has 0.5 times, ε3/ε4 3 times, and ε4/ε4 8 times more likely to develop Alzheimer's disease • 75% with one copy of ε4 allelle do not have Alzheimer's disease and 50% with the disease do not have a copy of ε4 • Routine testing for APOE genotype not recommended • ε4 is present more frequently in African Americans compared to European Americans, and the risk of AD caused by ε4 in this group is inconsistent

Table 13.3 Risk factors for Alzheimer's disease

Unmodifiable	Modifiable
Age	Low education level
Female sex: women living longer, survival bias of men, educational attainment, APOE interaction with estrogen	Hypertension Diabetes Obesity
APOE status	Physical inactivity
Race: African American 2 times likely to develop dementias and Hispanic 1.5 times more likely to develop dementias	Social engagement Cognitive inactivity

Pathophysiology, Biomarkers, and ATN Classification

The neuropathological hallmarks of AD are extracellular amyloid plaques and intracellular neurofibrillary tangles. Figure 13.5 depicts the pathological process by which plaques and tangles are formed [10]. It is now known that these abnormalities are detectable many decades before the onset of symptoms. There are a number of pathophysiological models of AD, with the amyloid hypothesis being one of the most prominent, which proposes β-amyloid (Aβ) as the primary driver of the disease [11]. Excess production or reduced clearance of Aβ leads to its gradual deposition, as well as toxicity due to Aβ oligomers, which drive the subsequent process of the disease, including the acceleration of tau pathology, subsequent neurodegeneration, and the emergence of cognitive symptoms. Figure 13.6 captures these biomarker changes over time [12]. While the amyloid hypothesis might explain the disease in early-onset cases, a number of observations to the contrary have challenged this notion in older-onset AD where other pathologies coexist or tau formation may precede amyloid pathology. Therefore, other mechanisms have been proposed such as the amyloid hastening the neocortical spread of preexisting lower levels of tau with or without age-related and non-AD pathologies and neurodegeneration leading to cognitive impairment [12].

In 2016, Jack et al. proposed A/T/N (amyloid/tau/neurodegeneration) as an unbiased, biomarker-based classification system for AD, independent of clinical status and any diagnostic criteria [13]. Figure 13.7 show images of FDG-PET, MRI scan of the brain, and amyloid PET scan of a patient with AD and a normal subject. There are other biomarkers that have been investigated [14]. Table 13.4 documents the validity of CSF, MR, FDG-PET, and amyloid PET imaging of the brain in diagnosing AD [14].

There are other biomarkers that have been investigated [14]. Amyloid PET scans are currently recommended only in difficult-to-diagnose cases and are not for use in routine clinical evaluation.

Treatment

While there is a great activity in the development of new treatments for AD, there is currently no disease-modifying treatment. The drugs available only offer symptomatic treatment. There is also much interest in strategies for the prevention and/or postponement of the onset of AD.

A recent systematic review and meta-analysis [15] demonstrated ten modifiable risk factors that had level A and

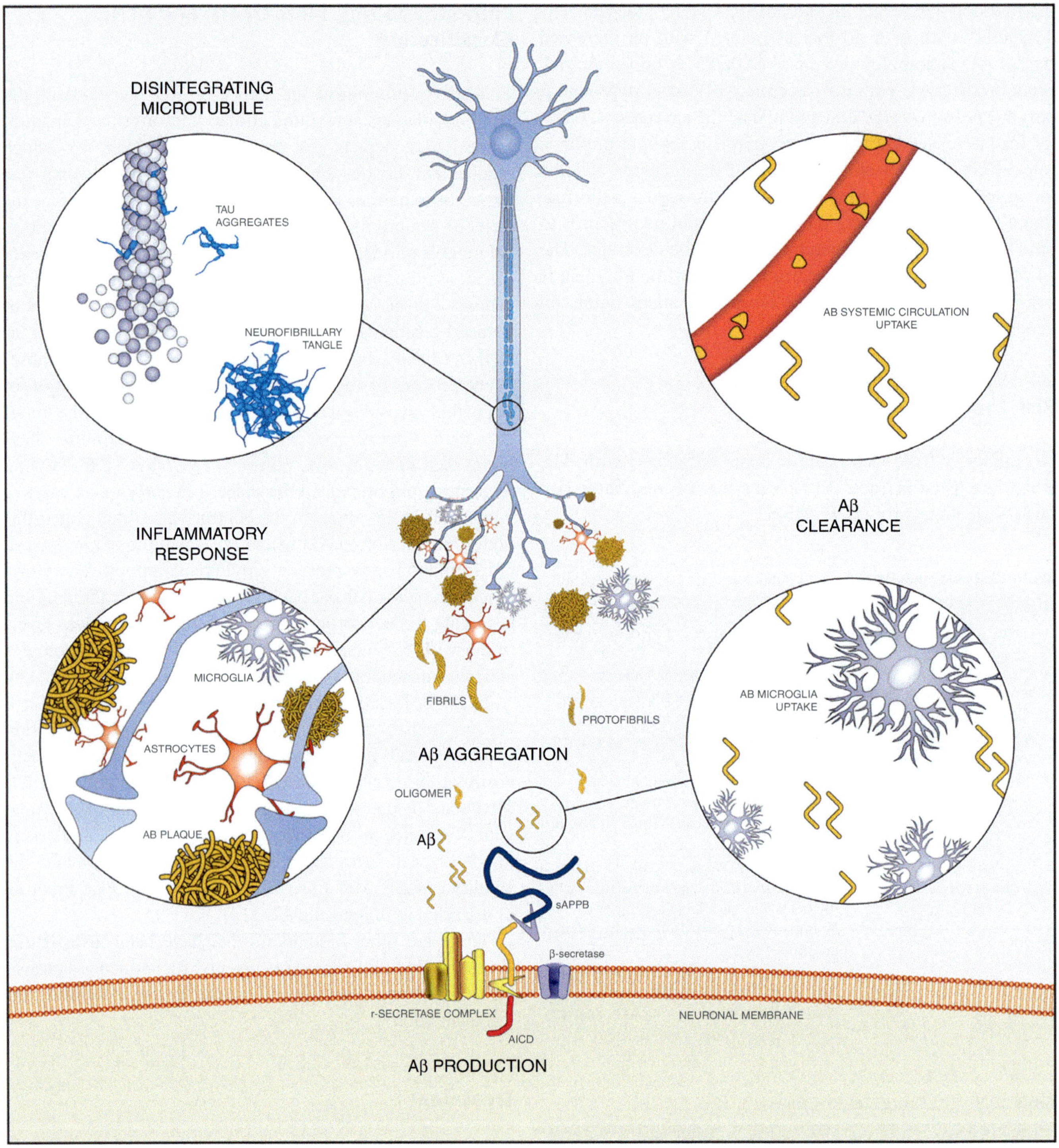

Fig. 13.5 Scheme of amyloid hypothesis in Alzheimer's disease. Amyloid precursor protein is neuronal membrane protein, and when cleaved by α-secretase, it produces a soluble extracellular fragment. However, when cleaved by β-secretase it forms a soluble extracellular fragment and a cell membrane-bound fragment, which is further cleaved by γ-secretase, releasing the intracellular domain and Aβ. Aβ aggregates to form oligomers, protofibrils, and plaques, which is one of the hallmarks of Alzheimer's disease (AD). The other hallmark neurofibrillary tangles are formed from hyperphosphorylation of intracellular tau protein, causing cytoskeleton changes and disrupting axonal transport. Amyloid is thought to accelerate tau phosphorylation leading to synaptic loss, neuronal death, and cognitive impairment. In early-onset AD, three genes have been identified which alter Aβ production leading to Aβ aggregation and deposition, and late-onset AD is believed to be due to defective clearance of Aβ and increased β-secretase activity. (*From* Panza et al. [10]; *with permission*)

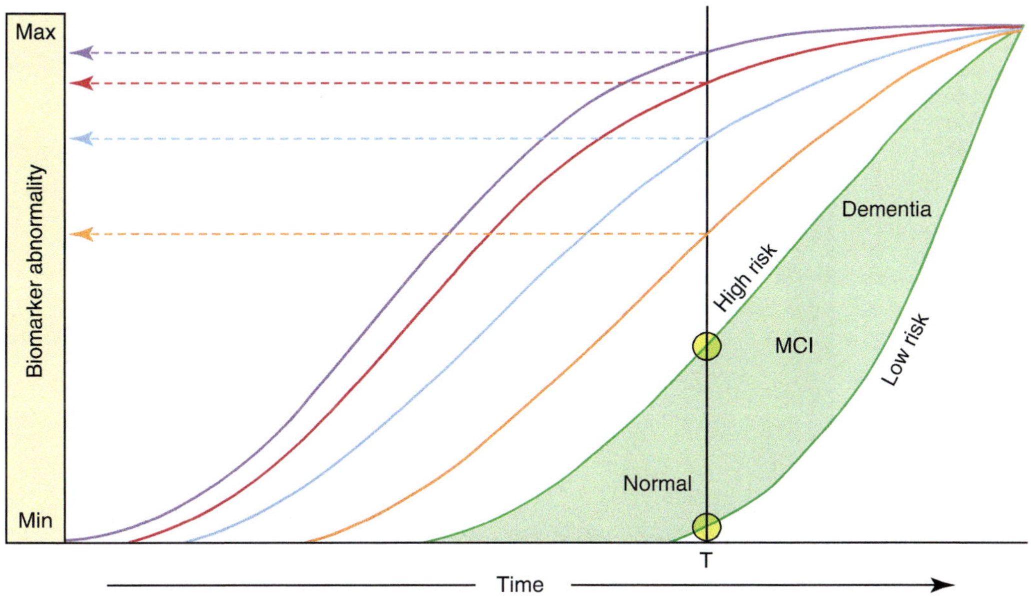

Fig. 13.6 Revised dynamic biomarkers of the AD pathological cascade model—2012. Aβ amyloid is identified by CSF Aβ42 (purple) or PET amyloid imaging (red). Elevated CSF tau (blue). Neurodegeneration is measured by fluorodeoxyglucose (FDG) PET and structural MRI, respectively, which are drawn concordantly (orange). By definition, all curves converge at the top right-hand corner of the plot, the point of maximum abnormality. The horizontal axis of disease progression is expressed as time. Cognitive response is illustrated as a zone (green-filled area) with low- and high-risk borders. The vertical black line denotes a given time (T). Projection of the intersection of time T with the biomarker curves to the left vertical axis (horizontal dashed arrows) gives values of each biomarker at time T, with the lead biomarker (CSF Aβ42) being most abnormal at any given time in the progression of the disease. Intersection of time T with the cognitive impairment zone gives cognitive impairment at that fixed point in time. Subjects who are at high risk of cognitive impairment due to AD pathophysiology are shown with a cognitive response curve that is shifted to the left. In contrast, the cognitive response curve is shifted to the right in subjects with a protective genetic profile, high cognitive reserve, and the absence of comorbid brain pathologies—illustrating that two subjects with the same biomarker profile (at time T) can have different cognitive outcomes (denoted by yellow circles at the intersection of time T and low- vs. high-risk cognitive profiles). (*From* Jack et al. [12]; *with permission*)

another nine with level B evidence (Table 13.5 and Fig. 13.8). The level of evidence was based on the credibility of meta-analysis, consistency of evidence, and directness of outcome for AD. Nearly two-third of the level A evidence points toward managing vascular risk factors and lifestyle. Lancet Commission have recently published their evidence-based recommendations, and air pollution has also been included as a target for reducing the risk of dementia [16]. A multimodal approach has been supported by the Finnish Geriatric Intervention Study to Prevent Cognitive Impairment and Disability (FINGER), evaluating the effectiveness of diet, exercise, cognitive training, and management of vascular risk factors compared to standard care in elderly patients at risk of developing dementia. Patients who received the active treatment did better in executive function, processing speed, and total scores on neuropsychological batteries except in memory tests [17].

Currently approved treatments of Alzheimer's are three cholinesterase inhibitors and an N-methyl-D-aspartate (NMDA) receptor antagonist, memantine. The review article by Grossberg [18] provides detailed information on the therapeutics of cholinesterase inhibitors. Table 13.6 details information on the pharmacology of the three cholinesterase inhibitors that are currently in use.

A Cochrane review and meta-analysis of ten RCTs studying the efficacy of cholinesterase inhibitors over 6 months demonstrated 2.4 points slower decline in cognitive outcome with a range of 0–70, which is similar to about 6 months of decline [19]. These medications tend to stabilize cognitive performance and daily functioning in the first year, but continued treatment has been shown to be beneficial in some studies and individualized decisions have to be made. If a decision is made to stop, the medication should be gradually weaned and sometimes a deterioration is noticed, highlighting the apparent benefit.

Another Cochrane systematic review has found memantine to be helpful in moderate to severe AD as monotherapy or in combination with cholinesterase inhibitors [20].

Disease-modifying therapies so far have been disappointing. A number of studies have evaluated anti-amyloid therapies. Other interventions targeting Tau, neuroinflammation, and neuroprotective strategies have been studied [21].

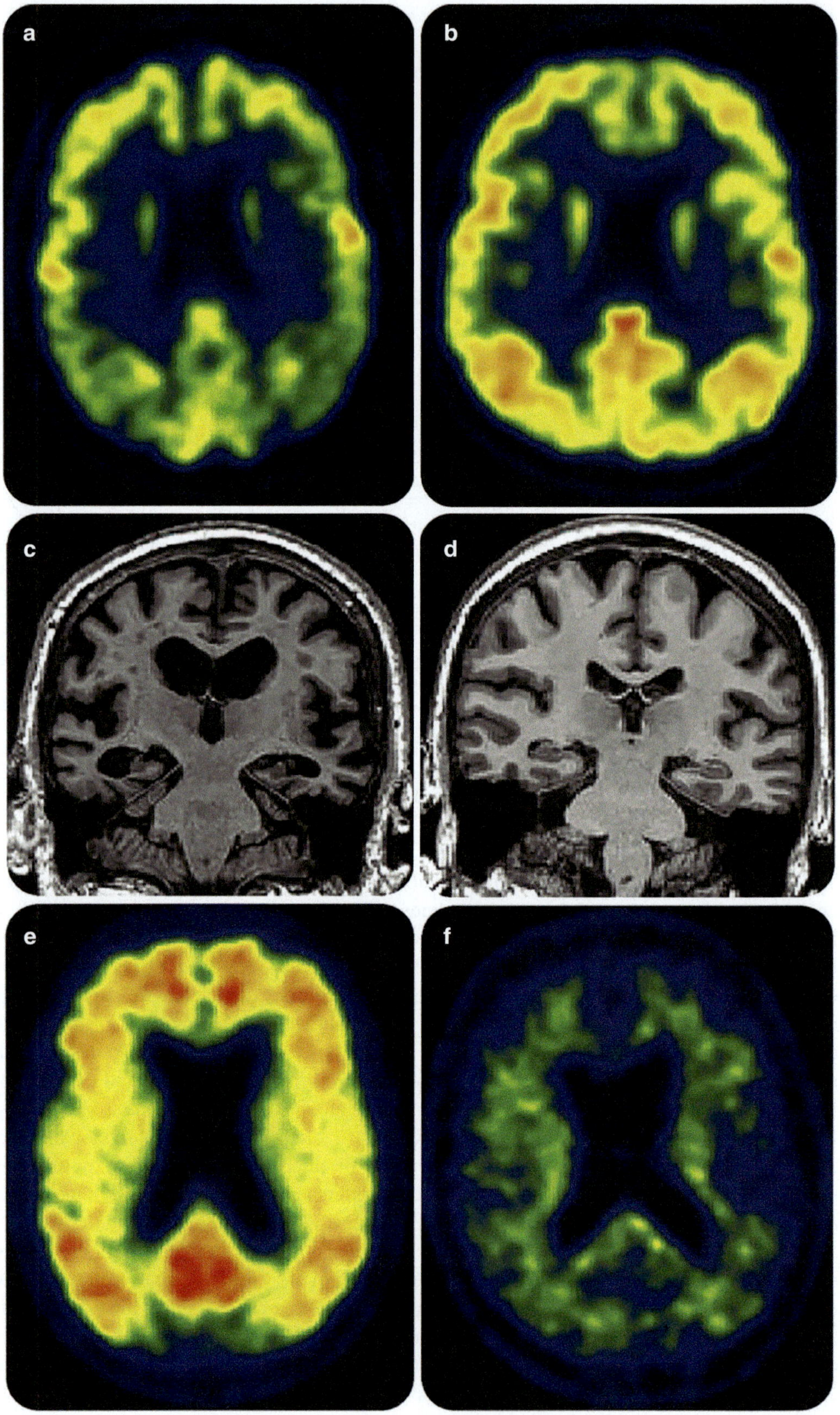

Fig. 13.7 Images of scans from patients with a clinical diagnosis of Alzheimer's disease (AD) and normal individuals. (**a**) fluorodeoxyglucose (FDG)-PET of 75-year-old man with AD dementia. Hypometabolism in medial parietal and lateral temporal-parietal isocortex with relative preservation of frontal metabolism, which is characteristic of typical (multidomain amnestic) AD. (**b**) FDG-PET of clinically normal 71-year-old man. Uniform FDG uptake is present throughout the isocortex. (**c**) MRI of a 71-year-old man with AD dementia. Atrophy is present in the medial temporal allocortex and the basal-lateral temporal isocortex, which is characteristic of typical (multidomain amnestic) AD. (**d**) MRI of a clinically normal 71-year-old woman without atrophy. (**e**) Amyloid PET with Pittsburgh compound B of a 71-year-old woman with AD dementia. Ligand uptake is seen throughout the isocortex. (**f**) Amyloid PET of a clinically normal 93-year-old man showing no ligand uptake in the isocortex. (*From* Jack et al. [12]; *with permission*)

Table 13.4 Biomarkers in Alzheimer's disease

	CSF	MR imaging of the brain	Functional imaging and amyloid PET
Discrimination from healthy controls	Aβ 42 sensitivity of 80% and specificity of 82% t-Tau sensitivity of 82% and specificity of 90% p-tau sensitivity of 80% and specificity of 83%	Hippocampal atrophy Sensitivity 95% and specificity 92% Atrophy of entorhinal cortex Sensitivity 90% and specificity 94%	FDG-PET reduced glucose uptake in temporoparietal and posterior cingulate cortex has sensitivity and specificity of over 90%
Discrimination from non-AD dementias	Aβ 42 sensitivity of 73% and specificity of 67% t-tau sensitivity of 78% and specificity of 75% p-tau sensitivity of 79% and specificity of 80% CSF Aβ42/Aβ40 ratio is more reliable with Sensitivity of 85% and specificity of 82%	Sensitivity 79% and specificity 81%	FDG-PET specificity 78%
MCI conversion to AD	Aβ 42 sensitivity of 81% and specificity of 64% t-tau sensitivity of 51–90% and specificity of 48–88% p-tau sensitivity of 40–100% and specificity of 22–86% p-tau/Aβ ratio sensitivity of 80–96% and specificity of 33–95%	Alzheimer's Disease Neuroimaging Initiative (ADNI) study (late MCI) Atrophy of temporal lobe predicted 72% conversion to AD in 2 years compared to MRI of entorhinal cortex and hippocampus predicting 68%	ADNI study—PET using PiB of lateral temporal cortex predicted 68% of comparison to AD Meta-analysis of PET scan using PiB Sensitivity of 80–100% but poor specificity of 46–88% Florbetapir—poor sensitivity of 67% and 89% and specificity of 71% and 58% for progression to AD in 4 and 2 years, respectively Florbetaben—sensitivity of 100% and specificity of 81% Flutemetamol—sensitivity of 89% and specificity of 80% progression to AD in 2 years Strong correlation with csf Aβ 42 and p-tau levels in patients with a clinical diagnosis of AD. Better concordance with clinical diagnosis when there was discordance between PET scan and csf Aβ 42 levels FDG-PET Sensitivity 88.8% and specificity 84.9%

Adapted from Khoury et al. [14];

Table 13.5 Guideline for prevention of AD: preliminary clinical suggestions

Factors/interventions	Suggestion
Lifestyle	
BMI and weight management	• Adults aged <65 years should maintain or lose weight through an appropriate balance of physical activity, caloric intake and formal behavioural programmes when indicated to maintain/achieve a BMI between 18.5 and 24.9 kg/m^2 (*Class I, level B*)
	• Adults aged >65 years should not to be too skinny (*Class I, level A4*)
	• Adults aged >65 years with a trend of weight loss should be closely monitored for their cognitive status (*Class I, level B*)
Physical exercise	• Individuals, especially those aged ≥65 years, should stick to regular physical exercise (*Class I, Level B**)
Cognitive activity	• Mentally stimulating activities should be encouraged, such as reading, playing chess, etc. (*Class I, Level A4*)
Smoking	• People should not smoke and should avoid environmental tobacco smoke. Counselling, nicotine replacement and other pharmacotherapy as indicated should be provided in conjunction with a behavioural programme or formal smoking cessation programme (*Class I, Level B*)
Sleep	• Get sufficient and good quality sleep and consult a doctor or receive treatment when you have problem with sleep (*Class I, Level B*)
Comorbidities	
Diabetes	• Stay away from diabetes via a healthier lifestyle and diabetic patients should be closely monitored for their cognitive decline (*Class I, Level A4*)

(continued)

Table 13.5 (continued)

Factors/interventions	Suggestion
CVD	• Maintain a good condition of the cerebral vessels via a healthier lifestyle or medications to avoid atherosclerosis, low cerebral perfusion and any CVD. Individuals with stroke, especially cerebral microbleeding, should be carefully monitored for their cognitive change and take preventative measures as indicated to protect cognition *(Class I, level B)*
Head trauma	• Protect your head from injuries *(Class I, level A4)*
Frailty	• Stay healthy and strong in late life. Those with increasing frailty should be especially monitored for their cognition *(Class I, Level B)*
Blood pressure	• Individuals aged <65 years should avoid hypertension via a healthier lifestyle *(Class I, Level A4)*
	• Individuals with OH should be closely monitored for their cognition *(Class I, Level A4)*
Depression	• Maintain a good condition of mental health and closely keep an eye on the cognitive status for those with depressive symptoms *(Class I, Level A4)*
AF	• Maintain a good cardiovascular condition and manage AF using pharmaceuticals *(Class I, level B)*
Stress	• Relax your mind and avoid daily stress *(Class I, Level A4)*
Other domains	
Education	• Receive as much education as possible in early life *(Class I, level A4)*
Hyperhomocysteinaemia	• Have a regular blood examination for homocysteine level. Individuals with hyperhomocysteinaemia should be treated with vitamin B and/or folic acid and be followed with a focus on their cognition *(Class I, Level A2)*
Vitamin C	• Vitamin C in the diet or taken as supplements might help *(Class I, Level B)*
Not recommended	
ERT	• Oestrogen replacement therapy should not be specifically used for AD prevention in postmenopausal women *(Class III, Level A2)*
ACI	• ACI should not be used for AD prevention in cognitively impaired individuals *(Class III, Level B)*

ACI acetylcholinesterase inhibitors; *AF* atrial fibrillation; *BMI* body mass index; *CVD* cerebrovascular disease; *ERT* estrogen replacement therapy; *IMT* intima-media thickness; *NSAIDs* nonsteroidal anti-inflammatory drugs; *OH* orthostatic hypotension. (From Yu et al. [15]; Creative Commons; http://creativecommons.org/licenses/by-nc/4.0/)

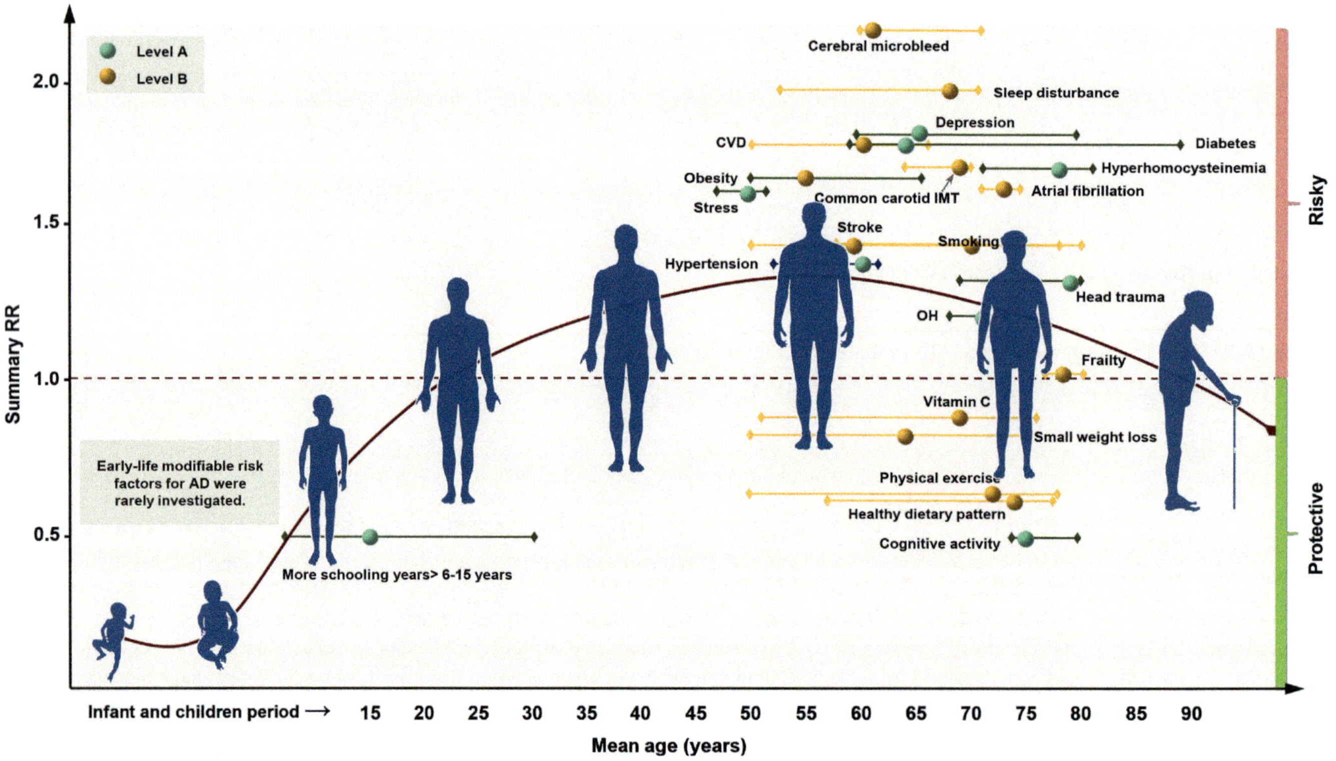

Fig. 13.8 Distribution of modifiable factors with Class I recommendation throughout the course of life. Class I suggestion (benefit >> risk due to intervention) risk factors include ten factors with Level A evidence (cognitive activity, hyperhomocysteinaemia, increased BMI in late life, depression, stress, diabetes, head trauma, hypertension in midlife, orthostatic hypotension and education) and nine factors (obesity in midlife, weight loss in late life, physical exercise, smoking, sleep, CVD, frailty, atrial fibrillation, and vitamin C) with Level B evidence. The x-axis represents the mean age of the total sample (solid circle) with a range of mean age (short horizontal line) for observational prospective studies included. The y-axis represents the summary relative risk (RR). *AD* Alzheimer's disease; *BMI* body mass index; *OH* orthostatic hypotension; *CVD* cerebrovascular disease; *IMT* intima-media thickness. (From Yu et al. [15]; Creative Commons; http://creativecommons.org/licenses/by-nc/4.0/)

Table 13.6 Overview and pharmacokinetic characteristics of cholinesterase inhibitors

	Donepezil	Rivastigmine	Galantamine
Chemical class	Piperidine	Phenylcarbamate	Phenanthrene alkaloid
Enzymes inhibited			
AChE	Yes	Yes	Yes
BuChe	Negligible	Yes	Negligible
nAChR modulation	Uncertain	Not studied	Yes
Brain vs. peripheral selectivity	Uncertain	Yes	No
Selectivity for AChE isoforms	None	G_1	None
Sustained inhibition of ChEs during long-term treatment	No	Yes	No
Metabolism by CYP450 isozymes	Yes	Minimal	Yes
Plasma protein binding, %	~96	~40	~18
Recommended dose, mg/day	5–10	6–12	16–24

AChE acetylcholinesterase; *BuChE* buttyrylcholinesterase; *nAChR* nicotinic ACh receptor; *CYP450* cytochrome P450

Table 13.7 Ongoing phase 3 trials on anti-amyloid therapy in AD in 2019

Agent	Mechanism of action	Target type and therapeutic purpose	ClinicalTrials.gov identifier	Status
Plasma exchange with albumin 1 immunoglobulin	Plasma exchange	Remove amyloid	NCT01561053	Completed
ALZT-OP1a + ALZT-OP1b	Mast cell stabilizer, anti-inflammatory	Amyloid-related and antineuroinflammatory	NCT02547818	Active, not recruiting
ANAVEX2-73	Anti-tau, Anti-amyloid	Anti-tau, anti-amyloid, and antineuroinflammatory	NCT03790709	Recruiting
Crenezumab	Monoclonal antibody directed at oligomers	Remove amyloid	NCT02670083. NCT03114657. NCT03491150	Completed
E2609 (elenbecestat)	BACE inhibitor	Reduce amyloid production	NCT02956486. NCT03036280	Active, not recruiting
Gantenerumab	Monoclonal antibody	Remove amyloid	NCT02051608. NCT01224106. NCT03444870. NCT03443973	NCT02051608.NCT01224106 Active, not recruiting, NCT03444870.NCT03443973 Recruiting
Gantenerumab and Solanezumab	Monoclonal antibody	Remove amyloid/reduce amyloid production	NCT01760005	Recruiting
GV-971 (sodium oligomannurarate)	Aβ aggregation inhibitor	Amyloid-related	NCT02293915	Completed
Solanezumab	Monoclonal antibody	Remove amyloid and prevent aggregation	NCT02008357	Active, not recruiting

Aducanumab is a human monoclonal antibody that selectively binds to amyloid β fibrils and soluble oligomers and has been claimed to reduce amyloid load and cognition. The analysis and the interpretation of the studies have been challenged by some, FDA are due to review the application for approval of aducanumab, and the outcome is being eagerly awaited. The article by Huang et al. reviews the studies in progress for AD. Table 13.7 contains anti-amyloid therapies and Table 13.8 non-anti-amyloid therapies that are being investigated [22].

Table 13.8 Ongoing phase 3 trials on non-anti-amyloid therapy in AD in 2019

Agent	Mechanism of action	Target type and therapeutic purpose	NCT number	Status
AC-1204	Induction of ketosis	Metabolic; symptomatic cognitive enhancer	NCT01741194	Completed
AGB101 (levetiracetam)	SV2A modulator	Amyloid-related and neuroprotective; disease-modifying therapy	NCT03486938	Recruiting
Aripiprazole	Partial agonist at dopamine D2 and 5-HT 1A receptors	Neurotransmitter based; symptomatic cognitive enhancer	NCT02168920	Terminated
AVP-786	Sigma-1 receptor agonist, NMDA receptor antagonist	Neurotransmitter based; BPSD (agitation)	NCT03393520	Recruiting
			NCT02446132	Recruiting
			NCT02442765	Completed
			NCT02442778	Completed
AXS-05	Sigma-1 receptor agonist; NMDA receptor antagonist and dopamine-norepinephrine reuptake inhibitor	Neurotransmitter based; BPSD (agitation)	NCT03226522	Recruiting
Azeliragon	Microglial activation inhibitor, antagonist of the receptor for advanced glycation end products	Amyloid-related and antineuroinflammatory; disease-modifying therapy	NCT02916056	Terminated
			NCT02080364	Terminated
			NCT03980730	Recruiting
OPC-34712 (brexpiprazole)	A partial agonist at serotonin 5-hydroxytryptamine1A and dopamine D2 receptors and an antagonist at serotonin 5-hydroxytryptamine2A	Neurotransmitter based; BPSD (agitation)	NCT01922258	Completed
			NCT01862640	Completed
			NCT03620981	Recruiting
			NCT03548584	Recruiting
			NCT03594123	Recruiting
			NCT03724942	Recruiting
Coconut oil	Reduction in ADP-ribosylation factor 1 protein expression	Anti-amyloid, antineuroinflammatory, anti-oxidative, and neuroprotective; symptomatic cognitive enhancer	NCT01883648	Terminated
COR388	Bacterial protease inhibitor	Antineuroinflammatory; disease-modifying therapy	NCT03823404	Recruiting
Escitalopram	Serotonin reuptake inhibition	Neurotransmitter based; BPSD (agitation)	NCT03108846	Recruiting
Gabapentin Enacarbil	Glutamate receptor-independent mechanisms	Neurotransmitter based and neuroprotective; symptomatic cognitive enhancer	NCT03082755	Recruiting
Ginkgo biloba	Antioxidant and anti-amyloid aggregation	Antioxidant and anti-amyloid; symptomatic cognitive enhancer	NCT03090516	Recruiting
Guanfacine	Alpha-2A-adrenoceptor agonist, a potent 5-HT2B receptor agonist	Neurotransmitter based; symptomatic cognitive enhancer	NCT03116126	Recruiting
Icosapent ethyl (IPE)	Omega-3 fatty acids protect neurons from disease	Neuroprotective; disease-modifying therapy	NCT02719327	Recruiting
Idalopirdine	5-HT6 receptor antagonist	Neurotransmitter based; symptomatic cognitive enhancer	NCT02006641	Completed
			NCT01955161	Completed
			NCT02006654	Completed
			NCT02079246	Completed
RVT-101 (intepirdine)	5-HT6 receptor antagonist	Neurotransmitter based; symptomatic cognitive enhancer	NCT02586909	Terminated
			NCT02585934	Completed
Insulin (Humulin® R U-100)	Metabolic	Metabolic; symptomatic cognitive enhancer	NCT01767909	Completed
ITI-007 (lumateperone)	A potent 5-HT2A antagonist	Neurotransmitter based; symptomatic cognitive enhancer	NCT02817906	Terminated
Losartan, amlodipine, aerobic exercise training, and others	Angiotensin II receptor blocker, calcium channel blocker, cholesterol agent	Antineuroinflammatory and metabolic; symptomatic cognitive enhancer	NCT02913664	Recruiting

Table 13.8 (continued)

Agent	Mechanism of action	Target type and therapeutic purpose	NCT number	Status
Masitinib	Selective tyrosine kinase inhibitor	Antineuroinflammatory; disease-modifying therapy	NCT01872598	Active, not recruiting
Methylphenidate	Dopamine reuptake inhibitor	Neurotransmitter based; behavioral and psychological symptoms of dementia or BPSD (apathy)	NCT03811847	Recruiting
			NCT02346201	Recruiting
Mirtazapine	Alpha-1 antagonist	Neurotransmitter based; BPSD (agitation)	NCT03031184	Recruiting
MK-4305 (suvorexant)	Orexin antagonist	BPSD (sleep)	NCT02750306	Completed
EVP-6124	Selective α7 nicotinic acetylcholine receptor partial agonist	Cholinergic system; symptomatic cognitive enhancer	NCT02004392	Terminated
			NCT01969136	Terminated
			NCT01969123	Terminated
Nabilone	Agonists at cannabinoid receptors 1 and 2 (CB1/2)	Neurotransmitter based; BPSD (agitation)	NCT02351882	Completed
Nilvadipine	Dihydropyridine calcium channel blocker	Amyloid-related, neuroprotective, and antineuroinflammatory; disease-modifying therapy	NCT02017340	Completed
AVP-923 (nuedexta)	Uncompetitive NMDA glutamate receptor antagonist, a sigma-1 receptor agonist, and a serotonin and norepinephrine reuptake inhibitor	Neurotransmitter based and neuroprotective; symptomatic cognitive enhancer	NCT01832350	Unknown
Pioglitazone	Peroxisome proliferator-activated receptor gamma (PPAR-γ) agonists	Antineuroinflammatory and neuroprotective; symptomatic cognitive enhancers	NCT02284906	Terminated
			NCT01931566	Terminated
Troriluzole	Glutamate modulator	Neuroprotective; disease-modifying therapy	NCT03605667	Recruiting
TRx0237 (LMTX)	Tau stabilizers and aggregation inhibitors	Anti-tau; disease-modifying therapy	NCT01689233	Completed
			NCT02245568	Terminated
			NCT03446001	Recruiting
Vitamin D3 (cholecalciferol)	Agonist of vitamin D receptor and other membrane-based receptors such as MARRS	Metabolic; symptomatic cognitive enhancer	NCT01409694	Completed
Zolpidem Zoplicone	Allosteric modulator of GABA-A receptors	Neurotransmitter based; BPSD (sleep)	NCT03075241	Recruiting

Dementia with Lewy Bodies

Dementia with Lewy bodies is the third most common type of NCD but is under-recognized in clinical practice.

Revised consensus criteria for DLB were published in 2017 by the DLB consortium in which clinical symptoms and signs were classified as core and supportive and biomarkers as indicative and supportive categories. They further defined the criteria for possible and probable DLB as in Box 13.8 [23].

Box 13.8 Revised Criteria for the Clinical Diagnosis of Dementia with Lewy Bodies (DLB)

Essential for a diagnosis of DLB is dementia, defined as a progressive cognitive decline of sufficient magnitude to interfere with normal social or occupational functions, or with usual daily activities. Prominent or persistent memory impairment may not necessarily occur in the early stages but is usually evident with progression. Deficits on tests of attention, executive function, and visuoperceptual ability may be especially prominent and occur early.

Core clinical features (The first three typically occur early and may persist throughout the course)

Fluctuating cognition with pronounced variations in attention and alertness.

Recurrent visual hallucinations that are typically well formed and detailed.

REM sleep behavior disorder, which may precede cognitive decline.

One or more spontaneous cardinal features of parkinsonism: these are bradykinesia (defined as slowness of movement and decrement in amplitude or speed), rest tremor, or rigidity.

Supportive clinical features

Severe sensitivity to antipsychotic agents; postural instability; repeated falls; syncope or other transient episodes of unresponsiveness; severe autonomic dysfunction, e.g., constipation, orthostatic hypotension, urinary incontinence; hypersomnia; hyposmia; hallucinations in other modalities; systematized delusions; apathy, anxiety, and depression.

Indicative biomarkers

Reduced dopamine transporter uptake in basal ganglia demonstrated by SPECT or PET.

Abnormal (low uptake) ^{123}iodine-MIBG myocardial scintigraphy.

Polysomnographic confirmation of REM sleep without atonia.

Supportive biomarkers

Relative preservation of medial temporal lobe structures on CT/MRI scan.

Generalized low uptake on SPECT/PET perfusion/metabolism scan with reduced occipital activity +/– the cingulate island sign on FDG-PET imaging.

Prominent posterior slow-wave activity on EEG with periodic fluctuations in the pre-alpha/theta range.

Probable DLB can be diagnosed if:

(a) Two or more core clinical features of DLB are present, with or without the presence of indicative biomarkers, or
(b) Only one core clinical feature is present, but with one or more indicative biomarkers.

Probable DLB should not be diagnosed on the basis of biomarkers alone.

Possible DLB can be diagnosed if:

(a) Only one core clinical feature of DLB is present, with no indicative biomarker evidence, or
(b) One or more indicative biomarkers is present but there are no core clinical features.

DLB is less likely:

(a) In the presence of any other physical illness or brain disorder including cerebrovascular disease, sufficient to account in part or in total for the clinical picture, although these do not exclude a DLB diagnosis and may serve to indicate mixed or multiple pathologies contributing to the clinical presentation, or
(b) If parkinsonian features are the only core clinical feature and appear for the first time at a stage of severe dementia.

Clinical Presentation

Patients with DLB present with fluctuations in attention and arousal that prevail over a long period. This can appear as vacant staring, incoherent speech, daytime drowsiness, and behavioral inconsistency. Visual hallucinations occur early in about 80% of the patients and are typically well-formed, complex hallucinations presenting as people, children, and animals. One of the cardinal features of parkinsonism—bradykinesia, tremor, or rigidity—is present in over 85% of patients and not secondary to antipsychotic medication or cerebrovascular disease. For a diagnosis of Parkinson's disease dementia, parkinsonism should have been present for at least a year before the emergence of cognitive decline. REM sleep behavior disorder (RBD) has assumed more prominence as a core feature in the revised criteria since it is present in 76% of autopsy-confirmed cases of DLB vs 4% in non-DLB cases. It presents as recurrent dream enactments due to the absence of atonia during the REM phase of sleep. Supportive clinical features individually lack diagnostic specificity and when present with others over time might raise suspicion for DLB.

Biomarkers

In the revised consensus criteria, biomarkers have assumed a prominent role in the diagnosis. Reduced dopamine transporter (DaT) ligand uptake in basal ganglia demonstrated by SPECT or PET imaging, reduced uptake on metaiodobenzylguanidine (MIBG) myocardial scintigraphy (see Table 13.9 for validity measures), and polysomnographic confirmation of REM sleep without atonia are indicative biomarkers, which have a greater volume of quality evidence and specificity. Figure 13.9 shows Coronal T1-weighted MRI and ^{123}iodine FP-CIT SPECT images demonstrating preserved medial temporal lobe structures and reduced tracer uptake in the caudate nucleus, and Fig. 13.10 shows ^{18}F-FDG-PET images in Alzheimer's disease (AD), dementia with Lewy bodies (DLB), and normal controls (NC) demonstrating the hypometabolism in the occipital cortex, which distinguishes DLB from AD.

Table 13.9 Validity measures of dopamine transporter (DaT) scan and iodine-MIBG myocardial scintigraphy in DLB

Biomarker	Sensitivity	Specificity
Reduced DAT uptake in basal ganglia	78%	90%
Reduced uptake in iodine-MIBG myocardial scintigraphy.	69%	87%
In milder cases MMSE >21	77%	94%

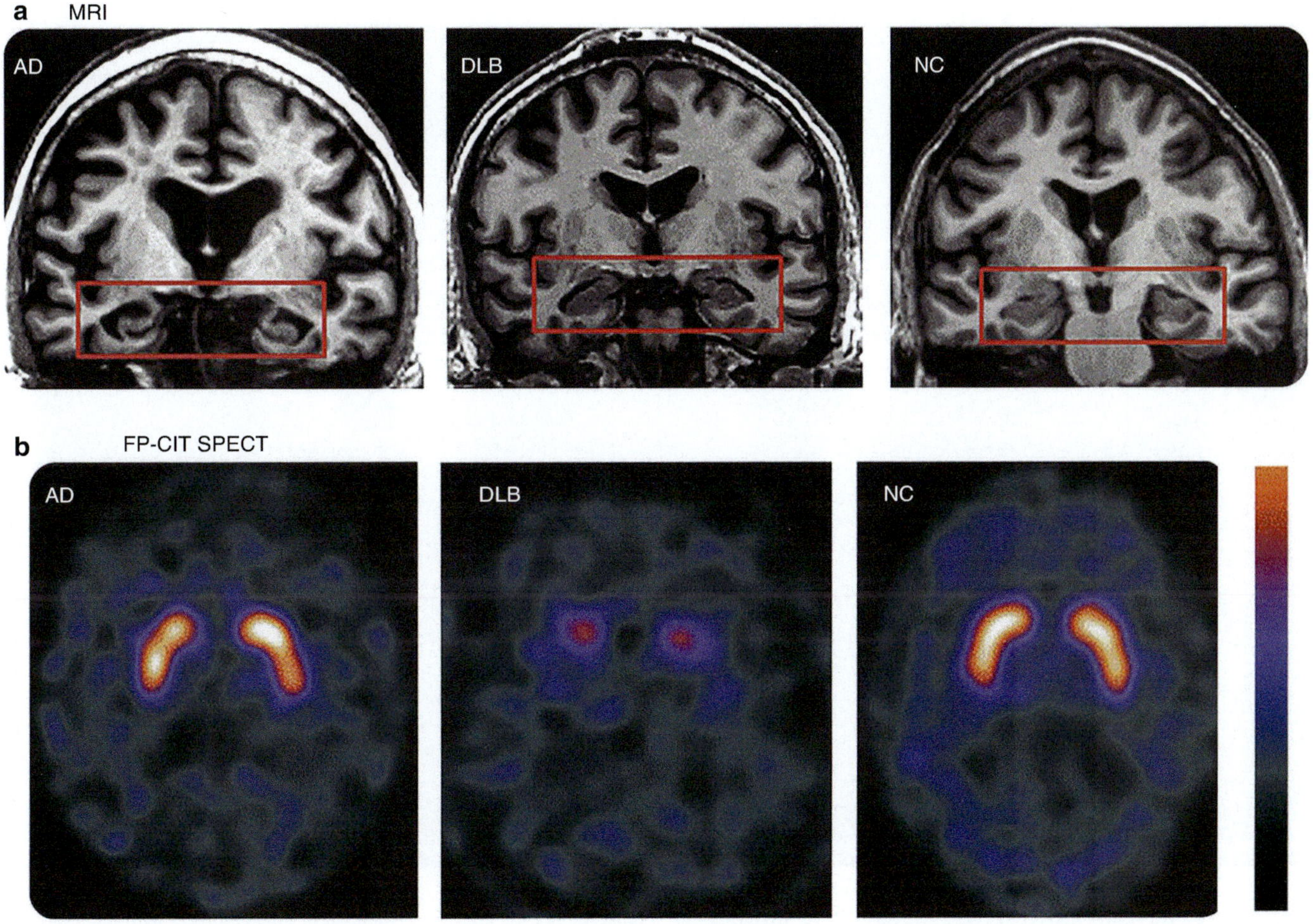

Fig. 13.9 Coronal T1-weighted MRI and ^{123}iodine FP-CIT SPECT images in Alzheimer disease (AD), dementia with Lewy bodies (DLB), and normal controls (NC). (**a**) On the MRI, note the relative preservation of medial temporal lobe volume (rectangles) in DLB, which is similar to NC, whereas atrophy is obvious in AD. (**b**) On the FP-CIT SPECT images, there is minimal uptake due to reduced dopamine transporter activity in DLB, which is restricted to the caudate (period or full-stop appearance) compared to the robust uptake in the caudate and putamen in AD and NC (comma appearance). (*From* McKeith et al. [23]; *with permission*)

Pathophysiology

Lewy bodies (LB) are the pathological hallmark of DLB and are formed from pathologic aggregation of alpha-synuclein in presynaptic terminals. Braak and his colleagues hypothesized that the LB pathology has a prion-like spread starting in the brainstem and progressing to the striatum and then the cortex. This has recently been challenged by studies suggesting that early pathology develops from the gut and olfactory cells [24]. However, whether Lewy bodies cause the disease has also been questioned as the LB densities do not always correlate with duration of disease, symptom severity, or individual symptoms. AD pathology is also commonly found in patients with DLB and is associated with a rapid decline in cognition, which has raised the possibility of synergistic effects of these pathologies.

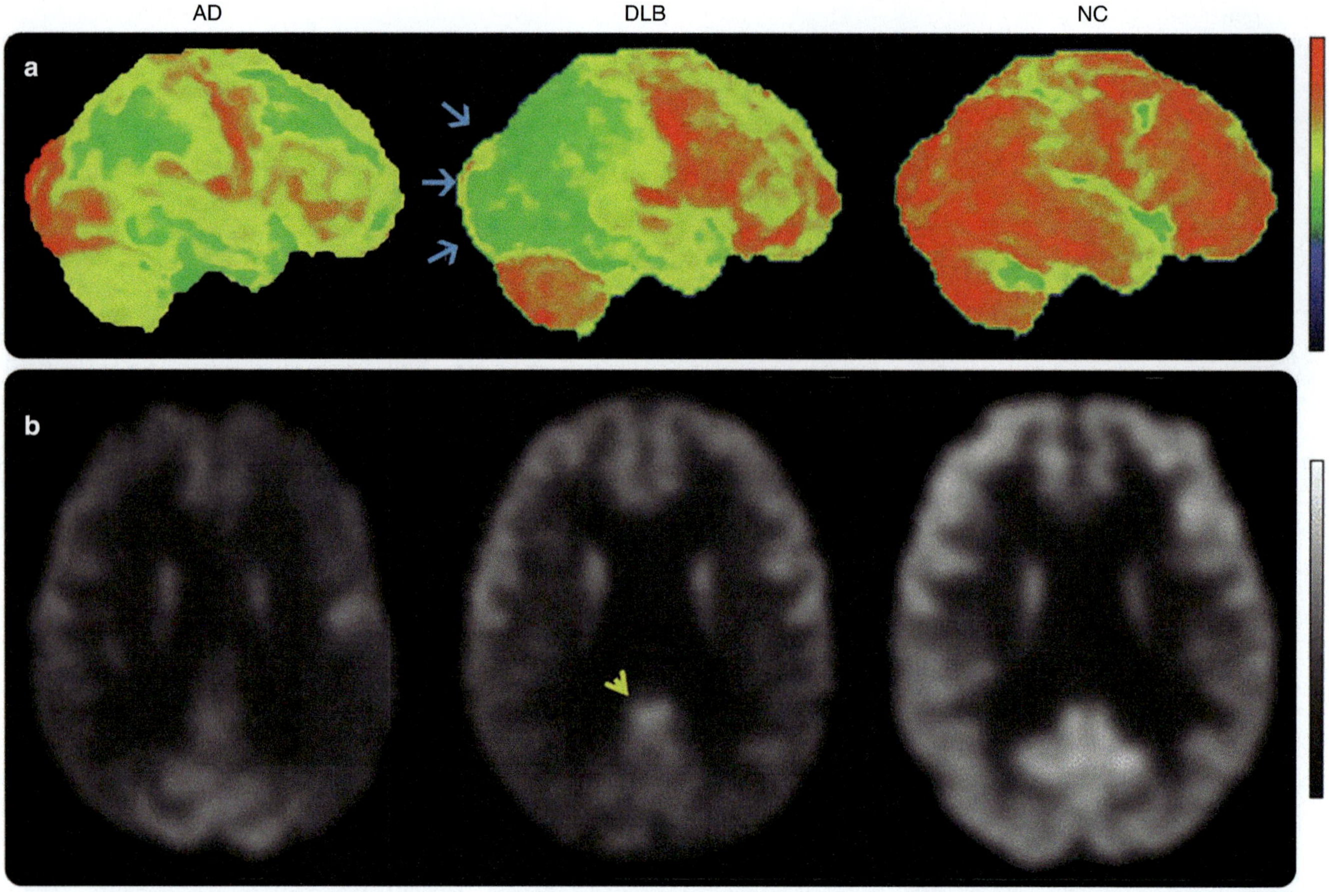

Fig. 13.10 18F-fluorodeoxyglucose (FDG)-PET images in Alzheimer's disease (AD), dementia with Lewy bodies (DLB), and normal controls (NC). (**a**) Right lateral metabolic surface map projection. (**b**) Standard axial view transecting the posterior cingulate region. Occipital lobe metabolism is preserved in AD and NC but reduced (blue arrows) in DLB. Hypometabolism in AD is predominantly in the temporal, parietal, and frontal regions. There is normal metabolism as reflected by the normal 18F-FDG uptake (lighter shade of gray) in the posterior cingulate region (yellow arrowhead) surrounded by reduced 18F-FDG uptake (darker gray) in the adjacent occipital cortex in DLB, representing the cingulate island sign. This contrasts with the relatively reduced 18F-FDG uptake in the posterior cingulate and relatively preserved 18F-FDG uptake in the occipital cortex regions in AD. In the control, there is normal 18F-FDG uptake in the posterior cingulate, occipital, and other neocortical regions. Color and grayscale sidebars show increasing degrees of deviation from normal as the signal trends lower in the sidebars (red is normal while black is maximally abnormal in color images; white is normal while black is maximally abnormal in grayscale images). (*From* McKeith et al. [23]; *with permission*)

Treatment

Most of the studies on nonpharmacological interventions have been carried out in AD or vascular dementia. However, there is some evidence for cognitive training, caregiver-oriented training for the management of psychiatric symptoms, and exercise as being beneficial in DLB. Cholinesterase inhibitors donepezil and rivastigmine have Class 1 evidence for improving cognition, global function, and activities of living. It is also shown to improve visual hallucinations, apathy, and delusions. Table 13.10 outlines the general approach to the treatment of various symptoms, but the evidence base is rather meager or absent.

Table 13.10 Treatment of symptoms of DLB

Cognition	Nonmotor symptoms	Motor symptoms
Class 1 level evidence for donepezil and rivastigmine Memantine-evidence less clear but well tolerated	CHEIs for visual hallucinations, apathy, and delusions Low-dose quetiapine and clozapine can be cautiously used for psychotic symptoms RBD—bedtime use of clonazepam and melatonin might be more tolerable Depression—SSRIs, SNRIs, and mirtazapine	Less responsive to dopaminergic agents Increased risk of psychosis with dopaminergic agents Low doses titrated slowly might be helpful with motor symptoms

Frontotemporal Neurocognitive Disorder

Frontotemporal dementia comprises a heterogeneous group of disorders with the endophenotype of degeneration of frontal and temporal lobes. DSM-5 classification recognizes two variants: behavioral variant (bvFTLD) and the language variant, which has semantic (svFTLD) and nonfluent subtypes (nfvFTLD).

FTLD is the third most common cause of degenerative dementias and constitutes 5–10% of all pathologically confirmed cases. The incidence is 3–4 per 100,000 person-years. It is the second most common dementia in those under 65 s after AD.

Classification and Subtypes

Classification of subtypes of frontotemporal dementia is based on symptoms that present early in the course of the disease. Box 13.9 contains the DSM-5 diagnostic criteria for the subtypes of FTLD [21].

Box 13.9 DSM-5 Criteria for Diagnosis of Frontotemporal Dementia

1. The criteria are met for major or mild neurocognitive disorder.
2. The disturbance has an insidious onset and gradual progression.
3. Either (a) or (b);
   (a) Behavioral variant:
      (i) Three or more of the following behavioral symptoms:
         - Behavioral disinhibition.
         - Apathy or inertia.
         - Loss of sympathy or empathy.
         - Perseverative, stereotyped or compulsive/ritualistic behavior.
         - Hyperorality and dietary changes.
      (ii) Prominent decline in social cognition and/or executive abilities.
   (b) Language variant:
      (i) Prominent decline in language ability, in the form of speech production, word finding, object naming, grammar, or word comprehension.
4. Relative sparing of learning and memory and perceptual-motor function.
5. The disturbance is not better explained by cerebrovascular disease, another neurodegenerative disease, the effects of a substance, or another mental, neurological, or systemic disorder.

Probable frontotemporal neurocognitive disorder is diagnosed if either of the following is present; otherwise, possible frontotemporal neurocognitive disorder should be diagnosed:

1. Evidence of a causative frontotemporal neurocognitive disorder genetic mutation, from either family history or genetic testing.
2. Evidence of disproportionate frontal and/or temporal lobe involvement from neuroimaging.

Possible frontotemporal neurocognitive disorder is diagnosed if there is no evidence of a genetic mutation, and neuroimaging has not been performed.

The subtypes have variable impairment in behavioral, executive, language, and motor functions and distinct atrophic changes in neuroimaging due to proteinopathies starting in specific hubs and spreading across the respective network in a prion-like manner (see Fig. 13.11) [25]. Motor neuron disease and parkinsonism are more common with bvFTLD, while corticobasal syndrome and progressive supranuclear palsy present with nfvFTLD.

Behavioral variant: Early degeneration affects the paralimbic structures of the ventromedial prefrontal cortex (VMPFC), anterior cingulate cortex (ACC), and anterior insula predominantly on the right lobe; this further progresses to involve the temporal lobes and then the dorsolateral prefrontal cortex.

Nonfluent primary progressive aphasia: Neuroanatomical network affected includes dominant frontal operculum, its connections to the supplementary motor area (SMA) through the frontal aslant tract, the premotor area, and the insular cortex.

Semantic primary progressive aphasia: Neuroanatomical distribution of pathology initially starts with the anterior temporal pole, spreading further to the uncinate fasciculus, frontal lobes, insula, and anterior hippocampus.

Histopathological Types and Genetics

There are three commonly recognized histopathological changes observed in FTD. Tau aggregation and transactive

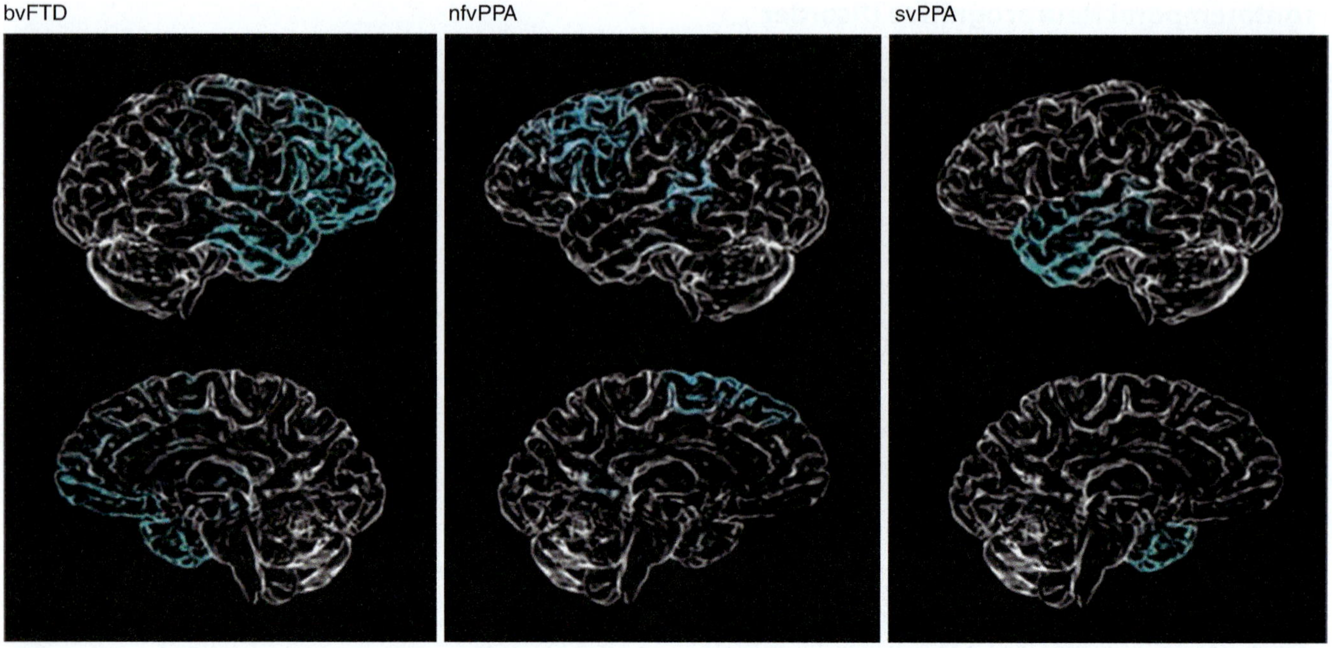

Fig. 13.11 Patterns of brain atrophy in frontotemporal dementia syndromes. . The images show the patterns of atrophy observed on structural imaging in various frontotemporal dementia (FTD) syndromes, which arise from frontotemporal lobar degeneration. The core neuropsychiatric symptoms of behavioral variant FTD (bvFTD), such as apathy, disinhibition, eating disorders, and aberrant motor behavior, localize to right frontal structures. Patients with nonfluent/agrammatic variant primary progressive aphasia (nfvPPA) present with fluency impairment and/or agrammatism. These deficits localize to the fronto-insular language network, with atrophy noted most frequently in the left inferior frontal and insular cortices (the entire network is not depicted in this figure). In semantic variant PPA (svPPA), degeneration of the anterior temporal lobes disrupts access to semantic memory. (*From* Elahi and Miller et al. [25]; *with permission*)

response DNA-binding protein of 43 kDa (TDP-43) accumulation account for the majority of the cases, and the remainder are caused by abnormal fused in sarcoma (FUS) inclusions. A small number of cases with ubiquitinated inclusions who are negative for both TDP and FUS are classified as FTD—ubiquitin proteasome system [26].

Histopathology correlates better with certain gene mutations than with phenotypic features. As illustrated in Fig. 13.12, bvFTD can have any one of the pathological changes and therefore can be caused by a number of genetic mutations. There are three commonly identified genes from Mendelian families with FTD: MAPT, C9orf72, and GRN. MAPT gene mutation expresses as tau pathology while C9orf72 and GRN as well as TAR DNA-binding protein (TARDBP) and valosin-containing protein (VCP) mutations present as TDP-43 pathology.

Treatment

There are no FDA-approved treatments for FTD. A number of SSRIs have been shown to improve stereotypies, disinhibition, apathy, problematic sexual and eating behaviors, and irritability. Atypical antipsychotics can be used in low doses to treat behavioral agitation, but they have to be balanced against the risk of an increase in mortality and extrapyramidal side effects. Cholinesterase inhibitors can worsen cognition in patients with FTD, and memantine has not been shown to be effective either. Gene therapies are being developed for FTD with known genetic mutations. Nonpharmacological interventions such as family education, respite care, diversional strategies, and speech therapy should be tailored to the individual.

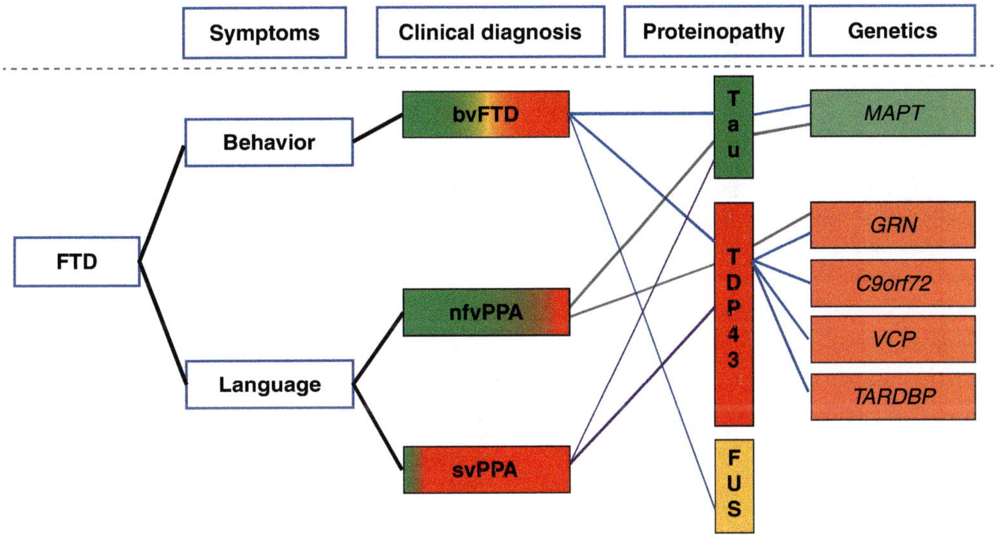

Fig. 13.12 Clinical, pathological, and genetic associations in FTD. Clinical symptoms are shown on the left, and colored regions of clinical diagnosis represent relative percentages of patients found to have each underlying neuropathological diagnosis. Blue line, genetic and pathological aspects of bvFTD; gray line, genetic and pathological aspects of nfvPPA; purple line, genetic and pathological aspects of svPPA. *bvFTD* behavioral-variant frontotemporal dementia; *svPPA* semantic-variant primary progressive aphasia; *nfvPPA* nonfluent variant primary progressive aphasia; *FUS* fused in sarcoma; *TDP-43* transactive response (TAR) DNA-binding protein of 43 kDa; *C9orf72* chromosome 9 open reading frame 72; *GRN* progranulin mutations; *MAPT* microtubule-associated protein tau; and *VCP* valosin-containing protein. (*From* Liu et al. [26]; *Creative Commons;* https://creativecommons.org/licenses/by/4.0/)

Vascular Neurocognitive Disorder

Vascular neurocognitive disorder is caused by cerebrovascular disease resulting from a number of diseases and risk factors. Our understanding of this condition has evolved over time from vasoparalysis and insufficiency to multi-infarct dementia to the prevailing view of multiple vascular factors, contributing to a spectrum of cognitive impairment in which vascular major NCD lies at the severe end of the spectrum.

Prevalence of vascular dementia (VaD) is estimated to be around 16% of all dementias and is considered the second most common cause of dementia. Autopsy studies of dementia cases show that one-third of cases have significant vascular pathology and up to three fourth have some vascular pathology.

Classification

Box 13.10 lists the DSM-5 criteria for vascular neurocognitive disorders.

Box 13.10 DSM-5 Criteria for Vascular Neurocognitive Disorders

1. The criteria are met for major or mild neurocognitive disorder.
2. The clinical features are consistent with a vascular etiology, as suggested by either of the following:
   (a) Onset of the cognitive deficits is temporally related to one or more cerebrovascular events.
   (b) Evidence for decline is prominent in complex attention (including processing speed) and frontal-executive function.
3. There is evidence of the presence of cerebrovascular disease from history, physical examination, and/or neuroimaging considered sufficient to account for the neurocognitive deficits.
4. The symptoms are not better explained by another brain disease or systemic disorder.

Probable vascular neurocognitive disorder is diagnosed if one of the following is present; otherwise, possible vascular neurocognitive disorder should be diagnosed:

1. Clinical criteria are supported by neuroimaging evidence of significant parenchymal injury attributed to cerebrovascular disease (neuroimaging-supported).
2. The neurocognitive syndrome is temporally related to one or more documented cerebrovascular events.
3. Both clinical and genetic (e.g., cerebral autosomal dominant arteriopathy with subcortical infarcts and leukoencephalopathy) evidence of cerebrovascular disease is present.

Possible vascular neurocognitive disorder is diagnosed if the clinical criteria are met, but neuroimaging is not available and the temporal relationship of the neurocognitive syndrome with one or more cerebrovascular events is not established.

Vascular Impairment of Cognition Classification Consensus Study (VICCCS) guidelines subdivides major VCD into four categories: post-stroke dementia (PSD), subcortical ischemic vascular dementia, multi-infarct (cortical dementia), and mixed dementias (with a variety of possible comorbid neuropathologies).

Clinical Presentation and Course

In PSD or multi-infarct dementia, the onset of cognitive impairment is temporally associated with one or more cerebrovascular events. This is usually acute in onset, followed by a stepwise decline with periods of stability in between cerebrovascular events. The clinical presentation is determined by the location and extent of the pathology caused by the stroke. There is a notable decline in complex attention and frontal-executive dysfunction in subcortical ischemic vascular dementia, which has an insidious onset and progresses gradually. The clinical profile is further characterized by dysexecutive syndrome, attentional deficits, and psychomotor slowing; memory deficits, if present, are mostly due to retrieval deficits. Personality change, apathy, and depression are often present.

Table 13.11 Vascular neurocognitive disorder: features in history, physical examination, and neuroimaging

History	Physical examination	Neuroimaging
Vascular risk factors Hypertension Hyperlipidemia Diabetes mellitus Obesity Alcohol use Smoking Physical inactivity Urinary incontinence unexplained by urinary pathology Gait disturbance Peripheral vascular disease	Arrhythmias Hypertension Psychomotor slowing Focal neurological deficits Hemiparesis Visual field defects Pseudobulbar syndrome	One or more large vessel infarcts or hemorrhage Single strategically placed infarct or hemorrhage in angular gyrus, thalamus, basal forebrain, etc. Two or more lacunar infarcts outside the brainstem or extensive or confluent white matter lesions

In addition, there should be evidence of cerebrovascular disease from the clinical history, physical examination, and/or neuroimaging (see Table 13.11). Figure 13.13 shows MRI scans of the brain demonstrating various changes associated with small vessel disease. It should be noted that the prevalence of abnormalities found in neuroimaging associated with small vessel disease increases from middle age, even in asymptomatic individuals.

Pathophysiology

Various vascular risk factors, lifestyle, and vascular pathology are thought to cause parenchymal injury through a number of mechanisms (see Fig. 13.14) and cause ischemia or hemorrhage, which causes neuronal loss and network disruption leading to cognitive impairment. As shown in the proposed schema, AD pathology can further compound the process causing cognitive impairment, while other protective factors such as cognitive reserve and prior educational attainment might delay clinical expression [27].

Treatment

There are no treatments approved for symptomatic treatment of vascular NCDs. Cholinesterase inhibitors and memantine were only estimated to impart about half the gains seen in AD. Donepezil use in VaD has been, however, supported by some guidelines. Sertraline has also been shown to have a positive effect on executive dysfunction with vascular NCDs.

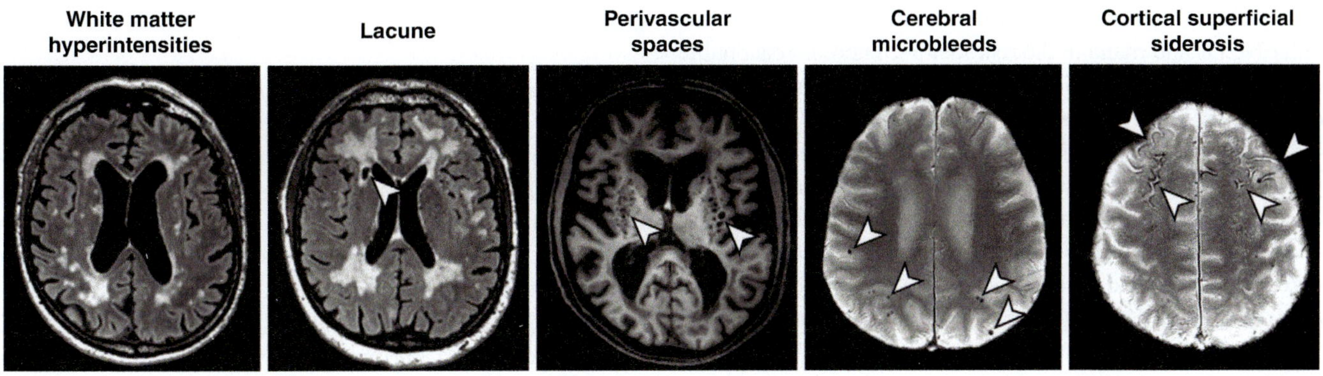

Fig. 13.13 Signal alterations on conventional magnetic resonance imaging (visible lesions) in small vessel disease (SVD). The arrowheads indicate the pathology mentioned at the top of each brain scan. (*From* Iadecola et al. [28]; *with permission*)

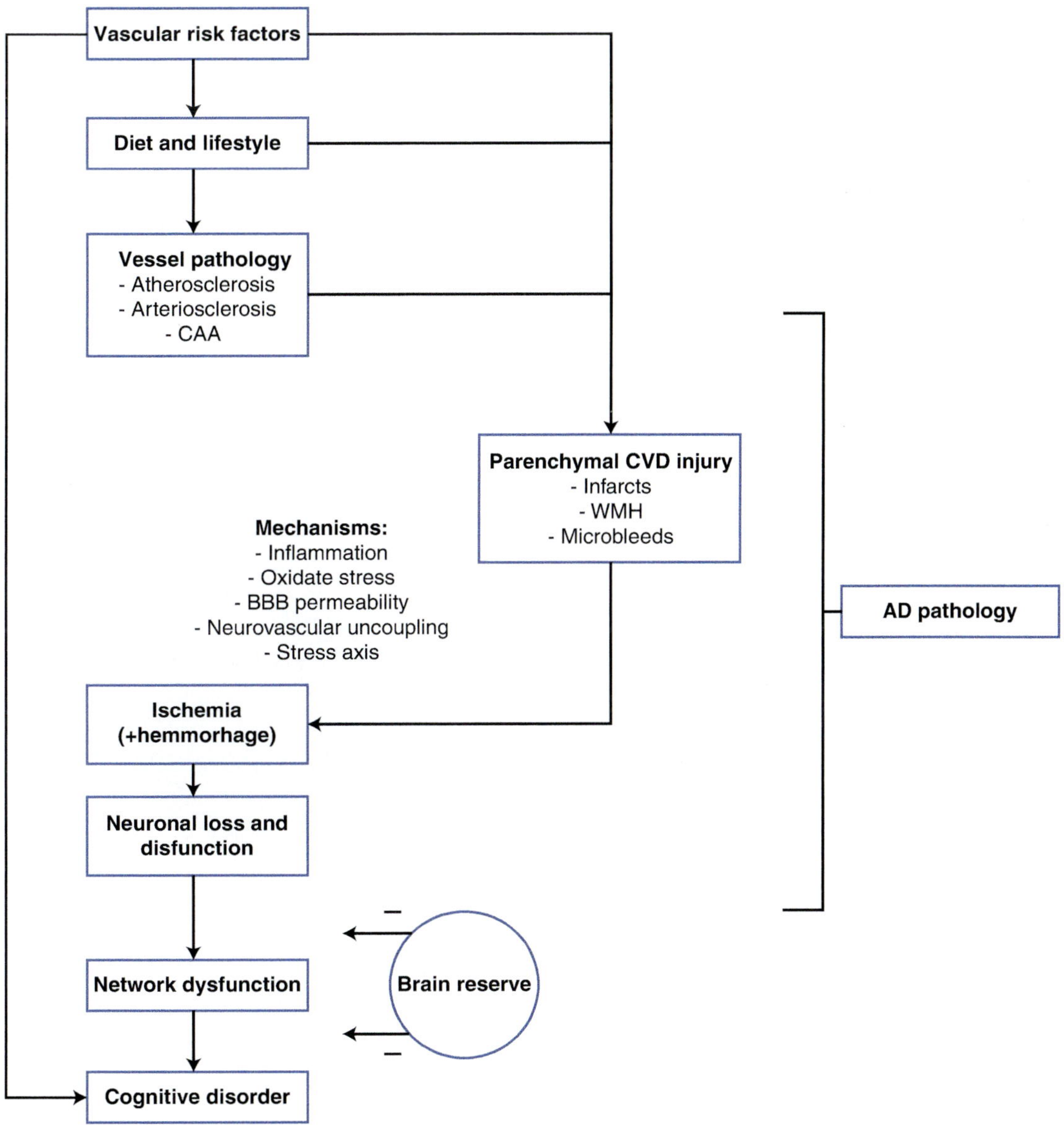

Fig. 13.14 Schema of proposed vascular cognitive disorder mechanisms. Multiple genetic, environmental, and vascular risk factors lead to vessel pathology, cerebrovascular disease (CVD) injury, and subsequent network dysfunction and cognitive impairment through multiple pathways. Brain/cognitive reserve can moderate the expression of this. Alzheimer's disease (AD) pathology interacts with CVD on a number of mechanistic levels. (*From* Paradise and Sachdev [27]; *with permission*)

It is therefore important to focus on the prevention of vascular NCDs and manage the risk factors. There is reasonable evidence for the beneficial effects of physical activity, weight control, smoking cessation, and moderation of alcohol intake. Complex cognitive activity has been examined as a protective factor against cognitive decline. Adequate management of hypertension and atrial fibrillation with oral anticoagulants have been shown to reduce incident dementia. Hyperglycemia and hypercholesterolemia should be adequately treated due to the broader benefits. The American Heart Association recommends "Life's simple 7" for brain health [28].

Delirium

Delirium is an acute neuropsychiatric condition secondary to a medical condition or toxic effects or withdrawal from substances or medications. It is characterized by deficits in awareness and the inability to direct, sustain, and shift attention. DSM-5 criteria for the diagnosis of delirium are presented in Box 13.11. Cognitive impairment is global and can manifest in any of the cognitive domains. In addition, patients can experience sleep–wake cycle disruption, hallucinations, delusions, and agitation [29]. Delirium has previously been classified as the hyperactive or hypoactive phenotypes. It generally develops within hours to days and can last for a variable amount of time, with some cases persisting for months (Fig. 13.15).

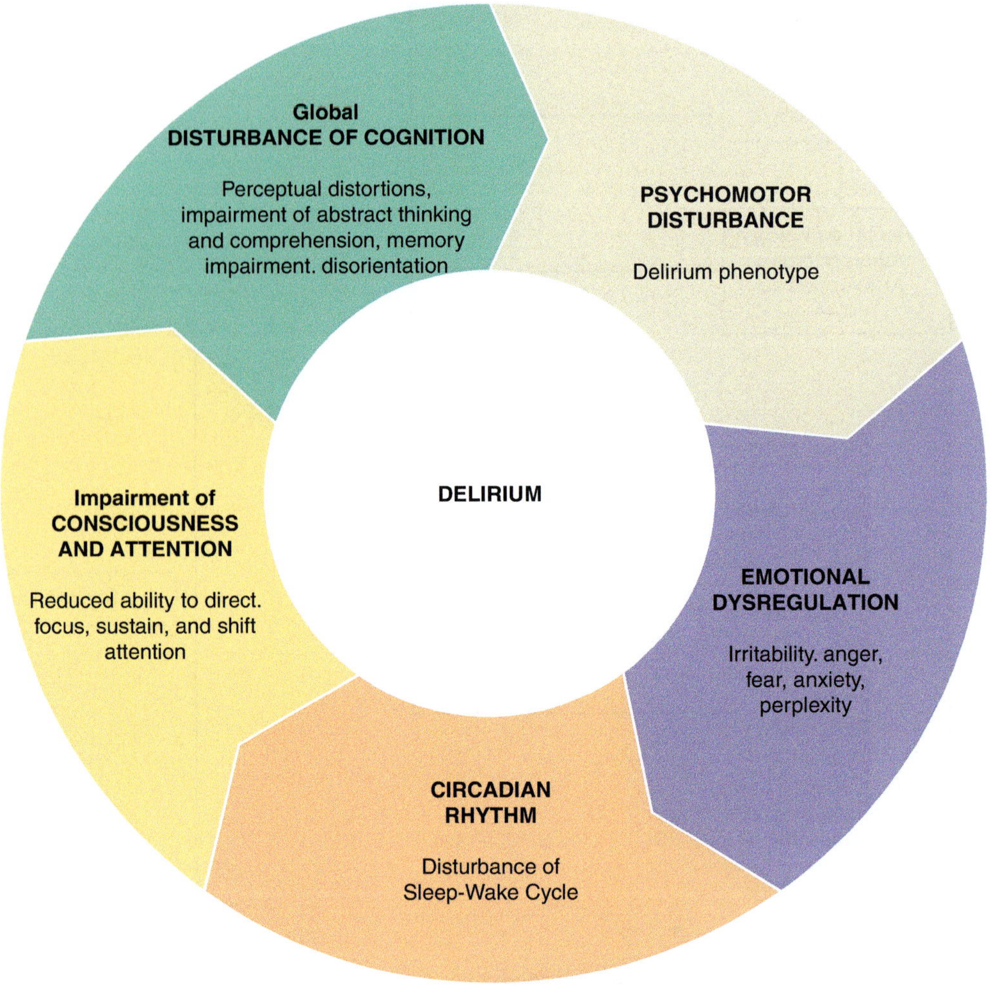

Fig. 13.15 Delirium core domains. The phenomenon of delirium has five core domains: cognitive deficits (characterized by perceptual distortions, impairment in memory, abstract thinking and comprehension, executive dysfunction, and disorientation), attentional deficits (characterized by disturbances in consciousness and a reduced ability to direct, focus, sustain, and shift attention), circadian rhythm dysregulation (characterized by fragmentation of the sleep–wake cycle), emotional dysregulation (characterized by perplexity, fear, anxiety, irritability, and/or anger), and psychomotor dysregulation (which confers the various phenotypic presentations). (*From* Maldonado [29]; *with permission*)

Box 13.11 DSM-5 Diagnostic Criteria for Delirium

1. A disturbance in attention (i.e., reduced ability to direct, focus, sustain, and shift attention) and awareness (reduced orientation to the environment).
2. The disturbance develops over a short period of time (usually hours to a few days), represents a change from baseline attention and awareness, and tends to fluctuate in severity during the course of a day.
3. An additional disturbance in cognition (e.g., memory deficit, disorientation, language, visuospatial ability, or perception).
4. The disturbances in Criteria A and C are not better explained by another preexisting, established, or evolving neurocognitive disorder and do not occur in the context of a severely reduced level of arousal, such as coma.
5. There is evidence from the history, physical examination, or laboratory findings that the disturbance is a direct physiological consequence of another medical condition, substance intoxication or withdrawal (i.e., due to a drug of abuse or to a medication), or exposure to a toxin, or is due to multiple etiologies.

Epidemiology

Delirium is more common in hospital settings, and the prevalence in the community has been estimated to be less than 0.5%. The incidence of delirium in hospitalized patients varies depending on the setting and risk factors, and the incidence and prevalence in the elderly are shown in Fig. 13.16 [30].

Risk Factors

Risk factors can be conceptualized as predisposing and precipitating factors. The vulnerability for delirium is high when there are a number of predisposing risk factors requiring only a minor insult to precipitate delirium and vice versa. Common risk factors are listed in Table 13.12.

Delirium is often underrecognized, and the impacts of delirium on the individual, families, and health care costs are enormous. These have been listed in Table 13.13.

Pathophysiology

Various pathogenetic mechanisms have been proposed. Inflammation is considered to increase exposure to toxins

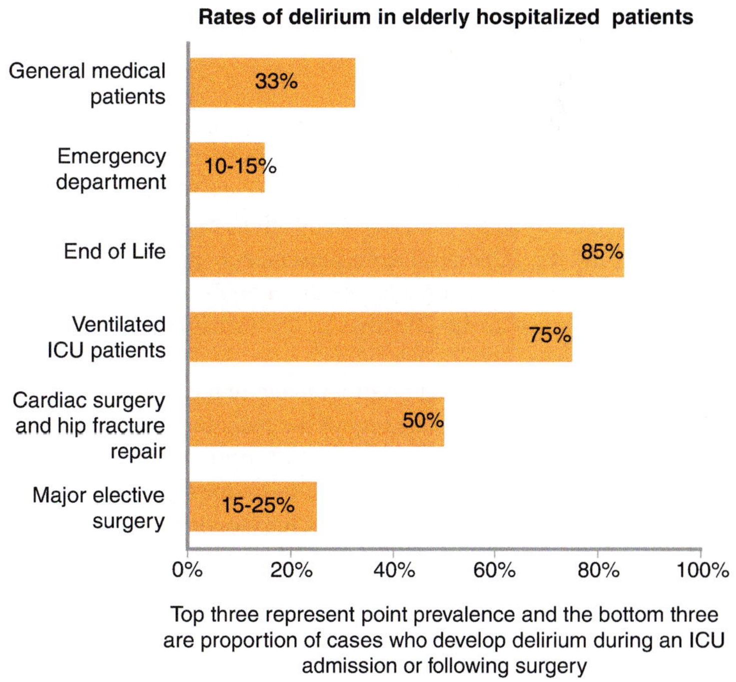

Fig. 13.16 Prevalence/incidence of delirium in elderly hospitalized patients

Table 13.12 Risk factors for delirium

Predisposing factors	Precipitating factors
Old age Major or minor NCD Preexisting medical conditions Male sex Poor vision Blood investigation abnormalities Alcohol use	Drugs—sedatives, anticholinergic Anesthetics Surgery Pain Infections Acute medical illness Exacerbation of preexisting condition Withdrawal or intoxication

Table 13.13 Impact of delirium

Individual and families	Health care costs
Risk of death doubles Risk of institutionalization increases 2.4 times Risk of dementia 12.5 times Loss of one ADL on average after an episode of delirium at 6 months of follow-up Persistence of delirium symptoms for 12 months	Increases length of stay by 5–10 days Cost of treating a person with delirium is 2.5 times more when compared to a nondelirious patient after adjusting for demographic and clinical factors In the United States, the annual national burden of delirium is in the range of $38 billion to $152 billion

through increased blood–brain barrier permeability, oxidative stress is known to increase dopamine, and hypoxia has been shown to reduce acetylcholine levels. In addition, melatonin levels have been low in delirious patients, which could be contributing to the sleep–wake cycle disturbances.

Treatment

The management of delirium requires a thorough evaluation for any reversible causes through a comprehensive history, physical examination, and relevant investigations. In particular, attention has to be given to any medications contributing to delirium and the withdrawal from substances or prescribed medication. Table 13.14 summarizes the models and treatments demonstrated to be effective in the management of delirium [31].

There has been significant progress made in the last couple of decades in our understanding of the pathological processes and our ability to measure these changes in vivo in NCDs. This has led to revisions of the criteria for diagnosis. More developments will make their way into routine clinical care improving diagnosis and our ability to provide targeted therapies and monitor response.

Table 13.14 Management of delirium

Prediction
The PRE-DELIRIC (PREdiction of DELIRium in Intensive Care patients) is a delirium prediction model for ICU patients, Delphi is a model for general surgical patients, and both of them have been shown to improve prediction
Prevention
Yale delirium prevention trial showed that addressing risk factors can reduce the incidence of delirium. The components of their intervention were Orientation Early mobilization Medication reconciliation Sleep–wake cycle preservation Addressing sensory impairment Dehydration Antipsychotics are shown to be helpful in reducing incidence in post-surgical patients, but routine use should be avoided Dexmedetomidine has been shown to reduce the incidence of delirium in ventilated patients
Treatment
Nonpharmacological approach is similar to prevention strategies. In ICU patients, the following ABCDEF bundle approach has been shown to reduce hospital death and coma. A—**A**ssess, prevent and manage pain B—spontaneous awakening and spontaneous **B**reathing trials C—**C**hoice of analgesia and sedation D—**D**elirium assessment, management, and prevention E—**E**arly mobility F—**F**amily engagement Pharmacological approaches Judicious use of antipsychotics for the treatment of agitation and psychotic phenomena. Sodium valproate Dexmedetomidine Melatonin Thiamine should be promptly administered when there is suspicion of alcohol misuse and when oral nutrition has been inadequate

References

1. Neurocognitive disorders. Diagnostic and statistical manual of mental disorders.
2. Diagnostic and statistical manual of mental disorders: DSM-IV: 4th edn. Washington, DC: American Psychiatric Association; 1994.
3. Mitchell AJ, Shiri-Feshki M. Rate of progression of mild cognitive impairment to dementia—meta-analysis of 41 robust inception cohort studies. Acta Psychiatr Scand. 2009;119(4):252–65.
4. Sachdev PS, Blacker D, Blazer DG, Ganguli M, Jeste DV, Paulsen JS, et al. Classifying neurocognitive disorders: the DSM-5 approach. Nat Rev Neurol. 2014;10(11):634–42.
5. Alzheimer's Disease International. World Alzheimer Report 2015: the global impact of dementia: an analysis of prevalence, incidence, cost and trends. 2015.
6. Alzheimer's Association Report. 2019 Alzheimer's disease facts and figures. Alzheimers Dement. 2019;15(3):321–87.

7. Barker WW, Luis CA, Kashuba A, Luis M, Harwood DG, Loewenstein D, et al. Relative frequencies of Alzheimer disease, Lewy body, vascular and frontotemporal dementia, and hippocampal sclerosis in the State of Florida Brain Bank. Alzheimer Dis Assoc Disord. 2002;16(4):203–12.
8. Crutch SJ, Lehmann M, Schott JM, Rabinovici GD, Rossor MN, Fox NC. Posterior cortical atrophy. Lancet Neurol. 2012;11(2):170–8.
9. Sims R, Hill M, Williams J. The multiplex model of the genetics of Alzheimer's disease. Nat Neurosci. 2020;23(3):311–22.
10. Panza F, Lozupone M, Seripa D, Imbimbo BP. Amyloid-β immunotherapy for alzheimer disease: is it now a long shot? Ann Neurol. 2019;85(3):303–15.
11. Hardy J, Selkoe DJ. The amyloid hypothesis of Alzheimer's disease: progress and problems on the road to therapeutics. Science. 2002;297(5580):353–6.
12. Jack CR Jr, Knopman DS, Jagust WJ, Petersen RC, Weiner MW, Aisen PS, et al. Tracking pathophysiological processes in Alzheimer's disease: an updated hypothetical model of dynamic biomarkers. Lancet Neurol. 2013;12(2):207–16.
13. Jack CR Jr, Bennett DA, Blennow K, Carrillo MC, Feldman HH, Frisoni GB, et al. A/T/N: an unbiased descriptive classification scheme for Alzheimer disease biomarkers. Neurology. 2016;87(5):539–47.
14. Khoury R, Ghossoub E. Diagnostic biomarkers of Alzheimer's disease: a state-of-the-art review. Biomarker Neuropsychiatr. 2019;1:100005.
15. Yu J-T, Xu W, Tan C-C, Andrieu S, Suckling J, Evangelou E, et al. Evidence-based prevention of Alzheimer's disease: systematic review and meta-analysis of 243 observational prospective studies and 153 randomised controlled trials. J Neurol Neurosurg Psychiatry. 2020;91(11):1201.
16. Livingston G, Huntley J, Sommerlad A, Ames D, Ballard C, Banerjee S, et al. Dementia prevention, intervention, and care: 2020 report of the *Lancet* Commission. Lancet. 2020;396(10248):413–46.
17. Ngandu T, Lehtisalo J, Solomon A, Levälahti E, Ahtiluoto S, Antikainen R, et al. A 2 year multidomain intervention of diet, exercise, cognitive training, and vascular risk monitoring versus control to prevent cognitive decline in at-risk elderly people (FINGER): a randomised controlled trial. Lancet. 2015;385(9984):2255–63.
18. Grossberg GT. Cholinesterase inhibitors for the treatment of Alzheimer's disease:: getting on and staying on. Curr Ther Res Clin Exp. 2003;64(4):216–35.
19. Birks JS. Cholinesterase inhibitors for Alzheimer's disease. Cochrane Database Syst Rev. 2006;(1).
20. McShane R, Westby MJ, Roberts E, Minakaran N, Schneider L, Farrimond LE, et al. Memantine for dementia. Cochrane Database Syst Rev. 2019;(3).
21. Bang J, Spina S, Miller BL. Frontotemporal dementia. Lancet. 2015;386(10004):1672–82.
22. Huang L-K, Chao S-P, Hu C-J. Clinical trials of new drugs for Alzheimer disease. J Biomed Sci. 2020;27(1):18.
23. McKeith IG, Boeve BF, Dickson DW, Halliday G, Taylor J-P, Weintraub D, et al. Diagnosis and management of dementia with Lewy bodies. Neurology. 2017;89(1):88.
24. Weil RS, Lashley TL, Bras J, Schrag AE, Schott JM. Current concepts and controversies in the pathogenesis of Parkinson's disease dementia and Dementia with Lewy Bodies. F1000Res. 2017;6:1604.
25. Elahi FM, Miller BL. A clinicopathological approach to the diagnosis of dementia. Nat Rev Neurol. 2017;13(8):457–76.
26. Liu M-N, Lau C-I, Lin C-P. Precision medicine for frontotemporal dementia. Front Psych. 2019;10:75.
27. Paradise MB, Sachdev PS. Vascular cognitive disorder. Semin Neurol. 2019;39(2):241–50.
28. Iadecola C, Duering M, Hachinski V, Joutel A, Pendlebury ST, Schneider JA, et al. Vascular cognitive impairment and dementia: JACC scientific expert panel. J Am Coll Cardiol. 2019;73(25):3326–44.
29. Maldonado JR. Delirium pathophysiology: an updated hypothesis of the etiology of acute brain failure. Int J Geriatr Psychiatry. 2018;33(11):1428–57.
30. Marcantonio ER. Delirium in hospitalized older adults. N Engl J Med. 2017;377(15):1456–66.
31. Thom RP, Levy-Carrick NC, Bui M, Silbersweig D. Delirium. Am J Psychiatr. 2019;176(10):785–93.

14 Substance-Related and Addictive Disorders

Mira Zein and Itai Danovitch

Introduction

The Substance-Related and Addictive Disorders section of the Diagnostic and Statistical Manual, 5th edition (DSM-5), encompasses ten substance classes and their disorders and gambling disorder [1]. These diagnostic criteria encompass maladaptive patterns of substance use and gambling behaviors with loss of control, compulsivity, and harmful biological and psychosocial consequences. These are syndromes with common, core symptoms and wide-ranging features depending on the substance, the environment, and the intrinsic characteristics of the individual [2].

Substance-Related Disorders and Gambling Disorder

Introduction

The DSM-5 divides substance-related disorders into substance-use disorders and substance-induced disorders, focusing on ten major substance categories (Fig. 14.1). A substance-use disorder (SUD) is defined as "a problematic pattern of substance use leading to "clinically significant impairment or distress," manifest by at least 2 of 11 criteria over a given year" [1]. Substance-induced disorders consist of substance intoxication, substance withdrawal, and "other substance-induced disorders," which encompass a variety of substance-induced mental disorders covered in other DSM-5 chapters (e.g., opioid-induced anxiety disorders are covered under "Anxiety Disorders"). Note that substance withdrawal is both a substance-induced disorder and a diagnostic criterion for substance-use disorders (see Table 14.3 in the Phenomenology Section).

The nine specific classes (the tenth class is "other") of intoxicating substances identified in the DSM-5 are shown in Fig. 14.1, and the diagnostic conditions are shown in Table 14.1. Of note, while caffeine is recognized as a substance class, the DSM-5 chapter defines caffeine-induced disorders (caffeine intoxication and caffeine withdrawal), but has not yet included caffeine use disorder as an official diagnosis (see section "Future Directions"). Gambling disorder is defined as "persistent and recurrent problematic gambling behavior leading to clinically significant impairment or distress, as indicated by the individual exhibiting at least 2 of 9 criteria in a 12 month period" [1].

Epidemiology of Substance-Related Disorders and Gambling Disorder

According to the 2020 United Nations World Drug Report, on an annual basis, approximately 269 million people globally use intoxicating substances other than alcohol (Fig. 14.2), 35 million people have a substance-use disorder, and 500,000 die because of their substance use [3]. In addition, approximately 38% of the population drinks alcohol, with 3.5–14.8% having an alcohol use disorder, and harmful use resulting in three million deaths and 131 million disability-adjusted life years (DALYs) each year (Fig. 14.3) [4].

The National Survey on Drug Use and Health (NSDUH) provides detailed information about SUD in the United States [5]. As Fig. 14.4 demonstrates, in 2019, among people over the age of 12, over 165 million people (60% of the pop-

M. Zein (✉)
Department of Psychiatry and Behavioral Sciences, Department of Primary Care and Population Health, Stanford University School of Medicine, Stanford, CA, USA
e-mail: mzein@stanford.edu

I. Danovitch
Department of Psychiatry and Behavioral Neurosciences, Cedars-Sinai Medical Center, Los Angeles, CA, USA
e-mail: Itai.Danovitch@cshs.org

W. W. IsHak (ed.), *Atlas of Psychiatry*, https://doi.org/10.1007/978-3-031-15401-0_14

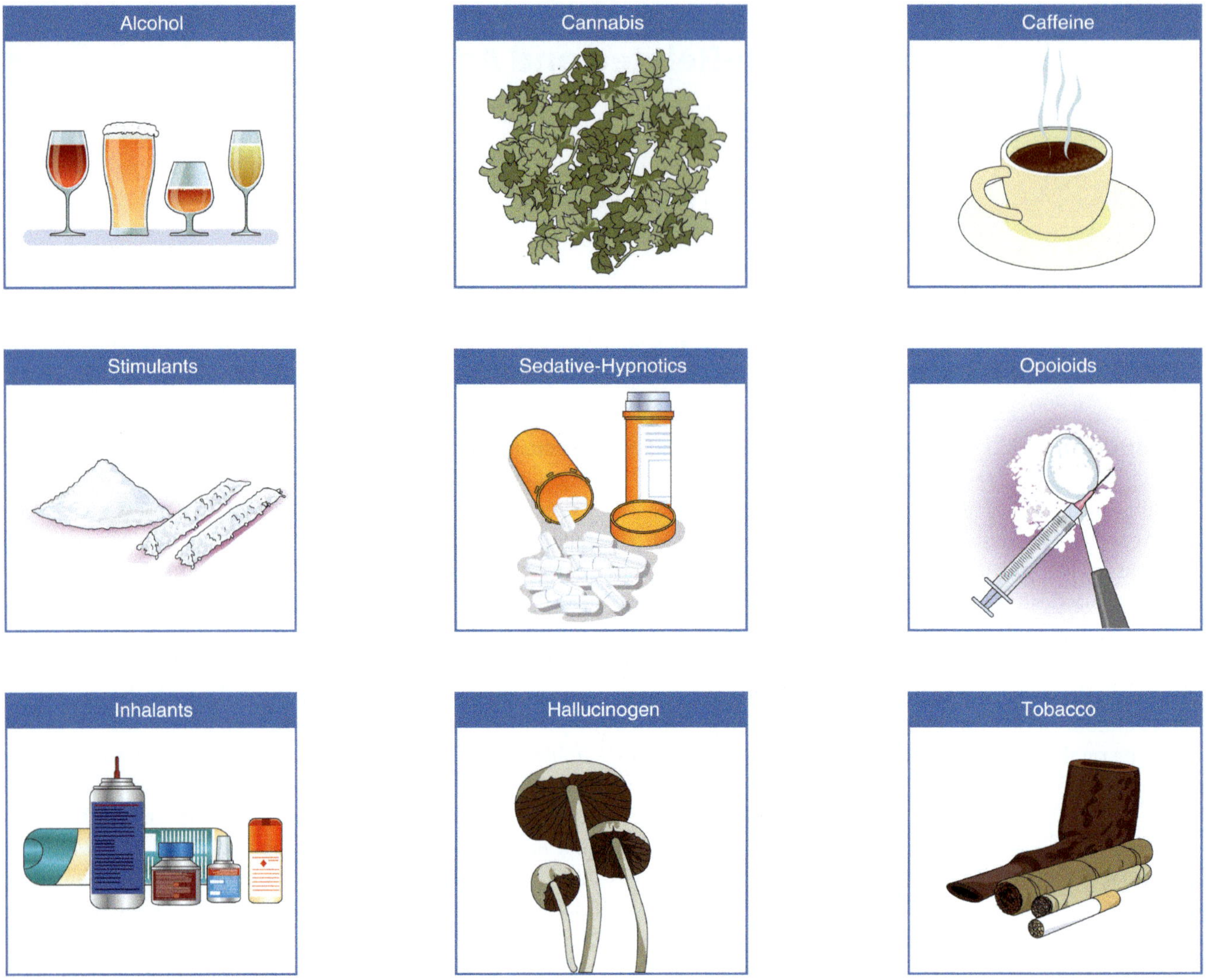

Fig. 14.1 DSM-5 defined substance classes for substance-related disorders

Table 14.1 Substance-related and addictive disorders

Class	Related disorder
Alcohol	Alcohol use disorder
	Alcohol intoxication
	Alcohol withdrawal
Caffeine	Caffeine intoxication
	Caffeine withdrawal
Cannabis	Cannabis use disorder
	Cannabis intoxication (with or without perceptual disturbances)
	Cannabis withdrawal
Hallucinogen	Phencyclidine use disorder
	Other hallucinogen use disorder
	Phencyclidine intoxication
	Other hallucinogen intoxication
	Hallucinogen persisting perception disorder
Inhalant	Inhalant use disorder
	Inhalant intoxication
	Other inhalant-induced disorders

Table 14.1 (continued)

Class	Related disorder
Opioid	Opioid use disorder
	Opioid intoxication (with or without perceptual disturbances)
	Opioid withdrawal
	Other opioid-induced disorders
Sedative, hypnotic, or anxiolytic	Sedative, hypnotic, or anxiolytic use disorder
	Sedative, hypnotic, or anxiolytic intoxication
	Sedative, hypnotic, or anxiolytic withdrawal (with or without perceptual disturbances)
	Other sedative-, hypnotic-, or anxiolytic-induced disorders
Stimulant	Stimulant use disorder E.g., amphetamine-type substance; cocaine
	Stimulant intoxication E.g., amphetamine or other stimulants (with or without perceptual disturbances); cocaine (with or without perceptual disturbances)
	Stimulant withdrawal E.g., amphetamine or other stimulants; cocaine
	Other stimulant-induced disorders
Tobacco-related disorders	Tobacco use disorder
	Tobacco withdrawal
	Other tobacco-induced disorders
Other (or unknown) substance	Other (or unknown) substance-use disorder
	Other (or unknown) substance intoxication
	Other (or unknown) substance withdrawal
	Other (or unknown) substance-induced disorders
	Unspecified other (or unknown) substance-related disorder
Nonsubstance	Gambling disorder

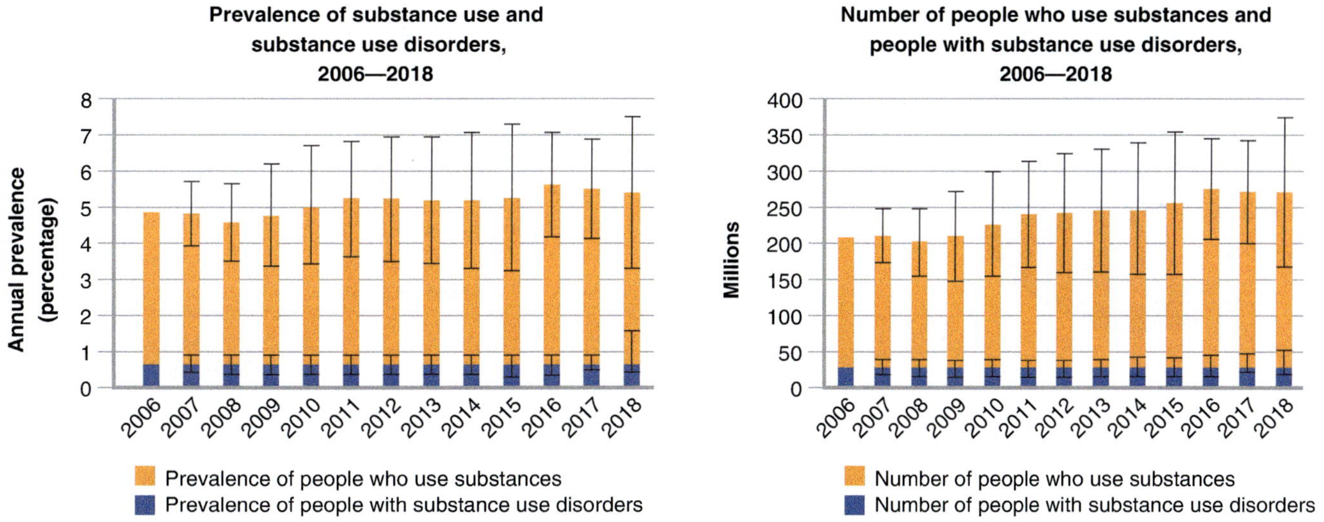

Fig. 14.2 Global prevalence and number of people (in millions) who use substances and have substance-use disorders

ulation) reported using an intoxicating substance in the past month (80% in the past year). Among these, 140 million people used alcohol, 58 million used tobacco, and 31 million used cannabis in the past month. Among illicit drugs, use of prescription opioids was most common, followed by cocaine, sedative-hypnotics, hallucinogens, and stimulants [5].

Additionally, 20 million people (7.4% of the US adult population) had a SUD in the past year. Figure 14.5 shows the breakdown of specific SUDs. The total number is greater than 20 million because over a third of individuals have two or more SUDs. Only 11% of those people actually received treatment at a hospital, a drug or alcohol rehabilitation program, or a mental health center [5].

Figure 14.6 demonstrates how SUD, mental illness, and medical conditions often co-occur as each category of illness can predispose and perpetuate illness in the other categories.

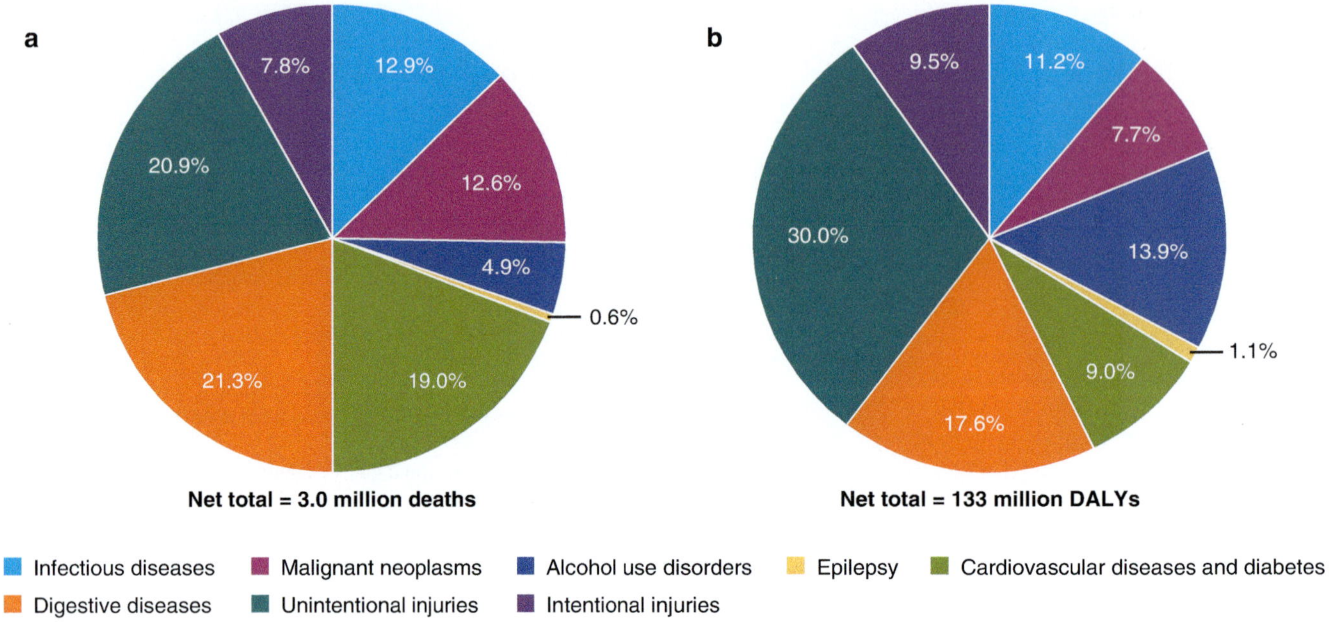

Fig. 14.3 (**a**) Percentage of alcohol-attributable deaths and (**b**) percentage of alcohol-attributable disability-adjusted-life years (DALYs) globally, by broad disease category, as of 2016

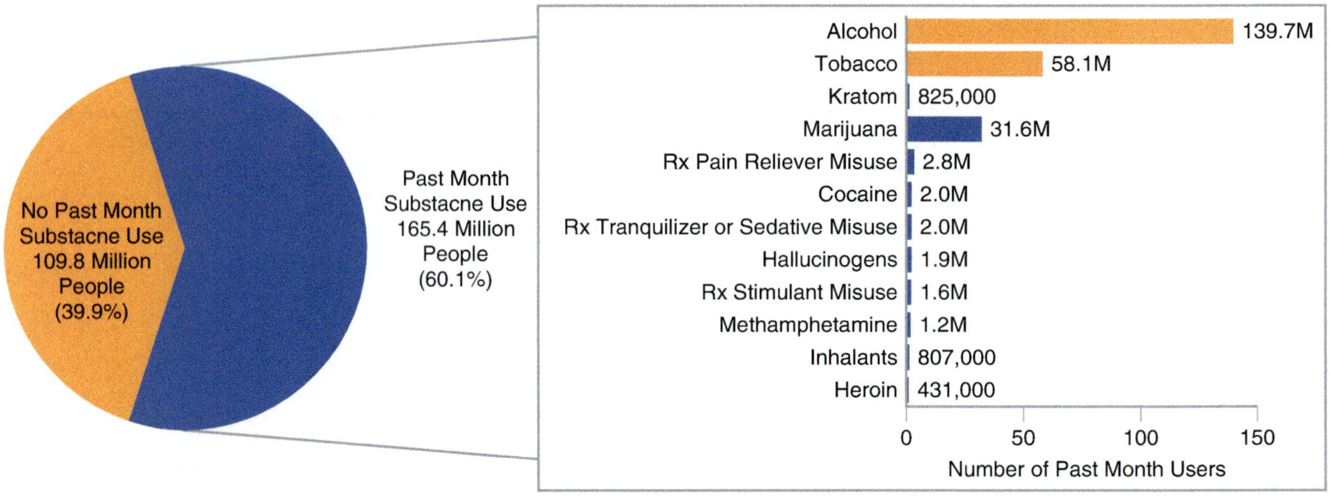

Fig. 14.4 Past month substance use among persons over the age of 12 in the United States in 2019

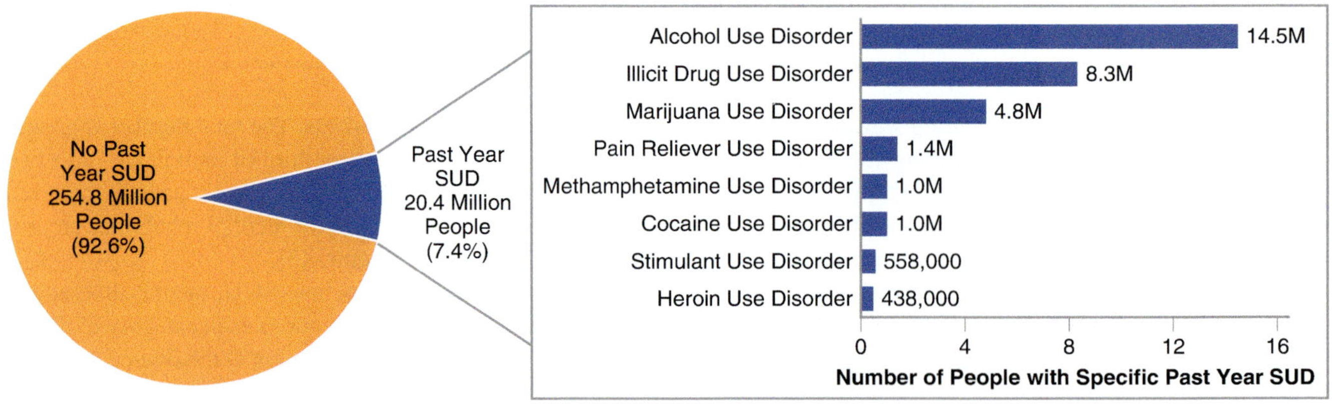

Fig. 14.5 Past year substance-use disorder among persons over the age of 12 in the United States in 2019

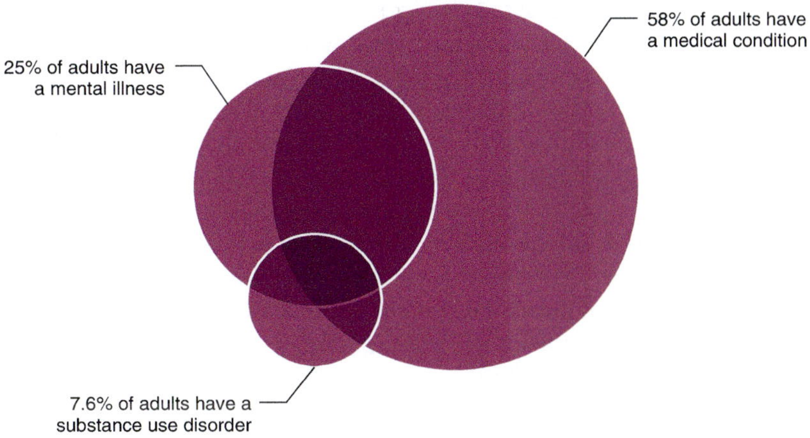

Fig. 14.6 Comorbidity of medical conditions, mental illness, and substance-use disorder in the United States

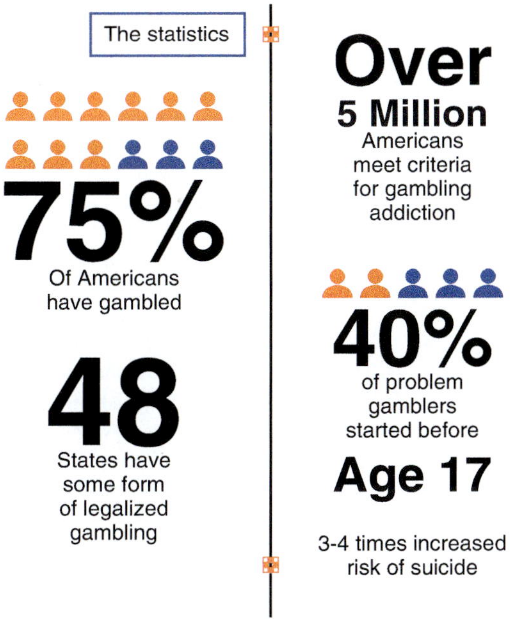

Fig. 14.7 Facts on gambling and gambling disorder in the United States

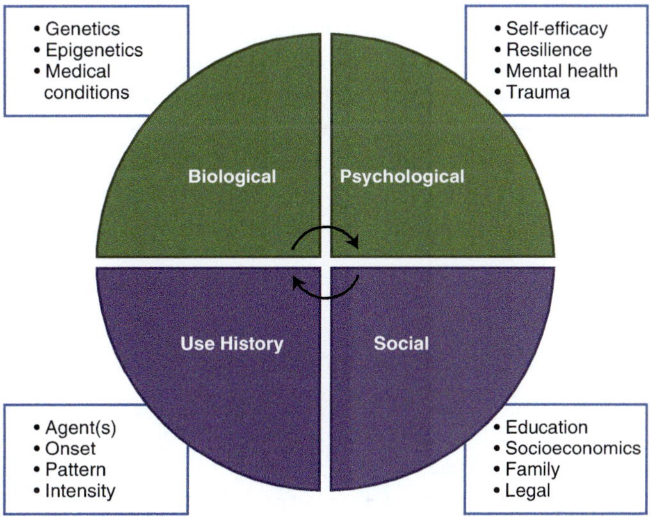

Fig. 14.8 Overview of the biological, psychological, social, and use factor domains that impact the development of a substance-use disorder

Approximately, 8.5 million adults (3.4%) had both a mental health condition and an alcohol or SUD in the past year. Among people with a SUD, 15 million (73%) had an alcohol use disorder, eight million (40%) had an illicit drug use disorder, and 2.7 million (13%) had both [5].

The lifetime prevalence of gambling disorder ranges globally between 0.2% and 2% depending on country and study, with a US average lifetime prevalence of 0.5% [6, 7]. According to the WHO, there are 350 million people worldwide who display problematic gambling behavior, with a 12-month prevalence of 0.1–5.8% [8]. As of 2015, over five million Americans met the criteria for gambling use disorder. Approximately two-thirds of persons with gambling disorder have a comorbid substance-use disorder, and gambling disorder is associated with an elevated risk of suicide attempts and completion (Fig. 14.7) [6].

Etiology

Substance-related and gambling disorders are paradigmatic biopsychosocial diseases. The etiology of these disorders encompasses complex interactions between biological factors (genetic vulnerability, physiological and behavioral responses to substance use, epigenetic changes to neurocircuits governing addiction), environmental factors (legality and criminalization, cultural perceptions, availability), psychological factors (personality traits such as novelty seeking), and substance factors (dose, route, biological action). Figure 14.8 summarizes the domains and factors that confer protective effects or vulnerability to substance-related and gambling disorders.

Genetics

Early family-based studies pointed to alcohol and other substance-use disorders clustering in families. Adoption studies further demonstrated genetic predisposition, with the presence of SUD among biological parents associated with increased risk in their offspring regardless of the adoptive environment [9]. As shown in Fig. 14.9, large cohort studies of monozygotic twins have provided heritability estimates for several different substance-use disorders [11]. These ranges indicate a significant genetic contributor to substance-use disorders. For gambling disorder, familial and twin studies have reported a higher presence of gambling disorder in family members of individuals diagnosed with gambling disorder, with one study finding a lifetime prevalence of up to 20% of first-degree relatives [6].

Animal studies and different candidate gene association studies (CGAS) have implicated genes that underlie the neurobiology of substance-related disorders. For instance, underlying all substances with addiction potential is their ability to activate the brain's reward pathway and increase dopamine levels in the nucleus accumbens. In addition to dopamine, other neurotransmitters including serotonin, opioid peptides such as dynorphins, gamma-aminobutyric acid (GABA), acetylcholine, endocannabinoids, and glutamate also contribute to reward pathway activation [11]. Several of the genetic polymorphisms related to SUDs have also been linked to gambling disorder [6, 7]. Table 14.2 demonstrates a small sample of different genes implicated in various substance-related disorder phenotypes, including the involvement of different neurotransmitter systems and substance metabolism.

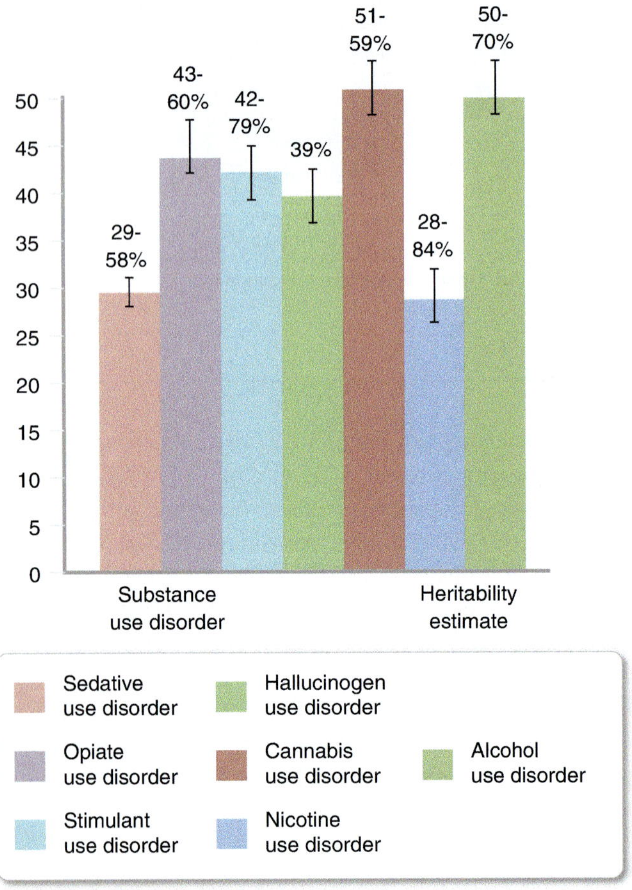

Fig. 14.9 Heritability estimates of substance-use disorders from monozygotic twin, adoption, and family studies. (Adapted from Ho et al. [10] with permission)

Neurodevelopment

Influencing the neurodevelopment of substance use and gambling behaviors are not only genetic polymorphisms but also epigenetic changes generated through early life stressors, such as insecure attachments; physical, emotional, and

Table 14.2 CGAS studies revealing genes implicated in substance-use disorder and gambling disorder phenotypes (Adapted from Ho et al. [10] with permission)

Target	Gene	Phenotype
Dopamine		
Receptors	*DRD2*	Smoking initiation, persistence, cigarette consumption, cessation
		Heroin use, cocaine use disorder
		Psychostimulant polysubstance-use disorder (mild)
		Alcoholism
	DRD3	Gambling disorder
	DRD4	Smoking risk, time to first cigarette, craving and response to smoking cues, nicotine use disorder
		Heroin, cocaine use disorder
		Methamphetamine use
		Gambling disorder
Transporters	*SLC6A3 (DAT1)*	Smoking risk
		Cocaine use disorder
Metabolism	*MAO-A*	Cigarette consumption, smoking risk, nicotine use disorder
		Gambling disorder
	TH	Smoking risk
	DBH	Smoking risk, nicotine use disorder
	COMT	Smoking risk, treatment response to nicotine spray and patch, nicotine use disorder
		Heroin, cocaine use disorder
		Alcohol use disorder
		Methamphetamine use
		Gambling disorder
Serotonin		
Transporters	*SLC6A4 (5HTT, SERT)*	Smoking risk, cigarette consumption, use disorder
		Alcohol use disorder
		Heroin use disorder
		Gambling disorder
Metabolism	*TPH1, 2*	Age of smoking initiation, risk of smoking
		Heroin use disorder
		Alcohol use disorder

Table 14.2 (continued)

Target	Gene	Phenotype
Receptor	*HTR2A*	Gambling disorder
Opioid		
Receptor (μ, δ, κ)	*OPRM1*	Heroin, opiate use disorder Alcohol use disorder
	OPRK1	Heroin, opiate use disorder Alcohol use disorder
	OPRD1	Heroin, cocaine use disorder
Acetylcholine		
Receptor	*CHRNA4*	Nicotine use disorder
	CHRNA5, A3, B4 gene cluster on chromosome 15	Nicotine use disorder, cigarette consumption, lung cancer, and COPD risk Alcohol, cocaine use disorder
Gamma-aminobutyric acid (GABA)		
Receptor	*GABRG2*	Heroin use disorder, methamphetamine use
	GABRA2	Alcohol use disorder
	GABBR2	Nicotine use disorder
Non-neurotransmitter enzyme targets		
Cytochrome P450 2A6	*CYP2A6*	Smoking risk, cigarette consumption, smoking cessation
Alcohol dehydrogenase 2	*ADH2, ADH4, ADH1B, ADH1C*	Alcohol use disorder
Aldehyde dehydrogenase 2	*ALDH2*	Alcohol use disorder
Cytochrome P450 2E1	*CYP2E1*	Alcohol use disorder

DRD2 D2 dopamine receptor; *DRD3* D3 dopamine receptor; *DRD4* D4 dopamine receptor; *SLC6A3 (DAT1)* dopamine transporter type 1; *MAO-A* monoamine oxidase A; *TH* tyrosine hydroxylase; *DBH* dopamine β hydroxylase; *COMT* catechol-*O*-methyltransferase; *SLC6A4 (5HTT, SERT)* serotonin transporter; *TPH1,2* tryptophan hydroxylase 1 and 2; *HTR2A* 2A serotonin receptor; *OPRM1/K1/D1* opioid receptor M1/K1/D1 subtypes; *CHRNA3/A4/A5/B4* nicotinic cholinergic receptor, α3, α4, α5, β4 subunit; *GABRG2* $GABA_A$ receptor, γ2 subunit; *GABRA2* $GABA_A$ receptor, α2 subunit; *GABBR2* $GABA_B$ receptor, subunit 2

sexual abuse; neglect; household instability; and poverty. These stressors lead to epigenetic changes that will alter circuits, influencing future substance use [12, 13]. Brain regions that are central to drug reward and reinforcement of behavior are part of the dopaminergic system [12, 14]. While dopaminergic circuits govern the robust drug reward response in substance use, recent publications review nondopaminergic circuits that also contribute to the development of substance-related disorders [14].

Figure 14.10 demonstrates the interconnectedness between the dopaminergic (DA) reward pathway, the hypothalamic–pituitary–adrenal (HPA) axis, and oxytocin (OT) circuits in the brain. Adverse childhood experiences lead to epigenetic changes in dopamine, oxytocin, and glucocorticoid production and receptor expression, which then changes brain reward pathways and how the brain responds to external cues. These alterations lead to higher-risk behaviors and development of mental health disorders that increase an individual's susceptibility to substance-use disorders [13].

The Dopamine Reward System

Figure 14.11 visualizes the main DA pathways in the brain. Most cerebral DA neurons are located in the ventral midbrain where the mesolimbic, mesocortical, and nigrostriatal DA systems begin. The mesolimbic DA system, known for its roles in reward and motivation, arises from the ventral tegmental area (VTA) and projects to the nucleus accumbens (NAc) (part of the ventral striatum) and amygdala (AMY); the mesocortical pathway projects from the VTA to the prefrontal cortex (PFC). The nigrostriatal DA system coordinates voluntary movement and regulates habit formation; it originates from the substantia nigra (SN) and projects to the dorsal striatum (DS) [14].

DA-related dysfunction has been associated with the pathophysiology of many psychiatric disorders, including depression, psychosis, substance-related, and gambling disorders. A growing body of research has established associations between early life experiences and DA changes. Figure 14.10 summarizes collated findings on dopaminergic changes at the molecular, neuroendocrine, and behavioral levels [6, 14].

The Hypothalamic–Pituitary–Adrenal Axis

The hypothalamic-pituitary-adrenal (HPA) axis governs the body's stress response and influences continued drug use, withdrawal, and relapse. Figure 14.12 outlines the HPA axis and its connection to the dopaminergic reward pathway. Stress activates the paraventricular nucleus (PVN) of the hypothalamus to release corticotropin-releasing factor (CRF). CRF binds to receptors in the pituitary to stimulate adrenocorticotropic hormone (ACTH) production [11]. ACTH is then transported to adrenal glands, leading to cortisol secretion. Once released, cortisol acts at glucocorticoid receptors (GRs) in the hypothalamus, pituitary, and hippocampus, to suppress further CRF and ACTH production (Fig. 14.12) [13]. The amygdala also produces CRF and mobilizes the HPA axis. Cortisol will stimulate the VTA, which leads to the activation of reward-seeking behaviors to mitigate stress (Fig. 14.12) [13].

As discussed below, in the withdrawal/negative affect stage of substance misuse, HPA axis dysregulation impacts SUD. Additionally, stress exposure precipitates substance use onset, decreases motivation to discontinue use, and enhances the risk of relapse [13]. The right column of Fig. 14.10 depicts how early childhood adversities increase HPA expression and stress sensitivity at a molecular level, leading to an individual's impaired capacity to respond effectively to stress and increasing susceptibility to substance use [13].

Oxytocin Pathways

Oxytocin's multiple functions are reflected in Fig. 14.13, which depicts modulatory interactions with systems impli-

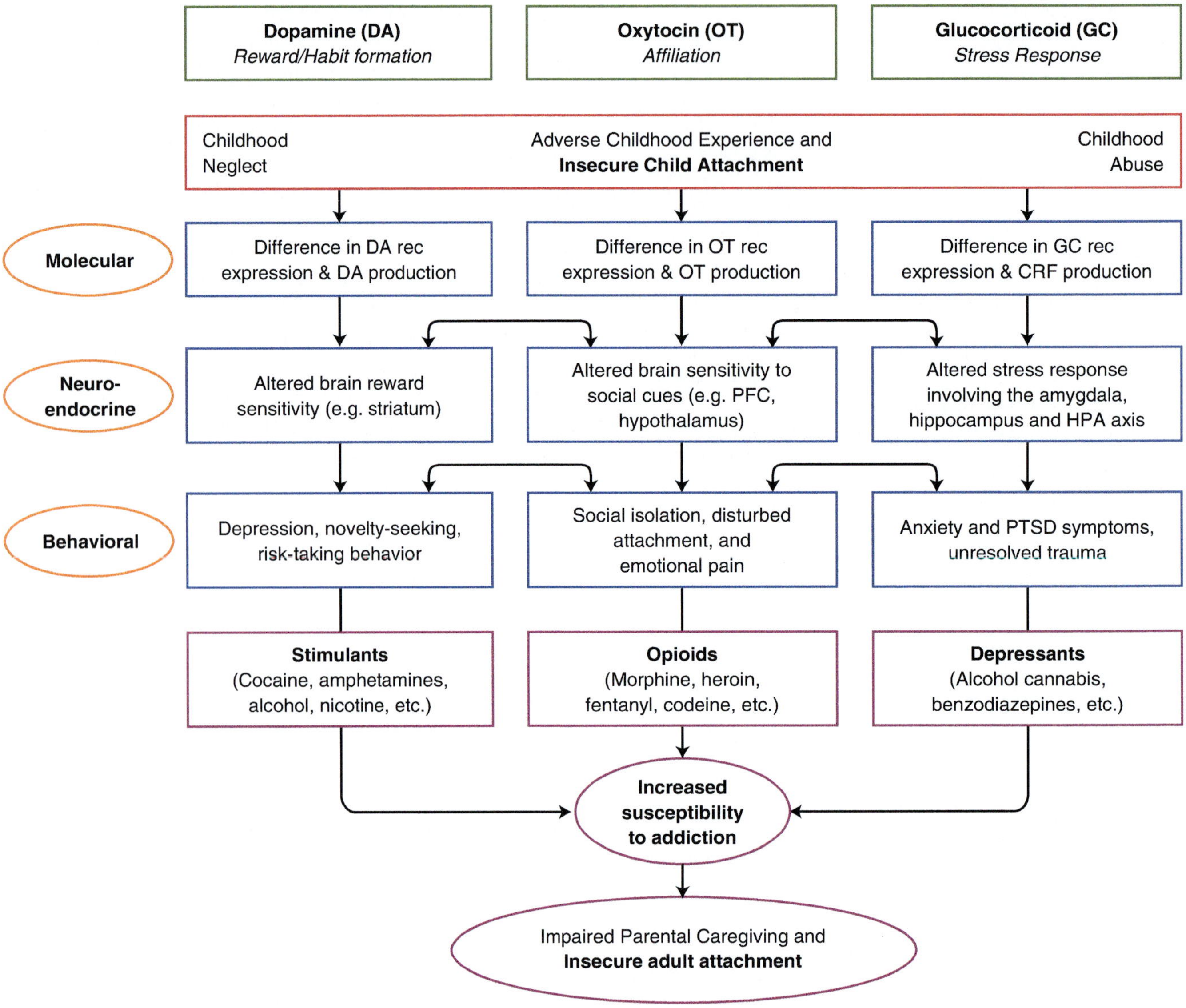

Fig. 14.10 Developmental and neurobiological pathways linking adverse childhood experience to susceptibility to addiction, due to modifications in the dopamine, oxytocin, and hypothalamic–pituitary–adrenal systems at molecular, neuroendocrine, and behavioral levels. *DA* dopamine; *OT* oxytocin; *GC* glucocorticoid; *rec* receptor; *CRF* corticotropin-releasing factor; *PFC* prefrontal cortex; *HPA* hypothalamic–pituitary–adrenal; *PTSD* post-traumatic stress disorder. (*Reproduced from* Strathearn et al. [13]; https://www.frontiersin.org/articles/10.3389/fpsyt.2019.00737/full. Creative Commons Attribution License [CC BY 4.0])

cated in mood, stress, immune function, and addiction. Oxytocin is synthesized in the PVN and supraoptic nuclei. It is transported to the posterior pituitary gland. Oxytocin-producing neurons project to brain regions involved in social interactions, including the amygdala, ventral tegmental area, and the ventral striatum [13, 15].

As Fig. 14.13a demonstrates, oxytocin inhibits the HPA and dopamine reward systems. Studies have demonstrated oxytocin-mitigated inhibition of substance consumption, substance reward response, emotional impairments in withdrawal, and stress-induced relapse [15]. In early childhood adversity, all of the systems in Fig. 14.13 are dysregulated, including suboptimal development of the oxytocin system. As depicted in the middle column of Fig. 14.10, oxytocin dysfunction leads to changes in social behaviors that increase the risk of substance-use disorders [13, 15]. In early childhood adversity, the modulatory role of oxytocin on the other systems is also reduced. As oxytocin levels and reactivity are reduced, the negative feedback loops it regulates become dysfunctional. The associated outcome is an increased susceptibility to substance-related disorders through increased expression of dopaminergic and HPA systems, as seen in Fig. 14.13b [15].

Comorbidities with Personality, Psychiatric, and Medical Conditions

The genetic and epigenetic changes that alter different neurobiological systems not only impact vulnerability to

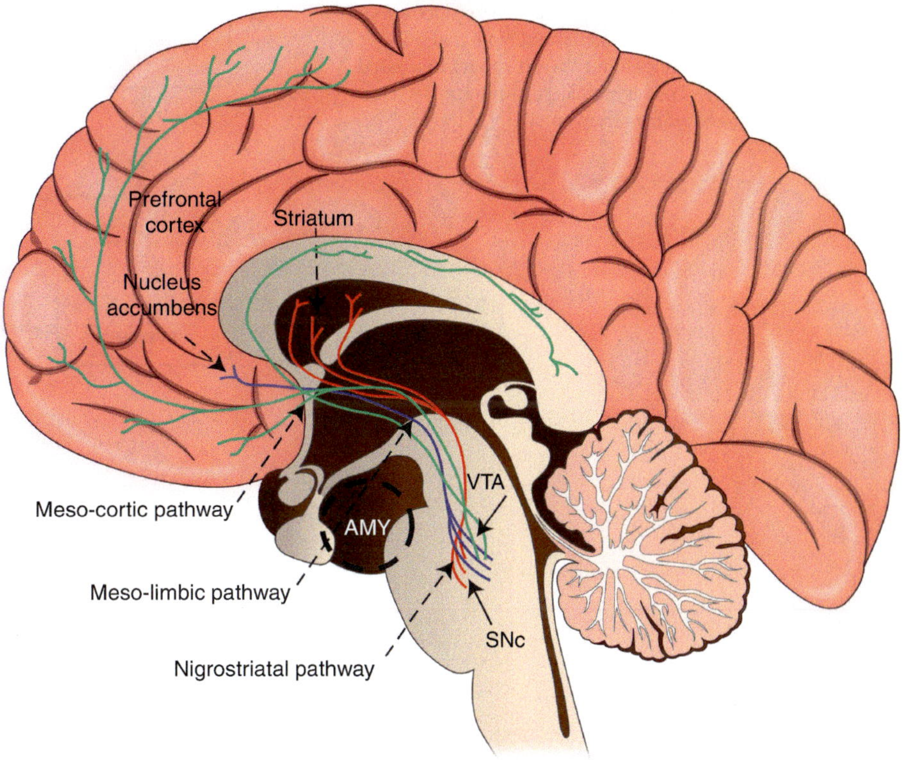

Fig. 14.11 Major dopaminergic pathways in the brain. *VTA* ventral tegmental area; *SN_c* substantia nigra pars compacta, *AMY* amygdala

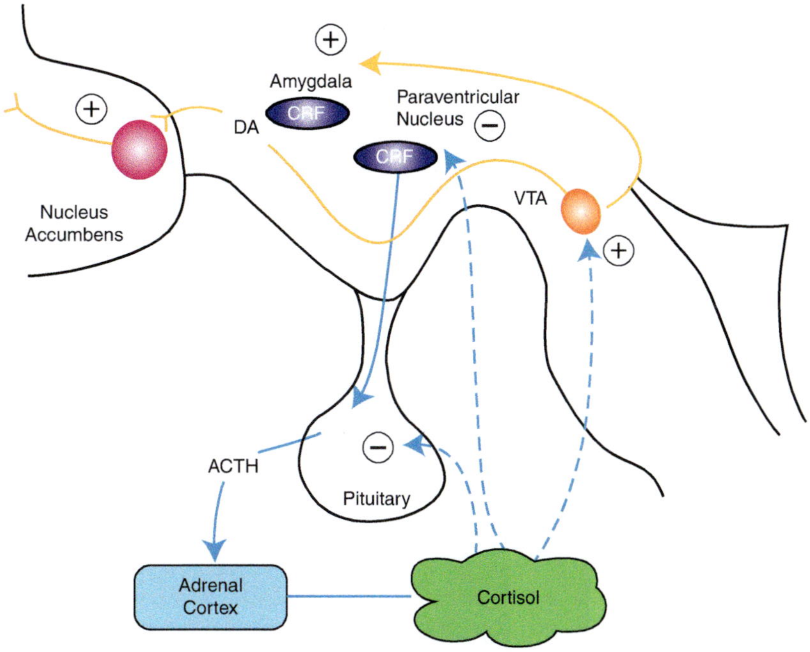

Fig. 14.12 The hypothalamic–pituitary–adrenal axis in relation to dopaminergic circuits. *CRF* cortico-tropin releasing factor; *ACTH* adrenocorticotropin hormone; *VTA* ventral tegmental area; *DA* dopamine

substance-related and gambling disorders but also influence an individual's development of personality traits, medical disorders, and psychiatric illness. In Fig. 14.14, genome-wide association studies (GWAS) mapped correlations between cigarette smoking and alcohol use parameters and various medical and psychiatric illnesses, with purple shading corresponding to negative correlations, orange to positive correlations, and intensity of color mapping to strength. The result was a network of interconnected correlations between alcohol- and nicotine-related behavior and a multitude of comorbidities [16].

Personality Traits

Figure 14.15 depicts three studied systems of personality.

Image (A) depicts the positive emotionality/extroversion (PEM/E) personality trait, which correlates with increased

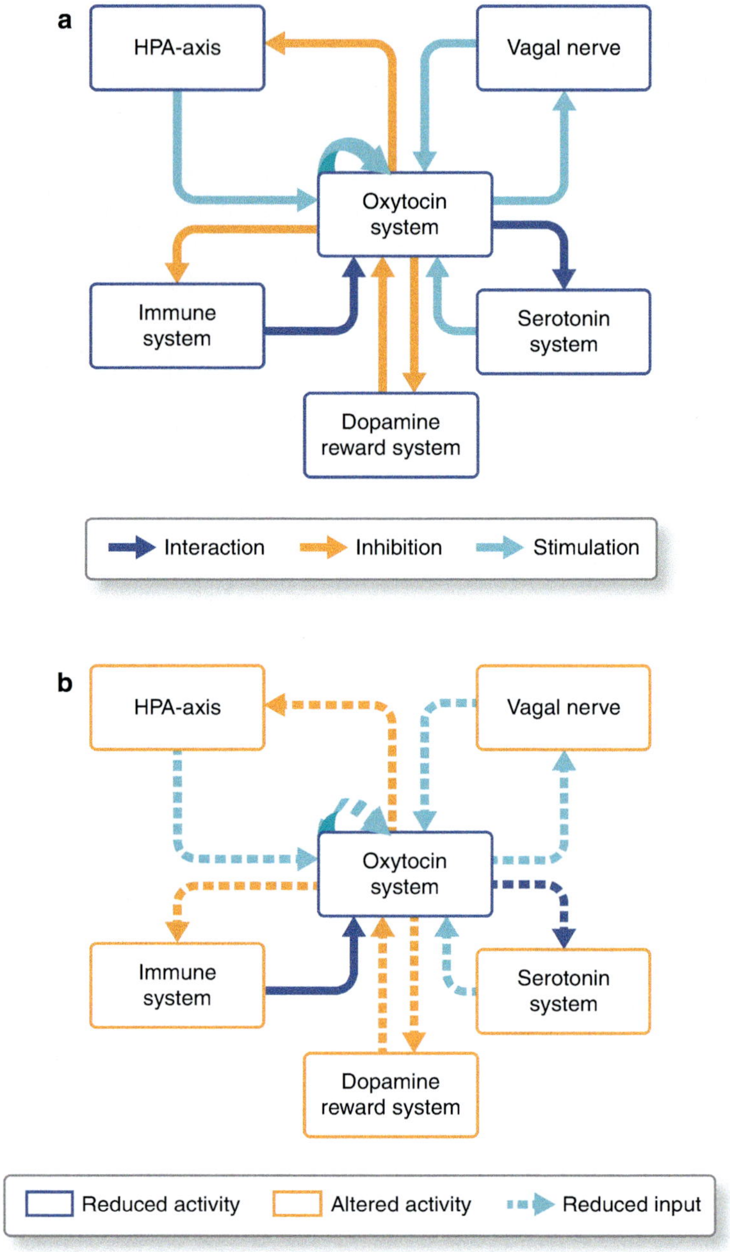

Fig. 14.13 Bidirectional interactions between oxytocin and other systems implicated in addiction. Note that only oxytocin, HPA-axis, and dopamine reward system discussed in detail in this chapter. *HPA* hypothalamic–pituitary–adrenal axis. (*Reproduced from* Bowen et al. [15]; *with permission*)

Fig. 14.14 Summary of GWAS studies correlations with cigarettes and alcohol markers and chronic physical and mental disorders. (*Reproduced from* Liu et al. [16]; *with permission*)

AgeSmk	CigDay	SmkInit	SmkCes	DrnkWk	
h2 = 0.05	-0.38**	-0.71**	-0.31**	-0.10*	Age of smoking initiation (AgeSmk)
-0.38**	h2 = 0.08	0.33**	0.42**	0.07*	Cigarettes per day (CigDay)
-0.71**	-0.33**	h2 = 0.08	0.40**	0.34**	Smoking initiation (SmkInit)
-0.31**	-0.42**	-0.40**	h2 = 0.05	0.11**	Smoking cessation (SmkCes)
-0.10*	-0.07*	-0.34*	0.11*	h2 = 0.04	Drinks per week (DrnkWk)
0.04	-0.01	-0.03	-0.10**	-0.02	Height
0.22**	-0.09*	-0.04	-0.02	-0.08*	Age at menarche
0.67**	-0.40**	-0.48**	-0.46**	-0.01	Age of first birth
0.55**	0.26**	-0.40**	-0.51**	-0.01	Years of education
-0.21	0.63*	0.16*	0.43*	-0.02	Cotinine
-0.32**	0.15**	0.28**	0.12**	0.20**	General risk tolerance
-0.43**	0.09	0.60**	0.06	0.36	Lifetime cannabis use
-0.31*	0.20*	0.41*	0.17*	0.17	ADHD
-0.06	-0.04	0.01	-0.08	-0.03	Autism spectrum disorder
-0.02	0.06	0.06	-0.10*	-0.04	Bipolar disorder
-0.17*	0.12*	0.19*	0.26**	-0.06	Major depressive disorder
-0.17**	0.13**	0.20**	0.20**	0.02	Neuroticism
-0.05	0.10**	0.14**	0.06*	0.01	Schizophrenia
-0.05	-0.02	-0.06	0.08	0.13	Alzheimer's
-0.03	-0.01	-0.04	0.04	0.03	Multiple sclerosis
-0.02	0.02	0.02	0.01	-0.10*	Parkinson's
-0.16**	0.19**	0.12**	0.12**	0.08*	Body mass index
-0.20**	0.24**	0.13**	0.17**	-0.11**	Obesity class I
0.03	-0.04	-0.08*	0.02	0.03	Bone density: femoral neck
0.03	0.01	-0.06	0.04	0.02	Lumbar spine
0.16**	-0.17**	-0.09**	-0.15**	0.17**	Cholesterol: HDL
-0.06	0.07*	0.02	0.10*	-0.03	LDL
-0.03	0.07	0.03	0.08*	-0.01	Total
0.01	0.05	-0.08	0.16*	-0.11	Chronic kidney disease
-0.27**	0.25**	0.19**	0.21**	_0.01	Coronary artery disease
-0.16*	0.15*	0.07*	0.06	-0.08*	Diabetes: type 2
-0.13*	0.17*	0.07*	0.11*	-0.01	Fasting main effect: glucose
-0.24*	0.16*	0.09*	0.10	-0.24**	Insulin
-0.17	0.22*	0.11	0.20	-0.01	Proinsulin
-0.03	0.14*	0.04	0.11*	-0.04	Heart rate
0.04	0.03	0.01	-0.05	-0.06*	Inflammatory bowel disease
0.08	-0.01	-0.03	-0.13*	-0.06	Ulcerative colitis
-0.04	0.08	0.08	0.02	-0.07	Primary biliary cirrhosis
0.06	0.07	0.01	0.06	-0.06	Systemic lupus erythematosus
AgeSmk	CigDay	SmkInit	SmkCes	DrnkWk	

reward sensitivity, demonstrated as positive affect, strong motivation, desire, enthusiasm, and optimism. The PEM/E personality is modulated by the dopaminergic systems previously discussed and connected to changes in the D2 receptor gene, and in studies, high PEM/E expression decreases the risk of SUD development and low PEM/E increases risk [17]. The blue arrows indicate the PEM/E brain system, with circuits from the ascending dopaminergic system originating from the mesencephalon and innervating the striatum, rostral anterior cingulate (rACC) cortex, and ventromedial prefrontal cortex.

Image (B) depicts the negative emotionality/neuroticism (NEM/N) personality trait, which represents underlying sensitivity to punishment and stress signals. Individuals with high NEM/N are more likely to have anger, anxiety, guilt, and depression. The NEM/N trait is modulated by connections between the frontal cortex and the amygdala. Individuals with high NEM/N have decreased prefrontal control over the amygdala, which increases substance-use risk [17]. The green arrows indicate the NEM/N system, with glutamatergic outputs from the rACC and vmPFC to the amygdala and insula (insula not shown).

Image (C) depicts the constraint (CON) personality trait, which is thought to be a more complex personality expression that encompasses behavioral restraint via intentional and volitional control versus impulsivity, and as such involves more complex circuits in the brain. Low CON in studies is consistently associated with SUD [17]. The green arrows indicate the CON brain system, with circuits from the pre-supplementary motor area (preSMA) and right inferior frontal gyrus (rIFG) to the striatum and the subthalamic nucleus (STN).

Psychiatric and Medical Comorbidities

Multiple national population surveys have found that about half of those who experience a mental illness during their lives will also experience a SUD and vice versa [5]. Figure 14.16, taken from the 2019 NSDUH survey, shows

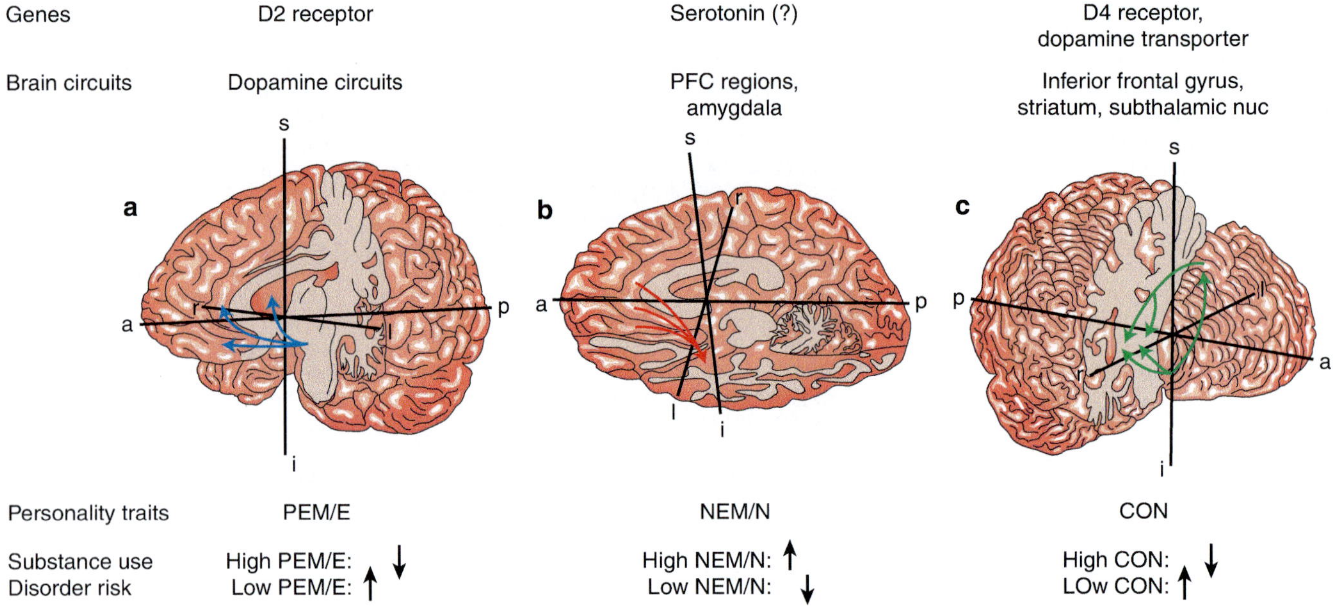

Fig. 14.15 Genes and correlated brain systems involved in the phenotypic expression of personality traits, *PFC* prefrontal cortex; *PEM/E* positive emotionality/extroversion; *NEM/N* negative emotionality/neuroticism; *CON* constraint. (*Adapted from* Belcher et al. [17]; *with permission*). The arrows indicate major input and output regions (see text) for the involved brain systems

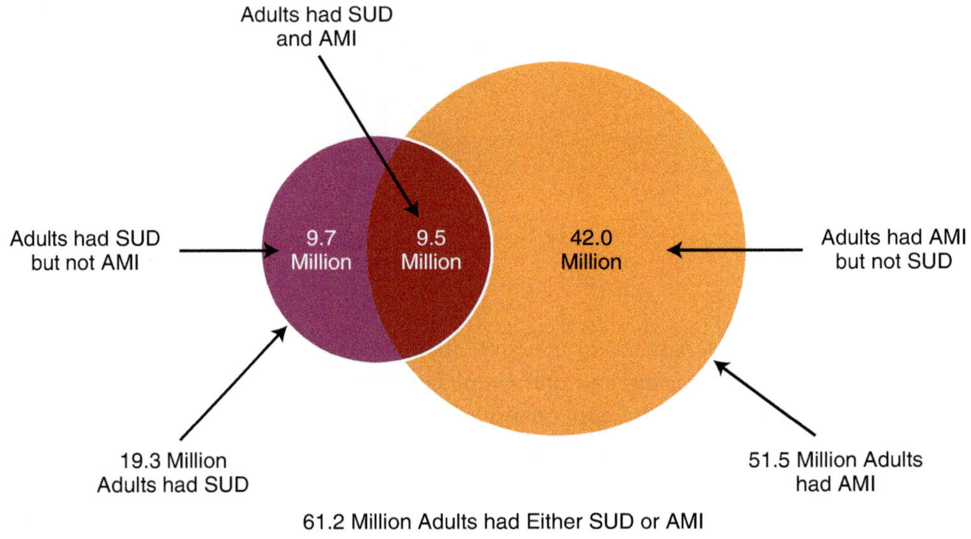

Fig. 14.16 Past year substance-use disorder (SUD) and mental illness among adults aged 18 or older in 2019 [5]. SUD, substance-use disorder

that out of 61.2 million adults who had either SUD or a mental illness diagnosis, 9.5 million people experienced both [4]. Reciprocal co-occurrence, as demonstrated in Fig. 14.16, is hypothesized to occur due to (1) overlapping genetic, neurobiological, developmental, and environmental influences, (2) increased risk of substance use as a way to self-medicate a mental illness, and/or mental illness and neurological changes increase substance use propensity, and (3) substance use may alter neural pathways that increase a person's propensity to develop a mental illness [5, 9].

In the US National Comorbidity Survey Replication study, 96% of individuals with disordered gambling were estimated to have one or more psychiatric disorder and 64% have been estimated to have three or more psychiatric disorders [6]. As seen in Fig. 14.17, major comorbidities included substance-use disorders, anxiety and trauma disorders, mood disorders, and impulse control disorders [6].

Figure 14.18 demonstrates that patients with SUD had a higher prevalence of 19 major health problems. Chronic pain, chronic obstructive pulmonary disease, congestive heart failure, and hepatitis C are among the most elevated prevalence. Patients with SUD also had a heightened 10-year mortality risk. Patients with opioid use disorder exhibited the highest elevation in 10-year mortality risk, with average disease-burden scores that were nearly twice as high as patients without opioid use disorder [18].

The reciprocal co-occurrence between SUD and medical disorders is due to direct damaging effects of the substances themselves on target organs (i.e., alcohol and hepatic cirrhosis or nicotine inhalation and lung diseases), consequences of the method of use (i.e., HIV and hepatitis C and injectable substances), links between mental illness, substance use, and decreased self-care, and epigenetic impacts of early adversity not only on substance use but also on the risk for concurrent physical illnesses (i.e., chronic pain, heart disease, diabetes [18, 19]).

Social and Structural Determinants

Figure 14.19 models the complex interaction between physical, economic, and sociocultural factors that contribute to substance use and gambling patterns and consequences [6, 20]. These social and structural determinants influence behavioral patterns but also shape how attitudes and policies impact the treatment of these disorders.

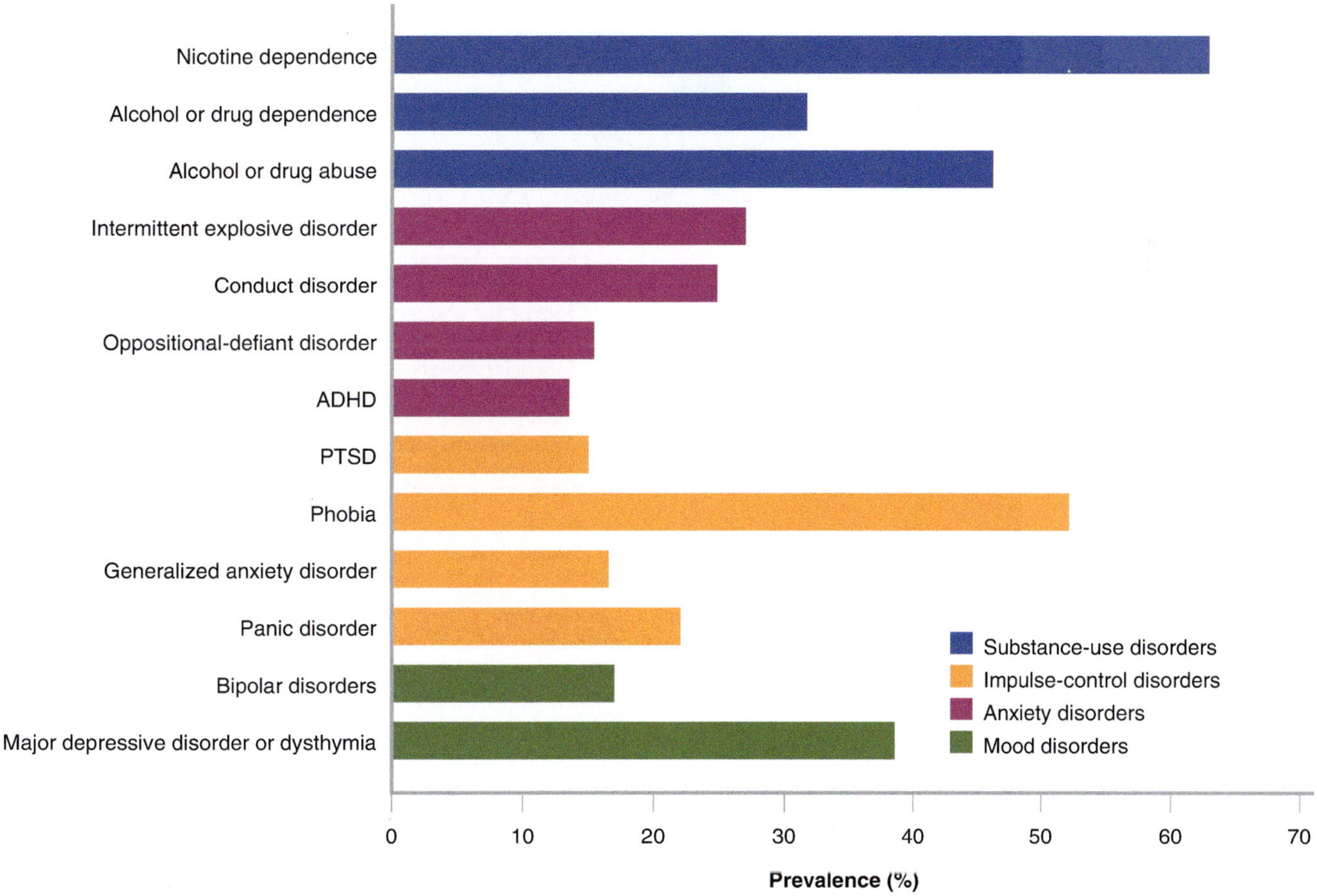

Fig. 14.17 Percent prevalence of substance-use disorders and mental health conditions co-occurring gambling disorder. (Data from the National Comorbidity Survey Replication; reproduced from Potenza et al. [6]; *with permission*)

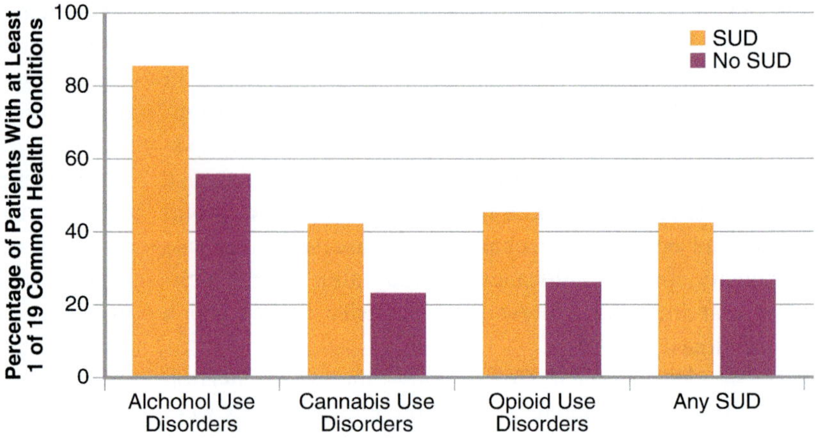

Fig. 14.18 Prevalence of major health problems co-occurring with substance-use disorders

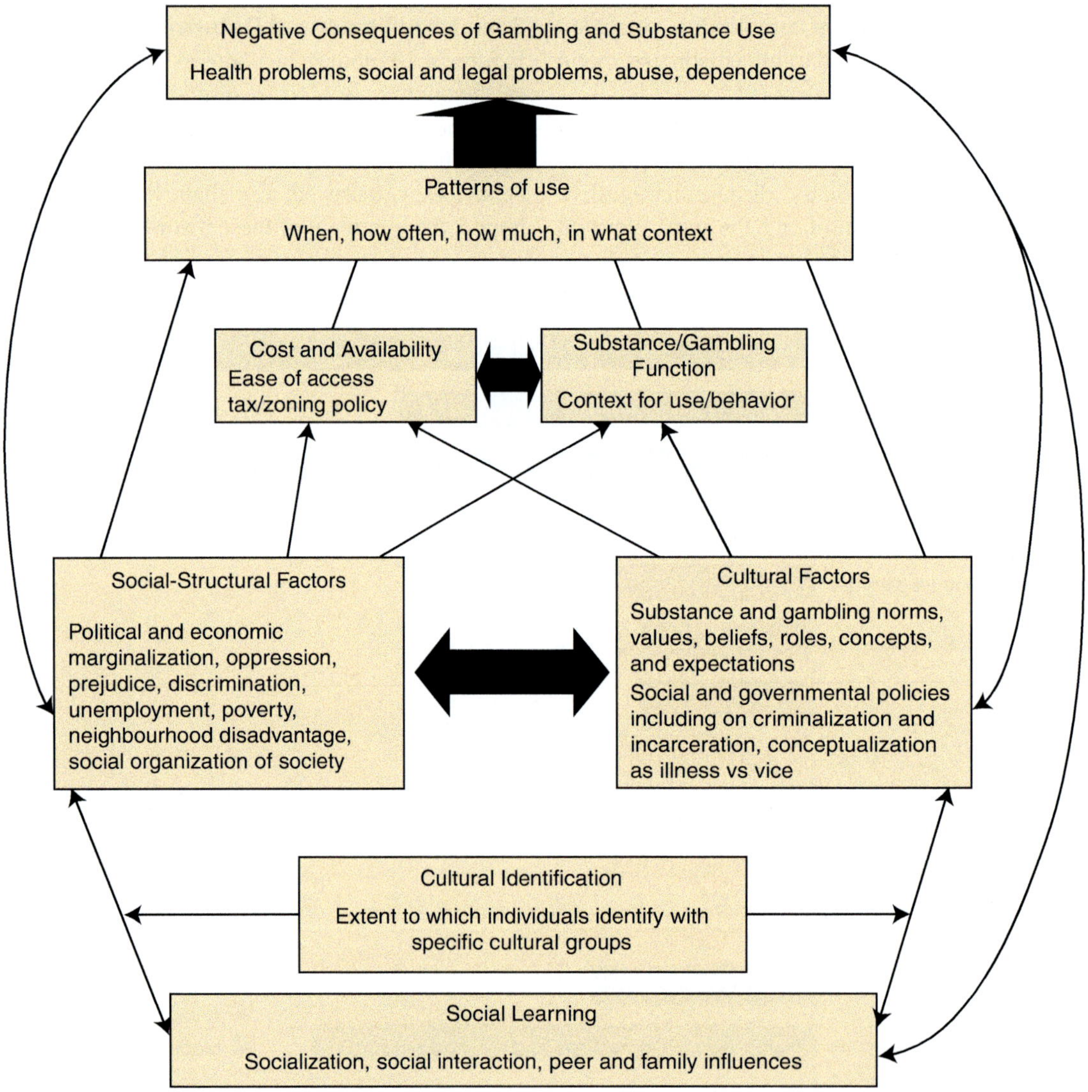

Fig. 14.19 Social and structural determinants contributing to the risk of developing a substance use or gambling disorder

There is budding research studying how structural vulnerabilities impact different stages of substance use and gambling disorders. In one study, increased illicit opiate and stimulant use in a population of HIV-positive women was associated with discrimination/stigma, economic hardship, and a summation of multiple adversities [21]. In another study, low rates of treatment for Hispanic men with alcohol use disorder mapped to poor access, lack of culturally and linguistically appropriate treatment, lack of cultural and community awareness and stigmatization, and education [22]. A study surveying US adults nationally found that adults living in disadvantaged neighborhoods and with lower educational status had higher rates of gambling disorder [23]. Thus, these environmental factors become just as important and complex in shaping the stages of substance misuse as an individual's biological underpinnings.

Pathophysiology

Stages of Substance Misuse and Gambling Leading to Substance-Related and Gambling Disorders

As Fig. 14.20 illustrates, substance-use and gambling disorders begin with an initial exposure and an associated reward response. The reward signaling in the brain positively reinforces substance use and/or gambling. Repeat stimulus/reward and positive reinforcement lead to an individual associating the addictive substance or gambling behavior—including its places, items, emotional states, and people—with an incentivized positive stimulus. This phenomenon, known as incentive salience, motivates the individual to continue substance use. Over time, an individual loses their ability to control their behavior. With continued use, neuroadaptations occur, the reward signals and positive reinforcement decrease, and the expression of stress systems increases. The negative emotional and physical states of substance withdrawal lead to negative reinforcement of continued use and eventually to dependence [12, 14]. Research on gambling disorder suggests a similar pattern of initial conditioning stimuli to perpetuate gambling use and reward impulsive behaviors, with decreased changes in reward signaling over time and stress dysregulation [6].

The pathophysiology of substance-related and gambling disorders is conceptualized in three stages of an ever-worsening cycle, which include the binge/intoxication, withdrawal/negative affect, and preoccupation/anticipation stages (Fig. 14.21). In the binge/intoxication stage, an individual consumes an intoxicating substance or engages in gambling behaviors and experiences the pleasurable reward that reinforces use. In the withdrawal/negative affect stage, the individual will experience a negative physical and emotional state without the substance/gambling behavior, and in the preoccupation/anticipation stage, the individual feels compelled to use the substance/gamble again after a period of abstinence [6, 12, 14].

There are at least 18 discrete neuro-circuits in the brain that mediate these pathophysiologic stages [14]. The three major brain regions involved in the development and persistence of SUD and gambling disorders are the basal ganglia, the amygdala and its extended structures, and the prefrontal cortex (Fig. 14.21) [6, 12, 14]. The major neurotransmitters and structures involved in the various stages are discussed here.

Neuroanatomy

The ventral tegmental area and basal ganglia structures, including the nucleus accumbens and dorsal striatum (DS), are discussed in the section on the dopaminergic pathways (Fig. 14.11) [14].

The extended amygdala, including the amygdala (CeA), and the bed nucleus of the stria terminalis (BNST) regulate

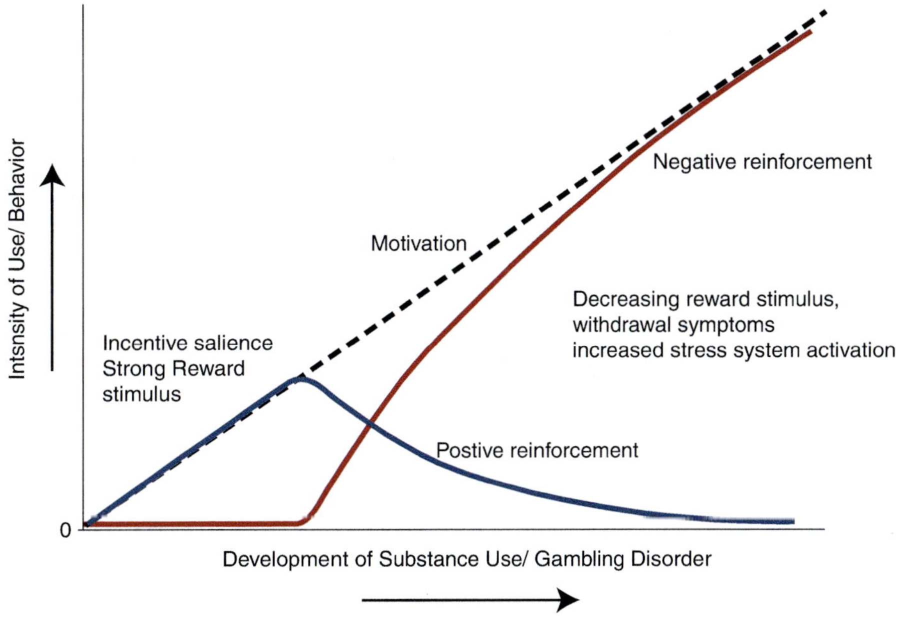

Fig. 14.20 Transition from positive to negative reinforcement in the development of a substance-use disorder

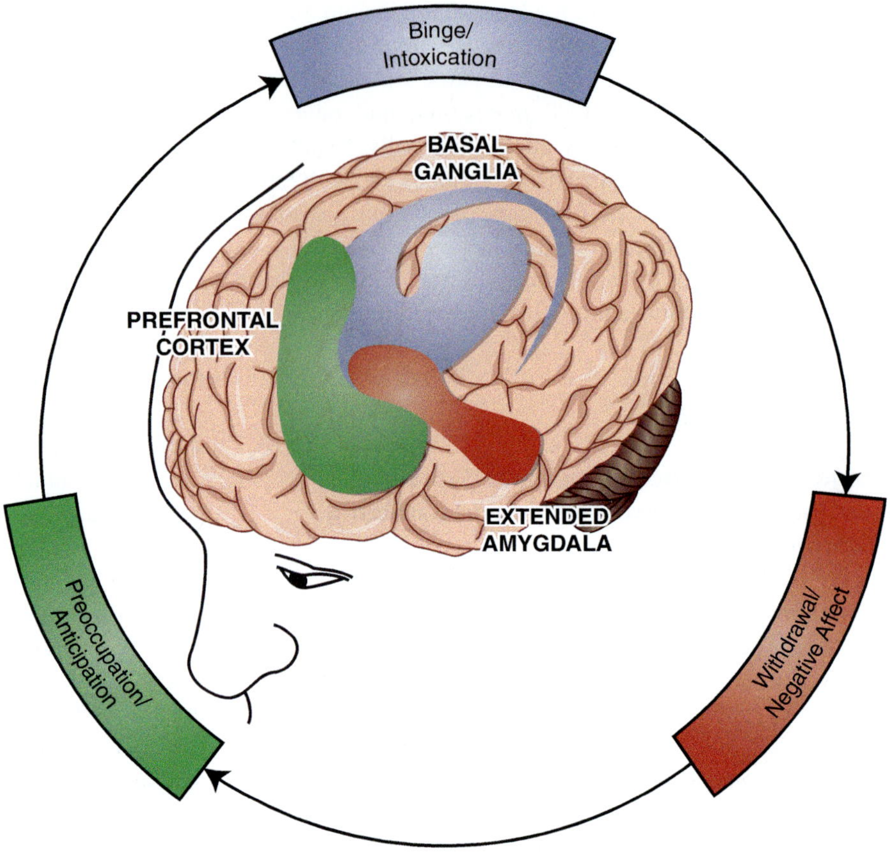

Fig. 14.21 The three stages and major brain regions involved in the substance and gambling misuse cycle

the brain's stress response and associated behavioral and emotional responses to stress (Fig. 14.21). As part of the stress circuitry, the extended amygdala has connections to the hippocampus to influence memory formation around substance use and the hypothalamus to activate the HPA axis and regulate cortisol release. The extended amygdala's functions play a role both initially in incentive salience and positive reinforcement but also in the negative reinforcement and withdrawal aspects of the misuse cycle leading to habituation and dependence [12, 14, 24].

The prefrontal cortex (PFC) (Fig. 14.21) is responsible for complex cognitive functions, including organization and prioritization of thoughts, activities, and behaviors; time management; complex decision-making; and regulation of action, emotions, and impulses. In substance use and gambling, the structures of the PFC (including the anterior cingulate cortex, the medial-orbitofrontal cortex, and the ventrolateral PFC) initially exert inhibitory control over substance use, but these circuits are downregulated with repeated, excess use [6, 12, 14].

Binge/Intoxication Stage

The main neuroanatomical structures and circuits involved in the binge intoxication stage are demonstrated in Fig. 14.22. Imaging studies such as Fig. 14.23 demonstrate that intoxicating doses of alcohol and drugs, as well as repeated wins and near-losses in gambling, release dopamine and opioid peptides from the VTA either directly or indirectly into the nucleus accumbens [6, 12, 14]. Dopaminergic projections from the VTA to the extended amygdala, the hippocampus, and insula create the positive emotional affiliations that lend to incentive salience (Fig. 14.22).

As Fig. 14.24 demonstrates, intoxicating substances lead to a much higher release of dopamine in the synapses of the reward pathway than natural rewards, encouraging repeat use to obtain a greater reward stimulus. Projections to the dorsal striatum (DS) encourage substance- and gambling-seeking behaviors; repeat DS signaling leads to habit formation and contributes to compulsive use (Figs. 14.11 and 14.22) [6, 12, 14]. While the prefrontal cortex provides inhibitory control to the basal ganglia and the extended amygdala through inhibitory gamma-aminobutyric acid (GABA) projections, these inhibitory signals begin to weaken as repeated stimulation of the reward circuits strengthen the incentive salience of the substance [6, 12, 14, 25] (Fig. 14.22, PFC projections).

Withdrawal/Negative Affect Stage

With chronic substance exposure, there are changes in the reward pathways that lead to diminished reward responses; in particular, decreased dopaminergic transmission in the nucleus accumbens and decrease opioid peptide signalling leads to decreased reward experience [6, 12, 14, 25] (Fig. 14.22). These changes in dopaminergic signaling

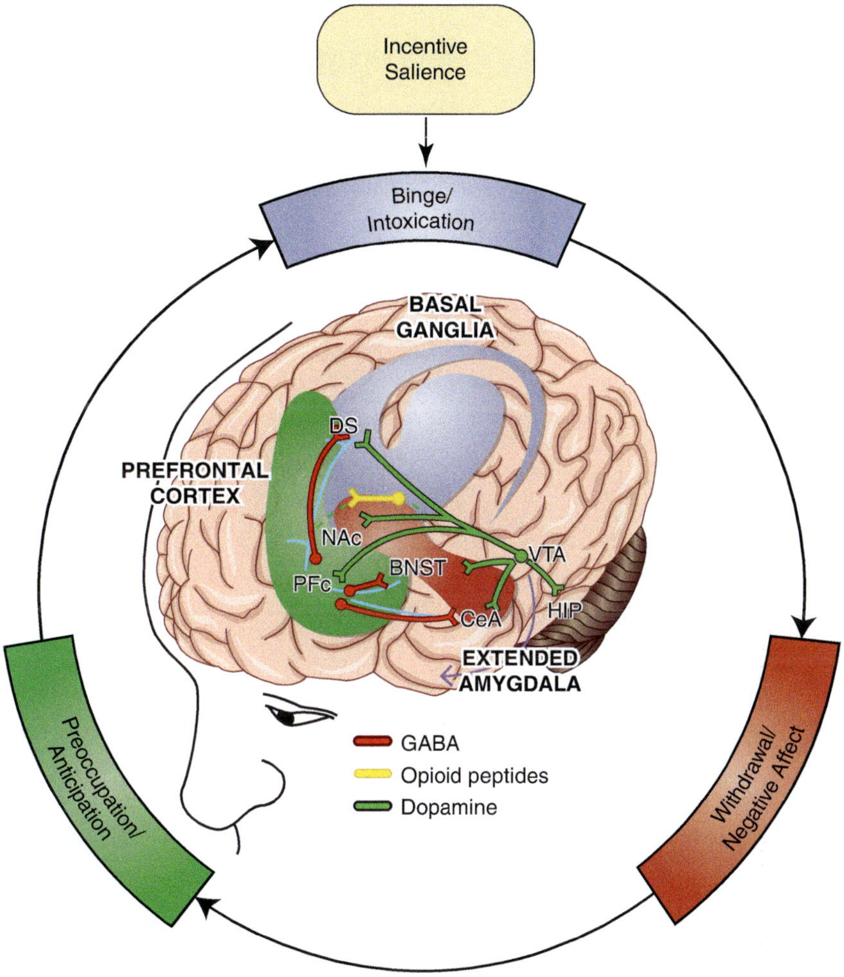

Fig. 14.22 Positive reward reinforcement and increased incentive salience in the binge/intoxication phase. *PFC* prefrontal cortex; *DS* dorsal striatum; *Nac* nucleus accumbens; *BNST* bed nucleus of the stria terminalis; *CeA* amygdala; *Hyp* hypothalamus; *VTA* ventral tegmental area; *HIP* hippocampus

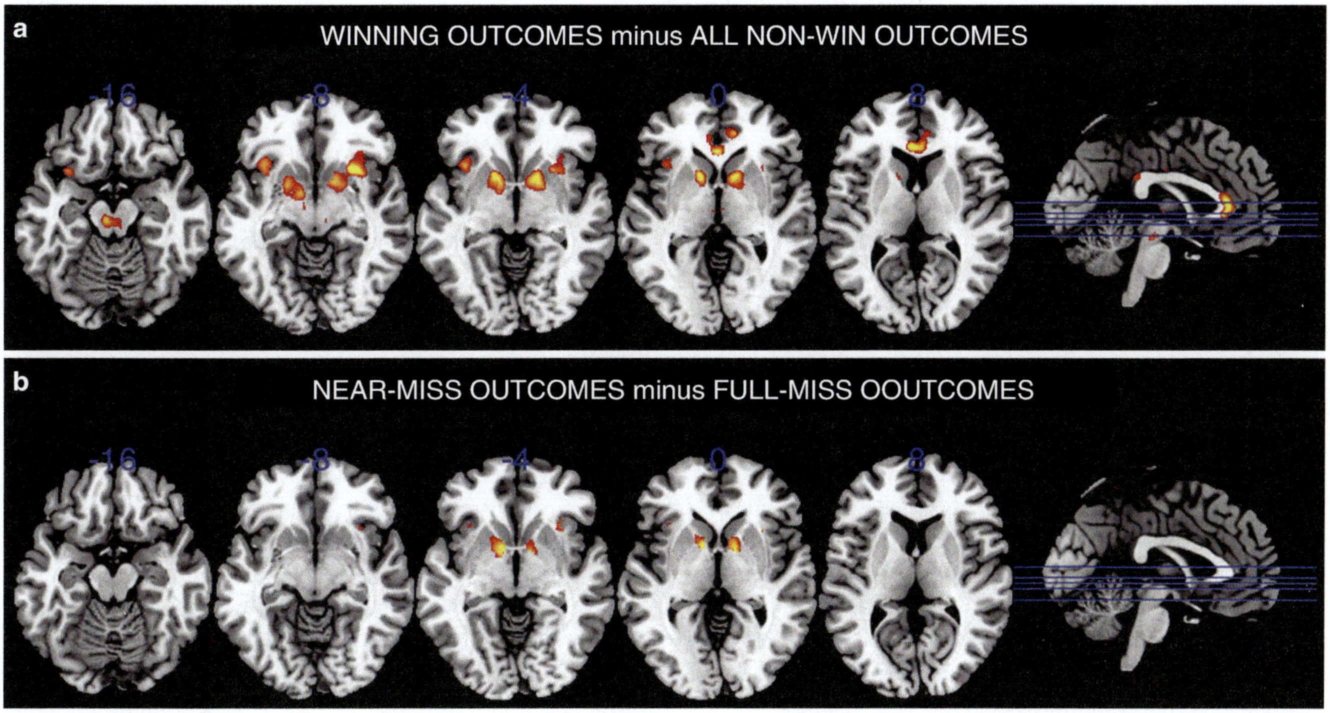

Fig. 14.23 Neural activity to winning and near-miss outcomes. (**a**) Neural responses to monetary wins compared to all non-wins, modeled to the onset of the outcome phase, with significant win-related activity in the striatum, ventral tegmental area, anterior insula, and prefrontal cortex (anterior cingulate). (**b**) Neural responses to near-miss compared to full miss outcomes, with significant activity in the bilateral striatum and anterior insula. (*Reproduced from* Clark [32]; https://doi.org/10.1016/j.neuron.2008.12.031. [CC BY 3.0])

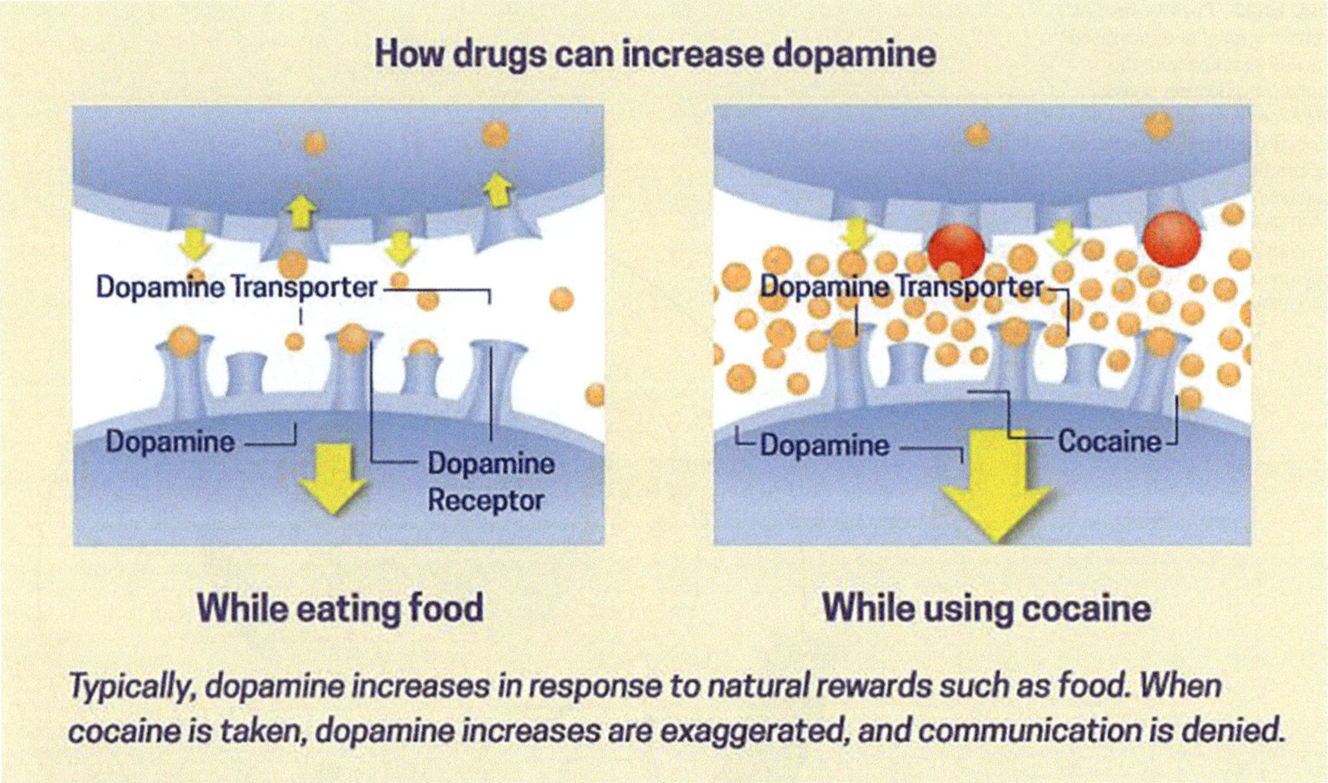

Fig. 14.24 Dopamine release in reward circuitry with food/other natural reward stimulus vs intoxicating substance or gambling (example of cocaine). (*Reproduced from* Ambre et al. [33]; *with permission*)

include a decrease in the expression of D2 receptors in reward circuitry. Figure 14.25 demonstrates changes in D2 dopamine receptors in the basal ganglia with repeated substance exposure. Studies of gambling disorder show decreased activation of the ventral striatum (nucleus accumbens) in response to gambling regard, which mirrors decreased activation of the reward circuitry in substance-use disorder at this stage [6, 14].

The emotional dysregulation associated with the withdrawal/negative affect stage involves the HPA axis and brain stress system. These systems, mediated by corticotropin-releasing factor (CRF), norepinephrine, and dynorphins, are recruited and then dysregulated by chronic exposure to gambling or a substance of abuse leading to increased HPA and central stress system expression in the extended amygdala (Fig. 14.26) [6, 12, 14].

Thus, an individual experiences both increased irritability and negative emotional states and decreased pleasure responses at baseline, with heightened negative and physical states in withdrawal and abstinence, known as "stress surfeit" [12, 14]. Thus, motivation increases to escalate substance use to regain the pleasurable effect, which becomes increasingly difficult to experience, but also to avoid uncomfortable withdrawal, leading to negative reinforcement of substance use and gambling behaviors (Fig. 14.20).

Preoccupation/Anticipation Stage

In the preoccupation/anticipation stage, an individual experiences craving and substance/gambling-seeking impulses during a period of abstinence. These drives are generated by increases in habitual behavior and incentive through reinforced circuits to the dorsal striatum, extended amygdala, and hippocampus, and negative reinforcement through stress-system expression, all of which lead to chronic downregulation of executive function control over substance use behavior [6, 12, 14] (Fig. 14.27). As seen in the PET imaging in Fig. 14.28, decreased brain metabolism in regions of the prefrontal cortex reflects the decrease in behavioral regulation of the PFC that occurs with chronic use of intoxicating substances.

With respect to the activity of neurotransmitters, there is prominent dysregulation of glutamate, the brain's primary excitatory neurotransmitter that drives actions/response throughout the brain, and GABA, the brain's primary inhibitory neurotransmitter that regulates the expression and prioritization of behavior. GABA also regulates the HPA axis, the brain's stress systems, the extended amygdala, and reward circuitry [6, 12, 14]. In chronic substance use and disordered gambling, there is a disruption in both glutamate and GABA signaling in the prefrontal cortex and throughout the brain, leading to executive function deficits

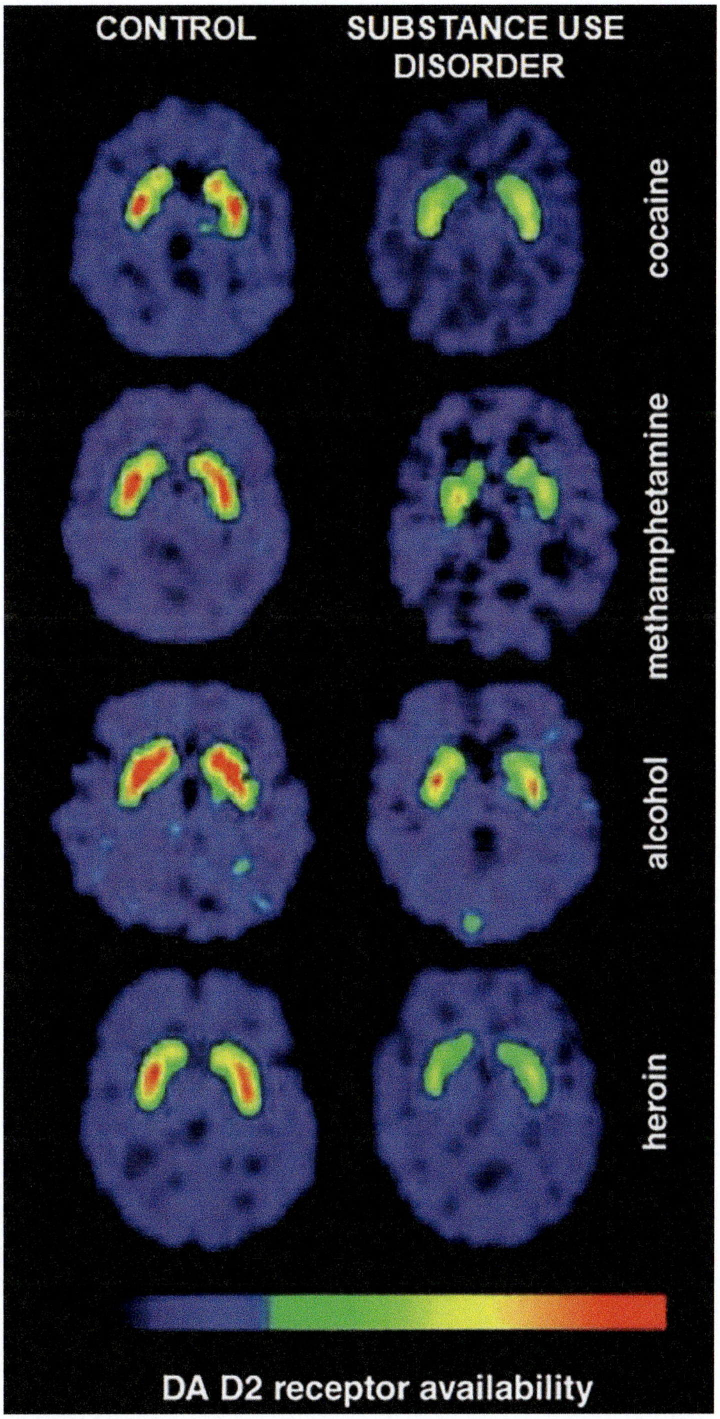

Fig. 14.25 Decreased D2 dopamine receptor expression in patients with various substance-use disorders as compared with controls. (*Adapted from* Volkow et al. [34]; *with permission*)

in the control of disordered behaviors and reactions (Fig. 14.27). The over-activation of glutamate in the prefrontal cortex promotes craving as impulsive/compulsive substance seeking, and over-activation throughout the brain leads to worsening of withdrawal/negative affect stage, encouraging relapse and return to the binge/intoxication stage [6, 12, 14].

Phenomenology

Table 14.3 presents the DSM-5 criteria for substance-use disorders, two of the substance-induced disorders—substance intoxication and substance withdrawal—and gambling disorder. Tolerance and withdrawal alone do not establish a diagnosis of SUD, and if a substance is prescribed

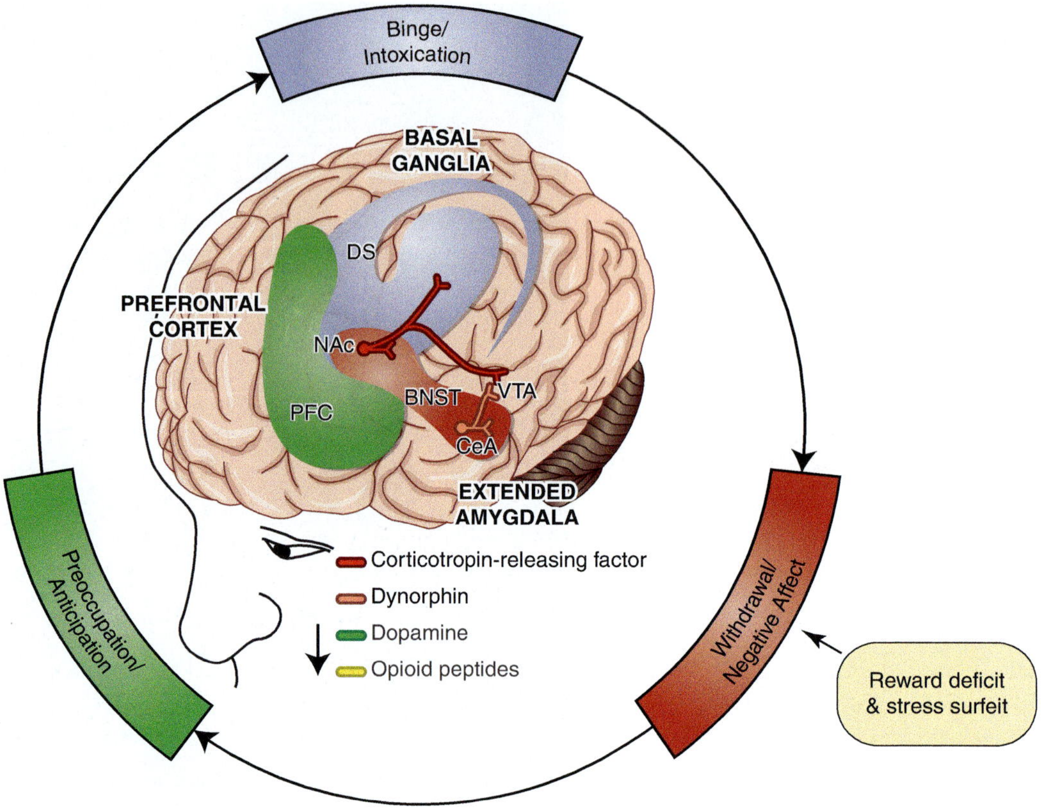

Fig. 14.26 Decreased reward and increased stress response in the withdrawal/negative affect stage. *PFC* prefrontal cortex; *DS* dorsal striatum; *Nac* nucleus accumbens, *BNST* bed nucleus of the stria terminalis; *CeA* amygdala; *Hyp* hypothalamus; *VTA* ventral tegmental area

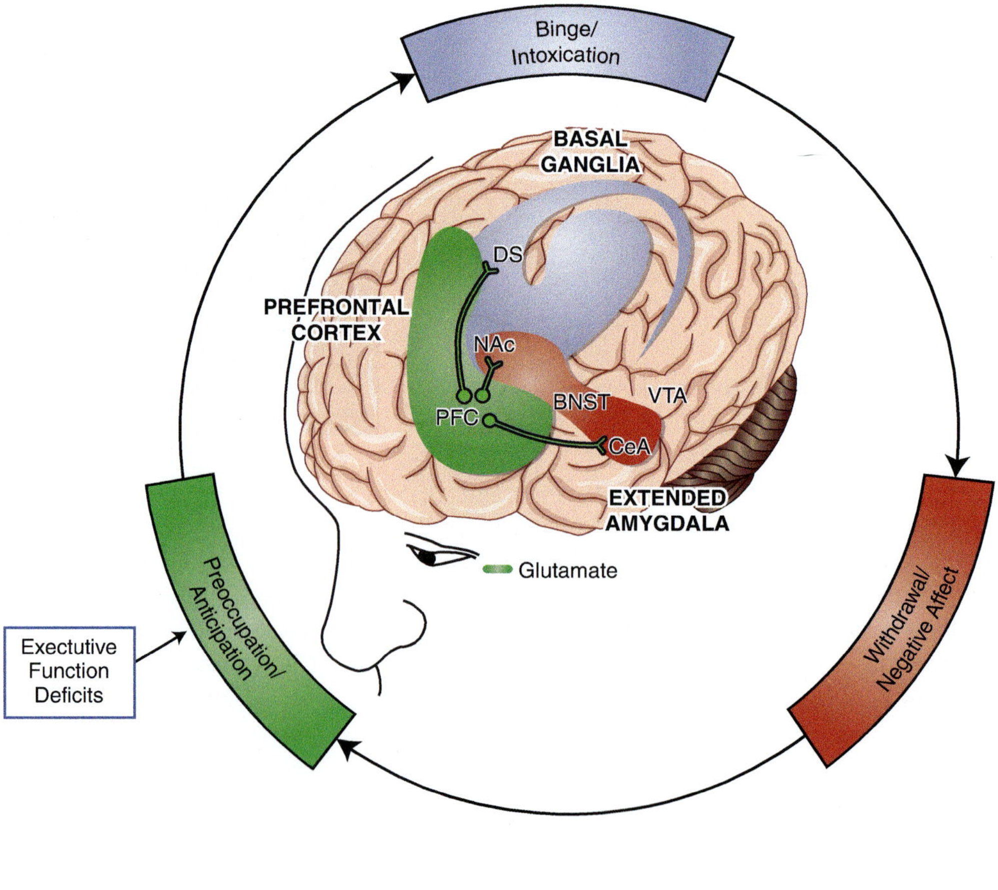

Fig. 14.27 Increased craving, compulsive use, and decreased control in preoccupation/anticipation stage. *PFC* prefrontal cortex; *DS* dorsal striatum; *Nac* nucleus accumbens; *BNST* bed nucleus of the stria terminalis; *CeA* amygdala; *VTA* ventral tegmental area

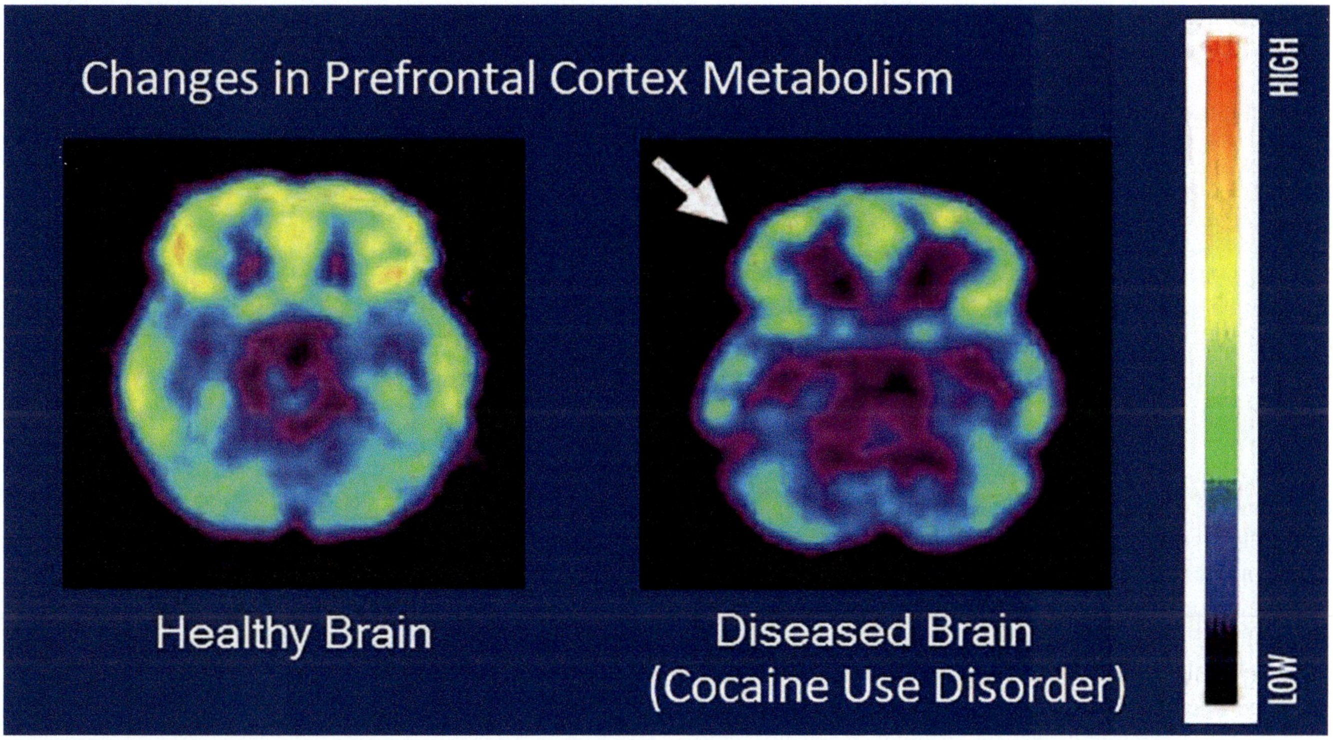

Fig. 14.28 Decrease in regional brain metabolism in the orbital frontal cortex, control vs cocainse use disorder. (*Adapted from* Volkow et al. [34]; *with permission*)

Table 14.3 DSM-5 criteria for substance use, disorders, substance-induced disorders, and gambling disorder

<table>
<tr><td colspan="2">Substance-use disorder</td></tr>
<tr><td colspan="2">A. A problematic pattern of substance use leading to clinically significant impairment or distress, as manifested by at least two of the following, occurring within a 12-month period:
1. Use in larger amounts or over a longer period than was intended
2. Persistent desire or unsuccessful effort to cut back or control use
3. A great deal of time is spent in activities necessary to obtain, use, or recover effects
4. Cravings or persistent desire to use
5. Failure to fulfill major role obligations at work, school, or home
6. Persistent use despite recurrent social or interpersonal problems
7. Important social, occupational, or recreational activities are given up or reduced
8. Recurrent use in situations in which it is physically hazardous
9. Persistent use despite knowledge of physical or psychological problems caused or exacerbated by using
10. Tolerance
11. Withdrawal (refer to Criteria A and B of the criteria set for cannabis withdrawal)</td></tr>
<tr><td colspan="2">Substance-induced disorders
(substance-induced psychiatric disorders covered in other sections)</td></tr>
<tr><td>Substance intoxication</td><td>Substance withdrawal</td></tr>
<tr><td>A. Recent use of substance
B. Clinically significant problematic behavioral or psychological changes (e.g., inappropriate behavior, mood lability, impaired sensory-motor function, impaired judgment) that developed during, or shortly after, substance use
C. One (or more) substance-specific signs or symptoms developing during or shortly after use (e.g., incoordination; altered speech; impaired cognition; altered vital signs; altered arousal)
D. The signs or symptoms are not attributable to another medical condition and are not better explained by another mental disorder, including intoxication with another substance</td><td>A. Cessation of substance use that has been heavy and prolonged
B. Two (or more) substance-specific signs and symptoms develop within approximately 1 week after Criterion A: (e.g., autonomic hyperactivity; tremor; insomnia; perceptual disturbances; affective dysregulation; seizures…)
C. The signs or symptoms in Criterion B cause clinically significant distress or impairment in social, occupational, or other important areas of functioning
D. The signs or symptoms are not attributable to another medical condition and are not better explained by another mental disorder, including intoxication or withdrawal from another substance</td></tr>
</table>

(continued)

Table 14.3 (continued)

Substance-use disorder
Gambling disorder
A. Persistent and recurrent problematic gambling behavior leading to clinically significant impairment or distress, as indicated by the individual exhibiting four (or more) of the following in a 12-month period:
1. Needs to gamble with increasing amounts of money in order to achieve the desired excitement
2. Is restless or irritable when attempting to cut down or stop gambling
3. Has made repeated unsuccessful efforts to control, cut back, or stop gambling
4. Is often preoccupied with gambling (e.g., having persistent thoughts of reliving past gambling experiences, handicapping or planning the next venture, thinking of ways to get money with which to gamble)
5. Often gambles when feeling distressed (e.g., helpless, guilty, anxious, depressed)
6. After losing money gambling, often returns another day to get even ("chasing" one's losses)
7. Lies to conceal the extent of involvement with gambling
8. Has jeopardized or lost a significant relationship, job, or educational or career opportunity because of gambling
9. Relies on others to provide money to relieve desperate financial situations caused by gambling
B. The gambling behavior is not better explained by a manic episode

(as in an opioid analgesic), they are discounted from the criteria. The severity of a SUD or gambling disorder is specified by the number of criteria that are present. The presence of 2–3 symptoms is specified as mild, 4–5 symptoms as moderate, and 6 or more symptoms as severe. Once criteria for a SUD or gambling disorder are met, early remission may be specified when no symptoms are present for at least 3 months, and sustained remission may be specified when no symptoms are met for 12 months [1].

Treatment

Substance-related and gambling disorders are complex conditions that are influenced by and impact multiple dimensions of an individual's life. Treatment plans are predicated on both a specific and accurate diagnosis of the disorder, as well as a multidimensional assessment of the person who is suffering from the disorder [25]. The purpose of a multidimensional assessment is to ensure that treatment is tailored to the needs of the specific individual, addressing not just drug use, but the other biomedical and psychosocial health problems that they face (Table 14.4).

To be effective, treatment must be integrated with interventions that address medical conditions, mental health, environmental factors, family dynamics, occupational challenges, and legal problems. Treatment duration and intensity must be tailored to the patient's evolving recovery status and relapse risk, rather than predetermined or fixed doses. Evidence-based interventions are prioritized, including psychotherapies and/or indicated medication treatments. Care plans must be modified over time and reflect that these disorders are chronic relapsing conditions, for which extended monitoring and support are essential to achieving sustained remission and recovery [26].

Table 14.4 illustrates the American Society of Addiction Medicine's (ASAM) multidimensional assessment framework, which may be used to make informed decisions about appropriate levels of care, wherein specific psychosocial and biomedical treatment interventions can be offered consistent with the standard of care for the patient's health conditions [26].

Table 14.4 ASAM multidimensional assessment framework

Dimension	Description	Focus of assessment
Dimension 1	Acute intoxication and/or withdrawal potential	Past and current experiences of substance use and withdrawal
Dimension 2	Biomedical conditions and complications	Health history and current physical conditions
Dimension 3	Emotional, behavioral, or cognitive conditions	Psychiatric conditions, psychological strengths and vulnerabilities
Dimension 4	Readiness to change	Insight, readiness, and interest in changing
Dimension 5	Relapse, continued use, or continued problem potential	Predisposing, perpetuating, precipitating triggers to problem substance use
Dimension 6	Recovery/living environment	Living situation, and the surrounding people, places, and things

The multidimensional assessment integrates a patient's needs, obstacles, and vulnerabilities, as well as their strengths, assets, resources, and support structure. This information is then used to determine the appropriate level of care across a continuum, from early interventions to increasing levels of outpatient support, to residential and finally inpatient treatment options (Fig. 14.29) [21].

Treatment of Substance Intoxication and Withdrawal

Intoxication

Intoxication syndromes are generally self-limited. As the substance is eliminated from the body, the syndrome

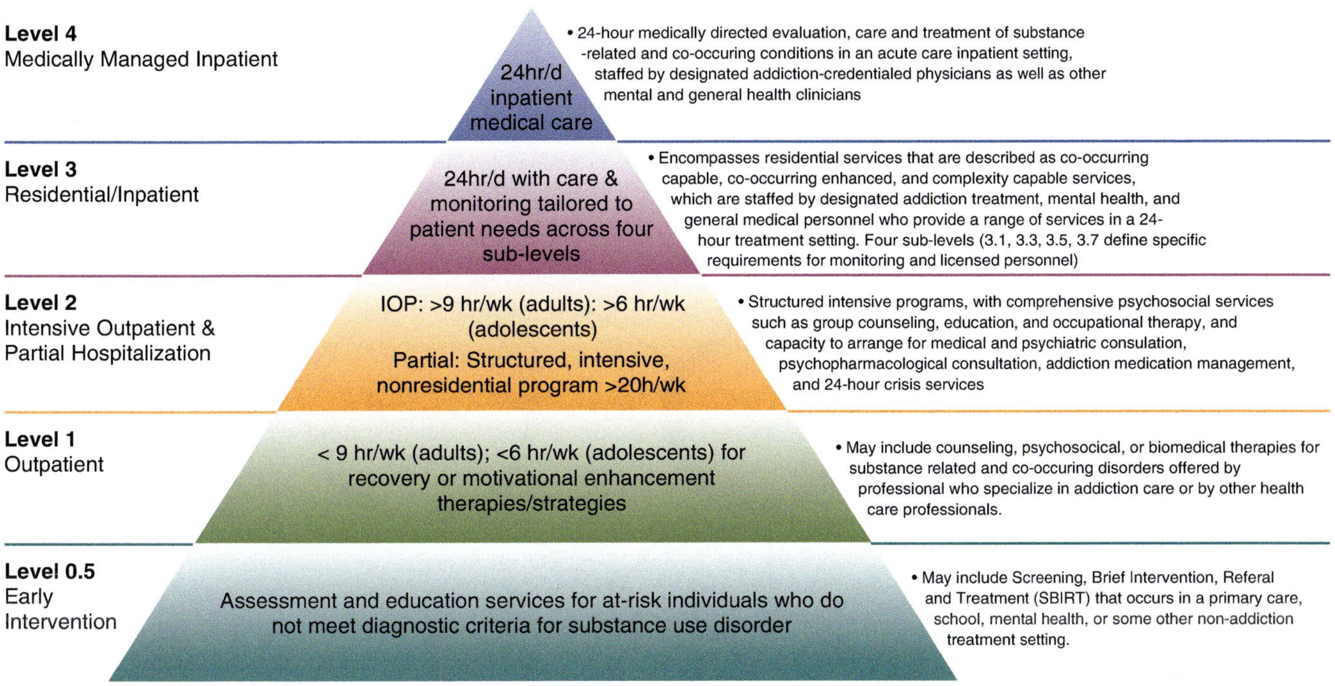

Fig. 14.29 American Society of Addiction Medicine (ASAM) levels of care for treatment

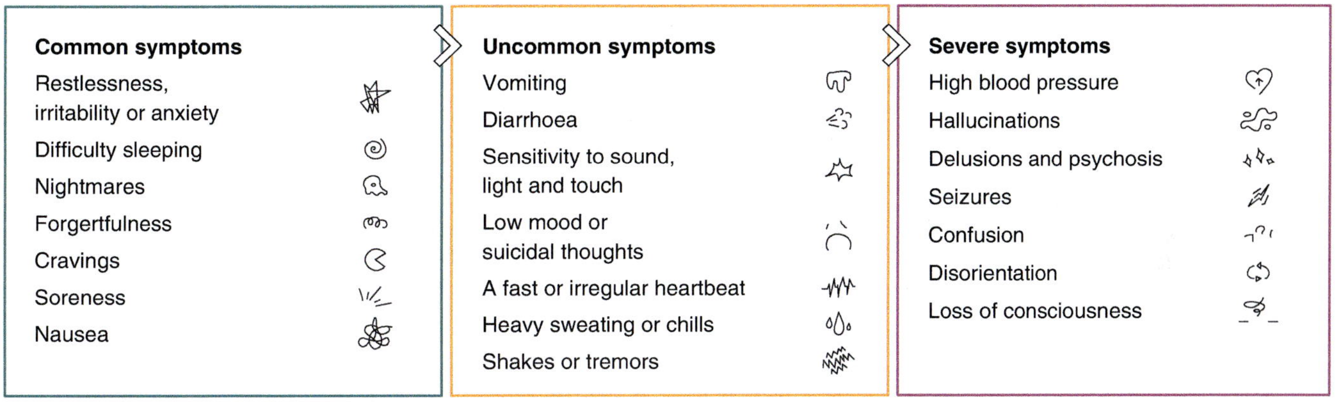

Fig. 14.30 Alcohol and other substance withdrawal symptoms

resolves. Thus, medical management of intoxication involves providing supportive measures to ensure safety (monitoring, hydration, nutrition, safe environment, support, and reassurance) and targeted interventions when the symptoms of intoxication pose a behavioral or physiological threat [12]. In the case of severe impairments or an acute overdose that is life threatening, treatment generally follows one of three approaches: increasing drug clearance, blocking the neuronal site at which the drug acts (e.g., naloxone for opioid intoxication), and pharmacologically counteracting drug effects with symptomatic management [12].

Withdrawal

While mild withdrawal syndromes may not require medical management, moderate to severe withdrawal syndromes are a major source of morbidity, and alcohol withdrawal is potentially fatal. Figure 14.30 summarizes various withdrawal symptoms people experience. The more severe symptoms occur primarily with alcohol and benzodiazepine withdrawals.

Pharmacologic treatment of any drug withdrawal syndrome generally follows one of the two approaches: suppression by a cross-tolerant medication from the same pharmacologic class—usually a longer-acting one to provide a milder, controlled withdrawal (i.e., methadone or buprenorphine for opioid medically supervised withdrawal)—and/or reducing the signs and symptoms of withdrawal by targeting the neurochemical or receptor systems that mediate withdrawal (i.e., clonidine, an alpha 2 agonist, to treat opioid withdrawal syndrome). Withdrawal treatment may be done

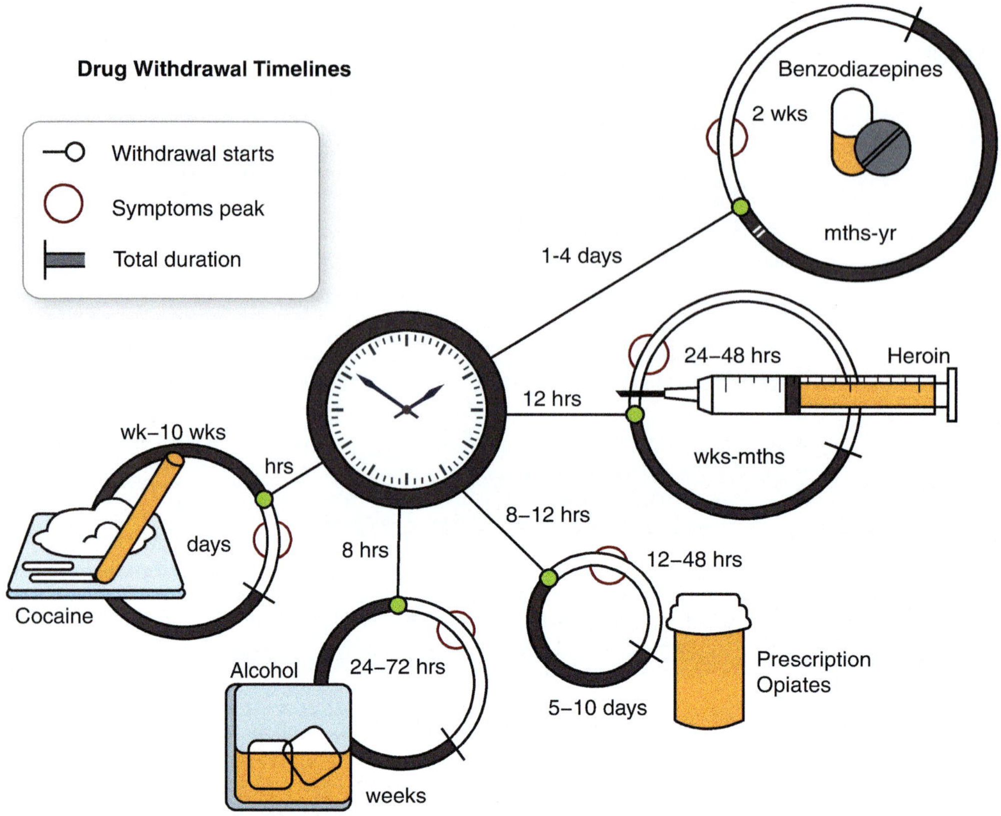

Fig. 14.31 Drug withdrawal timelines, including time to withdrawal from the cessation of substance, peak severity of symptoms, and total average duration. Withdrawal management can occur anywhere on the ASAM levels of care, from level 1 to level 4, depending on the severity and complexity of the withdrawal picture

on an outpatient or inpatient basis, depending on the withdrawal timeline of a substance (Fig. 14.31) and the severity of symptoms [12, 27].

Successful treatment of acute intoxication, overdose, or withdrawal can facilitate entry into substance use treatment by reducing uncomfortable withdrawal symptoms that negatively reinforce substance use. Even when successful, these early stages of treatment often are followed by relapse to substance use, with patients potentially reentering a "revolving door" of repeated detoxification programs. Short-term treatment of acute intoxication or withdrawal does not obviate the need for long-term treatment of substance-related disorders. Relapse rates for substance-related and addictive disorders are comparable to other medical illnesses, encouraging the utilization of a chronic disease model to implement multimodal interventions (Fig. 14.32).

Treatment to Promote Relapse Prevention, Remission, and Recovery

As shown in Fig. 14.33, prolonged abstinence from substance use (and gambling) can lead to improvements in neural circuitry, with returns to levels of dopamine transporters and other markers closer to control subject comparisons

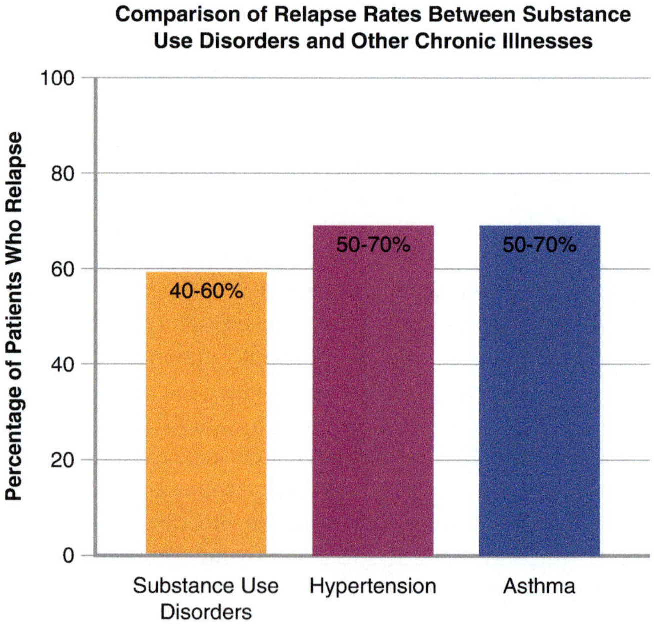

Fig. 14.32 Relapse rates for people treated for substance-use disorder as compared with relapse rates for people treated for hypertension and asthma

without a history of substance use. Thus, utilizing pharmacotherapy and nonmedication interventions is important to maximize the possibility of remission and recovery [25, 28].

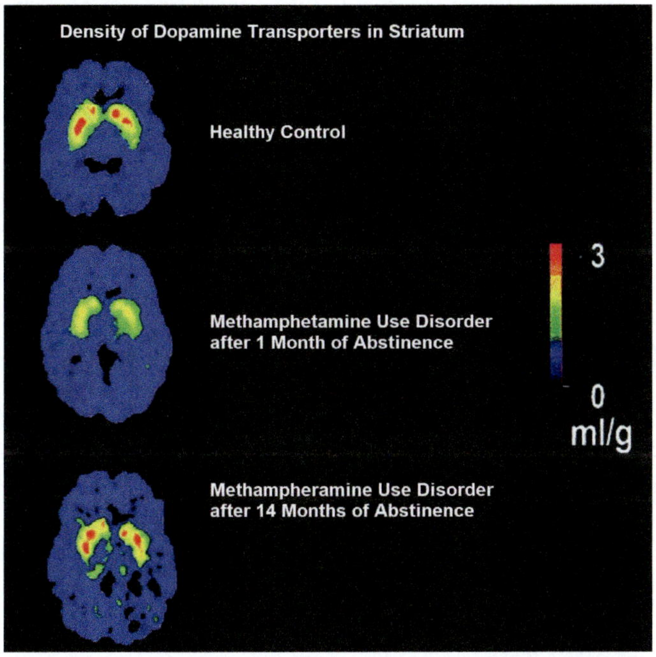

Fig. 14.33 Recovery of striatal D2 dopamine receptors after prolonged substance abstinence (example of methamphetamine). (*Adapted from* Volkow et al. [28]; *with permission*)

Pharmacological Interventions

The primary aim of pharmacological interventions for SUD and gambling disorder is to prevent relapse after abstinence, remission, or recovery has been achieved. Pharmacological interventions should be delivered in conjunction with psychosocial interventions, though if a patient is willing to start an appropriate pharmacological treatment, initiation should not be predicated on participation in a psychosocial intervention [12]. A range of established and proposed mechanisms are thought to underlie the efficacy of medication treatments for SUD and gambling disorders. Substance-specific, evidenced-based, medications approved by the US Food and Drug Administration (FDA) for opioid and alcohol relapse prevention and recovery are summarized in Table 14.5 [12]. Figure 14.34 illustrates the relative receptor activity of three FDA-approved medication treatments for opioid use disorder, while Fig. 14.35 demonstrates the mechanism of action for the three medications approved for alcohol use disorder.

To date, no FDA-approved medications are available to treat marijuana, cocaine, methamphetamine, or other SUDs [12]. Similarly, there are no FDA-approved medications for gambling disorder, though opioid-receptor antagonists have the best evidence so far and may reduce gambling urges and behaviors [6]. For all substance-related and gambling disorders, pharmacotherapy to treat comorbid mental and medical conditions is encouraged to minimize additional biological contributors to the disordered behaviors [12, 29].

Table 14.5 Pharmacological treatments for substance-use disorder

Indication	Medication	Form	Dosing	Mechanism
Opioid use disorder	Methadone	Oral	20–200 mg daily	Stimulates opioid receptor, preventing withdrawal and reducing craving
	Buprenorphine	SL; depot; implant	2–16 mg sublingual every day	Partially stimulates opioid receptor, preventing withdrawal and reducing craving
	Naltrexone	Oral; depot	50 mg once daily orally; 380 mg once every 4 weeks intramuscularly	Blocks opioid receptor, reducing reinforcing effects of substance use
Alcohol use disorder	Disulfiram	Oral	250 mg once daily (range: 125–500 mg/day; maximum: 500 mg/day)	Blocks metabolism of alcohol, leading to an aversive increase in toxic metabolites
	Acamprosate	Oral	666 mg three times daily	Blocks NMDA receptor, thought to attenuate post-acute withdrawal symptoms
	Naltrexone	Oral; depot	25–50 mg once daily orally; 380 mg once every 4 weeks intramuscularly	Blocks opiate receptors involved in the rewarding effects of drinking and craving for alcohol
Tobacco use disorder	Nicotine replacement therapy	Gum; lozenge; patch; spray	Varies with formulation; gum 2–4 mg every 1–2 h; patch 7–21 mg once daily	Stimulates nicotine receptors, preventing nicotine withdrawal and reducing craving
	Bupropion	Oral	150–300 mg daily	Inhibits reuptake of dopamine and norepinephrine, thought to influence cravings
	Varenicline	Oral	1 mg twice daily	Partial nicotine receptor agonist, preventing nicotine withdrawal and reducing craving

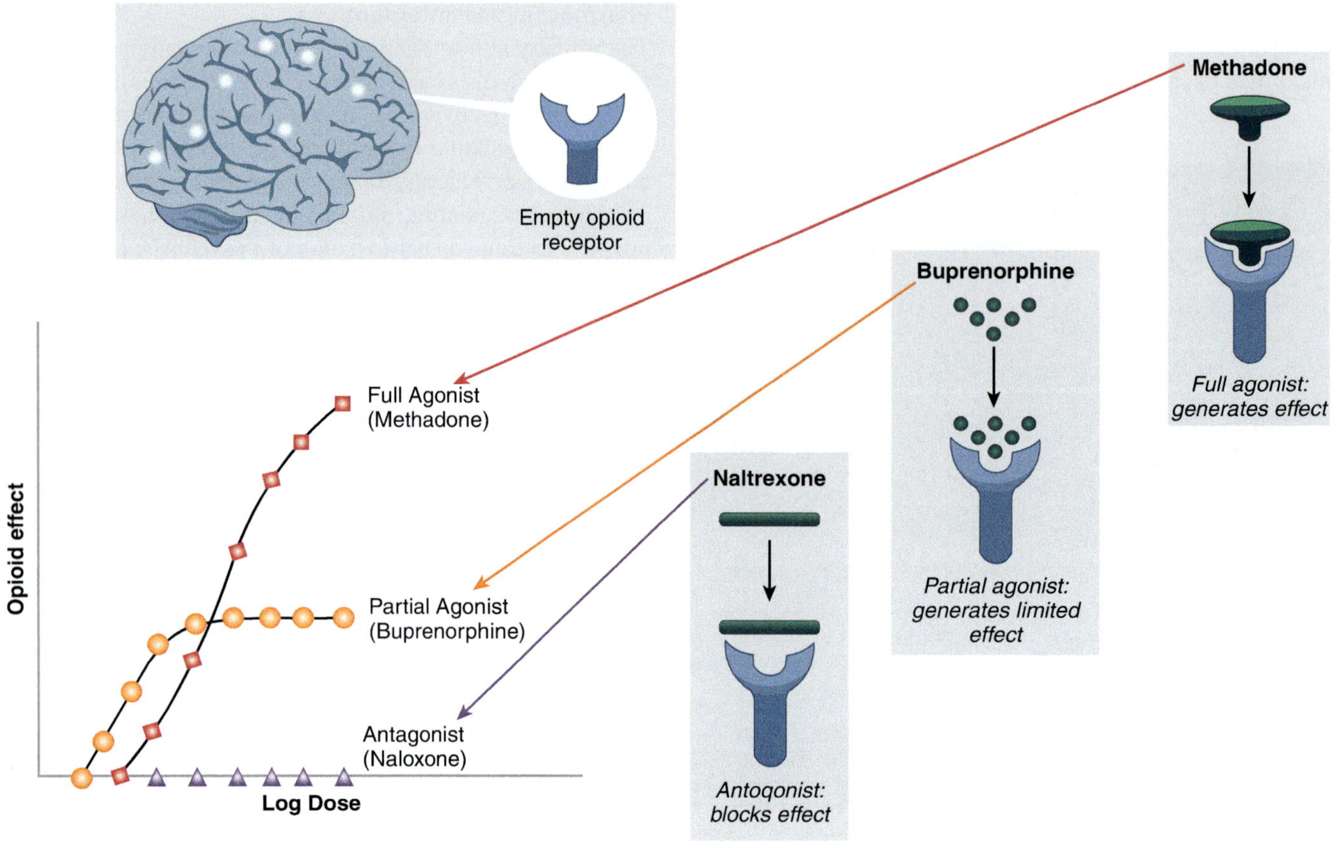

Fig. 14.34 Opioid receptor activities of naltrexone, buprenorphine, and methadone in treatment of opioid use disorder

Nonpharmacological Interventions

Whereas pharmacological interventions for SUD and gambling disorder are typically tailored, psychosocial interventions tend to have shared characteristics across the disorders. Most randomized trials of psychosocial treatment for SUDs, as well as behavioral addictions such as gambling disorder, have used manualized treatment methods to study various iterations of motivational enhancement therapy (MET), cognitive behavioral therapy (CBT), or contingency management (CM), as well as community and family interventions [6, 12, 29]. Because the underpinnings of these therapeutic models are complementary, research effort has focused as much on identifying effective combinations than on establishing the superiority of a single method.

Figure 14.36 lists psychosocial interventions focusing on the individual, their immediate support systems, and larger support communities. For gambling disorder, the best evidence exists thus far for CBT, MET, and 12-step programs, particularly when MET or 12-step programs are used in conjunction with CBT [6]. Well-supported scientific evidence shows that behavioral therapies are effective in treating substance-related and addictive disorders, but most evidence-based behavioral therapies are often implemented with limited fidelity and are underused [12, 29]. Figure 14.37 illustrates a recommended treatment algorithm for gambling disorder that integrates current evidence for pharmacologic and nonpharmacologic therapies for gambling disorder and common comorbid conditions [6].

To address the spectrum of substance-related and addictive disorders, a phase of care approach provides individuals an array of service options based on need, including prevention, early interventions, and more involved treatment to achieve sustained and recovery support [9, 22]. Figure 14.38 summarizes therapeutic objectives or interventions that are typically a focus within each phase of care. Every patient should have a tailored approach to their treatment plan based on a multidimensional assessment framework in order to

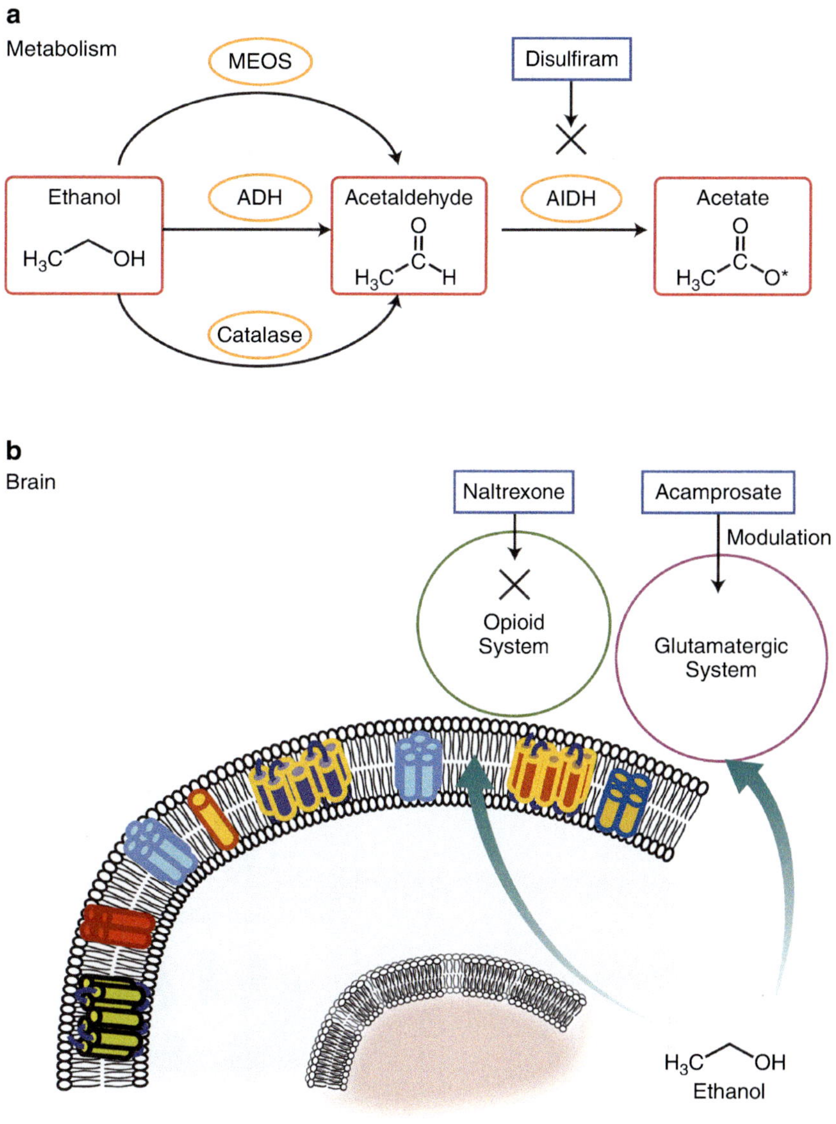

Fig. 14.35 Mechanisms of action of acamprosate (**b**-purple circle), naltrexone (**b**-green circle), and disulfiram (**a**) in the treatment of alcohol use disorder. Acamprosate inhibits aldehyde dehydrogenase (*AIDH*) leading to building up of acetaldehyde. *ADH* alcohol dehydrogenase; *MEOS* microsomal ethanol oxidizing system, and alternate first step in alcohol metabolism

integrate the unique biopsychosocial understanding of their substance use. Furthermore, the actual duration of each phase of care should be based on an assessment of clinical progress and evolving goals of care.

Over the last decade, a series of innovative care models have been developed with the objective of increasing access to evidence-based treatment services. These care models include, but are not limited to, collaborative care models to facilitate the integration of substance use treatment in primary care, telehealth services, technological applications, and consultative models.

Figure 14.39 illustrates addiction consultation teams, a model of care intended to enhance initiation of treatment for hospitalized patients with substance-use disorders. A common aim of these models is to integrate historically fragmented clinical services to create a seamless and patient-centered experience.

In conclusion, substance-related and gambling disorders are chronic diseases that have neurobiological underpinnings and are intertwined with the physical, psychological, and societal health of an individual. By utilizing a multidimensional framework to evaluate patients, a personalized assess-

Fig. 14.36 Selected psychosocial interventions for substance use and gambling disorders

Intervention	Theory of Change
Motivational Enhancement Therapy (MET) 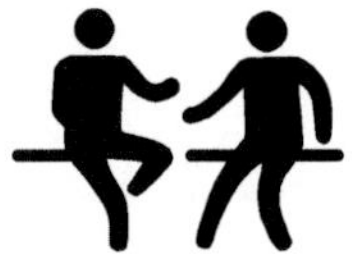	Patient-centered therapy that helps individuals resolve ambivalence in order to generate commitment to change. Views readiness to change as a dynamic process involving multiple stages: pre-contemplation, contemplation, preparation, action, and maintenance, and proposes that the role of the therapist is to create the conditions that promote the patient's intrinsic motivation.
Cognitive Behavior Therapy (CBT) 	Views drug use as a learned behavior. CBT posits that by identifying the associative links and chain of events precipitating substance use, patients can identify opportunities to alter their behavioral repertoire and use alternative, healthy coping mechanisms.
Contingency Management (CM) 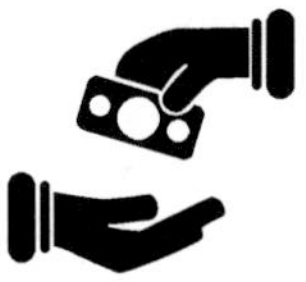	Based on operant conditioning theory, posits that behaviors will increase or decrease as a function of immediate and directly associated consequences (reward or punishment, respectively). By modifying the quality and immediacy of external consequences, contingency management attempts to systematically increase the likelihood of desired behaviors and minimize undesired behaviors.
Supportive Expressive Therapy (SEP) 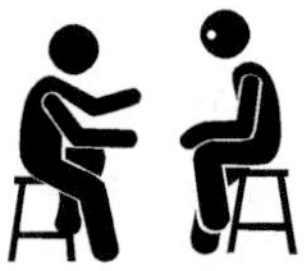	Aims to cultivate a strong therapeutic alliance to enable an expressive component, in which the therapist utilizes reflective listening and interpretation to explore the patient's subjective experience, point out patterns that manifest within the therapeutic relationship, and facilitate development of self-awareness, insight, and adaptive coping.
12-Step Facilitation (TSF) 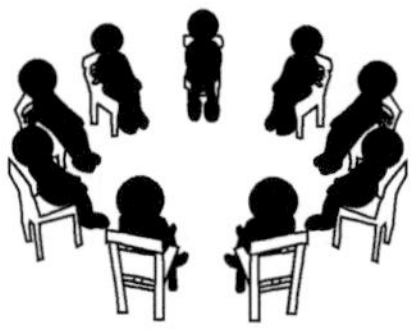	Semi-structured therapy that encourages and systematically supports active involvement in community-based 12-step meetings, such as Gamblers Anonymous, Alcoholics Anonymous ,and Narcotics Anonymous. Sessions involve discussion of common themes from 12-step meetings, exploring patient attitudes, and overcoming obstacles.
Adolescent Community Reinforcement Approach (ACRA) 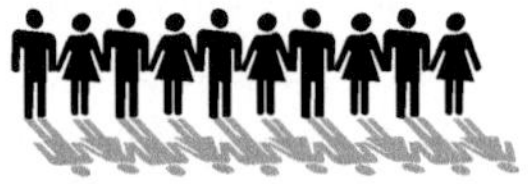	Multi-system behavioral therapy that seeks to integrate cognitive behavioral skills training with collaborative community support, and contingency management. Utilizes a community-based approach to assist youth in promoting the structures of a healthy lifestyle.
Multidimensional Family Therapy (MDFT) 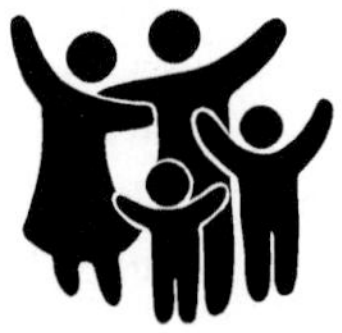	Comprehensive systems therapy that targets the functioning of the individual within the context of his or her environment by integrating individual therapy, parent coaching, family systems therapy, and engagement of key community stakeholders, such as school, medical supports, juvenile justice, and social services.

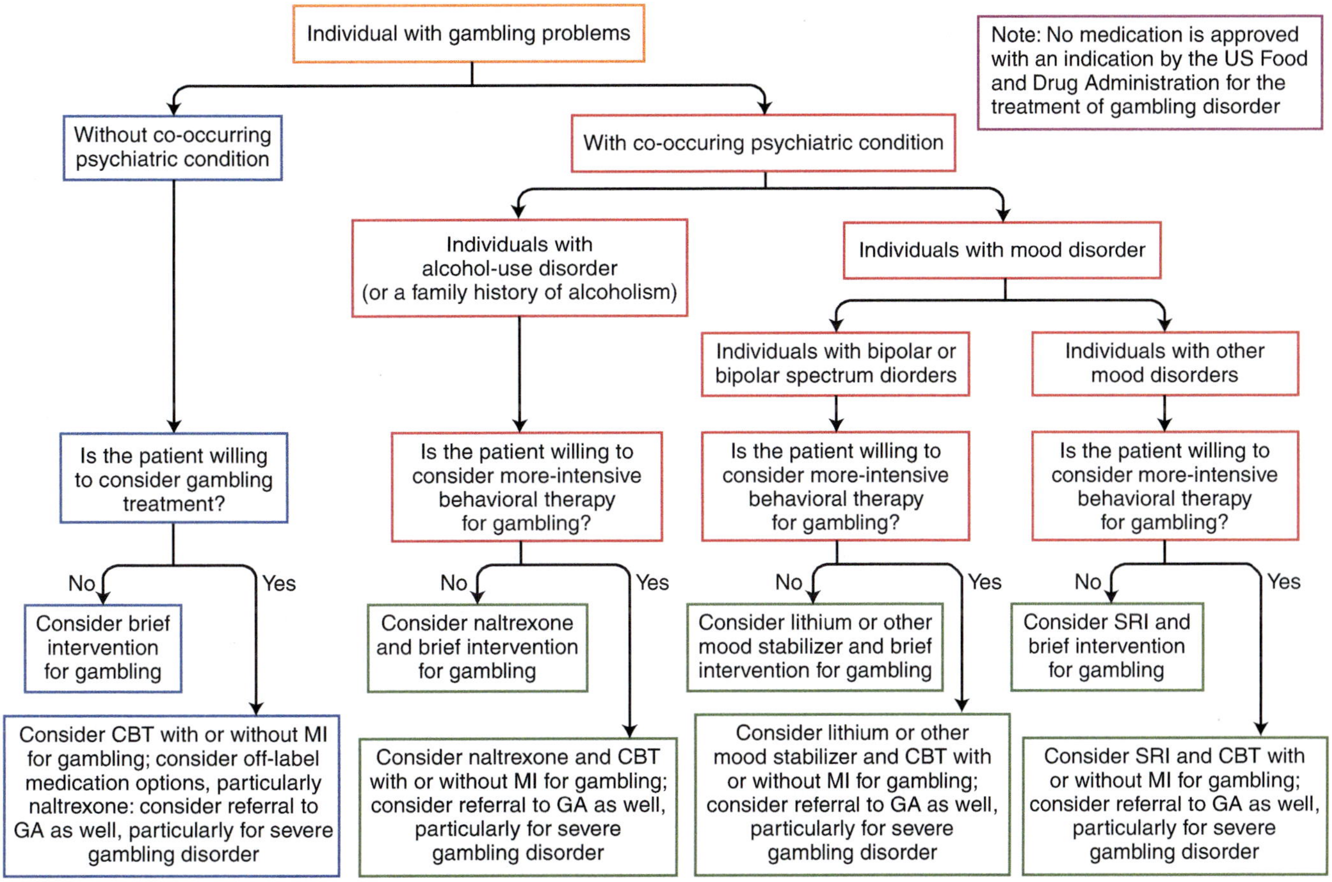

Fig. 14.37 Proposed algorithm for treatment of gambling disorder taking into account the presence of co-occurring mental health and/or substance-use disorders. (*Reproduced from* Potenza et al. [6]; *with permission*)

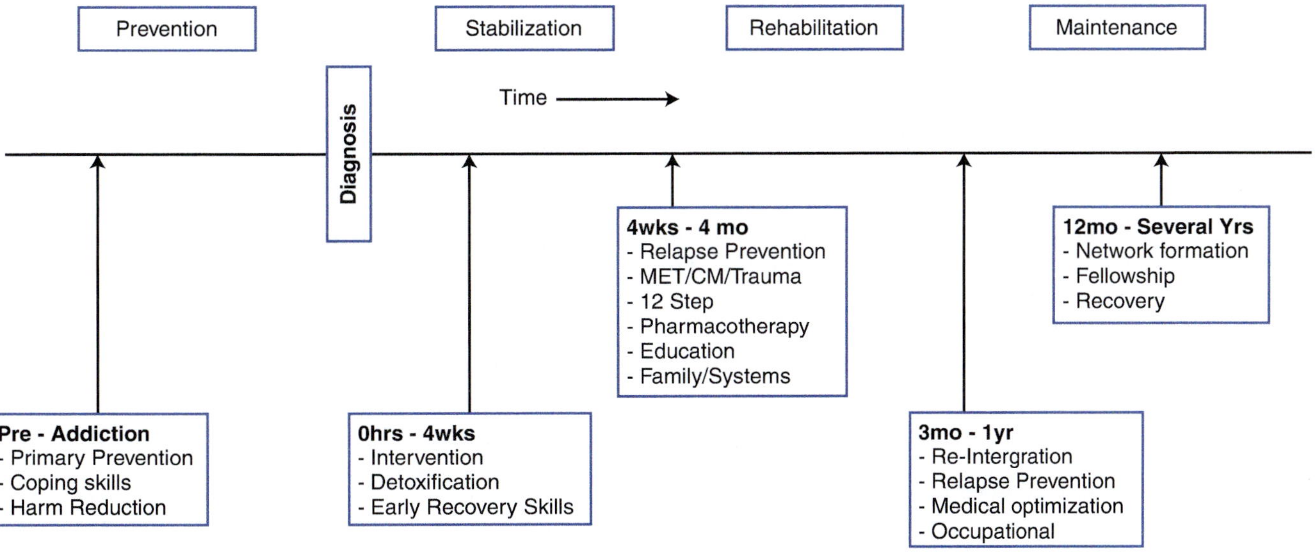

Fig. 14.38 Phases of recovery and the role of treatment interventions

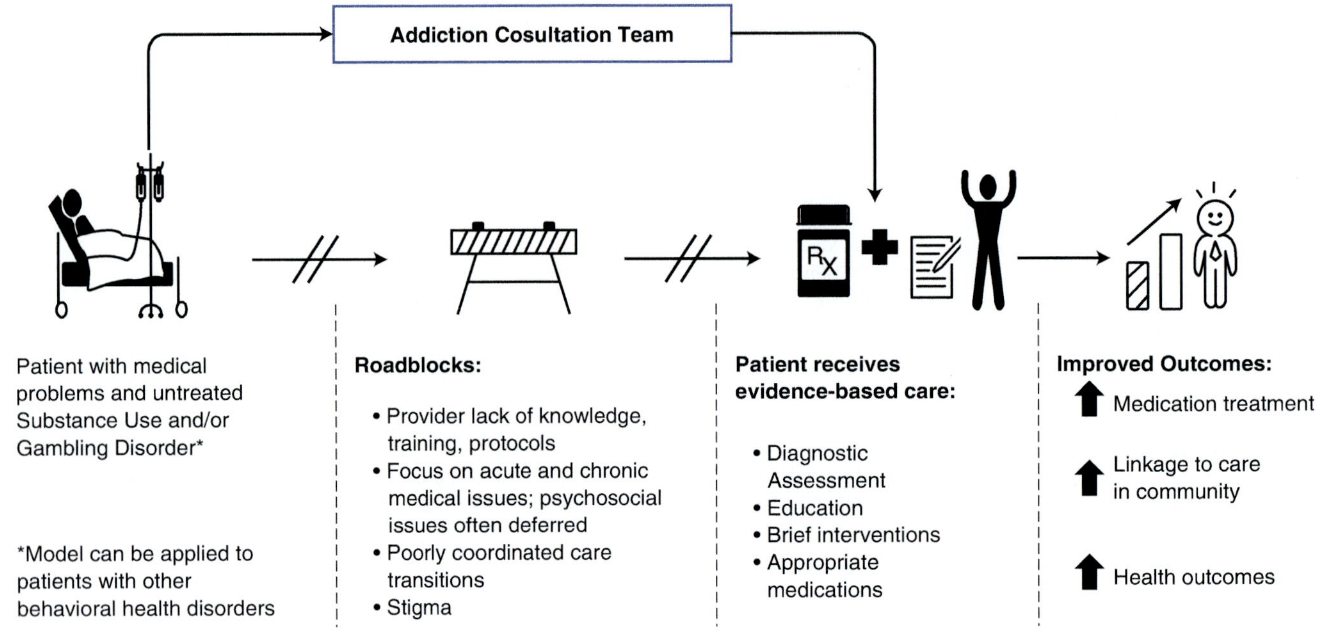

Fig. 14.39 Inpatient consultation model for treatment of substance use and gambling disorder

ment can be generated to guide a comprehensive treatment plan. With effective treatment, delivered within an appropriate continuum of care, prevention of relapse and sustainment of recovery can be achieved.

Future Directions

Additional disorders such as Internet Gaming Disorder and Caffeine Use Disorder are listed under "Conditions for Further Study" in the DSM-5 [30]. The conditions have proposed criteria similar to the other disorders listed in the Substance Related and Addictive Disorders section of the DSM-5 [30]. There was a similar discussion for inclusion of Hypersexual Disorder in the DSM-5 with criteria proposed in 2010 [31]. However, the proposed criteria were deemed to have insufficient evidence to be included in the DSM-5. The American Psychiatric Association has identified these two disorders as areas of further research.

References

1. American Psychiatric Association (APA). Substance-related and addictive disorders. Diagnostic and statistical manual of mental disorders. 5th ed. DSM library. Arlington, VA: American Psychiatric Association; 2013.
2. National Institute on Drug Abuse (NIDA). The National Institute on Drug Abuse Media Guide: how to find what you need to know about drug use and addiction. Washington DC: National Institute on Drug Abuse. Contract No.: October 1; 2020.
3. United Nations Office on Drugs and Crime (UNODC) World Drug Report 2020. Vienna, Austria: United Nations. Contract No.: Sales No. E.20.XI.6; 2020.
4. World Health Organization (WHO). Global Status Report on Alcohol and Health 2018. Geneva: World Health Organization. Contract No.: License: CC BY-NC-SA 3.0 IGO; 2018.
5. Substance Abuse and Mental Health Services Administration (SAMHSA). Key Substance Use and Mental Health Indicators in the United States: results from the 2019 National Survey on Drug Use and Health. Rockvile, MD: Substance Abuse and Mental Health Services Administration. Contract No. PEP20-07-01-001; 2020.
6. Potenza MN, Balodis IM, Derevensky J, Grant JE, Petry NM, Verdejo-Garcia A, et al. Gambling disorder. Nat Rev Dis Primers. 2019;5(1):51. https://doi.org/10.1038/s41572-019-0099-7.
7. Nautiyal KM, Okuda M, Hen R, Blanco C. Gambling disorder: an integrative review of animal and human studies. Ann N Y Acad Sci. 2017;1394(1):106–27. https://doi.org/10.1111/nyas.13356.
8. WHO. Addictive behaviors. In: Health topics. World Health Organization; 2020. https://www.who.int/health-topics/addictive-behaviours#tab=tab_1. Accessed Dec 2020.
9. Agrawal A, Lynskey MT. Are there genetic influences on addiction: evidence from family, adoption and twin studies. Addiction. 2008;103(7):1069–81. https://doi.org/10.1111/j.1360-0443.2008.02213.x.
10. Ho MK, Goldman D, Heinz A, Kaprio J, Kreek MJ, Li MD, et al. Breaking barriers in the genomics and pharmacogenetics of drug addiction. Clin Pharmacol Ther. 2010;88(6):779–91. https://doi.org/10.1038/clpt.2010.175.
11. Agrawal A, Verweij KJH, Gillespie NA, Heath AC, Lessov-Schlaggar CN, Martin NG, et al. The genetics of addiction—a translational perspective. Transl Psychiatry. 2012;2(7):e140. https://doi.org/10.1038/tp.2012.54.
12. U.S. Department of Health and Human Services (HHS) Office of the Surgeon General. Facing Addiction in America: the surgeon general's report on alcohol, drugs, and health. Washington, DC; 2016.

13. Strathearn L, Mertens CE, Mayes L, Rutherford H, Rajhans P, Xu G, et al. Pathways relating the neurobiology of attachment to drug addiction. Front Psych. 2019;10:737. https://doi.org/10.3389/fpsyt.2019.00737.
14. Koob GF, Volkow ND. Neurobiology of addiction: a neurocircuitry analysis. Lancet Psychiatry. 2016;3(8):760–73.
15. Bowen MT, Neumann ID. Rebalancing the addicted brain: oxytocin interference with the neural substrates of addiction. Trends Neurosci. 2017;40(12):691–708. https://doi.org/10.1016/j.tins.2017.10.003.
16. Liu M, Jiang Y, Wedow R, Li Y, Brazel DM, Chen F, et al. Association studies of up to 1.2 million individuals yield new insights into the genetic etiology of tobacco and alcohol use. Nat Genet. 2019;51(2):237–44. https://doi.org/10.1038/s41588-018-0307-5.
17. Belcher AM, Volkow ND, Moeller FG, Ferré S. Personality traits and vulnerability or resilience to substance use disorders. Trends Cogn Sci. 2014;18(4):211–7. https://doi.org/10.1016/j.tics.2014.01.010.
18. Sarlin E. Substance use disorders are associated with major medical illnesses and mortality risk in a large integrated health care system. In: NIDA Notes. National Institute of Drug Abuse; 2017. https://www.drugabuse.gov/news-events/nida-notes/2017/10/substance-use-disorders-are-associated-major-medical-illnesses-mortality-risk-in-large-integrated#figure2. Accessed May 2020.
19. NIDA. Common Comorbidities with Substance Use Disorders Research Report. National Institute on Drug Abuse; 2020. https://www.drugabuse.gov/publications/research-reports/common-comorbidities-substance-use-disorders/part-1-connection-between-substance-use-disorders-mental-illness.
20. Spooner C, Hetherington K. Social determinants of drug use. Sydney, Australia: National Drug and Alcohol Research Centre; 2005. Contract No.: 228.
21. Shokoohi M, Bauer GR, Kaida A, Logie CH, Lacombe-Duncan A, Milloy MJ, et al. Patterns of social determinants of health associated with drug use among women living with HIV in Canada: a latent class analysis. Addiction. 2019;114(7):1214–24. https://doi.org/10.1111/add.14566.
22. Valdez LA, Garcia DO, Ruiz J, Oren E, Carvajal S. Exploring structural, sociocultural, and individual barriers to alcohol abuse treatment among hispanic men. Am J Mens Health. 2018;12(6):1948–57. https://doi.org/10.1177/1557988318790882.
23. Welte JW, Barnes GM, Tidwell M-CO, Wieczorek WF. Predictors of problem gambling in the U.S. J Gambl Stud. 2017;33(2):327–42. https://doi.org/10.1007/s10899-016-9639-1.
24. NIDA. Drugs, brains, and behavior: the science of addiction. Washington DC: National Institute on Drug Abuse; 2020.
25. Tabakoff B, Hoffman PL. The neurobiology of alcohol consumption and alcoholism: an integrative history. Pharmacol Biochem Behav. 2013;113:20–37. https://doi.org/10.1016/j.pbb.2013.10.009.
26. Ries RK, Fiellin DA, Miller SC. The ASAM principles of addiction medicine. 5th ed. Philadelphia: Wolters Kluwer Health; 2015.
27. New Zealand Drug Foundation. Managing withdrawal. https://www.drugfoundation.org.nz/info/helping-someone/managing-withdrawal.
28. Volkow ND, Chang L, Wang G-J, Fowler JS, Franceschi D, Sedler M, et al. Loss of dopamine transporters in methamphetamine abusers recovers with protracted abstinence. J Neurosci. 2001;21(23):9414. https://doi.org/10.1523/JNEUROSCI.21-23-09414.2001.
29. NIDA. Principles of drug addiction treatment: a research-based guide. 3rd edn. Contract No.: NIH Publication No. 12–4180; 2018.
30. APA. Conditions for Further Study. Diagnostic and statistical manual of mental disorders. 5th ed. DSM library. Arlington, VA: American Psychiatric Association; 2013. p. 783–808.
31. Kafka MP. Hypersexual disorder: a proposed diagnosis for DSM-V. Arch Sex Behav. 2010;39(2):377–400. https://doi.org/10.1007/s10508-009-9574-7.
32. Clark L, Lawrence AJ, Astley-Jones F, Gray N. Gambling near-misses enhance motivation to gamble and recruit win-related brain circuitry. Neuron. 2009;61(3):481–90. https://doi.org/10.1016/j.neuron.2008.12.031.
33. Ambre J, Fischman M, Ruo TI. Urinary excretion of ecgonine methyl ester, a major metabolite of cocaine in humans. J Anal Toxicol. 1984;8(1):23–5.
34. Volkow ND, Fowler JS, Wang GJ, Swanson JM. Dopamine in drug abuse and addiction: results from imaging studies and treatment implications. Mol Psychiatry. 2004;9(6):557–69. https://doi.org/10.1038/sj.mp.4001507.

Schizophrenia Spectrum and Other Psychotic Disorders

15

Alaina V. Burns and Stephen Marder

Introduction

Schizophrenia is a severe psychiatric disorder that can significantly alter cognition, perception, behavior, and the ability to think clearly and logically. Symptoms appear in late adolescence or early adulthood and are persistent throughout the lifespan. Schizophrenia is highly heritable, though the risk is also increased by several environmental factors, including maternal malnutrition, early cannabis use, and migration. Etiologically, schizophrenia is currently conceptualized as a neurodevelopmental disorder that produces changes in the brain through altered neurotransmission and neuroendocrine dysfunction. Impacted individuals frequently develop beliefs and perceptual experiences that do not correspond to reality as well as the inability to organize their thoughts. These symptoms, along with the social withdrawal that is common to the disorder, often cause profound impairments in social and occupational functioning. The treatment of schizophrenia includes antipsychotic medications, which alter pathways of neurotransmission, as well as individual-, group-, and family-based talk therapies.

Epidemiology

Schizophrenia affects nearly 1% of the world's population. The risk is similar in nearly every part of the globe; however, certain groups such as migrants, individuals who have been exposed to childhood trauma, and those living in urban areas are at somewhat greater risk. The economic burden of schizophrenia is enormous—due to the direct costs of treatment as well as to patients' decreased productivity and impairment in psychosocial functioning, including increased risk of unemployment and homelessness (see Table 15.1) [2, 3].

Table 15.1 Global economic burden of schizophrenia: breakdown of direct and indirect costs

Direct costs	Indirect costs
Healthcare provider fees (including psychiatrists, psychologists, and nurse practitioners)	Unemployment, permanent disability, and early retirement
Hospital inpatient fees	Morbidity
Long-term institutional care	Premature mortality
Rehabilitation care	Income assistance
Emergency room visits	Law enforcement
Pharmacy fees and medications	Morbidity
Homeless shelters	Legal fees

A review of studies about the global economic burden of schizophrenia named some of the direct and indirect costs associated with the illness. Indirect costs contributed to 50–85% of the total cost burden of schizophrenia, which was estimated to range between 0.02–1.65% of the gross domestic product [1]

The first signs of schizophrenia usually emerge in late adolescence or early adulthood (see Fig. 15.1). Men tend to develop schizophrenia earlier than women [5] and with a higher symptom burden. For both men and women, earlier onset of symptoms predicts greater illness severity. In women, a second peak of illness onset occurs during menopause, thought to be due to the loss of protective effects of estrogen (see Fig. 15.2) [6].

Compared to the general population, people with schizophrenia have a two- to threefold greater risk of dying from any cause. Although some of the increased mortality risk is associated with an increased risk for suicide, most of the risk is associated with cardiovascular disease. This is likely related to the increased prevalence of smoking, obesity, and type-II diabetes in schizophrenia (see Table 15.2) [8, 9].

A. V. Burns (✉)
Department of Psychiatry and Biobehavioral Sciences, Adult Division, UCLA-Semel Institute for Neuroscience and Human Behavior, Los Angeles, CA, USA
e-mail: avburns@mednet.ucla.edu

S. Marder
Semel Institute for Neuroscience at UCLA, VA Desert Pacific Mental Illness Research, Education, and Clinical Center (VISN 22 MIRECC), Los Angeles, CA, USA
e-mail: marder@ucla.edu

W. W. IsHak (ed.), *Atlas of Psychiatry*, https://doi.org/10.1007/978-3-031-15401-0_15

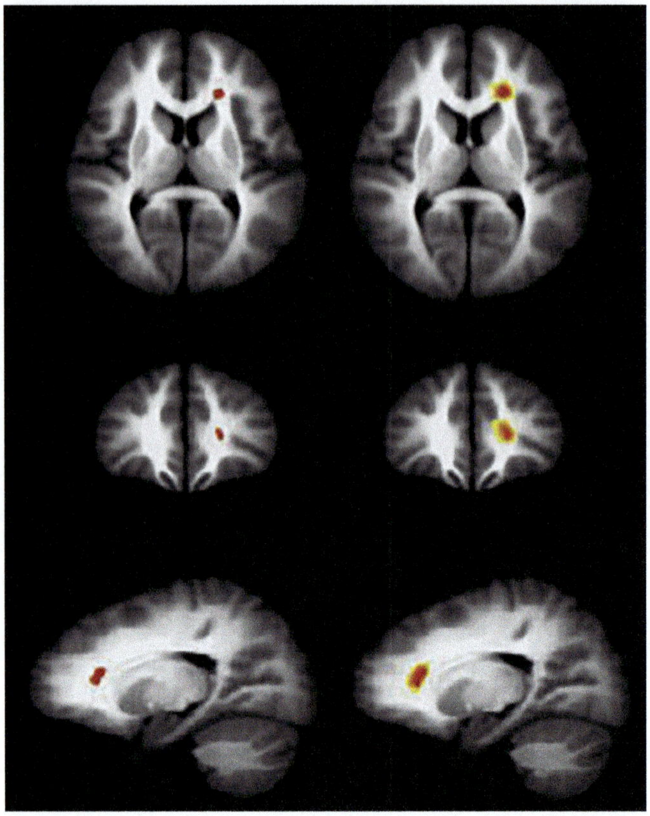

Fig. 15.1 Research suggests that much of the important structural maturation of fiber pathways connecting the frontal lobe to other brain regions takes place during adolescence. The pathophysiology of schizophrenia may involve abnormalities of frontal lobe white matter components, including oligodendrocytes and myelin, that impair these pathways of communication. Diffusion tensor imaging (DTI) is an MRI technique that can be used to measure fractional anisotropy (FA), a reduction of which may indicate structural impairment of white matter. One study compared DTI studies among patients with the onset of schizophrenia prior to age 18 years with healthy controls. Patients with schizophrenia showed significantly decreased FA in the subcortical white matter in the left anterior cingulate region, an area of the brain involved in higher-level functions, including affect regulation, attention, and motivation. (*From* Kumra et al. [4]; *with permission*)

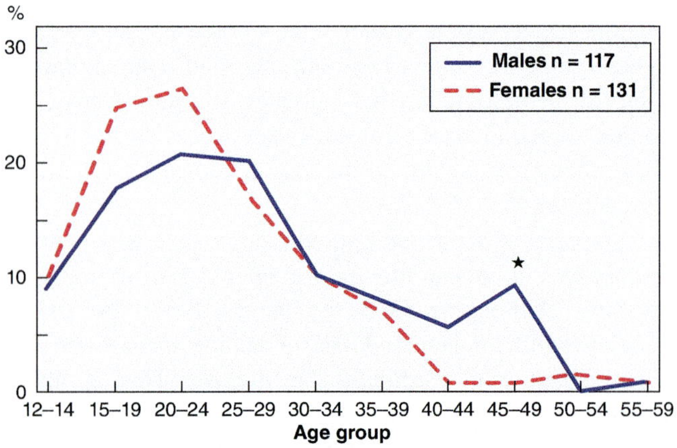

Fig. 15.2 The incidence of schizophrenia in men usually occurs during late adolescence and early adulthood, with incidence gradually declining over time. The incidence of schizophrenia in women is slightly later compared to men, with a second peak in onset occurring around menopause. (*From* Häfner et al. [6]; *with permission*)

Table 15.2 Leading causes of death among a sample of adults with schizophrenia, 2001–2007

Natural causes of death:
Cardiovascular disease
Cancer, especially lung cancer
Other: COPD, diabetes mellitus, pneumonia
Unnatural causes of death:
Suicide
Alcohol- and drug-induced deaths
Other: accidents, including accidental poisoning

A study by Olfson et al. [7] examined mortality rates and standardized mortality ratios among people diagnosed with schizophrenia between 2001 and 2007. Adults with schizophrenia were found to be more than 3.5 times as likely to die from any cause as adults without schizophrenia, highlighting the impact of metabolic syndrome and substance use, including tobacco use, in this population

Etiology

Schizophrenia is a syndrome that is thought to arise from a combination of genetic and environmental factors. For those with a genetic predisposition, events that occur during fetal development or during the perinatal period can increase the risk of developing schizophrenia. There is also evidence that drug use—particularly cannabis—as well as childhood abuse or neglect can increase risk.

Genetic Studies

Schizophrenia is one of the most highly heritable psychiatric illnesses. Twin studies show a heritability estimate of around 80%, suggesting that genetic makeup contributes a major proportion of the risk of developing schizophrenia. However, the concordance rate in both monozygotic and dizygotic twins emphasizes the importance of environmental factors (see Fig. 15.3) [10].

Genome-wide association studies (GWAS) have identified more than one hundred gene loci that are associated with schizophrenia. Each of these genes makes a relatively small contribution to risk. These include genes that are related to glutamatergic neurotransmission, synaptic plasticity, and voltage-gated calcium channel subunits. GWAS studies have also shown an association with schizophrenia and genes that are involved with key immune functions (i.e., B-lymphocyte lineages), suggesting that schizophrenia may be in part an illness of immune dysfunction [11]. Although single genes make very small contributions to risk, large deletions or duplications known as copy number variants can substantially increase risk [12].

Schizophrenia has been found to be genetically linked to other psychiatric and neurodevelopmental disorders, including bipolar disorder, intellectual disability, and autism spectrum disorder (see Fig. 15.4) [11, 14].

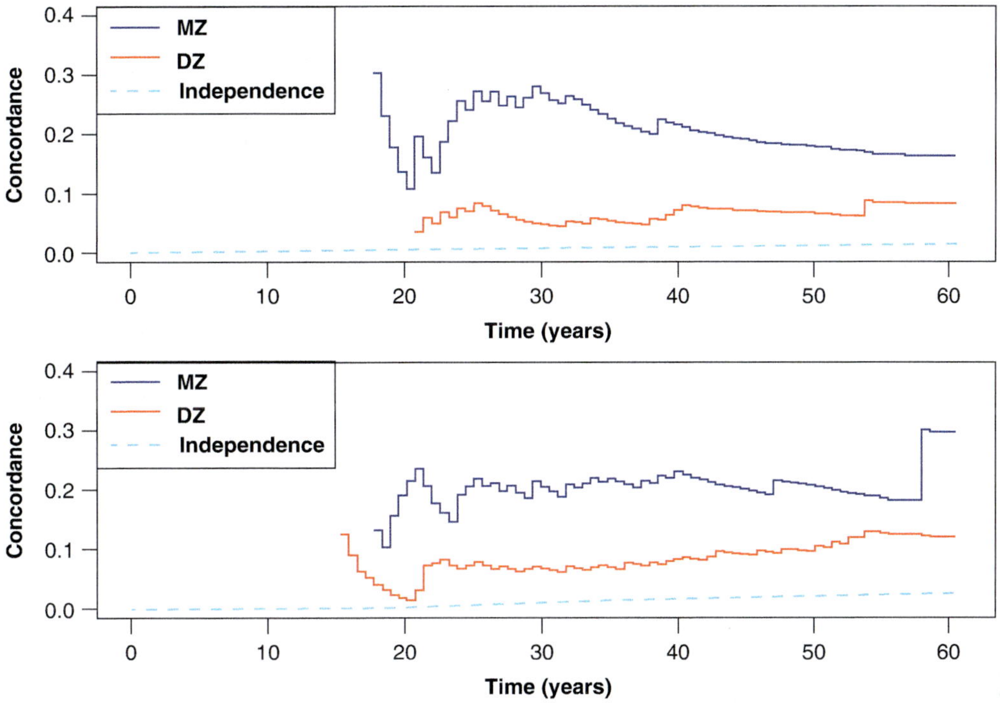

Fig. 15.3 In this Danish twin study, concordance rates of schizophrenia (top) and schizophrenia spectrum disorders (bottom) were 33% in monozygotic twins (MZ) and 7% in dizygotic twins (DZ), with an estimated heritability of schizophrenia of 79%. (*From* Hilker et al. [10]; *with permission*)

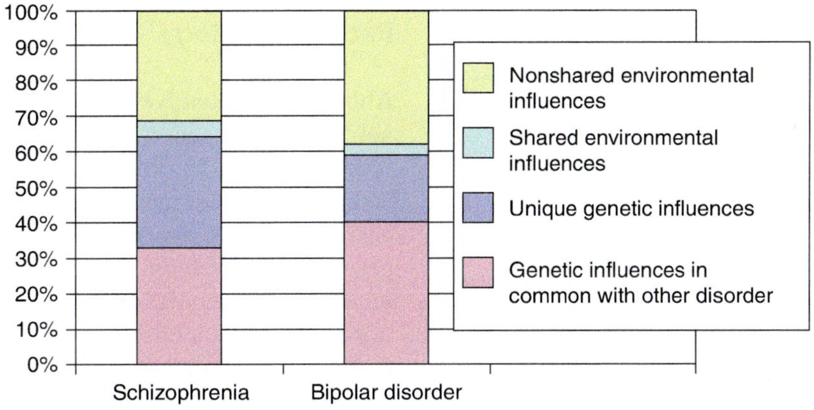

Fig. 15.4 A Swedish study examined the risk of schizophrenia or bipolar disorder among first-degree relatives of probands with either disorder. Heritability was found to be 64% for schizophrenia and 59% for bipolar disorder. Genetic relatives of a proband with bipolar disorder were found to be at increased risk for schizophrenia. In the figure above, the solid red portion of the lines represents the genetic variance for the disorder that is shared with the other disorder. These and other data suggest common genetic influences in schizophrenia and bipolar disorder. (*From* Lichtenstein et al. [13]; *with permission*)

Environmental Risk Factors

Obstetric Events

A variety of obstetric complications have been shown to increase the risk for schizophrenia. Fetal growth retardation, including low birth weight and smaller head circumference, as well as fetal hypoxia, have been linked to the later development of schizophrenia. There are also multiple prenatal exposures that are associated with schizophrenia risk. These exposures include maternal viral infections, including influenza A and other respiratory infections; maternal nutritional deficiency; and maternal stress, especially stress that occurs during times of war or natural disasters [15].

Advanced Paternal Age

The risk of schizophrenia rises with increasing paternal age, though not with increasing maternal age. One study showed an adjusted odds ratio of 1.3 for each ten-year increase in

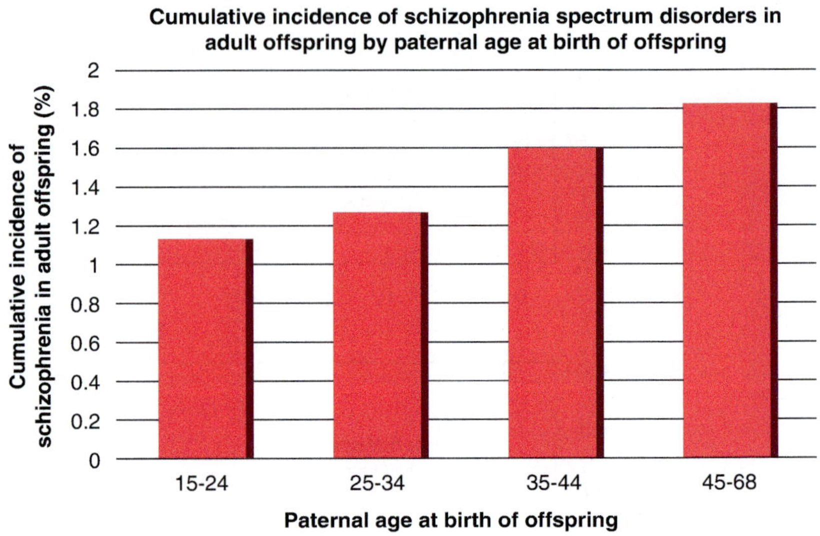

Fig. 15.5 Paternal age in years on the X axis (25–34, 35–44, 45–54, 55–64) and cumulative incidence of schizophrenia in adult offspring (%) on the Y axis (1.13, 1.27, 1.60, 1.83). Figure showing cumulative incidence of schizophrenia spectrum disorders by father's age [16]

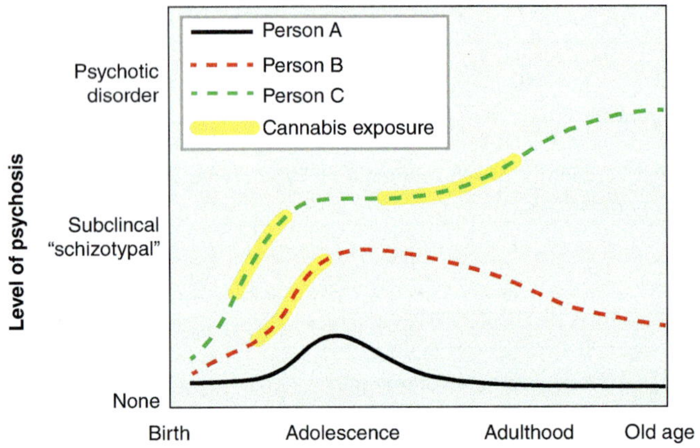

Fig. 15.6 A model showing how cannabis exposure throughout adolescence and early adulthood can influence the persistence of psychotic symptoms. Person A, who has no exposure to cannabis, develops subclinical and transient psychotic symptoms. Person B, who has some exposure to cannabis in adolescence, has subclinical symptoms that are more severe and persistent. Person C, with prolonged cannabis exposure during adolescence and young adulthood, develops clinical psychotic symptoms due in part to repeated exposure

paternal age, thought to be due in part to accumulated mutations in paternal germ cells (see Fig. 15.5) [17].

Cannabis Use

A large and growing number of studies implicate early cannabis use with an increased risk for schizophrenia. Cannabis use during adolescence and young adulthood is associated with an increased risk of incident psychotic experiences, while ongoing cannabis use has been shown to increase the severity and persistence of psychotic symptoms in a dose–response relationship (see Fig. 15.6) [18].

Migration Status

Decades of literature have revealed an increased incidence of schizophrenia in first- and second-generation immigrants; this is particularly marked among those who move from a country with a predominantly Black population to one with a predominantly white population [19].

Pathophysiology

Although the definitive pathophysiology of schizophrenia is not fully understood, it is currently conceptualized as a neurodevelopmental disorder that impacts the brain by altering neurotransmission, increasing inflammation, and producing changes in the neuroendocrine system. A combination of genetic predisposition and environmental stressors can impair the developing brain's ability to fine-tune neurotransmitter systems, stabilize synapses, and integrate brain structures (see Figs. 15.7 and 15.8) [21]. Imaging studies have shown evidence of brain changes including decreased cortical thickness and increased size of the lateral ventricles among individuals with schizophrenia as compared to controls (see Figs. 15.9 and 15.10).

Altered Dopamine Transmission

The dopamine hypothesis of schizophrenia is based on the observation that drugs such as antipsychotic medications that decrease dopamine neurotransmission or block dopamine receptors are effective for improving psychotic symptoms in schizophrenia and other illnesses. Drugs that increase dopamine transmission, including amphetamines, worsen

Working Model

Etiology: Multiple convergent factors such as

DNA ⇓ **Gene Expression** ⇓ **Viruses** ⇓ **Toxins** ⇓ **Nutrition** ⇓ **Birth Injury** ⇓ **Psychological Experiences** ⇓

Pathophysiology: Brain development from conception to early adulthood
(e.g., neuron formation, migration, synaptogenesis, pruning, apoptosis, activity dependent changes)

⇓

Anatomic and functional disruption in neruonal connectivity and communication

⇓

Impairment in a fundamental cognitive process

⇓

Impairment in one or more second-order cognitive processes (e.g., attention, memory, language, emotion)

⇓

Symptoms of schizophrenia (e.g., hallucinations, delusions, negative symptoms, disorganized speech)

Fig. 15.7 A conceptualization of how multiple factors, including viruses, toxins, and birth injuries, influence early and late brain development and the eventual generation of psychotic symptoms. (*From* Andreason [20]; *with permission*)

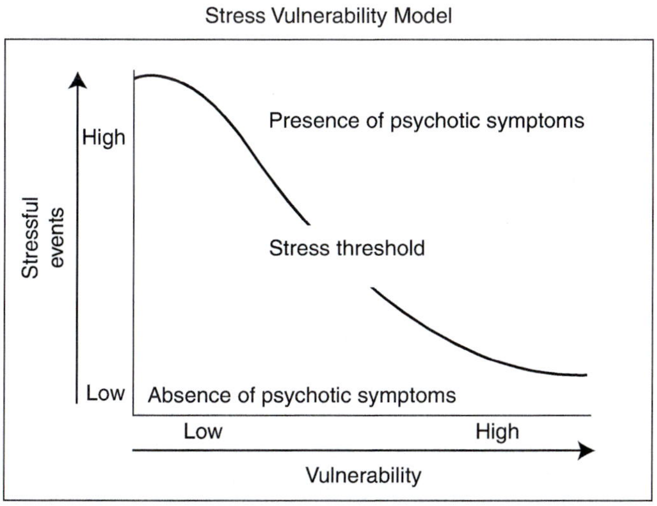

Fig. 15.8 The stress vulnerability model conceptualizes how genetic predisposition and environmental stressors, such as illicit drug use or trauma, interact and influence the development of psychotic symptoms. For those without a genetic predisposition, a very high level of stress is required to precipitate psychosis, whereas those with high genetic vulnerability may develop psychosis even in the absence of significant stress

psychosis in people with schizophrenia and can cause psychotic symptoms in others (see Fig. 15.11). While useful for researchers and drug developers, the original dopamine hypothesis is currently considered to be an oversimplification. It is likely that the effects of antipsychotic medications are related to neurochemical mechanisms that are adaptations to sustained blockade of D2 dopamine receptors. For example, dopamine interacts with both glutamate and GABA. These neurotransmitters are important in regulating excitatory and inhibitory interneurons in cortical circuits (see Fig. 15.12).

An aberrant salience hypothesis of schizophrenia provides an interesting explanation as to how abnormal dopamine signaling may lead to psychosis. Dopamine has an important role in attributing salience to information that reaches consciousness. If a disordered dopamine system gives excessive meaning to irrelevant information, it is possible that an affected individual will misinterpret this information. For example, an irrelevant sound may be interpreted as an indication of danger. This, in turn, may lead to the development of a delusion about the sound (see Fig. 15.13) [26, 28].

NMDAR Hypofunction

There is also evidence implicating the hypofunction of the excitatory glutamate-mediated *N*-methyl-D-aspartate receptor (NMDAR) in the development of schizophrenia. Drugs that block the NMDAR, including phencyclidine (PCP) and ketamine, produce psychotic states in otherwise healthy individuals. NMDAR encephalitis, in which autoantibodies are generated against an NMDAR subunit, produces schizophrenia-like symptoms. People with schizophrenia have been found to have lower in vivo glutamate concentrations in frontal brain regions. In addition, large-scale GWAS studies have identified genetic variants in the NMDAR gene that increase with the risk of schizophrenia [21].

Inflammation

Inflammation is a further mediator in the diathesis-stress model of schizophrenia. Genetic predisposition to schizophrenia causes increased response to negative stimuli, which

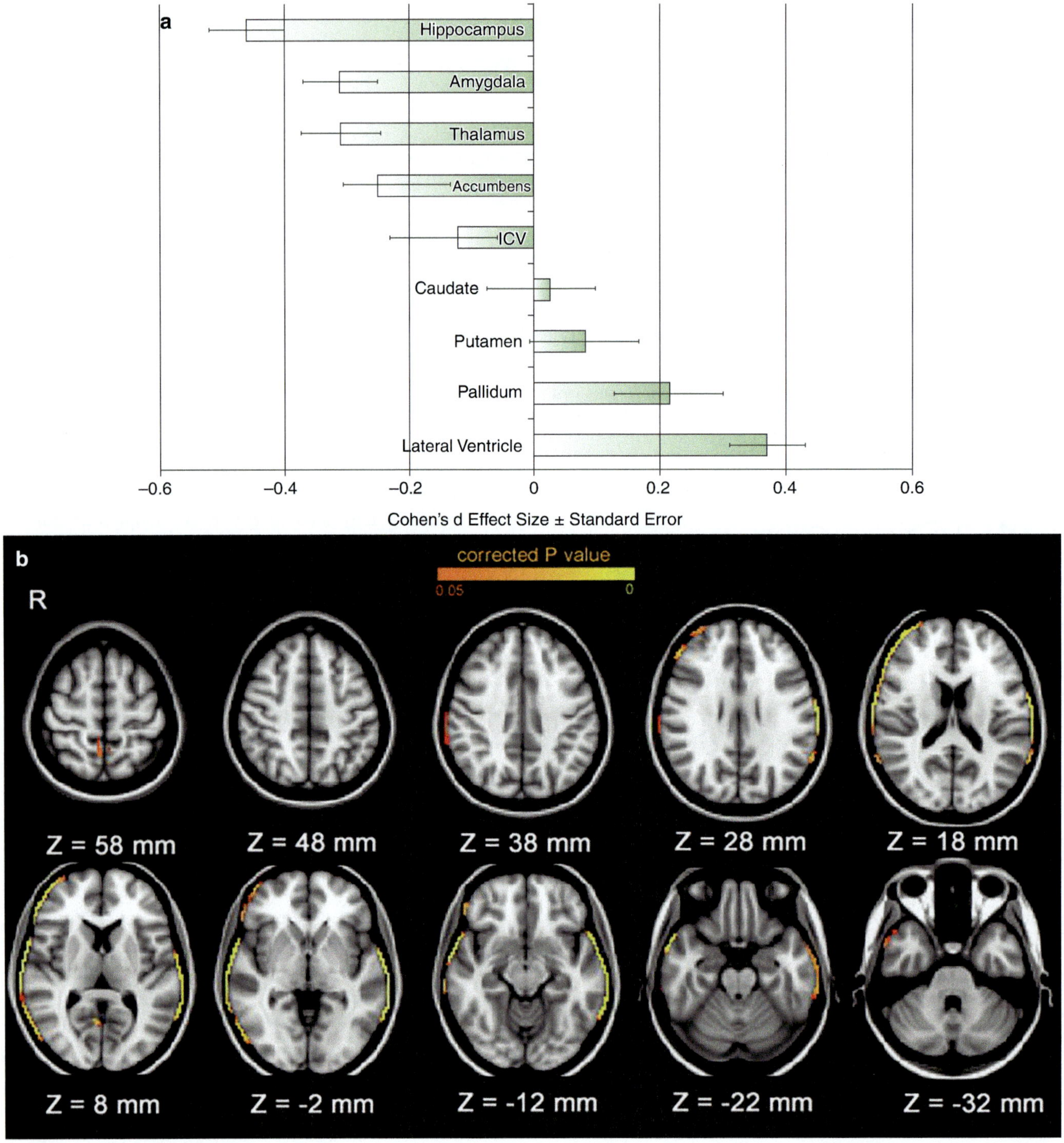

Fig. 15.9 MRI studies have shown that people with schizophrenia exhibit progressive changes in cortical and subcortical brain structures as well as ventricular enlargement relative to healthy controls. Pooled data from 15 worldwide brain imaging studies showed that subjects with schizophrenia had significantly smaller hippocampus, amygdala, thalamus, and accumbens volumes as well as larger lateral ventricle volumes, findings that were consistent with other studies that have shown smaller average intracranial brain volume in individuals with schizophrenia (**a**), *From* van Erp et al. [22]; *with permission*). Another study showed areas of atrophy in brain edge regions, including the right frontal lobe and the bilateral temporal lobes (**b**), From Guo et al. [23]; *with permission*). Patients with schizophrenia who experienced less deterioration of social and occupational functioning had greater volume preservation of the supramarginal gyrus, a structure involved in the mirror neuron system, highlighting the importance of parietal lobe structure in social functioning. Histological studies of the brain tissue of individuals with schizophrenia have shown no evidence of gliosis or the hypertrophy of glial cells in response to central nervous system damage. This has led to further support for the idea that schizophrenia is a disease of neurodevelopment rather than of neurodegeneration. Decreased cortical thickness seen in schizophrenia may be due to a lack of development of cell bodies, reduced length of dendritic spines, and decreased numbers of presynaptic terminals (**c**) [24]

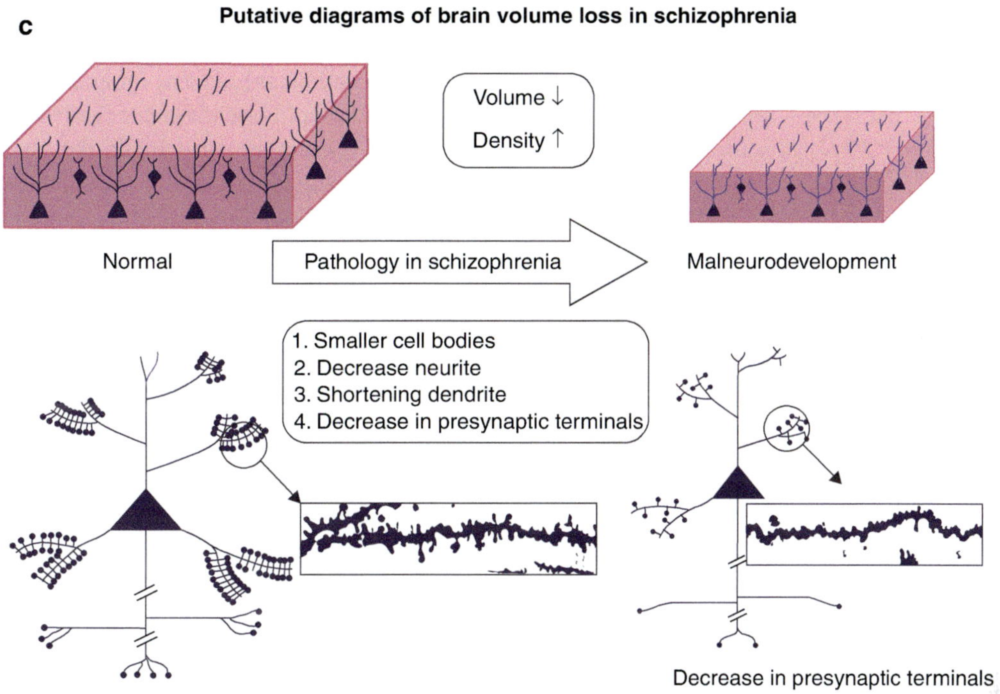

Fig. 15.9 (continued)

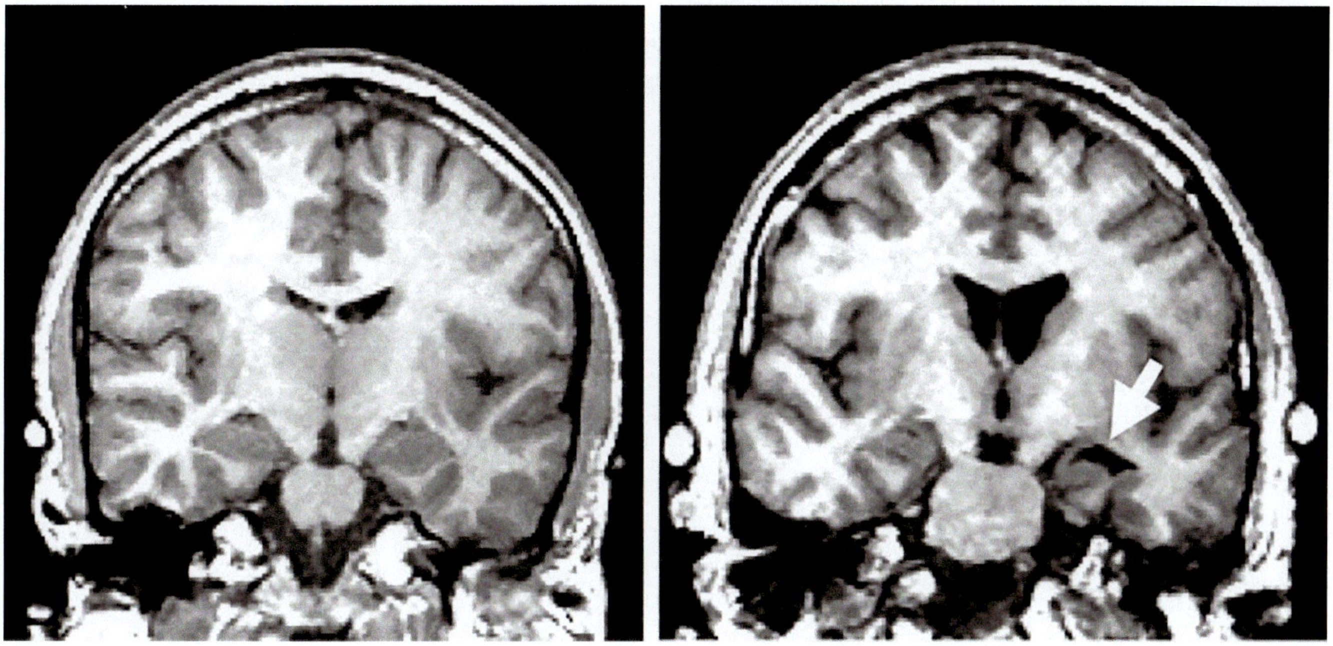

Fig. 15.10 The image on the left shows a coronal MRI section of the brain of a control subject, while the image on the right shows an analogous coronal section of the brain of a person with schizophrenia. Note on the right panel the increased cerebrospinal fluid surrounding the left temporal horn (indicated by the arrow), which surrounds the amygdala, as well as enlargement of the lateral ventricles (seen as black space in the middle of the image). (*From Shenton* et al. [25]; *with permission*)

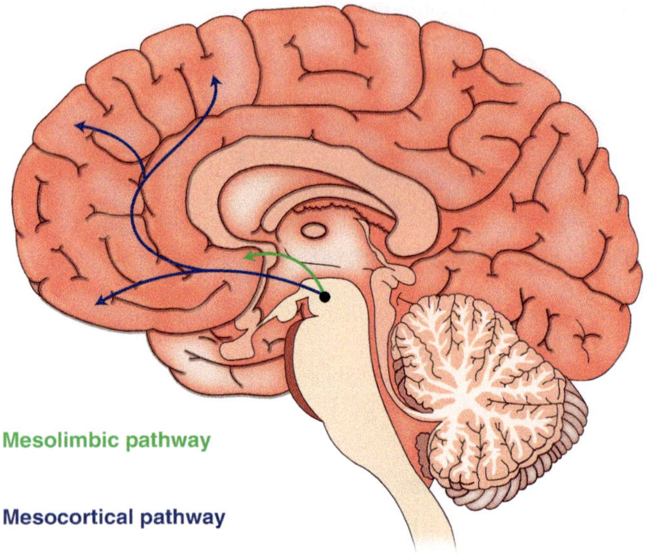

Fig. 15.11 Dopamine, a neurotransmitter produced in the substantia nigra and ventral tegmental regions of the brain, is projected through the nigrostriatal, mesolimbic, and mesocortical pathways. The mesolimbic pathway projects from the ventral tegmental area (VTA) in the brainstem to the nucleus accumbens in the ventral striatum, while the mesocortical pathway projects from the VTA to the prefrontal cortex. It is thought that positive symptoms of psychosis are caused by hyperactive dopamine transmission in the mesolimbic pathway, while negative symptoms of psychosis are caused by hypoactive dopamine transmission in the mesocortical pathway. In schizophrenia, dopamine dysfunction is also seen in other structures, including the hippocampus and the amygdala. (*Adapted from* Brisch et al. [26]; Creative Commons; https://creativecommons.org/licenses/by/3.0/)

in turn causes inflammation. In a process known as "kindling" or "sensitization," after an initial immune response to stress or infection, subsequent immune responses can occur at a lower threshold or with greater activation of the immune response. This may in part explain the association between prenatal exposure to viral infection and the later development of schizophrenia.

Studies have found an increase in the breakdown of products of inflammatory proteins in the cerebrospinal fluid (CSF) and brains of patients with schizophrenia. Higher levels of proinflammatory cytokines and lower levels of anti-inflammatory cytokines have been found in the CSF of subjects with schizophrenia versus healthy controls. Inflammation may also impact dopaminergic and glutamatergic neurotransmission [29, 30]. In addition, a history of any autoimmune disease has been found to increase the risk for schizophrenia by nearly 50% (see Fig. 15.14) [31].

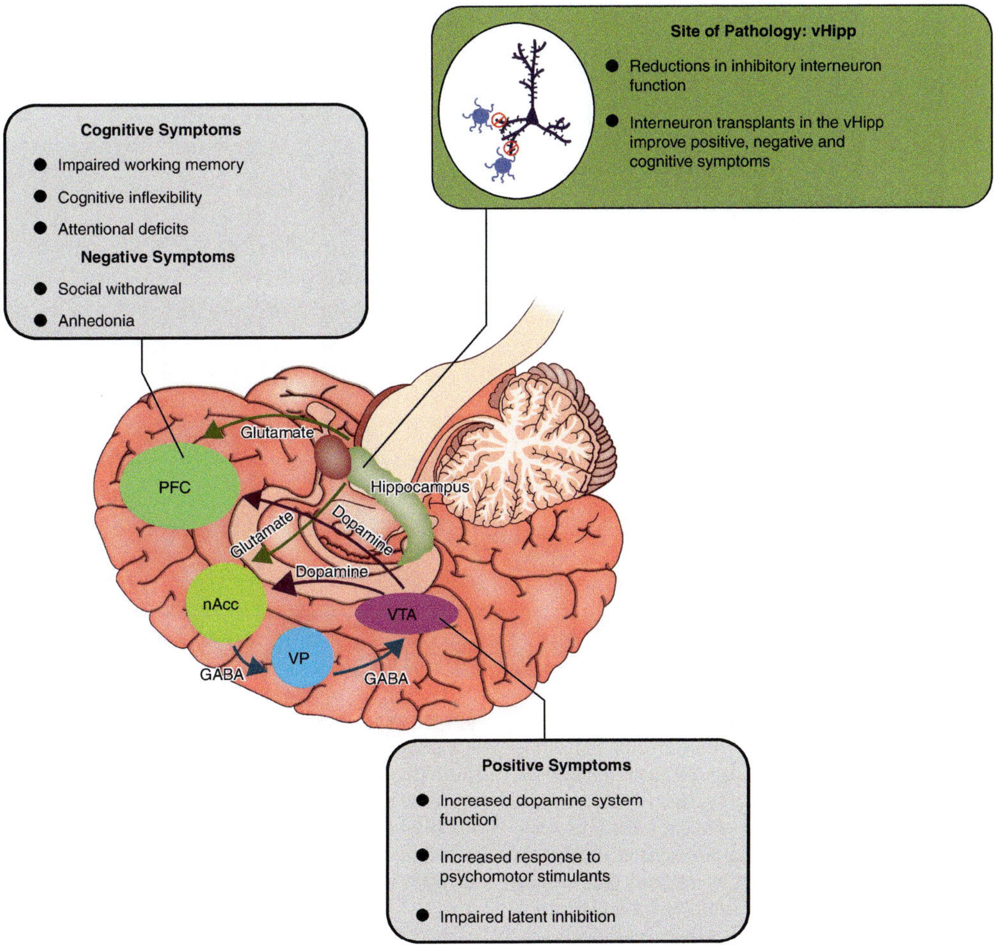

Fig. 15.12 The psychopathology associated with schizophrenia may be due to dysfunction in upstream brain regions that regulate the dopamine system. In animal models, the ventral hippocampus (vHipp) has been shown to regulate dopamine activity in the ventral tegmental area (VTA) via the nucleus accumbens (nAcc) and ventral pallidum (VP) and ultimately in the prefrontal cortex (PFC). Activation of the vHipp by a glutamate agonist can cause positive symptoms through activation of dopamine neurons in the ventral tegmental area. Inhibition of the nAcc by a glutamate antagonist causes the release of inhibitory GABAergic projections to the VP. Negative symptoms may be caused in part by deficits in connectivity between the vHipp and the PHC. Compared to controls, people with schizophrenia exhibit a decrease in hippocampal volume both in postmortem and in imaging studies. (*Adapted from* Donegan and Lodge [27]; *with permission*)

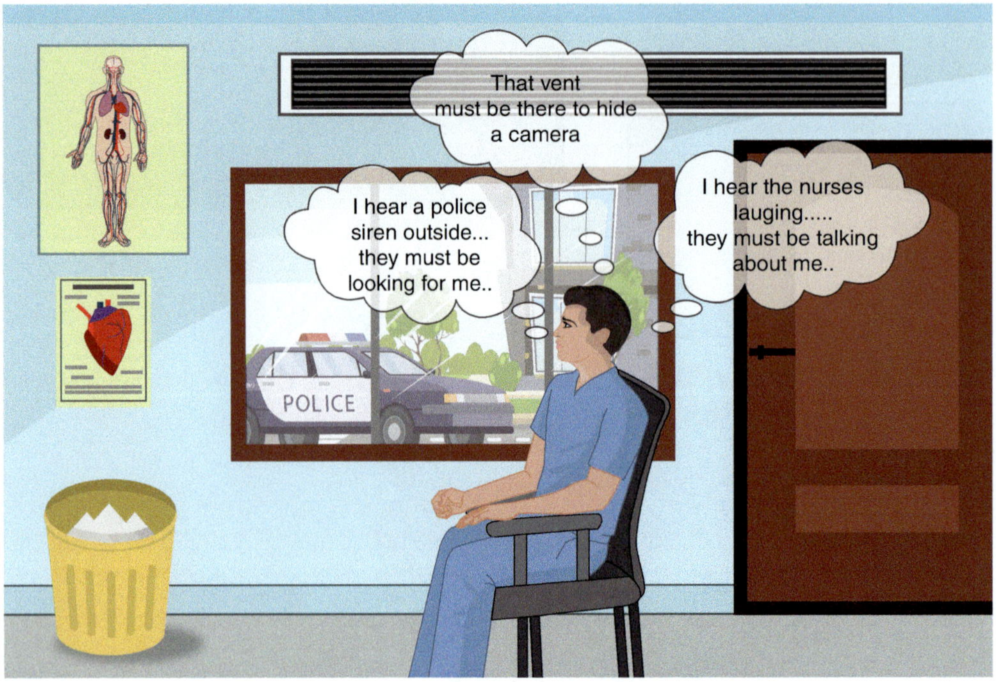

Fig. 15.13 Physiological or emotional disturbances cause anxiety that allows an organism to avoid danger or increase goal-directed behavior, a process mediated through the dopamine system. Research suggests that the dopamine system is hyper-responsive in patients with schizophrenia, thought to be due to dysregulation of afferent structures such as the hippocampus. A hyper-responsive dopamine system leads the individual to assign importance (salience) to minor stimuli that would otherwise be ignored. This condition, in which irrelevant stimuli are not "filtered out," is known as aberrant salience. This illustration shows how a state of aberrant salience may contribute to psychotic symptoms. The individual with schizophrenia experiences sensations—hearing a police siren outside or nurses talking in the hallway, seeing an air-conditioning vent in the wall—that, while objectively neutral, nonetheless seem important to the patient and are therefore interpreted in a way that feels personal and sinister

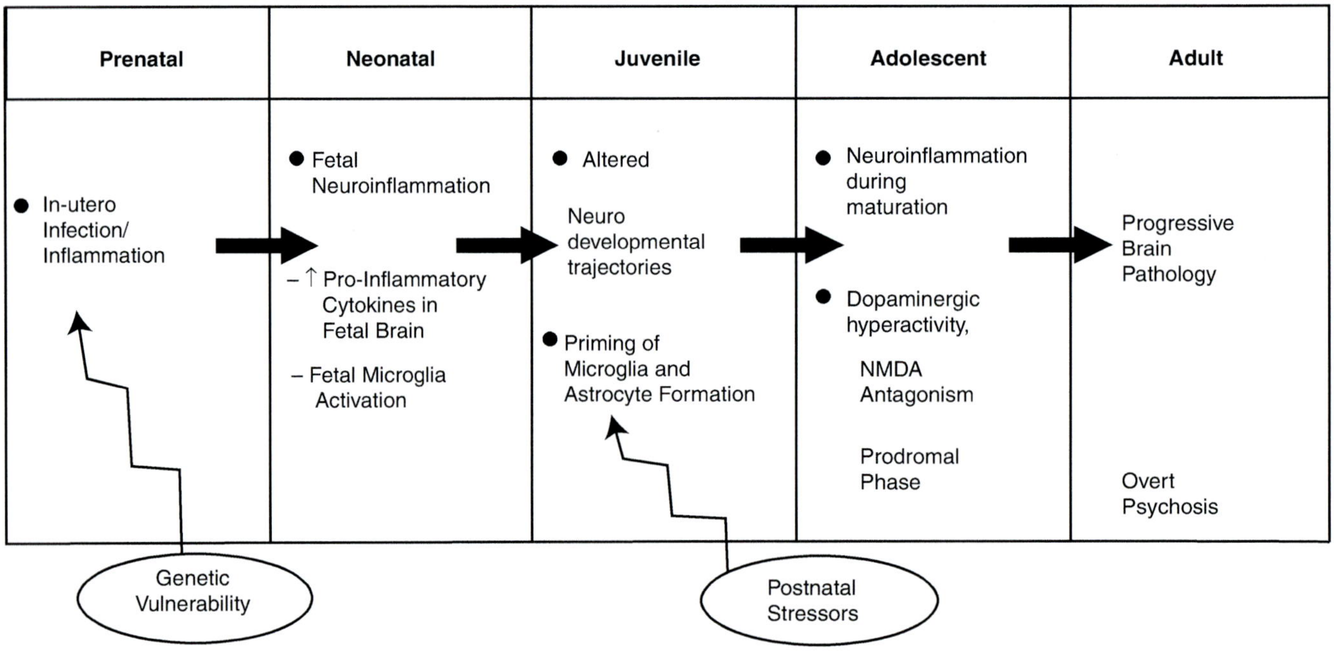

Fig. 15.14 This model conceptualizes how inflammation starting in the prenatal period contributes to the eventual development of psychotic symptoms in adulthood. Certain maternal exposures, including to stressors (such as famine) or illnesses (such as viral syndromes), can cause in-utero inflammation and associated neuropathological changes, including activation of proinflammatory cytokines and microglia. This may be potentiated by a genetic predisposition to psychosis. These changes, possibly in combination with postnatal stressors, including obstetric complications and early childhood trauma, can lead to further alterations in neurodevelopment. Over time, inflammation may cause disturbances in neurotransmission and ultimately contribute to clinically significant psychosis. (*From* Müller [29]; *with permission*)

Phenomenology

Psychosis is a psychological state characterized by a loss of contact with reality. It may be associated with disturbances in thought, perception, cognition, language, and behavior. Common symptoms of psychosis include hallucinations and delusions (defined below). Psychosis appears not only in schizophrenia but in other psychiatric and medical disorders.

The Schizophrenia Phenotype

The symptoms of schizophrenia can be broadly divided into three different domains: cognitive impairment, positive or psychotic symptoms, and negative symptoms (see Table 15.3). Although schizophrenia cannot be diagnosed without a history of psychotic symptoms, different individuals with schizophrenia have different combinations of symptoms. For this reason, there is no singular schizophrenia phenotype.

Table 15.3 Symptoms of psychosis can be loosely organized into positive, negative, and cognitive domains

Positive symptoms	Negative symptoms	Cognitive symptoms
Delusions	Emotional blunting	Short-term memory impairment
Hallucinations	Decreased speech production	Attentional deficits
Disorganized speech	Amotivation	Impairment in executive functioning
Disorganized behaviors	Social isolation	Language deficits

It is important to note that many people have mild psychotic symptoms without overt psychiatric illness. These symptoms exist on a continuum and can be a normal part of human experience. For example, it is common for someone who has experienced the death of a close loved one to hear that person's voice even after they are dead, and many people will relate to the experience of heightened awareness and fear that someone may be following them while walking alone at night in unfamiliar territory. Because of this, when evaluating for psychotic symptoms, it is important to focus on the patient's distress or functional impairment related to his or her symptoms so as not to pathologize normal psychological variance (see Fig. 15.15).

Cognitive Impairment

The first attempts to define schizophrenia as a distinct medical condition began in the late nineteenth century. Psychiatrists Emil Kraepelin and Eugen Bleuler made significant contributions to the field in their descriptions of the schizophrenia phenotype at the beginning of the twentieth century. Both emphasized schizophrenia as primarily a disorder of impaired cognition. Kraepelin referred to the illness as "dementia praecox," implying a dementing illness of early onset. Bleuler was the first to coin the term "schizophrenia," a word which in its Greek roots refers to a "splitting of the mind" [20].

Individuals with schizophrenia frequently have impairments in attention, short-term memory, and executive function. These deficits are considered a core feature of the illness. Cognitive deficits appear years before any other

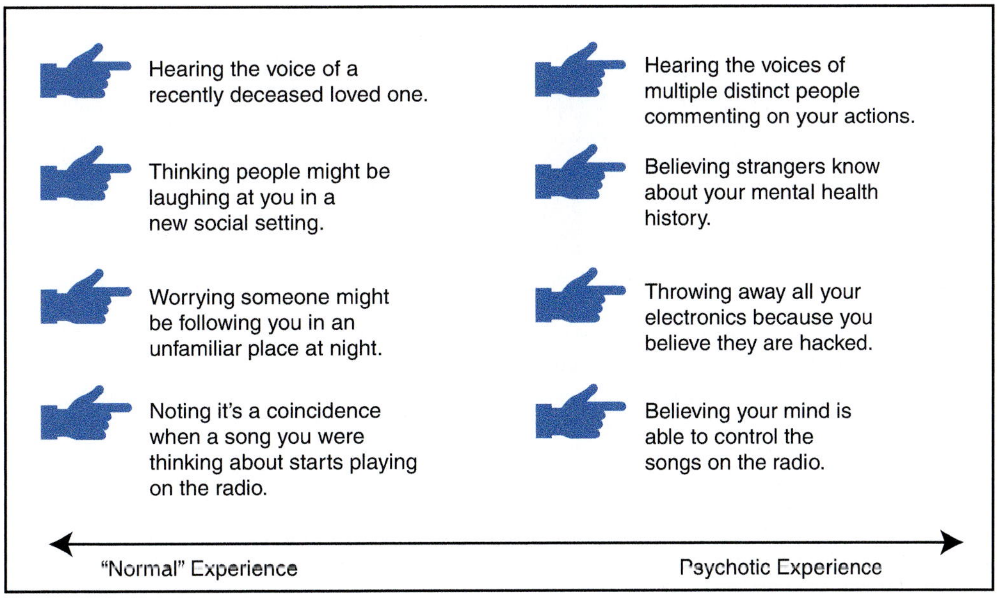

Fig. 15.15 Many, if not most, people have had perceptual abnormalities or mild paranoia considered to be within the realm of "normal" human experience. Above are some examples of these experiences and analogous psychotic symptoms [45]

symptoms and can predict the development of schizophrenia in high-risk individuals. Cognitive deficits worsen just before the onset of psychotic symptoms and are stable throughout the course of the illness, even when psychosis is considered to be in remission. Patients with schizophrenia have demonstrated deficits on almost all neuropsychological tests, performing approximately one to two standard deviations below controls (see Fig. 15.16). Cognitive impairment has been shown to be an important factor in whether or not an individual with schizophrenia is able to return to work or school (see Fig. 15.17) [34].

Schizophrenia patients commonly have impairments in the ability to process social information, referred to as social cognition. These impairments involve skills in detecting basic social cues, such as identifying emotions expressed in faces, and higher level skills involved in mentalizing, such as understanding the thoughts and feelings of others. These impairments are associated with poor community functioning, including the ability to work, succeed in educational activities, and sustain social relationships.

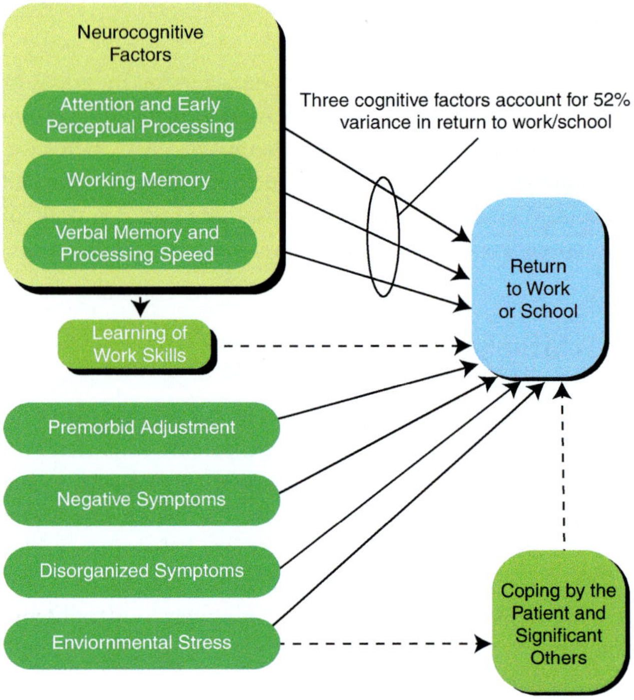

Fig. 15.17 Cognitive performance strongly influenced the functional outcome in one study of patients with first-episode psychosis, with three cognitive factors accounting for 52% of the variance in return to work or school 9 months after illness onset. (*From* Neuchterlein et al. [33]; *with permission*)

Positive Symptoms

Positive symptoms refer to the presence of disorganized speech, disorganized behavior, delusional thought content,

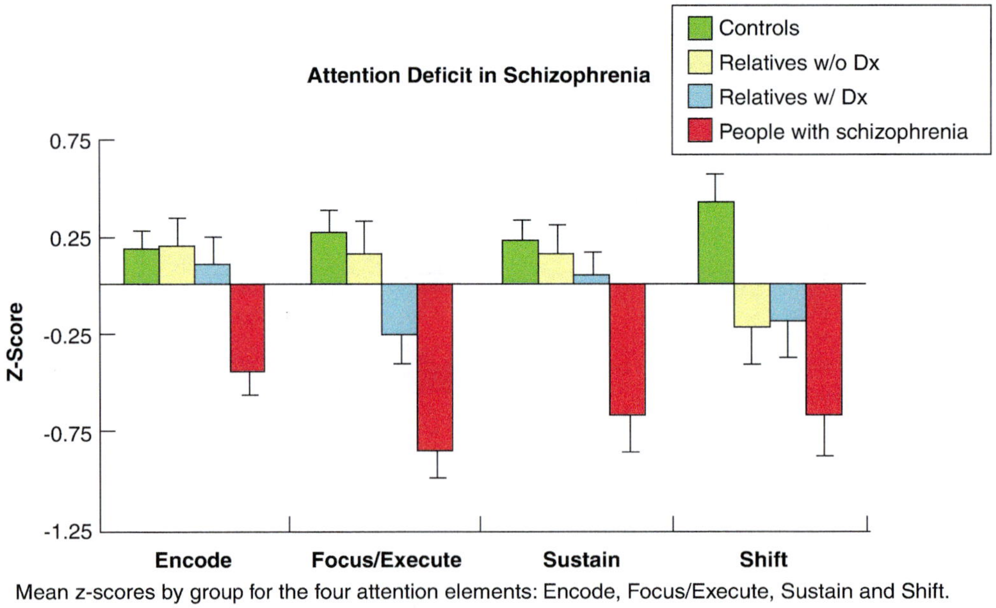

Fig. 15.16 Research has shown that individuals with schizophrenia exhibit impaired cognitive functioning, including attentional deficits. One study examined tests of attention among people with schizophrenia and their first-degree relatives, some with and some without psychiatric illness, as compared to a control sample without schizophrenia. Subjects were administered a battery of eight neuropsychological tests that measured four different elements of attention: encoding information; focusing on stimuli and executing tasks; sustaining focus of attention; and shifting attentional focus. Subjects with schizophrenia had the lowest test scores, while control subjects had the highest test scores and family members of those with schizophrenia had intermediate test scores. Evidence of schizophrenia's strong genetic basis is demonstrated through studies, such as this one, that reveal psychopathology not only in individuals with schizophrenia but in their nonaffected blood relatives as well [32]

or perceptual abnormalities, particularly auditory or visual hallucinations.

Delusions: Delusions are fixed, false beliefs that do not change despite evidence that they are untrue. Most common in schizophrenia are persecutory delusions, wherein an individual believes herself to be personally targeted by other people, groups of people, or entities such as the government. Ideas of reference, another common form of delusion, involve the belief that certain things in the environment (for example, a particular billboard, sound, or model of car) appear for some reason that is specific and meaningful to the individual. Grandiose delusions involve the belief that the individual has particular talents or powers that she does not actually have, while erotomanic delusions involve an individual's belief that someone, usually a person of fame or power, is in love with him. A person with nihilistic delusions believes that she does not exist or that the world does not exist. Somatic delusions involve the belief that the body is not functioning properly (for example, that the intestines are no longer working to move food through the body).

Some delusions involve a breakdown of boundaries between self and non-self, leading the individual to believe that he is being controlled by outside forces. This type of delusion may include thought insertion, the idea that thoughts are being placed in the mind by an external entity; thought withdrawal, the belief that thoughts are being removed from the mind; or delusions of control, the belief that the body or mind are being manipulated. Nonbizarre delusions are those that could plausibly occur in reality (i.e., the police are tracking my movements), while bizarre delusions could not plausibly occur (i.e., the police have inserted a microchip into my brain) [35].

Hallucinations: Hallucinations are experiences in perception that occur without a reality-based stimulus. In schizophrenia, these can occur in any sensory modality (sight, hearing, touch, smell, and taste), though auditory hallucinations are the most common. Auditory hallucinations can consist of the sound of bells, whistles, tones, thumps, whispers, or discernible voices that, for example, comment on the person's actions or tell her to do things she does not want to do (see Table 15.4). Visual hallucinations most commonly consist of seeing shapes, lights, or shadow-like figures out of the corner of one's eye. Fully formed people or animals are relatively uncommon visual hallucinations that might indicate the presence of a neurological, rather than psychiatric, disturbance.

Disorganization of thought and speech: People with schizophrenia frequently experience disorganization of thought content, which manifests outwardly as disorganized speech. This can include tangentiality, or moving from one topic to another closely-related topic; loosening of associations, or moving from one topic to another that is seemingly unrelated; or word salad, an incomprehensible jumble of words and phrases (see Fig. 15.18).

Disorganized or abnormal motor behavior: Disorganization of behavior, which can be viewed as a parallel to disorganization of thought content, can include any disturbance in a person's ability to carry out goal-directed behaviors. For example, this could manifest as generalized agitation, pacing, or inability to properly feed or clothe oneself (see Fig. 15.19).

Table 15.4 Characterizing voices

Origin:
Voices are experienced as originating from inside the mind
Voices are experienced as originating externally
Number of voices:
One voice
Multiple voices
Characterization:
Male voices
Female voices
Voices of people who are known to the patient
Voices of strangers
Quality of voices:
Loud
Soft
Mumbling
Whispering
Content:
Commanding the patient to do things or not to do things
Commenting on the patient's actions
Remarking kindly on the patient, including telling the patient she has special powers
Remarking negatively on the patient

No two people hear the same kinds of voices. This table lists some qualities of auditory hallucinations. Of note, auditory hallucinations may consist of sounds such as tones, whistles, bells, and thumps in addition to, or instead of, the sound of voices

Negative Symptoms

The term "negative symptoms" refers to the emotional, volitional, and social withdrawal that commonly occurs among individuals with schizophrenia. Negative symptoms may be characterized by two categories: diminished expressiveness including a decrease in emotional expression, gestures, and speech; and diminished motivation, including apathy, a lack of goal-directed behavior, and decreased social interest. Negative symptoms are responsible for a large portion of the impairments in functioning associated with schizophrenia [35].

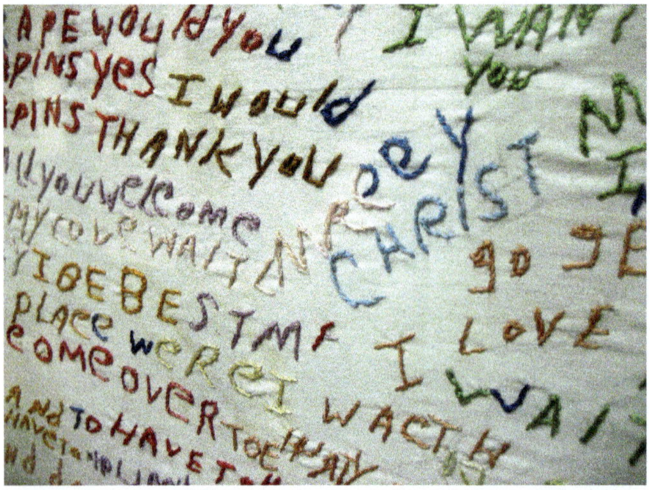

Fig. 15.18 Disorganization of thought is demonstrated by the confusing and unintelligible jumble of phrases and words embroidered onto this cloth by a person with schizophrenia. Both verbal and written language can show evidence of the so-called "word salad." The overall lack of coherent structure of the cloth's design may also be indicative of impairment in executive functioning, including difficulty with planning complex tasks. (*From* Wikimedia Commons; https://commons.wikimedia.org/wiki/File:Cloth_embroidered_by_a_schizophrenia_sufferer.jpg; Creative Commons Attribution 2.0 Generic license; https://creativecommons.org/licenses/by/2.0/deed.en)

Diagnostic Criteria for Schizophrenia Spectrum and Other Psychotic Disorders

Schizotypal (Personality) Disorder: Schizotypal disorder is a personality disorder characterized by discomfort with or reduced need for close interpersonal relationships. Schizotypal individuals are often mistrustful of others' intentions, misinterpreting neutral stimuli as personally directed. They may be superstitious, fixated on the supernatural, or believe that they have special powers, such as the ability to read minds or predict the future. Perceptual abnormalities may be present. People with schizotypal disorder are often eccentrically dressed and may exhibit odd mannerisms that do not fit social norms, and they may be unable to read common social cues. Speech may be odd, though not overtly disorganized. Social interactions are generally anxiety-producing, and schizotypal individuals often have few or no close friends (see Table 15.5) [37].

Delusional Disorder: A person with delusional disorder experiences a well-circumscribed and fixed delusion for a period of time greater than 1 month. Although the person's actions may change to accommodate or respond to the delusional belief, general psychosocial functioning remains relatively intact. The content of the delusion may be somatic,

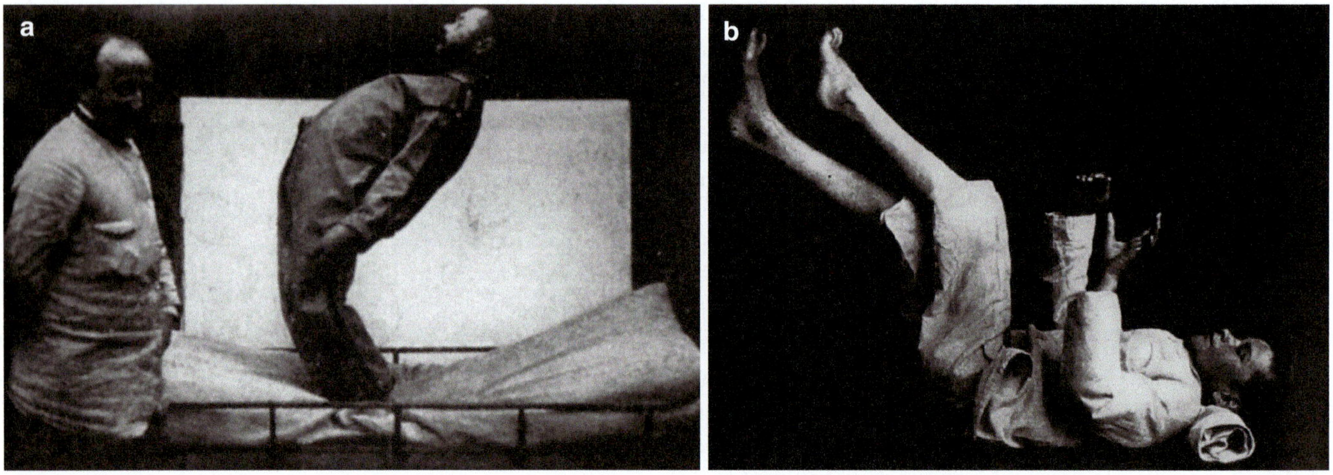

Fig. 15.19 Catatonia is a syndrome characterized by psychomotor abnormalities. It can occur in conjunction with a large variety of medical, neurological, and psychiatric disorders, including schizophrenia. Catatonia may involve several of the following: mutism, decreased spontaneous movement or stupor, muscular rigidity, resistance to movement, echolalia (repetition of another's words), and echopraxia (repetition of another's movements). If left untreated, catatonia may progress to abnormalities in blood pressure and temperature, and eventually coma and death. The rapid recognition and treatment of catatonia are essential. Catatonia was more commonly seen in schizophrenia prior to the development of antipsychotic medications. In (**a**), a photograph from the 1920s, shows a patient with catatonic rigidity. In (**b**), a man with catatonia can be seen demonstrating "waxy flexibility," a motor disturbance in which a person's limbs or other body parts demonstrate a mild and consistent resistance to repositioning, as if bending warm candle wax. Once repositioned, a person with waxy flexibility will generally maintain the new position [36]

Table 15.5 DSM-5 diagnostic criteria for schizotypal personality disorder

A.	A pervasive pattern of detachment from social relationships and a restricted range of expression of emotions in interpersonal settings, beginning by early adulthood and present in a variety of contexts, as indicated by four (or more) of the following:
	1. Neither desires nor enjoys close relationships, including being part of a family
	2. Almost always chooses solitary activities
	3. Has little, if any, interest in having sexual experiences with another person
	4. Takes pleasure in few, if any, activities
	5. Lacks close friends or confidants other than first-degree relatives
	6. Appears indifferent to the praise or criticism of others
	7. Shows emotional coldness, detachment, or flattened affectivity
B.	Does not occur exclusively during the course of schizophrenia, a bipolar disorder or depressive disorder with psychotic features, another psychotic disorder, or autism spectrum disorder and is not attributable to the physiological effects of another medical condition

Table 15.6 DSM-5 diagnostic criteria for delusional disorder

A.	The presence of one (or more) delusions with a duration of 1 month or longer
B.	Criterion A for schizophrenia has never been met
C.	Apart from the impact of the delusion(s) or its ramifications, functioning is not markedly impaired, and behavior is not obviously bizarre or odd
D.	If manic or depressive episodes have occurred, these have been brief relative to the duration of the delusional episode
E.	The disturbance is not attributable to the physiological effects of a substance or another medical condition and is not better explained by another mental disorder, such as body dysmorphic disorder or obsessive-compulsive disorder

persecutory, erotomanic, jealous, or grandiose. When not discussing the delusional belief, the individual may have no significant appreciable impairment. Disorganization of speech and behavior, negative symptoms, and hallucinations are not present (see Table 15.6) [35].

Brief Psychotic Episode, Schizophreniform Disorder, Schizophrenia, and Schizoaffective Disorder: A brief psychotic episode is a psychotic experience lasting greater than 1 day but less than 1 month. Brief psychotic episodes are characterized by the presence of delusions, hallucinations, and disorganization of speech and/or behavior. Although the episode may be severely impairing and might require psychiatric hospitalization, individuals will return to normal functioning following the episode (see Table 15.7) [35].

Schizophreniform disorder is a psychotic illness lasting between 1 and 6 months. It may include some or all of the features of a brief psychotic episode, plus the presence of negative symptoms. A person who experiences a psychotic episode of greater than 6 months' duration is considered to have schizophrenia. In addition to the presence of psychotic symptoms, the individual must have experienced a significant decline in one or more major functional areas, such as occupational, academic, or interpersonal (see Table 15.8). Schizoaffective disorder is diagnosed when a person with symptoms of schizophrenia also experiences a concurrent mood episode (either major depression or mania), though

Table 15.7 DSM-5 diagnostic criteria for brief psychotic episode

A.	Presence of one (or more) of the following symptoms. At least one must be (1), (2), or (3):
	1. Delusions
	2. Hallucinations
	3. Disorganized speech
	4. Grossly disorganized or catatonic behavior
B.	Duration of the episode is at least 1 day but less than 1 month, with eventual full return to premorbid level of functioning
C.	The disturbance is not better explained by major depressive or bipolar disorder with psychotic features or another psychotic disorder such as schizophrenia, and is not attributable to the physiological effects of a substance or another medical condition

Table 15.8 DSM-5 diagnostic criteria for schizophrenia

A.	Two (or more) of the following, each present for a significant portion of time during a 1-month period. At least one of these must be (1), (2), or (3):
	1. Delusions
	2. Hallucinations
	3. Disorganized speech
	4. Grossly disorganized or catatonic behavior
	5. Negative symptoms
B.	For a significant portion of the time since the onset of the disturbance, level of functioning in one or more major areas, such as work, interpersonal relations, or self-care, is markedly below the level achieved prior to the onset (or when the onset is in childhood or adolescence, there is failure to achieve expected level of interpersonal, academic, or occupational functioning)
C.	Continuous signs of the disturbance persist for at least 6 months. This 6-month period must include at least 1 month of symptoms (or less if successfully treated) that meet Criterion A (i.e., active-phase symptoms) and may include periods of prodromal or residual symptoms. During these prodromal or residual periods, the signs of the disturbance may be manifested by only negative symptoms or by two or more symptoms listed in Criterion A present in an attenuated form (e.g., odd beliefs, unusual perceptual experiences)
D.	Schizoaffective disorder and depressive or bipolar disorder with psychotic features have been ruled out because either (1) no major depressive or manic episodes have occurred concurrently with the active-phase symptoms or (2) if mood episodes have occurred during active-phase symptoms, they have been present for a minority of the total duration of the active and residual periods of the illness
E.	The disturbance is not attributable to the physiological effects of a substance (e.g., a drug of abuse, a medication) or another medical condition
F.	If there is a history of autism spectrum disorder or a communication disorder of childhood onset, the additional diagnosis of schizophrenia is made only if prominent delusions or hallucinations, in addition to the other required symptoms of schizophrenia, are also present for at least 1 month (or less if successfully treated)

Table 15.9 DSM-5 diagnostic criteria for schizoaffective disorder

A.	An uninterrupted period of illness during which there is a major mood episode (major depressive or manic) concurrent with Criterion A of schizophrenia
B.	Delusions or hallucinations for 2 or more weeks in the absence of a major mood episode (depressive or manic) during the lifetime duration of the illness
C.	Symptoms that meet criteria for a major mood episode are present for the majority of the total duration of the active and residual portions of the illness
D.	The disturbance is not attributable to the effects of a substance (e.g., a drug of abuse, a medication) or another medical condition
E.	Specify whether bipolar type (mania is part of the presentation; major depressive episodes may also occur) or depressive type (only major depressive episodes are part of the presentation)

Table 15.10 Medications that may cause psychosis [38]

Anticholinergics
Dopaminergic drugs
Interferon
Stimulants
Corticosteroids
Antiarrhythmics and digitalis
Anesthetics
Antimalaria drugs
Antituberculosis drugs
Antibiotics (ciprofloxacin)
Antivirals (HIV medications)
Antineoplastics
Sympathomimetics

with psychotic symptoms predominating throughout the course of the illness and present even when mood symptoms are absent (see Table 15.9) [35].

Substance- or Medication-Induced Psychotic Disorder: Many substances will produce psychotic symptoms, particularly hallucinations and delusional thought content, during or directly following ingestion, sometimes lasting as long as several weeks. A person is said to have a substance-induced psychotic disorder when these symptoms are severe enough to cause functional impairment. Methamphetamine, cocaine, and other illicit drugs are well known to cause psychosis. Some prescribed medications, including corticosteroids and antiparkinsonian drugs, can also precipitate psychotic symptoms, as can withdrawal from alcohol or benzodiazepines (see Table 15.10) [35].

Psychotic Disorder Due to a Medical Condition: Psychosis due to a medical condition occurs when a patient has prominent delusions and/or hallucinations with evidence that the psychological disturbance is due to a nonpsychiatric medical condition. Derangements in many different body systems can cause psychotic symptoms, though endocrine and autoimmune disorders, as well as epilepsy, are particularly implicated (see Table 15.11) [35].

Table 15.11 Medical conditions that may cause psychosis [38]

Parkinson's disease
Alzheimer's dementia
Hypoglycemia
Multiple sclerosis
Cushing's syndrome
Hyperthyroidism
Delirium (from any cause)
Syphilis
HIV/AIDS
Brain masses
Epilepsy
Huntington's disease
Prion diseases

Treatment

Pharmacotherapy: Antipsychotics

Antipsychotic medications are the mainstay of treatment for psychotic disorders. The first antipsychotic, chlorpromazine, was synthesized in 1950 as a potential anesthetic agent. Due to its sedative properties, it was initially marketed as a tranquilizer and was used nonspecifically to treat an array of neuropsychiatric illnesses. It was not until the 1970s that dopamine receptors were identified, and the efficacy of antipsychotic medications was then linked with their dopamine receptor-blocking properties. The antipsychotics that have been developed in subsequent decades have incorporated the essential properties of the earliest antipsychotics [39].

All of the current antipsychotic medications are antagonists at dopamine D2 receptors. With the exception of clozapine and quetiapine, their potency is related to their affinity for these receptors. Antipsychotics also act on a variety of additional receptors, including histamine H1, serotonin 5-HT2, and muscarinic M1 receptors. Some newer antipsychotics have a reduced affinity for dopamine D2 receptors and in some cases are partial dopamine D2 agonists [39].

All antipsychotic medications are significantly more effective than placebo for reducing psychotic symptoms in acute schizophrenia, with effect sizes in the medium range, similar to those seen in medications used to treat nonpsychiatric medical conditions including hypertension and type 2 diabetes (see Fig. 15.20). Compared to patients with multiple prior episodes, patients in their first episode of psychosis generally require lower doses of medication. Although approximately 15.–20% of patients with a single psychotic episode will not go on to have another one, it is not possible to predict with certainty which patients will have a subsequent episode and which will not. For this reason, it is generally recommended that patients continue antipsychotic medications for at least 1 year after a first episode and for at least

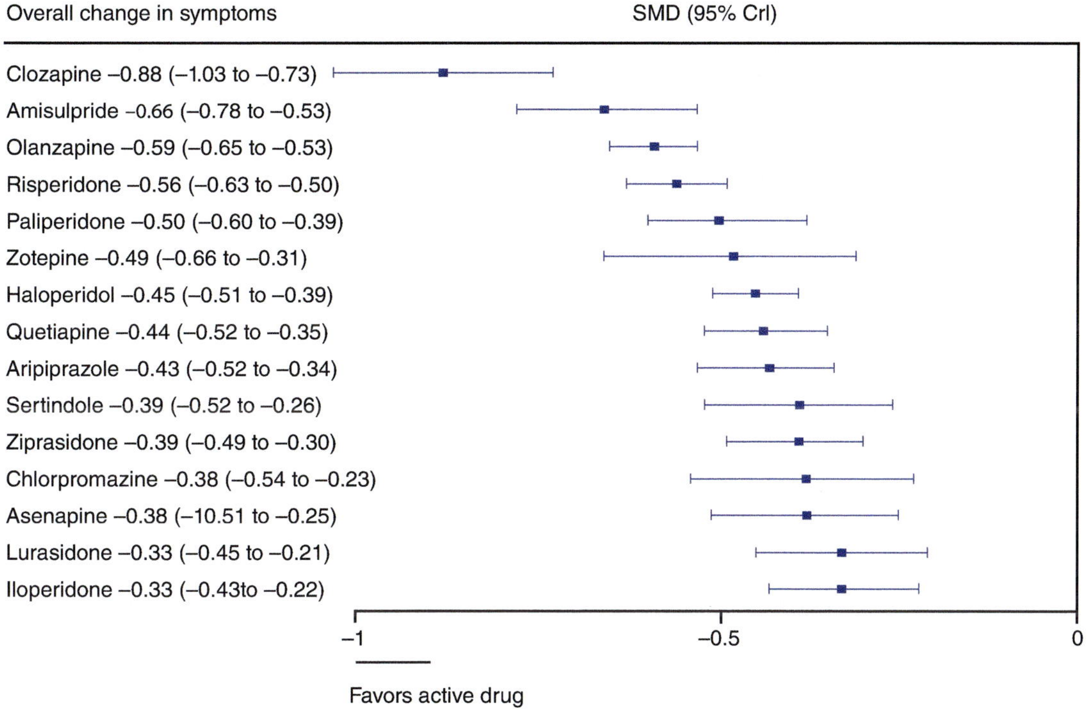

Fig. 15.20 Results from a meta-analysis comparing 15 antipsychotic medications and placebo in the acute treatment of schizophrenia. All medications studied were more effective than placebo. Clozapine was significantly more effective than all other medications. Generally, a standardized mean difference of −0.2 is small, −0.5 is medium, and −0.8 is large; the range of mean effect sizes for these drugs was −0.33 to −0.88. *SMD* standardized mean difference; *CrI* credible interval. (*From* Leucht et al. [40]; *with permission*)

Table 15.12 Factors that may impact a person's decision to take antipsychotic medication

Level of insight into illness
Family and cultural beliefs about mental illness
Quality of the patient–doctor relationship
Level of distress and functional impairment caused by the illness
Access to medical care, including ability to pay for medication
Side effect profile of the medication

5 years after subsequent episodes; however, patients with particularly severe illnesses, including those at high risk for violence against self or others, may be advised to continue medications indefinitely. The early discontinuation of antipsychotics after acute treatment is linked to an increased risk of symptom recurrence, hospitalization, and suicide [41, 42].

Because delays in treating psychosis are associated with poorer outcomes, all patients with psychotic symptoms that are causing distress or functional impairment should be offered treatment with antipsychotic medication (see Table 15.12). To establish effectiveness, the medication should be continued at a therapeutic dose for a period of approximately 4–6 weeks (see Table 15.13). However, if there is no evidence of improvement after 2 weeks, it is unlikely that the patient will improve if the medication is continued. If the medication is ineffective, medication nonadherence and illicit drug use should be explored as potential confounders. Efficacy is similar among all antipsychotics with the exception of clozapine, an antipsychotic that exceeds others in overall effectiveness. Clozapine is indicated for patients who have less than optimal responses to other antipsychotics. Although about 50–60% of treatment-resistant patients will respond to clozapine, it also has a number of serious side effects including agranulocytosis, which necessitates regular monitoring of white count [41, 42].

Table 15.13 Some commonly used antipsychotics with typical dosing ranges

Antipsychotic	Typical dosing range	Long-acting depot form available
Chlorpromazine	200–800 mg/day	No
Haloperidol	5–10 mg/day	Yes
Clozapine	200–600 mg/day	No
Quetiapine	200–800 mg/day	No
Risperidone	2–6 mg/day	Yes
Olanzapine	5–30 mg/day	Yes
Ziprasidone	40–160 mg/day	No
Abilify	5–20 mg/day	Yes
Lurasidone	40–120 mg/day	No

All antipsychotic medications are available in pill form for oral administration. Some medications can be administered intramuscularly for use in situations where emergent behavioral control is needed for patients who are unable or unwilling to accept oral medications. In addition, several antipsychotic medications are available in a long-acting depot injection. These medications, which are injected into the muscle at intervals between 2 and 8 weeks, are useful for patients who have difficulty remembering to take medications on a daily basis.

Side Effects

Antipsychotics cause a wide variety of side effects related to their impact on multiple pathways of neurotransmission. Many of these side effects are very unpleasant for patients and are a major barrier to treatment adherence (see Fig. 15.21).

Metabolic syndrome, the triad of obesity (particularly abdominal obesity), hypertension, and hypercholesterolemia, is a common side effect of many antipsychotic medications. Clozapine is among the most likely to cause weight gain, with over 50% of those who take clozapine gaining at least 10% of their baseline weight. Antipsychotics can also lead to insulin resistance and for some patients, type 2 diabetes. Due to the risk of metabolic syndrome and type 2 diabetes, all patients starting an antipsychotic medication should have regular monitoring of blood glucose, lipid panel, weight (including abdominal circumference), and blood pressure [42, 43].

Extrapyramidal symptoms (EPS) are another common side effect of antipsychotic medications. These side effects are thought to arise from the blockade of dopamine D2 receptors in the mesolimbic and mesocortical pathways. Several symptoms fall under the umbrella of EPS. Pseudoparkinsonism manifests as resting tremor, rigidity, masked facies, psychomotor retardation, emotional blunting, and anhedonia. Akathisia is a subjective feeling of physical restlessness and difficulty sitting still, sometimes coupled with anxiety, that can be very distressing for patients and may even lead to suicidality if not treated. Acute dystonias are involuntary, painful muscle contractions, especially of the head and neck, and are associated with first-generation antipsychotics and the intramuscular route of administration. Lastly, tardive dyskinesia (TD) is a disorder that causes uncontrollable, repetitive movements, generally of the lips, tongue, and hands. TD is often irreversible (see Fig. 15.22 and Table 15.14) [43].

Antipsychotics sometimes cause other side effects that can negatively impact a patient's quality of life. Many antipsychotics cause constipation, sedation, and orthostatic hypotension. Hyperprolactinemia can cause gynecomastia in men; galactorrhea, menstrual cycle dysfunction, and decreased bone density in women; and sexual dysfunction and infertility in both sexes. Antipsychotics generally lower the seizure threshold and can precipitate seizures in those who are predisposed or who overdose (see Table 15.15).

Nonpharmacological Management of Thought Disorders

While antipsychotic medications are the mainstay of treatment for psychotic disorders, they are often only partially effective, leaving patients with residual symptoms that are chronically present and distressing. In addition, the so-called negative symptoms of psychosis, including social withdrawal and emotional blunting, significantly limit psychosocial functioning and often make it very difficult for people with psychotic illnesses to maintain relationships and jobs. Nonpharmacological interventions have been developed to help address these lingering impairments, and there are several evidence-based treatments that should be offered as adjunctive treatment to pharmacotherapy (see Fig. 15.23).

Cognitive behavioral therapy (CBT) for psychosis, a form of talk therapy that focuses on recognizing and changing unhelpful thoughts and behaviors, has been proven to reduce the severity of positive symptoms or the distress associated with these symptoms. Patients are asked to identify particular problems or symptoms that are then addressed through therapy, which can be delivered either in individual or group-based format (see Figs. 15.24 and 15.25). Social skills training, which is sometimes combined with CBT, assists patients with improving social interactions by practicing skills such as maintaining appropriate eye contact or making small talk. Family-based therapy provides psychoeducation, emotional support, and training for symptom management for people with psychosis and their immediate support system, and it can reduce the risk of rehospitalization and relapse.

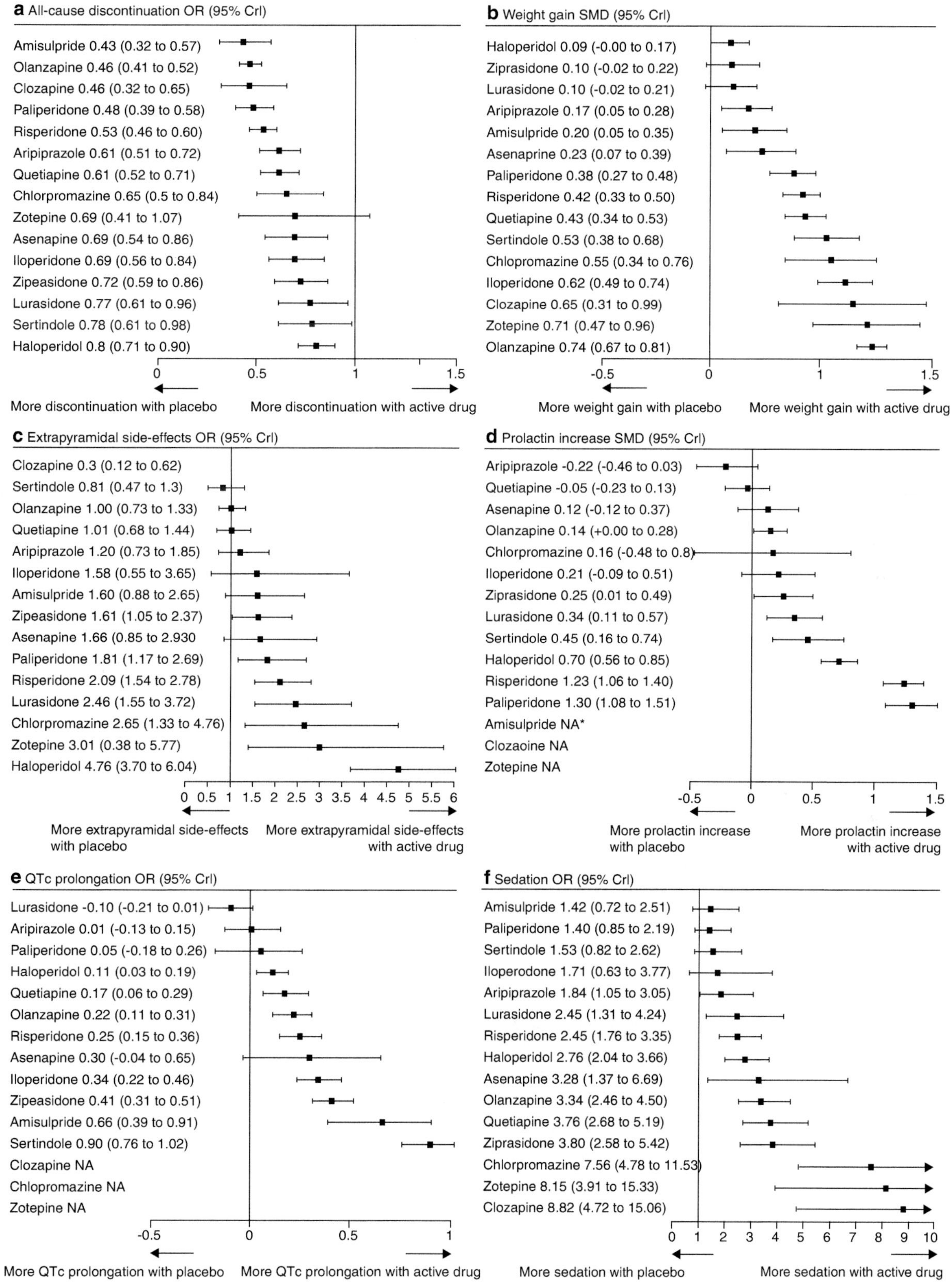

Fig. 15.21 This figure shows discontinuation rates of antipsychotic medications compared to placebo. All medications studied except haloperidol, ziprasidone, and lurasidone caused more weight gain than placebo. Risperidone and paliperidone were associated with the most significant elevation in prolactin level, while clozapine, zotepine, and chlorpromazine were most sedating. Haloperidol was associated with the highest rate of extrapyramidal symptoms. *OR* odds ratio; *CrI* credible interval; *SMD* standardized mean difference. (*From* Leucht et al. [40]; *with permission*)

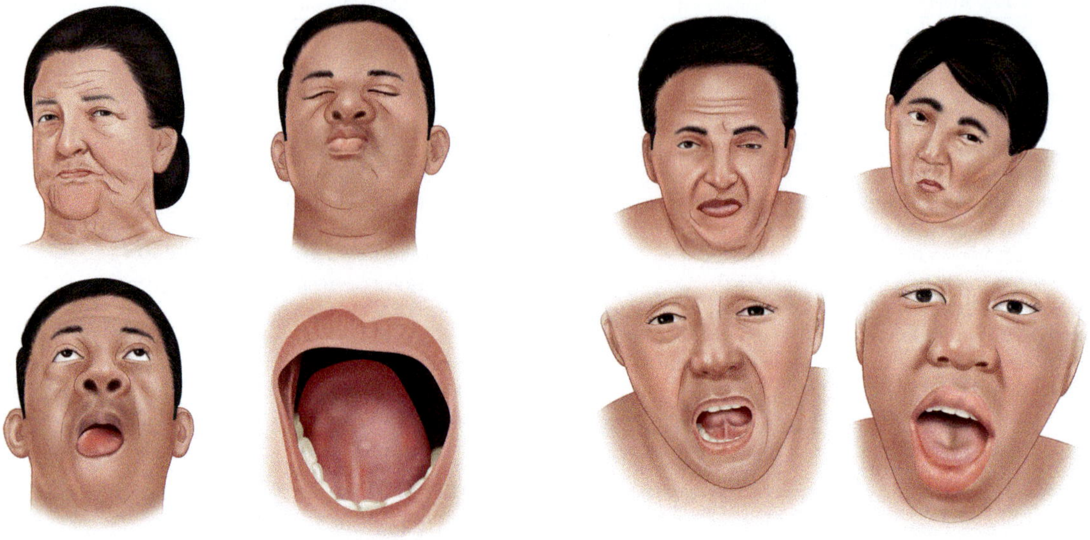

Fig. 15.22 Tardive dyskinesia (TD) is a movement disorder characterized by repetitive, involuntary muscle movements. TD commonly affects the mouth and face, causing grimacing, lip-smacking, or intermittent tongue protrusion. TD may also cause writhing movements of the fingers or jerking of the extremities. These movements can be disfiguring and can impair daily functioning. The risk of developing TD is highest within the first 5 years of treatment with antipsychotic medications, and older adults are more susceptible. TD may be permanent though it can be treated with pharmacotherapy

Table 15.14 Brief clinical assessment of movement disorders for patients on antipsychotic medication

Side effect and examination procedure
Akathisia
Observe for restless movements
Ask about difficulty sitting still and subjective need to pace
Rigidity and tremor
Observe for spontaneous movements and tremor
Examine for cogwheeling
Observe arm swing and gait while patient is walking
Tardive dyskinesia
Observe abnormal face and extremity movements while patient is sitting still with feet flat and again while patient is distracted with alternating thumb and finger tapping
Observe truncal, pelvic, and arm/hand movements while patient is walking

Monitoring guidelines recommend a complete examination for tardive dyskinesia (TD) and other abnormal movements at least every 6–12 months, depending on the medication prescribed and patient risk factors. The 12-item Abnormal Involuntary Movement Scale (AIMS) is a clinician-rated scale that is considered the standard for TD evaluation, though it may not be feasible for completion in a high-volume outpatient practice. Above is an alternative examination that can be completed in under 3 min

Supported employment services should be offered to provide assistance in finding and keeping employment, while assertive community treatment provides a multidisciplinary team to provide wraparound services and outreach to patients in the community in order to prevent rehospitalization or homelessness (see Fig. 15.26) [48].

Table 15.15 Sample monitoring schedule for patients taking antipsychotic medications [44]

	Baseline	During titration	At 3 months	Quarterly	Every 6 months	Annually
Weight	X	X		X		
Tardive dyskinesia	X	X			X	
Parkinsonism, akathisia	X	X				X
Glucose metabolism (fasting blood sugar, HbA1c)	X		X			X
Lipid metabolism (fasting lipids)	X		X			X
Heart rate	X	X	X			X
Sexual function	X	X				X
Sedation		X				
EKG (based on history and symptoms)	X					
Prolactin	If symptoms of hyperprolactinemia develop (galactorrhea, reduced frequency of menses, gynecomastia)					

Adapted from Stroup and Gray [45]; *with permission*

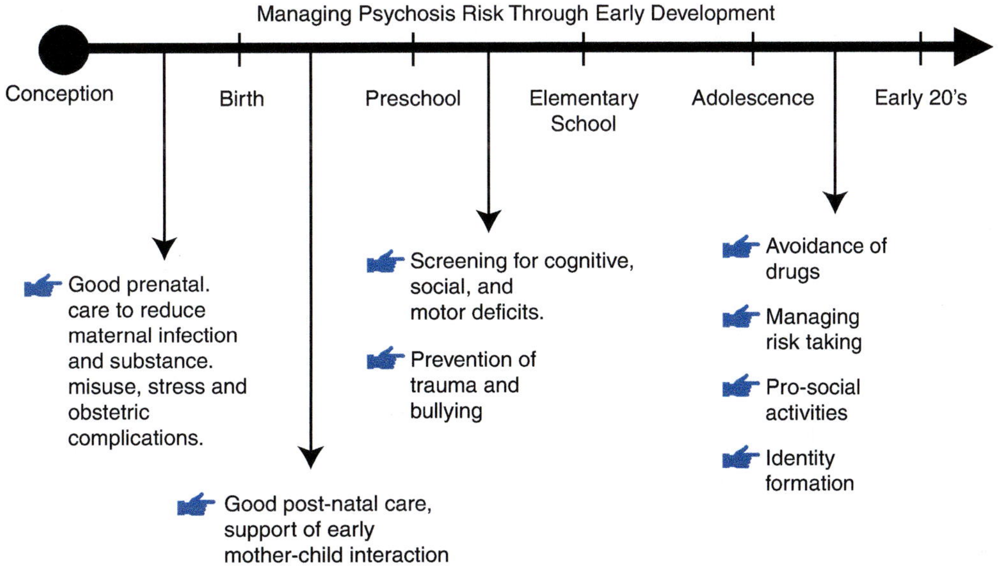

Fig. 15.23 Genetic predisposition, gene–environment interactions, stress, and risk and protective factors all play a role in determining the onset and severity of schizophrenia. The term "clinical high risk" is used to refer to individuals who exhibit prodromal, or sub-threshold, psychotic symptoms, some of whom go on to develop schizophrenia and some of whom do not. Cognitive abnormalities, for example, can manifest years before symptoms such as paranoia or hallucinations, and children who later develop schizophrenia may show evidence of socio-emotional, cognitive, neuromotor, and speech-language impairment. Early detection of prodromal symptoms allows for interventions that may delay the onset of a psychotic disorder or otherwise minimize the severity of the illness. These interventions can begin at conception, with access to high-quality prenatal care, and extend through early adulthood. (*From* Seidman and Mirsky [46]; *with permission*)

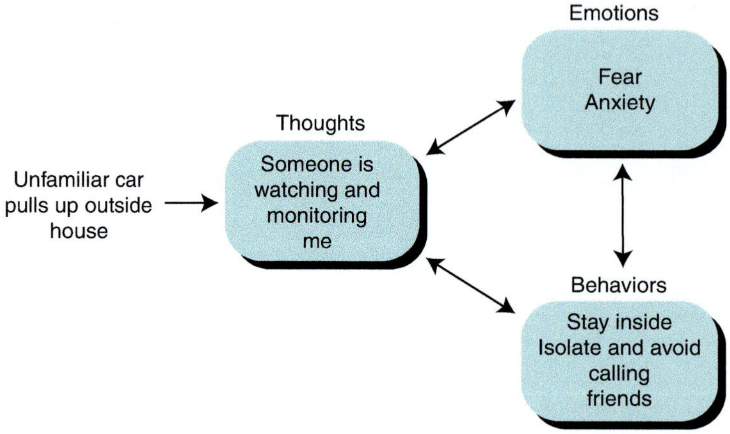

Fig. 15.24 Cognitive behavioral therapy (CBT) is a form of talk therapy that focuses on understanding how thoughts, behaviors, and emotions are linked, with the goal of recognizing and changing unhelpful patterns. Although first developed to target anxiety and depression, CBT can be applied to psychotic disorders as well. In the example above, a CBT framework is used to understand how assumptions about an objectively neutral stimulus (in this case, an unfamiliar car parked in front of the house) lead to paranoid thoughts, fear, and isolation. A CBT-focused therapist would assist the patient in coming up with alternative thoughts about the car that are less personalized and less malicious, with the goal of promoting more helpful behaviors and more positive emotions

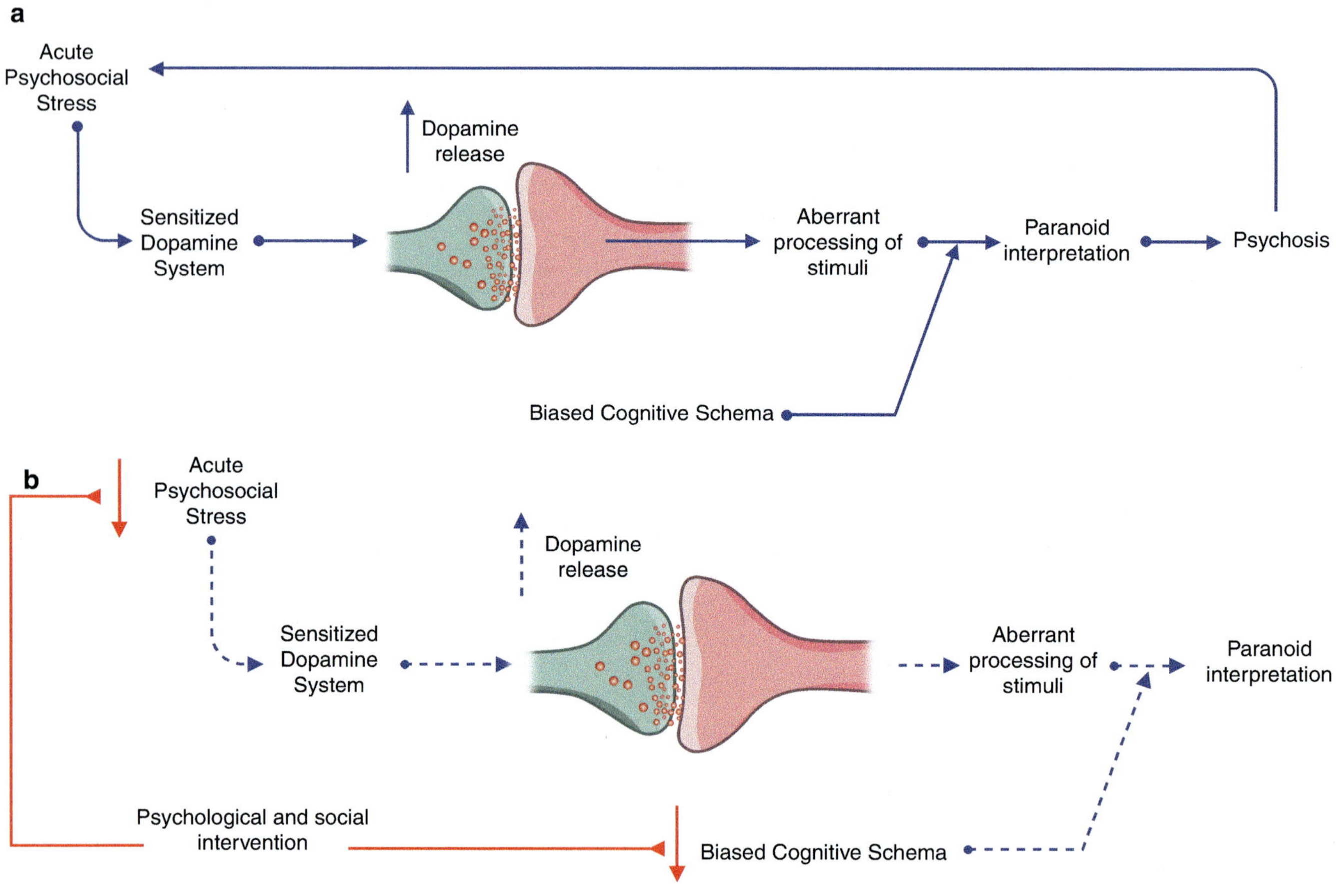

Fig. 15.25 (**a**) In those with schizophrenia, acute stressors and a hyperactive dopamine system contribute to the individual's inability to filter out neutral stimuli, a condition known as aberrant salience. Biased cognitive schema, such as a fundamental belief that the world is a dangerous place, then cause the individual to interpret the neutral stimuli in a personalized and malicious way. (*From* Howes and Murray [47]; *with permission.*) (**b**) Points in the process that can be revised through psychosocial interventions. Interventions such as family therapy or housing services can assist in reducing acute stressors, while cognitive therapy can help modify biased cognitive schema so that interpretations are less personal and more benign

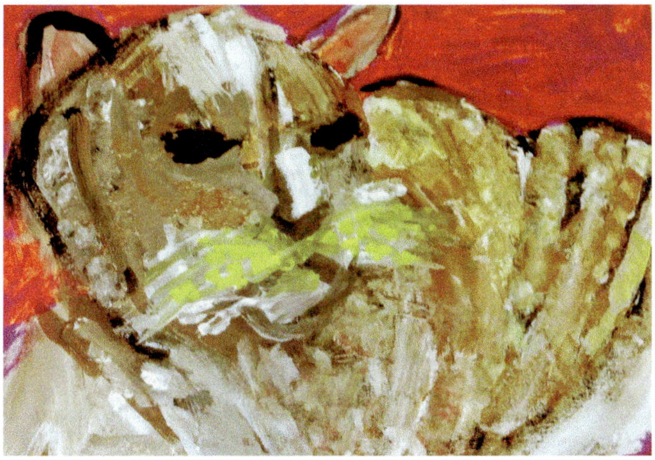

Fig. 15.26 This is a painting created by a man with schizophrenia who was undergoing integrated day treatment that consisted of group-based CBT and social skills training as well as individual visits with a psychiatrist for medication management. This individual was particularly interested in painting, which he considered to be an important creative outlet

References

1. Chong HY, Teoh SL, Wu DB, Kotirum S, Chiou C-F, Chaiyakunapruk N. Global economic burden of schizophrenia: a systematic review. Neuropsychiatr Dis Treat. 2016;12:357–73.
2. Charlson FJ, Ferrari AJ, Santomauro DF, Dominic S, Stockings E, Scott JG, et al. Global epidemiology and burden of schizophrenia: findings from the Global Burden of Disease Study 2016. Schizophr Bull. 2018;44:1195–203.
3. McGrath J, Saha S, Welham J, El Saadi O, MacCauley C, Chant D. A systematic review of the incidence of schizophrenia: the distribution of rates and the influence of sex, urbanicity, migrant status and methodology. BMC Med. 2004;2:13.
4. Kumra S, Ashtari M, Cervellione KL, Henderson I, Kester H, Roofeh D, et al. White matter abnormalities in early-onset schizophrenia: a voxel-based diffusion tensor imaging study. J Am Acad Child Adolesc Psychiatry. 2005;44:934–41.
5. Naqvi H, Khan MM, Faizi A. Gender differences in age at onset of schizophrenia. J Coll Physicians Surg Pak. 2005;15:345–8.
6. Häfner H, Heiden W, Behrens S, Gattaz WF, Hambrecht M, Löffler W, et al. Causes and consequences of the gender difference in age at onset of schizophrenia. Schizophr Bull. 1998;24:99–113.
7. Olfson M, Gerhard T, Huang C, Crystal S, Stroup TS. Premature mortality among adults with schizophrenia in the United States. JAMA Psychiat. 2015;72:1172–81.
8. McGrath J, Saha S, Chant D, Welham J. Schizophrenia: a concise overview of incidence, prevalence, and mortality. Epidemiol Rev. 2008;30:67–76.
9. Hennekens CH. Increasing global burden of cardiovascular disease in general populations and patients with schizophrenia. J Clin Psychiatry. 2007;64:4–7.
10. Hilker R, Helenius D, Fagerlund B, Skytthe A, Christensen K, Werge TM, et al. Heritability of schizophrenia and schizophrenia spectrum based on the nationwide Danish twin register. Biol Psychiatry. 2018;83:492–8.
11. Schizophrenia Working Group of the Psychiatric Genomics Consortium. Biological insights from 108 schizophrenia-associated genetic loci. Nature. 2014;511:421–7.
12. Stefansson H, Rujescu D, Cichon S, Pietiläinen OPH, Ingason A, Steinberg S, et al. Large recurrent microdeletions associated with schizophrenia. Nature. 2008;455:232–6.
13. Lichtenstein P, Yip BH, Björk C, Pawitan Y, Cannon TD, Sullivan PF, Hultman CM. Common genetic influences for schizophrenia and bipolar disorder: a population-based study of 2 million nuclear families. Lancet. 2009;373:9659.
14. Prata DP, Costa-Neves B, Cosme G, Vassos E. Unravelling the genetic basis of schizophrenia and bipolar disorder with GWAS: a systematic review. J Psychiatr Res. 2019;114:178–207.
15. Clark MC, Harley M, Cannon M. The role of obstetric events in schizophrenia. Schizophr Bull. 2006;32:3–8.
16. Brown AS, Schaefer CA, Wyatt RJ, Begg MD, Goetz R, Bresnahan MA, et al. Paternal age and risk of schizophrenia in adult offspring. Am J Psychiatry. 2002;159:1528–33.
17. Zammit S, Allebeck P, Dalman C, Lundberg I, Hemmingson T, Owen MJ, et al. Paternal age and risk for schizophrenia. Br J Psychiatry. 2003;183:405–8.
18. Kuepper R, van Os J, Lieb R, Wittchen H-U, Höfler M, Henquet C. Continued cannabis use and risk of incidence and persistence of psychotic symptoms: 10 year follow-up cohort study. BMJ. 2011;342:d738.
19. Selten J-P, Cantor-Graae E, Kahn RS. Migration and schizophrenia. Curr Opin Psychiatry. 2007;20:111–5.
20. Andreason NC. Schizophrenia: the fundamental questions. Brain Res Brain Res Rev. 2000;31:106–12.
21. Balu DT. The NMDA receptor and schizophrenia: from pathophysiology to treatment. Adv Pharmacol. 2016;76:351–82.
22. van Erp TGM, Hibar DP, Rasmussen JM, Glahn DC, Pearlson GD, Andreassen OA, et al. Subcortical brain volume abnormalities in 2028 individuals with schizophrenia and 2540 healthy controls via the ENIGMA consortium. Mol Psychiatry. 2016;21:547–53.
23. Guo JY, Huhtaniska S, Miettunen J, Jääskeläinen E, Kiviniemi V, Nikkinen J, et al. Longitudinal regional brain volume loss in schizophrenia: relationship to antipsychotic medication and change in social function. Schizophr Res. 2015;168:297–304.
24. Iritani S. What happens in the brain of schizophrenia patients? An investigation from the viewpoint of neuropathology. Nagoya J Med Sci. 2013;75:11–28.
25. Shenton M, Dickey C, Frumin M, McCarley R. A review of MRI findings in schizophrenia. Schizophr Res. 2001;49:1–52.
26. Brisch R, Saniotis A, Wolf R, Bielau H, Bernstein H-G, Steiner J, et al. The role of dopamine in schizophrenia from a neurobiological and evolutionary perspective: old fashioned, but still in vogue. Front Psych. 2014;5:47.
27. Donegan JJ, Lodge DJ. Cell-based therapies for the treatment of schizophrenia. Brain Res. 2017;1655:262–9.
28. Grace AA. Dysregulation of the dopamine system in the pathophysiology of schizophrenia and depression. Nat Rev Neurosci. 2016;17:524–32.
29. Müller N. Inflammation in schizophrenia: pathogenetic aspects and therapeutic considerations. Schizophr Bull. 2018;44:973–82.
30. Meyer U. Developmental neuroinflammation and schizophrenia. Prog Neuro-Psychoph. 2013;42:20–34.
31. Eaton WW, Byrne M, Ewald H, Mors O, Chen C-Y, Agerbo E, et al. Association of schizophrenia and autoimmune diseases: linkage of Danish national registers. Am J Psychiatry. 2006;163:521–8.
32. Mirsky AF, Yardley SL, Jones BP, Walsh D, Kendler KS. Analysis of the attention deficit in schizophrenia: a study of patients and their relatives in Ireland. J Psychiat Res. 1995;29:23–42.
33. Neuchterlein KH, Subotnik KL, Green MF, Ventura J, Asarnow RF, Gitlin MJ, et al. Neurocognitive predictors of work outcome in recent onset schizophrenia. Schizophr Bull. 2011;37:S33–40.

34. Neuchterlein KH, Ventura J, Subotnik KL, Bartzokis G. The early longitudinal course of cognitive deficits in schizophrenia. J Clin Psychiatry. 2014;75:25–9.
35. American Psychiatric Association. Schizophrenia Spectrum and Other Psychotic Disorders. In: Diagnostic and statistical manual of mental disorders. 5th ed; 2013.
36. Bumke O. Lehrbuch der Geisteskrankheiten. 2nd ed. Munich: Bergmann; 1924.
37. American Psychiatric Association. Personality disorders. In: Diagnostic and statistical manual of mental disorders. 5th ed; 2013.
38. American Psychiatric Association. Chapter 9. Psychosis, mania, and catatonia. In: The American Psychiatric Association publishing textbook of psychosomatic medicine and consult-liaison psychiatry. 3rd ed; 2019.
39. Kapur S, Mamo D. Half a century of antipsychotics and still a central role for dopamine D2 receptors. Prog Neuropsychopharmacol Bio Psychiatry. 2003;27:1081–90.
40. Leucht S, Cipriani A, Spineli L, Mavridis D, Örey D, Richter F, et al. Comparative efficacy and tolerability of 15 antipsychotic drugs in schizophrenia: a multiple-treatments meta-analysis. Lancet. 2013;382:951–62.
41. Haddad PM, Correll CU. The acute efficacy of antipsychotics in schizophrenia: a review of recent meta-analyses. Ther Adv Psychopharmacol. 2018;8:303–18.
42. Lally J, MacCabe JH. Antipsychotic medication in schizophrenia: a review. Br Med Bull. 2015;114:169–79.
43. Shirzadi AA, Ghaemi SN. Side effects of atypical antipsychotics: extrapyramidal symptoms and the metabolic syndrome. Harv Rev Psychiatry. 2006;14:152–64.
44. Bratti IM, Kane JM, Marder SR. Chronic restlessness with antipsychotics. Am J Psychiatry. 2007;164:1648–54.
45. Stroup TS, Gray N. Management of common adverse effects of antipsychotic medications. World Psychiatry. 2018;17:341–56.
46. Seidman LJ, Mirsky AF. Evolving notions of schizophrenia as a developmental neurocognitive disorder. J Int Neuropsychol Soc. 2017;23:881–92.
47. Howes OD, Murray RM. Schizophrenia: an integrated sociodevelopmental-cognitive model. Lancet. 2014;383:1677–87.
48. Dixon LS, Dickerson F, Bellack AS, Bennett M, Dickinson D, Goldberg RW, et al. The 2009 schizophrenia PORT psychosocial treatment recommendations and summary statements. Schizophr Bull. 2010;36:48–70.

Bipolar and Related Disorders

16

Ashley Ngor, Alexander J. Steiner, Sarin Pakhdikian, David Okikawa, Demetria Pizano, Lidia Younan, Samantha Cohen, and Waguih William IsHak

Until recent advancements made just over this past decade, bipolar and related disorders were once multifaceted mental health conditions that lacked comprehensive understanding and standardized diagnoses. While the categorization of these disorders will continue to advance with future research, the most recent Diagnostic and Statistical Manual of Mental Disorders (DSM–V) defines the category of "bipolar and related disorders" as the intermediate form between that of psychotic disorders and depressive disorders [1]. The three main bipolar disorders are bipolar I (BP-1) disorder, bipolar II (BP-2) disorder, and cyclothymic disorder: this category also encompasses substance/medication-induced bipolar and related disorder, bipolar and related disorder due to another medical condition, other specified bipolar and related disorder, and unspecified bipolar and related disorder. This chapter aims to provide an all-encompassing review of the bipolar disorder spectrum through the consideration of epidemiology, etiology, pathophysiology, phenomenology, and treatment interventions.

A. Ngor (✉)
University of California, Los Angeles, Los Angeles, CA, USA
e-mail: angor@g.ucla.edu

A. J. Steiner
Executive Mental Health, Inc., Los Angeles, CA, USA

S. Pakhdikian
Kirk Kerkorian School of Medicine, University of Nevada, Las Vegas, Las Vegas, NV, USA
e-mail: Sarin.pakhdikian@unlv.edu

D. Okikawa
David Geffen School of Medicine, University of California, Los Angeles, Los Angeles, CA, USA
e-mail: DOkikawa@mednet.ucla.edu

D. Pizano
University of Alabama at Birmingham, Birmingham, AL, USA
e-mail: Dpizano@uab.edu

L. Younan
Cedars-Sinai Medical Center, Los Angeles, CA, USA

S. Cohen
Department of Psychiatry and Behavioral Neurosciences, Cedars-Sinai Medical Center, Los Angeles, CA, USA

W. W. IsHak
Cedars-Sinai Health System, Department of Psychiatry and Behavioral Neurosciences, University of California Los Angeles, David Geffen School of Medicine, Los Angeles, CA, USA
e-mail: Waguih.IsHak@cshs.org

Epidemiology

Bipolar and related disorders are considered to be one of the most prevalent mental illnesses worldwide (Fig. 16.1). Lifetime prevalence varies among the three main types of bipolar disorder, with BP-I having a prevalence of 1%, BP-II with a prevalence of 0.4-2%, and cyclothymic disorder with a prevalence of 2.5% [2].

These disorders are ranked 17th out of the 20 leading causes of global burden of disease (GBD), as measured by age-standardized DALYs (disability-adjusted life years) that account for both the years of life lost and years lived with a disability (Fig. 16.2) [2].

Around 1–2% of the general population will experience bipolar and related disorders at some point in their lifetime, with estimates of their lifetime prevalence rates varying from 2.8 to 6.5% [3, 4]. When compared to other mental disorders common in adulthood by the 2013 Global Burden of Disease Study, bipolar disorder was associated with lower prevalence rates than other disorders such as major depressive disorder, dysthymia, and anxiety disorder (Fig. 16.3) [5].

Demographic Considerations (Age, Sex, Race/Ethnicity)

The onset of bipolar disorders is most commonly seen in adolescents and young adults, with early onset usually

W. W. IsHak (ed.), *Atlas of Psychiatry*, https://doi.org/10.1007/978-3-031-15401-0_16

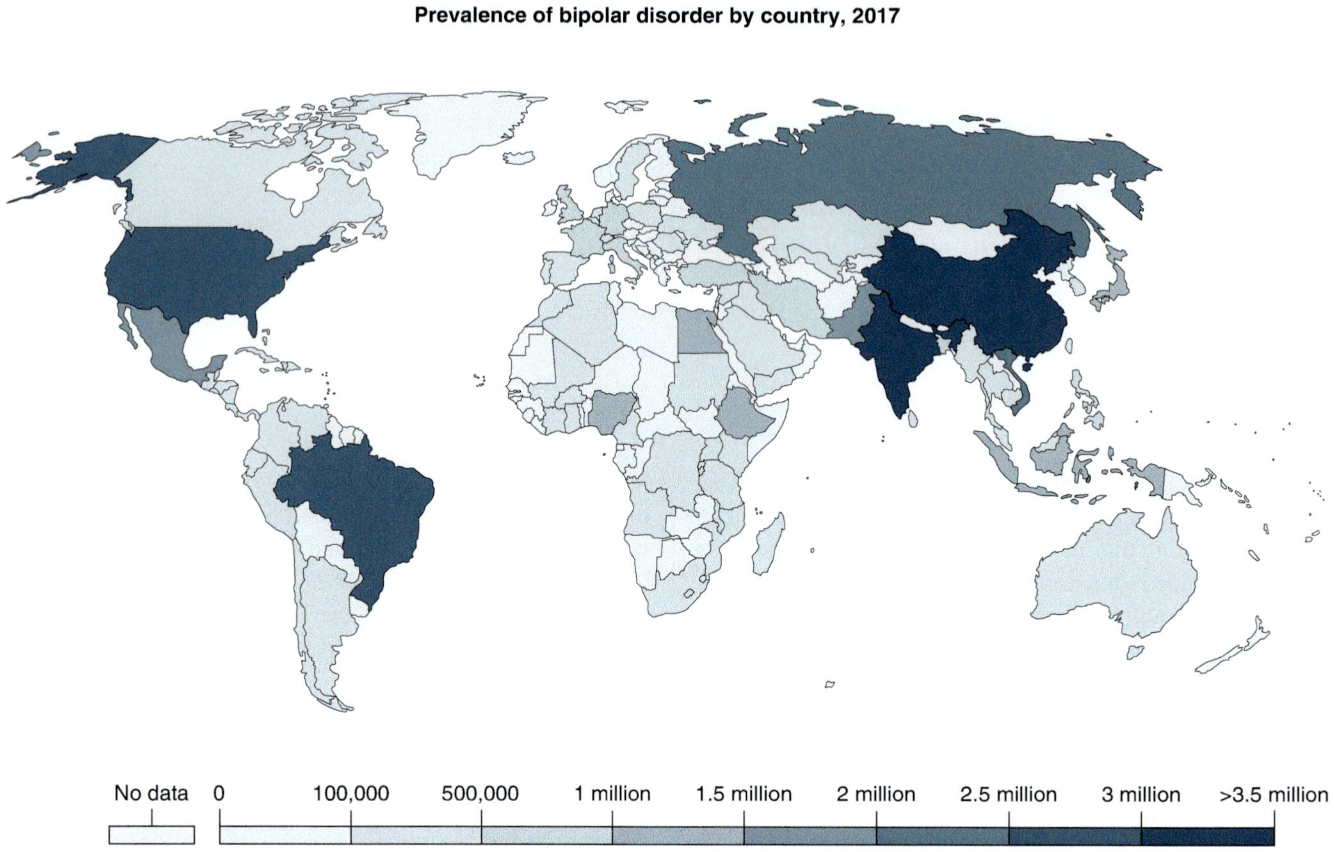

Fig. 16.1 The total number of individuals in 2017 with bipolar disorder across both sexes and all ages based on medical data, epidemiological data, surveys, and meta-regression modeling. (Wikimedia Commons; Creative Commons Attribution 3.0 Unported; https://creativecommons.org/licenses/by/3.0/)

appearing between the ages of 15 and 19 and full onset developing around the age of 20 [3, 6]. According to the Institute for Health Metrics and Evaluation (IHME), the greatest prevalence rates of bipolar disorder by age is seen in the 20- to 24-year-old age group, 15- to 49-year-old age group, and the 25- to 29-year-old age group (Fig. 16.4).

Past studies have shown that the likelihood of developing bipolar or related disorders is equal between females and males; however, recent findings demonstrate a greater proportion of females than males within the overall bipolar spectrum (Figs. 16.5 and 16.6). On a more specific basis, females have shown greater lifetime prevalence of BP-II than their male counterparts, while greater lifetime prevalence of BP-I was seen in males rather than females [7].

Although little research has been conducted in regard to the correlation between race/ethnicity and the bipolar disorder spectrum, Boyd et al. concluded that white mothers had a lower lifetime prevalence rate and 12-month prevalence rate of bipolar disorder than those recorded for African American mothers [8].

Environmental Considerations/Stressors

Environmental considerations in relation to the bipolar spectrum have increasingly become a topic of increasing interest over recent years. Stressful life events, obstetric complications, and physical illness are more likely to occur in the

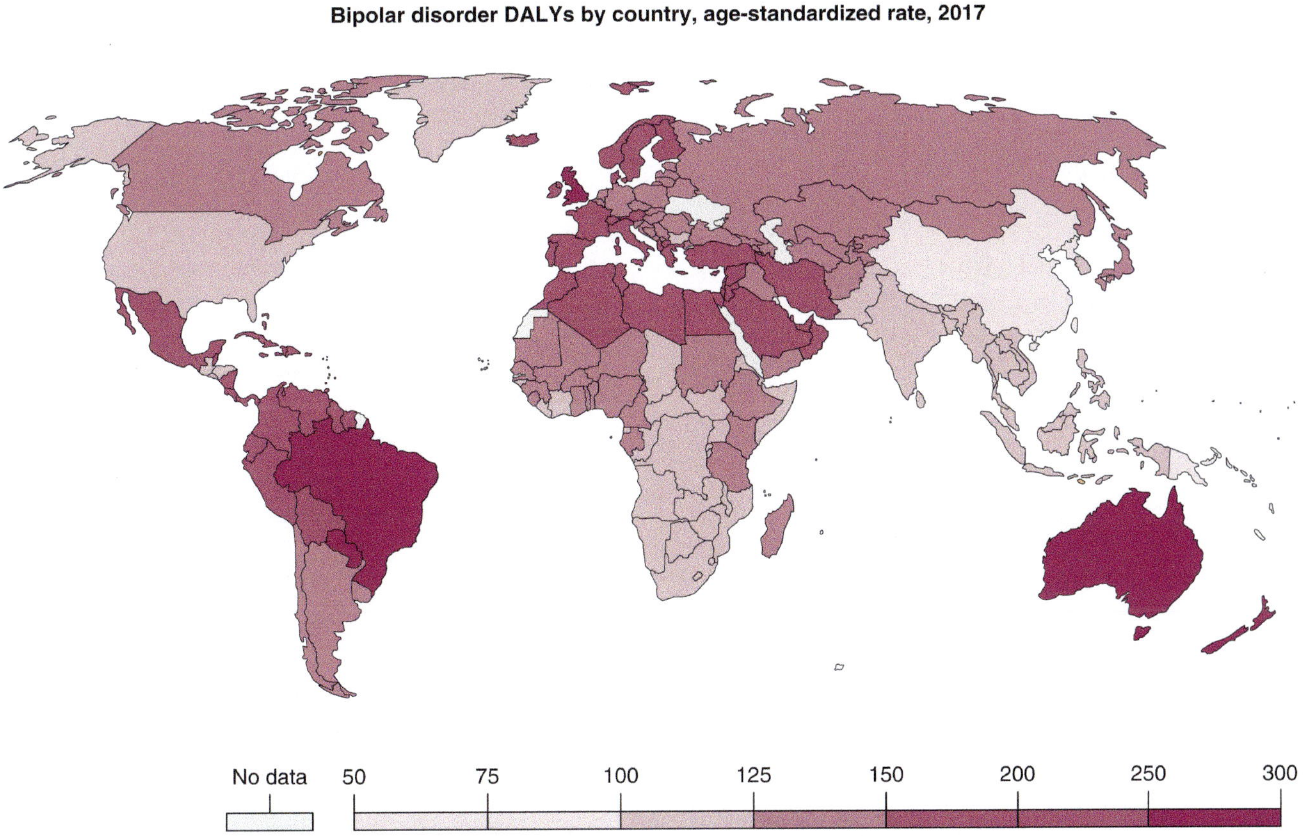

Fig. 16.2 Age-standardized DALYs (disability-adjusted life years) from bipolar disorder per 100,000 individuals. DALYs are used to measure the total burden of disease from both the lost years of life and the years lived with a disability. One DALY equals one lost year of healthy life. (Wikimedia Commons; Creative Commons Attribution 3.0 Unported; https://creativecommons.org/licenses/by/3.0/)

lives of people with bipolar and other related disorders [9, 10]. Bipolar spectrum disorder is more likely to occur in those who have experienced stressors such as a loss of a parent, childhood abuse and neglect, physical abuse, sexual abuse, and economic hardship (Fig. 16.7) [10].

Specific stressors may include altercations with loved ones, alcohol and drug misuse, changes in season, and certain antidepressants and medications [11]. Arguments can arise when the individual is irritable, which could be related to stress from personal and professional influences. The abuse of alcohol and drugs may worsen the underlying illness, not necessarily causing the disorder. Cocaine and amphetamines are known to worsen manic episodes, whereas the withdrawal of these drugs trigger depressive symptoms. When used alone, antidepressants are known to trigger a manic phase. Therefore, it is best to couple antidepressants with mood stabilizers. It is also important to consider the diagnosis of bipolar I versus bipolar II, as antidepressants alone have shown to be beneficial for bipolar II, but strongly discouraged as monotherapy for bipolar I. Mood can fluctuate with changing of the seasons. In the case of bipolar disorder, early winter poses a threat for depression, while mania or hypomania occurs more commonly in the spring or summer [12].

The DSM-5 notes that childbirth can contribute to a hypomanic episode in 10–20% of females within nonclinical settings and postpartum major depressive episodes in 3–6% of females [1]. Females with peripartum onset are likely to experience a change in mood from feelings of elation to that of depression, loss of interest or please, reduced sleep, and irritability (Fig. 16.8).

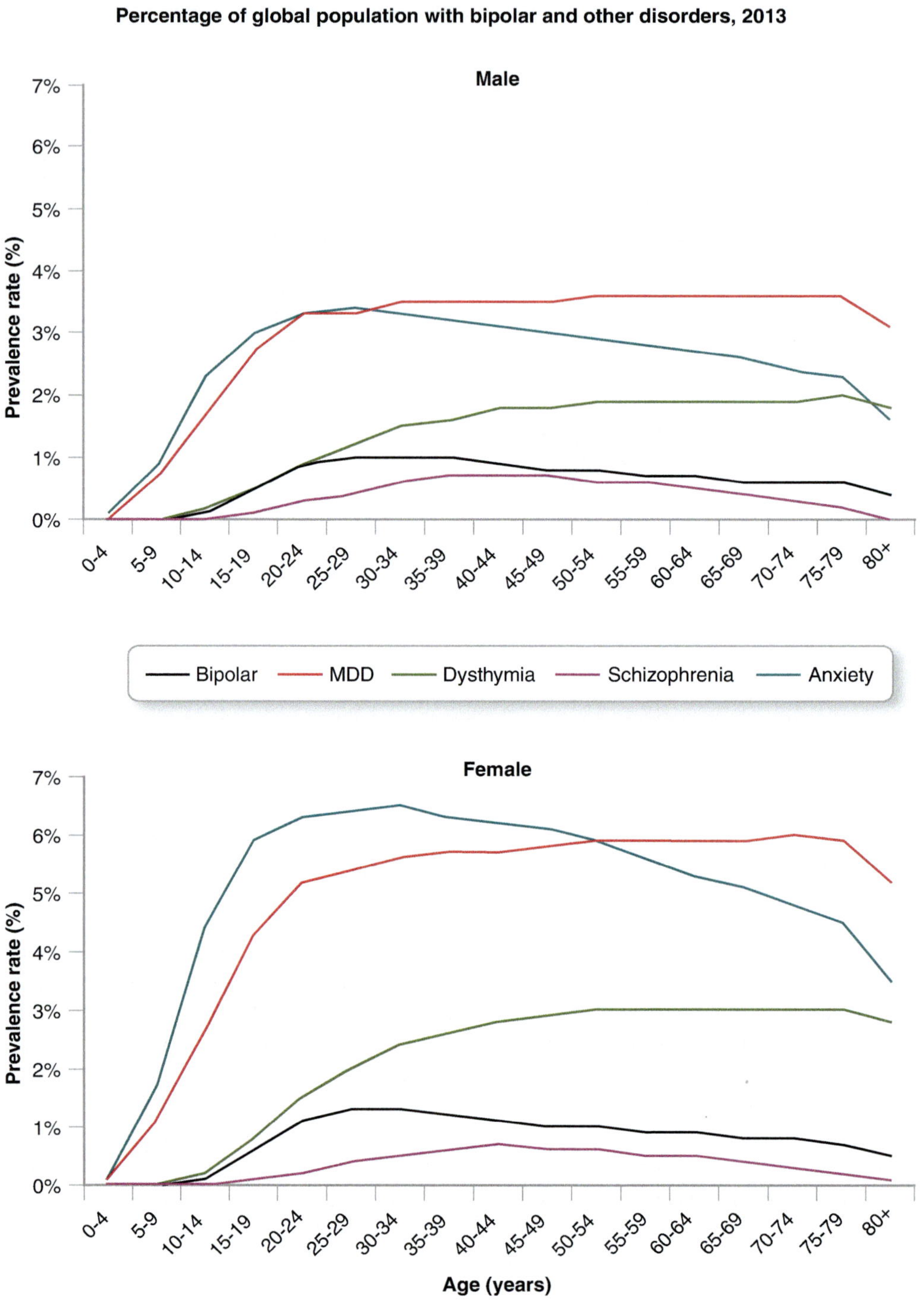

Fig. 16.3 Bipolar disorder prevalence rates in 2013 categorized by age and sex, as compared to other Global Burden of Disease Study 2013 mental disorders common in adulthood. *MDD* major depressive disorder. (Wikimedia Commons; Creative Commons Attribution 3.0 Unported; https://creativecommons.org/licenses/by/3.0/)

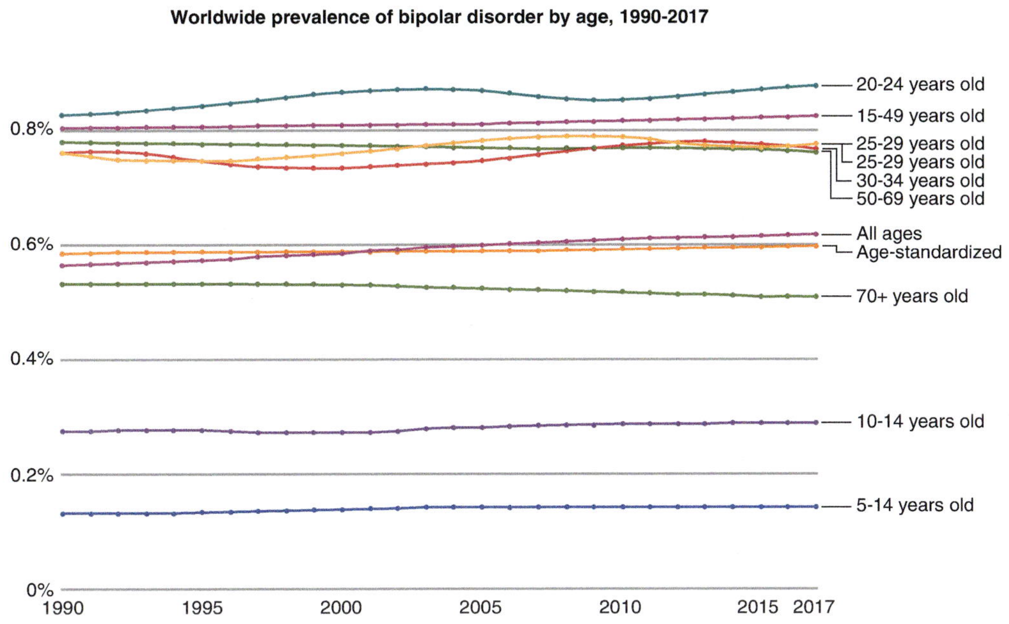

Fig. 16.4 The estimated total number of people worldwide suffering from bipolar disorder, organized by sex and across all ages. Based on medical data, epidemiological data, surveys, and meta-regression modeling. (Wikimedia Commons; Creative Commons Attribution 3.0 Unported; https://creativecommons.org/licenses/by/3.0/)

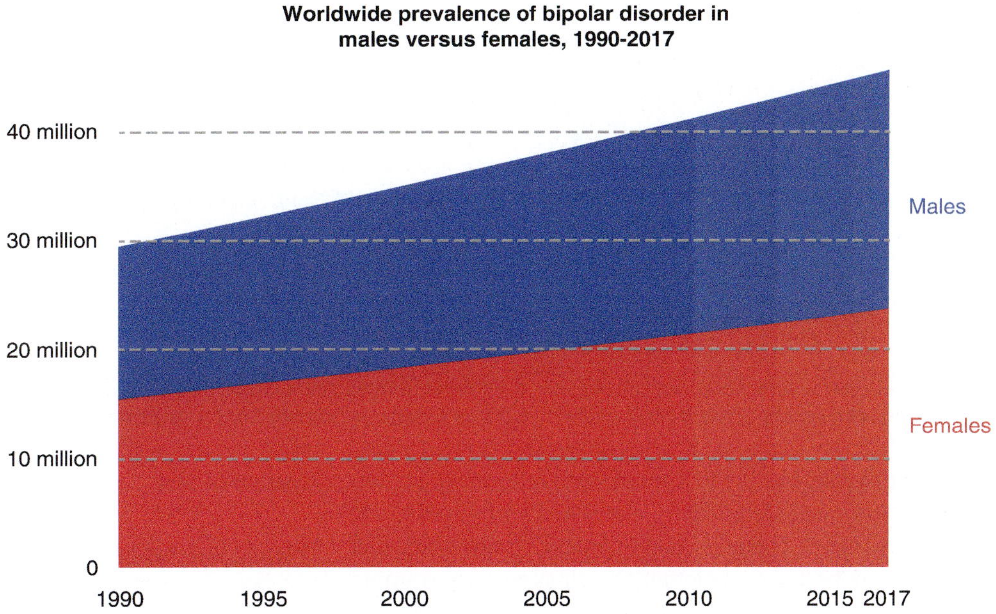

Fig. 16.5 Estimated population suffering from bipolar disorder, organized by different age groups and across both sexes. Based on medical data, epidemiological data, surveys, and meta-regression modeling. (Wikimedia Commons; Creative Commons Attribution 3.0 Unported; https://creativecommons.org/licenses/by/3.0/)

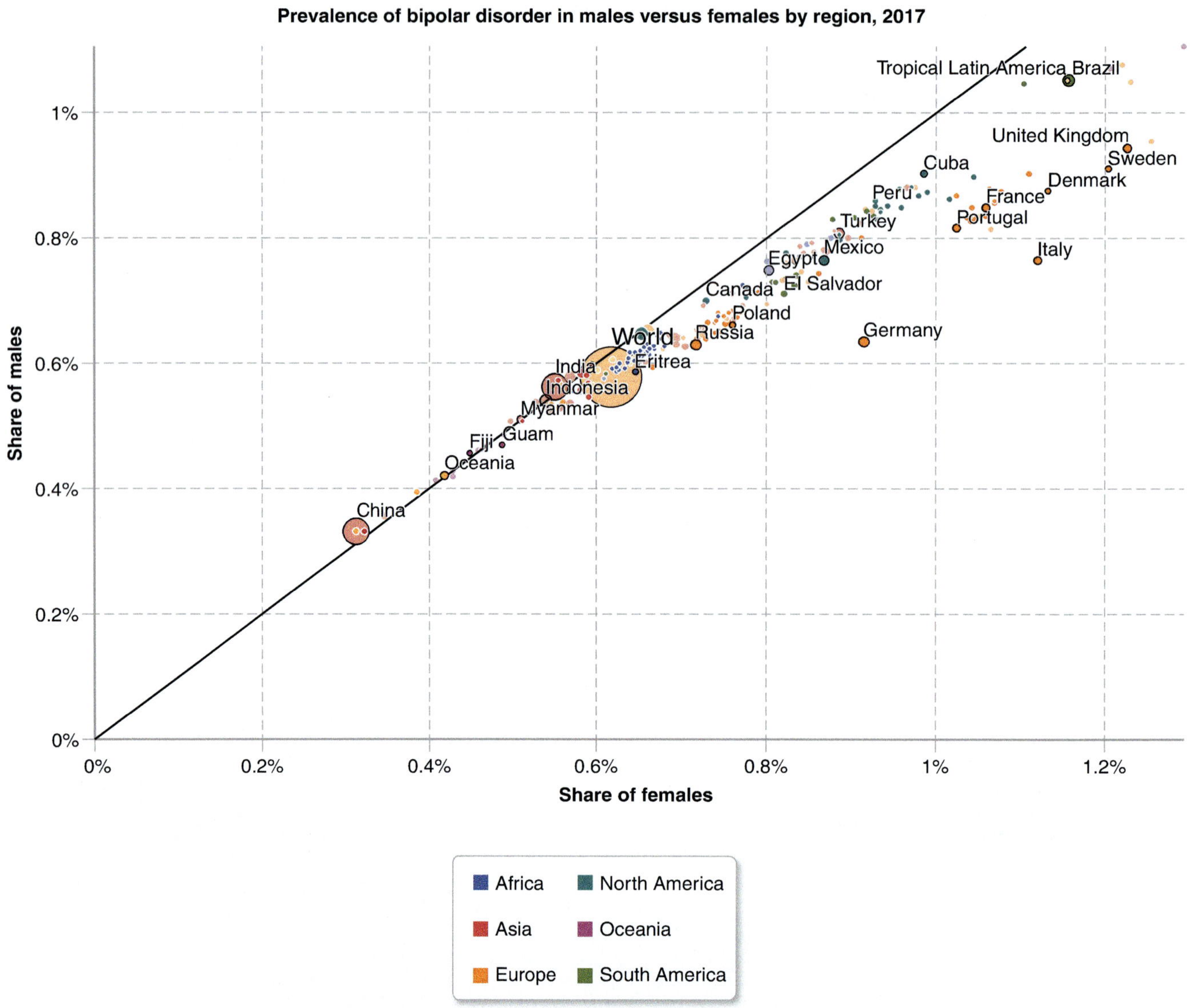

Fig. 16.6 Estimated male versus female population suffering from bipolar disorder. Based on medical data, epidemiological data, surveys, and meta-regression modeling. (Wikimedia Commons; Creative Commons Attribution 3.0 Unported; https://creativecommons.org/licenses/by/3.0/)

Sleep disturbances in the form of varying forms of insomnia have also been significantly correlated with bipolar and related disorders. There is much evidence suggesting that sleep loss can be a core symptom as well as an early warning sign in triggering a mood episode [13]. In a 10-year longitudinal study, difficulties in both falling asleep and waking up early were able to predict the onset of bipolar disorder in individuals (Fig. 16.9) [14].

Comorbidity

Bipolar and related disorders are often accompanied by a number of comorbidities, such as other mental disorders and physical disorders [10]. Those with bipolar disorder and related diseases are likely to have other psychiatric conditions such as anxiety (71% of bipolar population), substance abuse (56%), personality disorders (36%), and attention

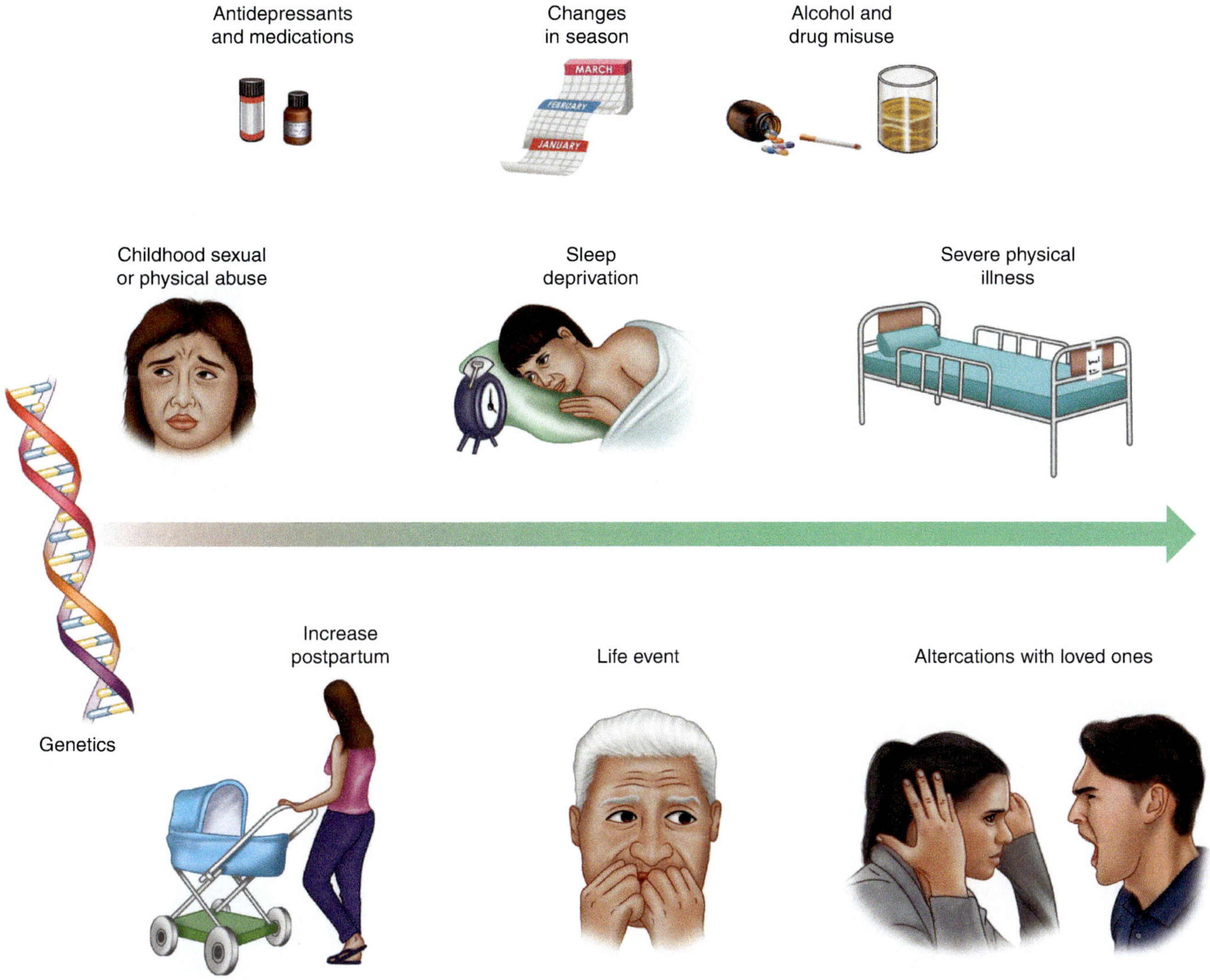

Fig. 16.7 Environmental considerations and bipolar disorder. (*From* Katona et al. [6]; *with permission*)

deficit-hyperactivity disorders (10–20%) [4]. A variety of studies, a few of which are included in Table 16.1, have also concluded that generalized anxiety disorder, phobias, separation anxiety, panic disorders, post-traumatic stress disorder (PTSD), disruptive behavior disorders, conduct disorder, impulsivity, criminal behavior, and attention deficit hyperactivity disorder (ADHD) are comorbidities in bipolar and related disorders [1, 4, 15].

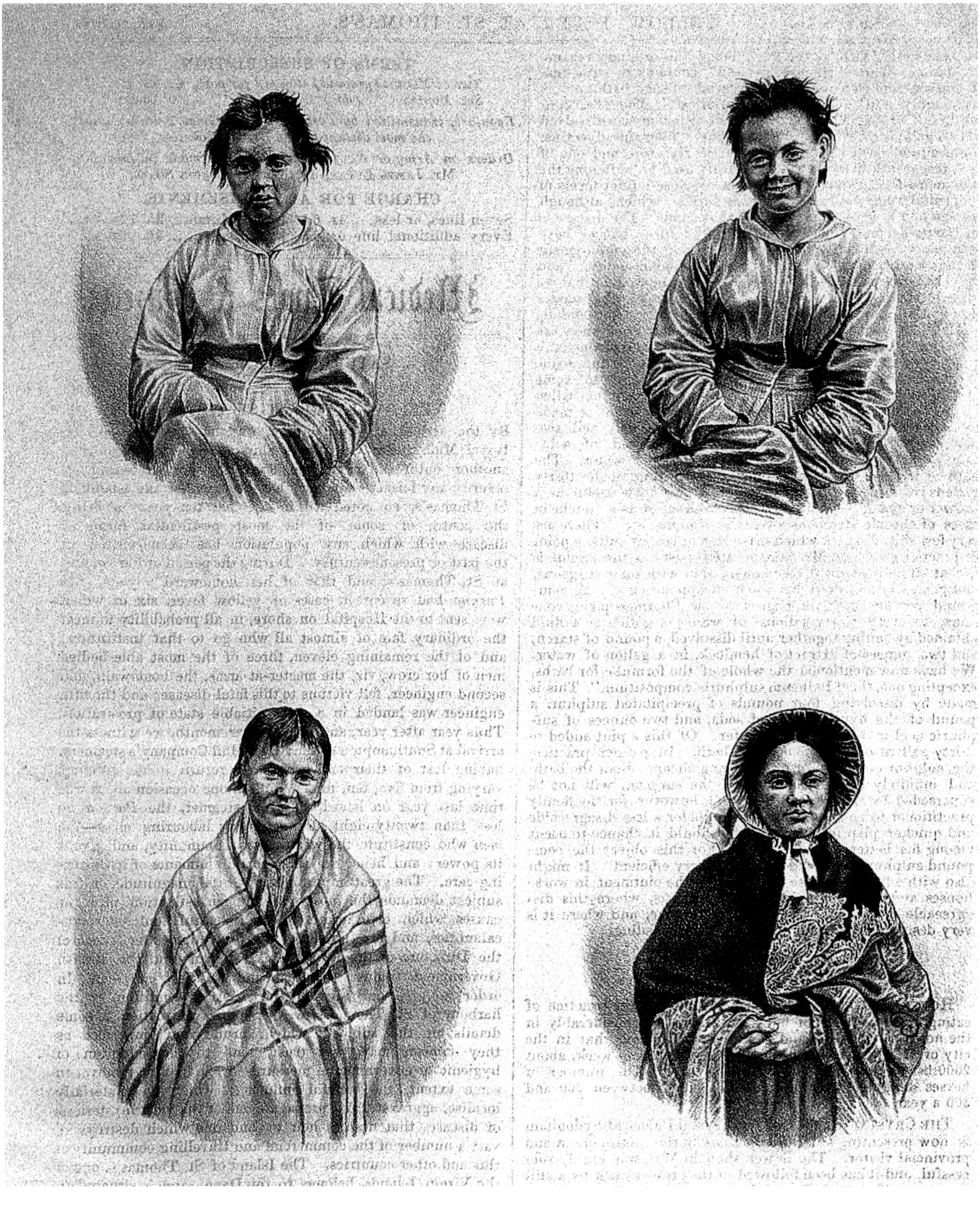

Fig. 16.8 An example of the stages in which the diagnostic features of a postpartum hypomanic episode or postpartum major depressive episode may be exhibited in a bipolar mother. (Wikimedia Commons; Creative Commons Attribution 3.0 Unported; https://creativecommons.org/licenses/by/3.0/)

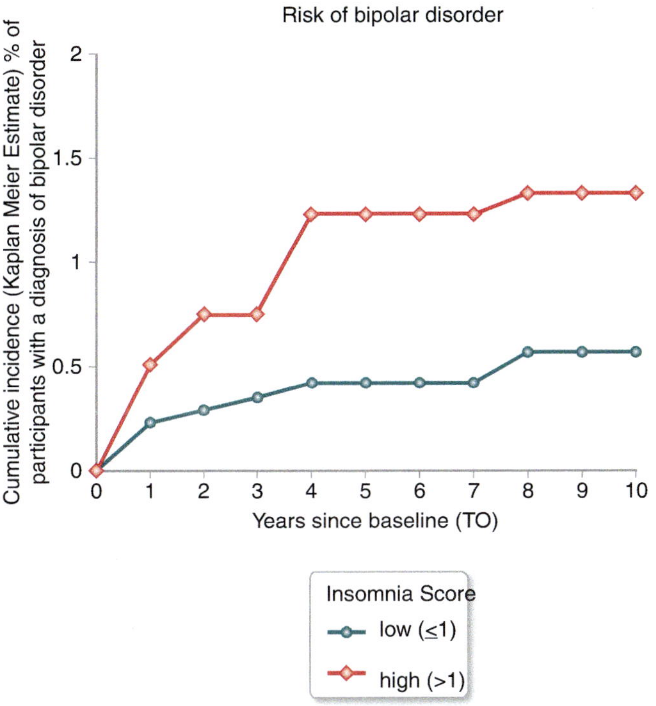

Fig. 16.9 The cumulative incidence of bipolar disorder for participants with both a low and high insomnia score, both indicating a progressively greater risk of bipolar disorder over the course of 10 years. (*From* Ritter et al. [14]; *with permission*)

Table 16.1 Anxiety disorder comorbidity and prevalence in bipolar disorder

Prevalence	Author
Anxiety disorder Current: 38% Lifetime: 43%	Bauer et al. (2005)
Generalized anxiety disorder 31%	Boylan et al. (2004)
Social phobia Lifetime: 47%	Kessler et al. (1997)
Panic disorder Lifetime: 38%	Dilsaver and Chen (2003)
Post-traumatic stress disorder Lifetime: 39%	Kessler et al. (1997)
Obsessive-compulsive disorder Lifetime: 39%	Tamam and Ozpoyraz (2002)

Etiology and Pathophysiology (Figs. 16.10 and 16.11)

Genetics

Bipolar disorder (BD) is highly heritable and inherited gene factors account for variation of its risk. It has been rather difficult to pinpoint exactly which genetic factors impose a risk for this disorder. To date, genome-wide association studies (GWAS) have been the most conclusive in identifying genes associated with BD.

Family studies both in the observational and systemic settings have found a lifetime risk of first degree relatives to be 5–20-fold. These studies have been excellent to define the range of clinical manifestation of underlying risk genotypes. The best-known study was published by Gershon et al. (1982) and Weissman et al. (1984), who showed that bipolar disorder, major depressive disorder, dysthymia, cyclothymia, and schizoaffective bipolar disorder were increased among first-degree relative probands with bipolar disorder (when compared to schizophrenia and other nonaffective psychotic illnesses) [16, 17]. Electronic medical records have made it easier to study families who are within these risk factors. Population-based studies are advantageous due to large sample size, reduced risk of misreporting or recall bias, and the ability to link distance relatives. The downfalls, however, include less detailed and precise information compared to a research grade analysis.

The most prominent genetic feature of bipolar disorder is the clear lack of Mendelian pattern of inheritance because the disorder is unable to exclude polygenic or multifactorial models to its etiology. Families of probands demonstrate assertive mating, genetic anticipation, parent origin effects (such as genomic imprinting), and mitochondrial inheritance.

Twin studies demonstrated the majority of variation in risk attributed to inherited genetic variation. The debate of overestimation due to gene–environment correlation proposes that genetic risk factors increase due to the likelihood of exposure to environmental risks. For example, true heritability can be overestimated if one was to propose that alcohol is a trigger for the onset of bipolar disorder if the individual is raised in a household of easy access to alcohol and parents who abuse the substance. Adoption studies help determine genetic factors; however, some nongenetic familial contributions are observed in adoptive parents with bipolar disorder.

Linking studies have helped distinguish genetic heterogeneity, with small effect sizes, and non-Mendelian inheritance patterns. They have culminated support for loci on chromosomes 6q, 8q, 13q, 18q, and 22q. Candidate gene studies directly measure the genetic differences between groups of unrelated individuals who differed for traits such as bipolar disorder. Genetic markers were used to identify differences, and there was little consensus around the main findings. Selecting candidate genes is more difficult than presumed as there are over 20,000 genes and genetic markers that have little effect on a trait. The power to detect true association was low, and no commonly accepted catalogs of genetic variants exist to help.

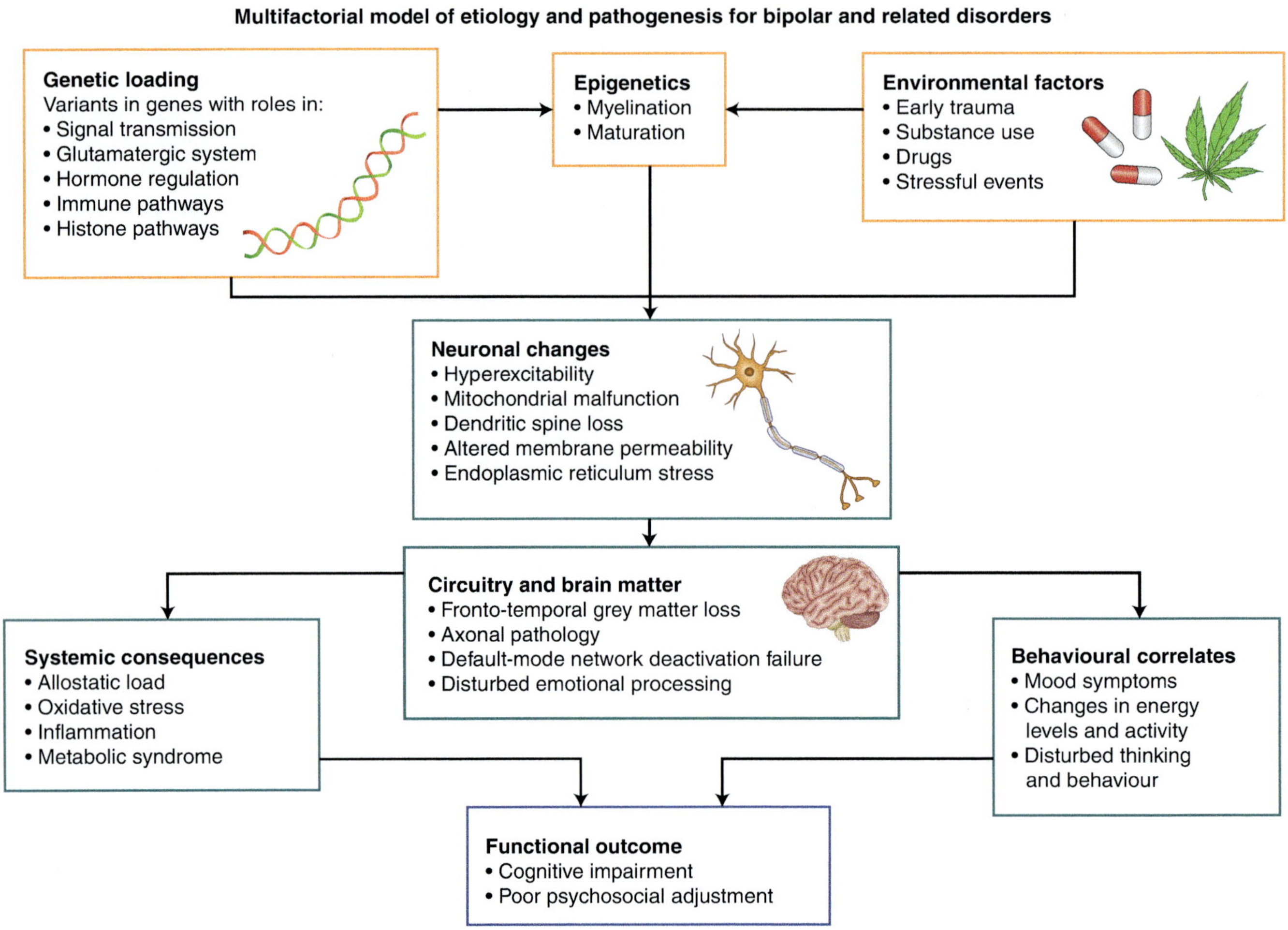

Fig. 16.10 Although bipolar disorders are among the most heritable psychiatric disorders, both genetic and environmental factors contribute to disease development. Gene–environment interactions might be mediated by epigenetic alterations. Genetic and environmental factors might contribute to the development of bipolar disorders through neuronal changes that modify brain circuitry. These changes systematically and behaviourally affect the body, leading to psychosocial and cognitive impairment

Genome-wide association studies (GWAS) involve several hundred thousand single nucleotide polymorphisms that are rapidly scanned across the complete genome of a larger number of case and control individuals, which are selected based on informativeness (thus, they are hypothesis-free studies). Many GWAS have been published for schizophrenia, obsessive-compulsive disorder, major depressive disorder, autism, ADHD, and bipolar disorders. Association signals have been found and replicated [18] (Fig. 16.12). The sophistication of meta-analysis has helped build the confidence to point out several loci with reproducible effects.

Although these genomes cannot make confident statements about etiologic pathways, they can speak to calcium signaling, neuronal transmission, and neuronal development. Despite high heritability, there is no common set of genetic markers that have a large effect on risk: all together, they encompass a risk of 2%, which 1–3% increased risk in carriers [19] (Table 16.2). The inheritance pattern is much more similar to a polygenic threshold model, where many alleles are assumed to play a role in risk [18] (Fig. 16.13).

Gene expression studies in the postmortem brain have begun to help us identify large sets of genes whose expression is consistently abnormal in bipolar disorder. The limitations lie in distinguishing between gene expression changes that play an etiologic role compared to those that arise as a consequence of bipolar disorder or its treatment. Epigenetics can play a role in the future of relating stressful life experiences, drug exposure, and other post-conception events that can influence gene expression.

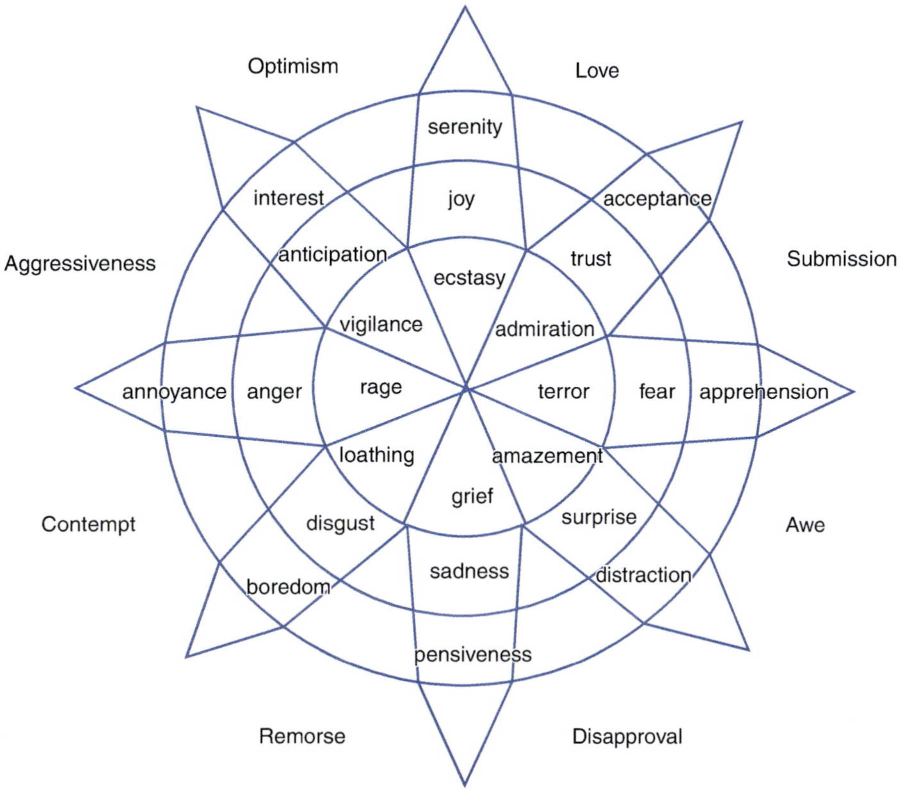

Fig. 16.11 The "wheel (cone) of emotions" according to Robert Plutchik [20]

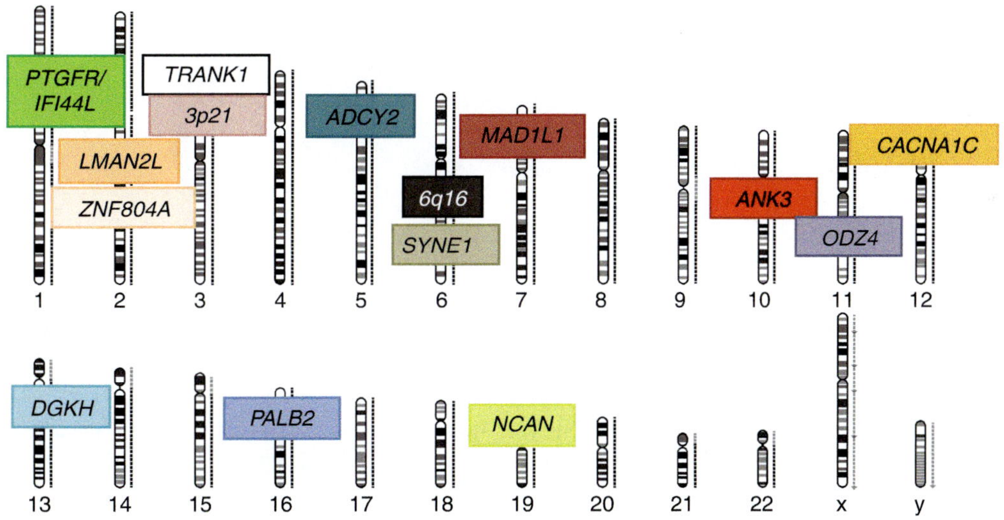

Fig. 16.12 The association signals found by genome-wide association studies that have associations with schizophrenia, obsessive-compulsive disorder, major depressive disorder, autism, ADHD, and bipolar disorders

Neurobiology and Pathophysiology

The most consistent neuropathological findings include structural, cellular, and functional changes in cortical and limbic regions. Many explanations involve pathways that ultimately result in cerebral atrophy and cell loss. Current leading hypotheses revolve around mitochondrial involvement, oxidative stress, role of inflammation, and neurotrophic factors.

Neural bases of affective states involve the subcortical limbic system and cortical regions (i.e., anterior cingulate cortex and dorsolateral prefrontal cortex). The limbic system includes primitive structures, amygdala, hippocampus, and

Table 16.2 Prospective gene expression of bipolar disorder from genome-wide association studies

Gene	Possible function
DAOA	Glutamate neurotransmission
BDNF	Neurogenesis and brain development
DISC1	Neuron microtubule formation
5HTT	Serotonergic neurotransmission
COMT	Monoamine metabolism
MAOA	Monoamine metabolism
TPH1&2	Serotonin synthesis
ANK3	Impacts on sodium channel structure
CACNA1C	Calcium channel function

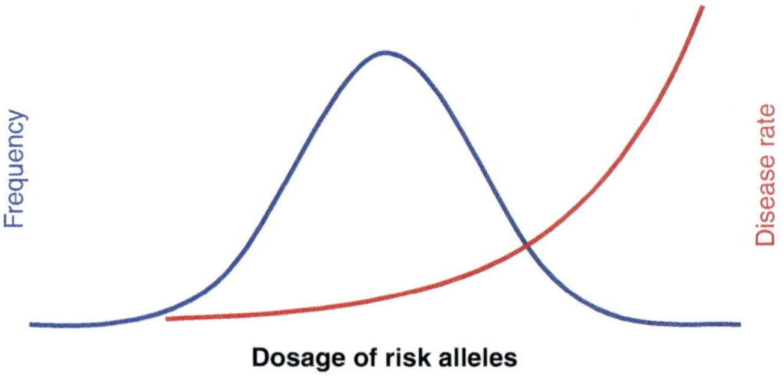

Fig. 16.13 The inheritance pattern of bipolar disorders is similar to that of a polygenic threshold model, where many alleles are assumed to play a role in risk

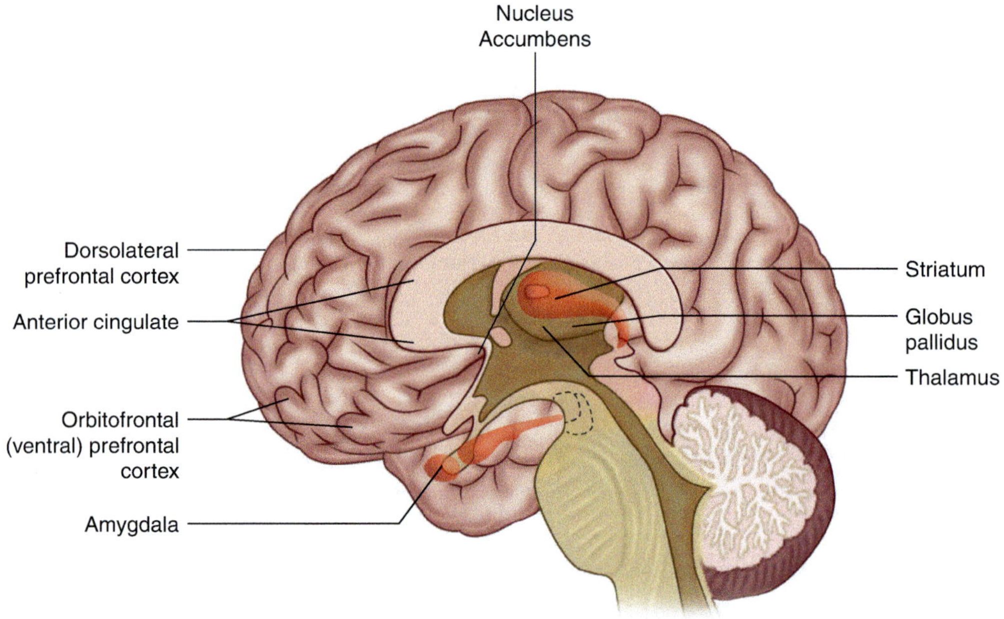

Fig. 16.14 Neuroanatomical abnormalities found in affective states are observed in both limbic and cortical areas (i.e., anterior cingulate cortex and dorsolateral prefrontal cortex)

thalamus—all of which perceive, process, and create memories about emotions and experiences with emotional valence. The cerebral cortex is a complex sensory information center processing, connecting, and modulating one's experience of emotion. Neuroanatomical abnormalities are observed in both limbic and cortical areas (Figs. 16.14 and 16.15) (Table 16.3) [18, 21, 22].

The most evident findings in physical changes of the brain in patients with bipolar disorder is the volume of the amygdala. Studies have shown a decrease in size when comparing healthy adolescent brains with adolescents diagnosed with BD. In contrast to adult populations, amygdala enlargement has been observed in BD patients. It is important to note that lithium has shown to have neuroprotective effects, and these findings may be due to treatment with this drug beginning in adolescence (Figs. 16.16 and 16.17) [18].

Table 16.3 Components of the limbic system and their function

Cortex	Amygdala	Hippocampus	Hypothalamus
Abstract thinking and insight Planning Conscious thought Judgment Hearing Vision Taste	Emotions: Rage Fear	Memories: Access to most brain signals Acquires knowledge or information from interactions between person and social world	Appetite for food Sexual arousal Body temperature Sleep cycle

During manic episodes and at depressive states, there have been changes observed in the ventral prefrontal cortex. Decreased activation in the lateral and medial regions has been reported. Loss of compensation by these centers in the

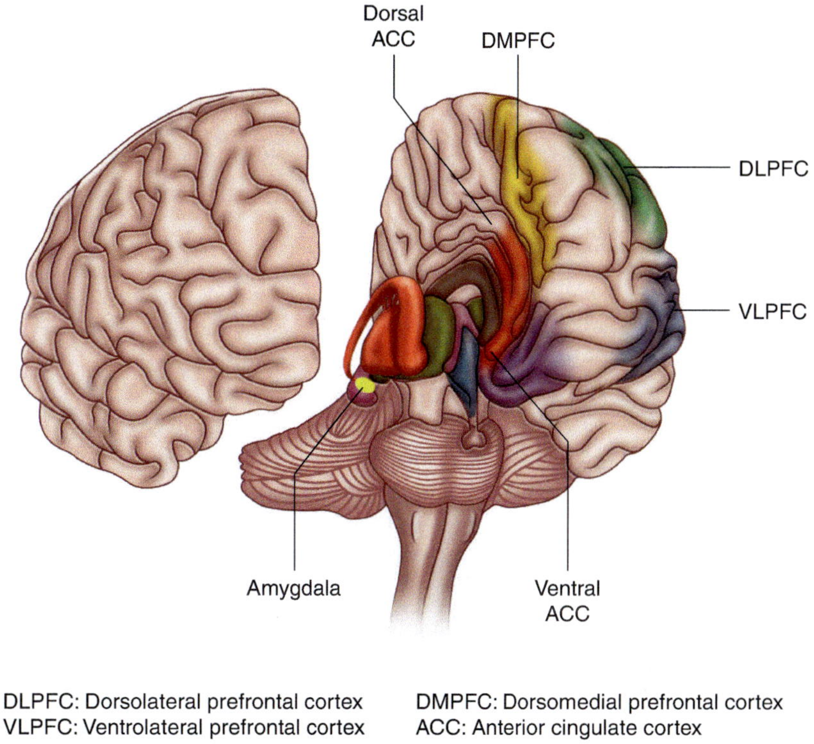

Fig. 16.15 Functional brain changes in bipolar disorder. Imaging studies of euthymic bipolar patients provide evidence of compromised cognitive control, combined with increased responsiveness of limbic and paralimbic brain regions involved in emotional regulation. Brain areas associated with cognitive control, which manifest reduced responsiveness, are labeled blue (dorsal ACC, DMPFC, and DLPFC). By contrast, limbic and paralimbic brain areas involved in emotional regulation, associated with greater responsiveness, are labeled in red (amygdala, VLPFC, and ventral ACC) [22]. (*From* Maletic and Raison [22]; Creative Commons CC BY 3.0; https://creativecommons.org/licenses/by/3.0/)

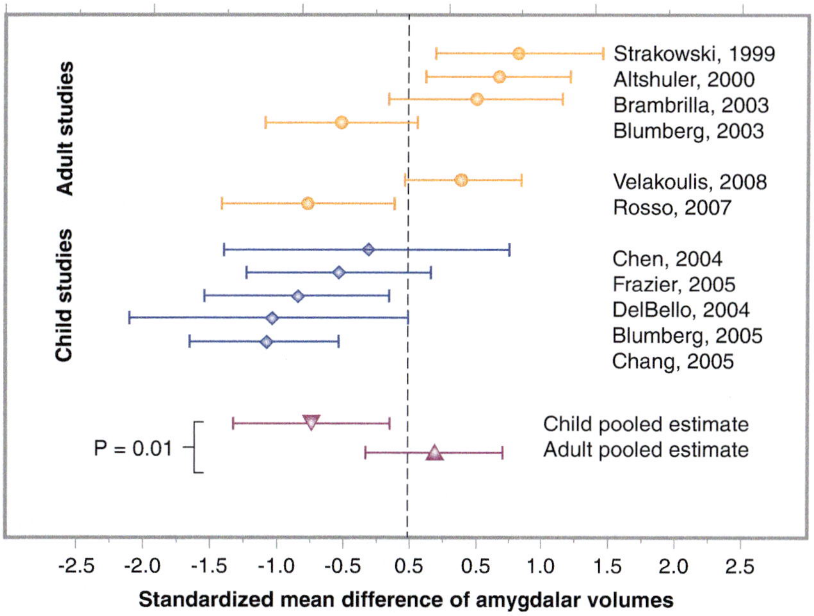

Fig. 16.16 In contrast to adult populations, amygdala enlargement in the adolescent brain has been observed in bipolar patients

setting of stress or other factors may lead to mood episodes (Fig. 16.18) [18]. The abnormalities occur over time, and loss of prefrontal volume is observed in recurrent affective episodes into adulthood. During remission, increased activity of the ventral prefrontal cortex has been observed with overactivation of the amygdala as well (Fig. 16.19).

There have been hypotheses developed in regard to the involvement of neurotransmitter dysregulation in bipolar disorder, specifically serotonin, dopamine, and norepinephrine. Dopamine and norepinephrine irregularities have been difficult to study and understand in terms of their influence on pathogenesis (Fig. 16.20). The evidence of increased dopamine concentration in BD has been inconsistent. Researchers have hypothesized that supersensitivity to dopamine receptors versus excess dopamine are causal factors of BD. Lithium has been shown to prevent this supersensitivity. Some studies have found that relative increases in norepinephrine are found in states of mania, compared to depres-

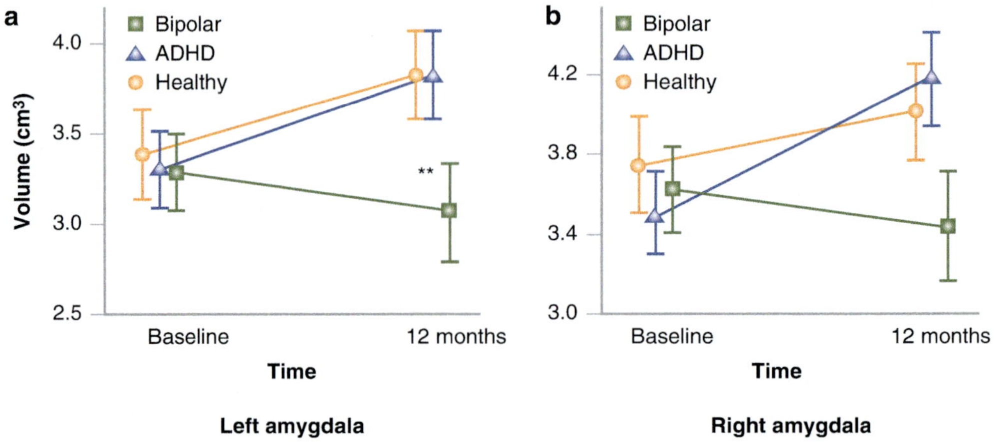

Fig. 16.17 Comparison of left amygdala (**a**) and right amygdala (**b**) volume between the bipolar brain, ADHD brain, and healthy brain

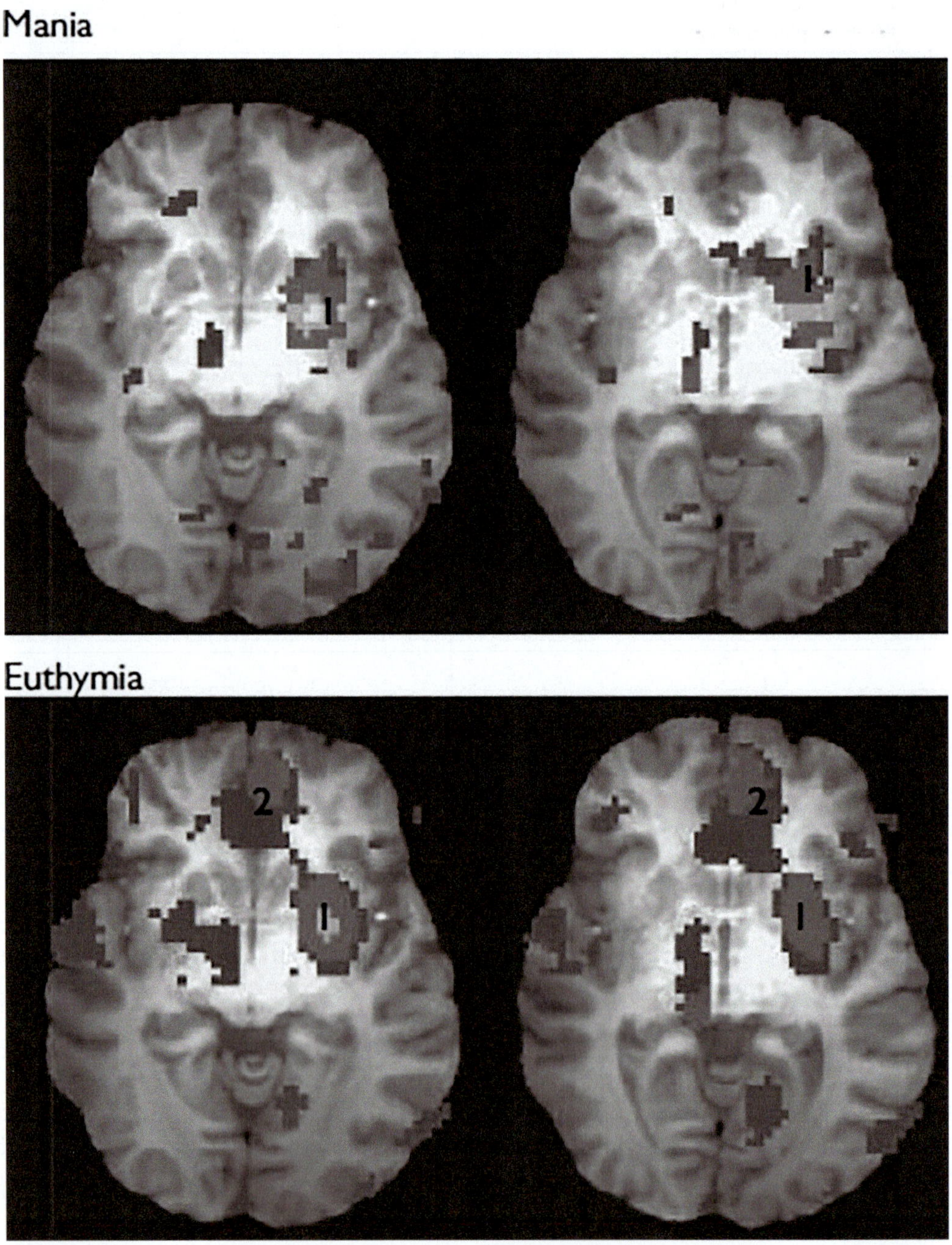

Fig. 16.18 Decreased activation in the lateral and medial regions during settings of stress or other factors may lead to mood episodes

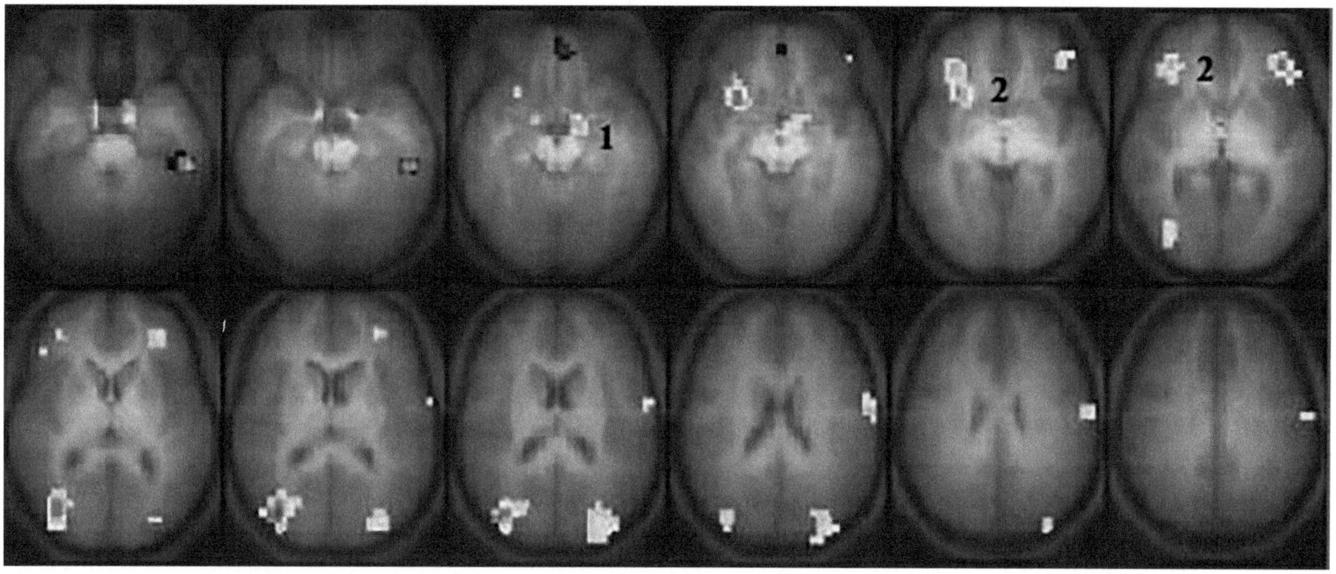

Fig. 16.19 During remission, increased activity of the ventral prefrontal cortex has been observed with overactivation of the amygdala

sive or eurythmic states. The serotonin permissive hypothesis describes that primary lesion producing low serotonergic tone results in dysregulation of both noradrenergic and dopaminergic pathways. The reduced function of serotonin pathways modulates the release of neurotransmitters, leading to an increase in norepinephrine and dopamine levels. Glutamate and gamma aminobutyric acid (GABA) have also been of interest in understanding neurotransmitter dysregulation as they are important in the communication pathways in the networks that modulate emotion; however, their role in BD has remained unclear.

The human brain tissue is susceptible to reactive oxygen species (ROS) damage because of high oxygen content and ROS overproduction, which can overwhelm endogenous antioxidants and create neuronal damage targeting lipids, proteins, and DNA. ROS are found to be elevated in BD, which reflect a deficiency of energy metabolism due to mitochondrial dysfunction. Decreased expression of certain mitochondrial subunits and downregulation of mitochondrial genes have been noted in BD. Lactate is the byproduct of anaerobic glycolysis, a route that is taken when the function of mitochondria is reduced. Increased lactate levels with decreased intracellular pH correspond to depressive states, as the brain attempts to correct this imbalance. Decreased levels of phosphocreatine (PCr) are associated with mitochondrial dysfunction and low focal levels of PCr in the left frontal lobe of patients in bipolar depressive states.

There have been various proposed mechanisms for brain atrophy and decreased cell density in this patient population. The association remains unknown as it is uncertain if the atrophy and reduced density are due to bipolar disorder, or these mechanisms cause bipolar disorder. Thiobarbituric acid reactive substances are byproducts of lipid peroxidation that can be quantified in serum samples. They have been found to be elevated in BD in various states. Lithium can reduce markers of lipid peroxidation. 4-hydroxy-2-nonenal (4-HNE) is another marker for lipid peroxidation, which is significantly increased in cells of the anterior cingulate cortex. Malondialdehyde (MDA) is created when ROS degrade cellular lipid components, and it is elevated in the peripheral serum in BD. Treatment with antidepressants and antipsychotics showed a reduction of these effects. 3-nitrotyrosine (3-NT) is increased in bipolar depressive states and corresponds to protein carboxylation. DNA damage is measured via 8-hydroxy-2-deoxyguanosine (8-OHdG) and elevated during manic episodes. Inflammation is also linked with affective episodes, oxidative stress, and medical comorbidities. Elevated CRP and circulating cytokines (IL-4, IL-2, TNF-alpha) are evident during these states of inflammation (Figs. 16.21, and 16.22).

Brain Imaging

Cortical thinning has been detected in bipolar disorder patients, especially with increased duration of illness, as well as cortical thickening as a result of treatment with lithium, but not antiepileptics or antipsychotics (Figs. 16.23, 16.24, and 16.25) [23].

Findings from SPECT brain imaging in adults with bipolar disorder adults showed significant cognitive impairment, correlated to neocortical decreased perfusion, during moderate-severe manic episodes. Alarmingly, at the 6-month follow-up, cognitive improvement was not observed despite the clinical improvement, related to an increase in perfusion only at orbitofrontal areas (Fig. 16.26) [24].

Fig. 16.20 Summary of dopamine molecular imaging findings in bipolar disorder

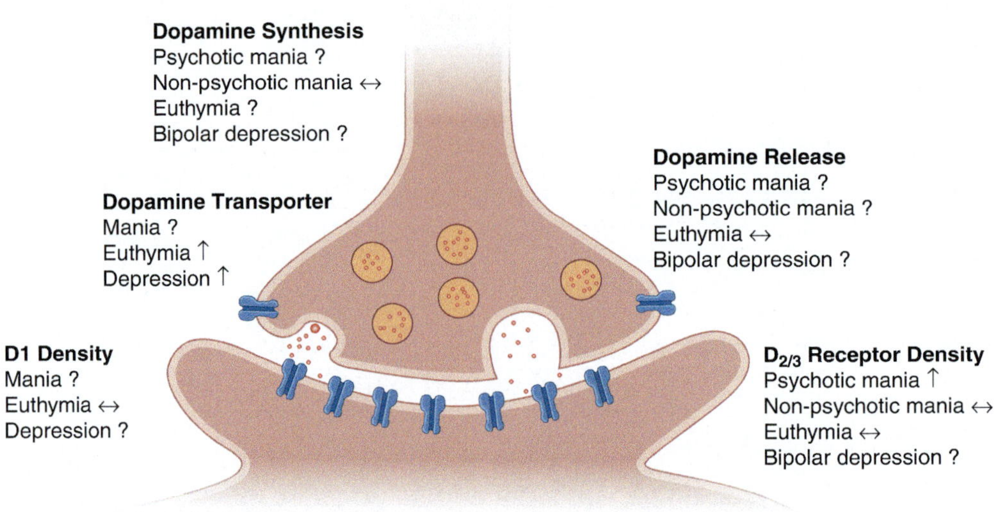

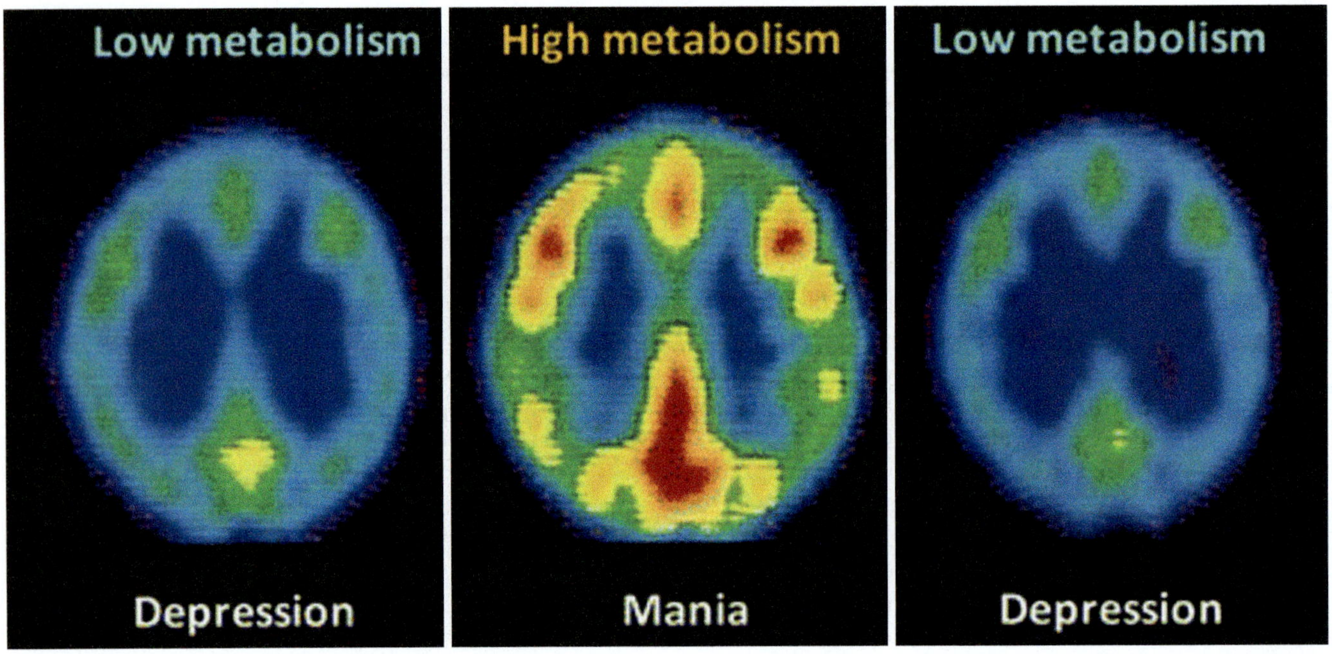

Fig. 16.21 PET imaging showing changes in brain energy consumption with the switch between mood states. The blue and yellow/red colors indicate areas of low and high energy consumption, respectively

Fig. 16.22 Proposed role of activated microglia in the modulation of inflammatory mediators, neurotransmitter synthesis, and synaptic plasticity in bipolar disorder (BD). *CRP* C-reactive protein; *IDO* indoindoleamine 2,3-dioxygenase; *5-HT* serotonin; *RNS* reactive nitrogen species; *ROS* reactive oxygen species

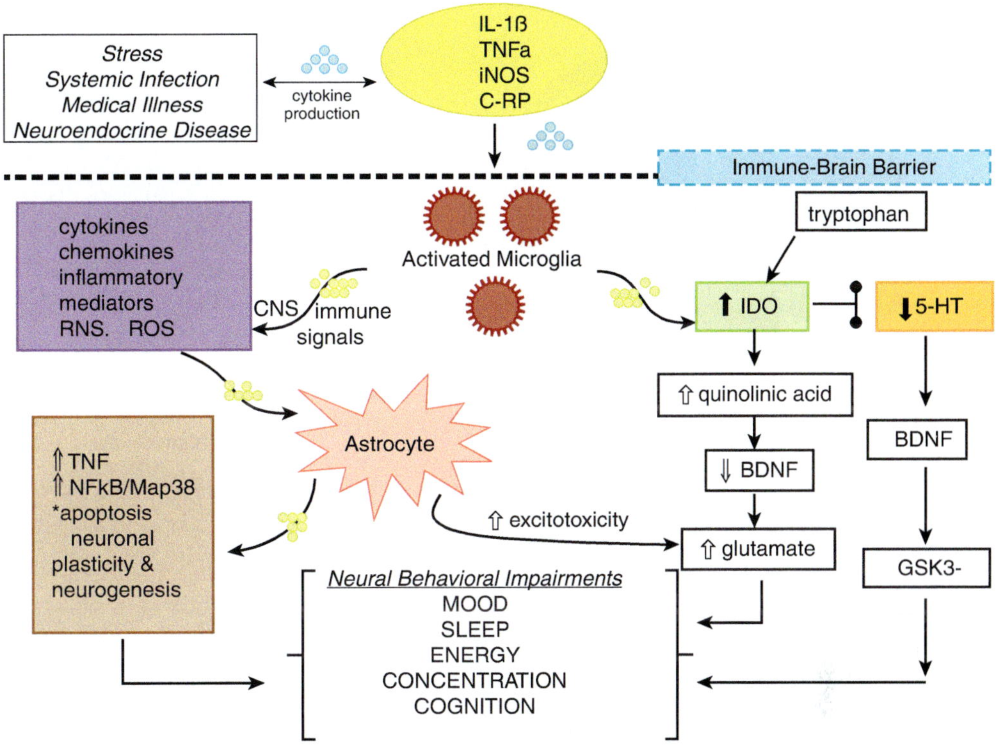

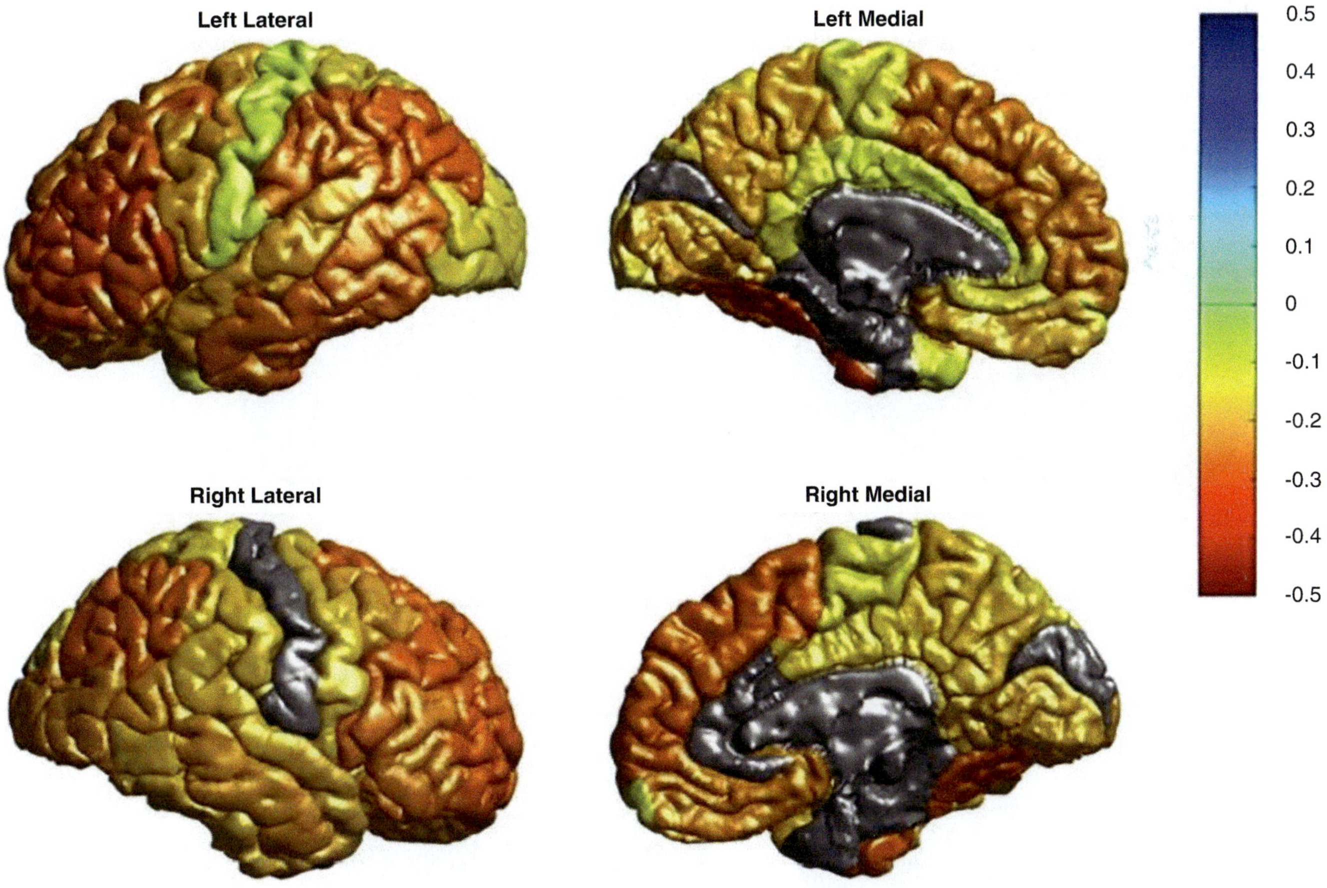

Fig. 16.23 Cortical thinning in adult patients with bipolar disorder compared with healthy controls. Cohen's d effect sizes are plotted for each region of interest on the cortical surface of a template image. Only significant regions are shown; nonsignificant regions are colored in gray. (*From* Hibar et al. [23]; Creative Commons CC-BY 4.0; http://creativecommons.org/licenses/by-nc-nd/4.0/)

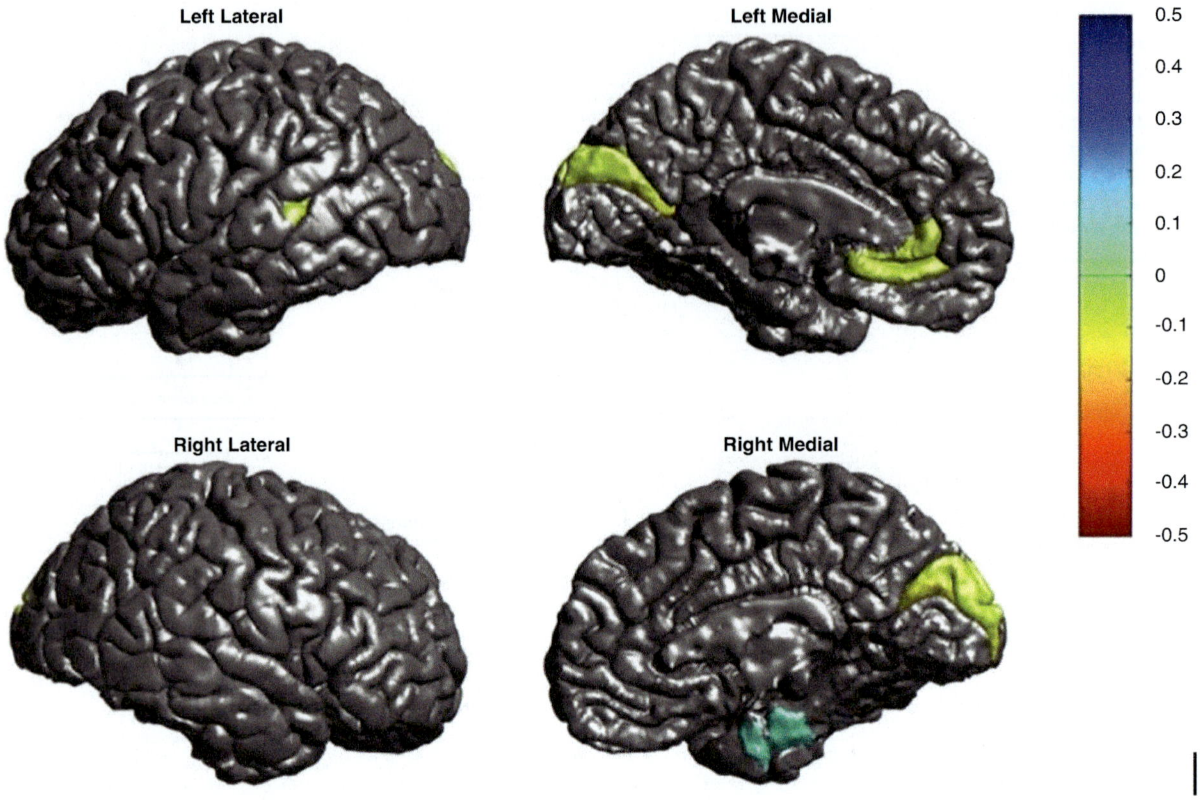

Fig. 16.24 Cortical thinning in adult patients with bipolar disorder associated with duration of illness. Pearson's correlation r effect sizes are plotted for each region of interest on the cortical surface of a template image. Only significant regions are shown; nonsignificant regions are colored in gray. (*From* Hibar et al. [23]; Creative Commons CC-BY 4.0; http://creativecommons.org/licenses/by-nc-nd/4.0/)

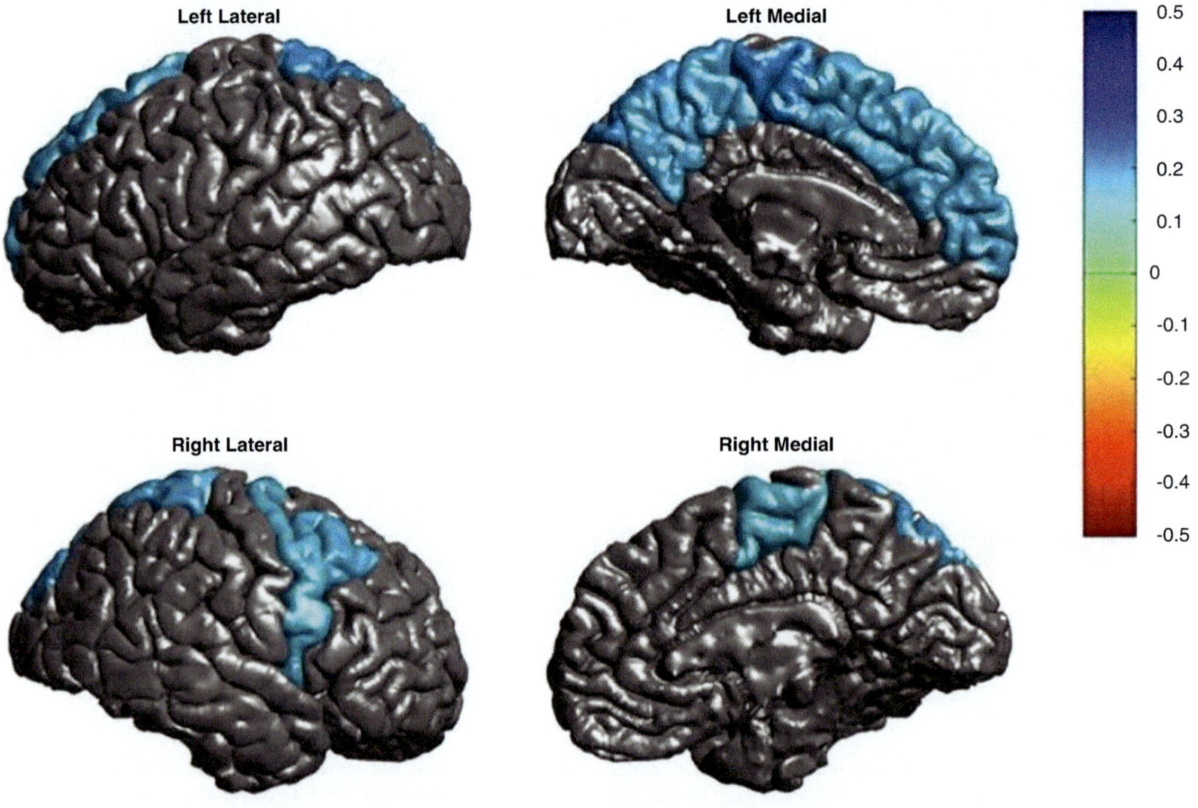

Fig. 16.25 Cortical thickening in adult patients with bipolar disorder associated with lithium treatment. Cohen's d effect sizes are plotted for each region of interest on the cortical surface of a template image. Only significant regions are shown; nonsignificant regions are colored in gray. (*From* Hibar et al. [23]; Creative Commons CC-BY 4.0; http://creativecommons.org/licenses/by-nc-nd/4.0/)

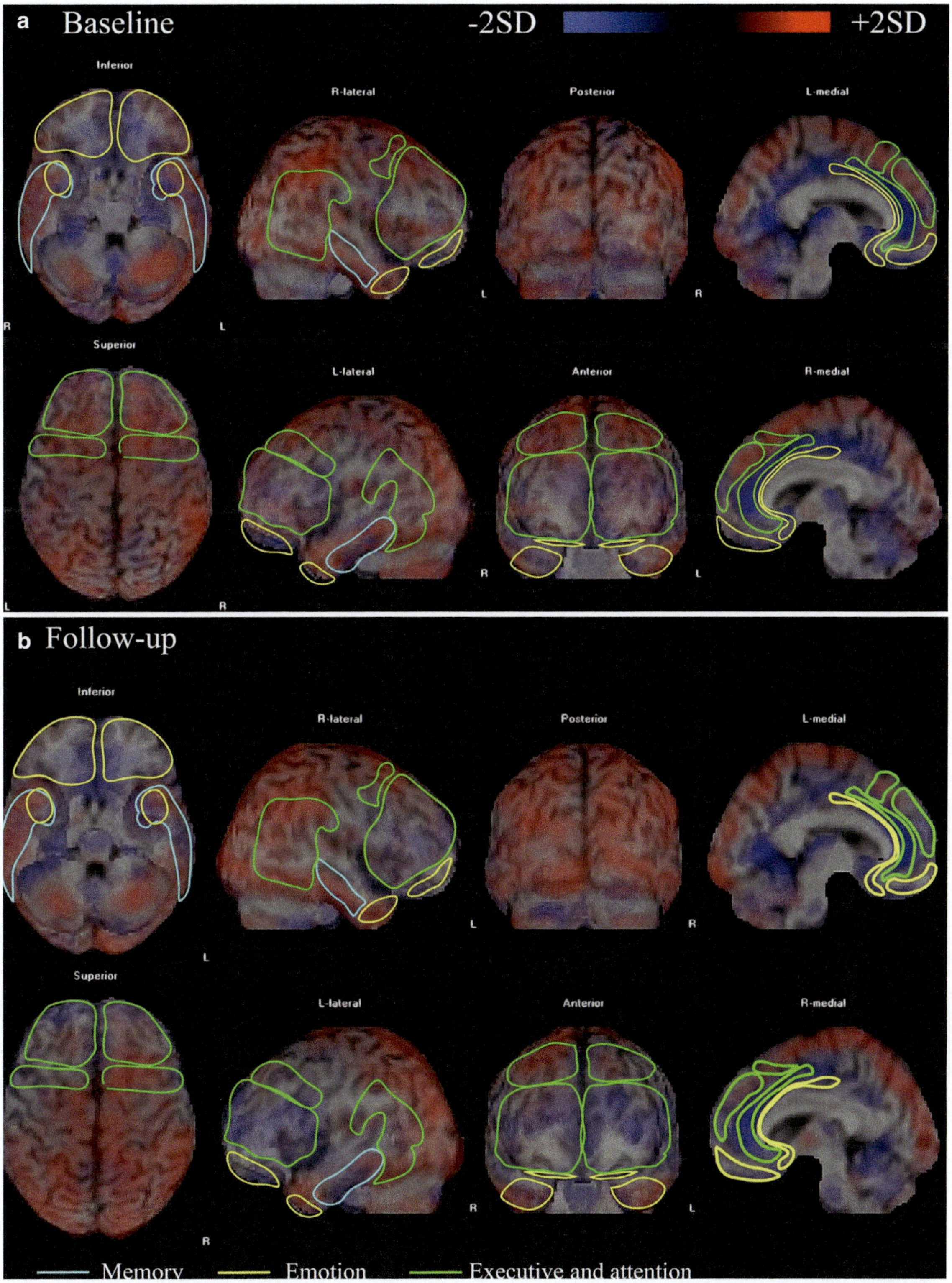

Fig. 16.26 SPECT findings. The following images show anterior, posterior, medial, and lateral cortex of a volumetric image of the brain of patients, in mania (**a**), and in their 6-month follow-up (**b**). The identification of the color scheme is based on the standard deviation of perfusion compared with a group of healthy controls. Noting that blue shows decreased flow in specific cortical areas, and red, cortical hyperperfusion. Also, the gray areas represent no significant changes in relation to the flow of healthy controls. According to the Brodmann areas, memory includes 21 (middle temporal gyrus—MTG), 28 (ventral entorhinal cortex); emotion network: 11 (orbitofrontal cortex—OFC), 24 (anterior cingulate cortex—ACC), 25 (subgenual cingulate cortex—sACC), 28 (ventral entorhinal cortex—vEC) and attention and executive networks: 7 (parietal cortex—PaC), 8 (oculomotor cortex), 9 (dorsolateral prefrontal cortex—DLPFC), 10 (frontopolar prefrontal cortex—FPC), and 32 (dorsal anterior cingulate cortex—dACC). (*From* Estudillo-Guerra et al. [24]; Creative Commons CC BY)

Phenomenology and Course

Clinicians and researchers alike encounter the daunting challenge of accurately clarifying one's psychiatric history with the ultimate goal of rendering a robust and scientifically sound clinical diagnosis. Throughout the years, the nomenclature, diagnostic criteria, and terminology for the collection of separate but related psychiatric disorders that fall under the broad umbrella of diagnoses that comprise "bipolar and related disorders" have changed. In the not-so-recent past, the term "manic depression" encompassed the constellation of psychiatric symptoms and associated features that reflect what is now viewed as several distinct subtypes within the spectrum of bipolar and related disorders. In 2000, the Diagnostic and Statistical Manual of Mental Disorders-IV-TR combined both major depressive disorder and the spectrum of bipolar and related disorders into one section titled, "Mood Disorders" [25]. Yet, the updated fifth edition of the Diagnostic and Statistical Manual of Mental Disorders (DSM-V) introduced two distinct sections, dividing bipolar and related disorders into one section, followed by a separate section for depressive disorders [1].

Of great importance, regardless of the evolving characterization of bipolar and related disorders, the first initial and primary target of clinicians or researchers should be to identify whether any current or past manic, hypomanic, or depressive episodes have occurred [26]. Once this crucial information is elucidated, then, and only then, can an accurate diagnosis be rendered. Table 16.4 provides a visual outline of essential criteria and additional symptom criteria derived from the DSM-V for major depressive episodes and manic or hypomanic episodes with additional user-friendly clinical probes to assess psychiatric symptomatology.

Once a well-defined psychiatric history has determined whether any current or previous depressive, manic, or hypomanic episodes have occurred, the next step that follows is to determine which specific diagnosis is most appropriate (i.e., bipolar I disorder, bipolar II disorder, cyclothymic disorder, other specified bipolar and related disorders, substance/medication-induced bipolar and related disorders, or bipolar and related disorders due to another medical condition). The reader is encouraged to review the DSM-V for expanded discussion of differential diagnoses between the group of bipolar and related disorders relative to other psychiatric disorders (i.e., personality disorders, schizophrenia, and other psychotic spectrum disorders) (Table 16.5) (Fig. 16.27) [1].

There are two additional points that necessitate greater deliberation. First, as described in the previous section on comorbid psychiatric disorders, many individuals with a disorder falling under the larger classification system of bipolar and related disorders commonly meet diagnostic criteria for one or more co-occurring psychiatric disorders.

Table 16.4 Diagnostic criteria and aids to diagnosing the basic subtypes of bipolar mood episodes

Major depressive episode[a] • **At least 1 essential criterion (depressed mood or anhedonia) persisting for ≥2 weeks and** • **Essential criteria and additional symptoms add up to ≥5 total diagnostic criteria being met**	
Essential criteria	**Clinical probes**
Persisting depressed mood	Have you been feeling depressed or down most of the day, nearly every day? How long has this lasted?
Persisting anhedonia	Have you lost interest or pleasure in things that you usually enjoy? How long has this lasted?
Additional symptom criteria	Clinical probes
Increase or decrease in appetite or body weight	Has your appetite changed from normal during the time you have been feeling depressed? Have you started eating more/less than usual? Has your weight changed? Did you intend to gain/lose weight?
Persisting insomnia or hypersomnia	Has there been a change in the amount of your sleep while feeling depressed? How many hours a night compared to normal? Do you have problems falling asleep, staying asleep, or waking up too early (or a combination of these)?
Persisting fatigue or energy loss	Have you felt tired or run down all the time (or nearly every day) while feeling depressed?
Psychomotor agitation or slowing	Have you been so fidgety or restless that you could not sit still? Have others noticed? Have you or others noticed that you have been talking or moving more slowly than usual?
Feelings of worthlessness or excessive guilt	Have you felt like you were less deserving than other people while feeling so depressed? Why? Have you been feeling worthless on a daily or near-daily basis while feeling depressed? Have you been feeling more guilty than usual about mistakes, things you have done, or even things you have not done? How so?
Problems concentrating or making decisions	Has it been harder for you to maintain your focus or think through things while feeling depressed? Has it been harder to make everyday decisions?
Recurring thoughts of death or suicide	Have you been thinking a lot about death or that you may be better off dead? Have you been thinking of hurting yourself and how you might do that? Have you done anything to hurt yourself? Are you having these thoughts now?
Manic or hypomanic episodes[a] • **At least 1 essential criterion persisting for ≥7 days (mania)[b] or ≥4 days (hypomania) and** • **Essential criteria and additional symptoms add up to ≥3 diagnostic criteria being met (≥4 if mood is irritable)[c]** • **Assess the threshold level of severity needed to distinguish between manic and hypomanic episodes[d]**	

Table 16.4 (continued)

Essential criteria	Clinical probes
Persisting elevated, expansive, or irritable mood[b]	Have you had a time in your life where your mood was so excited, energized, or high that others thought you were not your normal self? What was that like? How long did it last? How about feeling so irritable or angry for several days in a row that others thought you were not your usual self? Was that different than how you normally are when you get upset? How so? How long did that last? Did you need to be in the hospital because of any of this?
Additional symptom criteria	Clinical probes
Abnormally elevated self-esteem	When your mood was abnormally elevated/irritable, how did you feel about yourself? Did you feel more confident or smarter than usual? Did you think you had special capabilities or insights? What was that like? Do you recall feeling more attractive to others than usual? Do you remember having a lot more sexual energy or interest than usual?
Decreased need for sleep	When your mood was abnormally elevated/irritable, did you seem to need much less sleep than usual? How much is normal for you? How much were you getting by on when your mood was abnormally elevated/irritable? Did you still feel rested, or even more energized than usual, despite getting so little sleep?
Increased talkativeness	When your mood was abnormally elevated/irritable, were you more talkative than usual? Did others point it out to you? What did they say? Did others have problems understanding you because you talked too fast or too much? Did they have trouble interrupting you? Is that different than how you normally are or how you normally talk?
Flight of ideas or racing thoughts	When your mood was abnormally elevated/irritable, did your thoughts race or seem to go faster than normal? Did your head seem to become overcrowded with thoughts? What was that like?
Abnormal distractibility	When your mood was abnormally elevated/irritable, did you have problems staying focused on one thing? Were you really prone to being distracted? What was that like? Is that different than how you normally are? How so?
Increased energy or goal-directed activity	When your mood was abnormally elevated/irritable, were you unusually hyper or wired because you had an unusual amount of energy? What was that like? Do you recall being unusually restless, not being able to sit still, or pacing excessively? Were you unusually productive (or unproductive) during that time? How so? What was a typical day for you like when your mood was abnormally elevated/irritable? How does that compare with normal?
Abnormally risky behaviors[e]	When your mood was abnormally elevated/irritable, do you think you lost control of your impulses and judgment? Did you do things that were unusually risky or caused problems for you? Can you give me some examples?

Reprinted from Bobo [26]; *with permission*

[a]Can use the diagnostic probes to guide clinical history taking from patients and collateral historians, such as family members or significant others

[b]Psychiatric hospitalization is often needed to manage acute manic episodes to prevent patients from harming themselves or others, to prevent behaviors that could cause serious financial or legal problems, or to address psychotic symptoms. If hospitalization is required, then diagnostic criteria for a manic episode can be satisfied even if the defining symptoms have been present for less than 7 days

[c]If the mood state (essential criterion) is irritable instead of elevated, then four or more of the eight diagnostic criteria must be met to satisfy the diagnostic criteria for a manic episode

[d]Manic episodes are diagnosed if the defining symptoms are severe enough to result in psychiatric hospitalization, cause marked impairment in social or occupational functioning, or are associated with psychotic features (hallucinations or delusions)

[e]This can include any type of behavior stemming from a loss of impulse control or judgment. It can be helpful to provide examples of specific behaviors for patients, emphasizing that they must be behaviors that would not fall within the range of normal for that individual. These behaviors include excessive overspending, engaging in highly pleasurable but also high-risk activities (such as high-risk sexual encounters, gambling, and substance use), engaging in thrill-seeking types of behaviors (such as reckless driving or spending more money than usual), and making decisions impulsively to such a degree that it would be considered unusual for the patient

Some of the more commonly occurring comorbidities include social anxiety disorder, panic attack, specific phobia, AD/HD, substance use disorders, and disruptive, impulse-control, or conduct disorders [1]. Second, there are a number of pertinent etiological rule-outs that must ensure prior to rendering a diagnosis of any of the bipolar and related disorders. For example, a broad array of medical conditions or treatments can mimic "manic-like" symptoms that may be interpreted as a manic or hypomanic episode, including but not limited to a range of neurodegenerative conditions (particularly frontotemporal dementia, behavioral variant subtype), central nervous system insult/degradation (i.e., traumatic brain injury, cerebrovascular accident, epilepsy, brain tumor) that can negatively attenuate frontal "executive" control, which can result in residual and pervasive behavioral dysregulation, impulsivity, or decreased homeostasis of behavioral activation/arousal, as well as select medical treatments (e.g., use of corticotropic steroids or dopaminergic agents) (Fig. 16.28).

Table 16.5 Diagnostic criteria for major forms of bipolar disorder

Bipolar I disorder	Bipolar II disorder	Cyclothymic disorder (cyclothymia)
Essential diagnostic features:	Essential diagnostic features:	Essential diagnostic features:
(a) At least 1 lifetime manic episode	(a) At least 1 lifetime hypomanic episode	(a) Numerous hypomanic and depressive symptoms for ≥2 years
(b) The manic episode was not due to the effects of medication, substances, or medical illness	(b) At least 1 lifetime major depressive episode	(b) Diagnostic criteria for hypomanic episodes and for major depressive episodes not met
Diagnostic note: an episode of depression is not required to make a diagnosis of bipolar I disorder	(c) Neither the hypomanic nor the depressive episode(s) was due to effects of medication, substances, or medical illness	(c) No symptom-free period lasting ≥8 weeks during the 2-years period
Other specified bipolar and related disorders	**Substance/medication-induced bipolar and related disorders**	**Bipolar and related disorders due to another medical condition**
Examples include:	Clues to the diagnosis:	Clues to the diagnosis:
• Major depressive episodes + short episodes of hypomanic symptoms (2–3 days) that do not meet duration criteria for hypomanic episodes • Major depressive episodes + episodes of hypomanic symptoms that do not meet symptomatic criteria for hypomanic episodes • Hypomanic episodes with no previous major depressive episodes • Short-duration cyclothymia, with symptoms persisting for <2 years	• Mood disturbance (mania, hypomania, depression) develop during or soon after exposure to (or withdrawal from) the implicated substance/medication • The implicated substance/medication is capable of producing the mood disturbance • Mood disturbance abates soon after exposure to the implicated substance/medication ends • Reemergence of mood disturbance during rechallenge with the same substance/medication or a pharmacologically related alternative implicates the exposure as being causal, absent other factors	• Mania, hypomania, or depression develops in the context of existing or newly diagnosed medical illness • The medical illness is capable of causing the mood disturbance

Reprinted from Bobo [26]; *with permission*

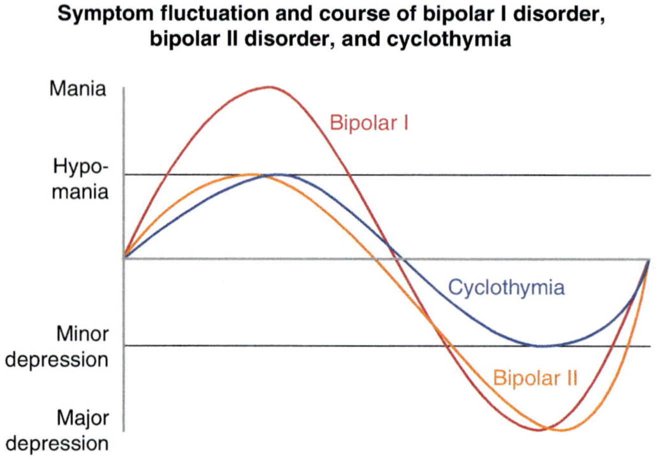

Fig. 16.27 This image displays the frequent course and range of symptom severity between bipolar I disorder, bipolar II disorder, and cyclothymia. Notice that the fluctuation and course of bipolar I disorder is the only diagnosis that includes a full mania episode, whereas bipolar II disorder and cyclothymia do not reach the threshold for a manic episode, per definition and diagnostic criteria. Furthermore, cyclothymia is characterized by mild depressive episodes, commonly fluctuating between subclinical hypomania and minor depression with the requirements of not meeting the criteria for hypomanic episodes or major depressive episodes over numerous periods for at least 2 years (at least 1 year in children and adolescents). (Wikimedia Commons; Creative Commons Attribution 3.0 Unported; https://creativecommons.org/licenses/by/3.0/)

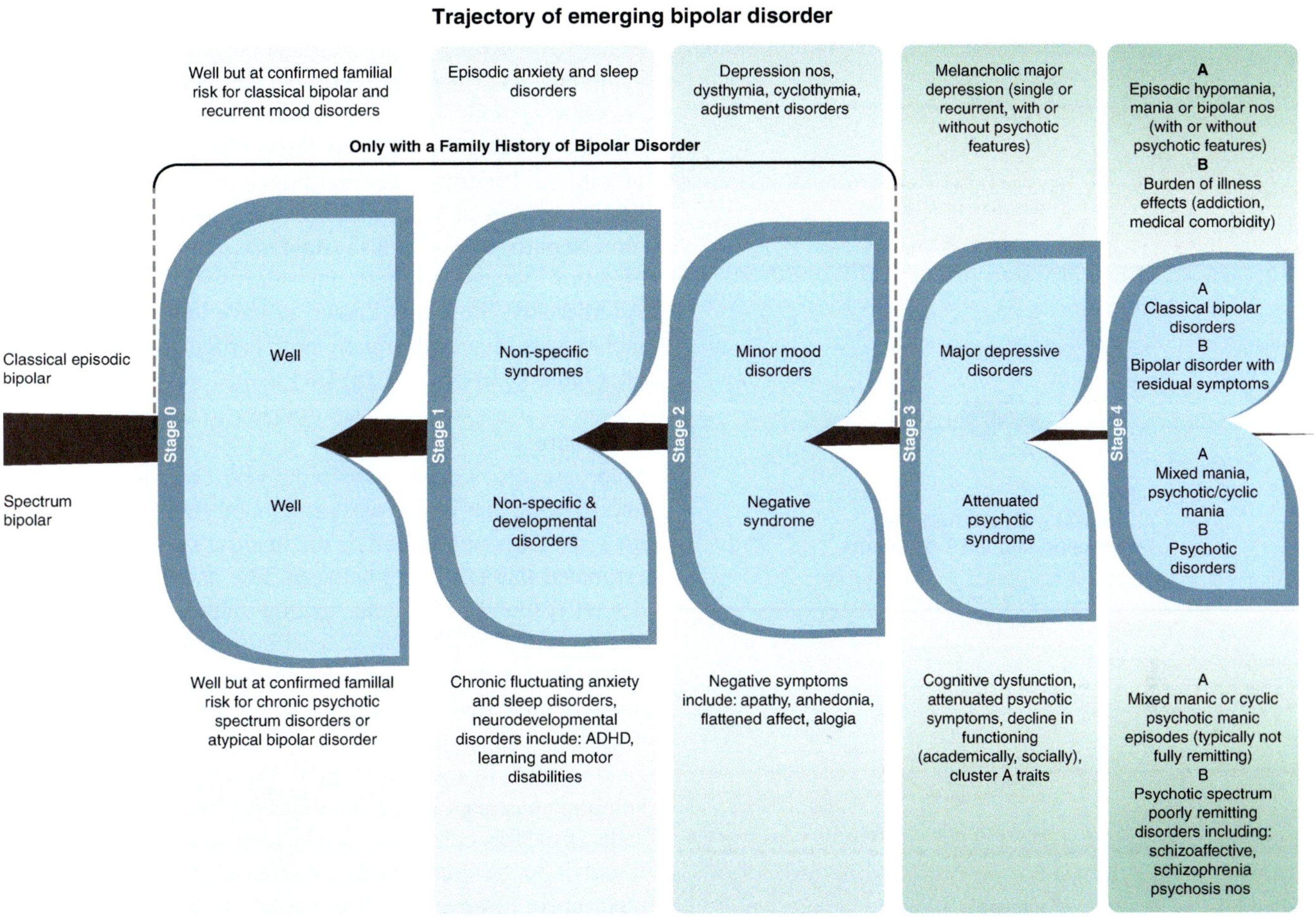

Fig. 16.28 The trajectory of emerging bipolar disorder in two subtypes of high-risk offspring

Biopsychosocial Treatments in Bipolar Disorder

Biological Interventions

The goal of treatment for bipolar disorder centers around either acute stabilization of a manic or depressive episode with recovery to a euthymic state or on maintenance therapy with prevention or reduction of symptoms and episodes. Even with therapies however, nearly 40% of patients relapse into a manic or depressive episode within a year and 60% will relapse within 2 years [27]. Various classes of pharmacologic interventions exist including mood stabilizers, antipsychotics, antidepressants, benzodiazepines, and novel therapies. Mood stabilizers are a particular class unique to bipolar disorder, and their use, mechanisms, and adverse effects are discussed. We also will examine the evidence for efficacy and indications for the use of each medication class. Additionally, approaches to treatment based on the treatment goals are presented along with special populations and considerations.

Mood Stabilizers: Lithium, Valproate, Lamotrigine, and Carbamazepine

Mood stabilizers were originally a drug class characterized by the ability to resolve and prevent mania. This class of drugs can further be described as treating or preventing both spectrums of mood disorders either from above or from below. "Above" in this instance refers to symptoms of mania and "below" to symptoms of depression. Mood stabilizers therefore can treat or stabilize from above, or treat mania and stabilize symptoms of mania, and, treat and stabilize from below, or treat and stabilize symptoms of depression (Fig. 16.29) [28].

In this section, we will examine the mood stabilizers with the most evidenced-based efficacy: lithium, valproate, lamotrigine, and carbamazepine. The mechanism of action and adverse effects of each will be briefly discussed (Fig. 16.30).

Lithium is the most widely studied treatment for the maintenance of bipolar disorder and is classified as a mood stabilizer. Introduced in 1949, it has the most robust evidence for long-term relapse prevention and can also be used in the acute mania setting. Lithium is considered the most efficacious medication for treating bipolar disorder. A meta-analysis of

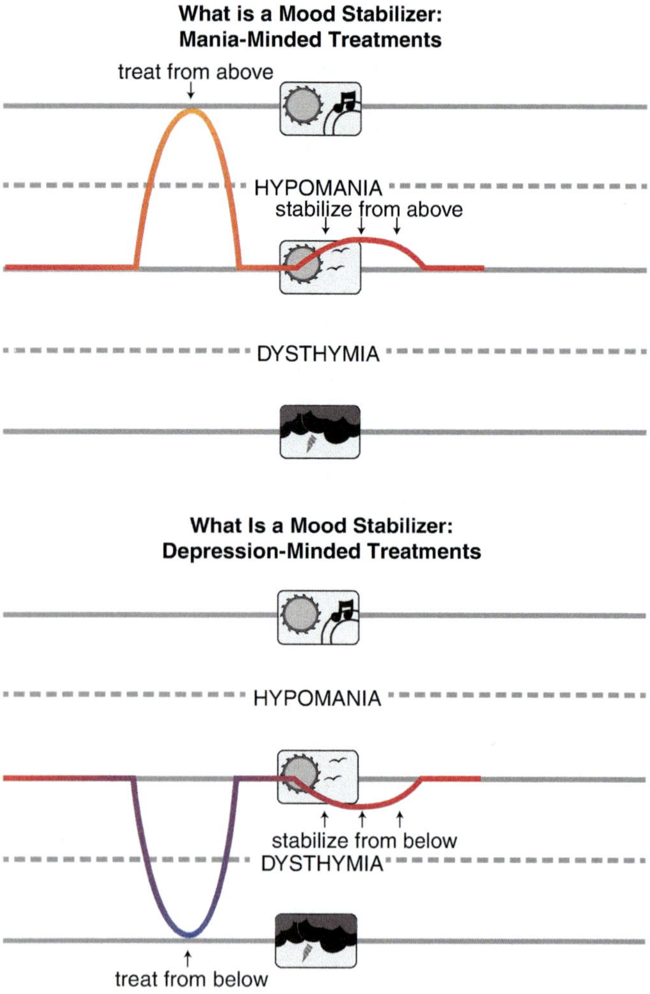

Fig. 16.29 Mood stabilizers treat and stabilize from above and below. Mood stabilizers are characterized by the ability to treat or stabilize symptoms of mania ("from above") and to treat or stabilize symptoms of depression ("from below")

five placebo-controlled maintenance studies found that reduction of manic relapses was decreased by 38% and depressive relapses by 28% for patients on maintenance lithium [29, 30]. In addition, lithium has been shown to reduce the risk of death by suicide by over 50% and is the only medication in the treatment of bipolar disorder with randomized evidence for suicide reduction (Fig. 16.31) [30, 31].

Lithium

Mechanism of action. The mechanism of action for lithium is not well characterized. Various mechanisms have been proposed, including inhibition of the inositol monophosphate system, which increases neuronal growth cone spreading at therapeutic concentrations. Lithium may also be neuroprotective through the mediation by inhibition of GSK-3 and protein kinase C pathway (Fig. 16.32) [28].

Adverse effects. Lithium's limitations come in the range of negative adverse events with maintenance therapy. These symptoms can range from nonspecific complaints to multiple other systems. Hypothyroidism is a known side effect of lithium therapy, and thyroid levels must be continuously monitored. Patients with renal impairments must also avoid lithium therapy as kidney injuries are possible while on lithium. Nephrogenic diabetes insipidus is another potential side effect of therapy as lithium interferes with ADH signaling. Additionally, lithium is known to have teratogenic effects, including cardiac malformations, in particular Ebstein anomaly (Table 16.6) (Fig. 16.33) [31].

Valproate

Valproate, also known as valproic acid or divalproex, is an antiepileptic that is also used as a mood stabilizer in bipolar disorder. Although lithium is the mainstay of treatment, it is estimated that anywhere between 20% and 40% of patients do not respond to lithium, making valproate an important alternative [31]. Valproate is used in similar settings as lithium to treat both acute and maintenance bipolar. Although its use has increased significantly in the treatment of bipolar disorder recently, placebo-controlled trials with valproate are lacking [30]. In the two studies that have been conducted, valproate has been shown to reduce any recurrent mood episodes by 30% compared to placebo, and four trials have found it to be comparable to lithium in effectiveness on recurrence; however, valproate seems to be better tolerated than lithium [31].

Mechanism of action. Similar to lithium, the mechanism of valproate is not well understood. It is thought that the mood stabilizing effects come from possibly the inhibition of GABA transaminase, which therefore increases the concentration of GABA in the synapse or by the inactivation of sodium channels decreasing neuronal excitability (Fig. 16.34) [28].

Adverse effects. Valproate is a medication that does not affect the renal system and therefore can be used when patients are unable to tolerate lithium due to renal complications. Valproate, however, can cause hepatotoxicity (rare), and liver function tests must be ordered prior to initiation and monitored. Teratogenicity also exists with valproate as it can cause neural tube defects. Additional side effects include gastrointestinal upset, tremors, alopecia, weight gain, pancreatitis, sedation, ataxia, rash, thrombocytopenia, and agranulocytosis [31].

Lamotrigine

Lamotrigine is another antiepileptic drug classified as a mood stabilizer that is considered a second-line treatment for maintenance of bipolar disorder. Notably, lamotrigine is not indicated in the acute treatment of mania [32]. Although evidence is more mixed and uncertain of the effectiveness

Fig. 16.30 FDA-approved treatment for bipolar disorder

U.S. Food and Drug Administration—approved treatments for bipolar disorder

Year of approval	Drug
Acute mania	
1970	Lithium[P/A]
1973	Chlorpromazine
1994	Divalproex, divalproex ER (2005)
2000	Olanzapine [A/M, P/A]
2003	Risperidone[A/M, P/A]
2004	Quetiapine, quetiapine XR (2008)[A/M, P/A]
2004	Ziprasidone
2004	Aripiprazole[A/M, P/A]
2004	Carbamazepine ERC
2009	Asenapine[A/M]
Acute bipolar depression	
2003	Olanzapine + fluoxetine combination
2006	Quetiapine, quetiapine XR (2008)
2013	Lurasidone[A/M]
Bipolar maintenance	
1974	Lithium[P/A]
2003	Lamotrigine
2004	Olanzapine
2005	Aripiprazole[A/M, P/A]
2008	Quetiapine, quetiapine XR (adjunct)
2009	Risperidone LAI[A/M]
2009	Ziprasidone (adjunct)

Note. LAI=long-acting injectable formulation.
[A/M]Adjunctive and monotherapy.
[P/A]Pediatric and adult.
Source. Adapted from Ketter and Wang 2010b.

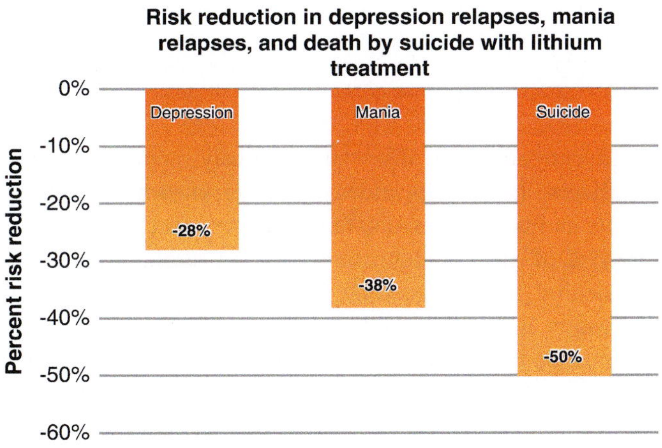

Fig. 16.31 Percent in risk reduction with lithium treatment. Lithium reduces the risk of depression relapse, mania relapse, and death by suicide with lithium treatment

of lamotrigine, a meta-analysis of three trials as well as a follow-up trial showed lamotrigine superior to placebo and comparable to lithium for maintenance relapse. Similar to valproate, a paucity of evidence exists on the effectiveness of lamotrigine in bipolar disorder. Additionally, lamotrigine appears to be better tolerated than lithium and could yield an acceptable alternative to lithium treatment and is possibly better than lithium at preventing depressive episodes [30, 33, 34].

Mechanism of action. Lamotrigine is also thought to stabilize mood by decreasing neuronal transmission. Lamotrigine inhibits sodium channels leading to decreased glutamate release and decreased neuronal excitability. Additionally, hypotheses exist that lamotrigine may have actions on other channels such as calcium and potassium. Overall, lamotrigine is an additional mood stabilizer thought to decrease neuronal excitation [28].

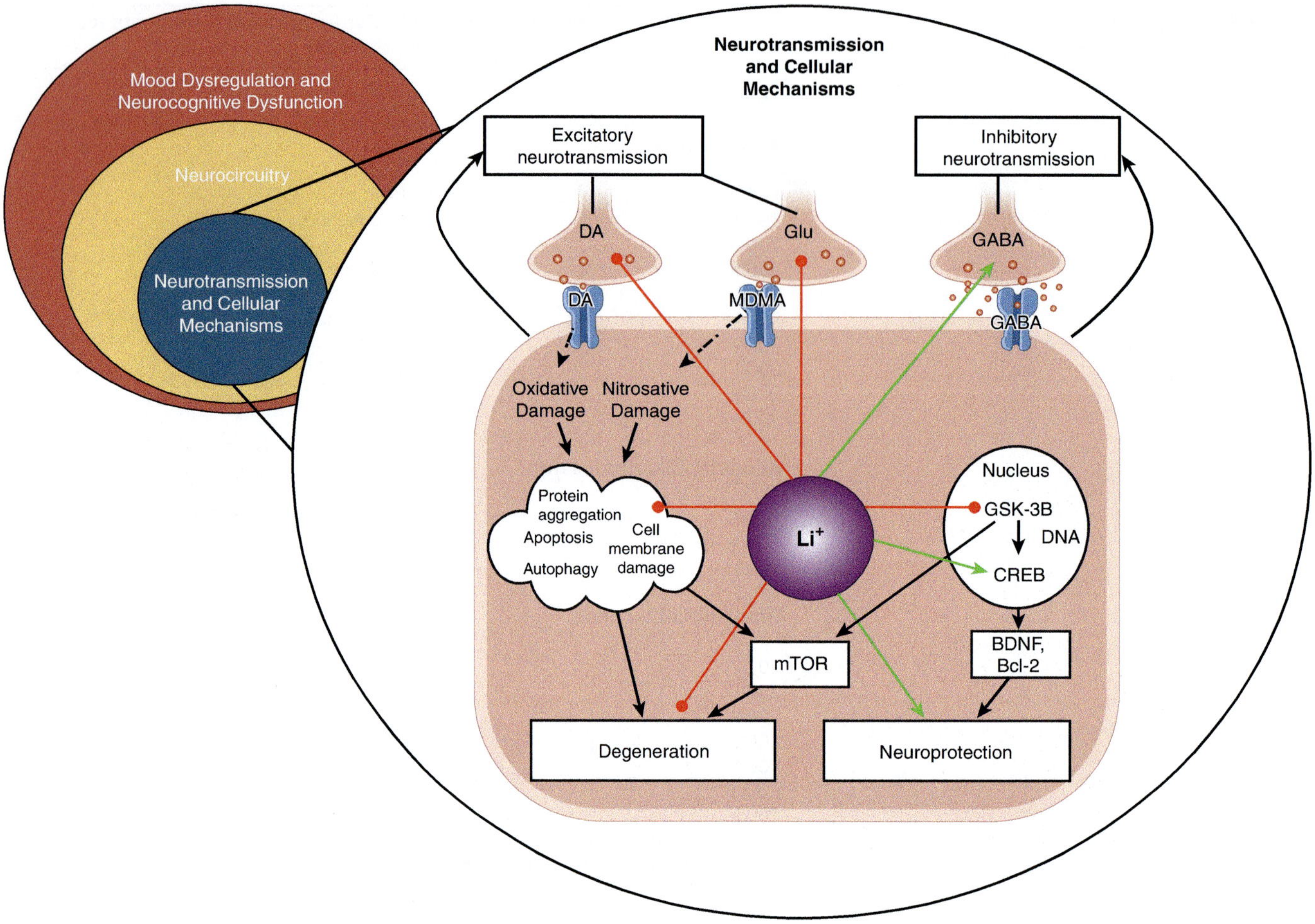

Fig. 16.32 A framework for understanding the impact of lithium treatment for bipolar disorder. Lithium inhibits (red arrows) and facilitates (green arrows) a number of neurotransmitter and cellular signal transduction mechanisms involved in degeneration and neuroprotection. In terms of key mechanisms, lithium inhibits neuroprogression through the excitotoxic damage-GSK-3β-mTOR and excitotoxic damage-GSK-3β-CREB-neurotrophin encoding pathways involved in neural degeneration and neuroprotection, where excitotoxic damage has occurred through oxidative and nitrosative damage pathways. These mechanisms are framed within the wider context of the therapeutic effects of lithium on the neurocircuitry dysfunction and mood dysregulation and neurocognitive dysfunction characteristic of bipolar disorder

Table 16.6 Summary of adverse effects of lithium therapy

General/GI	Nausea, diarrhea, weight gain, dry mucous membranes, leukocytosis
Motor	Nonprogressive tremor, muscle weakness
Dermatologic	Acne, worsening of psoriasis, thinning of hair
Cardiac	T wave depressions, U waves, dysfunction of sinus mode
Endocrine	Hypothyroidism, hyperparathyroidism, hypercalcemia, goiter
Renal	Nephrogenic diabetes insipidus, chronic interstitial nephritis
Pregnancy related	Cardiac malformations, Ebstein anomaly
Lithium toxicity (serum levels >1.5 mEq/L)	Nausea, vomiting, diarrhea, altered mental status, somnolence, acute kidney failure. Can be triggered by increased dose, intentional overdose, medication use (e.g., thiazide, NSAIDs, ACEi) [32]

Adverse effects. Unlike the previously mentioned mood stabilizers, lamotrigine does not have known teratogenic effects and is considered safe during pregnancy. It carries a rare risk of Stevens–Johnson syndrome (a potentially life-threatening immune-mediated skin reaction characterized by blisters and epidermal detachment). Therefore, lamotrigine must be titrated up slowly. Additional concerns are lymphohistiocytosis, hepatotoxicity (rare), nephrotoxicity (rare), blurry vision, and gastrointestinal symptoms (Fig. 16.35) [35].

Carbamazepine

Carbamazepine is yet another antiepileptic that can be used as a mood stabilizer and has been used for the treatment of trigeminal neuralgia. In fact, it was the first antiepileptic

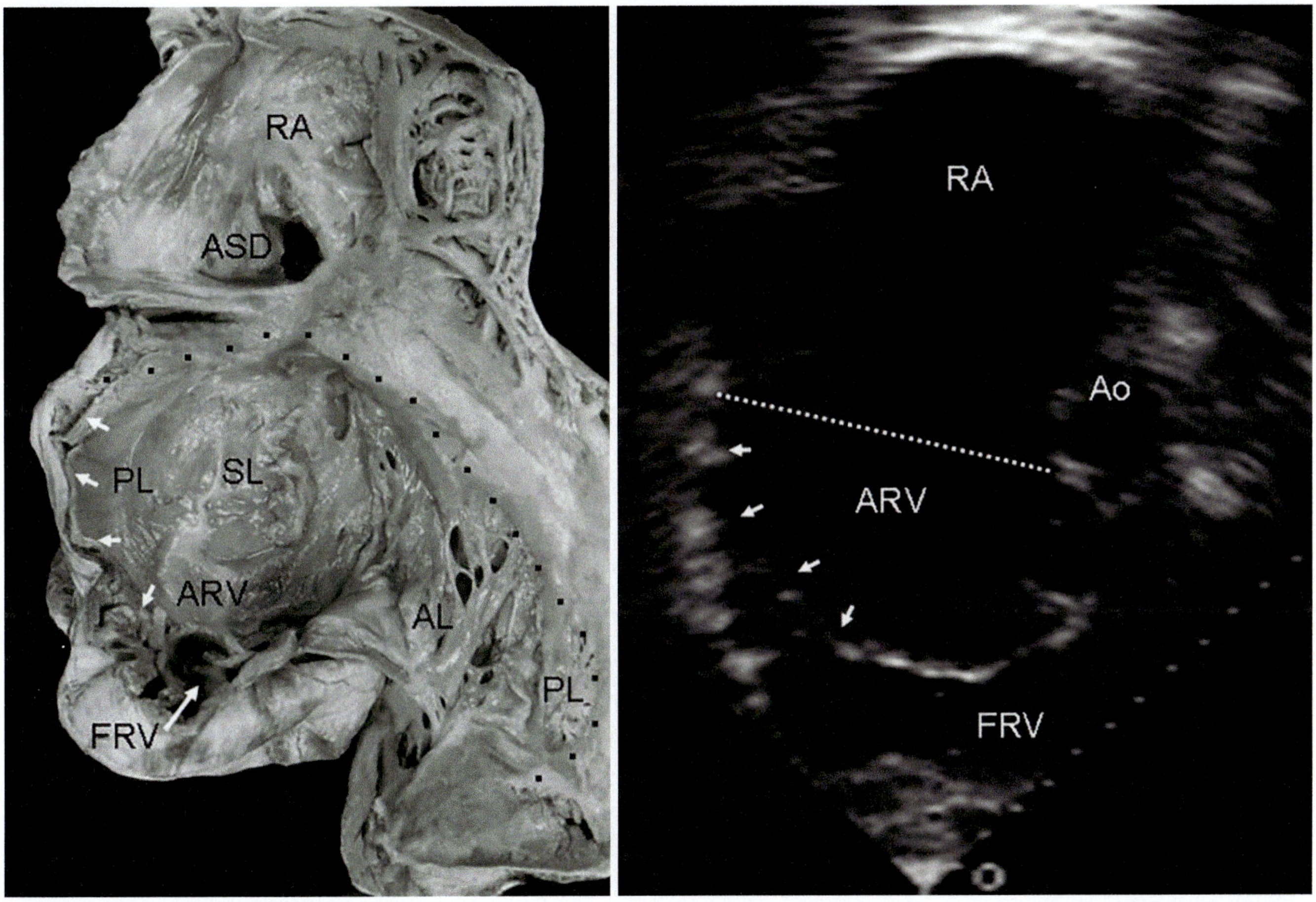

Fig. 16.33 Ebstein anomaly. Left: view of right heart chambers with tethering of tricuspid septal and posterior leaflets to the ventricular wall (short arrows). Long arrows demonstrate a reduction in the functional portion of the right ventricle. Right: echocardiogram demonstrating atrialized right ventricle. *RA* right atrium; *ARV* atrialized right ventricle; *FRV* functional right ventricle; *AL* anterior leaflet; *PL* posterior leaflet; *SL* septal leaflet; *ASD* atrial septal defect; *LA* left atrium; *LV* left ventricle; *AO* aorta. (Wikimedia Commons; Creative Commons Attribution 3.0 Unported; https://creativecommons.org/licenses/by/3.0/)

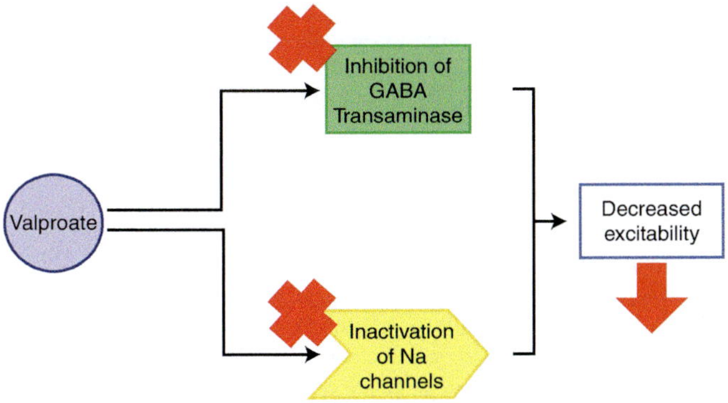

Fig. 16.34 Proposed mechanism of valproate. Valproate inhibits GABA transaminase leading to higher levels of GABA and more neuronal inhibition. Valproate inactivates Na channels, which additionally leads to decreased excitability

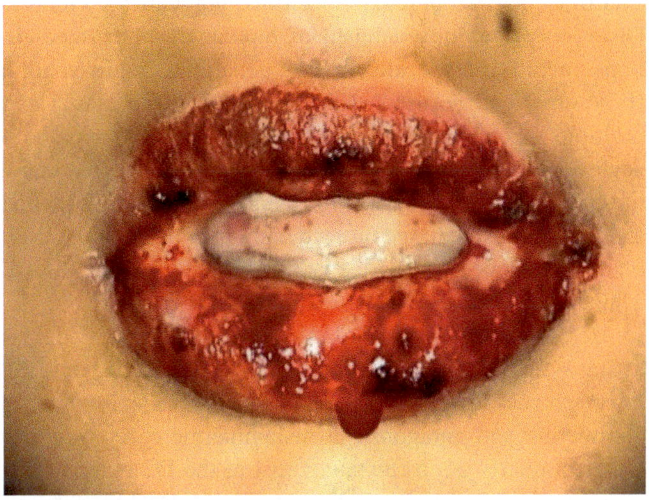

Fig. 16.35 Photograph of Stevens–Johnson syndrome. Lamotrigine carries a risk of Stevens–Johnson syndrome, depicted here on a patient's lips (Wikimedia Commons; Creative Commons Attribution 3.0 Unported; https://creativecommons.org/licenses/by/3.0/)

drug to be shown effective in treating mania. Evidence suggests carbamazepine may be useful in the acute manic phase and has been found to reduce recurrence and hospitalizations; however, these studies did not include a placebo arm [36]. It is thought to act similarly to valproate, inhibiting sodium channels; however, it may act on a different site on the channel [28]. For maintenance therapy, carbamazepine may be used as adjuvant therapy but is seldomly used as monotherapy.

Oxcarbazepine, as the name suggests, is structurally similar to carbamazepine. *Oxcarbamazepine* likely has fewer adverse events than carbamazepine; however, evidence suggests uncertainty or doubtful efficacy in the treatment of bipolar disorder [28].

Adverse effects. Carbamazepine carries multiple risks. Unique to other mood stabilizers, agranulocytosis and aplastic anemia are known possible effects of carbamazepine therapy, and blood levels should be continuously monitored. Carbamazepine can also be teratogenic, causing cleft lip/palate, especially with first-trimester use. Similar to lamotrigine, there is an increased risk for Stevens–Johnson syndrome as well with carbamazepine. Other effects include hyponatremia secondary to syndrome of inappropriate ADH (SIADH), drug reaction with eosinophilia and systemic symptoms (DRESS) syndrome (a rare hypersensitivity reaction), nausea, rash, diplopia, ataxia, hepatotoxicity, and induction of the cytochrome p-450 system, which may interact with other medications.

Antipsychotics

Antipsychotics are a heterogeneous class of substances used in the treatment of a variety of illnesses including bipolar disorder. Antipsychotics are discussed in further detail in Chap. 15 "Schizophrenia Spectrum and Other Psychotic Disorders". For the treatment of bipolar disorder, medications include haloperidol, a first-generation antipsychotic (FGA) that can be used in the setting of acute mania and multiple second-generation antipsychotics (SGA) for both acute and maintenance therapy. Evidence suggests that many of the SGAs are appropriate for the treatment of bipolar and should be adjusted based on each individual patient, although olanzapine appears to be the best tolerated with data that is available [37].

Mechanism of action. FGAs primarily has its effects by acting as a D2 antagonist. Although less pronounced than the lower potency FGAs, haloperidol also acts as an agonist at cholinergic and antagonist at histaminergic receptors. The SGAs similarly act as an antagonist at the D2 receptor but have an additional antagonism at the 5-HT2A receptor. Additionally, there are interactions with several other receptors with SGAs including D3, D4, alpha-adrenergic, and H1 receptors. Aripiprazole is a unique SGA as it is considered a partial agonist at the D2 receptor. The mood-altering effects of antipsychotics are poorly understood. It is hypothesized that a variety of serotonergic receptors as well as norepinephrine reuptake inhibition and alpha 2 antagonists play a role in the antidepressant effects, while D2 and 5-HT2A blockade are responsible for the antimanic effects [28].

Adverse effects. Generally speaking, SGA tends to have less severe side effects than FGA, making them more ideal for use in treatment, as summarized in Table 16.7 [28].

Clinical tips are provided to clinicians, as shown in Table 16.8.

Table 16.7 Summary of antipsychotic adverse effects

First-generation antipsychotics	Extrapyramidal symptoms, prolonged QT interval, neuroleptic malignant syndrome. Metabolic syndrome effects, hyperprolactinemia, anticholinergic effects, sedation
Second-generation antipsychotics	Metabolic syndrome effects (more so than FGA), prolonged QT interval, hyperprolactinemia (less than FGA), extrapyramidal symptoms (less than FGA), sedation, anticholinergic effects *Clozapine may cause agranulocytosis

*It is used as a specific clarification point for the adverse effects of clozapine as a second-generation antipsychotic.

Table 16.8 Principles in the treatment of bipolar disorders [65]

1. Maintain dual treatment focus: (a) acute short term and (b) prophylaxis
2. Chart illness retrospectively and prospectively
3. Mania as medical emergency; treat first; chemistries later
4. Load valproate and lithium (Eskalith); titrate lamotrigine (Lamictal) slowly
5. Careful combination treatment can decrease adverse effects
6. Augment rather than substitute in treatment-resistant patients
7. Retain lithium in the regimen for its antisuicide and neuroprotective effects
8. Taper lithium slowly, if at all
9. Educate patients and families about illness and risk-to-benefit ratios of acute and prophylactic treatments
10. Give statistics (i.e., 50% relapse in first 5 months of lithium)
11. Assess compliance and suicidality regularly
12. Develop an early warning system for the identification and treatment of emergent symptoms
13. Contract with the patient as needed for suicide and substance use avoidance
14. Use regular visits; monitor course and adverse effects
15. Arrange for interval phone contact when needed
16. Develop fire drill for mania reemergence
17. Inquire about and address comorbid alcohol and substance abuse
18. Targeted psychotherapy; use medicalization of illness
19. Treat the patient as a coinvestigator in the development of effective clinical approaches to the illness
20. If treatment is successful, be conservative in making changes, maintain the course, and continue full-dose pharmacoprophylaxis in the absence of side effects
21. If treatment response is inadequate, be aggressive in searching for more effective alternatives

Antidepressants: Benzodiazepines and Other Medications

Antidepressants are a class of medication used to treat a variety of psychiatric conditions, including depression, anxiety, and PTSD. Its role, however, in bipolar disorder remains controversial. Several classes of antidepressants exist, including selective serotonin reuptake inhibitors (SSRIs), serotonin-norepinephrine reuptake inhibitors (SNRIs), monoamine oxidase inhibitors (MAOIs), and tricyclic antidepressants (TCAs). Further details on antidepressants are discussed in Chap. 17 "Depressive Disorders". Use of antidepressants in bipolar is controversial for multiple reasons. For one, there is insufficient evidence to draw conclusions and understand the use of antidepressants in bipolar disorder [38]. In addition, the use of an antidepressant may induce a "switch" from a depressed state to manic or trigger the onset of rapid cycling. This switch seems to be more pronounced with the use of TCAs and SNRIs over other classes of antidepressants [38, 39]. Additionally, systematic reviews indicate that antidepressants do not appear to be effective in treating short-term bipolar depression and monotherapy with any antidepressant is not recommended. The only indication for use may be in second-line therapy for treatment-resistant bipolar depression (see treatment options below).

Benzodiazepines

Benzodiazepines are a class of sedative hypnotic drugs that target the GABA system creating central nervous system depression. As such, benzodiazepines are often used to treat anxiety disorders, seizures, insomnia, agitation, and alcohol withdrawal. Their use in bipolar disorder predominantly lies in the acute setting. Patients with mania symptoms may benefit from short-term use of a benzodiazepine such as clonazepam or lorazepam. Monotherapy is not common, and benzodiazepines are not used in the long-term maintenance of bipolar disorder. In fact, there may be an association between increased relapse and benzodiazepine use, or alternatively more severe bipolar disorder is associated with benzodiazepine use [40]. In addition, this class of medication carries a high risk of tolerance and overuse, with both intoxication and withdrawal as potential means for death.

Other Medications

Tamoxifen is a medication that is a selective estrogen receptor modulator used primarily in the treatment of estrogen-positive breast cancers. Recently, it has been investigated for use in treating mania. A systematic review and meta-analysis with five placebo randomized controlled trials concluded that tamoxifen was superior to placebo at reducing mania scale scores, suggesting a new potential treatment option for mania episodes in bipolar disorder [41].

Allopurinol is another novel treatment option for bipolar disorder. Typically, allopurinol is used to treat gouty arthritis and nephropathy. Studies suggest that it may be useful as add-on treatment for acute mania [42].

Choosing Treatment Options

Acute Mania

Acute mania can be separated into severe mania and mild to moderate mania [26, 43, 44]. In patients with severe mania, this can present as a medical emergency, often requiring hospitalization. First-line treatment involves the use of both a mood stabilizer (lithium or valproic acid) and a FGA or SGA. Although there is no data to suggest that one mood stabilizer is better than the other, individual patient factors should be taken into account. For example, if a patient has renal impairment, lithium should be avoided; if a patient has liver disease or is pregnant, avoid valproate. Antipsychotics are indicated in this instance due to the more rapid onset of action compared to mood stabilizers. Regarding the choice of antipsychotic, data is limited to providing efficacy comparisons. However, some data suggest that olanzapine is better tolerated and may provide better depressive symptom relief [45], and olanzapine, risperidone, and haloperidol seem to have the best efficacy and acceptability (Fig. 16.36) [30]. Should a patient fail this initial regimen, switching mood stabilizers is the next step in treatment (lithium to val-

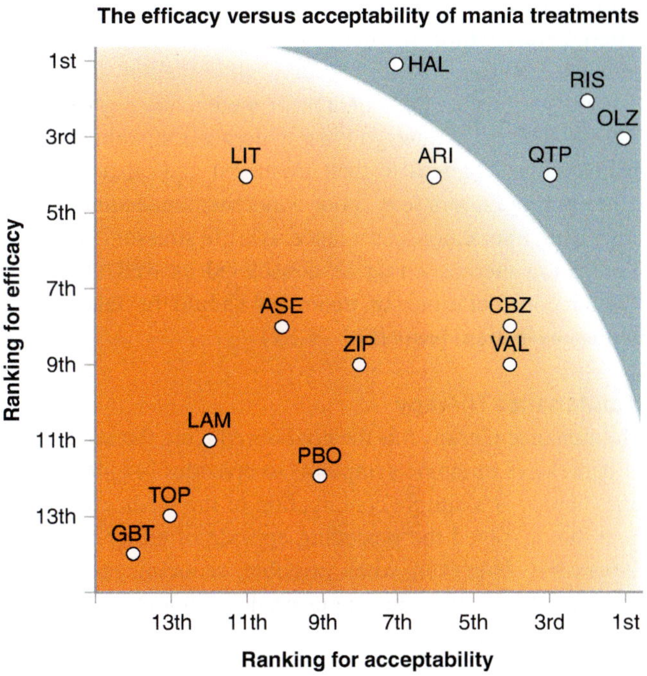

Fig. 16.36 Efficacy vs acceptability of mood stabilizers and antipsychotics in the treatment of mania

proate or valproate to lithium), followed by switching antipsychotics should desired results not be achieved. As discussed above, carbamazepine may also be trialed in the acute mania phase for resolution. In the acute severe manic stage, benzodiazepines may be indicated for use, for example, clozapine or lorazepam, especially if decreased sleep is being experienced by the patient or agitation and/or safety is a concern.

For less severe mania, monotherapy with either a mood stabilizer or antipsychotic is an option. Again, if the faster onset of action is desired, an antipsychotic would be preferable. Similar to severe mania, the choice in medication should examine a patient's medical history and individual circumstances. Should patients fail monotherapy treatment after multiple trials of different mood stabilizers and or antipsychotics, dual therapy with both a mood stabilizer and antipsychotic should be tried, similar to the recommendation for severe mania (Fig. 16.36).

Bipolar Depression

Treatment of bipolar depression is to reduce the severity and or frequency of depressive symptoms or cessation of suicidal ideation [26]. First-line therapy for bipolar depression involves monotherapy with either quetiapine or lurasidone, both SGAs. Quetiapine may be preferred as it has more evidence and may provide benefit in long-term maintenance therapy. Second-line therapy involves multiple options, including the combination of quetiapine or lurasidone plus lithium or valproate, olanzapine plus fluoxetine, or valproate monotherapy. Third-line therapy introduces lamotrigine and carbamazepine as well as other combination therapies. Patients who were stable on a prior medication regimen and present with breakthrough bipolar depression should be re-evaluated for changes to their treatment and other possible confounding factors (e.g., poor adherence, inadequate dose, other drug interactions, substance use, life stressors). Add-on medication therapy could be considered as well. As prior, special considerations in treatment should be taken on a patient-by-patient basis (Fig. 16.37).

Maintenance Therapy

Maintenance therapy has the goal of reducing the recurrence of depressive or manic symptoms or episodes [44, 46]. First-line therapy is a simple continuation of the medication regimen that resolved the preceding episode of either mania or depression. However, when possible, reducing medication regimens to monotherapy is desired to increase adherence and decrease potential adverse effects. Should patients find that their first-line therapy is not effective, moving to monotherapy second line is recommended. Medications for maintenance therapy may be decided upon based on preventing either manic or depressive relapses [46] (Fig. 16.38). In general, one of the mood stabilizers (lithium, valproate, or lamotrigine) or a SGA is acceptable second-line options. Third-line therapy involves monotherapy with a SGA such as risperidone or olanzapine. Considerations should be made based on patient circumstances and previously discussed adverse effects.

Special Considerations and Populations

Postpartum patients wishing to breastfeed: Unsurprisingly, postpartum patients are less likely to relapse into a manic or depressive state if taking medical therapy for bipolar disorder [47]. However, special consideration must be made when choosing a medication if the mother wishes to breastfeed. If possible, avoiding lithium and lamotrigine is preferred and can be replaced with valproate or carbamazepine [48]. In regard to antipsychotic use, a lack of evidence makes it difficult to draw conclusions. With the exception of clozapine and olanzapine, most antipsychotics are considered alternatives to mood stabilizers during breastfeeding [49].

Geriatric population: Recent evidence has implicated that the use of both FGAs and SGAs increases the risk of cerebrovascular accidents (CVAs), especially in an older population [50]. Given this increased risk, the pros and cons of treatment with an antipsychotic must be weighed. In general, similar treatment options exist for geriatric populations as for adults. Given the risk of CVA, this population should be taken into special consideration [51].

Psychosocial Interventions

A number of empirical and evidence-based psychosocial treatments for the population of bipolar and related disorders have been extensively researched to date [52]. Certainly, the greatest likelihood of a favorable treatment outcome is possible through a holistic and eclectic treatment approach that incorporates biological interventions (as discussed in the previous section), psychotherapeutic interventions, review of routine practices that both teach and reinforce optimal self-care/self-management techniques, and a variety of additional interventions to scaffold behavior.

While a detailed review of validated and randomized clinical trials for psychosocial treatments and interventions remains beyond the scope of this chapter [53], there are select treatment modalities worth favorable mention. Specifically, for adult populations, cognitive behavior therapy, family-focused therapy, mindfulness-based interventions, cognitive remediation, group psychoeducation, and interpersonal and social rhythm therapy (IPSRT) are among the most developed and appear to be beneficial in improving

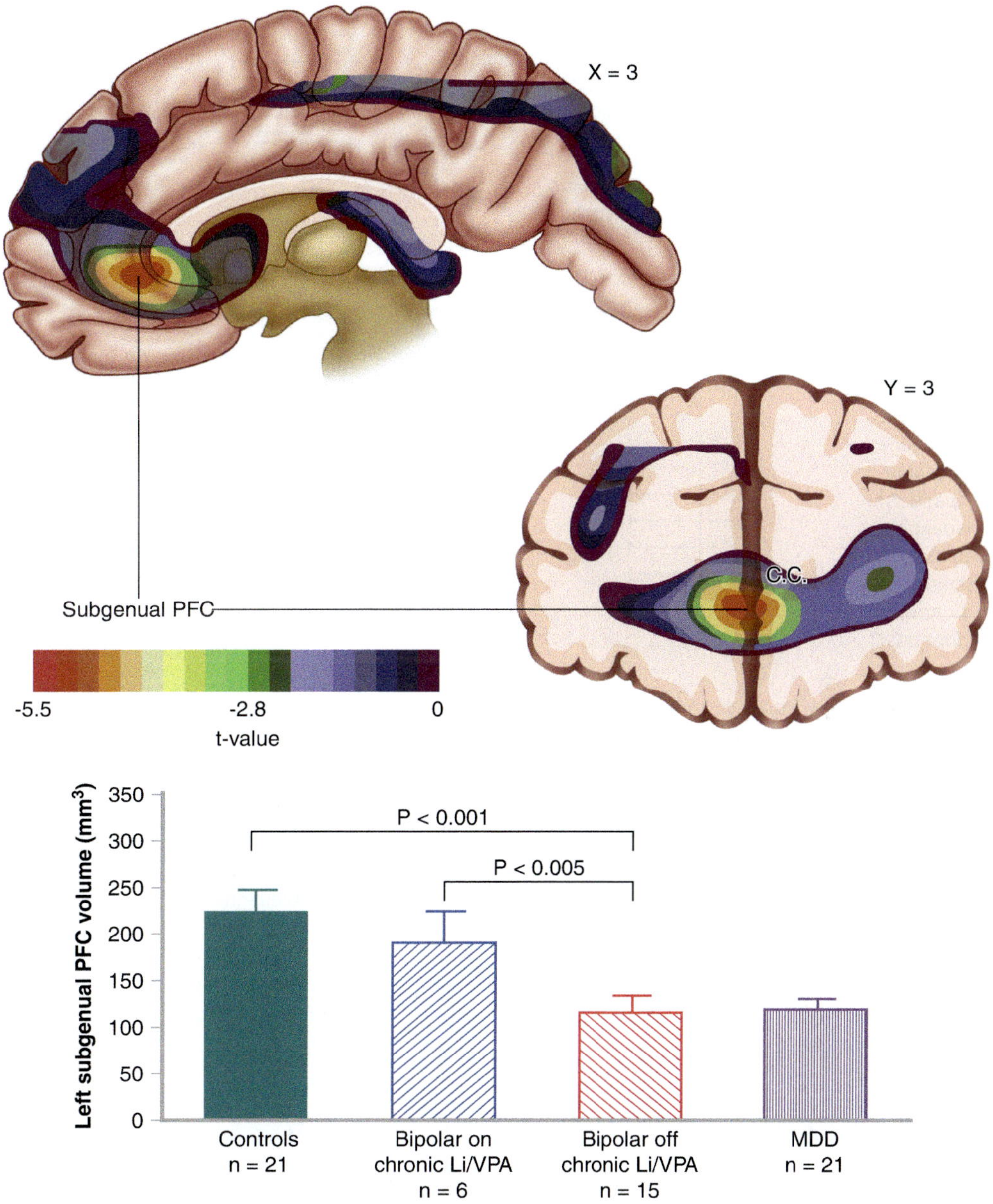

Fig. 16.37 Upper panel: Coronal (31 mm anterior to the anterior commissure; $y = 31$) and sagittal (3 mm left of midline; $x = -3$) sections showing negative voxel t-values where glucose metabolism is decreased in individuals with depression relative to controls. The reduction in activity in this prefrontal cortex (PFC) region located in the anterior cingulate gyrus ventral to the genu of the corpus callosum (i.e., subgenual) appeared to be accounted for by a corresponding reduction in cortex volume (Table 8.1; reproduced from Drevets et al. (1997)). Anterior or left is to the left. Lower Panel: Although the PET data shown in the upper panel were obtained exclusively in unmedicated subjects, the volumetric MRI data from this study were obtained in a larger sample that included six cases who had been chronically receiving lithium or valproate prior to scanning. The bar histogram shows the mean subgenual anterior cingulate cortex (sgACC) volumes in mm^3 for the healthy controls, individuals with major depressive disorder (MDD), unmedicated individuals with bipolar depression, and subjects with bipolar disorder (BD) chronically medicated with lithium or valproate

symptoms associated with any of the subtypes of bipolar disorder, as well as reducing rates of recurrence (Table 16.9) [26, 52, 53].

Notably, however, the treatment of this population is generally divided into two distinct phases, namely the acute phase of treatment, which focuses on the management of acute mood episodes, and the maintenance phase of treatment, which emphasizes a significant focus on preventing the recurrence of an acute episode [26]. Furthermore, the therapeutic alliance is an important cornerstone in the delivery of treatment for patients with bipolar disorders, as a strong therapeutic alliance will help increase the likelihood of treatment adherence, increase the likelihood of greater treatment engagement, and help reduce feelings of suicidal ideation [26]. In relation, the collective efforts of mutual treatment providers and collaborators (i.e., psychologists, psychiatrists, PCPs, case managers), as well as supplemental community resources (e.g., local support groups, substance use treatment centers, subsidized mental health centers, other community-based resources), are certainly of additional benefit to patients with bipolar disorders [26]. Furthermore, it is important for clinicians to determine what factors may be associated with psychotropic medication compliance/adherence among patients with bipolar disorders, as identification of reasons for non-compliance may be reviewed in psychotherapy (Fig. 16.39) [54].

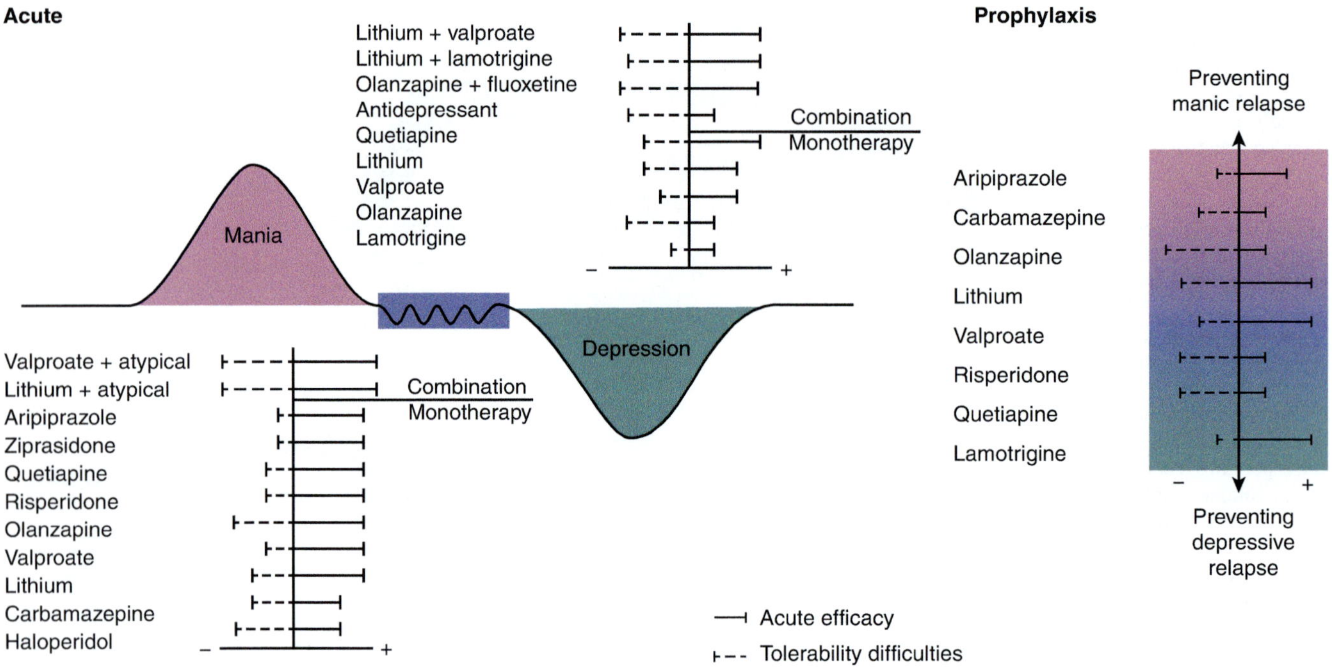

Fig. 16.38 Comparison of treatment options for acute vs prophylaxis (maintenance). The figure illustrates medication therapies for acute mania and depression as well as maintenance therapy with prevention targets

Table 16.9 Specific psychosocial interventions and their targeted therapeutic effect in bipolar disorder

Intervention	Efficacy					
	Relapse/ recurrence	Manic symptoms	Depressive symptoms	Anxiety	Neurocognition	Overall functioning
CBT	No	–	Yes	–	–	–
Psychoeducation	Yes	No	No	–	–	Yes
IPSRT	Eq	Eq	Eq	–	–	–
Family intervention	No	No	No	–	–	No
Intensive psychosocial intervention	–	–	–	–	–	–
Cognitive remediation	No	No	No	–	No	No
Mindfulness-based interventions	No	No	No	Yes	–	–

Eq equivocal

Reprinted from Miziou et al. [49]; Creative Commons Attribution 4.0 International License; https://creativecommons.org/licenses/by/4.0/

Other Interventions

Electroconvulsive Therapy

Electroconvulsive therapy (ECT) is another treatment proven useful in managing severe depressive, manic, and mixed states [55]. In a study of 522 individuals, 68.8% of the cases had a positive response to ECT across all phases of severe and drug-resistant BD.

Self-Management

The self-management of bipolar and related disorders is a vital practice that should be complementary to more formal means of psychotherapeutic care. As seen in Table 16.10, self-management can be accomplished by a variety of accessible means [56].

Many platforms such as workbooks, mobile technologies, and Internet-based/peer-led interventions utilize these strategies in bipolar management (Table 16.11) [56].

Limitations of the Biopsychosocial Model

Ever since Engel and Romano proposed the biopsychosocial model, it has achieved wide acceptance in psychiatry. Since its introduction, it has gained popularity both in teaching and in clinical practice, coming to be viewed as the overarching framework of the field. Despite its following, the model is not without its critics. The latter have been quick to point out its limitations, both in its scientific validity and in its usefulness in practice (Table 16.12).

Emotion Regulation Bipolar Disorder Handout

Reducing Vulnerability to a Manic Mood Episode in Bipolar Disorder

CAMERAS

C	**Check mood:** • When a mood episode is beginning, you may be starting to notice that your emotions are growing stronger or heightening, Pay attention to these cues. For a manic episode, you may be noticing that your confidence levels are rising, or it may be subtler, and you find yourself feeling happy or excited more often throughout the day. Whatever the signs are for you at this moment, try to describe and observe them nonjudgmentally. Notice if you have experienced these cues before.
A	**Analyze the pros and cons of goals:** • When beginning a manic or hypomanic episode, you may find that you start setting high goals for yourself. It could be work related, for example agreeing to take on five projects at once, or perhaps socially related, such as making several plans with friends. Before you begin working on your goal, it is important to weigh the pros and cons to decide if it is a realistic goal in this moment. It also will help you detect whether these goals are contributing to your hypomanic or manic symptoms.
M	**Minimize stimulation:** • If you have walked through the steps and determined that a hypomanic or manic episode may be coming on, it is important to create an environment for yourself that does not increase these symptoms. Maybe take some time to yourself instead of going out to a party or perhaps take some time off work.
E	**Evaluate confidence levels:** • Individuals with bipolar disorder may experience times of extreme confidence where they think they are on top of the world. Both low and high levels of confidence can increase vulnerabflity to developing a mood episode. If you are feeling high in confidence it can be a good idea to check back on your past successes and shortcomings when approaching a goal. If you cannot think of anything on your own, you could ask a friend/family member for their opinions.
R	**Relax:** • Now that you have lessened stimulation, you want to promote relaxation. This can be done using progressive relaxation or deep breathing techniques. Progressive relaxation has been shown to benefit individuals struggling with hypomanic and manic symptoms. You could also brainstorm strategies that you think could work or have worked for you in the past (i.e. listening to calming music, gardening, taking a bath).
A	**Ask for help and feedback:** • When you begin to observe and label your behaviors as being typical of symptoms you experience before a mood episode, it is important to let someone know. Phone a friend, family member, or a mental health professional so that you are not alone in dealing with your symptoms, and they can assist you in getting the right help. Another person may also be a reliable source in providing you feedback if you are experiencing symptoms.
S	**Sleep: Monitor Schedule:** • People with bipolar disorder experience sleep disturbance in both manic and depressive episodes. In mania, a person may go several nights in a row without sleeping. Sleep disturbances can also trigger the onset of a mood episode. Interventions have been designed to target sleep problems in bipolar disorder and have been proven to be effective in reducing mood symptoms. Monitoring your sleep schedule and promoting healthy sleep patterns can be a beneficial tool towards regulating your symptoms.

Fig. 16.39 Dialectical behavioral therapy (DBT) skills handout and worksheet adapted for the treatment of bipolar disorder titled "CAMERAS." CAMERAS stands for: Check mood, Analyze the pros and cons of goals, Maximize/Minimize stimulation, Evaluate confidence levels, Relax, Ask for help, and Sleep monitoring

Table 16.10 Self-management strategies in bipolar disorder

1. Providing education on accurate diagnosis, symptoms, medication adherence, and side effects, and avoidance of substance use
2. Self-monitoring mood, depression, and energy daily
3. Optimizing sleep hygiene
4. Setting goals in the following domains: relationships, employment, education, health, recreation, house/homecare, and self-management
5. Prioritizing a healthy lifestyle: regular physical activity, healthy eating, and weight loss and/or weight management

Table 16.12 Summary of criticisms of the biopsychosocial model

1. Not a model: descriptive, not predictive
2. Vague, "fluffy," and lacks coherence
3. Vague conception of biology
4. Unclear boundaries between "bio," "psycho," and "social"
5. Fails to curtail the advance of biomedical psychiatry
6. Fails to appropriately account for the patient's subjective experience
7. Unsophisticated approach to cultural identity
8. Shortcomings as a teaching tool

Table 16.11 Currently available self-management resources for bipolar disorder by mode of delivery

Mode of delivery	Psychoeducation	Mood monitoring	Sleep hygiene	Setting goals	Physical activity
Bipolar Education Programme—Cymru (BEP-C)		X	X		X
Wellness Self-Management Personal Workbook	X			X	X
Overcoming Bipolar Disorder Workbook	X			X	X
Beating Bipolar		X	X		X
Bipolar UK	X	X			

One criticism leveled against the biopsychosocial model is that it is, in fact, not a "model" in the rigorous scientific sense. The words "theory" and "model" are sometimes used interchangeably; however, in the strict sense, while a theory can be defined as an "unbodied concept or abstract notion," a model is required to meet certain criteria. It is a "formal, working representation of an idea" that is "real" and measurable. In practice, while a theory is a useful tool to explain a phenomenon post hoc, it does not have the predictive value of a model [57]. Another shortcoming of the biopsychosocial model, some argue, is its vagueness and lack of coherence. Its inclusive approach has been criticized as unscientific and "fluffy," giving equal weight and merit to different perspectives. To one author, this is reminiscent of the dodo in Alice in Wonderland, who declared: "Everybody has won, and all must have prizes" [58, 59].

Additionally, the biopsychosocial model has been criticized for its unbounded eclecticism. When the model was conceived, its creators sought to put an end to the strife that was brewing in psychiatry, between the psychoanalytic and biomedical dogmas. The goal was to combat dogmatism in psychiatry, by introducing some eclecticism into psychiatric practice and individualizing the treatment to the patient. Some argue that, in practice, this eclectic freedom has gone too far. Particularly, the boundaries and interrelationships of the "bio," "psycho," and "social" components become blurry at best when examined more closely [58]. Furthermore, in practice, practitioners chose to emphasize the "bio," the "psycho," or the "social," depending on their inclinations. If the goal of the proponents of the biopsychosocial model was to give an equal voice to the different approaches to treatment, then they have failed. By emphasizing one part over other, practitioners change the model's initial point in giving each section a certain weight. Instead of overcoming dogmatism, it allowed each clinician to enact their own dogmas [60]. This can be seen in clinical practice, where the biopsychosocial model has failed to curb the dominance of the biological approach in the past decades. This is most evident in the United States, where the vast majority of clinical research has been biomedically focused [61]. The proportion of biomedically focused articles in the American Journal of Psychiatry, for instance, has increased dramatically in the past half-century, in contrast to the British Journal of Psychiatry [62].

Another criticism leveled at the biopsychosocial model is that it does give due attention to the patient's subjective experience of illness, such as in matters of personal meaning and spirituality. Furthermore, it fails in its conceptualization of psychopathology of larger social units, such as community, culture, and society [61]. Even when cultural factors are considered—pegged under the "social" domain—it is exclusively conceptualized through a positivistic lens that assumes that the groups are homogeneous, ignoring each individual's unique lived experience of the cultural identity [63].

The biopsychosocial model is still regarded as a very useful tool in the teaching of psychiatry [57]. Nevertheless, some have questioned its value in medical education, pointing out that its vagueness and eclecticism may baffle and be rejected by medical students. As for psychiatry residents, they would be offered through their training a "confusing smorgasbord" of competing approaches to patient care [60].

Without the biopsychosocial "model" meeting the criteria or guidelines of a model, there is a loss of validity, which in turn takes away from its effectiveness in the psychiatry and medical realms. Ultimately, critics argue, the biopsychosocial model must move beyond the vague—albeit well-intentioned—inclusivity of its name, and to become a true model that is predictive as well as explanatory [64].

Proposal for Future Considerations of the Biopsychosocial Model

Use Within Healthcare Systems and Potential Pitfalls

Our current healthcare system is one in which patients, in all of their complexity, are reduced to checkboxes of billable codes and diagnoses. Documentation is increasingly geared toward meeting the criteria for those billable services rather than providing an informative and meaningful account of the clinician's observations and assessment. Clinicians often find it hard to record effective and thorough patient history. Consequently, neither the factors that make up the biopsychosocial model nor the identification of potentially valuable social or psychological interventions leads to the ability to provide to the patient. This is in part due to the inequities in our system. Physicians must be trained in not only how to use the biopsychosocial model but also how to advocate for its implementation within the systems in which they operate.

Inclusion of Structural and Cultural Factors

The intention of the BPS model is to conceptualize a patient holistically, with consideration of the factors that contribute to the development, expression, and progression of illness. Accordingly, our knowledge of how cultural and structural factors contribute to health and disease naturally leads to their inclusion. Cultures are systems of knowledge that can influence how illness is viewed, manifested, and maintained [1]. Cross-cultural evidence has highlighted how an illness such as depression is expressed and explained differently across the world [2]. Structural factors include the social, economic, and political conditions which contribute to a person's health. The result of all factors being considered in the conceptualization are interventions that target upstream forces on symptoms and diseases through advocacy and policy change [3]. For example, the inclusion of structural factors in the conceptualization of a patient with mental illness could lead to an increase in social support. Support could be given through a community organization that would assist the patient with medication affordability and larger advocacy efforts against unjust prescription drug pricing (Table 16.13).

Table 16.13 A proposal of the biopsychosocial model with the inclusion of structural and cultural factors

Structural factors	Experience of discrimination Ability to pay for treatment Incarceration Housing insecurity Access to: • Educational opportunities • Employment opportunities • Nutritional food • Outdoor spaces
Cultural factors	Language Spirituality and religion Family structures Customs and rituals Moral systems Explanatory models of illness Stigma resulting in barriers to treatment Cultural sources of strength and support Race/ethnicity
Biological	Age Sex Genetics/family history Other medical conditions Nutritional status Medications Exposure to toxins History of substances
Social factors	Educational history Relationship history (romantic and platonic) Support system Occupation history Living situation Economic status
Psychological factors	Personality traits Coping mechanisms Cognitive state (memory, negative thought patterns) Intrapersonal relationship Impulsivity History of treatment History of suicidal ideation/attempts Trauma history

References

1. American Psychiatric Association. Diagnostic and statistical manual of mental disorders. 5th ed. Washington, DC; 2013.
2. Katona C, Cooper C, Robertson M. Psychiatry at a glance. 6th ed. Chichester, West Sussex: Wiley; 2016. p. 20–1.
3. Vigo D, Thornicroft G, Atun R. Estimating the true global burden of mental illness. Lancet Psychiatry. 2016;3(2):171–8. https://doi.org/10.1016/S2215-0366(15)00505-2.
4. Bauer M, Pfennig A. Epidemiology of bipolar disorders. Epilepsia. 2005;46 https://doi.org/10.1111/j.1528-1167.2005.463003.x.
5. Ferrari AJ, Stockings E, Khoo JP, Erskine HE, Degenhardt L, Vos T, Whiteford HA. The prevalence and burden of bipolar disorder: findings from the Global Burden of Disease Study 2013. Bipolar Disord. 2016;18:440–50. https://doi.org/10.1111/bdi.1242.
6. Haack S, Pfennig A, Bauer M. Bipolare Depression. Epidemiologie, Etiopathogenesis und Verlauf [Bipolar depression. Epidemiology,

etiopathogenesis, and course]. Nervenarzt. 2010;81(5):525–30. https://doi.org/10.1007/s00115-009-2849-3.
7. Merikangas KR, Jin R, He JP, et al. Prevalence and correlates of bipolar spectrum disorder in the world mental health survey initiative. Arch Gen Psychiatry. 2011;68(3):241–51. https://doi.org/10.1001/archgenpsychiatry.2011.12.
8. Boyd RC, Joe S, Michalopoulos L, Davis E, Jackson JS. Prevalence of mood disorders and service use among US mothers by race and ethnicity: results from the national Survey of American life. J Clin Psychiatry. 2011;72(11):1538–45.
9. Misiak B, Stramecki F, Gawęda Ł, et al. Interactions between variation in candidate genes and environmental factors in the etiology of schizophrenia and bipolar disorder: a systematic review. Mol Neurobiol. 2018;55:5075–100.
10. Yildiz A, Ruiz P, Nemeroff C. The bipolar book: history, neurobiology, and treatment. Oxford; 2015. p. 21–8.
11. Madeline R. Vann M, Kathryn Keegan M. 9 most common triggers for bipolar mood episodes | Everyday Health. EverydayHealth.com. 2020. https://www.everydayhealth.com/bipolar-disorder-pictures/biggest-triggers-of-bipolar-mood-swings.aspx.
12. Geoffroy PA, Bellivier F, Scott J, Etain B. Seasonality and bipolar disorder: a systematic review, from admission rates to seasonality of symptoms. J Affect Disord. 2014;168:210–23. https://doi.org/10.1016/j.jad.2014.07.002. Epub 2014 Jul 10
13. Lewis KS, Gordon-Smith K, Forty L, et al. Sleep loss as a trigger of mood episodes in bipolar disorder: individual differences bases on diagnostic subtype and gender. Br J Psychiatry. 2017;211(3):169–74. https://doi.org/10.1192/bjp.bp.117.202259.
14. Ritter PS, Höfler M, Wittchen HU, Lieb R, Bauer M, Pfennig A, Beesdo-Baum K. Disturbed sleep as risk factor for the subsequent onset of bipolar disorder—data from a 10-year prospective-longitudinal study among adolescents and young adults. J Psychiatr Res. 2015;68:76–82. https://doi.org/10.1016/j.jpsychires.2015.06.005.
15. McIntyre RS, Soczynska JK, Bottas A, Bordbar K, Konarski JZ, Kennedy SH. Anxiety disorders and bipolar disorder: a review. Bipolar Disord. 2006;8:665–76. https://doi.org/10.1111/j.1399-5618.2006.00355.x.
16. Gerhson ES, Hamovit J, Guroff JJ, Dibble E, Leckman JF, Sceery W, Targum SD, Numberger JI Jr, Goldin LR, Bunney WE Jr. A family study of schizoaffective, bipolar I, bipolar II, unipolar, and normal control probads. Arch Gen Psychiatry. 1982;39(10):1157–67.
17. Weissman MM, Gershon ES, Kidd KK, Prusoff BA, Leckman JF, Dibble E, Hamovit J, Thompson WD, Pauls DL, Guroff JJ. Psychiatric disorders in the relatives of probands with affective disorders. The Yale University-National Institute of Mental Health Collaborative Study. Arch Gen Psychiatry. 1984;41(1):13–21.
18. Zarate C Jr, Manji H. Bipolar depression: molecular neurobiology, clinical diagnosis, and pharmacotherapy. 2nd ed. Cham: Springer International Publishing; 2016.
19. Strakowski S. Bipolar disorder. Oxford University Press; 2014.
20. Fountoulakis K. Bipolar disorder an evidence-based guide to manic depression. 1st ed. Berlin Heidelberg: Springer; 2015.
21. Taylor E. Atlas of bipolar disorders. London [UK]: Taylor & Francis; 2006.
22. Maletic V, Raison C. Integrated neurobiology of bipolar disorder. Front Psych. 2014;5:98. https://doi.org/10.3389/fpsyt.2014.00098.
23. Hibar DP, Westlye LT, Doan NT, Jahanshad N, Cheung JW, Ching CRK, Versace A, Bilderbeck AC, Uhlmann A, Mwangi B, Krämer B, Overs B, Hartberg CB, Abé C, Dima D, Grotegerd D, Sprooten E, Bøen E, Jimenez E, Howells FM, Delvecchio G, Temmingh H, Starke J, Almeida JRC, Goikolea JM, Houenou J, Beard LM, Rauer L, Abramovic L, et al. Cortical abnormalities in bipolar disorder: an MRI analysis of 6503 individuals from the ENIGMA Bipolar Disorder Working Group. Mol Psychiatry. 2017;23(4):932–42. https://doi.org/10.1038/mp.2017.73.
24. Estudillo-Guerra MA, Pacheco-Barrios K, Cardenas-Rojas A, Adame-Ocampo G, Camprodon JA, Morales-Quezada L, Gutiérrez-Mora D, Flores-Ramos M. Brain perfusion during manic episode and at 6-month follow-up period in bipolar disorder patients: correlation with cognitive functions. Brain Behav. 2020;10(6):e01615. https://doi.org/10.1002/brb3.1615. Epub 2020 May 1
25. American Psychiatric Association. Diagnostic and statistical manual of mental disorders. 4th ed. Washington, DC; 2000.
26. Bobo WV. The diagnosis and management of bipolar I and II disorders: clinical practice update. Mayo Clin Proc. 2017;92(10):1532–51.
27. Gitlin MJ, Swendsen J, Heller TL, Hammen C. Relapse and impairment in bipolar disorder. Am J Psychiatry. 1995;152(11):1635–40.
28. Stahl SM, Stahl SM. Stahl's essential psychopharmacology: neuroscientific basis and practical applications. Cambridge University Press; 2013.
29. Geddes JR, Burgess S, Hawton K, Jamison K, Goodwin GM. Long-term lithium therapy for bipolar disorder: systematic review and meta-analysis of randomized controlled trials. Am J Psychiatr. 2004;161(2):217–22.
30. Geddes JR, Miklowitz DJ. Treatment of bipolar disorder. Lancet. 2013;381(9878):1672–82.
31. Cipriani A, Pretty H, Hawton K, Geddes JR. Lithium in the prevention of suicidal behavior and all-cause mortality in patients with mood disorders: a systematic review of randomized trials. Am J Psychiatr. 2005;162(10):1805–19.
32. Cipriani A, Barbui C, Salanti G, Rendell J, Brown R, Stockton S, Purgato M, Spineli LM, Goodwin GM, Geddes JR. Comparative efficacy and acceptability of antimanic drugs in acute mania: a multiple-treatments meta-analysis. Lancet. 2011;378(9799):1306–15.
33. Smith LA, Cornelius V, Warnock A, Bell A, Young AH. Effectiveness of mood stabilizers and antipsychotics in the maintenance phase of bipolar disorder: a systematic review of randomized controlled trials. Bipolar Disord. 2007;9(4):394–412.
34. Licht RW, Nielsen JN, Gram LF, Vestergaard P, Bendz H. Lamotrigine versus lithium as maintenance treatment in bipolar I disorder: an open, randomized effectiveness study mimicking clinical practice. The 6th trial of the Danish University Antidepressant Group (DUAG-6). Bipolar Disord. 2010;12(5):483–93.
35. Katzung BG. Basic and clinical pharmacology. Mc Graw Hill. 2012;
36. Ceron-Litvoc D, Soares BG, Geddes J, Litvoc J, Lima MS. Comparison of carbamazepine and lithium in treatment of bipolar disorder: a systematic review of randomized controlled trials. Hum Psychopharmacol Clin Exp. 2009;24(1):19–28.
37. Yildiz A, Nikodem M, Vieta E, Correll CU, Baldessarini RJ. A network meta-analysis on comparative efficacy and all-cause discontinuation of antimanic treatments in acute bipolar mania. Psychol Med. 2015;45(2):299.
38. Pacchiarotti I, Bond DJ, Baldessarini RJ, Nolen WA, Grunze H, Licht RW, Post RM, Berk M, Goodwin GM, Sachs GS, Tondo L. The International Society for Bipolar Disorders (ISBD) task force report on antidepressant use in bipolar disorders. Am J Psychiatr. 2013;170(11):1249–62.
39. Gijsman HJ, Geddes JR, Rendell JM, Nolen WA, Goodwin GM. Antidepressants for bipolar depression: a systematic review of randomized, controlled trials. Am J Psychiatr. 2004;161(9):1537–47.
40. Perlis RH, Ostacher MJ, Miklowitz DJ, Smoller JW, Dennehy EB, Cowperthwait C, Nierenberg AA, Thase ME, Sachs

GS. Benzodiazepine use and risk of recurrence in bipolar disorder: a STEP-BD report. J Clin Psychiatry. 2010;71(2):194–200.
41. Palacios J, Yildiz A, Young AH, Taylor MJ. Tamoxifen for bipolar disorder: systematic review and meta-analysis. J Psychopharmacol. 2019;33(2):177–84.
42. Bartoli F, Crocamo C, Clerici M, Carra G. Allopurinol as add-on treatment for mania symptoms in bipolar disorder: systematic review and meta-analysis of randomised controlled trials. Br J Psychiatry. 2017;210(1):10–5.
43. Grunze H, Vieta E, Goodwin GM, Bowden C, Licht RW, Moeller HJ, Kasper S, WFSBP Task Force on Treatment Guidelines for Bipolar Disorders, Grunze H, Vieta E, Goodwin GM. The World Federation of Societies of Biological Psychiatry (WFSBP) guidelines for the biological treatment of bipolar disorders: update 2009 on the treatment of acute mania. World J Biol Psychiatry. 2009;10(2):85–116.
44. Canadian Network for Mood and Anxiety Treatments (CANMAT) and International Society for Bipolar Disorders (ISBD) 2018 guidelines for the management of patients with bipolar disorder.
45. Perlis RH, Baker RW, Zarate CA Jr, Brown EB, Schuh LM, Jamal HH, Tohen M. Olanzapine versus risperidone in the treatment of manic or mixed States in bipolar I disorder: a randomized, double-blind trial. J Clin Psychiatry. 2006;67(11):1747.
46. Malhi GS, Adams D, Cahill CM, Dodd S, Berk M. The management of individuals with bipolar disorder. Drugs. 2009;69(15):2063.
47. Wesseloo R, Kamperman AM, Munk-Olsen T, Pop VJ, Kushner SA, Bergink V. Risk of postpartum relapse in bipolar disorder and postpartum psychosis: a systematic review and meta-analysis. Am J Psychiatr. 2016;173(2):117–27.
48. ACOG Committee on Practice Bulletins–Obstetrics. ACOG practice bulletin: clinical management guidelines for obstetrician-gynecologists number 92, April 2008 (replaces practice bulletin number 87, November 2007). Use of psychiatric medications during pregnancy and lactation. Obstet Gynecol. 2008;111(4):1001–20.
49. Gentile S. Infant safety with antipsychotic therapy in breast-feeding: a systematic review. J Clin Psychiatry. 2008;69(4):666.
50. Aziz R, Lorberg B, Tampi RR. Treatments for late-life bipolar disorder. Am J Geriatr Pharmacother. 2006;4(4):347–64.
51. Gill SS, Rochon PA, Herrmann N, Lee PE, Sykora K, Gunraj N, Normand SL, Gurwitz JH, Marras C, Wodchis WP, Mamdani M. Atypical antipsychotic drugs and risk of ischaemic stroke: population based retrospective cohort study. BMJ. 2005;330(7489):445.
52. Miziou S, Tsitsipa E, Moysidou S, Karavelas V, Dimelis D, Polyzoidou V, Fountoulakis KN. Psychosocial treatment and interventions for bipolar disorder: a systematic review. Ann General Psychiatry. 2015;14(1):1–11.
53. Goldstein BI, Birmaher B, Carlson GA, DelBello MP, Findling RL, Fristad M, et al. The International Society for Bipolar Disorders Task Force report on pediatric bipolar disorder: knowledge to date and directions for future research. Bipolar Disord. 2017;19(7):524–43.
54. Peselow ED, Long R, Steiner AJ, Pizano DR, Naghdechi L, Akladios N, IsHak WW. Factors affecting long-term lithium compliance in bipolar patients. Int Neuropsychiatr Disease J. 2016;7(4):1–8.
55. Perugi G, Medda P, Toni C, Mariani MG, Socci C, Mauri M. The role of Electroconvulsive Therapy (ECT) in bipolar disorder: effectiveness in 522 patients with bipolar depression, mixed-state, mania and catatonic features. Curr Neuropharmacol. 2017;15(3):359–71. https://doi.org/10.2174/1570159X14666161017233642.
56. Miller TH. Bipolar disorder. Prim Care. 2016;43(2):269–84. https://doi.org/10.1016/j.pop.2016.02.003.
57. McLaren N. A critical review of the biopsychosocial model. Aust N Z J Psychiatry. 1998;2(1):86–92.
58. Henriques G. The biopsychosocial model and its limitations. Psychology Today. 2015. https://www.psychologytoday.com/us/blog/theory-knowledge/201510/the-biopsychosocial-model-and-its-limitations.
59. Carroll L. Alice's adventures in wonderland. New York: Macmillan; 1920.
60. Ghaemi N. The rise and fall of the biopsychosocial model. Br J Psychiatry. 2009;195:3–4.
61. Benning TB. Limitations of the biopsychosocial model in psychiatry. Adv Med Educ Pract. 2015;6:347–52.
62. Kecmanovic D, Hadzi-Pavlovic D. Psychiatric journals as the mirror of the dominant psychiatric model. Psychiatry Bull R Coll Psychiatry. 2010;34:172–6.
63. Hatala A. The status of the "biopsychosocial model" in health psychology: towards an integrated approach and a critique of cultural conceptions. Open J Med Psychol. 2012;1:51–62.
64. McManus C. Engel, Engels, and the side of the angels. Lancet. 2005;365:2169–217.
65. Sadock BJ, Sadock VA, Ruiz P. Kaplan & Sadock's synopsis of psychiatry: behavioral sciences/clinical psychiatry. 11th ed. Philadelphia: Wolters Kluwer; 2015.

Depressive Disorders

17

Eric L. Goldwaser and Scott T. Aaronson

Introduction

The *Diagnostic and Statistical Manual of Mental Disorders* (DSM) serves as a reference point for the mental health professional to categorically group symptoms into diagnoses. The fifth edition of the DSM (DSM-5) [1], the most recently revised one, cohorts eight disorders into the depressive disorders chapter. Often these different disorders share aspects of their presentation including symptomatology, diagnostic criteria, prognosis, treatment, etiology, course, and severity, but critical differences such as the presence of substance use, crippling environmental stresses, a cyclical pattern of symptoms, or relationship to hormonal cycles may help define optimal treatment strategies. Patients are best served when clinicians pay close attention to these defining aspects of the presentation which help clarify a working diagnosis and contribute to refining a treatment strategy which may include pharmacotherapy, psychotherapy, behavioral therapy, or rehabilitation.

Diagnostic Criteria and Features

Disruptive mood dysregulation disorder (DMDD) is a chronic (i.e., non-episodic), severe, persistent irritability marked by temper outbursts diagnosed in children up to 12 years of age who meet criteria shown in Table 17.1. It acknowledges the propensity for these children to develop unipolar depressive disorders later in youth and adulthood and is distinguished from more cyclical types of mood disor-

Table 17.1 Diagnostic criteria for disruptive mood dysregulation disorder

A.	Severe recurrent temper outbursts manifested verbally (e.g., verbal rages) and/or behaviorally (e.g., physical aggression toward people or property) that are grossly out of proportion in intensity or duration to the situation or provocation
B.	The temper outbursts are inconsistent with developmental level
C.	The temper outbursts occur, on average, three or more times per week
D.	The mood between temper outbursts is persistently irritable or angry most of the day, nearly every day, and is observable by others (e.g., parents, teachers, peers)
E.	Criteria A–D have been present for 12 or more months. Throughout that time, the individual has not had a period lasting 3 or more consecutive months without all of the symptoms in Criteria A–D
F.	Criteria A and D are present in at least two of three settings (i.e., at home, at schools, with peers) and are severe in at least one of these
G.	The diagnosis should not be made for the first time before age 6 years or after age 18 years
H.	By history or observation, the age at onset of Criteria A–E is before 10 years
I.	There has never been a distinct period lasting more than 1 day during which the full symptom criteria, except duration, for a manic or hypomanic episode have been met. **Note:** developmentally appropriate mood elevation, such as that occurs in the context of a highly positive event or its anticipation, should not be considered as a symptom of mania or hypomania
J.	The behaviors do not occur exclusively during an episode of major depressive disorder and are not better explained by another mental disorder (e.g., autism spectrum disorder, posttraumatic stress disorder, separation anxiety disorder, persistent depressive disorder [dysthymia]). **Note:** this diagnosis cannot coexist with oppositional defiant disorder, intermittent explosive disorder, or bipolar disorder, though it can coexist with others, including major depressive disorder, attention-deficit/hyperactivity disorder, conduct disorder, and substance use disorders. Individuals whose symptoms meet criteria for both disruptive mood dysregulation disorder and oppositional defiant disorder should only be given the diagnosis of disruptive mood dysregulation disorder. If an individual has ever experienced a manic or hypomanic episode, the diagnosis of disruptive mood dysregulation disorder should not be assigned
K.	The symptoms are not attributable to the physiological effects of a substance or to another medical or neurological condition

E. L. Goldwaser (✉)
Department of Psychiatry, Weill Cornell Medicine, New York, NY, USA
e-mail: bxt9001@med.cornell.edu

S. T. Aaronson
Sheppard Pratt Health System, Baltimore, MD, USA
e-mail: saaronson@sheppardpratt.org

W. W. IsHak (ed.), *Atlas of Psychiatry*, https://doi.org/10.1007/978-3-031-15401-0_17

ders in that DMDD presents with an ongoing, non-cyclic levels of irritability, with no evidence of relief from the irritability itself between outbursts as would be seen in bipolar disorder. Anxiety and bipolar disorder are also considerations for this presentation; however, they are less common than unipolar depression.

Major depressive disorder (MDD) denotes a discrete episode of major depression defined in Table 17.2, which lasts at least 2 weeks' duration (most of the day, nearly every day) involving a clear change in affect, cognition, and neurovegetative function alongside interepisode remissions. The depressed mood or anhedonia is present, persistent, and not linked specifically to one thought, preoccupation, or psychosocial stressor (e.g., loss of job/loved one [i.e., grief], financial difficulties, sudden disability). Often negative, self-hypercritical, and pessimistic ruminations are present in the major depressive episode, and thoughts surrounding death are usually tied to these feelings as are worthlessness and hopelessness about achieving relief from the emotional pains of the depression. Symptoms must be present nearly every day (except weight change and suicidal ideation) and may present initially as somatic complaints. In children, irritability may be the manifestation of sadness and can be regarded diagnostically as such. Milder symptoms along the depressive spectrum may be marked by a functional intactness that necessitated greater effort to accomplish similar tasks of being and activity.

Table 17.2 Diagnostic criteria for major depressive disorder

A. Five (or more) of the following symptoms have been present during the same 2-week period and represent a change from previous functioning; at least one of the symptoms is either (1) depressed mood or (2) loss of interest or pleasure. (Note: do not include symptoms that are clearly attributable to another medical condition)
1. Depressed mood most of the day, nearly every day, as indicated by either subjective report (e.g., feels sad, empty, hopeless) or observation made by others (e.g., appears tearful) (note: in children and adolescents, it can be irritable mood)
2. Markedly diminished interest or pleasure in all, or almost all, activities most of the day, nearly every day (as indicated by either subjective account or observation)
3. Significant weight loss when not dieting or weight gain (e.g., a change of more than 5% of body weight in a month) or decrease or increase in appetite nearly every day (note: in children, consider failure to make expected weight gain)
4. Insomnia or hypersomnia nearly every day
5. Psychomotor agitation or retardation nearly every day (observable by others, not merely subjective feelings of restlessness or being slowed down)
6. Fatigue or loss of energy nearly every day
7. Feelings of worthlessness or excessive or inappropriate guilt (which may be delusional) nearly every day (not merely self-reproach or guilt about being sick)
8. Diminished ability to think or concentrate, or indecisiveness, nearly every day (either by subjective account or as observed by others)
9. Recurrent thoughts of death (not just fear of dying), recurrent suicidal ideation without a specific plan, or a suicide attempt or a specific plan for committing suicide
B. The symptoms cause clinically significant distress or impairment in social, occupational, or other important areas of functioning
C. The episode is not attributable to the physiological effects of a substance or to another medical condition
Note: Criteria A–C represent a major depressive episode
D. The occurrence of the major depressive episode is not better explained by schizoaffective disorder, schizophrenia, schizophreniform d/o, delusional disorder, or other specified and unspecified schizophrenia spectrum and other psychotic disorders
E. There has never been a manic episode or a hypomanic episode. This exclusion does not apply if all the manic-like or hypomanic-like episodes are substance-induced or are attributable to the physiological effect of another medical condition
Specifiers: with anxious distress, mixed features, melancholic features, atypical features, mood-congruent psychotic features, mood-incongruent psychotic features, catatonia, peripartum onset, seasonal pattern

Persistent depressive disorder (PDD), previously known as dysthymia, features a depressed mood that occurs for at least 2 years in adults and 1 year in children, most of the day and more days than not, outlined in Table 17.3. The chronicity of the disorder and reduced severity separates it from MDD; however, it can co-occur with an MDD diagnosis if both criteria are met and is often referred to as a double depression.

Premenstrual dysphoric disorder (PMDD) is characterized by mood lability, irritability, dysphoria, and anxiety

Table 17.3 Diagnostic criteria for persistent depressive disorder

A. Depressed mood for most of the day, for more days than not, as indicated by either subjective account or observation by others, for at least 2 years (in children/adolescents, mood can be irritable and duration must be at least 1 year)
B. Presence, while depressed, of at least two of the following:
1. Poor appetite/overeating
2. Insomnia/hypersomnia
3. Low energy/fatigue
4. Low self-esteem
5. Poor concentration or difficulty making decisions
6. Feelings of hopelessness
C. During the 2-year period (1 year for children/adolescents) of the disturbance, the individual has never been without the symptoms in Criteria A and B for more than 2 months at a time
D. Criteria for a major depressive disorder may be continuously present for 2 years
E. There has never been a manic/hypomanic episode, and criteria have never been met for cyclothymic disorder
F. The disturbance is not better explained by a persistent schizoaffective disorder, schizophrenia, delusional disorder, or other specified or unspecified schizophrenia spectrum and other psychotic disorder
G. The symptoms are not attributable to the physiological effects of a substance (drug of abuse/medication) or another medical condition (hypothyroidism)
H. The symptoms cause clinically significant distress or impairment in social, occupational, or other important areas of functioning

symptoms that occur repeatedly during the premenstrual phase of the cycle and remit around the onset of menses or shortly thereafter. Behavioral and physical symptoms may accompany these disturbances and are defined in Table 17.4. Symptoms must be present in most of the menstrual cycles over the past year and must adversely impact work or social functioning. Sociocultural aspects should also be accounted for when consideration of this diagnosis is warranted, including the woman's family perspectives, religious beliefs, social tolerance, and gender role. Symptoms typically peak around menses onset and may linger days past menses as well, but there must be a symptom-free period correlating to the follicular phase after the beginning of the menstrual period. Daily prospective symptom ratings are also required for at least two symptomatic cycles, but preliminary diagnoses can be made on historical accounts alone.

Table 17.4 Diagnostic criteria for premenstrual dysphoric disorder

A. In the majority of menstrual cycles, at least five symptoms must be present in the final week before the onset of menses, start to improve within a few days after the onset of menses, and become minimal or absent in the week postmenses
B. One (or more) of the following symptoms must be present:
1. Marked affective lability (e.g., mood swings, feeling suddenly sad or tearful, or increased sensitivity to rejection)
2. Marked irritability or anger or increased interpersonal conflicts
3. Marked depressed mood, feelings of hopelessness, or self-deprecating thoughts
4. Marked anxiety, tension, and/or feelings of being keyed up or on edge
C. One (or more) of the following symptoms must additionally be present, to reach a total of five symptoms when combined with symptoms from Criterion B:
1. Decreased interest in usual activities (e.g., work, school, friends, hobbies)
2. Subjective difficulty in concentration
3. Lethargy, easy fatigability, or marked lack of energy
4. Marked change in appetite, overeating, or specific food cravings
5. Hypersomnia or insomnia
6. A sense of being overwhelmed or out of control
7. Physical symptoms such as breast tenderness or swelling, joint or muscle pain, a sensation of "bloating," or weight gain
Note: the symptoms in Criteria A–C must have been met for most menstrual cycles that occurred in the preceding year
D. The symptoms are associated with clinically significant distress or interference with work, school, usual social activities, or relationships with others (e.g., avoidance of social activities, decreased productivity and efficiency at work, school, or home)
E. The disturbance is not merely an exacerbation of the symptoms of another disorder such as MDD, panic disorder, PDD (dysthymia), or a personality disorder (although it may co-occur with any of these disorders)
F. Criterion A should be confirmed by prospective daily ratings during at least two symptomatic cycles (**Note:** the diagnosis may be made provisionally prior to this confirmation)
G. The symptoms are not attributable to the physiological effects of a substance (e.g., a drug of abuse, a medication, other treatment) or another medical condition (e.g., hyperthyroidism)

Substance/medication-induced depressive disorder and depressive disorder due to another medical condition are defined diagnostically in Tables 17.5 and 17.6, respectively. If depressive symptoms arise in relation to substance use, it should be specified whether the occurrence prevailed during the intoxication or the withdrawal phase of usage. Regarding timeframe, roughly 1 month after substance use has last occurred is typically long enough to consider that adequate metabolism and effects have worn off; however, physiological and psychologic effects can certainly prevail for several months afterward, blurring this line considerably. Complete abstinence may be difficult to obtain, and similarly, toxicology screens are infrequently available in all settings. Depressive disorder due to another medical condition simi-

Table 17.5 Diagnostic criteria for substance/medication-induced depressive disorder

A. A prominent and persistent disturbance in mood that predominates in the clinical picture and is characterized by depressed mood or markedly diminished interest or pleasure in all, or almost all, activities
B. Evidence from history, physical examination, or lab findings of both:
1. Symptoms in Criterion A developed during or soon after substance intoxication or withdrawal or after exposure to a medication
2. The involved substance/medication is capable of producing the symptoms in Criterion A
C. The disturbance is not better explained by a depressive disorder that is not substance/medication-induced. Such evidence of an independent depressive disorder could include the following: the symptoms preceded the onset of the substance/medication use; the symptoms persist for a substantial period of time (e.g., about 1 month) after the cessation of acute withdrawal or severe intoxication; or there is another evidence suggesting the existence of an independent non-substance/medication-induced depressive disorder (e.g., a history of recurrent no-substance/medication-related episodes)
D. The disturbance does not occur exclusively during the course of a delirium
E. The disturbance causes clinically significant distress or impairment in social, occupational, or other important areas of functioning

Table 17.6 Depressive disorder due to another medical condition

A. A prominent and persistent period of depressed mood or markedly diminished interest or pleasure in all, or almost all, activities that predominates in the clinical picture
B. There is evidence from the history, physical examination, or laboratory findings that the disturbance is the direct pathophysiological consequence of another medical condition
C. The disturbance is not better explained by another mental disorder (e.g., adjustment disorder with depressed mood, in which the stressor is a serious medical condition)
D. The disturbance does not occur exclusively during the course of a delirium
E. The disturbance causes clinically significant distress or impairment in social, occupational, or other important areas of functioning

larly must follow in response to another medical diagnosis not explained by an adjustment disorder. The resultant behavioral disturbance is marked by anhedonia or a diminished interest/pleasure in all or almost all activities. Of course, there should be a reasonable pathophysiologic connection between the substance or illness of interest and symptom development.

Other specified depressive disorder and unspecified depressive disorder are the remaining two categories of depressive disorder diagnoses as defined in Tables 17.7 and 17.8, respectively. When symptoms characteristic of a depressive disorder are unable to meet full criteria for any of the disorders in the depressive disorder diagnostic class, specifiers are used to classify this entity as recurrent brief

Table 17.7 Other specified depressive disorder

Recurrent brief depression	Concurrent presence of depressed mood and at least four other symptoms of depression for 2–13 days at least once per month (not associated with the menstrual cycle) for at least 12 consecutive months in an individual whose presentation has never met criteria for any other depressive or bipolar disorder and does not currently meet active or residual criteria for any psychotic disorder
Short-duration depressive episode (4–13 days)	Depressed affect and at least four of the other eight symptoms of a major depressive episode associated with clinically significant distress or impairment that persists for more than 4 days, but less than 14 days, in an individual whose presentation has never met criteria for any other depressive or bipolar disorder, does not currently meet active or residual criteria for any psychotic disorder, and does not meet criteria for recurrent brief depression
Depressive episode with insufficient symptoms	Depressed affect and at least one of the other eight symptoms of a MDE associated with clinically significant distress or impairment that persists for at least 2 weeks in an individual whose presentation has never met criteria for any other depressive or bipolar disorder, does not currently meet active or residual criteria for any psychotic disorder, and does not meet criteria for mixed anxiety and depressive disorder symptoms

Table 17.8 Unspecified depressive disorder

This category applies to presentations in which symptoms characteristic of a depressive disorder that cause clinically significant distress or impairment in social, occupational, or other important areas of functioning predominate but do not meet the full criteria for any of the disorders in the depressive disorder diagnostic class. The unspecified depressive disorder category is used in situations in which the clinician chooses *not* to specify the reason that the criteria are not met for a specific depressive disorder and includes presentations for which there is insufficient information to make a more specific diagnosis (e.g., in emergency room settings)	
With anxious distress	Presence of at least two (mild), three (moderate), four to five (moderate to severe), or four or five with motor agitation (severe) of the following symptoms during the majority of days of a MDE/PDD: feeling keyed up or tense, feeling unusually restless, difficulty concentrating because of worry, fear that something awful may happen, and feeling that the individual might lose control of himself or herself
With mixed features	At least three manic/hypomanic symptoms present nearly every day during the majority of days of a MDE: elevated, expansive mood, inflated self-esteem/grandiosity, more talkative than usual or pressure to keep talking, flight of ideas or subjective experience that thoughts are racing, increase in energy or goal-directed activity (either socially, at work or school, or sexually), increased or excessive involvement in activities that have a high potential for painful consequences (e.g., engaging in unrestrained buying sprees, sexual indiscretions, foolish business investments), decreased need for sleep (feeling rested despite sleeping less than usual; to be contrasted with insomnia). Mixed features are observable by others and represent a change from the person's usual behavior. These mixed symptoms are not attributable to the physiological effects of a substance
With melancholic features	One of the following is present during the most severe period of the current episode: loss of pleasure in all/almost all activities and lack of reactivity to usually pleasurable stimuli (does not feel much better, even temporarily, when something good happens); at least three of the following—(1) distinct quality of depressed mood characterized by profound despondency, despair, and/or moroseness or by the so-called empty mood, [2] depression that is regularly worse in the morning, [3] early morning awakening (at least 2 h before usual awakening), [4] marked psychomotor agitation or retardation, [5] significant anorexia/weight loss, and [6] excessive or inappropriate guilt
With atypical features	These features predominate during the majority of days with the current or most recent MDD or PDD. Mood reactivity (i.e., mood brightens in response to actual or potential positive events). At least two of the following: significant weight gain/increased appetite, hypersomnia, leaden paralysis (i.e., heavy, leaden feelings in arms or legs), and long-standing pattern of interpersonal rejection sensitivity (not limited to episodes of mood disturbance) that results in significant social or occupational impairment
With psychotic features	Delusions and/or hallucinations present. Can be mood-congruent (i.e., content is consistent with the typical depressive themes of personal inadequacy, guilt, disease, death, nihilism, or deserved punishment) or mood-incongruent
With catatonia	Refers to marked psychomotor disturbances like decreased motor activity, which can be observed as a decreased engagement during interview due to this psychomotoric slowing, or conversely, an excessive and peculiarity to motor activity
With peripartum onset	Most recent MDE onset of symptoms occurs during pregnancy or in the 4 weeks following delivery
With seasonal pattern	Recurrent MDD that has a regular temporal relationship between onset of MDE in MDD and a particular time of the year. This does not include seasonally related psychosocial stressors like unemployment every winter. Full remissions (or change to mania/hypomania) also occur at a particular time of the year. In the past 2 years, two MDEs have occurred that demonstrate the temporal seasonal relationships and no nonseasonal MDE during the same period. Seasonal MDEs substantially outnumber the nonseasonal MDEs over the lifetime

Table 17.9 Specifiers for depressive disorders

Severity	Defined as either mild, moderate, or severe, depending on the daily functional impairment
With anxious distress	Co-occurring anxiety is present and more likely to accompany suicidal thoughts and be more resistant to traditional antidepressants. Requires at least two of the following: a sense of being "keyed up" or tense, unusual restlessness, trouble concentrating secondary to worry, fear that awful things will happen, and worry about loss of self-control
With mixed features	Includes at least three of the following features of mania: elevated and expansive mood, heightened self-esteem or grandiosity, increased speech or pressure of speech, racing thoughts, increased energy or directed activity, excessive activity in behavior with possibly negative consequences, and reduced need for sleep
With melancholic features	Also referred to as "endogenous features"; includes anhedonia, lack of pleasure and loss of reactivity to positive stimuli, distinct quality of depressed mood (despair), depression worse in the morning, waking early in the morning, psychomotor disturbance, weight loss, and excessive guilty thoughts
With atypical features	Mood reactivity requires that mood brightens in response to actual or potential positive events, which is in contrast to the melancholic specifier. Also, atypical features require two of the following: significant increase in weight or appetite, increased sleep, sense of leaden paralysis, and interpersonal sensitivity
With psychotic features	Can be mood-congruent typical for depressive themes of personal inadequacy, guilt, disease, death, nihilism, and deserved punishment or can be mood-incongruent which typically portends a more severe/pervasive course
With catatonic features	Characterized by marked psychomotoric signs, like slowness or excessive and peculiar activity; can be observed as a decreased engagement during an interview or physical examination

depression, short-duration depressive episode (4–13 days), or depressive episode with insufficient symptoms. Unspecified depressive disorder applies similarly to when a full diagnostic criterion is unmet but significant impairment in social, occupational, or other important functional areas remains, and qualifiers, rather than specifiers, are used. In this entity, the depressive presentation can be qualified with anxious distress, mixed features, melancholic features, atypical features, psychotic features, catatonia, peripartum onset, or seasonal pattern.

Specifiers, also known as modifiers, can be added to the diagnosis to help capture the features of the depressive episode which may impact recommended interventions. The first specifier defines the severity (e.g., mild, moderate, or severe) as it relates to the daily functional impairment imparted by the current illness. Another specifier may be added similar to those described for other specified or unspecified depressive disorders, which are shown in Table 17.9. The presence of psychosis, catatonia, or mixed features may be particularly important for treatment considerations.

Epidemiology

Epidemiological considerations of major depressive disorder include prevalence, disease course, and burden.

Prevalence

The World Mental Health Surveys [2] demonstrate a 12-month prevalence of MDD to range from roughly 2 to 10%, with Japan showing the lowest and Brazil the highest, respectively. Similarly, income was only nominally related, in that high- and low-income countries were roughly 5.5–5.9% prevalence of MDD, as shown in Fig. 17.1. Median age of onset, severity, symptom profile, and basic sociodemographic and environmental correlates (like sex, education, and life events) all comparably aligned across countries and cultures [3]. Regarding gender differences, MDD occurs twice as often in women than men [4], with the median age of onset being 25 years and peak risk timeframe for the onset in the mid-to-late adolescent years through the early 40s [2].

Major depressive disorder 1-year prevalence in the United States is about 7%. However, stark differences exist as a function of age, in that between 18 and 29 years old, there is a threefold higher prevalence compared to those older than 60 years. Gender differences demonstrate a 1.5- to threefold higher rate in females than males beginning in early adolescents. Lifetime prevalence estimates roughly 20% cumulative prevalence overall [6].

Disease Course

Puberty typically is where depression first manifests most observably. Remission is said to occur when 2 or more months have passed with no symptoms or only one or two symptoms to a mild degree. When followed longitudinally, a chronic depressive trait points more toward an underlying personality, anxiety, or substance use disorder and limits the prognostic optimism for full and sustained resolution of symptoms following adequate treatment. To this point, it may be beneficial to learn when the last time that such a period of 2 months without symptom burden had appeared. Mean episode duration lasts roughly for 3 months in 40% of

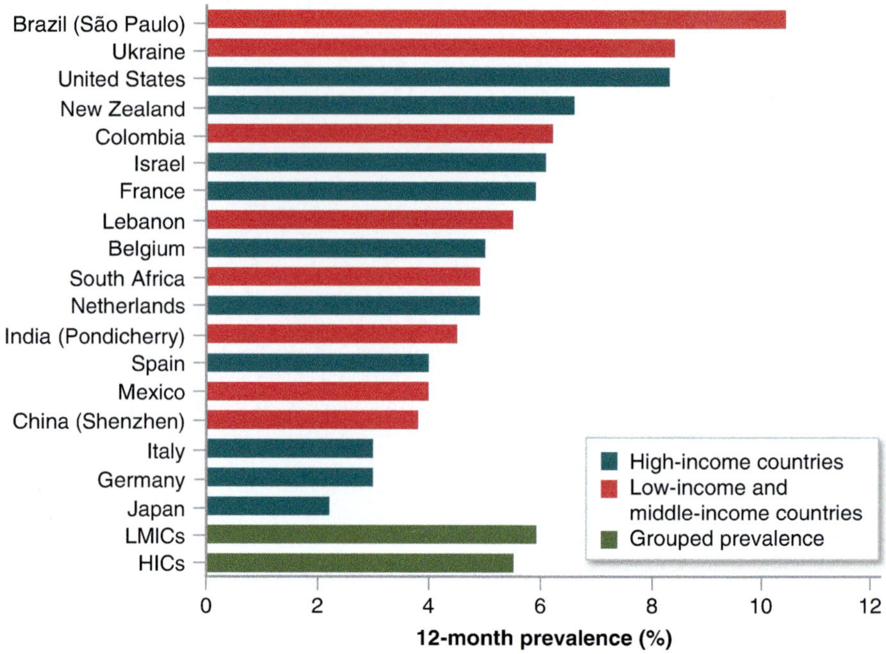

Fig. 17.1 Average 12-month prevalence of MDD. Although considerable variation in inter-country prevalence of major depressive disorder is noted, the overall estimates in high-income countries (5.5%) and low-income and middle-income countries (5.9%) are not different (*From* Otte et al. [5]; *with permission*)

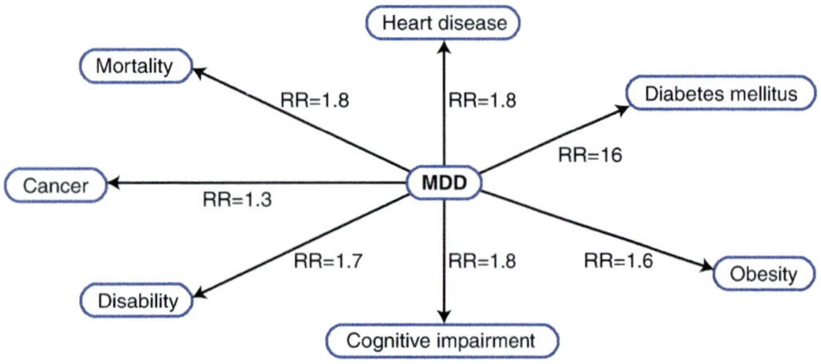

Fig. 17.2 Somatic consequences of MDD have shown through longitudinal analysis that the relative risk is increased to developing a range of seemingly unrelated manifestations to depressive symptoms alone. However, unhealthy lifestyle, poorer self-care, adverse medication effects, and a shared pathophysiology housed in perturbed immunologic and endocrine responses are all contributors to this observation (*From* Otte et al. [5]; *with permission*)

patients and up to 1 year in nearly 80% of patients and harbors a 70–90% 1-year recovery [7]; meanwhile, relapse may occur in up to 80% of the time at least once [8]. Harbingers of poor recovery include the length of episode, presence of psychotic features or prominence of anxiety, as well as symptom severity during this development. In fact, the persistence of mild depressive symptoms during a period of remission also portends to relapses with more severity.

Disease Burden

The Global Burden of Disease Consortium [9] found that MDD was the second leading contributor to global disease burden in disability-adjusted life years. The more systemic impact that MDD has on seemingly unrelated somatic illness [10] is detailed in Fig. 17.2 and includes an increased risk of diabetes mellitus, heart disease, stroke, hypertension, obesity, cancer, cognitive impairment, and Alzheimer's disease [10], with an all-cause mortality estimated at 10%. Indeed, depressed individuals admitted to nursing homes have an increased likelihood of death within the first year [1].

Etiology

Etiologic determinants of MDD span a wide range of temperamental, environmental, and genetic/physiological risks. Temperamental risks include negative affectivity also known as neuroticism, which can predict the likelihood of developing depressive symptoms as a response to stressful life events [1]. Environmental risks include an absence of a partner, negative life events [11], and social determinants like childhood adversities and early life traumatic events, low socioeconomic support, and low education, which all increase the risk of developing MDD [12]. Given the overlay on a heterogeneous and not yet fully identified genetic backdrop, the actual experience of a particularly traumatic event does not in and of itself harbor predictive value for an episode of depression onset. In terms of prognosis or treatment selection, however, childhood trauma has a twofold increased risk of developing MDD [13] and with higher symptom severity and worse prognostic outcome [14] than those without such a history. The genetic and physiological risks that are well-established include first-degree family members with MDD, which are two- to fourfold higher than the general population. Heritability estimates attempting to capture the genetic determinants of depression development from twin studies have found about 40% of the contribution attributed to neuroticism as a personality trait.

Pathophysiology

Biological systems involved in the pathophysiology and mechanism of MDD are complex and not fully understood. A perspective on depression that encompasses biology, psychology, and environment best captures the nature and treatment accepted in the field. Aspects regarding a generalized understanding of the more widely studied areas will be discussed, as shown in Fig. 17.3, that include the central nervous system, immune system, hypothalamic-pituitary-adrenal (HPA) axis and neuroendocrinological system with the autonomic nervous system, and cardiovascular and metabolic system that have all shown to be highly important factors in MDD.

Genetics and the Environment

The heritability of MDD is nearly 35% in first-degree relatives [15], although main genetic effects remain elusive among replication studies [16]. This may not be surprising given the fact that MDD is highly multifactorial and poly-

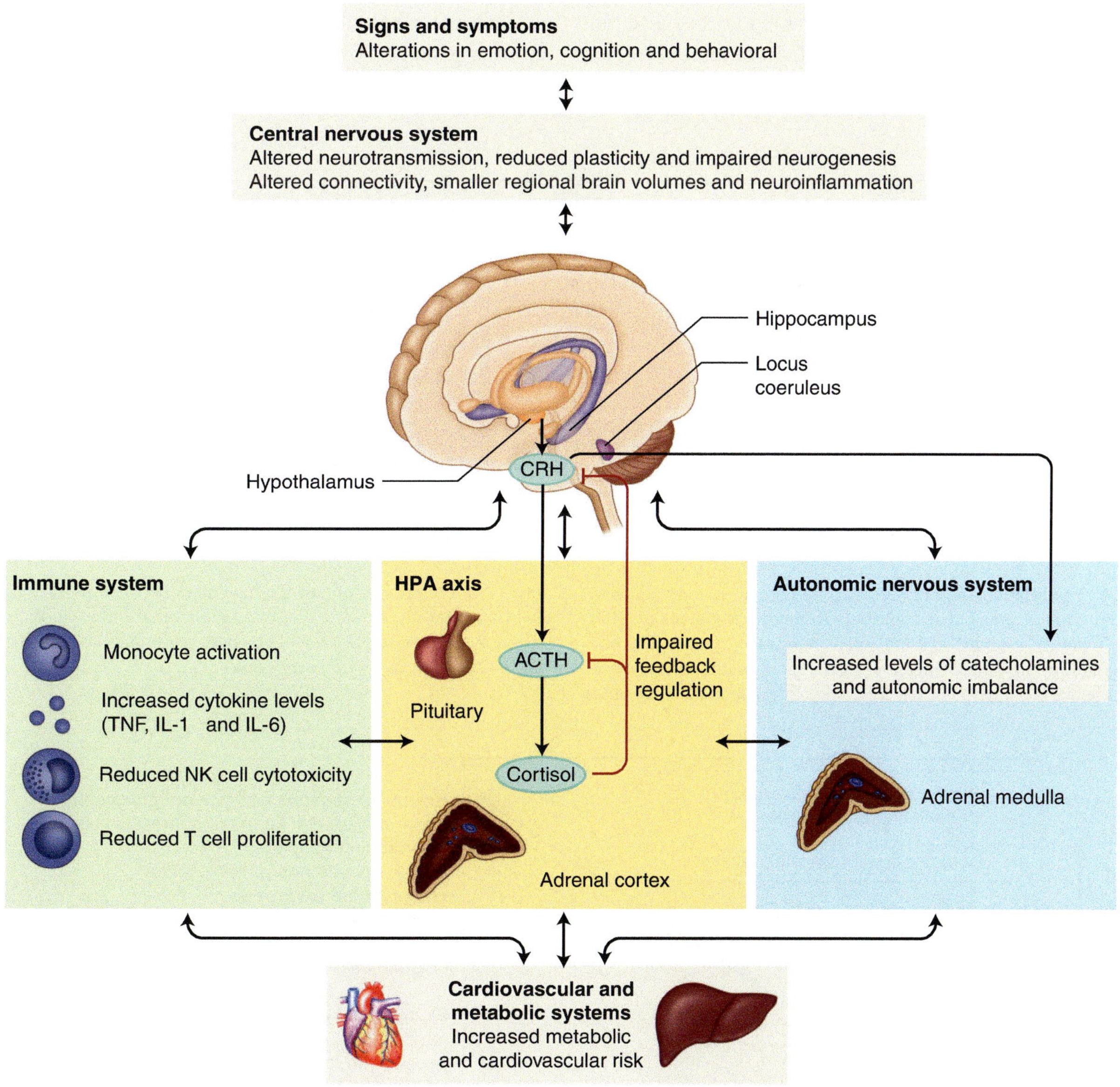

Fig. 17.3 Biological systems involved in the pathophysiology of MDD. Hypotheses governed by neurotransmission concentrate on alterations of monoamines like serotonin that appear downregulated in relevant cerebral structures, hypofunctioning circuitry, and connectivity from cortical to deep brain areas. Neuroinflammatory changes as well as basal peripheral inflammatory changes are evident in MDD as well. The effect that environmental and psychosocial determinants have on immediate and chronic levels of stress molecules also shares pathophysiologic impact in MDD. Inflammatory cells and effector chemicals distributed with an interplay with the HPA axis are of particular interest to MDD and its influence on a host of somatic illnesses espoused (*From* Otte et al. [5]; *with permission*)

genic whereby genes of interest typically only carry small effect sizes. A clear dose-response relationship does exist, however, in adverse life events in both number and severity toward the severity and course of MDD [17]. The lasting consequences of stressors from earlier in life are poorly understood from a mechanistic standpoint, but the impact on the HPA axis is perhaps well-suited to capture this influence. Persistent increases in corticotrophin-releasing hormone (CRH) by means of activated neural circuits relevant to these pathways may capture this interaction [18]. Childhood trauma in the form of abuse demonstrates enhanced HPA axis activation into adulthood in response to stressors [19]. Exposure to these hormonal and stress molecule effectors during perinatal, in utero life may also account for some of the environmentally loaded determinants seen in MDD [20].

The stress diathesis involves a vulnerability to developing MDD imparted by genes that interact with environmental circumstances in a way to produce the symptomatology. Candidate genes continue to grow with increased molecular technologies to study them, but ones that have borne out more repeatedly consistent associations in translational literature include several, albeit without definitive consensus reached in the field. The sodium-dependent serotonin transporter (*SLC6A4*), CRH receptor 1 (*CRHR1*), and peptidyl-prolyl *cis-trans* isomerase (*FKBP5*) have received significant attention in informing psychiatric studies given their impact on relevant neurotransmitter systems and circuits involved in what is known about mechanistic contributions. Figure 17.4 provides the progression of this crucially important interplay between genetics and psychosocial factors that culminate in proposed etiopathophysiology of MDD. Figure 17.5 repre-

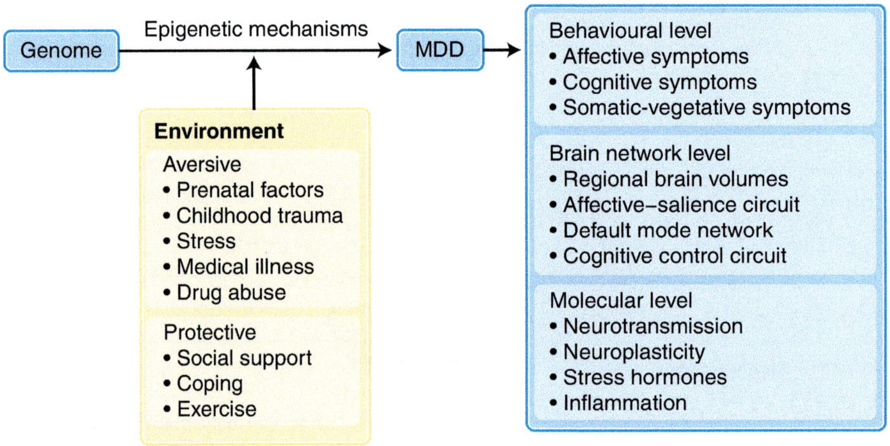

Fig. 17.4 The relationship between genetic predispositions and environmental circumstances that contribute to the development of MDD involves a highly complex and not fully understood system. The etiopathophysiology displayed in the textual representations here represents a schematic depiction of this trajectory. Epigenetic mechanisms at play are a reference to one of the mediators between psychosocial and environmental inputs with genomic outputs that influence the individual on a multitude of levels—behavior, brain, and cellular/molecular (*From* Otte et al. [5]; *with permission*)

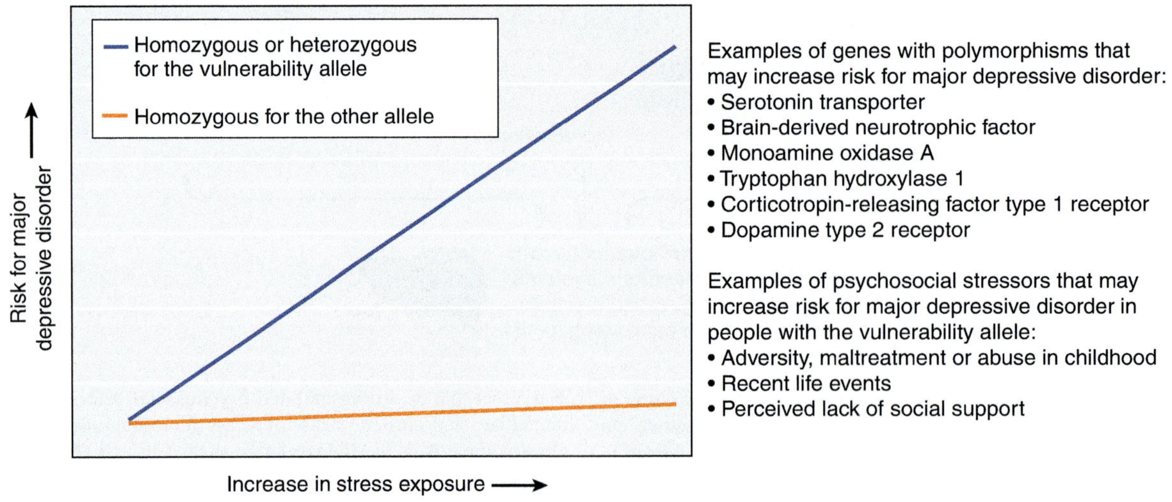

Fig. 17.5 Genetic predispositions exist in the form of polymorphisms that confer variable functionality, like increased transporter efficiency or reduced enzyme degradation, for instance. Psychosocial stressors similarly serve a major risk for development of MDD when superimposed on a genetically vulnerable background. The risk may even be more synergized than additive and remains a huge area of research

sents the schematic imposed by the gene x environment interaction, with some examples of both factors [21].

Neuroendocrinology

The adaptive role that stress plays is only observed when the compensatory mechanisms are in place to successfully navigate through it. In other words, stress has a differential effect depending on factors that allow an individual to acutely deal with the stressful situation. A multitude of pathways that stresses in many forms converge on is through the neuroendocrine system, by way of the production of cortisol. The reader is directed toward more detailed reviews on the topic for the physiologic role of stress as it relates to behavior [22], outside the scope of this text, but suffice it to say that repeated studies have implicated elevated cortisol levels among individuals with MDD [19], and even as a predictive factor for its development [23]. Figure 17.6 depicts this pathway [24] with Fig. 17.7 extending it to the downstream cellular targets under influence that also implicate neuroplastic contributions discussed in section “Neuroplasticity” [23]. Figure 17.3 provides a generalized overview of this central-peripheral dynamic whereby stress is related to and from the brain among other systems.

Inflammation

One of the means by which the periphery can communicate with deep brain structures both directly and indirectly is via the immune and inflammatory system. Cytokines and inflammatory signals may traverse endothelial vascular systems between the brain and the blood to influence receptor expression, neurogenesis, and plasticity [25] with effects toward behavioral outcomes. This multimodal circuit is also known as the neuro-immune axis, detailed in Fig. 17.8. Postmortem studies have even demonstrated increased levels of neuroinflammatory changes and microglial activation in the brains of patients with MDD [26].

Neuroplasticity

The “neurotrophin hypothesis” of depression holds factors that affect neuronal plasticity and growth as a critical mediator in the psychopathologic development of MDD [27]. This relates the ability for neurons to structurally adapt overtime, denoted as the brain’s plasticity, and is a crucially important component of dealing with stress. Indeed, molecules involved in neuroplasticity and growth, including serving as a protective factor, such as brain-derived neurotrophic factor (BDNF), have been studied in MDD [28, 29]. BDNF in the blood of patients with MDD was reduced, and levels even served for biomarker utility in the most severe symptoms of MDD, including suicidality [30]. Aside from direct impacts that BDNF may hold on synaptic changes, it also influences the HPA axis by reducing its activity and subsequently curbing neuroendocrine responses as well. The impact that stress has on neuroplasticity is graphically shown in Fig. 17.9, showing the effect that antidepressant medication has on combating stress-related pathophysiologic changes.

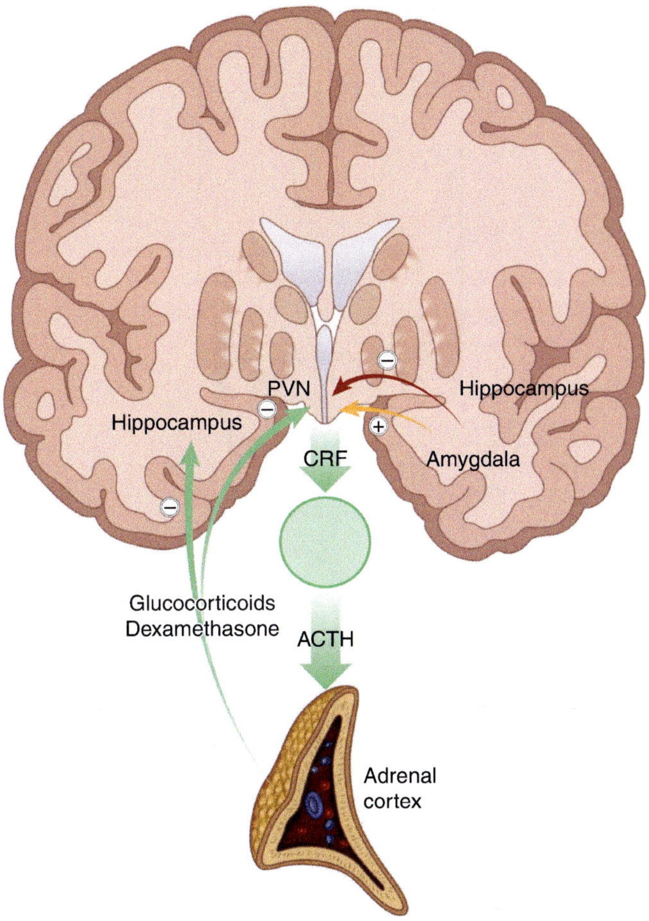

Fig. 17.6 Regulation of the hypothalamic-pituitary-adrenal (HPA) axis depends on central and peripheral inputs and outputs. Neural inputs include reciprocal activity between amygdalar and hippocampal structures, among others. The hypophyseal portal system conducts signaling molecules into the circulation to stimulate adrenal cortical activity, namely, release of glucocorticoids, in response to stress. Glucocorticoids in turn act in ways to stop aberrant overactivity or perpetuation of this system as a means of controlling the resources used during this process related to stress. With impaired resolution of stressors, in reality or perceived, this system can malfunction and maintain higher levels of glucocorticoids that causes damage to neural structures responsible for regulation

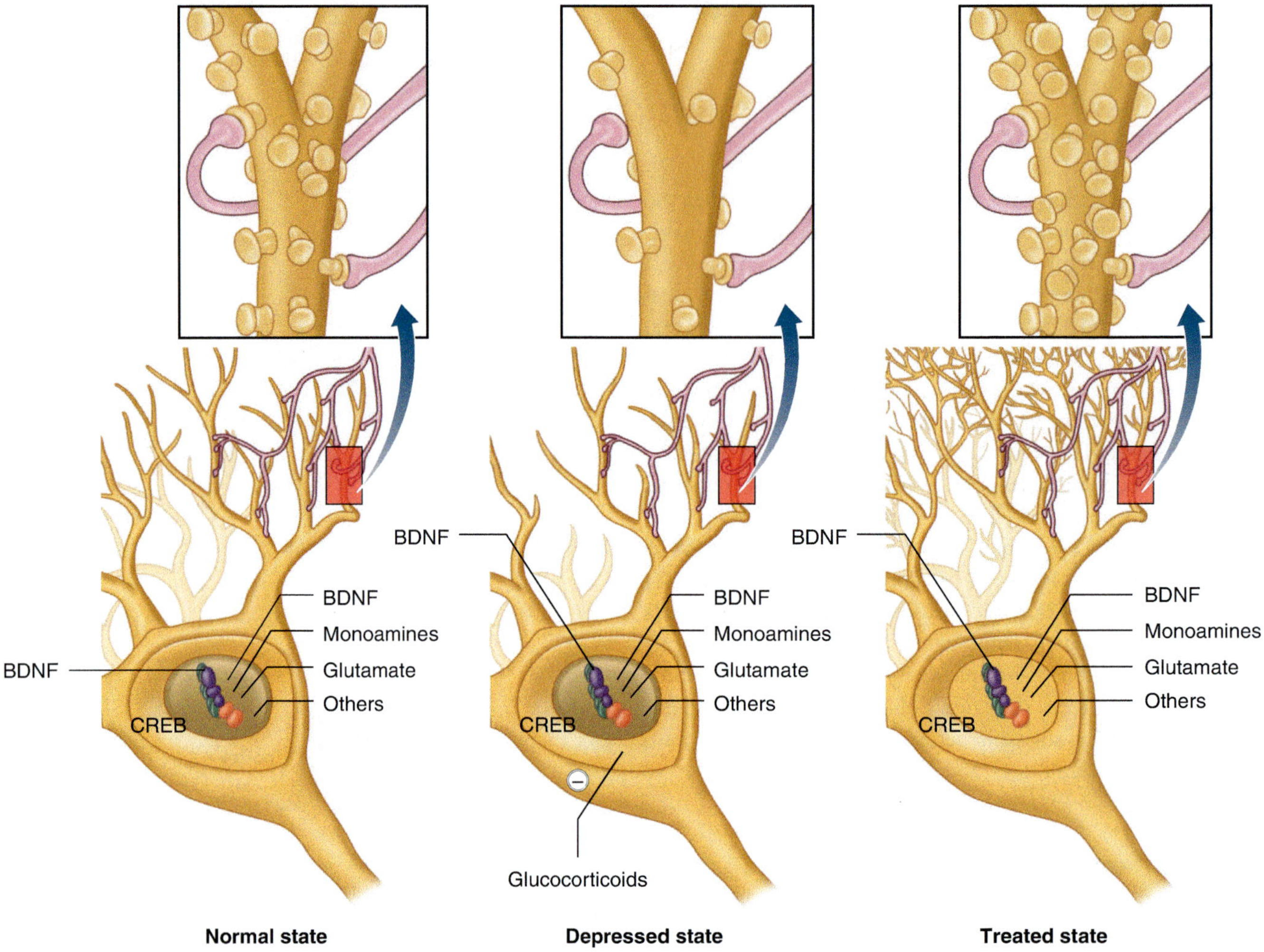

Fig. 17.7 Downstream effects and cellular targets implicated in the neurotrophic mechanism of depression. Panels demonstrate a normal hippocampal pyramidal neuron (left) and its innervation by glutamatergic, monoaminergic, and other neurons. Brain-derived neurotrophic factor (BDNF) levels are decreased in depression, with subsequent negative impacts on functions such as dendritic arborizations. Prolonged elevations of glucocorticoid levels are an established means by which BDNF levels may be reduced in a depressed state (middle), likely involved with damage to these hippocampal neurons involved in BDNF production and effect propagation, through intracellular mechanisms on a genomic transcriptional level (with mediators like CREB). Antidepressants may act by producing the opposite effects, increasing BDNF expression in the hippocampal neurons, and restoring dendritic arborization (right)

Monoamines

Early theories about depression pathophysiology were founded upon deficiencies of neurochemicals belonging to the amino acid-derived neurotransmitters norepinephrine, serotonin, and dopamine. Monoamines are reduced by antihypertensives like reserpine, which was shown to induce depression [31]. By directly targeting the monoaminergic systems, especially on postsynaptic receptor targets, a very quick onset of effect is observed after administration, but antidepressant effects (covered in more detail in section "Treatment") are often only evident after several weeks of treatment. Figure 17.10 displays a cartoon of the serotonin synapse with a focus on the presynaptic and postsynaptic areas for an overview of this most important neurotransmitter [21]. This scheme shares much overlap with other monoaminergic systems, but notable differences are present and often exploited for psychopharmacologic effects. Antidepressants developed target these monoaminergic systems in the brain, which are very widespread and interact in not yet fully understood ways. Hopes of better defining more specific pathways responsible for producing symptoms of MDD hold promise of resolution with advancements in the sophisticated technologies of neuroimaging.

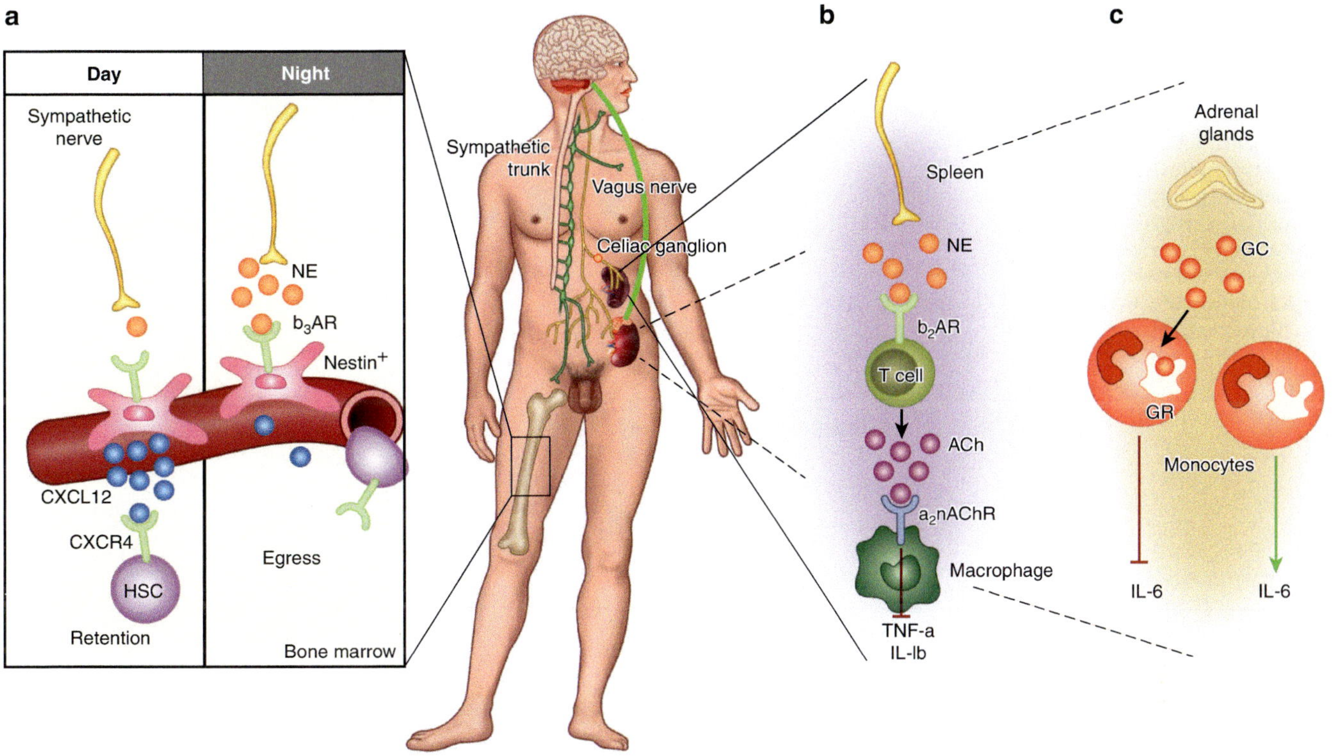

Fig. 17.8 The inflammatory system communicates reciprocally with the CNS via circuits and pathways spanning peripheral immune mediators and neural tissue, known as the neuro-immune axis. (**a**) Bone marrow innervations via sympathetic innervation act through norepinephrine release to stimulate stem cell circulation during rest. (**b**) Vagus nerve afferents survey circulating cytokines and communicate these signals to the brain stem in "the inflammatory reflex," which in turn can act back toward end organs in the periphery, including the enteric nervous system, or elsewhere in the deeper brain structures, including the limbic system. (**c**) The hypothalamic-pituitary-adrenal (HPA) axis secretes glucocorticoids to attenuate inflammatory responses throughout the body

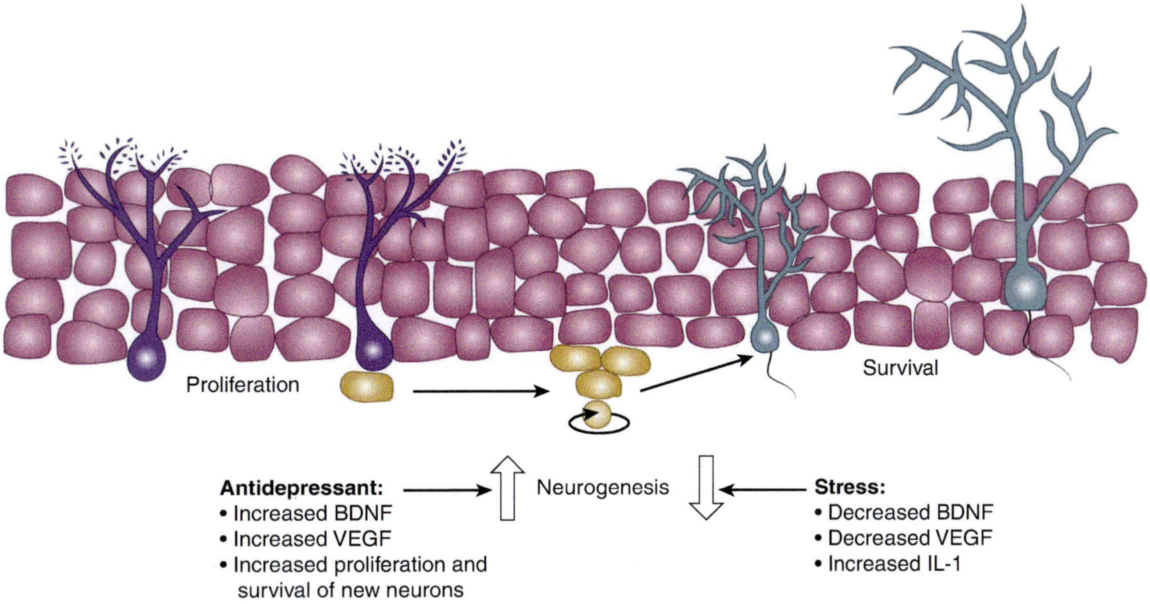

Fig. 17.9 Stress has opposing effects to antidepressants on neurogenesis, shown in the diagram. Neurotrophic molecules, like brain-derived neurotrophic factor (BDNF), have direct impacts on the synaptic and neural substrates

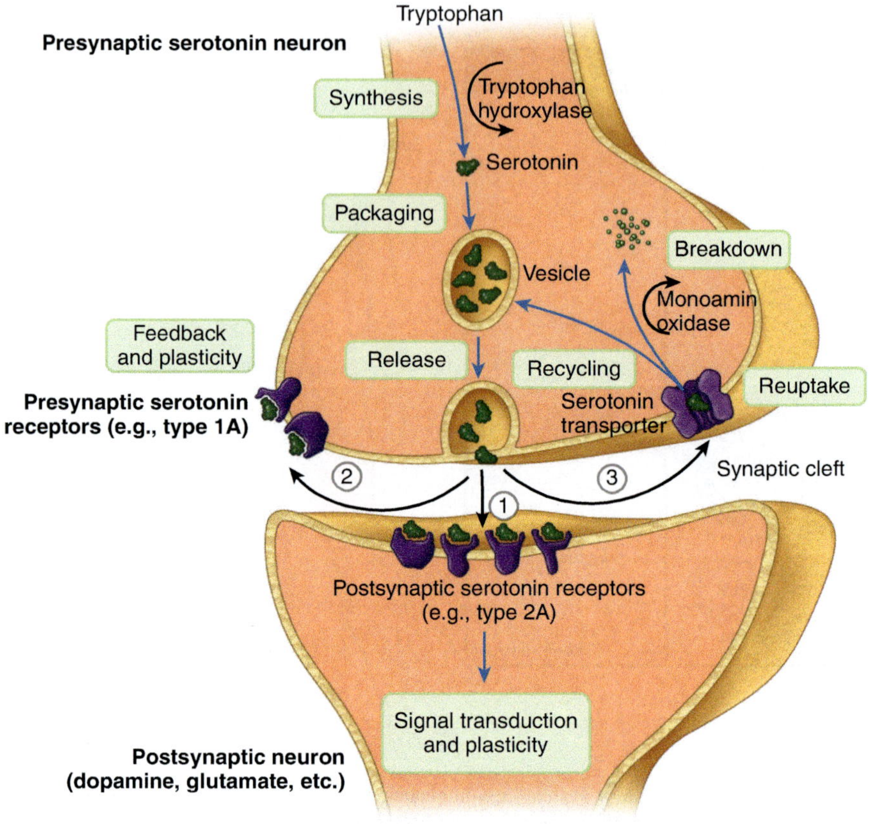

Fig. 17.10 The serotonin synapse shown here begins with the biochemical synthesis of serotonin from the essential amino acid tryptophan. Multiple enzymatic steps exist in its biosynthesis, but tryptophan hydroxylase catalyzes the early and important step that produces the hydroxylated version ultimately converted into 5-hydroxytryptamine, "5-HT"

Structural and Functional Brain Alterations

With sizable contributions to our understanding of the pathophysiology underwriting MDD, the neuroimaging field remains one of the most exciting areas of psychiatric neuroscience and has heralded in novel therapeutic paradigms aimed at targeting particular aberrancies in this population. A simplified version of the neural system and neuroanatomic structures and connections of interest most identified in MDD is shown in Fig. 17.11. Neural systems critically involved in emotional and reward processing and voluntary and automatic regulation of emotion are depicted in Fig. 17.12 similarly implicated in MDD with widespread enthusiasm.

Structural alterations nearly ubiquitously reference one of the most established findings of volumetric decreases in the hippocampus of MDD [33–35]. Figures 17.13 and 17.14 show one of the early works describing hippocampal atrophy on MRI as a function of time depressed, sparking much interest in both the neuroanatomic structure itself and areas of the brain it may operate with in sync.

Other findings on structural MRI have been shown with cortical thinning in the orbitofrontal cortex, anterior and posterior cingulate, insula, and temporal lobes in MDD [36, 37]. Figure 17.15 shows meta-analytic results of the comparative volume reduction of structures, including the hippocampus, in MDD. Microstructural integrity of white matter is further discerned using MRI technologies in the form of diffusion tensor imaging, implicating dysconnectivity within callosal and internal capsular fiber tracts [38], rendered in Figs. 17.16 and 17.17.

Functional neural circuits speak to the understanding that neural connections span widely throughout the brain, in seemingly distinct areas, and operate concordantly to produce an outcome, be it at "rest" or while performing a given "task," so defined in the two overarching variants of functional MRI studies describing "resting-state" or "task-based" findings. Functional MRI (fMRI) studies have delineated more broadly applied, but replicated, circuits in terms of networks relative to their behavioral manifestations. One of the fundamental principles of fMRI is that neuronal populations may work cooperatively, sequentially, and in pre-set ways,

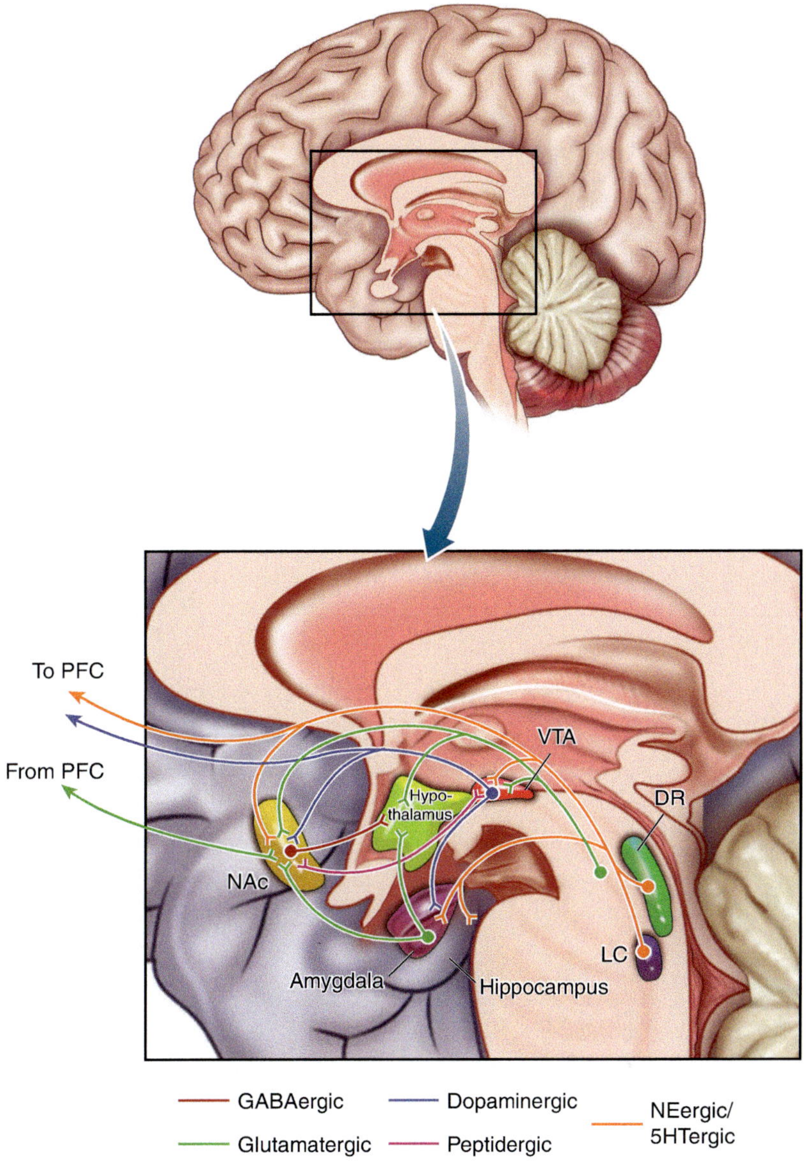

Fig. 17.11 Neural circuitry of depression involves pathways between the hippocampus and prefrontal cortex structures. The behavioral outputs served by these networks are implicated in reward, fear, and motivation, with other notable subcortical structures playing integral roles, including the nucleus accumbens, ventral tegmental area, and hypothalamus. Monoaminergic system interfaces within these limbic structures focally at the locus coeruleus and the dorsal raphe, the main sites of norepinephrine and serotonin production, respectively

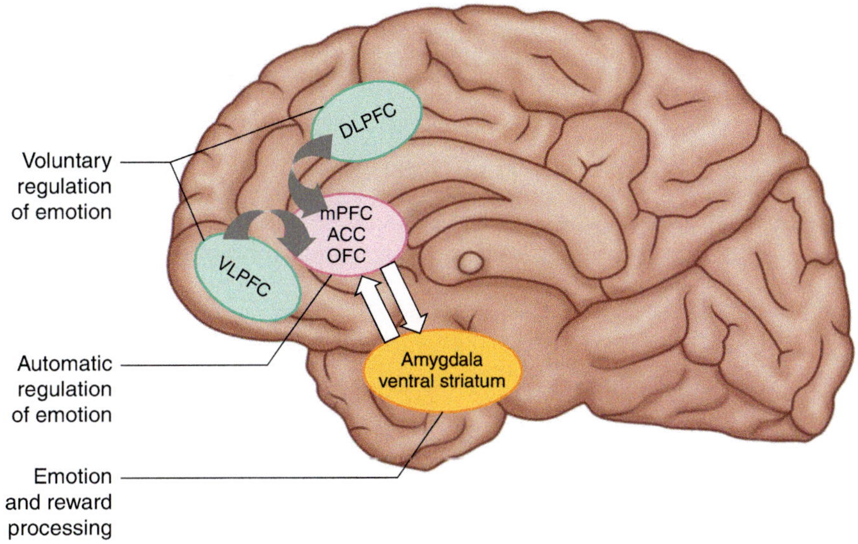

Fig. 17.12 Neural systems implicated in major depressive disorder are overlaid on a grayscale three-dimensional rendition of the human brain. Regions and circuits of interest are those involved in emotional and reward processing and voluntary and automatic regulation of emotion from various prefrontal cortical structures to medially subcortical and deeper brain structures

Fig. 17.13 Coronal section through the hippocampus (**a**) slices across the whole brain on conventional structural MRI. Hippocampal sections were volumetrically assessed in sagittal, axial, and coronal sections for greater clarity of anatomic localization (**b**). Analysis proceeded with depressed versus controls for group differences in hippocampal volumes, demonstrating reductions in bilateral neuromorphometric measures in the hippocampus in depressed subjects compared to normal controls

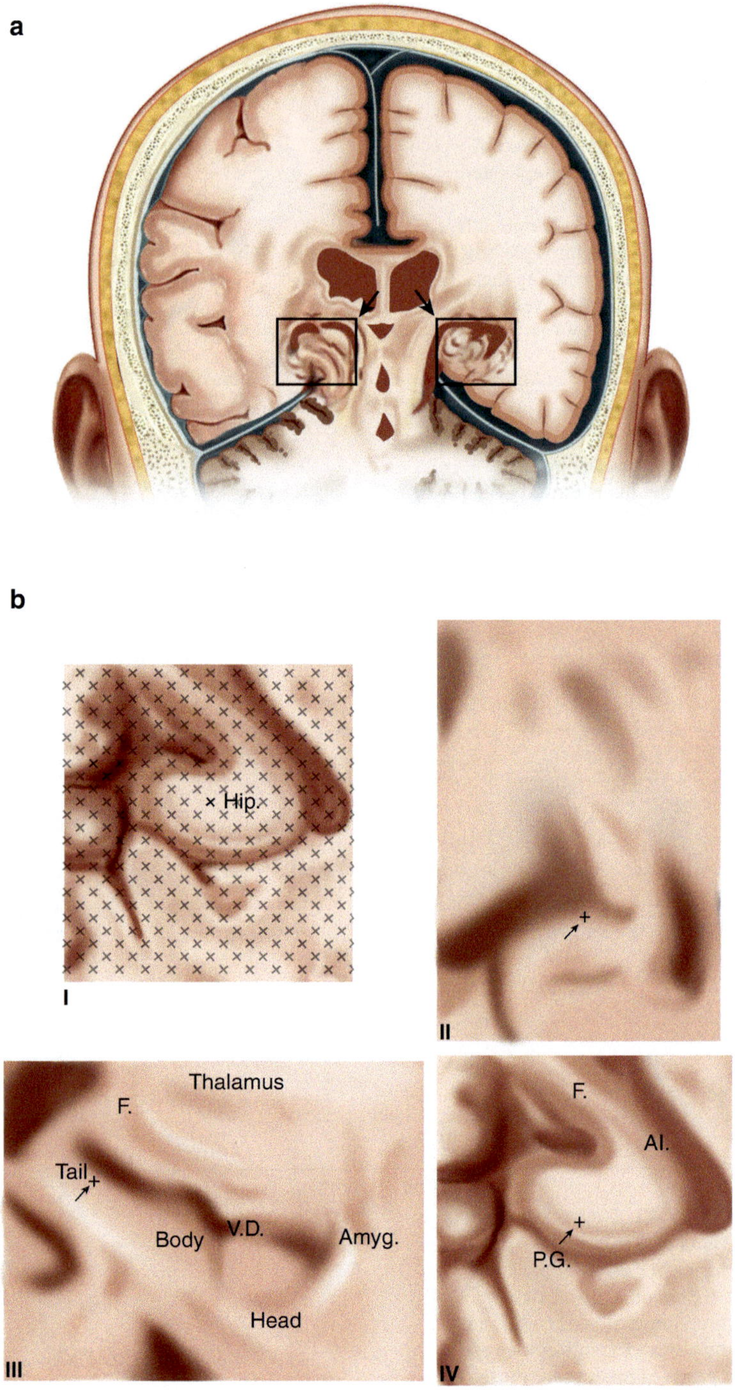

and when disturbed along this pathway, behavioral problems may ensue. The affective-salience circuit plays a central role in directing motivation secondary to an emotional or cognitive stimuli. Neurons within this network are located, partly, in the dorsal cingulate, anterior insula, ventral striatum, and amygdala and target areas within the hypothalamus and brain stem. In MDD, there is a reported increase in connectivity, reflecting a heightened activation pattern of the amygdala [39], disrupting the necessary balance needed between amygdalar activity within this circuit to achieve proper mood stability. Hypoactivity with concomitant reduced connectivity is observed in the ventral striatum of this network in MDD, causing impaired recruitment of dorsal cingulate and anterior insula [40], negatively impacting these regions with significance in the reward pathways [41]. Figure 17.18 presents a schematic model that incorporates an interplay between the neurobiological circuit-based findings and their associated mechanisms and triggers.

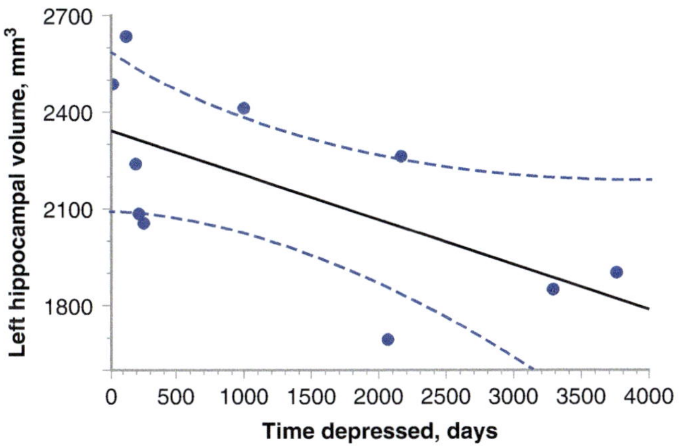

Fig. 17.14 Data from hippocampal sections of depressed and non-depressed control individuals showing the correlation between left hippocampal gray matter volumes and total days of major depression being inversely proportional

The default mode network, another functional neuronal connectivity pattern, is active during resting states when mental activity is predominantly of an internal or self-directed manner [42]. In MDD, symptoms of rumination [43] are due to a "hyperconnected" default mode network [39, 44], perpetuating these symptoms, due to an inability to tamper the excessive self-referential thoughts oftentimes coupled with negative thinking.

Lastly, the frontoparietal cognitive control circuit responsible for engagements in cognitive tasks is found to be hypoconnected in MDD as well. Most notably, this aberrancy is demonstrated in the region of the dorsolateral prefrontal cortex, which is implicated in goal-directed attention deficits seen in MDD [45]. Cognitively distorted negative appraisals of events known to occur in MDD are thought to be due to this dysfunctional network [46, 47] as well. The

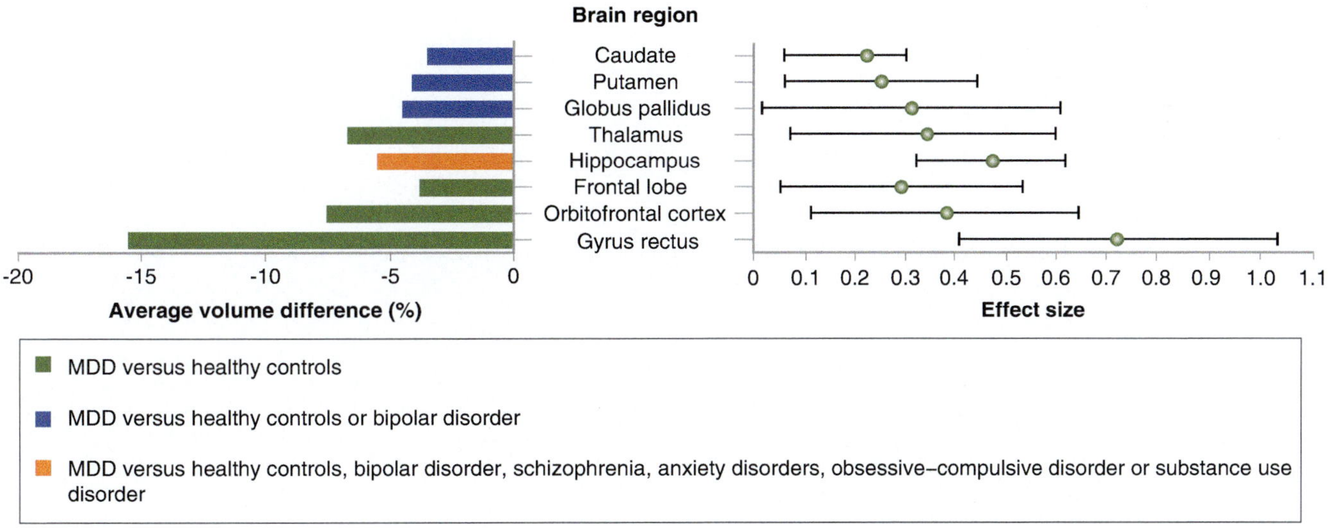

Fig. 17.15 Structural brain alterations in MDD from MRI studies compared to healthy controls, bipolar disorder, schizophrenia, anxiety disorders, obsessive-compulsive disorder, or substance use disorder, alongside respective effect sizes (*From* Otte et al. [5]; *with permission*)

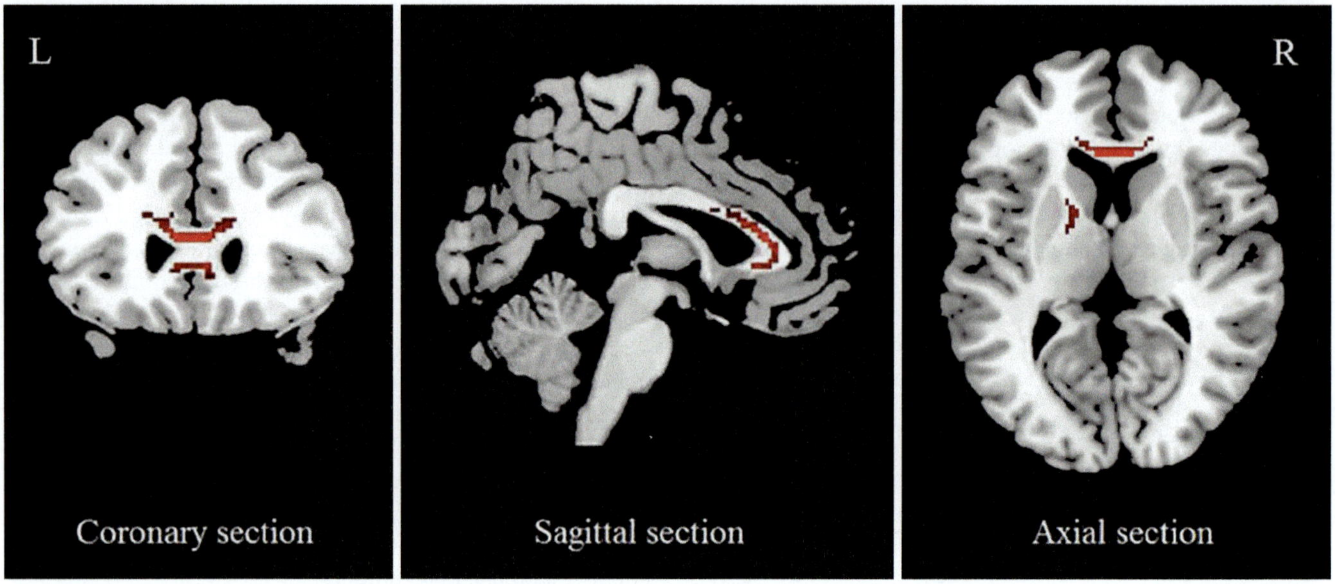

Fig. 17.16 Fractional anisotropy, a measure of microstructural connectivity, derived from diffusion tensor imaging MRI techniques, demonstrates reductions in the genu and body of the corpus callosum and the left anterior limb of the internal capsule in major depressive disordered patients compared with healthy control subjects. Clusters are overlaid in red color to delineate these structures. The main fibers passing through the corpus callosum are the interhemispheric tracts connecting prefrontal and orbitofrontal cortices. The anterior limb of the internal capsule serves as the major tract for the anterior thalamic radiation serving connections with the medial dorsal thalamic nuclei and prefrontal cortices. (From Chen et al. [38]; Creative Commons; http://creativecommons.org/licenses/by/4.0)

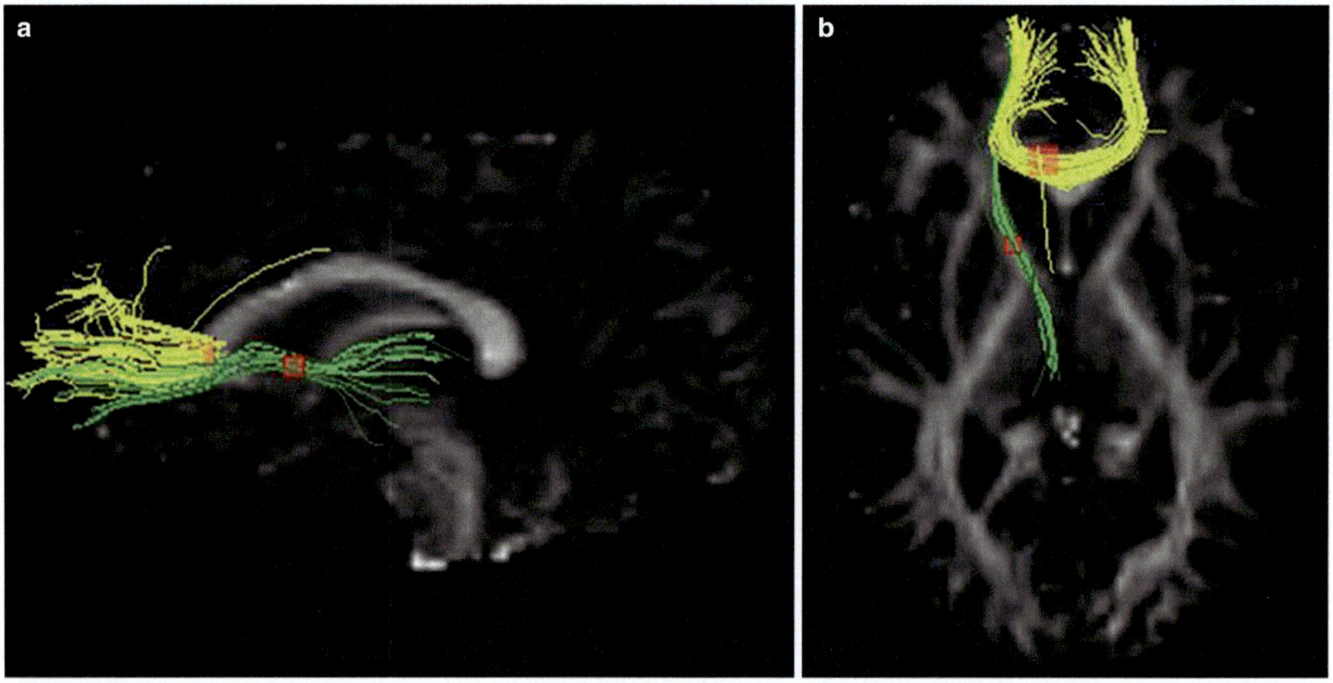

Fig. 17.17 This three-dimensional rendition of white matter tracts traversing frontally oriented fibers from the view of the left side of the brain (**a**) and from above (**b**). Tracts shown in yellow include the interhemispheric coursing fibers through the genu of the corpus callosum and the thalamic radiation traversing the left anterior limb of the internal capsule shown in green. Sagittal and axial slices mapping the fractional anisotropy values are also displayed (From Chen et al. [38]; Creative Commons; http://creativecommons.org/licenses/by/4.0)

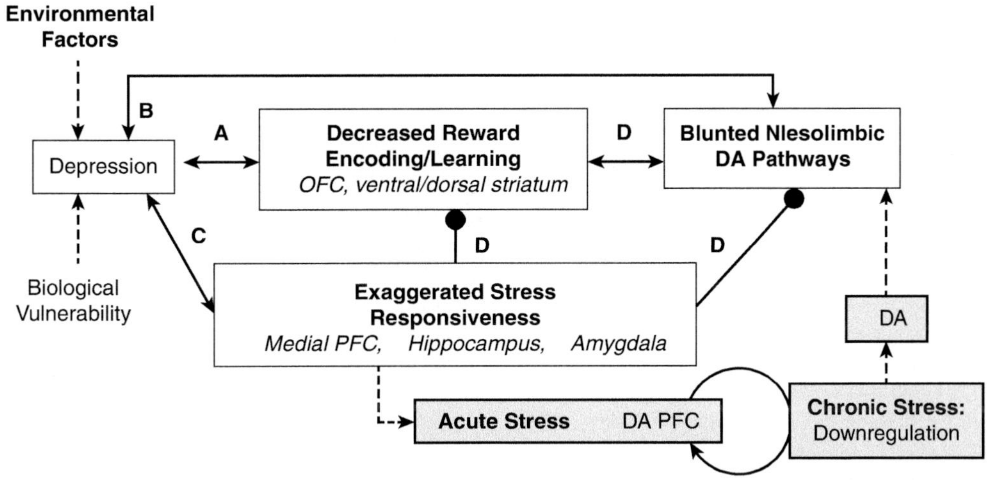

Fig. 17.18 Heuristic model that represents anhedonia arises from dysfunctional interactions between stress and brain reward systems. Reward-related decision-making and reinforcement learning are core features of depression interactions (*Link A*). Dopamine is closely linked to depression via reward processing when blunted (*Link B*). Environmental relationships between stress and depression, including early adverse events, are established to increase vulnerability to develop depression and stress sensitivity later in life (*Link C*). Preclinical work has suggested stress to negatively impact mesocorticolimbic dopaminergic pathways (*Link D*)

fMRI networks that display the most replicated findings on meta-analysis comparing MDD to healthy controls [45] are shown in Fig. 17.19, with neuroanatomic correlates juxtaposed as well for the important structures within the networks of interest. Similarly, Fig. 17.20 displays the interplay between these networks and deficit patterns in MDD [45] that may arise from these observations, across domains such as cognitions, ruminative thoughts, attentional/emotional dysregulation, and affective salience. An overview of pertinent neuroimaging findings is depicted in the diagram of Fig. 17.21, with certain areas and their implications for therapeutic interventions also noted.

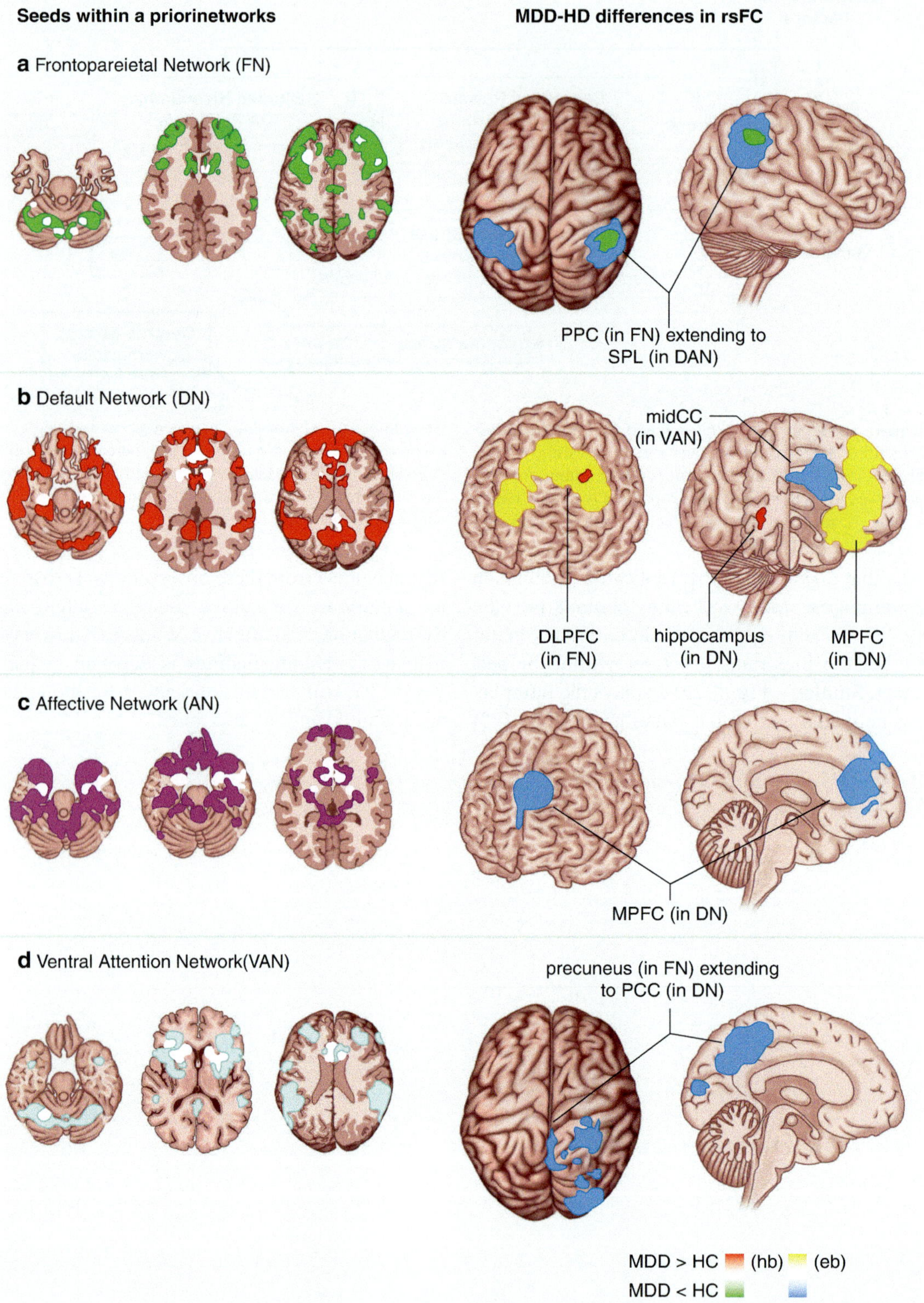

Fig. 17.19 Resting-state functional MR images of four major networks implicated in MDD with corresponding neuroanatomic structures found dysfunctional in MDD relevant to these networks. (**a**) MDD individuals exhibited hypoconnectivity within the frontoparietal network and a region of interest in the superior parietal lobule of the dorsal attention network. (**b**) MDD was associated with hyperconnectivity within the default network and areas in the prefrontal cortical regions. (**c**) MDD was linked to hypoconnectivity between areas in the affective network and regions of the medial prefrontal network. (**d**) MDD was related to activity changes between ventral attention network and precuneus extending to the occipital and posterior cingulate cortex; however, the direction remained unclear

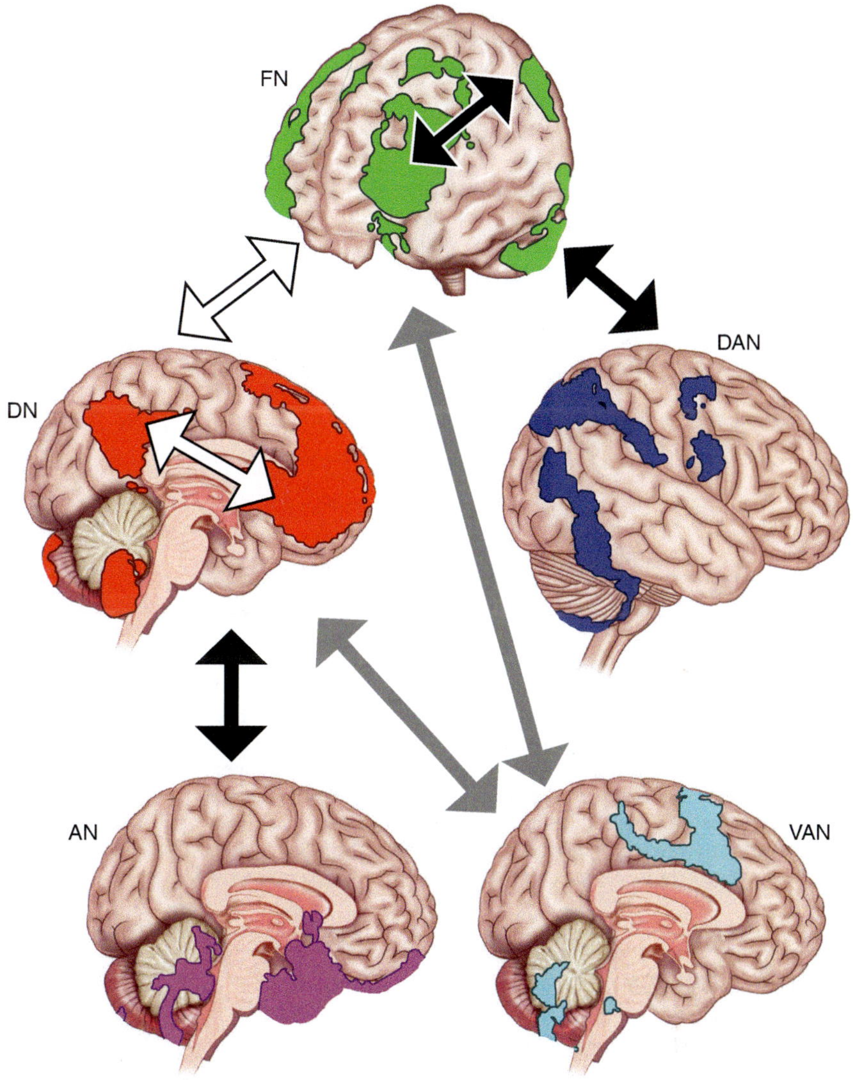

Fig. 17.20 The neurocognitive network model of major depressive disorder posits the interaction within and between four major functional connectivity networks with behavioral implications. Reduced connectivity among regions of frontoparietal network serves deficits in cognitive control, while increased connectivity between this network and the default network and reduced connectivity between frontoparietal network and dorsal attention network contribute toward ruminative thoughts. Meanwhile, reduced connectivity between the affective network and prefrontal cortical regions reflects the impairments in emotional and arousal regulation, whereas abnormal connectivity patterns between the ventral attention network and posterior regions implicated biased salience monitoring (black arrows represent hypoconnectivity; white arrows represent hyperconnectivity; and gray arrows represent abnormal connectivity in either direction)

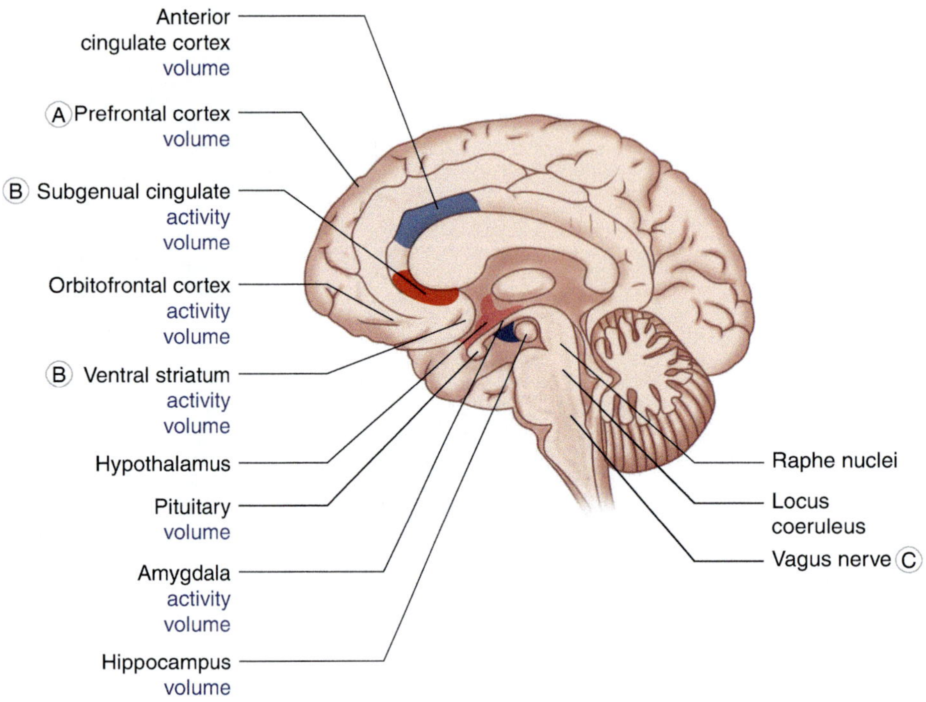

Fig. 17.21 Structural and functional brain abnormalities in patients with MDD are highlighted with a nod to sites of actions of novel neuromodulatory techniques. Structural patterns of abnormal findings include anterior cingulate volume reduction, in particular the subgenual cingulate, as well as related prefrontal cortical regions and subcortical regions like the amygdala, hippocampus, and ventral striatum. (**a**) Transcranial magnetic stimulation of the dorsolateral prefrontal cortex and (**b**) deep brain stimulation of the subgenual cingulate have antidepressant efficacy in subgroups of patients. (**c**) Vagus nerve stimulation similarly provides antidepressant properties by interacting with the locus coeruleus, the major site for norepinephrine production

Phenomenology

Symptomatology and RDoC Approach

Advances in the neurobiology of major depressive disorder have benefited from genetic, molecular, and neuroimaging technologies to further our understanding of these dynamic relationships and behavioral outputs. The schematic shown in Fig. 17.22 details an overview of these advances in the widening breadth of knowledge surrounding MDD with a much more research angle than previously applied to mental illnesses and their diagnoses based on phenomenology.

The Research Domain Criteria (RDoC) is not a diagnostic system but is helpful in organizing research questions that pertain to symptom categorization [48]. It was born out of efforts from the National Institutes of Health to reconcile a growing rift between neuroscience and psychiatry despite parallel hopes of better aligning the two in future iterations of the DSM. Figure 17.23 shows the matrix that is generated to help structure domains of inquiry into investigatory directions [49, 50]. The RDoC approach assumes a transdiagnostic paradigm that leans more heavily on psychobiological underpinnings than phenomenology, or symptom classification, that defines diagnosis and, ultimately, treatment.

DSM-5 criteria were outlined earlier in this chapter for each of the depressive disorders. A major depressive episode (MDE) is often described by the person as depressed, sad, hopeless, discouraged, or “down in the dumps.” Somatic complaints may be a chief complaint, like bodily aches and pains, but with careful interview, the underlying feelings of sadness can be gleaned. Irritability and anxiety can also be present or noted with persistent anger and a tendency to place blame or respond with outbursts or exaggerated frustration over minor matters. Loss of interest or anhedonia is always present, and fatigue may, in more milder or prodromal forms, appear as a greater effort required to perform similar tasks as one had previously been able to do. Changes in eating or sleeping in either direction may constitute MDE and at times will portend different treatment strategies depending on these “neurovegetative” symptoms. Psychomotor changes are also key indicators into disease course and must also be gathered from both the mental status and a physical examination, especially when concerns for catatonia may be present.

Memory complaints can often accompany elderly populations in a category known as “pseudodementia.” Here, attentional deficits beget the memory ones in depression and are reversible when the depression is appropriately treated [51] and attentional capacity is restored.

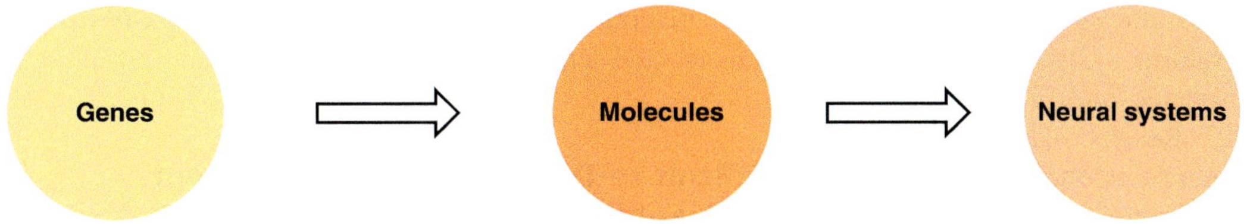

Genetic measures
- Candidate genes associated with MDD (ie, beyond the conventional monoamine focus)
- Candidate genes associated with biological mechanisms and metabolic pathways for antidepressant medications
- Serotonergic mechanisms
- Other mechanisms
- Genome-wide association studies

Molecular measures
- Neurotrophic factors and other growth factors
- Proinflammatory cytokines
- Impaired regulation of the hypothalamic-pituitary-adrenocortical axis

Neuroimaging measures
Abnormalities in anatomically-defined neural systems
- Subcortical neural systems for emotion and reward processing
- Medal prefrontal regions involved in processing and implicit regulation of emotion
- Lateral prefrontal cortical systems involved in cognitive control and voluntary or effortful regulation of emotion

Abnormalities in neurotransmitter-defined neural systems
- Medial prefrontal-limbic network, modulated by serotonin
- Reward network, centred on ventral striatum and medial prefrontal cortices, modulated by dopamine

Newer neuroimaging methodologies to study MDD
- Measurement of brain activity during rest

Neuroimaging and antidepressant treatment response

Fig. 17.22 Advances in studying MDD from vantage points of genes, molecules, neural systems, and behavior to better understand and ask pathophysiologic underpinnings and treatment response prediction profiles. (*From* Kupfer et al. [32]; *with permission*)

UNITS OF ANALYSIS								
DOMAINS/CONSTRUCTS	**Genes**	**Molecules**	**Cells**	**Circuits**	**Physiology**	**Behavior**	**Self-Reports**	**Paradigms**
Negative Valence Systems								
Acute threat ("fear")								
Potential threat ("anxiety")								
Sustained threat								
Loss								
Frustrative nonreward								
Positive Valence Systems								
Approach motivation								
Initial responsiveness to reward								
Sustained responsiveness to reward								
Reward learning								
Habit								
Cognitive Systems								
Attention								
Perception								
Working memo								
Declarative me								
Language behavior								
Cognitive (efforeful) control								
Systems for Social Processes								
Affiliatio attachment								
Social communication								
Perception/understanding of self								
Perception/understanding of others								
Arousal/ Modulatory Systems								
Arousal								
Biological rhythms								
Sleep-wake								

Fig. 17.23 The RDoC matrix. A two-dimensional organizational structure of functional constructs in rows, denoted by "genes," "molecules," "cells," "circuits," "physiology," "self-report," and "paradigms." Five higher-level domains of functioning are placed in columns as "negative valence systems" (encompassing fear, anxiety, loss), "positive valence systems" (reward seeking and consummatory behavior), "cognitive systems," "systems for social processes," and "arousal and regulatory systems" (generating activation of neural systems as appropriate for various actions and homeostatic control for energy, balance, and sleep)

A recent study using fMRI to address circuit-based symptom targets distinguished dysphoric symptoms, like sadness and anhedonia, from anxiosomatic ones like sleep, sexual interest, and irritability [52]. Results like that shown in Fig. 17.24 spark immense interest as one of the first of its kind in continuing to bolster a neurobiological approach to psychopathology as opposed to the vastly heterogeneous current scheme for classifying illness based on symptomatology. As will be explored in the section "Treatment", circuit abnormalities like these described have helped to inform novel neuromodulatory treatments that can non-invasively influence the activity of neuronal populations.

Difficult-to-Treat Depression (Treatment-Resistant Depression)

The long-term course of depression has been conceptualized to occur in phases, shown in Fig. 17.25. When depression persists despite adequate dose and duration of psychophar-

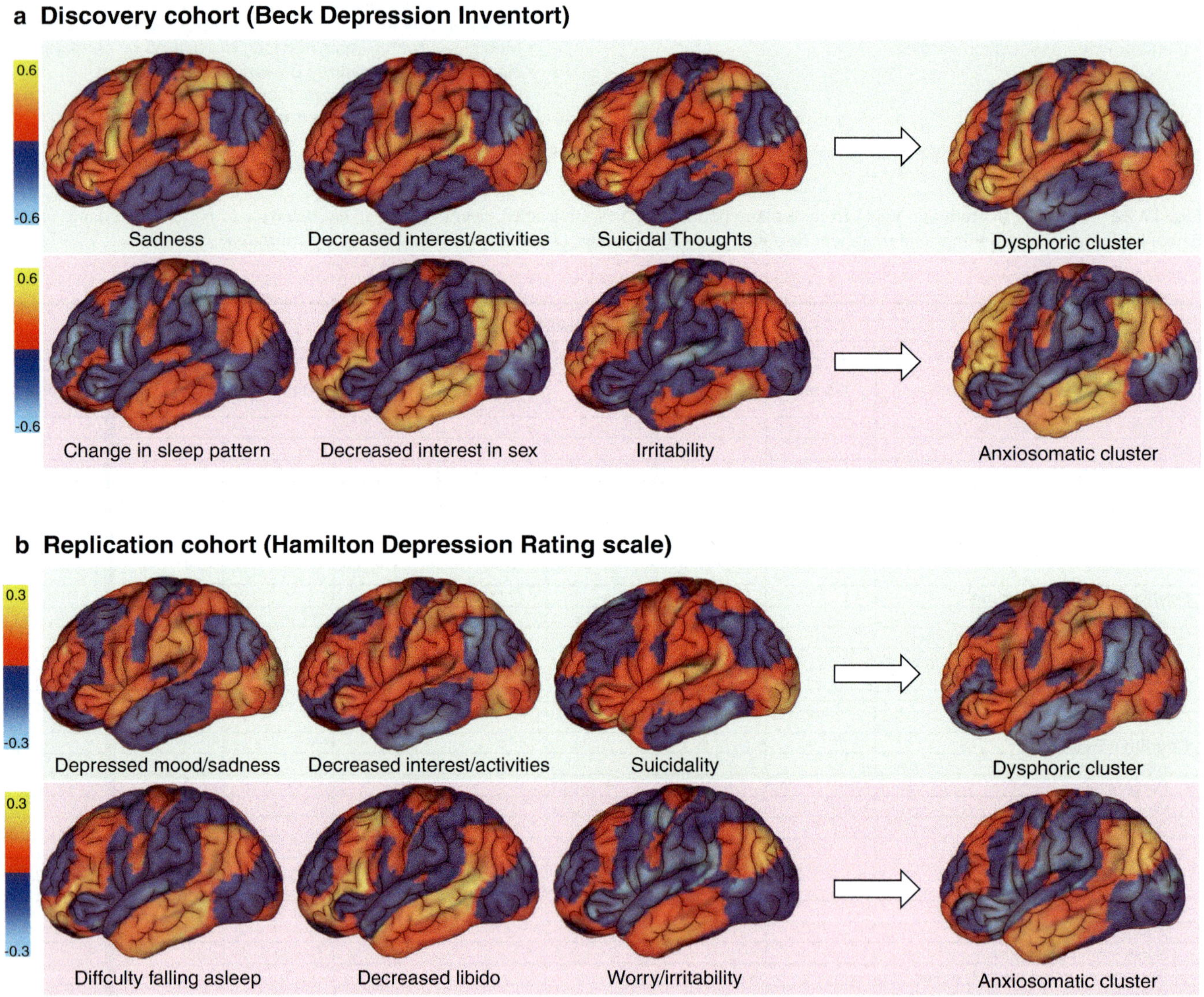

Fig. 17.24 Dysphoric vs anxiosomatic subtypes of depression based on neurobiological markers have sparked enormous interest in the field. In this high impact figure, the authors demonstrate a distinct set of improvements in symptoms as it relates to circuit-based neuromodulatory targets. (**a**) The Beck Depression Inventory, a commonly used clinical tool to measure depression, was used to correlate symptoms of sadness, decreased interest/activities, and suicidal thoughts, together grouped as the 'dysphoric cluster' to specific brain activity patterns. Similarly, changes in sleep pattern, decreased interest in sex, and irritability tracked together in the sonamed 'anxiosomatic cluster'. (**b**) This strategy was replicated using another commonly assessed clinical tool, the Hamilton Depression Rating Scale, to again parse out the 'dysphoric' and 'anxiosomatic' clusters, respectively. Note that the Hamilton Depression Rating Scale contains similar but not identical symptom domains, and so 'difficulty falling asleep', 'decreased libido', and 'worry/irritability' tracked in the same anxiosomatic cluster as its analogs in the Beck Depression Inventory

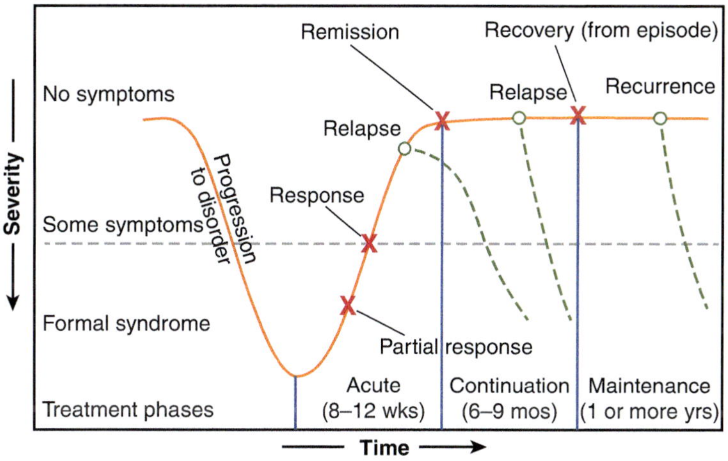

Fig. 17.25 Natural course of depression in phases and symptom severity as a function of time. The progression of MDD as outlined in this model was the basis for the design of the STAR*D trial, which found that about one-third of patients achieved remission following initial antidepressant medication

Table 17.10 A comparison of concepts

Term	Treatment-resistant depression (TRD)	Difficult-to-treat depression
Positioning	Opposition to…	Collaborative concept (patient, family, physician)
Model	Acute illness model	Chronic illness model
Approach	Mainly biological	Biopsychosocial
	Biomedical: cure	Capability approach
		Recovery movement
		Optimizing symptom control
		Minimizing impact of symptoms
Endpoint	Categorical (remission or not)	Dimensional (waxing and waning)

Fig. 17.26 Proposed workup of potential difficult-to-treat depression involves a concerted and often multidisciplinary effort

Proposed workup of potential difficult-to-treat depression.

Confirm primary psychiatric diagnosis
Assess adequacy of prior treatment recommendations (dose & duration)
Confirm adherence to prior treatment recommendations
Consider pharmacogenetics testing or therapeutic blood level monitoring
Assess concurrent psychiatric conditions that require remediation
Assess current general medical conditions that require remediation
Assess for undiagnosed general medical conditions that can cause depression
Evaluate current environmental stressors needing remediation

macologic interventions, the terminology "treatment-resistant" is broadly applied, which opens up options for more interventional and even off-label approaches to care, not limited to polypharmacy and neuromodulation discussed in the next section of this chapter. However, in 2019, clinician-researchers coined the term "difficult-to-treat" [53] as an alternative model for formulating therapeutic directions for this most marginalized and refractory demographic. A general overview of the main differences between these two systems is highlighted in Table 17.10 as well. Importantly, a proposed workup for depression unsatisfactorily managed with typical treatment strategies warrants more comprehensive consideration for a range of etiologic factors, as shown in Fig. 17.26.

Depression as a primary illness requires the exclusion of medical conditions that may present with such behavioral symptoms. Table 17.11 charts a non-exhaustive list of clinical laboratory tests that may be warranted in the basic workup for depression, especially if non-responsiveness is demonstrated to adequate psychopharmacologic trials [54]. A thorough review of medications taken is also warranted, as side effects of depression are well-established [54] in the list provided in Table 17.12.

Table 17.11 Laboratory studies in the workup to exclude medical illnesses that may present as depression

Complete blood cell count
Thyroid function test
Serum levels of vitamins B-12 and B-9 (folic acid)
Rapid plasma reagin
Electrocardiogram
HIV test
Electrolytes, including calcium, phosphate, and magnesium levels
Blood urea nitrogen and creatinine
Liver function tests
Blood alcohol level
Blood and urine toxicology screen
Arterial blood gas
Dexamethasone suppression test (Cushing disease, but also positive in depression)
Cosyntropin (ACTH) stimulation test (Addison disease)
Computed tomography (CT) scanning or magnetic resonance imaging (MRI) of the brain should be considered if organic brain syndrome or hypopituitarism is suspected, especially in the first episode of depression

Treatment

The treatment paradigm espoused posits that psychotherapy plus psychopharmacology works synergistically, that is, more beneficial than either component alone. However, with that idea comes the ability to properly assess and ascertain the most indicated forms of treatment, especially from the outset, based on severity and symptomatology. Figure 17.27 shows the stepwise progression in the management of MDD, assuming that all levels and intensities of care are available. It is not uncommon that real-world practice will face limitations on resources accessible. It is generally accepted that if psychotherapeutic interventions are available, milder forms of depression can be aptly managed without use of psychopharmacology initially, so long as close follow-up and properly tailored psychotherapy is able to be provided.

Table 17.12 Medications known to cause depression

Cardiovascular drugs	Anti-infective agents	Sedative and antianxiety drugs
• ACE inhibitors	• Ampicillin	• Barbiturates
• Calcium channel blockers	• Chloramphenicol	• Benzodiazepines
• Clonidine	• Chloroquine	• Chloral hydrate
• Digitalis	• Clofazimine	**Other drugs**
• Guanethidine	• Cycloserine	• Choline
• Hydralazine	• Cyclosporine	• Cimetidine
• Methyldopa	• Dapsone	• Disulfiram
• Procainamide	• Ethambutol	• Lecithin
• Propranolol	• Ethionamide	• Methysergide
• Reserpine	• Foscarnet	• Phenylephrine
• Thiazide diuretics	• Ganciclovir	• Physostigmine
• Guanabenz	• Griseofulvin	• Ranitidine
• Zolamide diuretics	• Isoniazid	• Statins
Chemotherapeutics	• Interferon	• Tamoxifen
• 6-Azauridine	• Metoclopramide	**Antiretroviral drugs**
• Asparaginase	• Metronidazole	• Atazanavir
• Azathioprine	• Nalidixic acid	• Efavirenz
• Bleomycin	• Nitrofurantoin	• Enfuvirtide
• Cisplatin	• Penicillin G procaine	• Saquinavir
• Cyclophosphamide	• Streptomycin	• Zidovudine
• Doxorubicin	• Sulfonamides	**Anticonvulsants**
• Vinblastine	• Tetracycline	• Ethosuximide
• Vincristine	• Trimethoprim	• Phenobarbital
Antiparkinsonian drugs	**Hormones**	• Phenytoin
• Amantadine	• Adrenocorticotropin	• Primidone
• Bromocriptine	• Anabolic steroids	• Tiagabine
• Levodopa	• Glucocorticoids	• Vigabatrin
Stimulants	• Oral contraceptives	**Anti-inflammatory agents**
• Amphetamines (withdrawal)	**Antipsychotic drugs**	• NSAIDs
• Caffeine	• Fluphenazine	
• Cocaine (withdrawal)	• Haloperidol	
• Methylphenidate (Ritalin)		

From Avasthi [54]; Creative Commons; https://creativecommons.org/licenses/by/3.0/

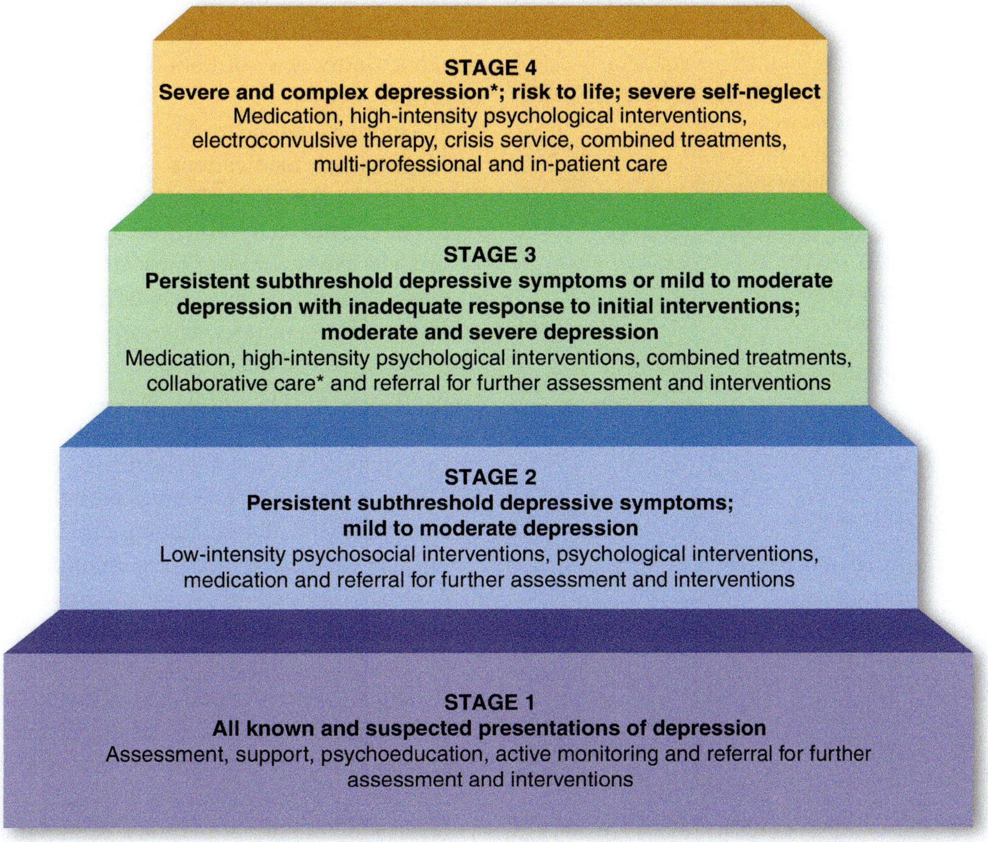

Fig. 17.27 Stepped care model in the management of MDD is aimed at guiding patients and providers in the treatment decisions that operates on a graded acuity to dictate the appropriateness of the intervention. The early steps in this model follow with the least intrusive, most effective strategies at the outset before proceeding in complexity of illness, responsiveness, and comorbidities or psychosocial complicating factors to success. (*From* Otte et al. [5]; *with permission*)

Psychotherapy

Several of the more popular psychotherapeutic interventions for MDD are listed in Table 17.13. Although comparable efficacy exists in the literature, theory and technique vary widely, and schools of thought have converged on the therapeutic alliance to subserve much of the benefit gained irrespective of the specific psychotherapeutic modality practiced [55].

The neurobiology of psychotherapy has taken shape with functional neuroimaging and ushered in a wave of research aimed at uncovering the mechanism behind the benefits in more depth and detail. Pivotal work toward this end identified the long theorized "top-down" approach to cognitive behavioral therapy, whereas antidepressant medication acted in a "bottom-up" fashion [57, 58], as shown in Fig. 17.28.

Psychopharmacology

An exhaustive review of the pharmacologic details surrounding MDD is outside the scope of this text; however, here we will review main psychopharmacologic considerations when approaching MDD in clinical practice. Major players of the antidepressant toolbox span several classes of drug families based on their predominate neurotransmitter targets, notably the monoamines, that is, serotonin, dopamine, and norepinephrine/epinephrine. Characteristics of these classes, including popularly used ones, side effects, and common considerations [59] are included in Table 17.14.

Crucial to grasping the mechanism behind psychopharmacologic benefit is the neurobiology of where the functional input takes hold, that is, at the level of the neuron and, more specifically, the neurotransmitter, receptor, and synap-

Table 17.13 Summary of study characteristics across the 198 studies included in the network meta-analysis

Descriptive categories	Study characteristics	Number of studies	Percent
Patient population	Regular depression	94	47%
	Geriatric depression	26	13%
	Student populations	8	4%
	Women with postpartum depression	16	8%
	General medical patients with depression	27	14%
	Miscellaneous	27	14%
Psychotherapeutic intervention[a]	Interpersonal therapy	27	14%
	Behavioral activation	26	13%
	Cognitive behavioral therapy	139	70%
	Problem-solving therapy	19	10%
	Social skills training	7	4%
	Psychodynamic therapy	16	8%
	Supportive counseling	37	19%
Control condition[b]	Placebo	27	14%
	Usual care	60	30%
	Waitlist	75	38%
Intervention format and setting	Individual and face to face	97	49%
	Others	98	50%
	Mixed	2	1%
Country	United States	115	58%
	United Kingdom	23	11%
	Continental Europe	27	13%
	Canada	8	4%
	Australia	13	6%
	Miscellaneous	15	8%

https://doi.org/10.1371/journal.pmed.1001454.t002

From Barth et al. [56]; Creative Commons Attribution License. https://creativecommons.org/licenses/by/3.0/us/

[a] The percentages do not add up to 100% because many studies contained more than one treatment

[b] The percentages do not add up to 100% because not all studies contained a control condition

tic sites (pre- and post-). Figure 17.29 depicts a cartoon of the main psychopharmacologic agents utilized in MDD and their sites of action. The complexity of the highly intricate system of the monoamine neurotransmitters which are influenced by these medications to target the depressive symptoms is far from clearly understood. Moreover, dynamics between receptor subtypes and neuronal functional networks are an active area of research that remains limited to the in vivo capabilities for investigation, leaving much still unknown in the way of definitive and singular mechanisms of action.

A landmark study to develop a treatment algorithm in antidepressant medications produced the scheme in Fig. 17.30 by which modern standard of practice is largely built upon. This study also provided evidence that psychopharmacologic benefit was most attained earlier in the course of treatment and that there may be dramatically reduced optimism for treatment responsiveness after the first augmentation strategy for antidepressants is utilized [60]. This notion is expressed in Fig. 17.31 and also suggests that other approaches to symptom relief may be warranted earlier on in disease course. A typical trajectory of what this course may look like as the patient traverses through treatment protocols en route to treatment non-response is shown in Fig. 17.32.

Difficult-to-treat depression emerges after a failure to achieve an adequate response or progression through the psychopharmacologic armamentarium, as previously stated. When this clinical entity is suspected, a variety of considerations are warranted to help formulate the patient and move forward with other forms of treatment that may still prove beneficial [61]. An overview of this concept with clinical implications and suggestions is provided in Fig. 17.33.

Neuromodulation, also called brain stimulation or interventional psychiatry, is a growing field, although also housing within it perhaps one of the oldest and most effective forms of treatment for depression, electroconvulsive therapy (ECT). Table 17.15 describes the neuromodulation methods commonly used in practice today [62]. Figure 17.21 provides a look at how ECT and transcranial magnetic therapy (TMS) are delivered, as well as deep brain stimulation, which is yet to achieve adequate and robust successes in depression but with much promise able to be seen in neurologic disorders with more observable and easily measurable phenotypes. The primary TMS target is the dorsolateral prefrontal cortex, given its functional connections to deeper brain structures also involved in MDD.

Emerging Therapy

With the technological advancements mentioned that are taking place within fields of genetics, neuroimaging, and novel treatments, abilities to predict response have come to the fore-

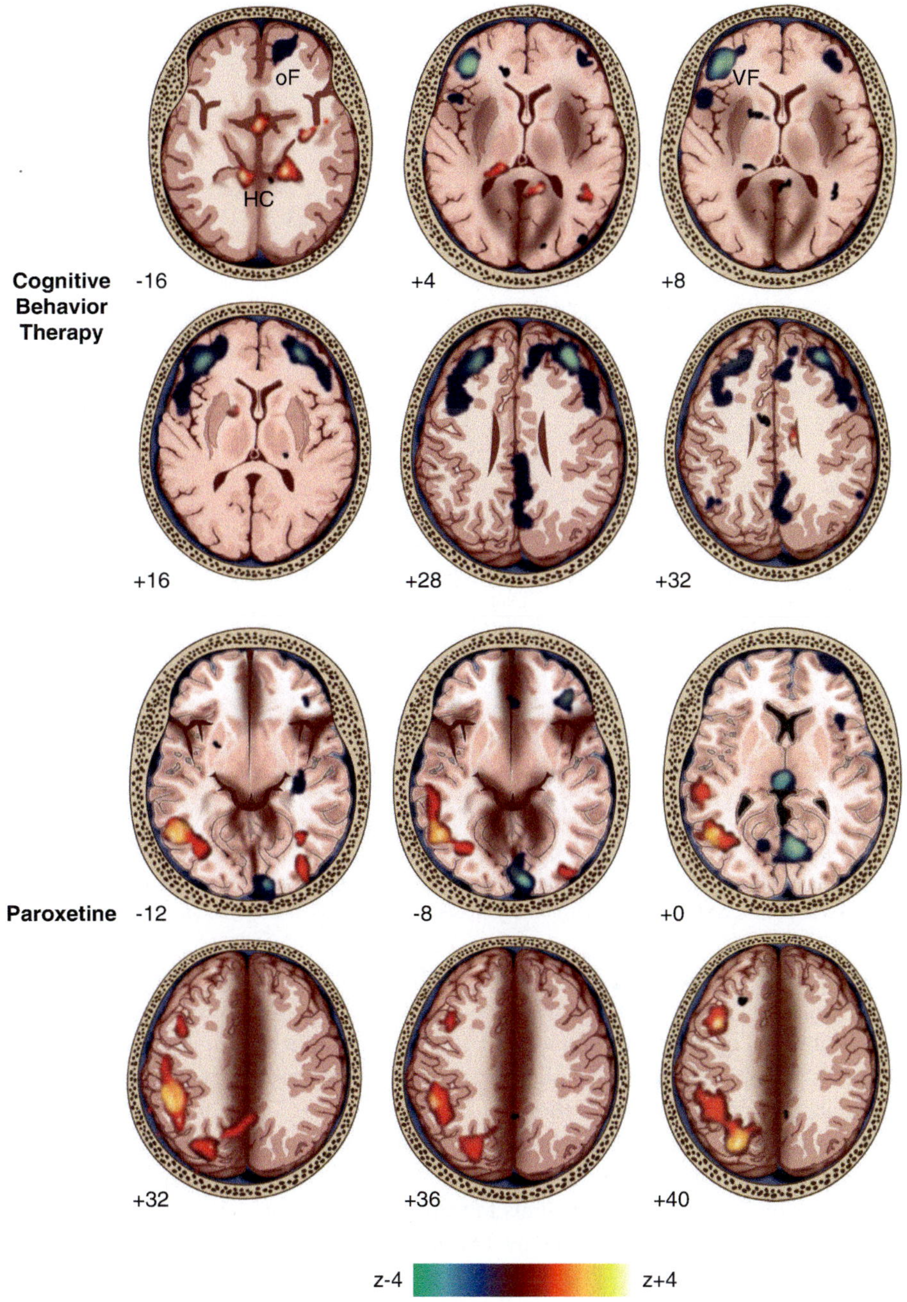

Fig. 17.28 Treatment with psychotherapy and antidepressant medication were each associated with significant regional metabolic changes. Changes in regional glucose metabolism in psychotherapy responders (top) and antidepressant responders (bottom) demonstrated differential patterns. Frontal and parietal decreases and hippocampal increases are seen with psychotherapy response, while the reverse pattern is observed with antidepressant psychopharmacology. Common to both treatments are decreases in ventral lateral prefrontal cortex

Table 17.14 Classes, SEs, and prescribing considerations for ADT

Class	Drugs	SE	Considerations
TCA	Imipramine Amitriptyline Doxepin Desipramine Nortriptyline	Weight gain, sedation, dry mouth, nausea, blurred vision, constipation, tachycardia	Generally not first-line therapy due to increased anticholinergic and cardiotoxic SE
MAOI	Isocarboxazid Phenelzine Tranylcypromine Selegiline	Weight gain, fatigue, sexual dysfunction, hypotension	Generally not first-line therapy due to serotonin syndrome and hypertensive crises
SSRI	Fluoxetine Paroxetine Sertraline Citalopram Escitalopram	Headaches, GI distress, insomnia, fatigue, anxiety, sexual dysfunction, weight gain	Often first-line treatment due to safer SE profile. Subtle SE differences must be weighed by the prescriber
SNRI	Venlafaxine Desvenlafaxine Duloxetine Levomilnacipran	Nausea, insomnia, dry mouth, headache, increased blood pressure, sexual dysfunction, weight gain	SEs are similar to but may be slightly more frequent than with SSRI
Atypical	Bupropion	Headache, agitation, insomnia, loss of appetite, weight loss, sweating	Increased seizure risk in eating disorder and epilepsy patients. No sexual dysfunction or weight gain. May also help to quit smoking
	Mirtazapine	Sedation, increased appetite, weight gain	Sedation may be less with higher dose. Much reduced nausea and sexual dysfunction compared with SSRI/SNRI. Some risk of reduced white blood cell count
	Trazodone	Sedation, nausea, priapism (rare)	Lower risk of weight gain and sexual dysfunction, but may cause priapism. Often used to induce sleep as a positive effect
	Vilazodone	Nausea, diarrhea, insomnia	Better SE profile than most ADTs with lower risk of sexual dysfunction or weight gain
	Vortioxetine	Nausea, diarrhea, dizziness	Similar SE profile to the SSRI. May have precognitive benefits in adults with MDD

ADT antidepressant treatment; *MAOI* monoamine oxidase inhibitor; *MDD* major depressive disorder; *SE* side effect; *SNRI* serotonin-norepinephrine reuptake inhibitor; *SSRI* selective serotonin reuptake inhibitor; *TCA* tricyclic antidepressant

front of what personalized delivery of psychiatric care has come to mean. To that end, the ability to custom blend management based on biomarkers has become an exciting area of research with wide reaching implications, and already available data toward this avenue is shown in Fig. 17.34.

An adaptation from the previously held standard of care that makes use of these response predictors may shape guidelines and directions for patients to utilize in the not so distant future, as conceptualized by researchers shown in Fig. 17.35.

The glutamatergic system, operating through a variety of receptors including the NMDA receptor, has heralded in a new age of mechanistic approaches to depression treatment. With it, ketamine and its derivative and related compounds, including esketamine, have recently received widespread attention and an FDA indication in this population. The mechanism is still being more fully investigated and likely operates widely through other means than was previously thought. The pharmaco-biologic understanding depicted in Fig. 17.36 attempts to detail some of the major pathways and means in which ketamine acts.

Psychedelic drugs have made their way into potential treatments for severe forms of depression, and benefits continue to yield promise. Mechanisms are beginning to be explored that juxtaposes their actions next to the predominantly serotonergic-acting compounds, given shared overlap in target neurotransmitter systems [65], as shown in Fig. 17.37. Perhaps most exciting of all prospects related to this model is that with it comes the necessity that psychotherapeutic targets are also addressed. Dosing of psilocybin as currently conceptualized requires that sessions of psychotherapy are paired in preparatory and integration sessions alongside the hallucinogenic experience. Hope for the coming wave of this and similar types of research will again seek concerted efforts between both arenas in psychiatry, that is, psychopharmacology and psychotherapy, as interventions with individual and synergized effects at mitigating this most marginalized population.

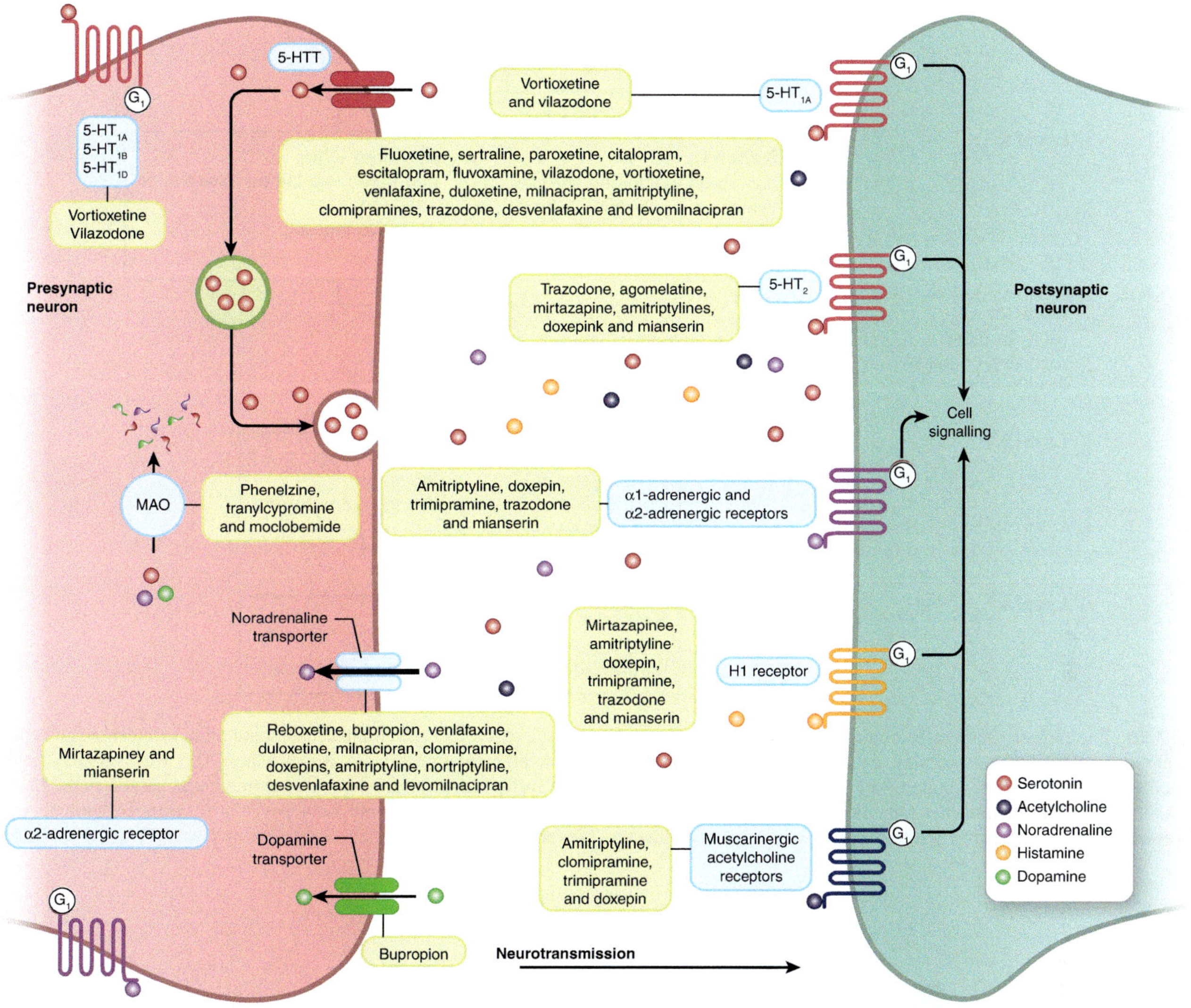

Fig. 17.29 Major psychopharmacologic agents utilized in MDD and their sites of action are shown in this cartoon. Mechanisms of action are illustrated for many commonly used medications, including selective serotonin reuptake inhibitors (SSRIs), which antagonize the serotonin transporter (5-HTT), preventing reuptake. Relatively selective noradrenaline reuptake inhibitors act similarly at the noradrenaline transporter. Tricyclic antidepressants (TCAs) and other cyclic antidepressants, as well as the serotonin-noradrenaline reuptake inhibitors (SNRIs), block the reuptake of serotonin and noradrenaline by opposing the respective transporter activity in varying ratios. Noradrenaline-dopamine reuptake inhibitors (NDRIs) act primarily to prevent the noradrenaline and dopamine reuptake. Alpha-2 adrenergic receptor antagonists enhance release of serotonin and noradrenaline by blocking these autoreceptors. Dual-action serotonin receptor antagonists/agonists primarily bind to serotonin 5-HT2 receptors, one of the many subtypes that exist. (*From* Otte et al. [5]; *with permission*)

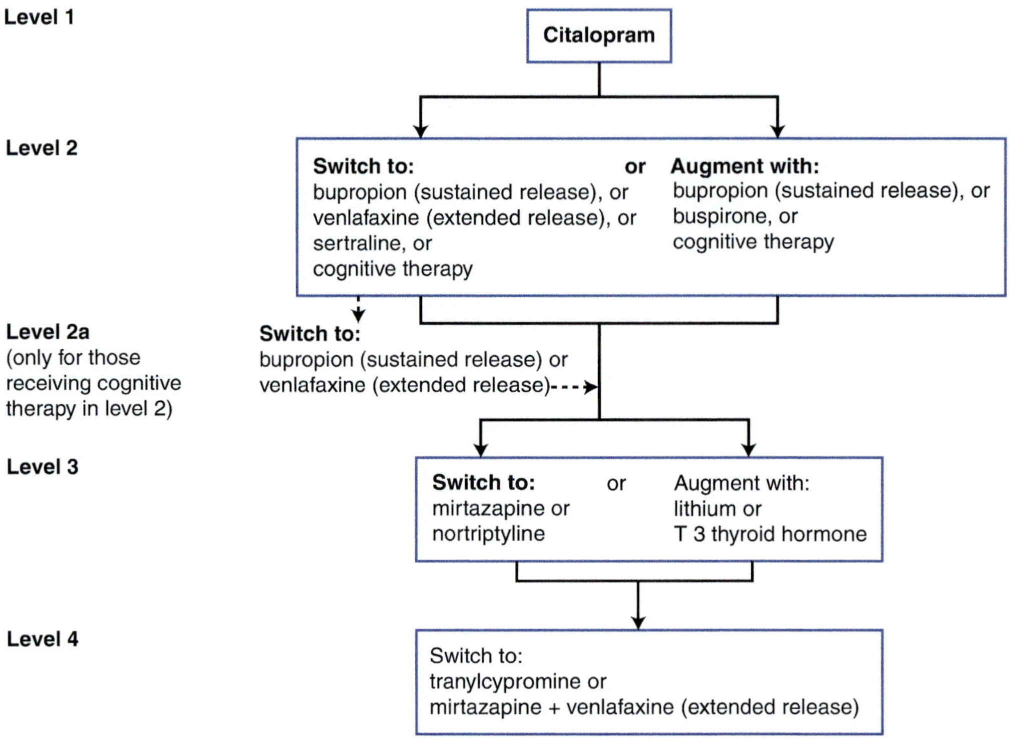

Fig. 17.30 The largest prospective clinical trial of major depressive disorder is captured by this diagram, called the STAR*D study. All enrolled patients began on a single SSRI (citalopram) for a 12-week course. If remission was not met after dose was increased, patients progressed to the next level of treatment provision whereby either a switch to another psychopharmacologic class or mechanism of action or an augmentative strategy was initiated. This was similarly followed into further levels of medication treatment and served as the basis for follow-up studies shaping how psychiatric practice evolved in this regard

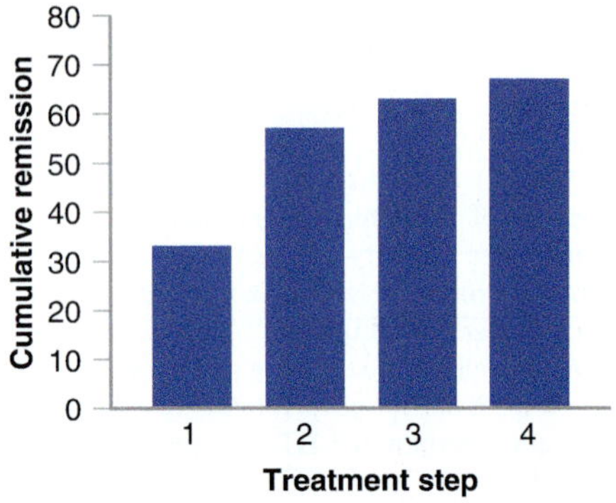

Fig. 17.31 An outcome of the STAR*D trial also revealed the cumulative remission rate at each treatment level. The cumulative remission rate was theorized at 67% but was found to be very dependent on the level of treatment the patient progressed through, such that remission was more likely to occur during the earlier trials at roughly 20–30% than during the later trials, roughly 10–20%

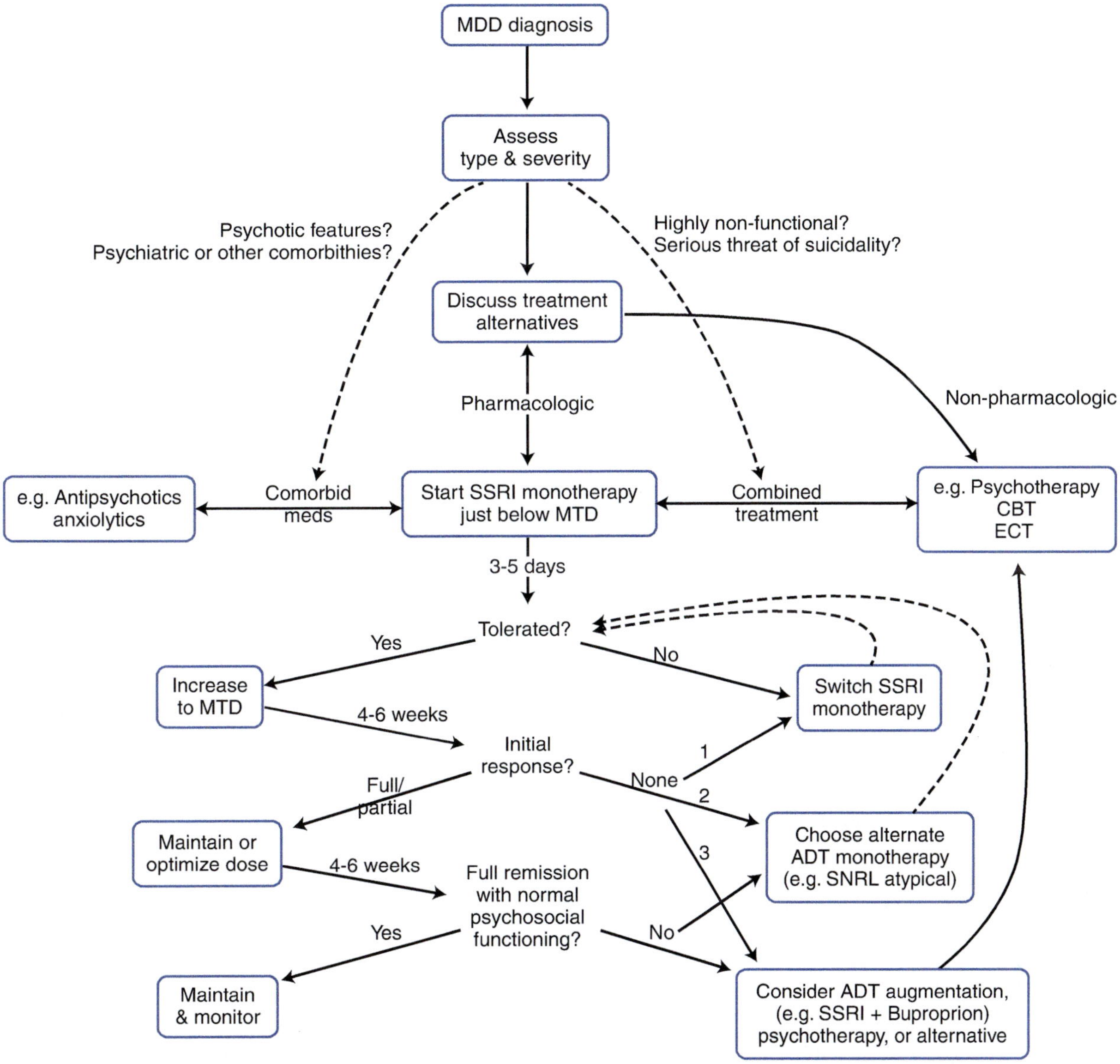

Fig. 17.32 Treatment algorithms have become more detailed by including other modalities available in addition to psychopharmacologic regimens. This figure illustrates the basic progression of patients with the combination of treatments, including psychotherapeutic and brain stimulation, especially if suicidality is present. *ADT* antidepressant treatment; *CBT* cognitive behavioral therapy; *ECT* electroconvulsive therapy; *GI* gastrointestinal; *MDD* major depressive disorder; *MID* minimum therapeutic dose; *SNRI* serotonin-norepinephrine reuptake inhibitor; *SSRI* selective serotonin reuptake inhibitor

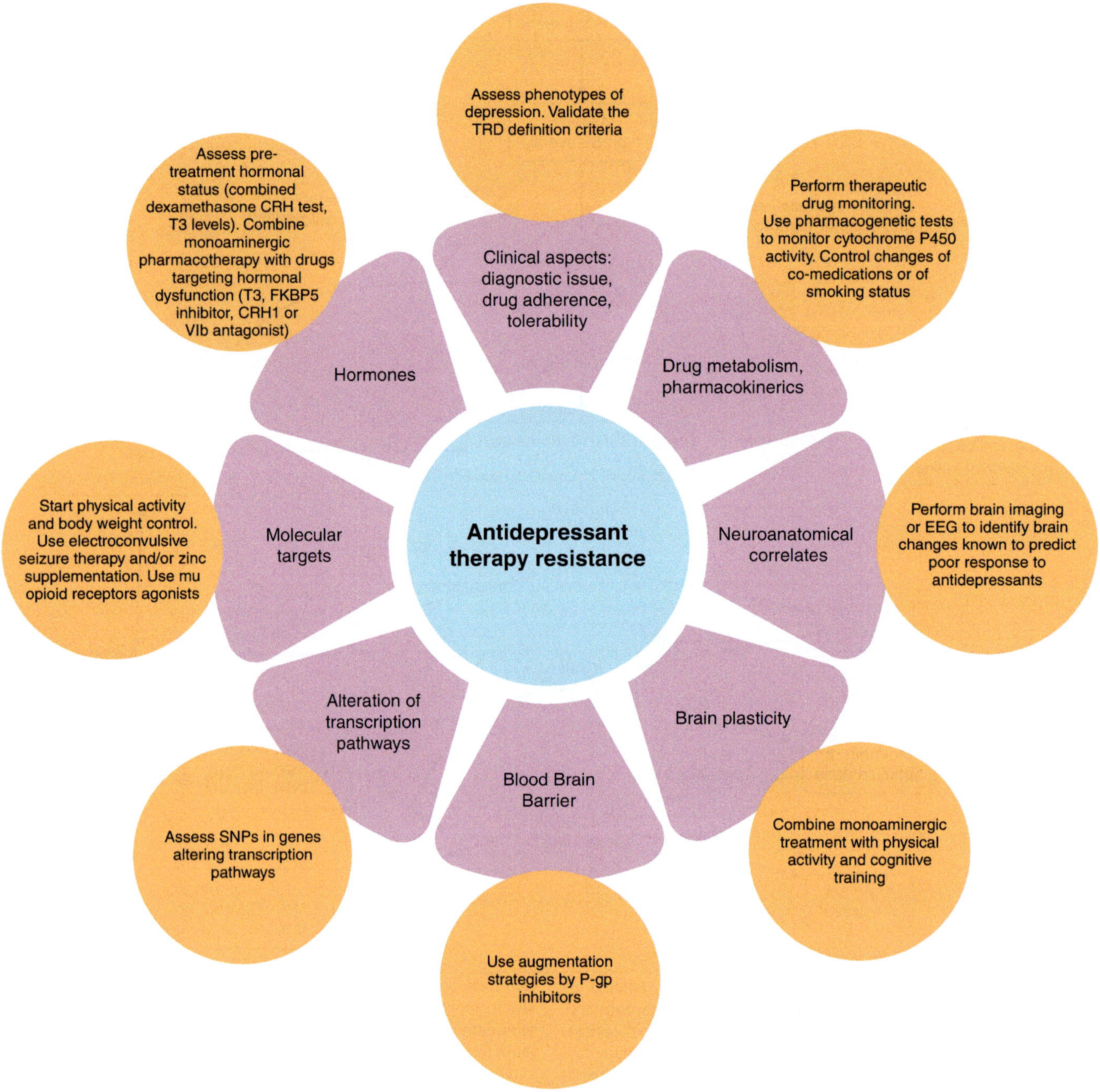

Fig. 17.33 Mechanisms associated with antidepressant therapy resistance (purple) and recommendations for clinical practice (orange). (*From* El-Hage [61]; Creative Commons; https://creativecommons.org/licenses/by/3.0/)

Table 17.15 The neuromodulation methods commonly used in practice

Method	Mechanism of action	Efficacy	Safety	Delivery method(s)
Electroconvulsive therapy (ECT)	Potent electric stimuli for inducing therapeutic seizures and increasing overall cortical activity.	Meta-analyses suggest strong effectiveness for severe MDD, psychotic MDD, TRD and MDD with suicidal ideation. It is also shown to be superior to simulated ECT and antidepressants.	Very low mortality rates, but caution with patients with cardiovascular disease. Short-term side effects are headache and myalgia. Long-term cognitive impairment is a consideration, especially in subgroup of patients and in some techniques.	Pulse vs. Sinewave Uni- vs. Bilateral Bifrontal vs. Bitemporal 2 vs. 3 times/week
Repetitive transcranial magnetic stimulation (rTMS)	Use of electromagnetic induction to focus induced current in brain; repetitive TMS modulates long-term cortical excitability.	Recent meta-analyses show it is as effective as antidepressant drugs in treating MDD and TRD (indirect comparison). One RCT showed rTMS and venlafaxine ER to have sim-ilar efficacy. One subgroup analysis suggests that rTMS has increased efficacy in TRD patients.	Induced seizures are the most severe adverse event, but only 16 cases were re-ported hitherto. Common side effects include head-ache and facial pain. No cognitive impairment reported.	High vs. Low frequency Left vs. Right DLPFC stimulation 80–120% MT 10–30 sessions
Transcranial direct current stimulation (tDCS	Weak direct currents are applied to the brain via scalp electrodes in a simple, painless manner; shifting up or down the cortical excitability according to the current polarity.	Mixed results so far (One positive and one negative RCT, two positive open-label studies).	No serious adverse events. Common side effects include skin irritation and itching sensation on the spot of stimulation.	Target area: left DLPFC Reference: right DLPFC or right supra-orbital area 1–2 mA / 15–30 min 5–10 sessions
Deep brain stimulation (DBS)	Electrodes connected to pulse generators are im-planted in some brain areas, the most studied is the subgenual cingulate region.	There are only open trials with small samples to date, studying patients with high degree of refractoriness and showing response rates of 50–60%.	Invasive brain stimulation procedure with the usual risks of a neurosurgical procedure. Long-term ad-verse events include trem-or and transient hypomania. No cognitive impairment reported.	Parameters of stimulation are adjusted individually.
Vagus nerve stimulation (VNS)	Electrodes connected to the left vagus nerve generate impulses further transmitted to subcortical areas.	Mixed results overall, but open-label studies are favorable. FDA-approved for patients who failed +4 antide-pressant treatments.	Usual risks of a head & neck surgery. Transient hypomania reported. No cognitive impairment reported.	Parameters of stimulation are adjusted individually.

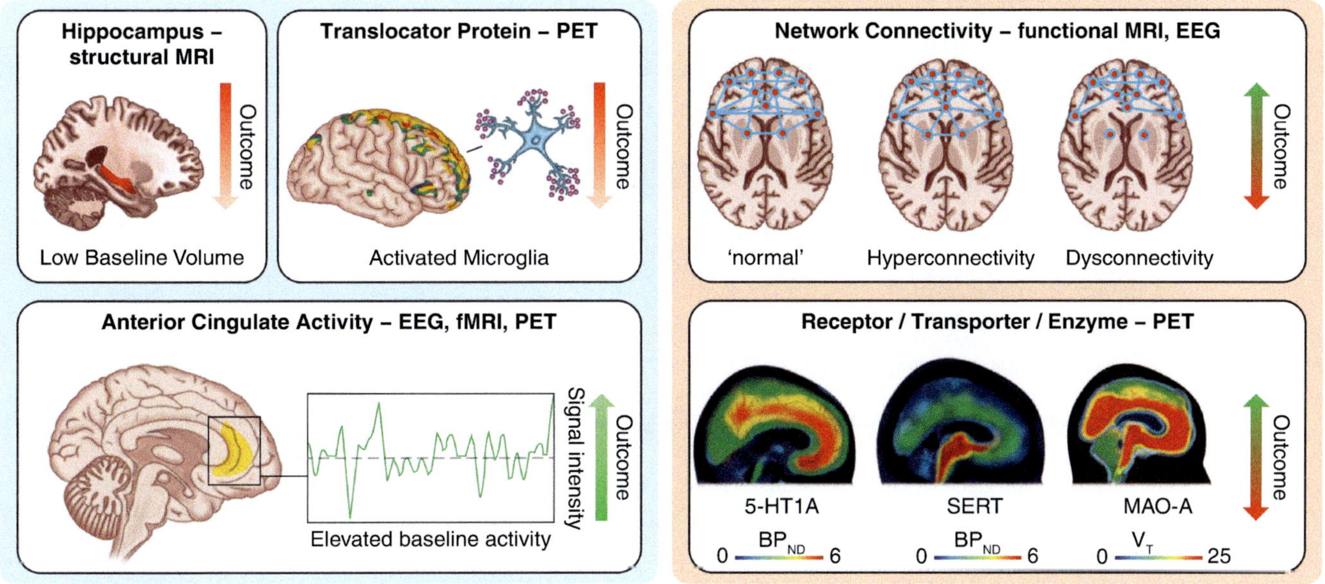

Fig. 17.34 Summary of findings from neuroimaging research and neurophysiologic correlates of depression-related pathology. (From Kraus [63]; Creative Commons; https://creativecommons.org/licenses/by/4.0/)

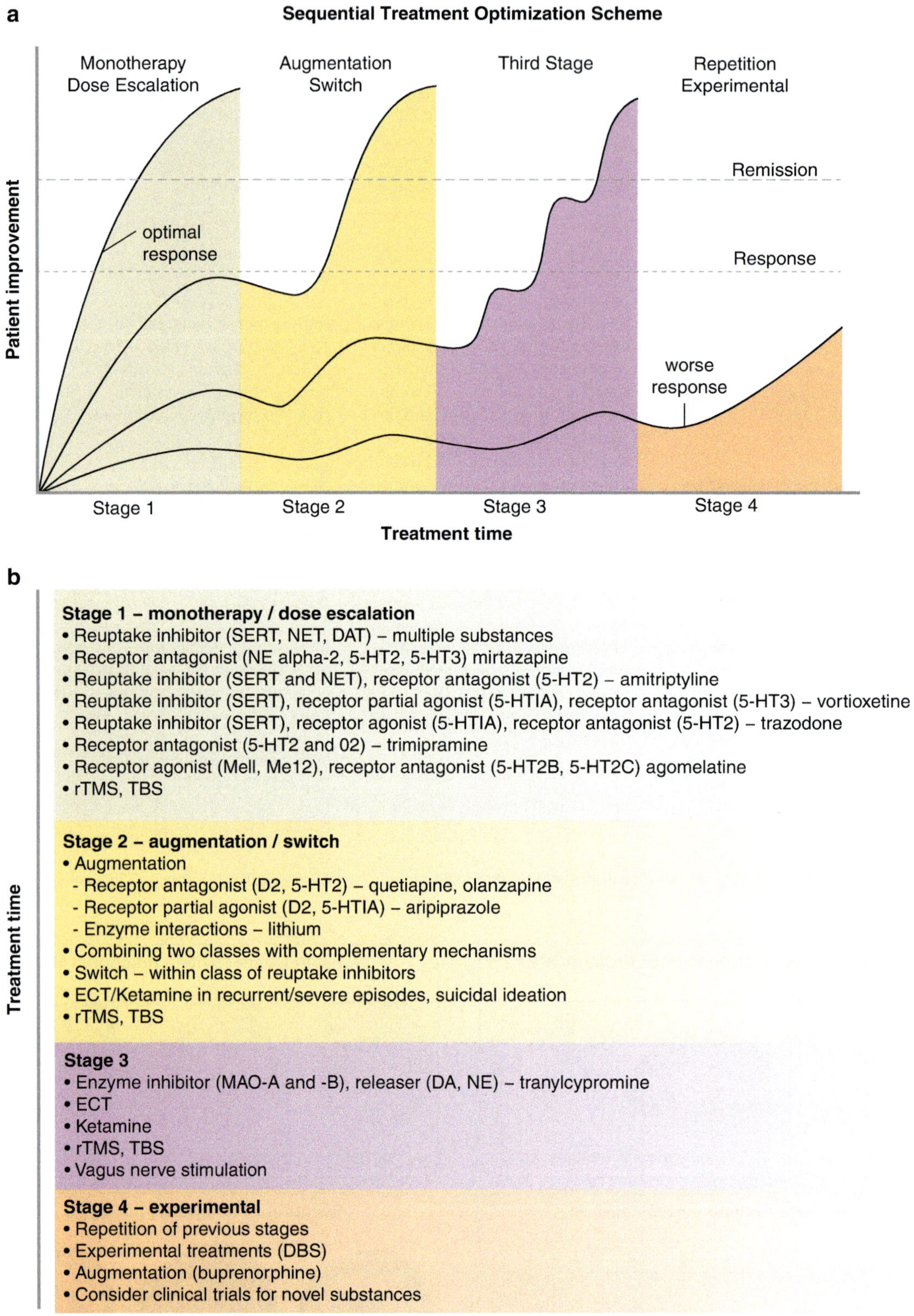

Fig. 17.35 Treatment optimization guidelines in the sequential scheme of recommended options for care of major depression. (**a**) Treatment response curves for four common response trajectories. (**b**) Listwise treatments available with relation to above response curves. (From Kraus [63]; Creative Commons; https://creativecommons.org/licenses/by/4.0/)

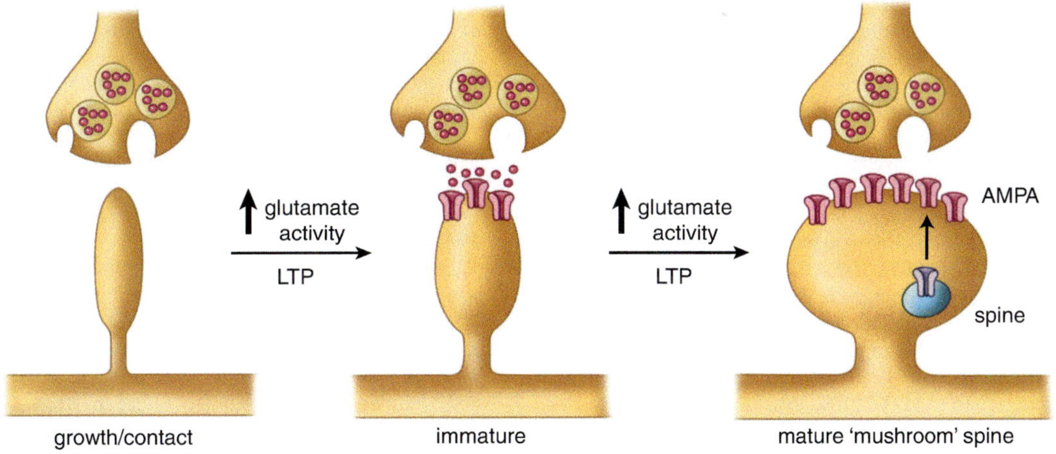

Fig. 17.36 Schematic model for the cellular mechanisms by which rapid-acting antidepressants and subsequent synaptic changes occur. Ketamine results in a glutamatergic burst that causes synaptic improvements in functioning directly opposed by the process of chronic stress and depression. (From Duman [64]; Creative Commons; https://creativecommons.org/licenses/by/4.0/)

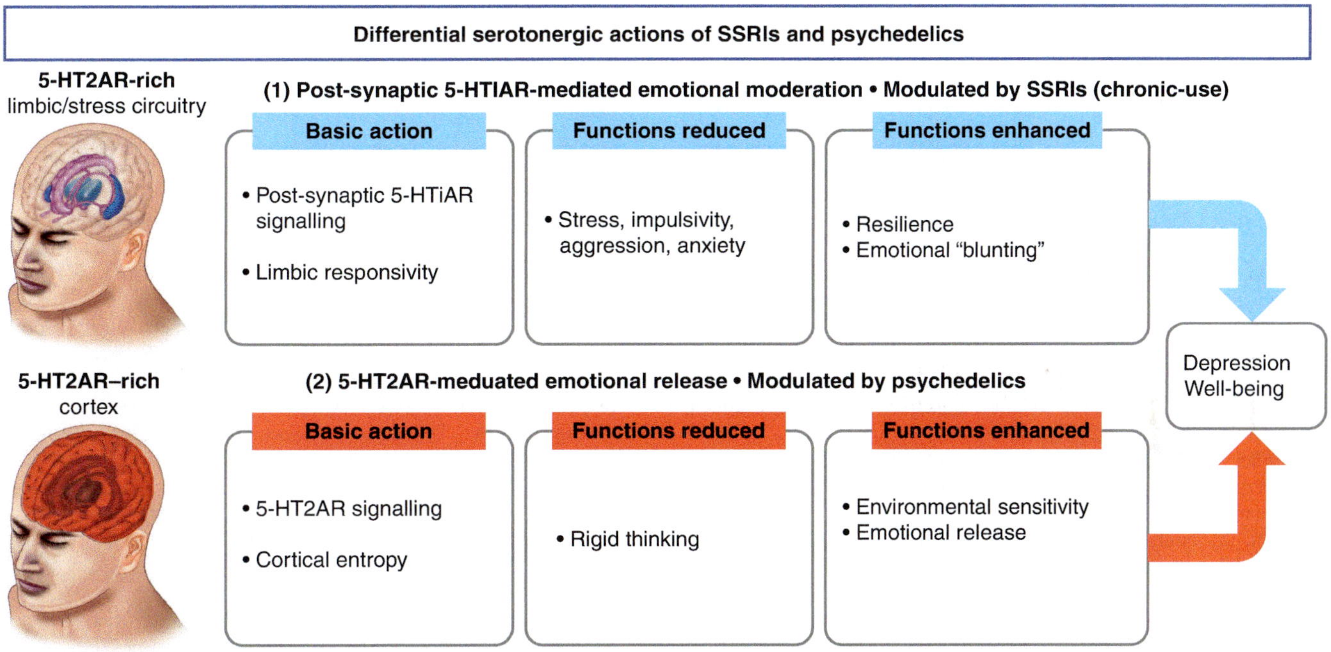

Fig. 17.37 A bipartite model of serotonergic functioning found on postsynaptic 5-HT1AR and 5-HT2AR action. SSRI use is thought to in part treat depression by decreasing stress and increasing pro-coping properties at the cost of a blunting of emotional responsiveness. Meanwhile, the psychedelic mechanism may act by enhancing sensitivity to the environment and subsequently facilitate emotional release. (*From* Carhart-Harris [65]; *with permission*)

References

1. Depressive disorders. In Diagnostic and statistical manual of mental disorders. Arlington, VA; 2013. https://doi.org/https://doi.org/10.1176/appi.books.9780890425596.dsm04.
2. Bromet E, Andrade LH, Hwang I, et al. Cross-national epidemiology of DSM-IV major depressive episode. BMC Med. 2011;9(1):90.
3. Kessler RC, Bromet EJ. The epidemiology of depression across cultures. Annu Rev Public Health. 2013;34:119–38.
4. Seedat S, Scott KM, Angermeyer MC, et al. Cross-national associations between gender and mental disorders in the World Health Organization World Mental Health Surveys. Arch Gen Psychiatry. 2009;66(7):785–95.
5. Otte C, Gold SM, Penninx BW, et al. Major depressive disorder. Nat Rev Dis Primers. 2016;2(1):16065.
6. Patten SB. Accumulation of major depressive episodes over time in a prospective study indicates that retrospectively assessed lifetime prevalence estimates are too low. BMC Psychiatry. 2009;9:19.

7. Keller MB, Lavori PW, Mueller TI, et al. Time to recovery, chronicity, and levels of psychopathology in major depression. A 5-year prospective follow-up of 431 subjects. Arch Gen Psychiatry. 1992;49(10):809–16.
8. Vos T, Haby MM, Barendregt JJ, Kruijshaar M, Corry J, Andrews G. The burden of major depression avoidable by longer-term treatment strategies. Arch Gen Psychiatry. 2004;61(11):1097–103.
9. Global, regional, and national incidence, prevalence, and years lived with disability for 301 acute and chronic diseases and injuries in 188 countries, 1990-2013: a systematic analysis for the Global Burden of Disease Study 2013. Lancet. 2015;386(9995):743–800.
10. Penninx BW, Milaneschi Y, Lamers F, Vogelzangs N. Understanding the somatic consequences of depression: biological mechanisms and the role of depression symptom profile. BMC Med. 2013;11:129.
11. Risch N, Herrell R, Lehner T, et al. Interaction between the serotonin transporter gene (5-HTTLPR), stressful life events, and risk of depression: a meta-analysis. JAMA. 2009;301(23):2462–71.
12. Lorant V, Deliège D, Eaton W, Robert A, Philippot P, Ansseau M. Socioeconomic inequalities in depression: a meta-analysis. Am J Epidemiol. 2003;157(2):98–112.
13. Heim C, Binder EB. Current research trends in early life stress and depression: review of human studies on sensitive periods, gene-environment interactions, and epigenetics. Exp Neurol. 2012;233(1):102–11.
14. Hovens JG, Giltay EJ, Wiersma JE, Spinhoven P, Penninx BW, Zitman FG. Impact of childhood life events and trauma on the course of depressive and anxiety disorders. Acta Psychiatr Scand. 2012;126(3):198–207.
15. Geschwind DH, Flint J. Genetics and genomics of psychiatric disease. Science. 2015;349(6255):1489–94.
16. Bosker FJ, Hartman CA, Nolte IM, et al. Poor replication of candidate genes for major depressive disorder using genome-wide association data. Mol Psychiatry. 2011;16(5):516–32.
17. Li M, D'Arcy C, Meng X. Maltreatment in childhood substantially increases the risk of adult depression and anxiety in prospective cohort studies: systematic review, meta-analysis, and proportional attributable fractions. Psychol Med. 2016;46(4):717–30.
18. Meaney MJ. Maternal care, gene expression, and the transmission of individual differences in stress reactivity across generations. Annu Rev Neurosci. 2001;24:1161–92.
19. Stetler C, Miller GE. Depression and hypothalamic-pituitary-adrenal activation: a quantitative summary of four decades of research. Psychosom Med. 2011;73(2):114–26.
20. Stein A, Pearson RM, Goodman SH, et al. Effects of perinatal mental disorders on the fetus and child. Lancet. 2014; 384(9956):1800–19.
21. aan het Rot M, Mathew SJ, Charney DS. Neurobiological mechanisms in major depressive disorder. CMAJ. 2009;180(3):305–13.
22. Holsboer F, Ising M. Stress hormone regulation: biological role and translation into therapy. Annu Rev Psychol. 2010;61(81–109):c101–11.
23. Goodyer IM, Herbert J, Tamplin A, Altham PM. Recent life events, cortisol, dehydroepiandrosterone and the onset of major depression in high-risk adolescents. Br J Psychiatry. 2000;177:499–504.
24. Nestler EJ, Barrot M, DiLeone RJ, Eisch AJ, Gold SJ, Monteggia LM. Neurobiology of depression. Neuron. 2002;34(1):13–25.
25. Hodes GE, Kana V, Menard C, Merad M, Russo SJ. Neuroimmune mechanisms of depression. Nat Neurosci. 2015;18(10):1386–93.
26. Steiner J, Bielau H, Brisch R, et al. Immunological aspects in the neurobiology of suicide: elevated microglial density in schizophrenia and depression is associated with suicide. J Psychiatr Res. 2008;42(2):151–7.
27. Duman RS, Li N. A neurotrophic hypothesis of depression: role of synaptogenesis in the actions of NMDA receptor antagonists. Philos Trans R Soc Lond Ser B Biol Sci. 2012;367(1601):2475–84.
28. Lee BH, Kim YK. The roles of BDNF in the pathophysiology of major depression and in antidepressant treatment. Psychiatry Investig. 2010;7(4):231–5.
29. Duman RS. Pathophysiology of depression: the concept of synaptic plasticity. Eur Psychiatry. 2002;17(Suppl 3):306–10.
30. Dwivedi Y. Brain-derived neurotrophic factor: role in depression and suicide. Neuropsychiatr Dis Treat. 2009;5:433–49.
31. Schildkraut JJ. The catecholamine hypothesis of affective disorders: a review of supporting evidence. Am J Psychiatry. 1965;122(5):509–22.
32. Kupfer DJ, Frank E, Phillips ML. Major depressive disorder: new clinical, neurobiological, and treatment perspectives. Lancet. 2012;379(9820):1045–55.
33. Kempton MJ, Salvador Z, Munafò MR, et al. Structural neuroimaging studies in major depressive disorder. Meta-analysis and comparison with bipolar disorder. Arch Gen Psychiatry. 2011;68(7):675–90.
34. Schmaal L, Veltman DJ, van Erp TG, et al. Subcortical brain alterations in major depressive disorder: findings from the ENIGMA Major Depressive Disorder working group. Mol Psychiatry. 2016;21(6):806–12.
35. Sheline YI, Wang PW, Gado MH, Csernansky JG, Vannier MW. Hippocampal atrophy in recurrent major depression. Proc Natl Acad Sci U S A. 1996;93(9):3908–13.
36. Schmaal L, Hibar DP, Sämann PG, et al. Cortical abnormalities in adults and adolescents with major depression based on brain scans from 20 cohorts worldwide in the ENIGMA Major Depressive Disorder Working Group. Mol Psychiatry. 2017;22(6):900–9.
37. Goodkind M, Eickhoff SB, Oathes DJ, et al. Identification of a common neurobiological substrate for mental illness. JAMA Psychiat. 2015;72(4):305–15.
38. Chen G, Hu X, Li L, et al. Disorganization of white matter architecture in major depressive disorder: a meta-analysis of diffusion tensor imaging with tract-based spatial statistics. Sci Rep. 2016;6:21825.
39. Hamilton JP, Etkin A, Furman DJ, Lemus MG, Johnson RF, Gotlib IH. Functional neuroimaging of major depressive disorder: a meta-analysis and new integration of base line activation and neural response data. Am J Psychiatry. 2012;169(7):693–703.
40. Pizzagalli DA. Depression, stress, and anhedonia: toward a synthesis and integrated model. Annu Rev Clin Psychol. 2014;10:393–423.
41. Satterthwaite TD, Kable JW, Vandekar L, et al. Common and dissociable dysfunction of the reward system in bipolar and unipolar depression. Neuropsychopharmacology. 2015;40(9): 2258–68.
42. Dutta A, McKie S, Deakin JF. Resting state networks in major depressive disorder. Psychiatry Res. 2014;224(3):139–51.
43. Cooney RE, Joormann J, Eugène F, Dennis EL, Gotlib IH. Neural correlates of rumination in depression. Cogn Affect Behav Neurosci. 2010;10(4):470–8.
44. Sheline YI, Barch DM, Price JL, et al. The default mode network and self-referential processes in depression. Proc Natl Acad Sci U S A. 2009;106(6):1942–7.
45. Kaiser RH, Andrews-Hanna JR, Wager TD, Pizzagalli DA. Large-scale network dysfunction in major depressive disorder: a meta-analysis of resting-state functional connectivity. JAMA Psychiat. 2015;72(6):603–11.
46. Pizzagalli DA, Holmes AJ, Dillon DG, et al. Reduced caudate and nucleus accumbens response to rewards in unmedicated individuals with major depressive disorder. Am J Psychiatry. 2009;166(6):702–10.
47. Hamilton JP, Chen MC, Gotlib IH. Neural systems approaches to understanding major depressive disorder: an intrinsic functional organization perspective. Neurobiol Dis. 2013;52:4–11.

48. Insel T, Cuthbert B, Garvey M, et al. Research domain criteria (RDoC): toward a new classification framework for research on mental disorders. Am J Psychiatry. 2010;167(7):748–51.
49. Lilienfeld SO, Treadway MT. Clashing diagnostic approaches: DSM-ICD versus RDoC. Annu Rev Clin Psychol. 2016;12:435–63.
50. Insel TR. The NIMH Research Domain Criteria (RDoC) project: precision medicine for psychiatry. Am J Psychiatry. 2014;171(4):395–7.
51. da Silva Novaretti TM, D'Ávila Freitas MI, Mansur LL, Nitrini R, Radanovic M. Comparison of language impairment in late-onset depression and Alzheimer's disease. Acta Neuropsychiatr. 2011;23(2):62–8.
52. Siddiqi SH, Taylor SF, Cooke D, Pascual-Leone A, George MS, Fox MD. Distinct symptom-specific treatment targets for circuit-based neuromodulation. Am J Psychiatry. 2020;177(5):435–46.
53. Rush AJ, Aaronson ST, Demyttenaere K. Difficult-to-treat depression: a clinical and research roadmap for when remission is elusive. Aust N Z J Psychiatry. 2019;53(2):109–18.
54. Avasthi A, Grover S. Clinical practice guidelines for management of depression in elderly. Indian J Psychiatry. 2018;60(Suppl 3):S341–s362.
55. Ardito RB, Rabellino D. Therapeutic alliance and outcome of psychotherapy: historical excursus, measurements, and prospects for research. Front Psychol. 2011;2:270.
56. Barth J, Munder T, Gerger H, et al. Comparative efficacy of seven psychotherapeutic interventions for patients with depression: a network meta-analysis. PLoS Med. 2013;10(5):e1001454.
57. Goldapple K, Segal Z, Garson C, et al. Modulation of cortical-limbic pathways in major depression: treatment-specific effects of cognitive behavior therapy. Arch Gen Psychiatry. 2004;61(1):34–41.
58. Kennedy SH, Konarski JZ, Segal ZV, et al. Differences in brain glucose metabolism between responders to CBT and venlafaxine in a 16-week randomized controlled trial. Am J Psychiatr. 2007;164(5):778–88.
59. Santarsieri D, Schwartz TL. Antidepressant efficacy and side-effect burden: a quick guide for clinicians. Drugs Context. 2015;4:212290.
60. Gaynes BN, Warden D, Trivedi MH, Wisniewski SR, Fava M, Rush AJ. What did STAR*D teach us? Results from a large-scale, practical, clinical trial for patients with depression. Psychiatr Serv. 2009;60(11):1439–45.
61. El-Hage W, Leman S, Camus V, Belzung C. Mechanisms of antidepressant resistance. Front Pharmacol. 2013;4:146.
62. Brunoni AR, Teng CT, Correa C, et al. Neuromodulation approaches for the treatment of major depression: challenges and recommendations from a working group meeting. Arq Neuropsiquiatr. 2010;68(3):433–51.
63. Kraus C, Kadriu B, Lanzenberger R, Zarate CA Jr, Kasper S. Prognosis and improved outcomes in major depression: a review. Transl Psychiatry. 2019;9(1):127.
64. Duman RS. Ketamine and rapid-acting antidepressants: a new era in the battle against depression and suicide. F1000Res. 2018;7.
65. Carhart-Harris RL, Goodwin GM. The therapeutic potential of psychedelic drugs: past, present, and future. Neuropsychopharmacology. 2017;42(11):2105–13.

Anxiety Disorders and Obsessive-Compulsive and Related Disorders

18

Sophie M. D. D. Fitzsimmons, Neeltje M. Batelaan, and Odile A. van den Heuvel

Introduction

Anxiety disorders (ADs) and obsessive-compulsive and related disorders (OCRDs) comprise multiple mental disorders, characterized by high levels of anxiety, dysfunctional catastrophic thoughts and most often substantial avoidance. These disorders contribute a significant burden to individual patients and society, due to high prevalence, early onset of symptoms, chronic course, high levels of impairment and high comorbidity. Although the various disorders have very specific symptom profiles, as described in the classification systems—the 5th edition of the *Diagnostic Statistical Manual of Mental Disorders* (DSM-5) [1] and the 11th edition of the International Classification of Diseases (ICD-11) (see Table 18.1) [2]—they share phenomenological characteristics and underlying etiology and pathophysiology.

In addition, therapeutic approaches are mostly disorder non-specific: pharmacological treatment options largely target the serotonergic system and the GABA-glutamate balance; psychotherapeutic strategies mainly focus on exposure-based extinction learning, reappraisal-based cognitive control and behavioural inhibition; and brain circuit-based targeted neurostimulation techniques are used to potentiate cognitive control and behavioural inhibition. The current classification systems (DSM-5/ICD-11) have proven very helpful in harmonized diagnosis of patients worldwide, crucial for reliable comparison of research results and use in evidence-based treatment guidelines. However, these classification systems lack a strong link to underlying disease mechanisms. In order to bring the field forward, for instance, by the development of etiology or pathophysiology-based treatments, it is useful to understand the various sources of dysfunction contributing to the symptom profiles. For this reason, the Research Domain Criteria (RDoC) [3] have been proposed. The RDoC framework is an evolving model attempting to integrate many levels of information (from genomics and brain circuit function to observable behaviours and self-report) to understand dimensions of functioning that span the full range of human behaviour from normal behaviour to disease during the various stages of development and in interaction with the environment (see Fig. 18.1). The current version of the framework is constructed on a grid with six major domains of human functioning (with, for instance, the domain 'negative valence' specifically relevant for anxiety disorders) on one axis and units of analysis on the other axis. Each domain consists of the so-called constructs, i.e. behavioural elements, that comprise different aspects of that specific domain of human behaviour (e.g. in the case of 'negative valence,' the differentiation between acute, potential and sustained threat). Units of analyses consist of neural systems (genes, molecules, cells) and behavioural dimensions (physiology, behaviour, self-report).

The aim of this atlas is to describe the various mental disorders within the anxiety and obsessive-compulsive and related disorders categories, using information from both the disorder-specific literature and the transdiagnostic research field.

S. M. D. D. Fitzsimmons (✉) · O. A. van den Heuvel
Department of Psychiatry and Department of Anatomy and Neurosciences, Amsterdam UMC, Vrije Universiteit Amsterdam, Amsterdam Neuroscience, Amsterdam, Netherlands
e-mail: s.fitzsimmons@amsterdamumc.nl; oa.vandenheuvel@vumc.nl

N. M. Batelaan
Department of Psychiatry, Amsterdam UMC, Vrije Universiteit Amsterdam, Amsterdam Public Health, Amsterdam, Netherlands
e mail: N.Batelaan@ggzingeest.nl

W. W. IsHak (ed.), *Atlas of Psychiatry*, https://doi.org/10.1007/978-3-031-15401-0_18

Table 18.1 Summary of DSM-5 criteria for OCRDs and ADs

Obsessive-compulsive and related disorders	Criteria
Obsessive-compulsive disorder	• Presence of obsessions, compulsions or both • Obsessions are defined by recurrent and persistent thoughts, urges or images that are experienced, at some time during the disturbance, as intrusive and unwanted and that in most individuals cause marked anxiety or distress • The individual attempts to ignore or suppress such thoughts, urges or images or to neutralize them with some other thought or action (i.e. by performing a compulsion) • Compulsions are defined by repetitive behaviours (e.g. hand washing, ordering, checking) or mental acts (e.g. praying, counting, repeating words silently) that the individual feels driven to perform in response to an obsession or according to rules that must be applied rigidly • The behaviours or mental acts are aimed at preventing or reducing anxiety or distress or preventing some dreaded event or situation; however, these behaviours or mental acts are not connected in a realistic way with what they are designed to neutralize or prevent or are clearly excessive* **Young children may not be able to articulate the aims of these behaviours or mental acts* • The obsessions or compulsions are time-consuming (e.g. taking >1 h/day) • Disorders are specified with (a) with good or fair insight, (b) with poor insight, (c) with absent insight of condition or (d) tic-related
Body dysmorphic disorder	• Preoccupation with one or more perceived defects in physical appearance that are not observable to others • The individual has performed repetitive behaviours or mental acts in response to the appearance concerns • A subtype includes muscle dysmorphia: the idea that his or her body build is too small or insufficiently muscular
Hoarding disorder	• Persistent difficulty discarding or parting with possessions, regardless of their actual value • The difficulty discarding possessions results in the accumulation of possessions that congest and clutter active living areas • The disorder is also specified if it exists with excessive acquisition of new items
Trichotillomania	• Recurrent pulling out of one's hair, resulting in hair loss
Excoriation disorder	• Recurrent skin picking resulting in skin lesions
Substance/medication-induced obsessive-compulsive and related disorder	• Obsessions, compulsions, skin picking, hair pulling, other body-focused repetitive behaviours or other symptoms develop during or soon after substance intoxication or withdrawal • Substance is capable of producing symptoms
Obsessive-compulsive and related disorder due to another medical condition	• Obsessions, compulsions, skin picking, hair pulling, other body-focused repetitive behaviours or other symptoms develop due to a medical condition • The disturbance does not occur exclusively during the course of a delirium • The condition must be specified if it exists with OCD-like symptoms, appearance preoccupations, hoarding or hair or skin pulling

Anxiety disorders	Criteria
Separation anxiety disorder	• Developmentally inappropriate and excessive fear or anxiety concerning separation from major attachment figure • Persistent and excessive worry about losing attachment figures • Persistent reluctance or refusal to go out, because of fear of separation • Repeated nightmares of separation • Repeated complaints of physical symptoms • The fear, anxiety or avoidance is persistent, lasting ≥4 weeks in children and adolescents and ≥6 months in adults
Selective mutism	• Consistent failure to speak in specific social situations, in which there is an expectation for speaking • The duration of the disturbance is ≥1 month
Specific phobia	• Marked fear or anxiety about a specific object or situation* • The phobic object or situation almost always provokes immediate fear or anxiety • The fear, anxiety or avoidance is persistent, typically lasting ≥6 months • Types of specific phobia include (a) animal, (b) natural environment and (c) blood-injection-injury **In children, the fear or anxiety may be expressed by crying, tantrums, freezing or clinging*
Social anxiety disorder (social phobia)	• Marked fear or anxiety about social situations in which the individual is exposed to possible scrutiny by others* • The fear, anxiety or avoidance is persistent lasting ≥6 months or more • A specific type includes performance anxiety when fear is restricted to speaking or performing in public **In children, the anxiety must occur in peer settings and adult interactions*
Panic disorder	• Recurrent unexpected panic attacks • A significant maladaptive change in behaviour related to the attacks
Agoraphobia	• Marked fear or anxiety about using public transportation or public places • The fear, anxiety or avoidance is persistent, typically lasting ≥6 months

Table 18.1 (continued)

Anxiety disorders	Criteria
Generalized anxiety disorder	• Excessive anxiety and occurring frequently for ≥6 months, about number of events/activities • The individual finds it difficult to control the worry • The anxiety and worry are associated with irritability, muscle tension, fatigue, lack of sleep or difficulty concentrating
Substance/ medication-induced anxiety disorder	• Panic attacks or anxiety is predominant where there is evidence of substance intoxication or withdrawal from a medication/substance • The disturbance does not occur exclusively during the course of a delirium

In this chapter, we use DSM-5 criteria summarized in this table to define ADs and OCRDs. These criteria largely overlap with the criteria in the ICD-11 [2] classification of mental disorders, though hypochondriasis and olfactory reference disorder are included in the ICD-11 classification but not in the DSM-5

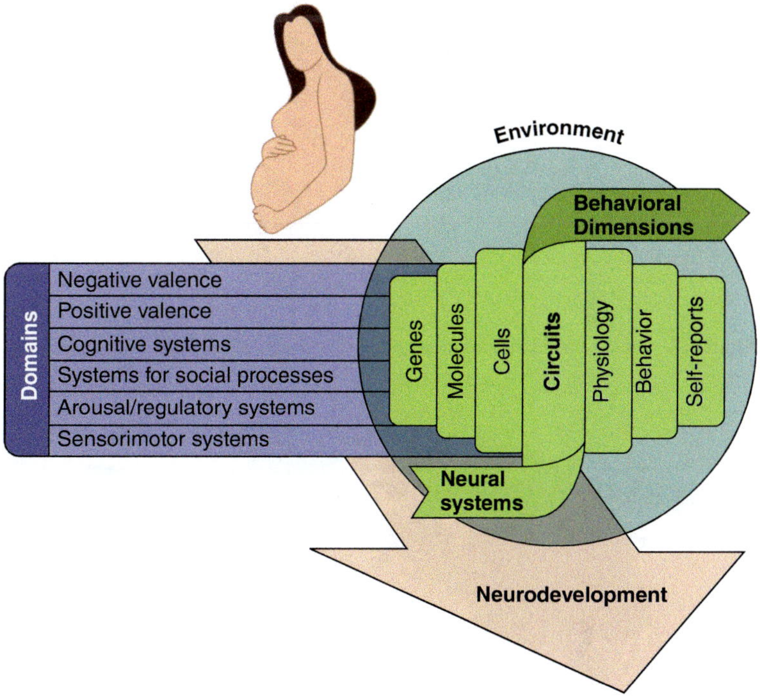

Fig. 18.1 Research Domain Criteria

Epidemiology

Prevalence

The group of disorders comprising ADs, OCRDs and post-traumatic stress disorder is the most prevalent class of mental disorder worldwide (Fig. 18.2).

Similar to many mental disorders, prevalence of ADs varies considerably across the world, and estimates are dependent on several factors, such as whether data is collected from inpatient or outpatient populations and the importance of ADs in a particular culture. Reported prevalence of these disorders is generally highest in North and South America, Australasia and Europe (Fig. 18.3), and figures have remained relatively stable for the past 20 years [4].

The most common type of AD in adults is specific phobia, followed by social phobia [5]. In addition, children frequently suffer from separation anxiety. The prevalence of all OCRDs together is estimated at 9.4%, with skin picking being the most common disorder (3%), followed by OCD (2–3%) [5, 6]. Variations in prevalence between countries may be due to differing cultural definitions. Culture-bound variants of anxiety disorders are common around the world (e.g. ataque de nervios, trúng gió, khyâl, taijin kyofusho). While symptoms of OCD and other OCRDs are remarkably consistent across cultures, the specific presentation of BDD can vary (such as in shubo-kyofu [1, 7]).

AD and OCRDs Throughout the Lifespan

Both ADs and OCRDs frequently begin early in life but can also emerge during early adulthood (especially generalized anxiety disorder and perinatal OCD). The course of ADs and

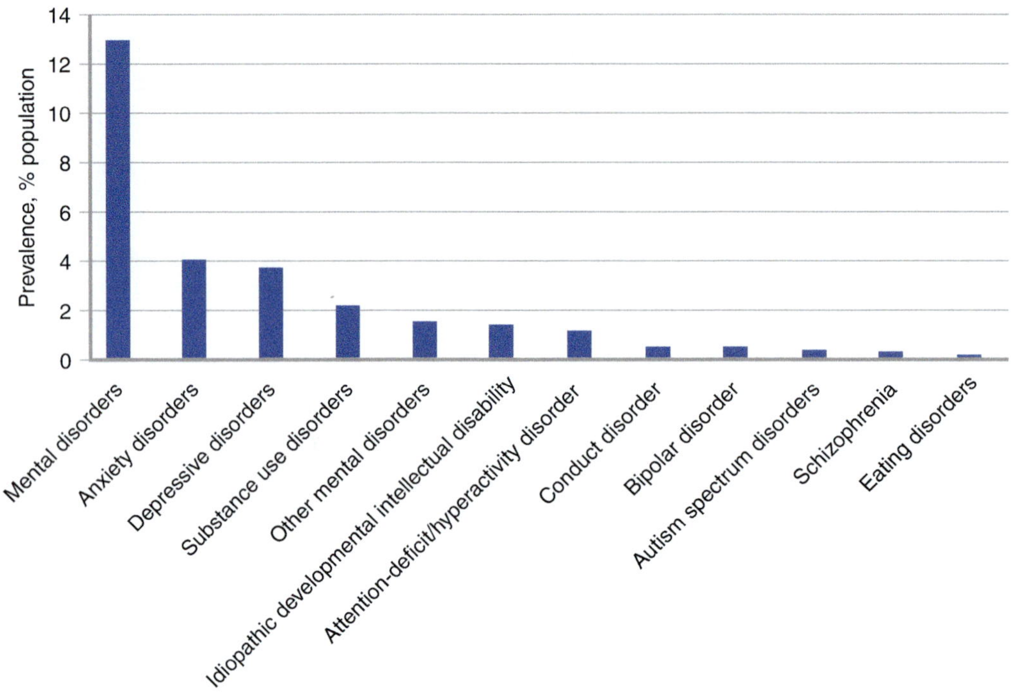

Fig. 18.2 Global prevalence of mental disorders, 2019. N.B. This dataset includes OCRDs and PTSD within anxiety disorders

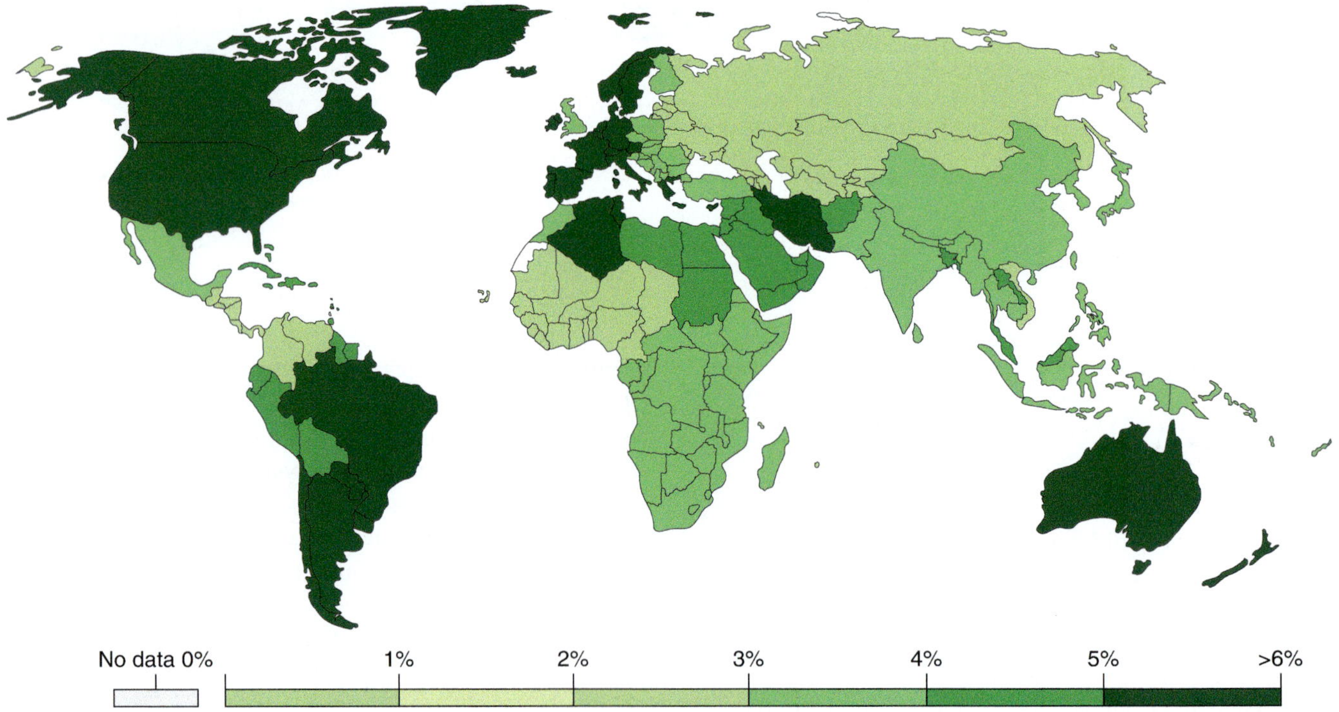

Fig. 18.3 Share of population with anxiety disorders, 2017. Anxiety disorders are most commonly reported in the Americas, Australasia and Europe, with a prevalence of more than 6%. N.B. This dataset includes OCRDs and PTSD within anxiety disorders

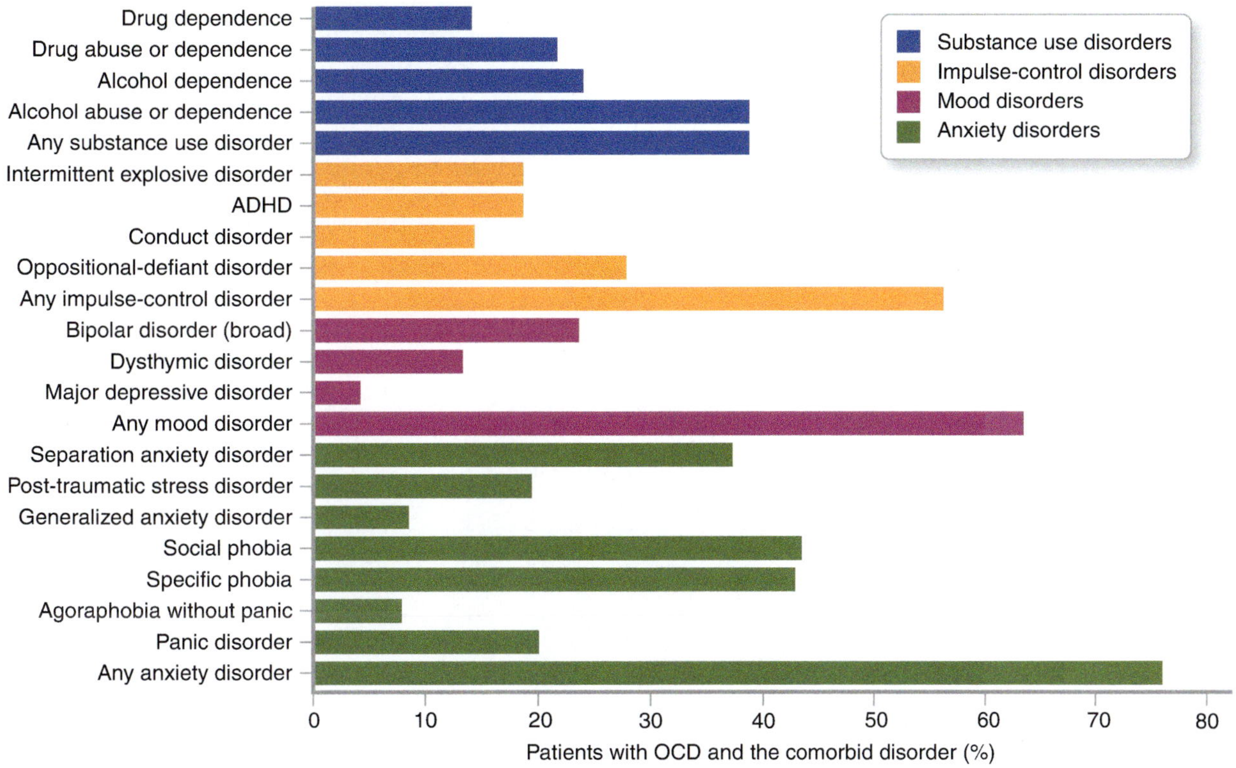

Fig. 18.4 In the general population, OCD is comorbid with a wide range of mental disorders, with anxiety and mood disorders being the most common comorbidities

OCRDs is heterogeneous. While remission rates of 23–40% are reported for ADs [7] and 53% for OCD [8], chronicity or recurrence after initial remission is common.

Impact

ADs and OCRDs have a significant impact on daily functioning and quality of life and therefore on society in general. They impact not only the ability to work but also relationships, family life and life satisfaction [5]. ADs are frequently underdiagnosed and undertreated and have been ranked as the third most burdensome group of disorders in the EU [7].

Comorbidities

Comorbidities are common in both OCRDs and ADs. Ninety percent of OCD patients meet the criteria for another DSM disorder, most frequently anxiety disorders [6], while ADs have similar levels of comorbidity (Fig. 18.4).

ADs are frequently comorbid with other ADs—more than 50% of patients with an anxiety disorder have multiple anxiety disorders [7]. Secondary depression is common in both groups of disorders [5].

Phenomenology

General Characteristics and Differential Diagnosis of Anxiety Disorders

Fear and anxiety are common, everyday emotions, experienced in healthy individuals in response to present or future threats. Anxiety is also experienced across several psychiatric disorders, for example, in schizophrenia, in response to hallucinations or delusions, or in post-traumatic stress disorder, which is no longer included in the DSM-5 classification of ADs. ADs themselves are characterized by excessive anxiety to either external or internal perceived threats [7]. As well as direct exposure to the perceived threat, even thinking of the threat may provoke anxiety. Extreme anxiety may lead to panic attacks. Alternatively, patients may avoid the anxiety-provoking situation altogether, which decreases the anxiety experienced, but only temporarily. The arousal associated with anxiety is frequently accompanied by physical symptoms (Fig. 18.5).

Both anxiety and avoidance behaviour may limit daily functioning substantially. In addition, patients with AD usually have good insight into the fact that their catastrophic thoughts, anxiety and avoidance are not realistic, which fuels self-stigma.

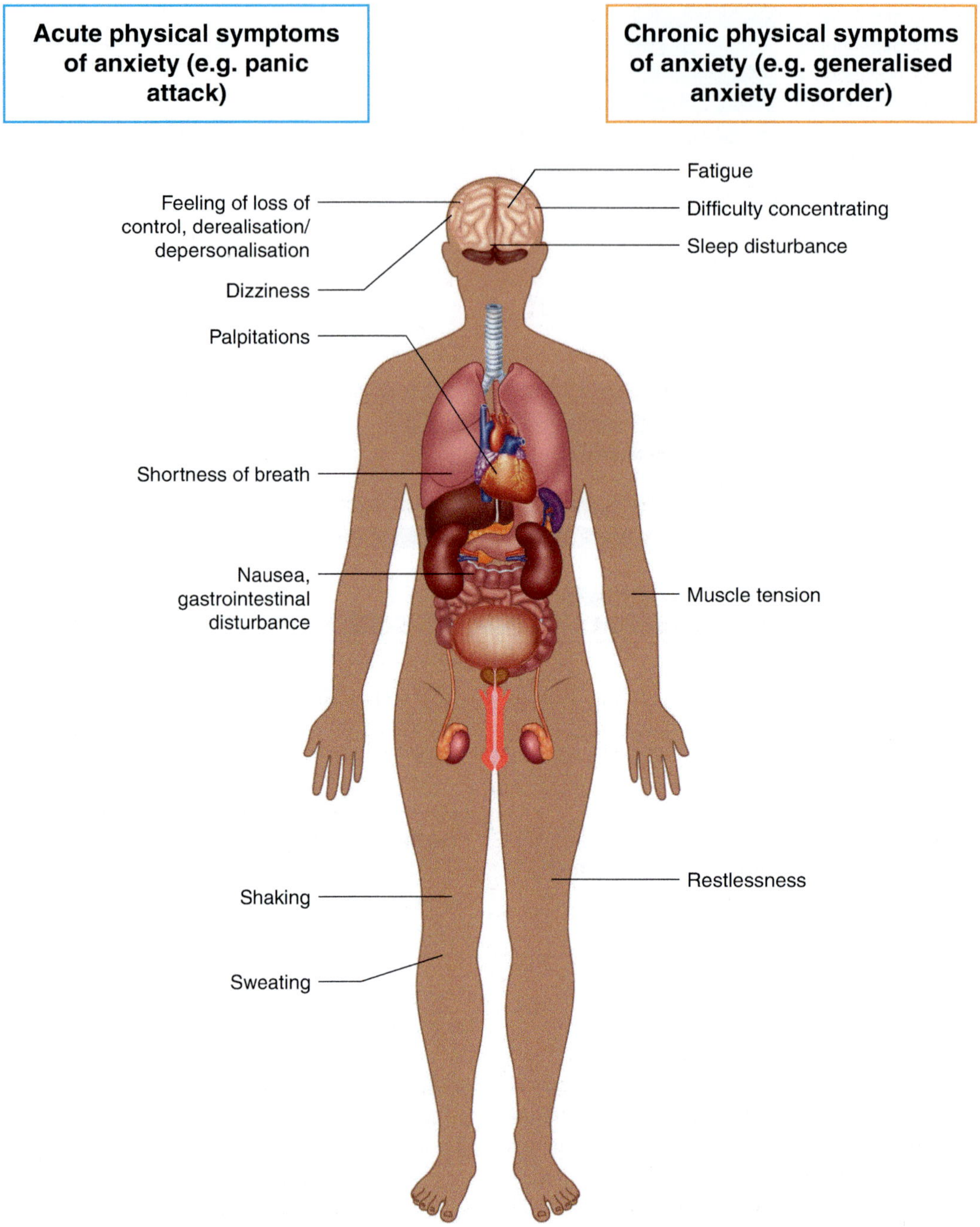

Fig. 18.5 Acute and chronic physical symptoms of anxiety

AD should be differentiated both from anxiety inherent to daily life and from other psychiatric disorders that are accompanied by symptoms of anxiety. Differentiation between the various ADs themselves can usually be achieved by elucidating the thoughts and beliefs accompanying the anxiety [7]. A description of the specific symptoms for each disorder can be found in Table 18.1.

It is also important to differentiate between anxiety due to an AD and anxiety due to another psychiatric disorder. Although trauma-related disorders, OCRDs and illness anxiety disorder are no longer part of ADs in the DSM-5, there are many overlapping symptoms between these disorders. Presence of a trauma, accompanying symptoms such as compulsions and the extensiveness of perceived threats may be helpful to adequately classify disorders.

Finally, drug intoxication/withdrawal and a wide range of disorders, including cardiopulmonary disorders, endocrine disorders (such as thyroid disease) and neurological disorders (such as complex partial seizures) [7], may all present with symptoms of anxiety. Somatic causes are more likely in

Table 18.2 OCD symptom dimensions

Symptom type	Obsession	Compulsion
Symmetry/ordering	Uncomfortable sensation that things do not feel right, for example, household objects are misaligned	Touching, tapping or rubbing things in special ways
Contamination/cleaning	Concern about developing cancer from environmental pollution	Repeated and excessive cleaning such as cleaning all household surfaces with bleach every day
Harm/aggression	I may be responsible for a murder	Checking that nothing bad happened, asking others if they are ok, checking the news for reports of murders
Sexual/religious	Unwanted images of violent sexual behaviour towards others	Praying over and over to prevent the sexual behaviour from occurring
Hoarding	Do not throw things away as they may be important in the future	Hoarding unusual items or excessive acquisition of objects like magazines
Miscellaneous	Intrusive nonsensical images, songs or words	Getting stuck performing everyday tasks such as getting dressed, eating and work tasks

cases of symptoms affecting a specific organ system or in cases of late-onset anxiety.

General Characteristics and Differential Diagnosis of Obsessive-Compulsive and Related Disorders (OCRDs)

The OCRDs, while fairly diverse in terms of phenomenology, all involve some form of repetitive thoughts or behaviours. Within obsessive-compulsive disorder (OCD), symptoms usually fall within a broad range of symptom dimensions (Table 18.2); the other OCRDs usually have a more specific focus for the obsessive and/or compulsive behaviour (see Table 18.1 for a description of all OCRDs).

BDD and OCD are both characterized by obsessional distressing thoughts and compulsions (which can take the form of compulsive, repetitive actions or thoughts) which are usually related to the obsession. The symptoms of the other disorders in the OCRD category are more compulsive/behavioural in nature, rather than specifically being associated with obsessive thoughts (see Fig. 18.6 for examples of trichotillomania and dermatotillomania).

OCRD symptoms can be related to medication/substance use or other medical conditions. Hoarding symptoms can be caused by a wide variety of conditions, including dementia, Prader-Willi syndrome, traumatic brain injury, brain surgery for tumour or seizure control or infections of the central nervous system. Hair loss/hair pulling and skin picking can be a result of skin inflammation or another dermatological condition rather than trichotillomania or excoriation disorder [5].

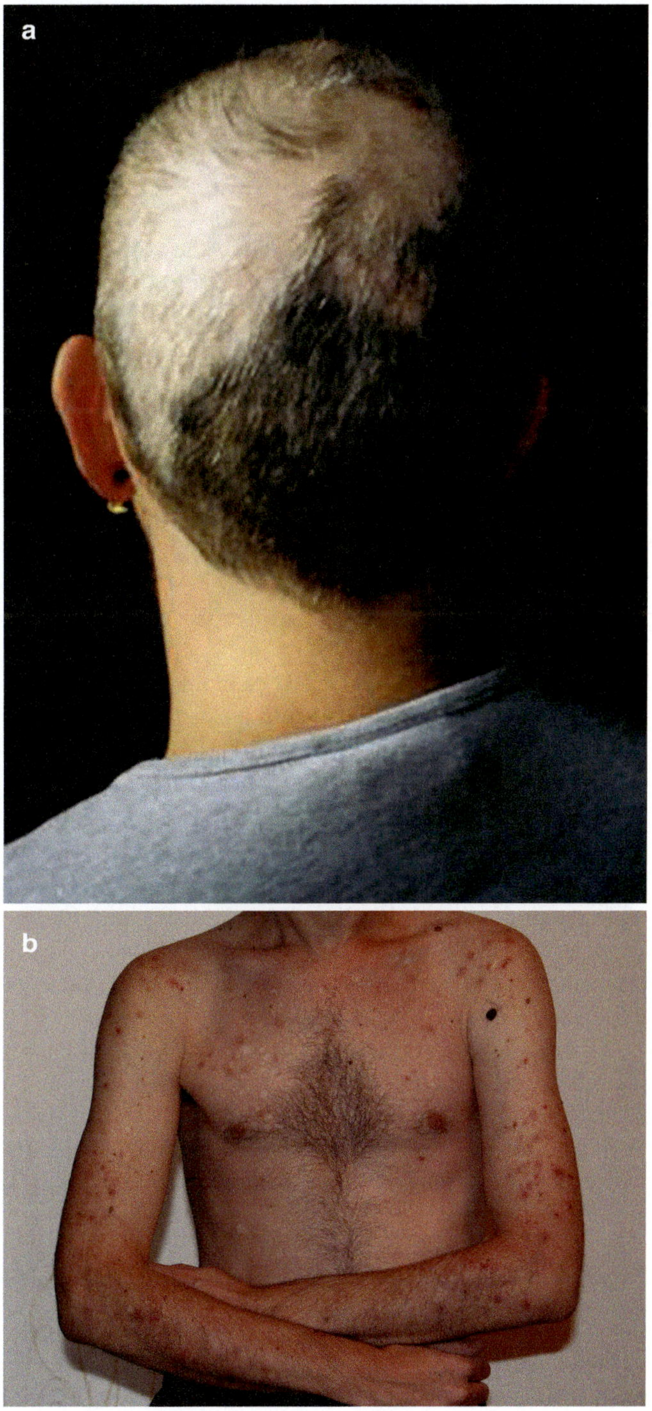

Fig. 18.6 (**a**) Trichotillomania. (**b**) Excoriation disorder

Insight is usually intact in most OCRDs. However, certain OCRDs can present with limited or even lack of insight, notably OCD, BDD and hoarding disorder [5].

Etiology and Pathophysiology

Note: we have chosen to combine the Etiology and Pathophysiology sections. While several physiological and environmental factors have been associated with ADs and OCRDs, it is sometimes unclear whether these are cause or consequence of the disorder (e.g. some neuroimaging differences identified in these disorders may be a result of genetic or congenital alterations and may predispose to the disorder, while others may develop as a result of disorder-related symptoms and behaviours or received treatments).

Risk Factors

The development of an AD/OCRD cannot usually be traced to a single cause per individual but is instead likely to be due to multiple interacting vulnerability and risk factors, both of genetic and environmental origin. If a critical level of stress/anxiety is reached as a result of these interacting factors, then a disorder will develop (see Fig. 18.7). For example, traumatic experiences early in life increase vulnerability for a wide range of mental disorders later, probably due to dysfunctional stress regulation as a direct consequence of early traumatic experiences and altered maturation of the prefrontal regions.

Various environmental and individual factors have been identified as risk factors for ADs and OCRDs. These can be broadly classified as stressful/traumatic life events, physical health factors, familial factors and temperament/personality factors (see Fig. 18.8) (see *Genetics* for genetic factors) [5]. These risk factors are fairly non-specific—there is considerable overlap in risk factors between OCRDs, ADs and other mental disorders—and therefore are of limited use in differentiating between disorders.

Genetics

Heritability estimates derived from twin studies demonstrate varying estimates of genetic contribution for ADs and OCRDs: as low as 32–38% for GAD and as high as 51–71% for hoarding disorder [10]. The specific genetic basis of this heritability has been researched with a number of different methods. The current evidence suggests that the etiology of ADs and OCRDs, like most psychiatric disorders, is a complex and heterogeneous combination of common genetic variants, all having relatively small effects, which cause vulnerability to environmental stressors (see *Risk Factors*), or a few rare variants giving a greater contribution of risk.

In the early days of genetic studies, several single gene mutations related to OCRDs and ADs were found in candidate gene studies and linkage studies. However, these were later found to be poorly replicated and are now believed to represent rare variants that are only related to specific cases of these disorders. Single gene mutations are now more relevant for the creation of animal models of ADs and OCRDs—for example, the Sapap3 knockout mouse (Fig. 18.9), which lacks a gene encoding for a scaffolding protein at excitatory synapses that is highly expressed in the striatum. This mouse model is frequently used in studies on compulsivity, since the grooming behaviour in the animals resembles (highly simplistically) the repetitive behaviours in OCD patients.

Genome-wide association studies (GWAS), in which relevant genetic variants are identified through examining polymorphisms throughout the genome in very large cohorts,

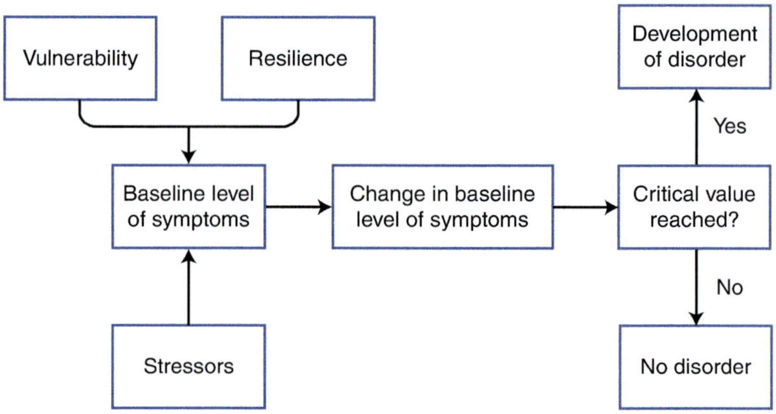

Fig. 18.7 Contribution of stress and vulnerability risk factors to the development of ADs/OCRDs [9]

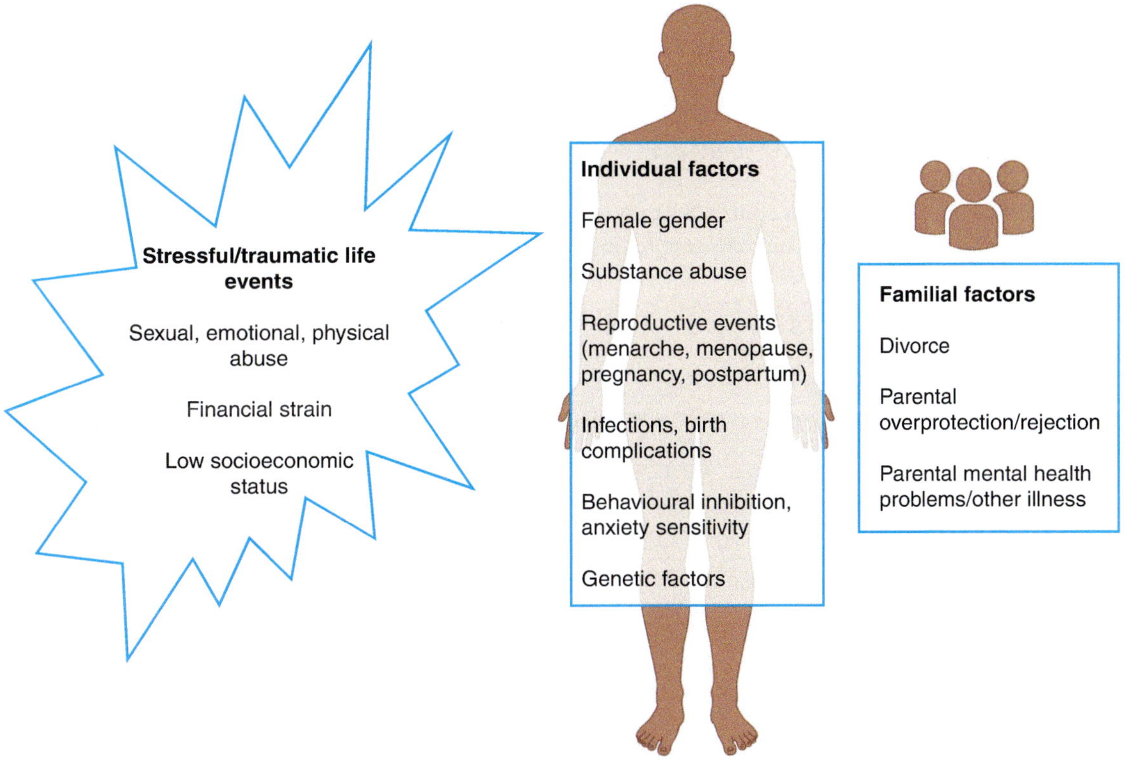

Fig. 18.8 Risk factors for OCD and AD. The two disorders share several risk factors. This is not intended to be an exhaustive list of all possible risk factors, but rather an overview of common examples

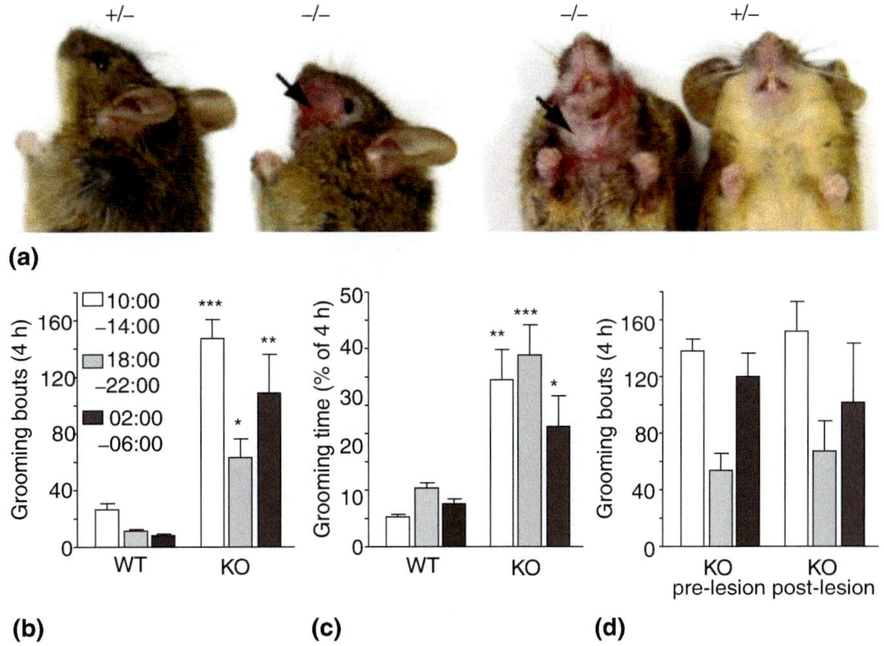

Fig. 18.9 OCD-like behaviours in Sapap3-mutant mice. Sapap3 knockout (KO) mice show increased grooming behaviours compared to wild types (WT) (**a–d**) and are frequently used as an experimental animal model of OCD and compulsive behaviour. (*Reprinted from* Welch et al. [11]; with permission)

have largely replaced candidate gene studies and linkage studies in recent years as more reliable ways of identifying polymorphisms that are relevant to complex disorders such as psychiatric disorders. Recent GWAS meta-analyses of OCD [12] have not identified any genome-wide significant single-nucleotide polymorphisms associated with OCD (though some variants in genes related to glutamatergic signalling in the basal ganglia and anterior cingulate cortex approached significance). A recent GWAS meta-analysis across ADs had more success, revealing an RNA polymorphism on chromosome 3q12.3, and on 2p21, related to calcium-dependent signalling [13].

Gene-environment interactions are particularly important in ADs and OCRDs, given their relationship to stressful life events and early life traumas. Examples of genes associated with or giving a vulnerability to ADs and OCD are listed in Table 18.3 (there have been few studies examining genetic associations with other OCRDs).

Epigenetic processes are processes that control the expression of a gene, such as methylation or histone acetylation, but without altering the DNA sequence, and are a possible mechanism of vulnerability to mental disorders following early life stress exposure. One example of this is illustrated in Fig. 18.10 and demonstrates how chronically high cortisol levels as a result of early life stress can epigenetically alter immune system function and future reactivity to stressful situations [14].

Table 18.3 Genes associated with ADs and OCRDs or with a vulnerability to these disorders

Gene/epigenetic process linked to gene	Function	Associated with
MAOA; hypomethylation	Gene encoding an enzyme that degrades amine neurotransmitters (NA, DA, 5HT)	PD, GAD, phobia
COMT	Gene encoding an enzyme that degrades catecholamines (DA, NA)	OCD, phobia, PD
SLC6A4, 5HT1D, 5HT2C	Gene encoding serotonin transporter protein; genes encoding serotonin receptors	PD, GAD, SAD, OCD
SNP within oxytocin gene	Social bonding, social functioning	SA, SAD
NPS, NPSR1	Encoding of neuropeptide S and neuropeptide S receptor; role in anxiety suppression	PD

MAOA monoamine oxidase A; *PD* panic disorder; *GAD* generalized anxiety disorder; *SA* separation anxiety; *SAD* social anxiety disorder; *OCD* obsessive-compulsive disorder; *SNP* single-nucleotide polymorphism; *DA* dopamine; *NA* noradrenaline; *5HT* serotonin; *NPS* neuropeptide S

Physiology

As described in the Phenomenology section, physical stress symptoms are a key component of many anxiety disorders, as well as stress and anxiety as part of everyday life. Long-term or aberrant activation of physiological moderators of the stress response is linked to both the experience of acute anxiety and the later development of anxiety disorders (as well as several other psychiatric disorders). Here, we describe three main components of the physiological anxiety response and their role in ADs and OCRDs: the autonomic nervous system, the hypothalamic-pituitary-adrenal axis and the immune system.

The autonomic nervous system mediates the acute stress response and is involved in producing the symptoms of panic attacks. This system innervates the viscera (Fig. 18.11) and consists of the sympathetic ('fight or flight') system, mediated by adrenaline, and the parasympathetic ('rest and digest') system, whose main neurotransmitter is acetylcholine.

As well as the physical symptoms of acute stress, alterations in heart rate variability and increased rates of heart dis-

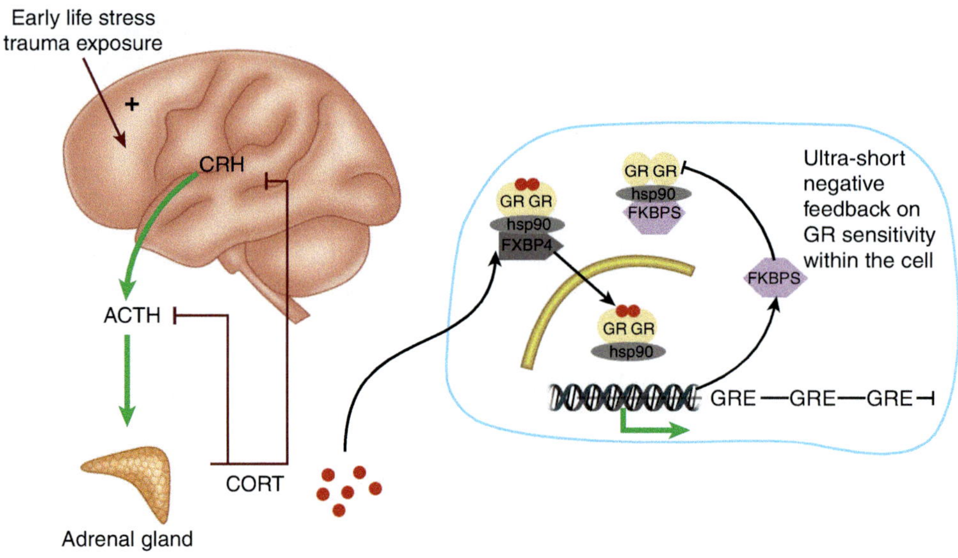

Fig. 18.10 Epigenetic consequences of stress and anxiety. The hypothalamic-pituitary-adrenal axis is activated in response to stress, producing cortisol (CORT). This binds to steroid receptors, such as glucocorticoid receptors (GR), that act as transcriptional activators or repressors in the nucleus. This influences the expression of numerous genes involved in the stress response, immune function and metabolism. For example, binding of cortisol to the GR leads to transcriptional activation of FKBP5. This is a protein involved in immunoregulation, but which also provides ultrashort negative feedback to the GR, terminating the stress response and secretion of cortisol

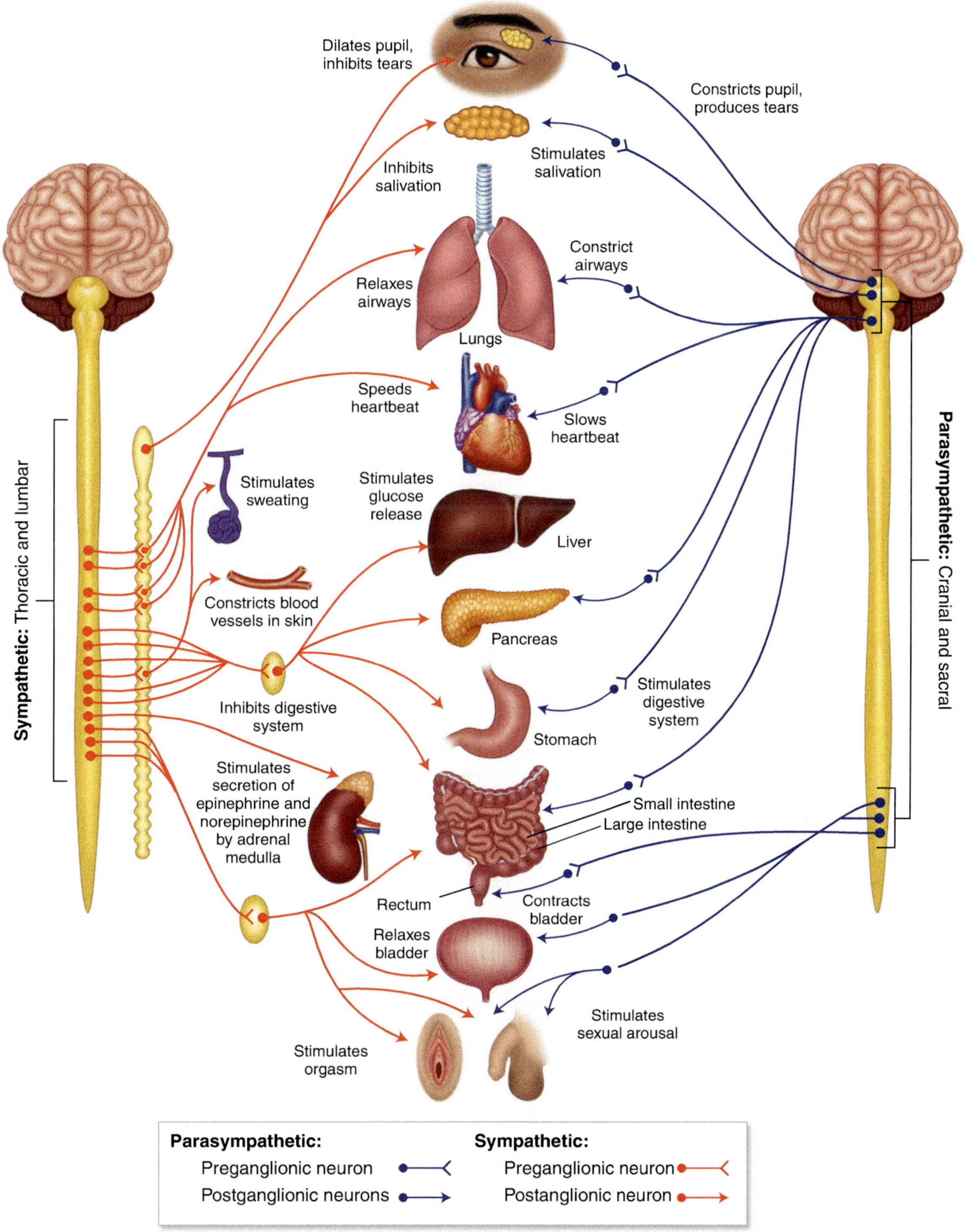

Fig. 18.11 The autonomic nervous system. Activation of the sympathetic nervous system is involved in many of the physical symptoms of acute anxiety as described in Fig. 18.7

ease have been linked to ADs, though this association may in fact be linked to the use of SSRIs in treatment [15].

A second key component of the physiological response to stress and anxiety is the hypothalamic-pituitary-adrenal (HPA) axis. This is a feedback loop between three hormone-releasing structures which controls the secretion of cortisol from the adrenal cortex (Fig. 18.12).

Cortisol is a regulator of several bodily systems, including metabolism, the immune system and the central nervous system. In the short term, it increases availability of glucose

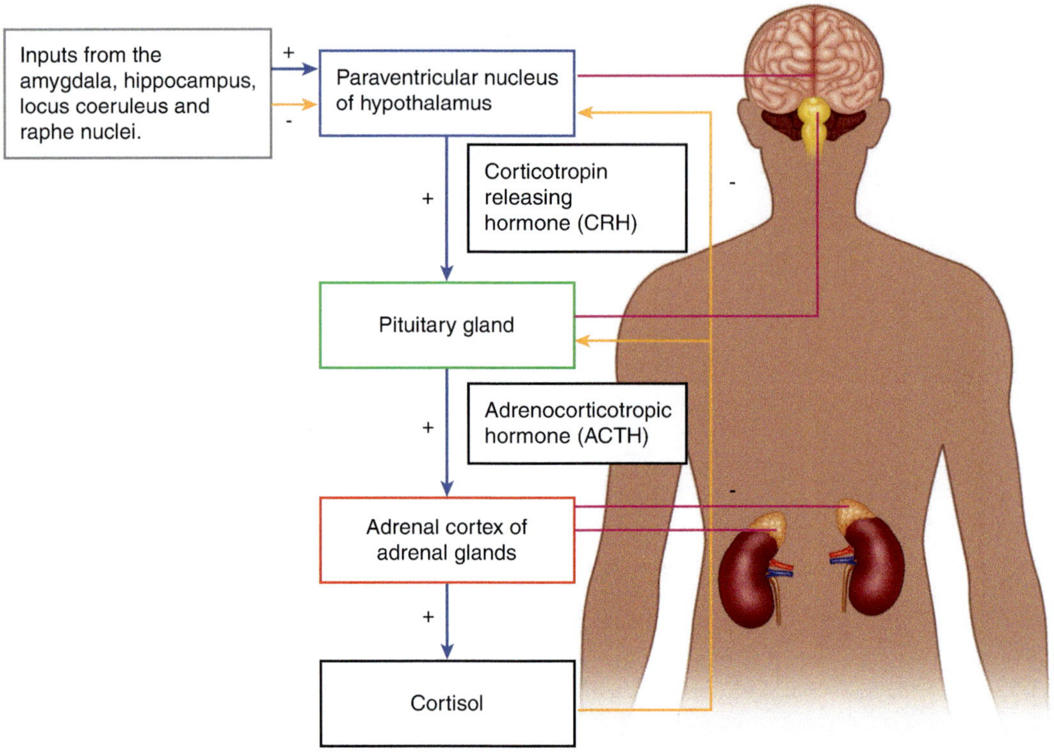

Fig. 18.12 Hypothalamic-pituitary-adrenal axis. The hypothalamic paraventricular nucleus releases corticotropin-releasing hormone in response to stress-induced inputs from other brain areas including the amygdala. This in turn stimulates the pituitary gland to synthesize and release adrenocorticotrophic hormone. This causes the production of cortisol from the adrenal glands. The production of cortisol is self-regulating, with cortisol providing negative feedback on both the hypothalamus and the pituitary gland. Prolonged stress results in sustained high levels of cortisol and disrupted negative feedback mechanisms

to help deal with stressful situations, but chronically raised cortisol can lead to suppression of hippocampal neurogenesis, aberrant immune function and epigenetic alterations such as suppression of BDNF translation [16] (see also *Genetics*). There is evidence for aberrant HPA activation across ADs: in panic disorder, both ACTH and cortisol levels are raised, while in social anxiety disorder and specific phobia, salivary cortisol is increased in response to stressors [16]. However, these alterations are common across psychiatric disorders and are unlikely to specifically differentiate ADs from other chronic stress-related disorders such as depression.

Long-term activation of the autonomic nervous system and HPA axis can alter immune system activity (Fig. 18.13).

Adrenaline release in acute stress can activate release of cytokines and inflammation. In OCD, cytokines IL1-beta and TNF-alpha have been found to be reduced [16], suggesting suppression of the immune system after long-term NA/HPA activation. While a link between possible autonomic attack of the basal ganglia following streptococcal infection in childhood and sudden-onset OCD/tic disorders has been hypothesized (paediatric autoimmune neuropsychiatric disorders associated with streptococcal infections, PANDAS), firm evidence for this is lacking, and this theory has largely been discredited as a cause of OCD [16].

Neurotransmitters and Neuropeptides

Various neurotransmitters and neuropeptides have been implicated in both the pathophysiology and the pharmacological treatment of ADs and OCRDs. Two of the most important are serotonin (5HT) and gamma-aminobutyric acid (GABA).

- Serotonin (5HT): this neurotransmitter mediates both fear response in the periaqueductal grey and anxiety response in the amygdala. There are various genetic links to 5HT in both ADs and OCRDs (see *Genetics*), and lower 5HT levels have been found in the plasma of panic disorder patients. Selective serotonin reuptake inhibitors (SSRIs), which delay the removal of serotonin from the synapse, are the main long-term psychopharmacological intervention for both ADs and OCRDs.
- Gamma-aminobutyric acid (GABA): it is the main inhibitory neurotransmitter in the brain. Benzodiazepines,

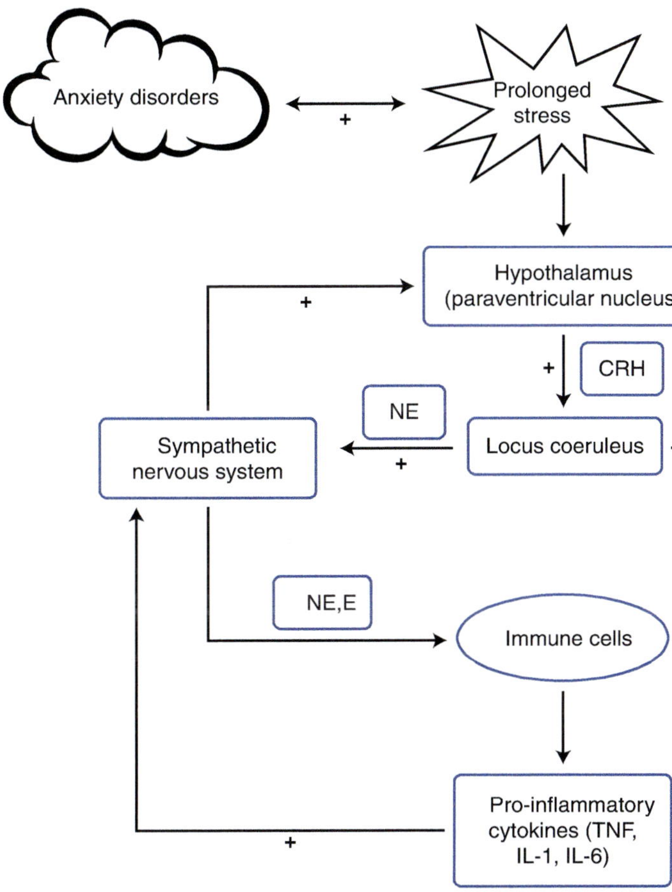

Fig. 18.13 The interaction between the HPA axis, autonomic nervous system and immune system

which are GABA agonists frequently used to treat acute anxiety symptoms in both ADs and OCRDs, act via the GABA-A receptor alpha-2 subunit (Fig. 18.14).

Behavioural Theories

Threat Processing

Confrontation with acute, prolonged or potential threats, i.e. stimuli that can harm the organism immediately or might in the future, activates the fear circuitry. The fear system in the brain functions similarly across mammals, reflecting the evolutionary advantages of an efficiently functioning threat-processing circuitry. Instead of a single fear system, which processes both the conscious feeling of threat and the behavioural and physiological responses to it (Fig. 18.15a), more recently the 'two systems' framework was proposed [17], consisting of one pathway for generating conscious feelings and a second pathway for controlling behavioural and physiological responses to threats (Fig. 18.15b).

The brain regions involved in threat processing depend on the defensive distance, i.e. how near the threat is (Fig. 18.16) [18], and it is therefore important to differentiate the mental states of fear and panic (feelings that occur when the source of harm, the threat, is either immediate or imminent) and anxiety (feelings that occur when the source of harm is uncertain or is distal in space or time). The more immediate and inevitable the threat is, the more the central nucleus of the amygdala and periaqueductal grey is involved; in the presence of anticipation or perceived uncertain or distal threat, the bed nucleus of the stria terminalis (BNST) and prefrontal regions play an important role (see Figs. 18.16 and 18.17) [19].

Pavlovian Fear Conditioning, Context Learning and Extinction Learning

Pavlovian (or classical) fear conditioning is based on the prediction of an aversive event based on previous experiences. Classical conditioning results from the coupling between an aversive stimulus, e.g. an electrical shock (= unconditioned stimulus (US)), and a neutral stimulus or context, e.g. a sound or a room (= conditioned stimulus (CS)). Eventually, the conditioned fear response (CR) will appear to the neutral conditioned stimulus only, even in the absence of the actual aversive event. After repeated presentation of the conditioned stimulus alone, so that it no longer predicts the coming of the uncondi-

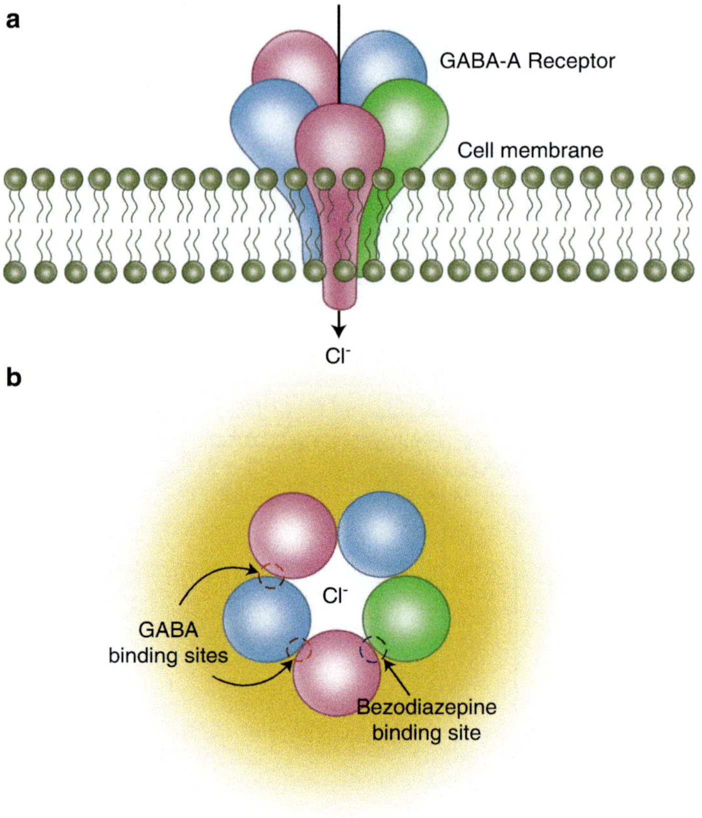

Fig. 18.14 Schematic representation of the GABA-A receptor (**a**) and GABA and benzodiazepine binding sites (**b**)

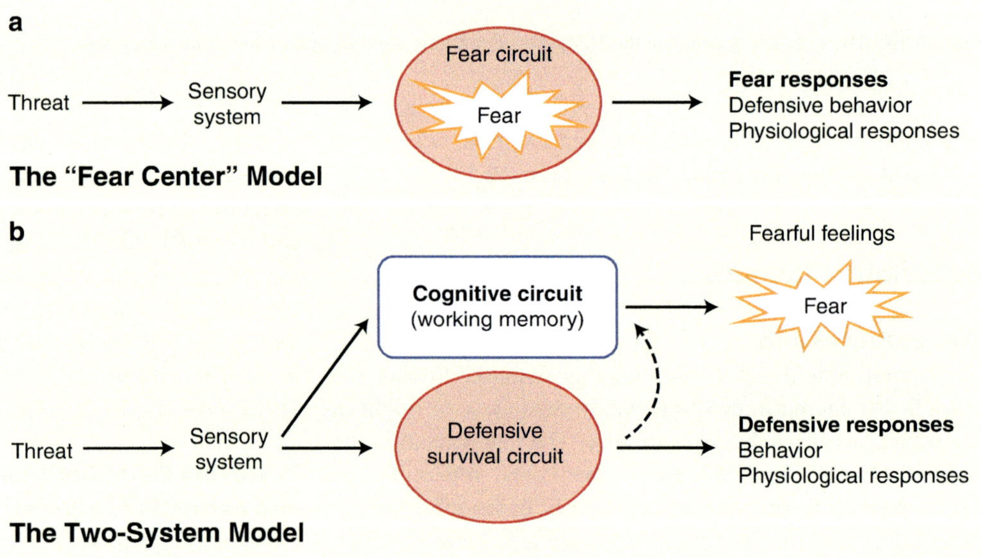

Fig. 18.15 Threat processing models: (**a**) the "Fear Center" model (**b**) The Two-System model

tioned stimulus, the conditioned response gradually decreases and fades away, a process called extinction learning [20].

Reconsolidation

Recently, more research has focused on reconsolidation. After the initial phase of learning (memory acquisition) which strongly relies on the hippocampus, the memory trace becomes stable (memory consolidation) and independent of the hippocampus. The consolidated memories can be made labile again through reactivation of the memory trace (e.g. during imaginary exposure). In this reactivated state, the memory can be manipulated by blocking reconsolidation using pharmacological agents (e.g. propranolol [21]) and facilitating extinction learning by psychological techniques (e.g. EMDR), leading to an altered memory trace that is less emotionally loaded (see Fig. 18.18).

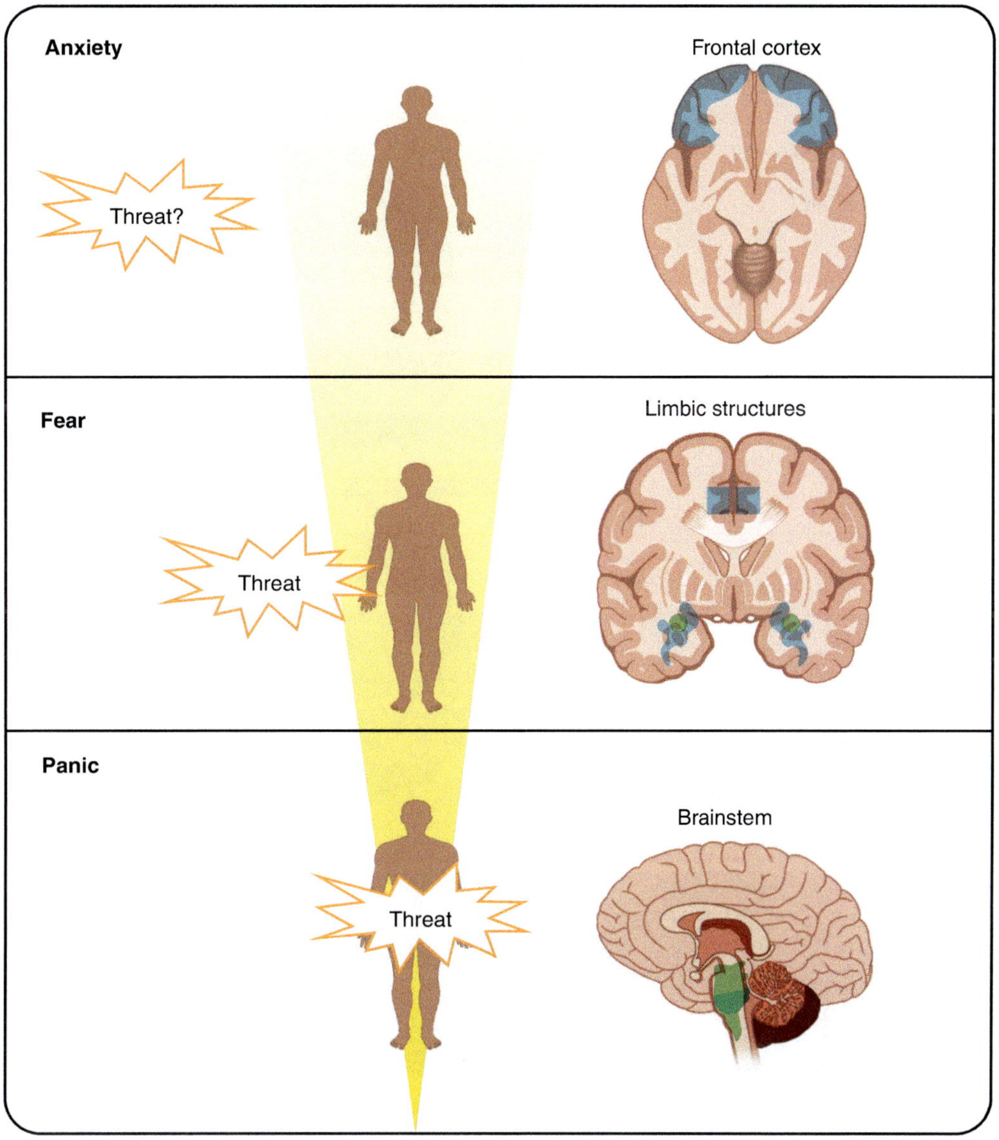

Fig. 18.16 Defensive distance

Emotion Regulation

The conscious processing of fear and anxiety largely depends on the higher-order association cortex, mainly frontoparietal regions, involved in extinction learning (ventromedial prefrontal and subgenual anterior cingulate cortex), error monitoring (dorsal anterior cingulate cortex), emotional reappraisal (dorsomedial and dorsolateral prefrontal cortices) and body awareness (anterior insula) (Fig. 18.19). Knowledge of basic threat processing mechanisms can contribute to innovative adaptations of exposure-based therapies, for instance, by increasing extinction learning and/or reconsolidation.

Goal-Directed Versus Habitual Learning

Another domain of knowledge, mostly relevant for OCRDs, comes from animal work in deficient goal-directed (action-outcome) behaviour and overreliance on habitual (stimulus-response) behaviour [23] as a model for compulsivity across diagnoses. Habits are automatic behaviours that do not require planning or organization. These behaviours result from historical experience of whether or not actions were rewarded in the past. In computational frameworks, habitual learning is also called model-free learning. Habits do not flexibly adjust to the changing environment or outcome devaluation (as seen in OCD patients who keep on washing their hands even when obviously clean, causing enormous negative impact on daily functioning). Ideally, the goal-directed system controls habitual behaviour, by using new information, e.g. the desirability of the outcome and changes to the contingency between action and outcomes (also called model-based learning; see Fig. 18.20).

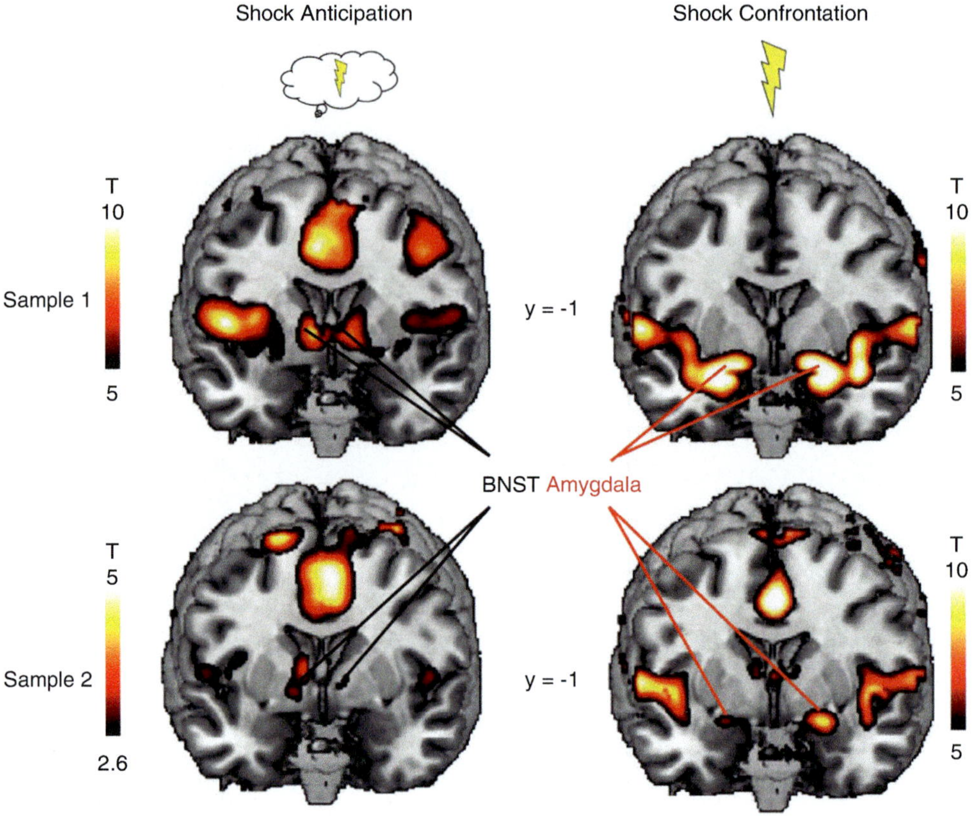

Fig. 18.17 Brain areas involved in anticipated vs immediate threat. (*Reprinted from* Klumpers et al. [19]; Creative Commons Attribution 4.0 International License; http://creativecommons.org/licenses/4.0/)

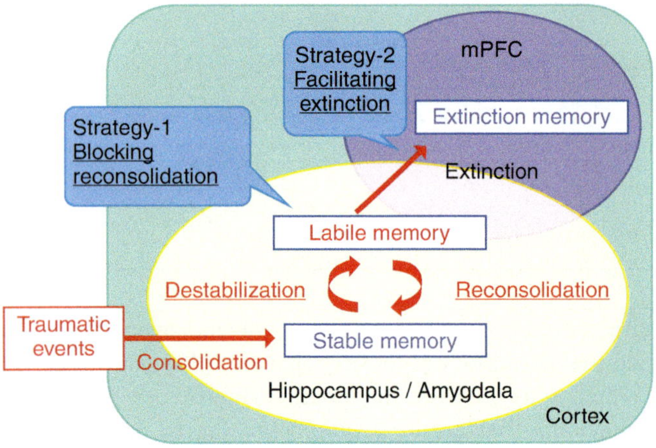

Fig. 18.18 Reconsolidation and extinction. (*From* Kida [22]; Creative Commons CC BY license; http://creativecommons.org/licenses/4.0/)

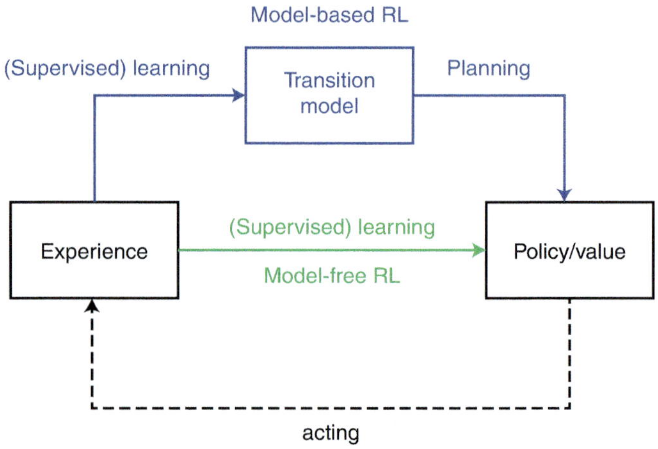

Fig. 18.20 Model-free and model-based reinforcement learning (RL)

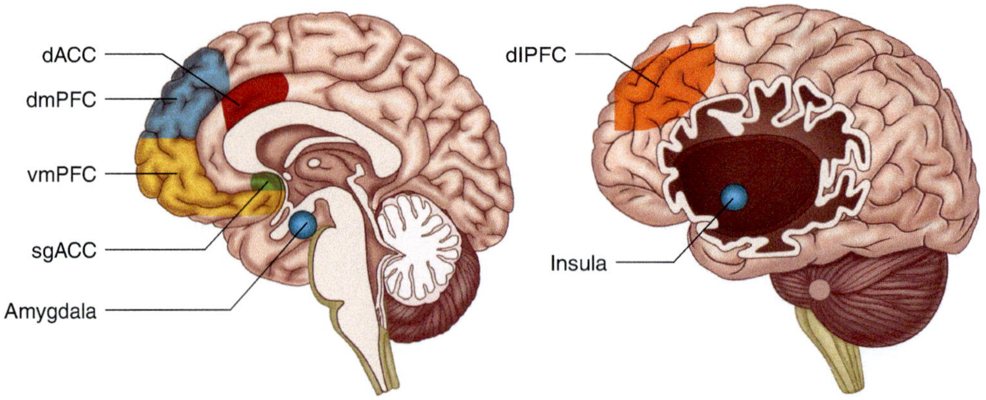

Fig. 18.19 Brain regions involved in fear and anxiety processing: ventromedial prefrontal cortex (vmPFC), subgenual anterior cingulate cortex (sgACC), dorsal anterior cingulate cortex (dACC), dorsomedial and dorsolateral prefrontal cortex (dmPFC, dlPFC), insula, amygdala

Disease Models

Where the classical fear conditioning and extinction learning models and the work on reconsolidation as discussed above are especially relevant for understanding of the trauma-related disorders and ADs [7], the repetitive behaviours as seen in OCRDs might be (at least partly) better explained by altered functioning of the so-called cortico-striato-thalamo-cortical circuits, in which dysfunctions within the parallel circuits explain cognitive deficits (see Fig. 18.21a) that contribute to the symptom level. Based on recent insights, 'the model' does not exist, since the involvement of the various brain circuits differs with developmental age and disease stage (see Fig. 18.21b). Disease models, although oversimplistic, can help to further develop treatment methods. Due to

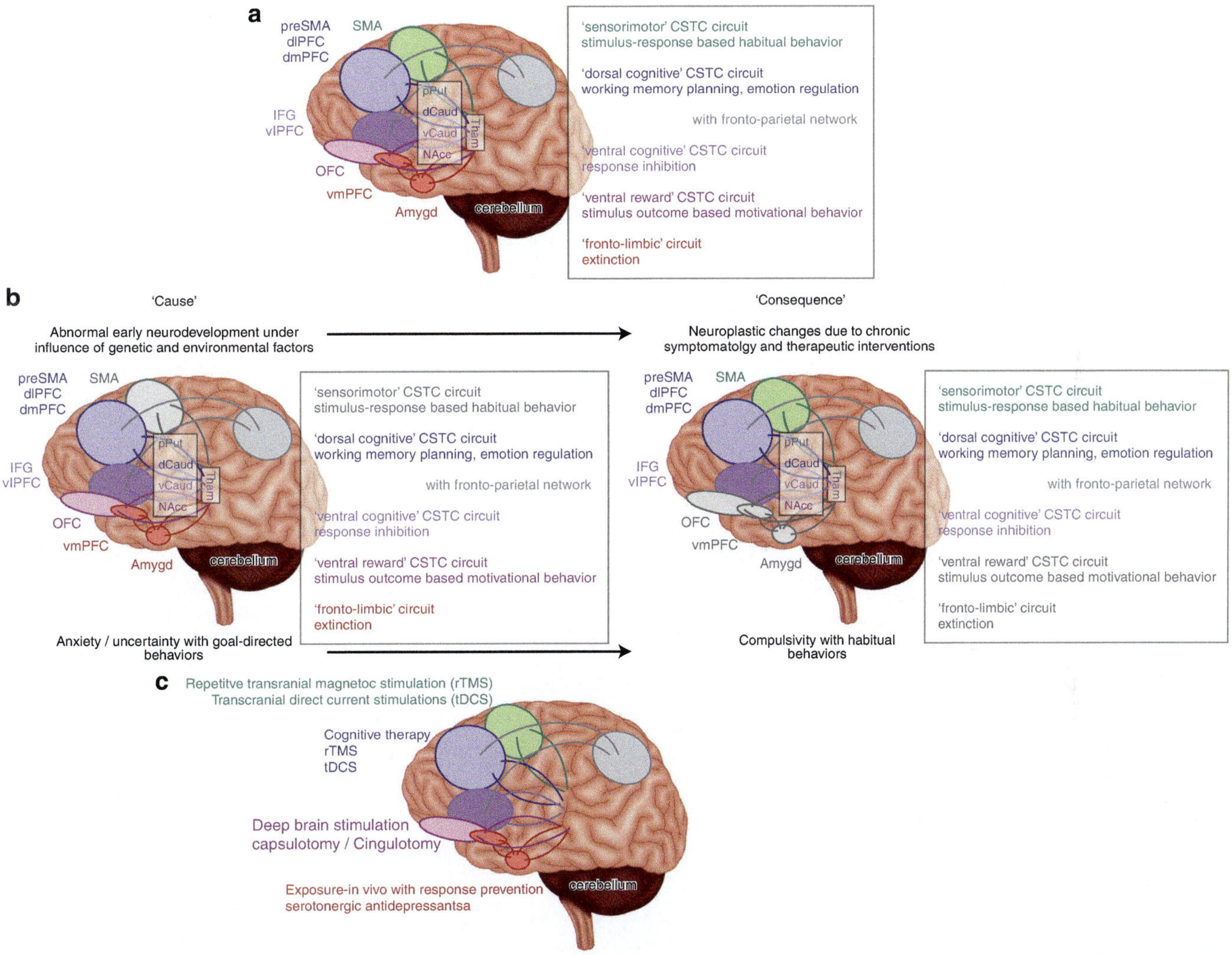

Fig. 18.21 (**a**) Circuits involved in OCD. Obsessive-compulsive disorder (OCD) is mediated by parallel, partly segregated, cortico-striato-thalamo-cortical (CSTC) circuits that are involved in sensorimotor, cognitive, affective and motivational processes. *dCaud* dorsal part of caudate nucleus; *dlPFC* dorsolateral prefrontal cortex; *dmPFC* dorsomedial prefrontal cortex; *IFG* inferior frontal gyrus; *NAcc* nucleus accumbens; *OFC* orbitofrontal cortex; *pPut* posterior part of putamen; *pre-SMA* pre-supplementary motor area; *SMA* supplementary motor area; *Tham* thalamus; *vCaud* ventral part of caudate nucleus; *vlPFC* ventrolateral prefrontal cortex; *vmPFC* ventromedial prefrontal cortex. (**b**) Brain changes as a cause and consequence of OCD. The involvement of these circuits is hypothesized to depend on the symptom profile and the disease stage. In early phases of obsessive-compulsive disorder (OCD), alterations within the dorsal cognitive, ventral cognitive and ventral reward cortico-striato-thalamo-cortical (CSTC) circuits and the frontolimbic circuit are hypothesized to be related to symptoms involving anxiety, uncertainty and goal-directed behaviours. In later phases of OCD, alterations within the sensorimotor, dorsal cognitive and ventral cognitive CSTC circuits are hypothesized to be related to symptoms involving habitual behaviours. *dCaud* dorsal part of caudate nucleus; *dlPFC* dorsolateral prefrontal cortex; *dmPFC* dorsomedial prefrontal cortex; *IFG* inferior frontal gyrus; *NAcc* nucleus accumbens; *OFC* orbitofrontal cortex; *pPut* posterior part of putamen; *pre-SMA* pre-supplementary motor area; *SMA* supplementary motor area; *Tham* thalamus; *vCaud* ventral part of caudate nucleus; *vlPFC* ventrolateral prefrontal cortex; *vmPFC* ventromedial prefrontal cortex. (**c**) Targets for treatment. Different treatment modalities, including neuromodulation, neurosurgery and pharmacological therapy, might target different neurocircuits that have been implicated in obsessive-compulsive disorder. *CSTC* cortico-striato-thalamo-cortical; *DBS* deep brain stimulation; *ERP* exposure and response prevention; *rTMS* repetitive transcranial magnetic stimulation; *SRI* serotonin reuptake inhibitor; *tDCS* transcranial direct current stimulation

the heterogeneity between patients (and their brains), ideally one would target the circuit that is most relevant for the individual patient (see Fig. 18.21c).

Brain Imaging in ADs and OCRDs

Imaging studies using magnetic resonance imaging (MRI) in ADs and OCRDs focus on morphometry, such as subcortical volume (e.g. bigger pallidum in adult OCD and bigger thalamus in paediatric OCD [24]) and cortical volume and/or thickness (e.g. smaller dorsomedial prefrontal and insular cortices in most mental disorders [25]), white matter integrity (e.g. reduced integrity in sagittal stratum and posterior thalamic radiation in OCD [26]), functional network connectivity (e.g. decoupling between the executive control network and the default mode network in ADs [27]) and activation patterns during emotional paradigms (e.g. showing increased amygdala response in GAD [28] and OCD [29]) (see Fig. 18.22) and cognitive paradigms (e.g. showing altered error monitoring network in OCRDs [30]).

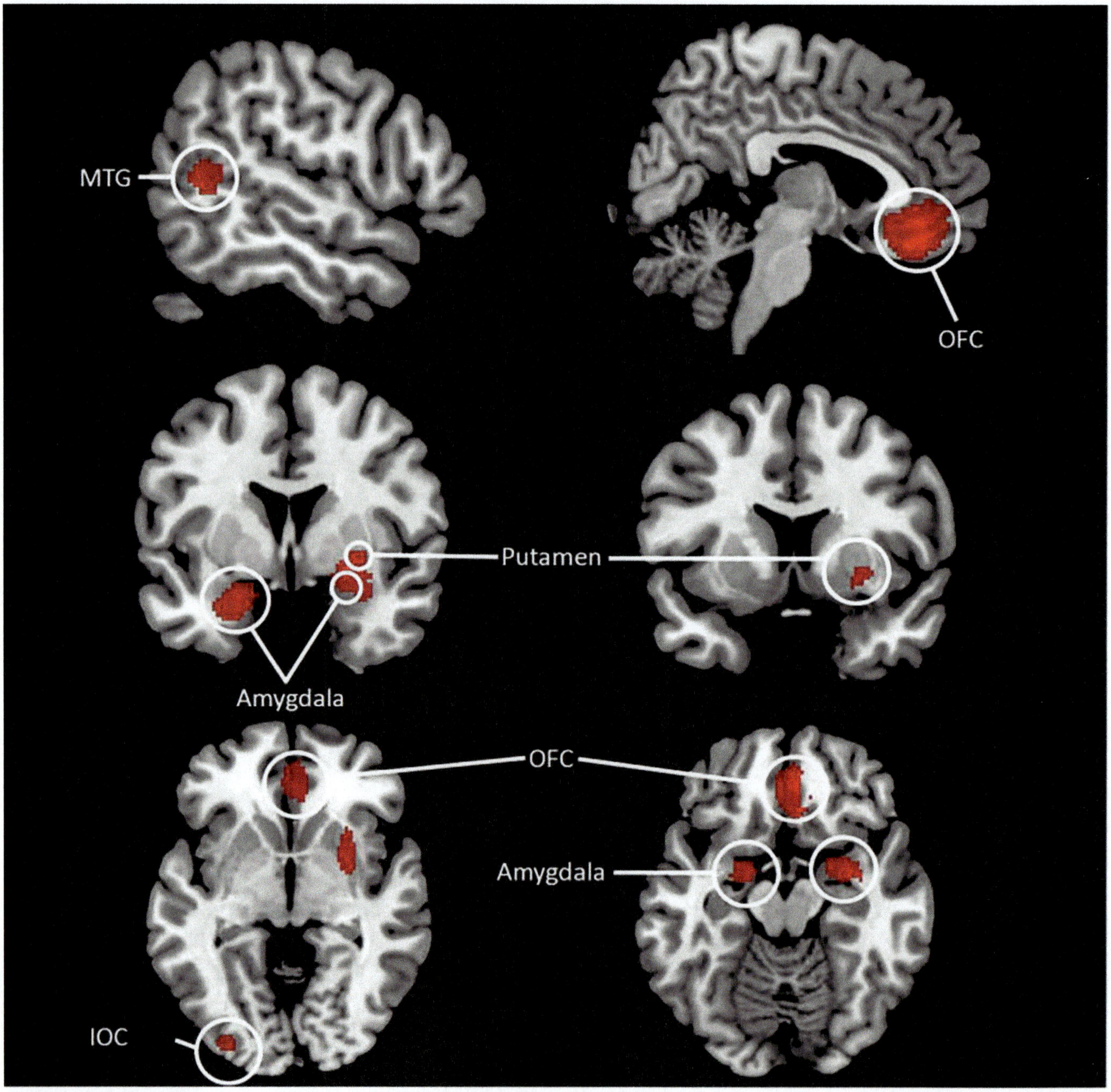

Fig. 18.22 Amygdala activation in response to symptom provocation in OCD. Regions of hyperactivation in OCD patients compared to healthy controls during emotional processing, showing a distributed affective circuit including frontal, limbic, striatal and ventral visual areas. Abbreviations: *IOC* inferior occipital cortex; *MTG* middle temporal gyrus; *OFC* orbitofrontal cortex. (*Reprinted from* Thorsen et al. [29]; *with permission*)

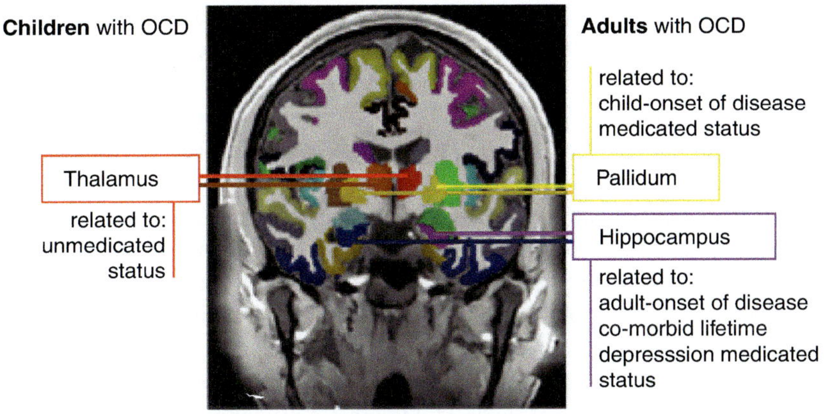

Fig. 18.23 Subcortical structural findings in OCD from the ENIGMA Consortium

Electroencephalography (EEG) is used mainly in OCD to investigate error-related negativity. Other relevant methods are magnetic resonance spectroscopy (MRS) to study neurometabolites, including the GABA and glutamate, and nuclear imaging using SPECT and PET ligands to test other neurotransmitter systems. Most imaging studies are small-sampled and cross-sectional and compare one single disorder with health. The field is moving towards more large-scale cross-disorder comparisons and longitudinal studies, also helped by worldwide collaborations such as the ENIGMA Consortium (Enhancing Neuroimaging Genetics through Meta-analysis) (see Fig. 18.23) [26].

Overall, imaging studies in ADs and OCRDs show structural, functional and chemical alterations within and between brain networks that are relevant for threat and emotional processing and cognitive control. The overlap across disorders is large, and specific alterations largely depend on developmental age, disease stage, medication status, comorbidity and experimental paradigms and imaging techniques used. In contrast to the ADs, OCRDs show more striatal alterations (both structural and functional), fitting with the disease model as described earlier.

Treatment

Treatments for anxiety and obsessive-compulsive and related disorders mostly include psychological interventions (mostly involving exposure-based therapies and cognitive reappraisal strategies) and pharmacotherapy (predominantly serotonergic antidepressants [31], with some recent developments targeting the glutamatergic system). Although most patients favour psychotherapy over medication, worldwide, most patients receive pharmacological therapy as first-line treatment as it is less resource intensive.

A meta-analysis comparing psychotherapies and pharmacotherapies in anxiety disorders and OCD found no significant difference in efficacy for panic disorder and social anxiety disorder between psychotherapy and pharmacotherapy [32]. However, both in the short-term (e.g. immediate side effects) and in the long-term perspective (e.g. unfavourable effects of chronic drug treatment at the cortical level [33] and risk of relapse after discontinuation of medication), evidence-based psychological treatments might have some advantages compared with medication. Also, for OCD, CBT has shown to be significantly more efficacious compared to pharmacological treatment [32]. Non-invasive and invasive neuromodulation techniques (such as repetitive transcranial magnetic stimulation and deep brain stimulation or brain surgery) are increasingly used as adjuvant treatment in patients with obsessive-compulsive and related disorders who do not sufficiently profit from psychological and/or pharmacological interventions.

Psychotherapy

The most extensively tested form of psychotherapy is cognitive behavioural therapy (CBT). Meta-analyses show that CBT is effective in the treatment of anxiety [32] and in obsessive-compulsive disorder [34]. Depending on the disorder and/or symptom profile, the treatment mainly consists of behavioural techniques, i.e. exposure in vivo with response prevention (in anxiety disorders and OCD) or behavioural inhibition (in other OCRDs, such as trichotillomania and excoriation disorder), or focuses on cognitive techniques, i.e. improving cognitive reappraisal and reducing attentional bias. Various modifications are being developed, including metacognitive therapy for GAD and inference-based approach for OCD. With the presence of a trauma component, combination with eye movement desensitization and reprocessing (EMDR) is useful. Psychological treatments should be delivered by well-trained therapists and/or supervised by senior staff. It is also important to limit avoidance by the patients and deviation from the evidence-based treatment protocols by the therapist. The success of the treatment in the short term largely depends on the motivation of the patient (who needs to practice on a daily basis using homework exercises) and in the long term by investment in relapse prevention and/or booster sessions after successful symptom reduction.

Psychotherapy results not only in better emotional processing and cognitive control but also results in normalized brain function. Extinction learning largely depends on appropriate inhibition of the amygdala response by activation of the ventromedial prefrontal and subgenual anterior cingulate cortices. Cognitive reappraisal mainly depends on the recruitment of dorsal prefrontal areas, such as the dorsomedial and dorsolateral prefrontal cortices (see Fig. 18.24).

Imaging studies comparing brain activation patterns pre- versus post-CBT show that successful treatment is accompanied by better recruitment of these control areas and reduced activation of the amygdala (see Fig. 18.25).

Pharmacology

Pharmacological treatment of anxiety disorders and OCRDs mainly relies on serotonergic antidepressants, including SSRIs, selective serotonin and noradrenaline reuptake inhibitors (SNRIs) and the predominantly serotonergic tricyclic antidepressants (TCAs) clomipramine and imipramine. These all increase the serotonergic neurotransmission in the brain, and due to a similar working mechanism, efficacy, latency until effect and side-effect profile are all largely similar (though the broader-acting TCAs have a risk of cardiotoxicity in case of overdose). The broader-acting MAO inhibitor phenelzine has also proven to be effective but is preserved for highly treatment-resistant patients given its unfavourable side-effect profile, the necessity to maintain a tyramine-free diet and the limited evidence for long-term efficacy. Benzodiazepines, working on the GABA-ergic system in the brain, have proven to be similarly effective to serotonergic antidepressants, have the advantage of working fast and result in fewer treatment dropouts. However, benzodiazepines are not regarded a first-choice treatment option because of the side effects, including cognitive effects, sedation, higher risk of falls and the risk of dependency. Moreover, benzodiazepines are not effective for the treatment of depression, a condition frequently comorbid with anxiety and OCD.

For specific disorders, other agents have proven to be effective. For instance, beta-blockers, which act peripherally to block the effects of stress hormones, can be used in the specific subtype of social anxiety disorder. Likewise, antipsychotics, blocking dopaminergic neurotransmission in the brain, can have an additive value as adjuvant to antidepressants in some OCD patients.

Serotonergic antidepressants [36], benzodiazepines and beta-blockers [37] all reduce the responsiveness of the limbic circuits in the brain (see Fig. 18.26). This explains their effect on anxiety and distress but also explains why these drugs give flattening of the affect, an often reported side effect of drug therapy.

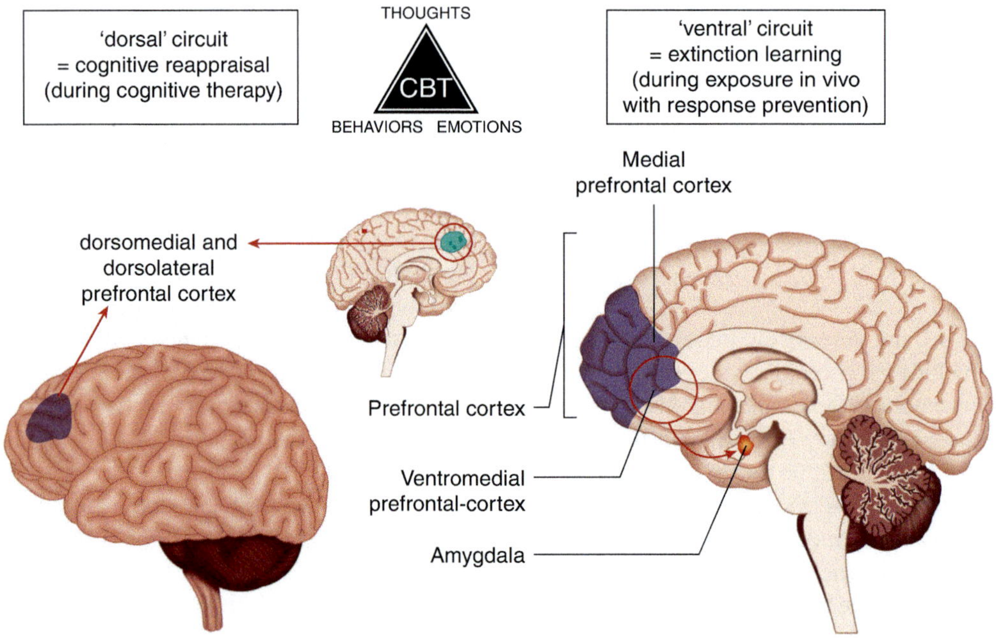

Fig. 18.24 Brain regions involved in exposure therapy and cognitive therapy

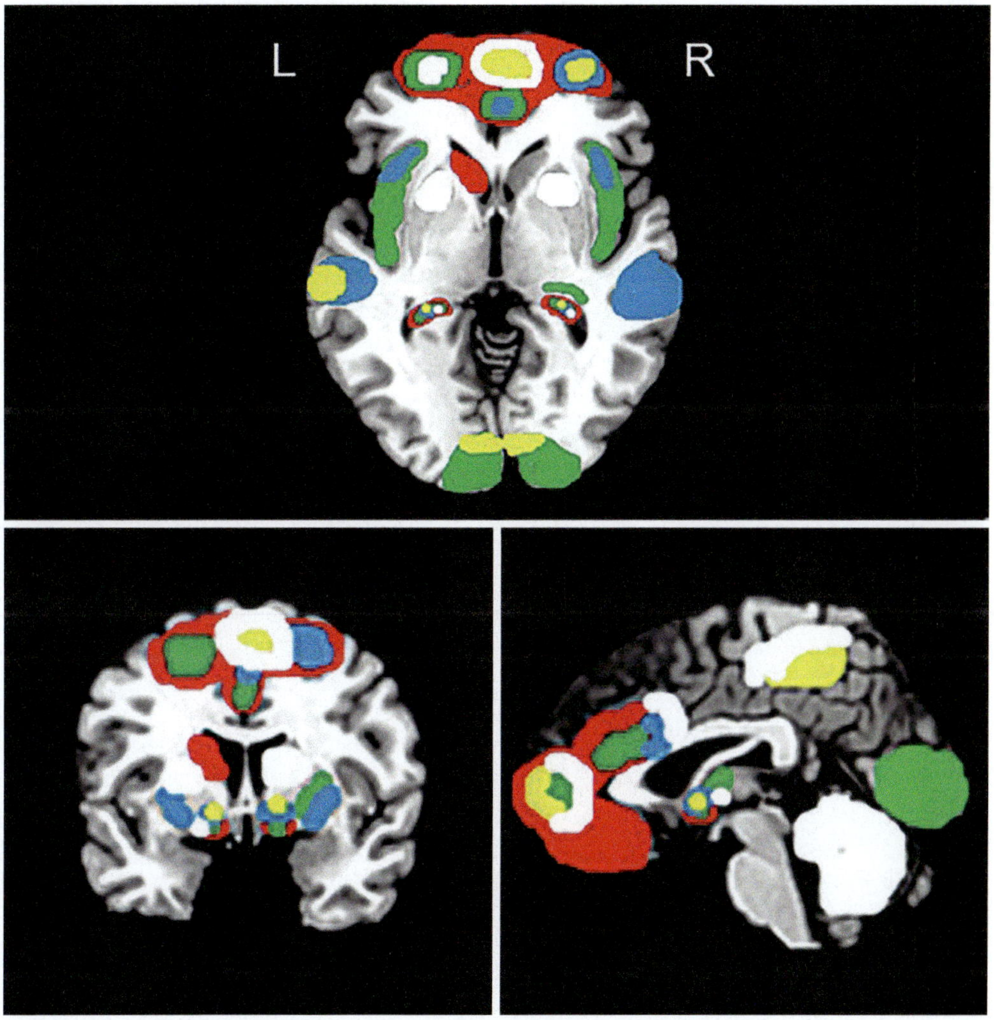

Fig. 18.25 A schematic brain activation map demonstrating regional activation most altered by CBT in ADs, OCD and trauma-related disorders. (*Reprinted from* Brooks and Stein [35]; Creative Commons Attribution License; http://creativecommons.org/licenses/4.0/)

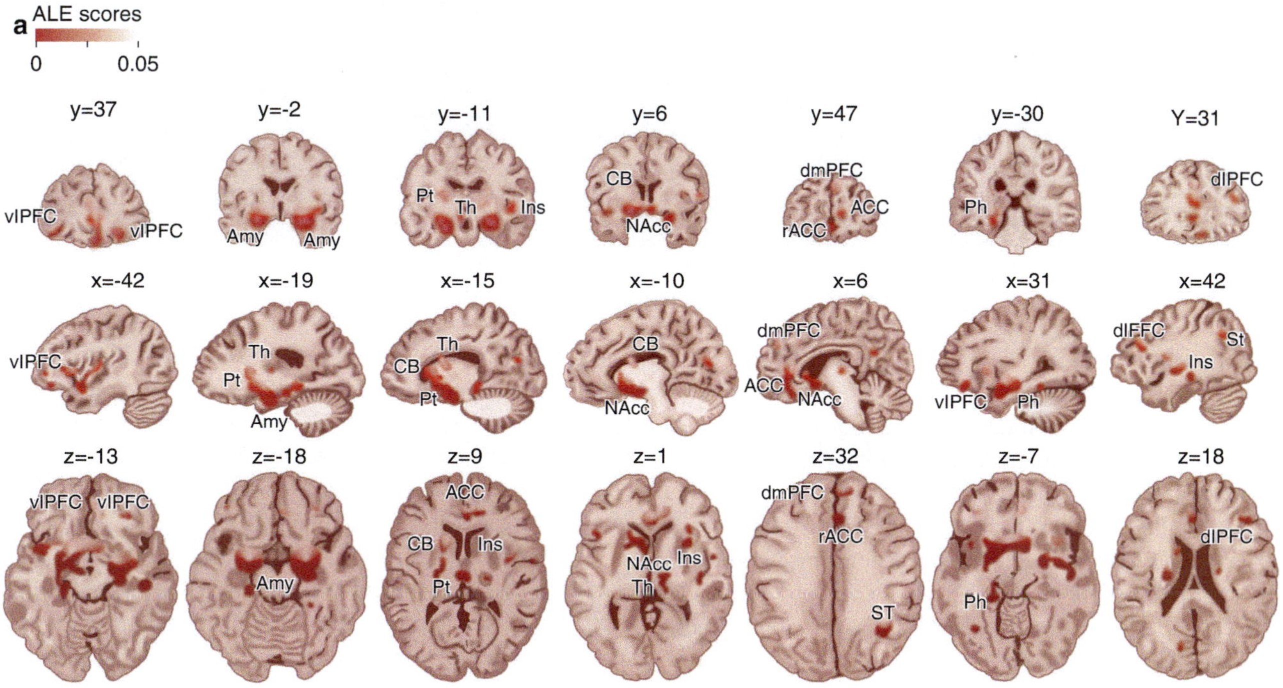

Fig. 18.26 Effects of antidepressants (**a**) and beta-blockers (**b**) on limbic circuit activation. (**b**, *Reprinted from* Hurlemann et al. [37]; with permission)

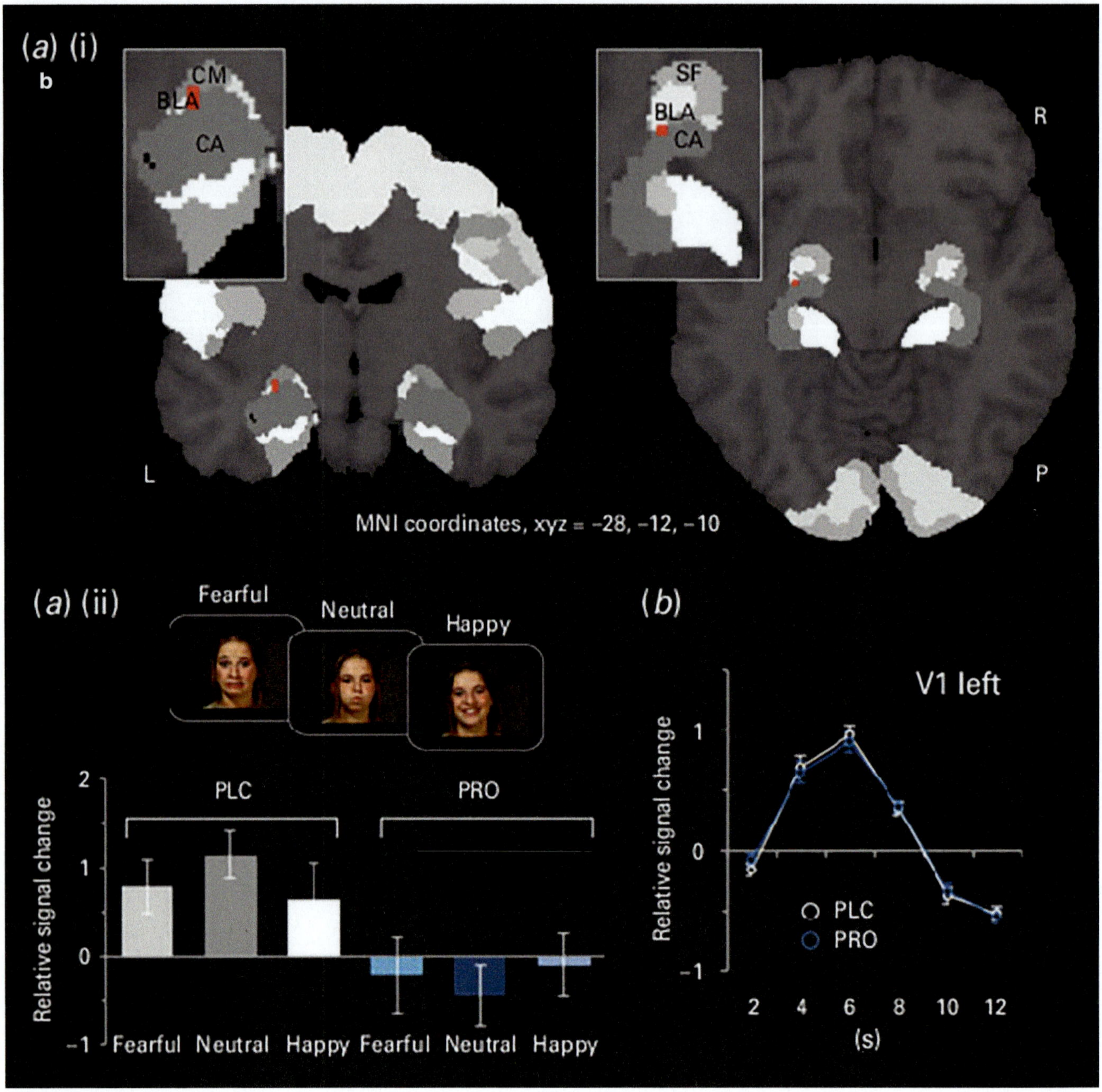

Fig. 18.26 (continued)

Neuromodulation

Various forms of neuromodulation techniques are increasingly used as adjuvant treatment in patients with anxiety disorders and obsessive-compulsive and related disorders [38].

Neurofeedback (or biofeedback) is based on the feedback from neural activity in targeted brain regions, mostly derived from functional MRI or electroencephalography (EEG) to allow the patient to learn to regulate the activation of these brain areas (Fig. 18.27).

The results of a recent systematic review (including a small meta-analysis) point to a positive effect of neurofeedback in OCD, but there is a serious lack of high-standard randomized controlled trials [39]. Although various forms of biofeedback (including EEG- and fMRI-based neurofeedback) appear generally efficacious for anxiety disorders, the specific effects of biofeedback cannot be distinguished from non-specific effects of treatment [40].

Non-invasive brain stimulation techniques, such as repetitive transcranial magnetic stimulation (rTMS) and transcranial direct current stimulation (tDCS), are increasingly used as adjuvant treatment for OCD. Using magnetic (Fig. 18.28a) and electrical stimulation (Fig. 18.28b), targeted brain regions (and interconnected networks) can be inhibited or

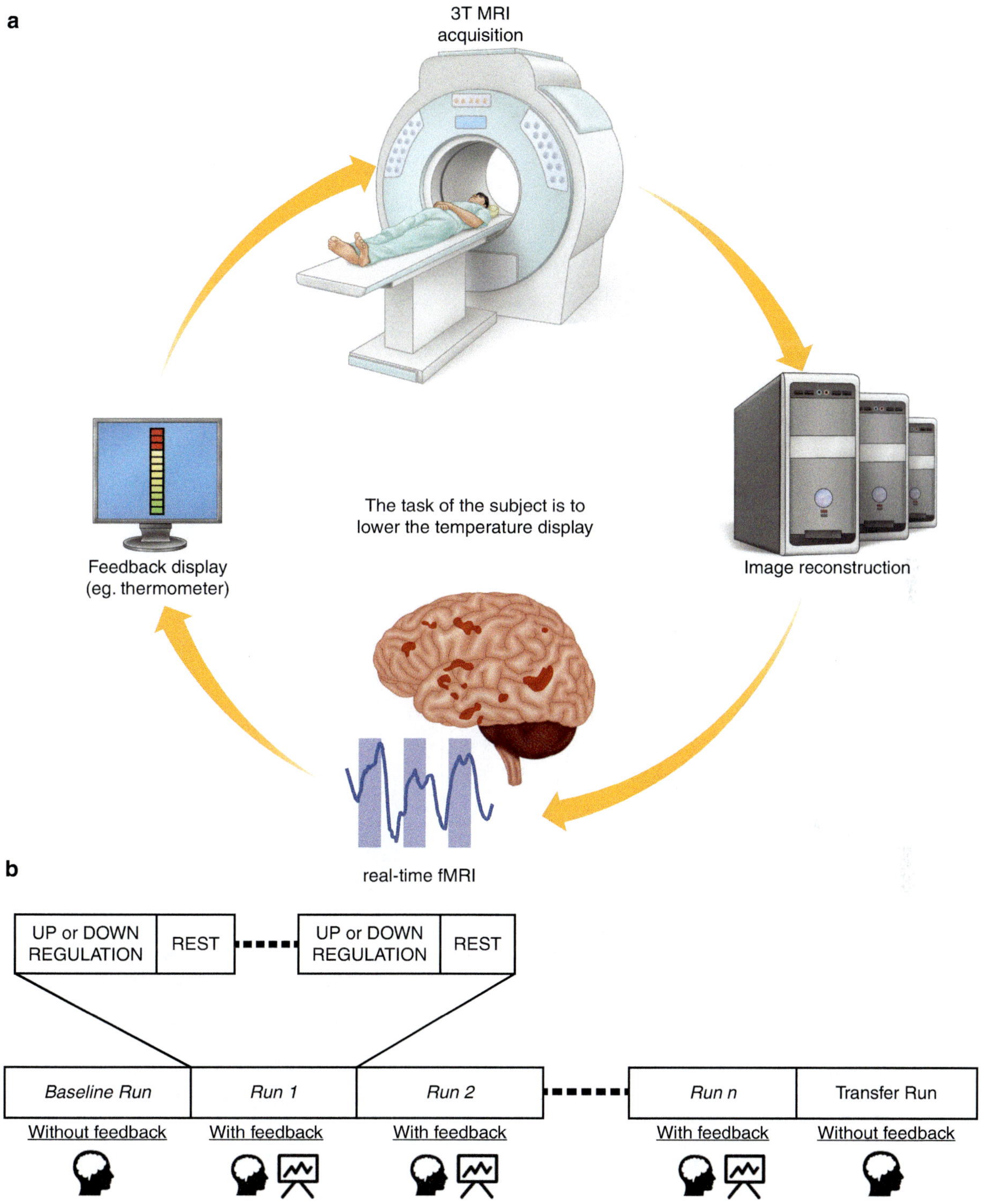

Fig. 18.27 Principles of fMRI-based neurofeedback: (**a**) Diagram of an fMRI-based neurofeedback system: subject lies in an MRI scanner where images of brain activation are acquired. The subject recieves visual feedback (here in the form of a thermometer) to let them know whether the desired brain activation patterns have been achieved. (**b**) A typical neurofeedback training protocol: first, baseline brain activation without regulation or feedback is acquired, followed by several imaging runs where the subject aims to up- or down-regulate their brain activation with feedback. Finally, when satisfactory regulation has been achieved, a final run is carried out without feedback

enhanced, dependent on the stimulation parameters. Meta-analysis of the size of the therapeutic effect shows a medium effect size for rTMS in OCD [41], and the first randomized controlled studies show potential efficacy for tDCS [42]. rTMS seems to have added value in generalized anxiety disorder as well, but the level of evidence is less clear [43].

In extreme cases of treatment resistance, deep brain stimulation (DBS) or brain surgery (i.e. capsulotomy and cingu-

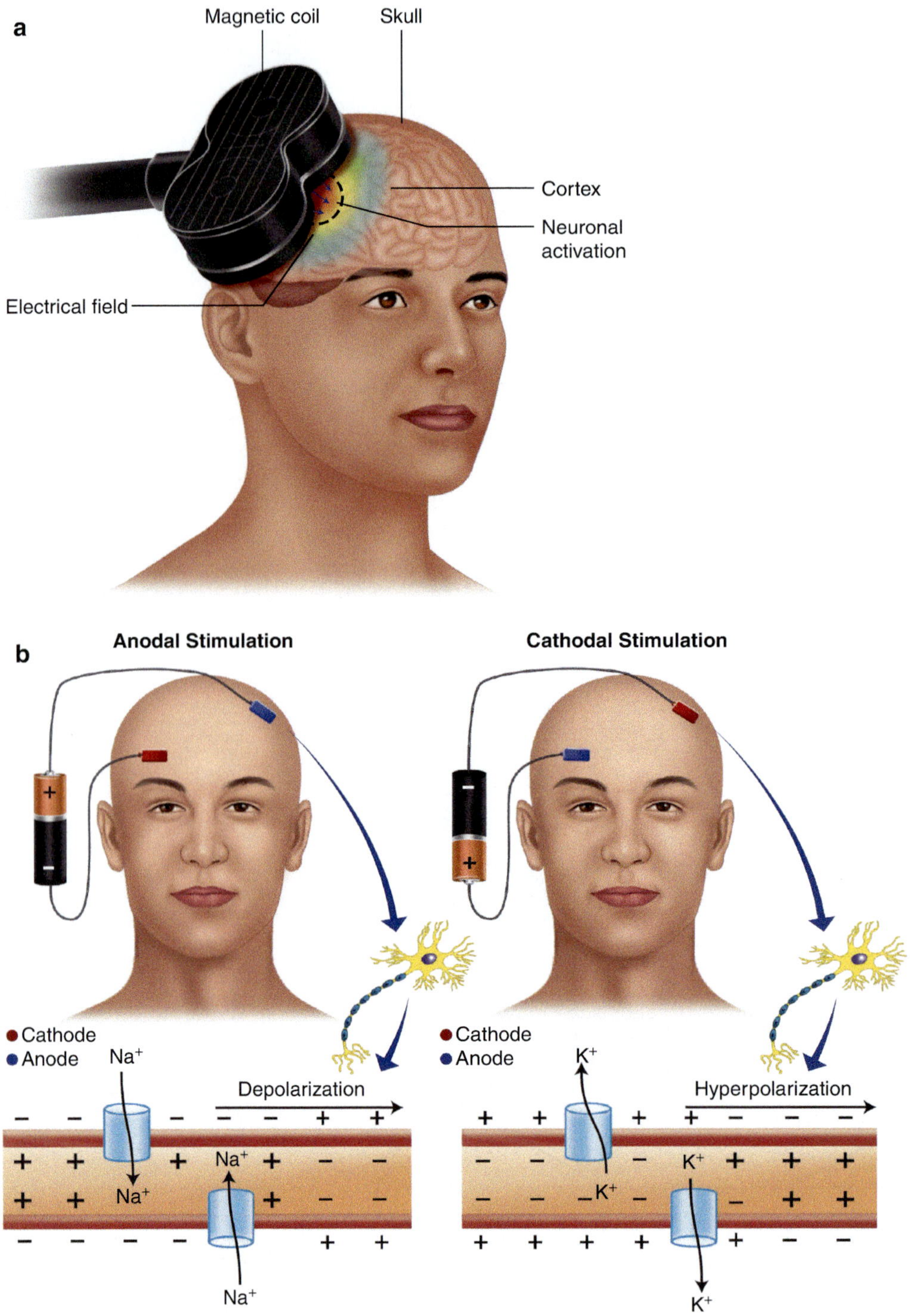

Fig. 18.28 (**a**) Transcranial magnetic stimulation. (**b**) Principles of transcranial direct current stimulation. Anodal stimulation depolarizes the neuronal membrane and enhances excitability. Cathodal stimulation hyperpolarizes the neuronal membrane and diminishes excitability

lotomy) is an option. DBS has been studied mostly for OCD, targeting the subthalamic nucleus, the nucleus accumbens, the anterior limb of the internal capsule or the bed nucleus of the stria terminalis (Fig. 18.29a) [41]. Recently case studies have also appeared for body dysmorphic disorder [44]. Current exciting technical developments concern non-invasive MRI-guided focused ultrasound with some initial open-labelled small-sampled studies that might give new opportunities for mainly OCRDs [45].

Vagus nerve stimulation (VNS) is not yet a well-studied treatment modality for anxiety disorders and OCRDs, but based on animal and experimental studies, VNS increases

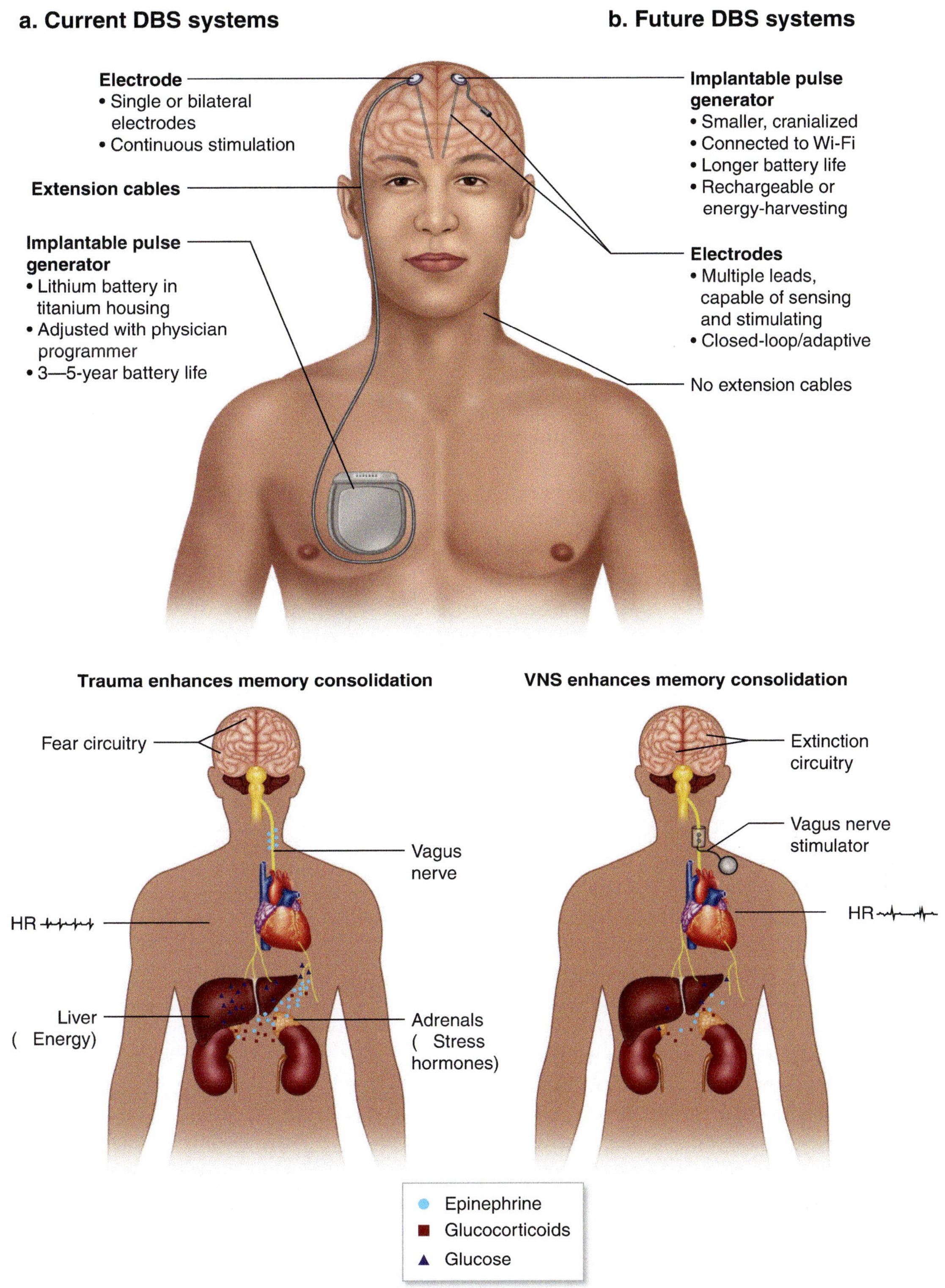

Fig. 18.29 (**a**) Deep brain stimulation. (**b**) Vagus nerve stimulation and extinction learning

extinction learning (Fig. 18.29b) [46] and might thus be of added value as adjuvant to exposure-based therapies in trauma-based and anxiety disorders.

Long-Term Effects of Therapy

Given the unfavourable course trajectories of anxiety disorders and OCRD, with high rates of chronicity and recurrences following remission, enduring treatment effects and relapse prevention are important. Continuing antidepressants appears to be efficacious. However, following discontinuation of antidepressants, relapse is common with more than one third of patients experiencing a relapse [47]. Effects of cognitive behavioural therapy last up till 12 months after treatment completion [48]. After 1 year, effects are still present for generalized anxiety disorder and social anxiety disorder, but absent for panic disorder. Long-term effects of CBT for OCD are unknown. Despite the importance, it is unknown whether psychotherapeutic relapse prevention is effective. Long-term effects of neuromodulation techniques have been poorly studied.

Concluding Remarks

This chapter aimed to summarize established knowledge and recent research in the fields of OCRDs and ADs. While advances in several areas have been made in recent years, especially in exploring the role of genetic and neuroimaging factors in the etiology/pathophysiology of these disorders, there are still several underexplored areas of pathophysiology, especially in the non-OCD OCRDs. Though current therapies have full efficacy in only half of patients, several emerging neuromodulation and neurofeedback interventions show promise for both ADs and OCRDs—a major research focus for the coming years will be the evaluation and optimization of these therapies. Finally, while the adoption of RDoC in clinical practice has been limited, evidence for common pathophysiological mechanisms across the ADs and OCRDs demonstrates the continuing relevance of this approach, which will hopefully continue to lead to new insights into these disorders and further development of effective treatments in the coming years.

References

1. American Psychiatric, A. Diagnostic and statistical manual of mental disorders: DSM-5. 5th ed. American Psychiatric Association; 2013. p. xliv, 947p.
2. World Health Organisation. International classification of diseases for mortality and morbidity statistics (11th Revision). 2018. https://icd.who.int/.
3. Insel T, et al. Research domain criteria (RDoC): toward a new classification framework for research on mental disorders. Am J Psychiatry. 2010;167:748–51. https://doi.org/10.1176/appi.ajp.2010.09091379.
4. Institute for Health Metrics and Evaluation. Global Health Data Exchange, Global Burden of Disease Results Tool. http://ghdx.healthdata.org/gbd-results-tool.
5. Geddes J, Andreasen NC, Goodwin G. New Oxford textbook of psychiatry. 3rd ed. Oxford University Press; 2020.
6. Stein DJ, et al. Obsessive-compulsive disorder. Nat Rev Dis Primers. 2019;5:52. https://doi.org/10.1038/s41572-019-0102-3.
7. Craske MG, et al. Anxiety disorders. Nat Rev Dis Primers. 2017;3:17024. https://doi.org/10.1038/nrdp.2017.24.
8. Sharma E, Thennarasu K, Reddy YC. Long-term outcome of obsessive-compulsive disorder in adults: a meta-analysis. J Clin Psychiatry. 2014;75:1019–27. https://doi.org/10.4088/JCP.13r08849.
9. Ormel J, Sytema S, Oldehinkel AJ. Epidemiologische aspecten van angststoornissen. In: den Boer JA, Westenberg HGM, editors. Leerboek Angststoornissen. Utrecht: De Tijdstroom; 1995.
10. Bandelow B, et al. Biological markers for anxiety disorders, OCD and PTSD—a consensus statement. Part I: neuroimaging and genetics. World J Biol Psychiatry. 2016;17:321–65. https://doi.org/10.1080/15622975.2016.1181783.
11. Welch JM, et al. Cortico-striatal synaptic defects and OCD-like behaviours in Sapap3-mutant mice. Nature. 2007;448:894–900. https://doi.org/10.1038/nature06104.
12. International Obsessive Compulsive Disorder Foundation Genetics, C. & Studies, O. C. D. C. G. A. Revealing the complex genetic architecture of obsessive-compulsive disorder using meta-analysis. Mol Psychiatry. 2018;23:1181–8. https://doi.org/10.1038/mp.2017.154.
13. Otowa T, et al. Meta-analysis of genome-wide association studies of anxiety disorders. Mol Psychiatry. 2016;21:1391–9. https://doi.org/10.1038/mp.2015.197.
14. Klengel T, Binder EB. Epigenetics of stress-related psychiatric disorders and gene x environment interactions. Neuron. 2015;86:1343–57. https://doi.org/10.1016/j.neuron.2015.05.036.
15. Licht CM, de Geus EJ, van Dyck R, Penninx BW. Association between anxiety disorders and heart rate variability in The Netherlands Study of Depression and Anxiety (NESDA). Psychosom Med. 2009;71:508–18. https://doi.org/10.1097/PSY.0b013e3181a292a6.
16. Bandelow B, et al. Biological markers for anxiety disorders, OCD and PTSD: a consensus statement. Part II: neurochemistry, neurophysiology and neurocognition. World J Biol Psychiatry. 2017;18:162–214. https://doi.org/10.1080/15622975.2016.1190867.
17. LeDoux JE, Pine DS. Using neuroscience to help understand fear and anxiety: a two-system framework. Am J Psychiatry. 2016;173:1083–93. https://doi.org/10.1176/appi.ajp.2016.16030353.
18. McNaughton N, Gray JA. Anxiolytic action on the behavioural inhibition system implies multiple types of arousal contribute to anxiety. J Affect Disord. 2000;61:161–76. https://doi.org/10.1016/s0165-0327(00)00344-x.
19. Klumpers F, Kroes MCW, Baas JMP, Fernandez G. How human amygdala and bed nucleus of the stria terminalis may drive distinct defensive responses. J Neurosci. 2017;37:9645–56. https://doi.org/10.1523/JNEUROSCI.3830-16.2017.
20. Lipp OV, Waters AM, Luck CC, Ryan KM, Craske MG. Novel approaches for strengthening human fear extinction: the roles of novelty, additional USs, and additional GSs. Behav Res Ther. 2020;124:103529. https://doi.org/10.1016/j.brat.2019.103529.

21. Kindt M, Soeter M, Vervliet B. Beyond extinction: erasing human fear responses and preventing the return of fear. Nat Neurosci. 2009;12:256–8. https://doi.org/10.1038/nn.2271.
22. Kida S. Reconsolidation/destabilization, extinction and forgetting of fear memory as therapeutic targets for PTSD. Psychopharmacology. 2019;236:49–57. https://doi.org/10.1007/s00213-018-5086-2.
23. Gillan CM, Robbins TW, Sahakian BJ, van den Heuvel OA, van Wingen G. The role of habit in compulsivity. Eur Neuropsychopharmacol. 2016;26:828–40. https://doi.org/10.1016/j.euroneuro.2015.12.033.
24. Boedhoe PS, et al. Distinct subcortical volume alterations in pediatric and adult OCD: a worldwide meta- and mega-analysis. Am J Psychiatry. 2017;174:60–9. https://doi.org/10.1176/appi.ajp.2016.16020201.
25. Goodkind M, et al. Identification of a common neurobiological substrate for mental illness. JAMA Psychiat. 2015;72:305–15. https://doi.org/10.1001/jamapsychiatry.2014.2206.
26. van den Heuvel OA, et al. An overview of the first 5 years of the ENIGMA obsessive-compulsive disorder working group: the power of worldwide collaboration. Hum Brain Mapp. 2020;43(1):23–36. https://doi.org/10.1002/hbm.24972.
27. Xu J, et al. Anxious brain networks: a coordinate-based activation likelihood estimation meta-analysis of resting-state functional connectivity studies in anxiety. Neurosci Biobehav Rev. 2019;96:21–30. https://doi.org/10.1016/j.neubiorev.2018.11.005.
28. Kolesar TA, Bilevicius E, Wilson AD, Kornelsen J. Systematic review and meta-analyses of neural structural and functional differences in generalized anxiety disorder and healthy controls using magnetic resonance imaging. Neuroimage Clin. 2019;24:102016. https://doi.org/10.1016/j.nicl.2019.102016.
29. Thorsen AL, et al. Emotional processing in obsessive-compulsive disorder: a systematic review and meta-analysis of 25 functional neuroimaging studies. Biol Psychiatry Cogn Neurosci Neuroimaging. 2018;3:563–71. https://doi.org/10.1016/j.bpsc.2018.01.009.
30. Norman LJ, et al. Error processing and inhibitory control in obsessive-compulsive disorder: a meta-analysis using statistical parametric maps. Biol Psychiatry. 2019;85:713–25. https://doi.org/10.1016/j.biopsych.2018.11.010.
31. Slee A, et al. Pharmacological treatments for generalised anxiety disorder: a systematic review and network meta-analysis. Lancet. 2019;393:768–77. https://doi.org/10.1016/S0140-6736(18)31793-8.
32. Cuijpers P, et al. The efficacy of psychotherapy and pharmacotherapy in treating depressive and anxiety disorders: a meta-analysis of direct comparisons. World Psychiatry. 2013;12:137–48. https://doi.org/10.1002/wps.20038.
33. Boedhoe PSW, et al. Cortical abnormalities associated with pediatric and adult obsessive-compulsive disorder: findings from the ENIGMA Obsessive-Compulsive Disorder Working Group. Am J Psychiatry. 2018;175:453–62. https://doi.org/10.1176/appi.ajp.2017.17050485.
34. Ost LG, Havnen A, Hansen B, Kvale G. Cognitive behavioral treatments of obsessive-compulsive disorder. A systematic review and meta-analysis of studies published 1993-2014. Clin Psychol Rev. 2015;40:156–69. https://doi.org/10.1016/j.cpr.2015.06.003.
35. Brooks SJ, Stein DJ. A systematic review of the neural bases of psychotherapy for anxiety and related disorders. Dialogues Clin Neurosci. 2015;17(3):261–79. https://doi.org/10.31887/DCNS.2015.17.3/sbrooks.
36. Ma Y. Neuropsychological mechanism underlying antidepressant effect: a systematic meta-analysis. Mol Psychiatry. 2015;20:311–9. https://doi.org/10.1038/mp.2014.24.
37. Hurlemann R, et al. Human amygdala reactivity is diminished by the beta-noradrenergic antagonist propranolol. Psychol Med. 2010;40:1839–48. https://doi.org/10.1017/S0033291709992376.
38. Freire RC, Cabrera-Abreu C, Milev R. Neurostimulation in anxiety disorders, post-traumatic stress disorder, and obsessive-compulsive disorder. Adv Exp Med Biol. 2020;1191:331–46. https://doi.org/10.1007/978-981-32-9705-0_18.
39. Ferreira S, Pego JM, Morgado P. The efficacy of biofeedback approaches for obsessive-compulsive and related disorders: a systematic review and meta-analysis. Psychiatry Res. 2019;272:237–45. https://doi.org/10.1016/j.psychres.2018.12.096.
40. Tolin DF, Davies CD, Moskow DM, Hofmann SG. Biofeedback and neurofeedback for anxiety disorders: a quantitative and qualitative systematic review. Adv Exp Med Biol. 2020;1191:265–89. https://doi.org/10.1007/978-981-32-9705-0_16.
41. Schruers K, et al. The effects of deep-brain non-stimulation in severe obsessive-compulsive disorder: an individual patient data meta-analysis. Transl Psychiatry. 2019;9:183. https://doi.org/10.1038/s41398-019-0522-6.
42. Gowda SM, et al. Efficacy of pre-supplementary motor area transcranial direct current stimulation for treatment resistant obsessive compulsive disorder: a randomized, double blinded, sham controlled trial. Brain Stimul. 2019;12:922–9. https://doi.org/10.1016/j.brs.2019.02.005.
43. Cui H, et al. Efficacy and safety of repetitive transcranial magnetic stimulation for generalised anxiety disorder: a meta-analysis. Gen Psychiatr. 2019;32:e100051. https://doi.org/10.1136/gpsych-2019-100051.
44. Baldermann JC, et al. Deep brain stimulation of the ventral capsule/ventral striatum reproducibly improves symptoms of body dysmorphic disorder. Brain Stimul. 2016;9:957–9. https://doi.org/10.1016/j.brs.2016.09.003.
45. Kinfe T, Stadlbauer A, Winder K, Hurlemann R, Buchfelder M. Incisionless MR-guided focused ultrasound: technical considerations and current therapeutic approaches in psychiatric disorders. Expert Rev Neurother. 2020;20:687–96. https://doi.org/10.1080/14737175.2020.1779590.
46. Noble LJ, Souza RR, McIntyre CK. Vagus nerve stimulation as a tool for enhancing extinction in exposure-based therapies. Psychopharmacology. 2019;236:355–67. https://doi.org/10.1007/s00213-018-4994-5.
47. Batelaan NM, et al. Risk of relapse after antidepressant discontinuation in anxiety disorders, obsessive-compulsive disorder, and post-traumatic stress disorder: systematic review and meta-analysis of relapse prevention trials. BMJ. 2017;358:j3927. https://doi.org/10.1136/bmj.j3927.
48. van Dis EAM, et al. Long-term outcomes of cognitive behavioral therapy for anxiety-related disorders: a systematic review and meta-analysis. JAMA Psychiat. 2020;77:265–73. https://doi.org/10.1001/jamapsychiatry.2019.3986.

Trauma- and Stressor-Related Disorders and Dissociative Disorders

19

Samoon Ahmad

Introduction

Trauma- and stressor-related disorders and dissociative disorders are distinct diagnostic classes of disorders with symptoms that can severely impair one's ability to function, particularly in a social environment. In the case of the former, a traumatic event or stressor antecedes the symptoms, and symptomology is defined by a combination of avoidant behavior, hypervigilance, negative mood, re-experiencing of the trauma, and dissociative experiences such as amnesia, depersonalization/derealization, and flashbacks (one of the most common symptoms associated with the trauma- and stressor-related disorder posttraumatic stress disorder (PTSD)). In extreme cases, individuals may also report difficulties regulating emotion, a diminished sense of self, and severe interpersonal problems. For the latter, trauma is not necessarily an antecedent of the disorder, but some form of trauma is common. Dissociative symptoms are characterized by a discontinuity in normal cognitive functioning that may affect memory, identity, behavior, emotion, or even one's sense of proprioception (as in depersonalization or derealization disorder).

To highlight the close relationship between trauma- and stressor-related disorders and dissociative disorders, the DSM-5 and ICD-11 have each placed the two conditions next to each other. Though they share many similarities, disorders in these two groups each possess distinct symptoms and prognoses and therefore demand unique and specific treatments. These will be explored below.

Trauma- and Stressor-Related Disorders

Exposure to trauma is a diagnostic criterion for each trauma- and stressor-related disorder explored in this chapter. These conditions include acute stress disorder (ASD), posttraumatic stress disorder (PTSD), complex PTSD (CPTSD), adjustment disorder (AjD), reactive attachment disorder (RAD), disinhibited social engagement disorder (DSED), prolonged grief disorder (PGD), and other disorders both specified and non-specified. The 5th edition of the American Psychiatric Association's *Diagnostic and Statistical Manual of Mental Disorders* (DSM-5) and 11th edition of the World Health Organization's International Classification of Diseases (ICD-11) have classified these disorders within the category of either "trauma- and stressor-related disorders" (DSM-5) or "disorders specifically associated with stress" (ICD-11) because they are categorically distinct from other disorders, including anxiety or fear-related disorders [1] (Tables 19.1 and 19.2).

The most well-known of these disorders is PTSD, which is more common among combat veterans than the general public. They tend to re-experience wartime trauma via intrusive memories either as nightmares or "flashbacks" (Fig. 19.1). While events that take place during such conflicts often serve as a source for severe psychological stress and trauma, PTSD and other trauma- and stressor-related disorders can be linked to traumatic events that occur in less violent settings. Moreover, symptom profiles of disorders like PTSD, ASD, and AjD can take on many forms. There are

S. Ahmad (✉)
Department of Psychiatry, NYU Grossman School of Medicine, New York, NY, USA
e-mail: samoon@samoonmd.com

W. W. IsHak (ed.), *Atlas of Psychiatry*, https://doi.org/10.1007/978-3-031-15401-0_19

Table 19.1 Prevalence of trauma exposure and PTSD diagnosis

Region	Trauma exposure	PTSD lifetime prevalence total	PTSD lifetime prevalence with trauma exposure	PTSD 12-month prevalence with trauma exposure	12-month prevalence among lifetime PTSD	30-day prevalence among 12-month PTSD	Sample size
The United States	82.7% (0.9)	6.9% (0.4)	8.3% (0.5)	4.3% (0.3)	52.4% (2.9)	49.3% (4.1)	5692
High-income nations	72.4% (0.4)	5.0% (0.1)	6.9% (0.2)	3.6% (0.1)	52.1% (1.2)	51.3% (1.8)	42,308
Middle-income nations	63.2% (0.6)	2.3% (0.1)	3.6% (0.2)	1.6% (0.1)	43.5% (2.7)	44.3% (4.5)	16,913
Lower-income nations	69.1% (0.7)	2.1% (0.2)	3.0% (0.2)	1.5% (0.2)	47.8% (3.9)	43.2% (5.4)	11,862
Total	69.7% (0.3)	3.9% (0.1)	5.6% (0.1)	2.8% (0.1)	50.5% (1.0)	49.8% (1.6)	71,083

The high-income nation group included Australia, Belgium, France, Germany, Israel, Italy, Japan, New Zealand, Northern Ireland, Portugal, Spain, Spain (Murcia), the Netherlands, and the United States. The middle-income nation group included Brazil, Bulgaria, Colombia (Medellin), Lebanon, Mexico, Romania, and South Africa. The lower-income nation group included Colombia, Iraq, Peru, People's Republic of China, and Ukraine

Table 19.2 Trauma clusters and specific events

Trauma cluster	Specific event
Collective violence	Civilian in a war zone; refugee from a war zone; civilian in a terrorized region; relief worker in a war zone; kidnapping victim
Caused/ witnessed bodily harm	Accidentally caused injury or death; purposefully tortured, maimed, or killed another; combat experience; saw atrocities; witnessed death/dead body/gruesome injury
Interpersonal violence	Battered by caregiver; witnessed physical fights at home; assault by a non-caregiver
Intimate partner/ sexual violence	Rape; sexual assault; battered by spouse/partner; stalked; traumatic event to loved one; private event; other events
Accident/injuries	Child with serious illness; natural disaster; life-threatening illness; toxic chemical exposure; auto accident; other life-threatening accidents
Other traumas	Unexpected death of loved one; mugged or threatened with a weapon; man-made disaster

Exposure to a traumatic or stressful event is a necessary feature of all disorders described in this section, and a variety of experiences or events may be properly referred to as "traumatic" in the colloquial sense. However, DSM-5 has included specific conditions for this term as outlined in Criterion A. Experiences that fail to satisfy these conditions are, therefore, not considered "traumatic" as per DSM-5, which precludes a diagnosis of either acute stress disorder (ASD) or posttraumatic stress disorder (PTSD). This describes the types of trauma that do meet those conditions and that may warrant a diagnosis of either ASD or PTSD, provided the patient's symptoms meet additional diagnostic criteria

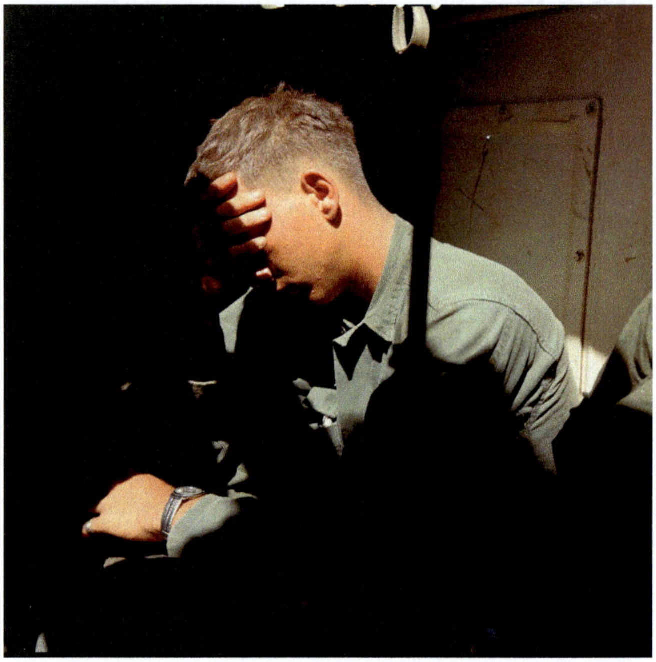

Fig. 19.1 PTSD has long been associated with veterans who see combat and the horrors of war. Image of 25th Infantry Division soldier resting inside an M113 armored personnel carrier during Operation Cedar Falls in January 1967. (*From the* National Archives [local identifier: 111-CCV-345-CC37978])

phenotypes in which avoidant, hypervigilant, dissociative, anhedonic, or even aggressive symptoms can also be more pronounced than others [1].

PTSD, CPTSD, ASD, AjD, and PGD are distinct disorders with their own symptom profiles, but all share some core symptom patterns to be elucidated below. Diagnostic criteria within DSM-5, for example, describe AjD as distinct from ASD and PTSD because the stressor fails to meet the definition of Criterion A (see Table 19.3) for both ASD and PTSD and/or because symptom severity does not meet additional criteria for either ASD or PTSD (see Figs. 19.2 and 19.3) [3]. A more abstract visualization of how these disorders are related can be found in Figs. 19.4 and 19.5. RAD and DSED, meanwhile, share a diagnostic requirement and etiology (childhood neglect), but symptom manifestations are vastly dissimilar [4].

Table 19.3 Evolution of posttraumatic stress disorder from DSM-III through DSM-5

	DSM-III	DSM-III-R	DSM-IV and DSM-IV-TR	DSM-5
Experience of traumatic event/ Criterion A	A recognizable stressor that would evoke significant symptoms of distress in almost everyone	An event transcending typical human experience that is experienced with intense fear or helplessness and would be distressing to almost anyone	• A1: a traumatic event that involves: – Threat of death – Death of others – Serious injury – Threat to "physical integrity" • A2: intense fear, horror, or sense of helplessness	A traumatic event that involves threat of death or death of others, serious injury, or sexual assault
Examples of traumatic experiences	• **Natural disaster**: tsunami, earthquake, mudslide • **Accidental incident**: serious car accident, airplane crash, destructive fire • **Deliberate incident**: terrorist attack, rape, assault, military combat	• **Natural disaster**: tsunami, earthquake, mudslide • **Accidental incident**: serious car accident, airplane crash, destructive fire • **Deliberate incident**: terrorist attack, rape, assault, military combat	• **Direct experience**: military combat, physical assault, accident, sexual assault, natural or man-made disaster, kidnapping, terrorist attack, incarceration as prisoner of war or in concentration camp, diagnosis of life-threatening illness • **Witnessed**: war, disaster, violent assault, accident, unexpected viewing of dead body or body parts • **Indirect experience**: learning that one's child has a life-threatening disease and that a close friend or relative experienced sudden or violent death or suffered a serious injury from assault or accident	• **A1: direct experience**—military combat, physical assault, accident, sexual assault, natural disaster, kidnapping, terrorist attack, incarceration as prisoner of war or in concentration camp, catastrophic medical event • **A2: witnessed**—unnatural death, serious injury, physical or sexual assault, catastrophic medical event • **A3: indirect experience**—learning that a close friend or relative has committed suicide or been involved in either a serious accident or an assault and has suffered severe injuries or unnatural death • **A4: repeated exposure to consequences of traumatic events**—police officers documenting details of child abuse; first responders arriving on scenes of carnage
Experiences that do not qualify as traumatic events	Simple bereavement, business failure, chronic illness, marital problems	Simple bereavement, business failure, chronic illness, marital problems		A4 precludes exposure via media unless the exposure is work related
Exposure criteria		• **Direct exposure**: threat to life or "physical integrity" • **Witnessing**: seeing another maimed, injured, or killed via natural disaster, accident, or violence • **Indirect exposure**: learning of an incident to one's child, spouse, or close friend/relative • **Property destruction**: abrupt obliteration of home or community	Experienced, witnessed, or "was confronted" with trauma. Includes trauma to self or to others • **Direct exposure**: lived personal experience • **Witnessing**: seeing another maimed, injured, or killed • **Indirect exposure**: learning of a traumatic incident to a family member or close friend	Same as above: • A1: direct exposure • A2: witnessed • A3: indirect exposure via others (restricted to close friends and family) • A4: repeated/extreme exposure to gruesome details
Number of potential symptoms	12	17	17	20

(continued)

Table 19.3 (continued)

	DSM-III	DSM-III-R	DSM-IV and DSM-IV-TR	DSM-5
Number of groupings in diagnostic criteria	3: B, C, D	3: B, C, D	3: B, C, D	4: B, C, D, E
Criterion B	**Re-experiencing** (at least one of the following): • Intrusive recollections of event • Dreams of event • Feeling that event is reoccurring (flashbacks)	**Re-experiencing** (at least one of the following): • Intrusive recollections of event[a] • Dreams of event • Feeling that event is reoccurring (flashbacks) • Intensification of symptoms from reminders, including anniversaries	**Re-experiencing** (at least one of the following): • Intrusive recollections of event[a] • Dreams of event[b] • Feeling that event is reoccurring (flashbacks)[c] • Intensification of symptoms from reminders, including anniversaries, from internal or external cues pertaining to event • Physiologic symptoms from internal or external cues	**Re-experiencing** (at least one of the following): • Intrusive and involuntary recollections of event[a] • Upsetting dreams related to event[b] • Dissociative reactions in which the patient feels the event is reoccurring (flashbacks)[c] • Intense and protracted psychological distress from internal or external cues pertaining to event • Physiologic symptoms from internal or external cues
Criterion C	**Numbing** (at least one of the following): • Diminished interest • Sense of estrangement from others • Constricted affect	**Avoidance/numbing** (at least three of the following): • Diminished interest[a] • Sense of estrangement from others • Constricted affect • Avoidance of phenomena/activities associated with event • Avoidance of thoughts or feelings associated with event • "Psychogenic amnesia" pertaining to the event in part or in its entirety • Despair about future opportunities [a]Symptoms may manifest as development backslides in some young children	**Avoidance/numbing** (at least three of the following): • Diminished interest or participation in significant activities[d] • Sense of estrangement from others • Constricted affect • Avoidance of activities, places, and people associated with event • Avoidance of thoughts, feelings, or conversations associated with event • Amnesia pertaining to the event in part or in its entirety • Despair about future opportunities	**Avoidance** (at least one of the following): • Avoidance of activities, places, and people associated with event • Avoidance of thoughts, feelings, or conversations associated with event
Criterion D	**Arousal/avoidance** (at least two of the following): • Avoidance of phenomena/activities associated with event • Intensification of symptoms from reminders • Exacerbated startle response • Sleep disturbance • Memory impairment/ difficulty concentrating • Survival guilt	**Hyperarousal** (at least two of the following): • Physiologic symptoms from reminders • Exacerbated startle response • Sleep disturbance • Difficulty concentrating • Irritability • Hypervigilance	**Hyperarousal** (at least two of the following): • Exacerbated startle response • Sleep disturbance • Difficulty concentrating • Irritability • Hypervigilance	**Negative mood or cognition** (at least two of the following): • Dissociative amnesia pertaining to the event in part or in its entirety • Distorted perception leading patient to blame self/others for cause or consequences of the event • Diminished interest or participation in significant activities[d] • Negative beliefs about self, others, or world • Persistent negative emotions • Inability to feel positive emotions • Sense of estrangement from others

Table 19.3 (continued)

	DSM-III	DSM-III-R	DSM-IV and DSM-IV-TR	DSM-5
Criterion E				**Hyperarousal** (at least two of the following): • Exacerbated startle response • Sleep disturbance • Difficulty concentrating • Irritability • Hypervigilance • Recklessness or overtly self-destructive behavior
Duration of symptoms (Criterion E prior to DSM-5; Criterion F in DSM-5)	Not specified	At least 1 month	More than 1 month	More than 1 month
Clinical impairment	Not specified	Not specified	Yes. Criterion F	Yes. Criterion G
Criteria for exclusion	N/A	N/A	N/A	Criterion H: symptoms cannot be attributable due to the effects of a substance or other medical condition
Broader category	Anxiety disorders	Anxiety disorders	Anxiety disorders	Trauma- and stressor-related disorders

The above follows the evolution of the diagnostic criteria of PTSD from its first appearance in DSM-III to its conception in DSM-5. The most notable change between DSM-IV and DSM-5 is the placement of PTSD under the newly created category of trauma- and stressor-related disorders instead of under the category of anxiety disorders [2]. Other notable changes include the removal of the intense sense of fear or helplessness condition in Criterion A; the inclusion of only work-related media depicting traumatic violence; and the reconfiguring of criteria to include a separate criterion (Criterion D) specifically pertaining to symptoms affecting mood, perception of self, and cognition. Additionally, DSM-5 notes in Criterion H that the "disturbance" cannot be attributable to another condition or the use of a substance such as alcohol. The causal language between stressor event and symptoms is removed from DSM-5, whereas it had been present in previous editions of DSM

[a]Symptoms may manifest as repetitive play related to event in some young children

[b]Children may experience frightening dreams without recognizing an association with the event

[c]Trauma-specific reenactments may occur in young children

[d]Symptoms may manifest as development backslides in some young children

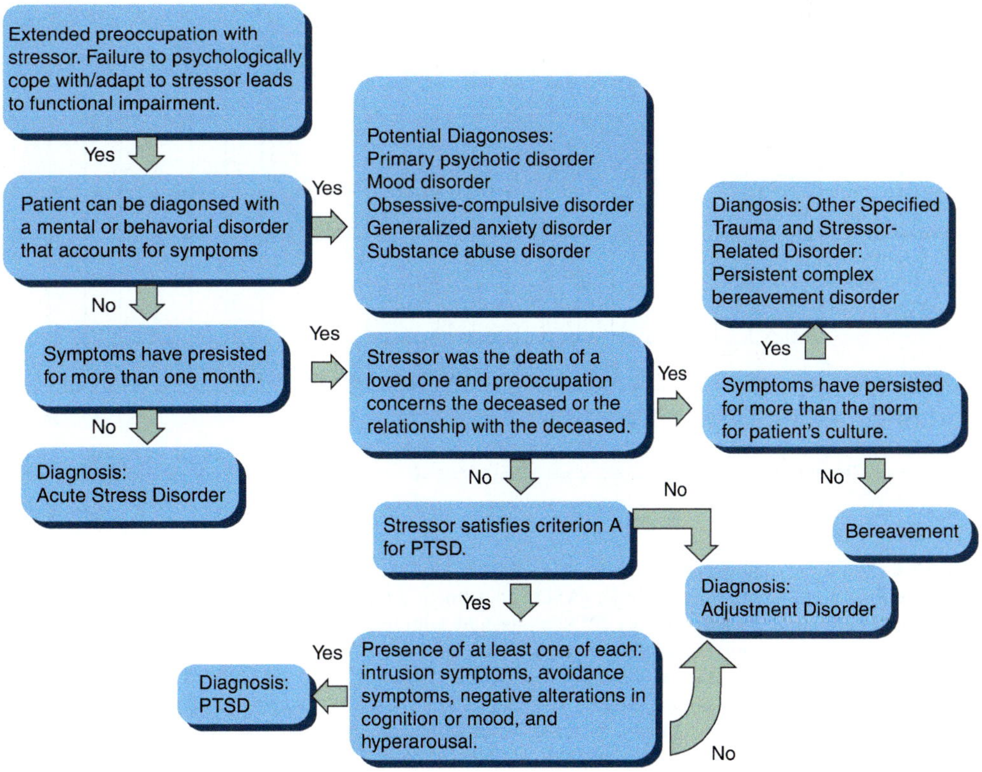

Fig. 19.2 This flow diagram traces how clinicians can distinguish between trauma- and stressor- related disorders given different symptoms via the diagnostic system within the DSM-5

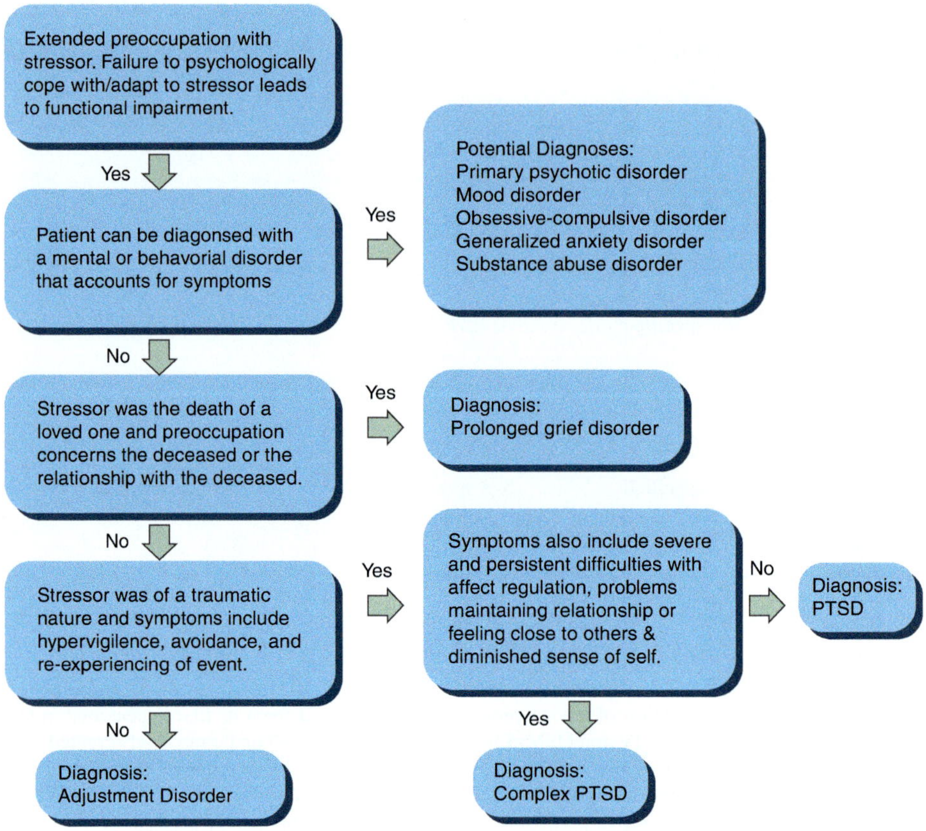

Fig. 19.3 This flow diagram uses the diagnostic system within ICD-11 to arrive at similar but slightly different conclusions. Note that acute stress disorder does not appear in the diagram because ICD-11 views the symptoms associated with acute stress disorder as described in DSM-5 to be normative responses to stressful events. Meanwhile, complex PTSD (CPTSD) is included. Another key distinction is that ICD-11 is less focused on strict criteria or time frames than DSM-5, though some rough approximations are provided. Specifically, ICD-11 does note that adjustment disorder symptoms typically arise within a month of the appearance of the stressor; that a grief response should persist for at least 6 months to qualify as prolonged grief disorder; and that a diagnosis of PTSD is appropriate only if symptoms persist for a bare minimum of several weeks. ICD-11 also notes that a diagnosis of PTSD and complex PTSD cannot be given simultaneously

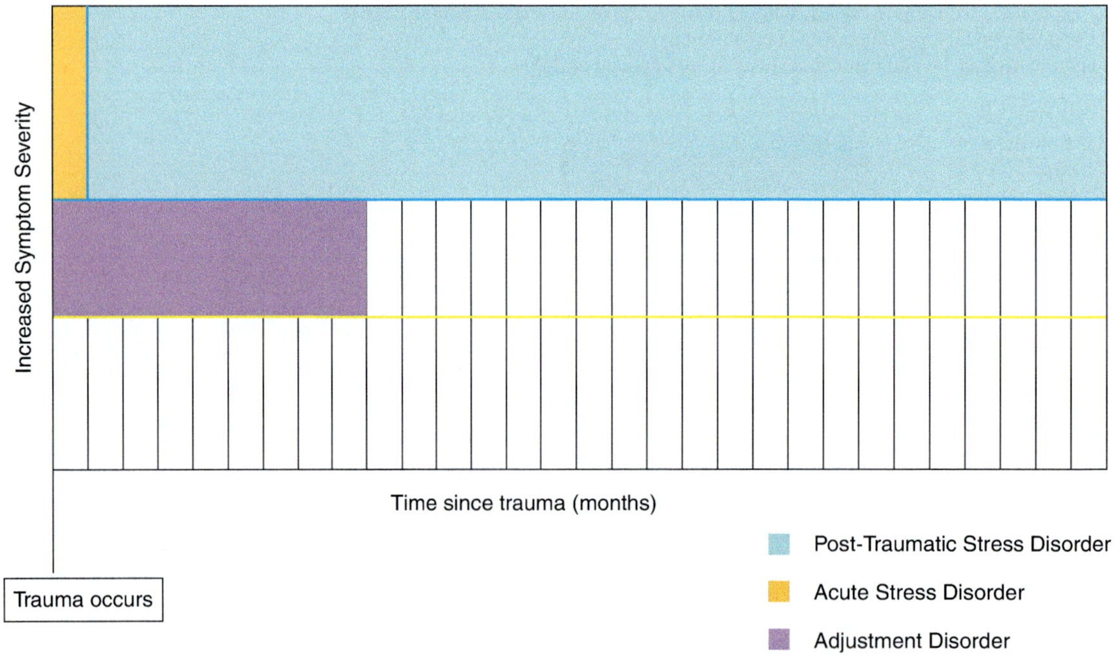

Fig. 19.4 The figure below is an imprecise visualization of the space that three disorders—acute stress disorder (ASD), adjustment disorder (AjD), and posttraumatic stress disorder (PTSD)—occupy with respect to symptomology following a traumatic event that meets Criterion A in DSM-5. A greater value on the x axis indicates more time (in months) have passed since the traumatic experience. A greater value on the y axis indicates more severe symptoms. A lower value indicates less severe symptoms. A y value below the blue line indicates a constellation of symptoms that would not be severe enough to meet Criteria B, C, D, and E for PTSD or any of the categories within Criterion B for ASD. A y value below the yellow line indicates a constellation of symptoms that would not be severe enough to meet Criterion B for AjD. DSM-5 allows for symptoms to emerge within 3 months of the stressor (Criterion A) even if it places a 6-month limit on symptoms of AjD (Criterion E). Consequently, the diagram indicates that AjD symptoms may be discernible as many 9 months following the stressor event

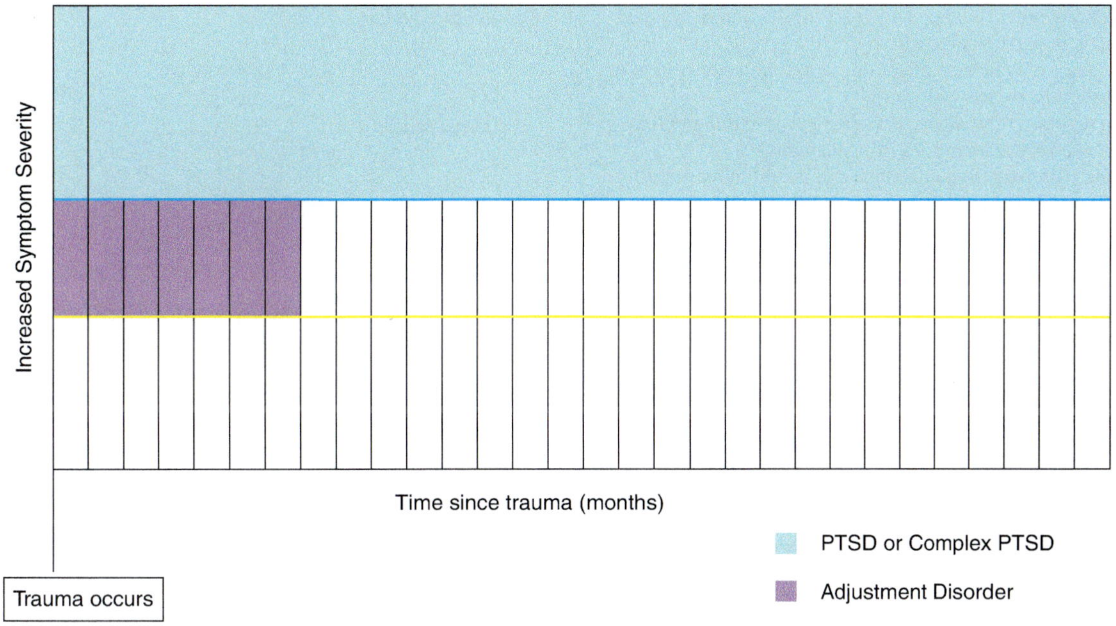

Fig. 19.5 The figure below is an imprecise visualization of the space that three disorders—adjustment disorder (AjD), posttraumatic stress disorder (PTSD), and complex PTSD (CPTSD)—occupy with respect to symptomology following a traumatic event according to ICD-11. A greater value on the x axis indicates more time (in months) have passed since the traumatic experience. A greater value on the y axis indicates more severe symptoms. A y value below the blue line indicates a symptom profile less severe than PTSD or CPTSD. A y value below the yellow line indicates distress levels that do not meet diagnostic requirements for any disorder recognized in ICD-11. Differences from Fig. 19.4: acute stress disorder is not included and CPTSD has been added. Though individuals diagnosed with CPTSD may have more severe symptoms than individuals with PTSD, the two are distinct because of the addition of symptoms associated with disturbances in self-organization to the three necessary symptoms of PTSD as noted in ICD-11 (see below). ICD-11 also proposes that symptoms of AjD usually emerge within 1 month of the stressor and typically resolve themselves within 6 months, meaning that AjD symptoms generally dissipate within 7 months following the stressor event

Trauma and Stress

Stress is a normal part of everyday life, especially when we use the term in a colloquial sense to describe the feeling of being overwhelmed by responsibilities or tense because of difficult situations. We may conceive of it as a figurative sense of pressure, but it does have clear neurophysiological correlates. Stress responses involve the limbic system (Figs. 19.6 and 19.7), the sympathetic nervous system, and (once the threat has passed) the parasympathetic nervous system (Fig. 19.8) [6].

Traumatic stress is distinct from everyday stress because it involves extreme situations (e.g., rape, threat of death, serious injury), and it can provoke severe responses that lead to functional impairment and disorders like the ones discussed in the remainder of this chapter. What constitutes a sufficiently traumatic event is not defined in ICD-11. In DSM-5, the definition of a "traumatic event" is far more clearly elucidated in Criterion A of PTSD and ASD (see below) [1]. The majority of those exposed to examples of trauma or stress that meet Criterion A experience a brief period of clinical distress and then quickly recover [7]. This type of resilience appears to be influenced by various pre-traumatic, peri-traumatic, and posttraumatic factors to be explored below. When these mitigating factors are wanting, there is a higher probability that a patient will develop one of these disorders.

Exposure to Trauma and Stressors

Exposure to trauma is unfortunately quite common, though rates of exposure vary widely between nations (see Table 19.1) and even within nations [8]. Likewise, different studies have found vastly different exposure rates to potentially traumatic events despite surveying similar populations. In the United States, for example, estimates of the average exposure rate have ranged from 40.8 to 82.7% [8, 9], while estimates that focus on severely disadvantaged communities, such as parts of Atlanta, GA, have been as high as 90% [10]. Figures 19.9 and 19.10 explore the prevalence of traumatic events by type worldwide [11].

Gender, age, race, ethnicity, sexual orientation, marital status, education level, and neighborhood of residence are just some of the predictors associated with different types of trauma, but making blanket statements about specific predictors and trauma as a uniform concept can be problematic due

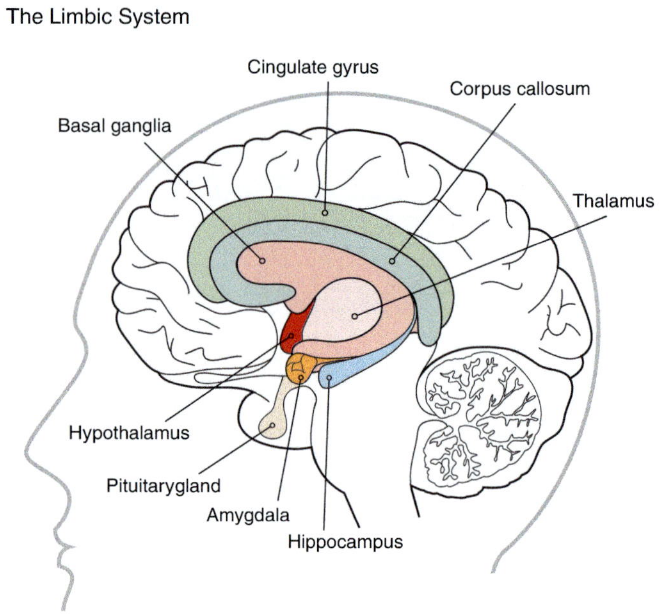

Fig. 19.6 Among other functions, the parts of the limbic system identified below are responsible for:

- Communicating with other parts of the central nervous system or beyond (thalamus, corpus callosum)
- Regulating emotion (amygdala, cingulate gyrus, basal ganglia)
- Forming new episodic memories (hippocampus)
- Make up the HPA axis (hypothalamus and the pituitary gland)

Of key importance is the amygdala, which is responsible for recognizing a threat to specific stimuli. Known as fear conditioning, the amygdala works in concert with the hippocampus to color the emotional content of memories and assign emotional valences to stimuli. Learning to separate the stress response/fear from conditioned stimuli is known as fear extinction. The medial prefrontal cortex, which includes the cingulate gyrus, subcallosal gyrus, and orbitofrontal cortex, attenuates the fear response that is mediated by the amygdala [26]. Research has shown a correlation between impaired fear extinction circuitry and trauma-related disorders, particularly PTSD [73]. Image courtesy of Tim Shaner

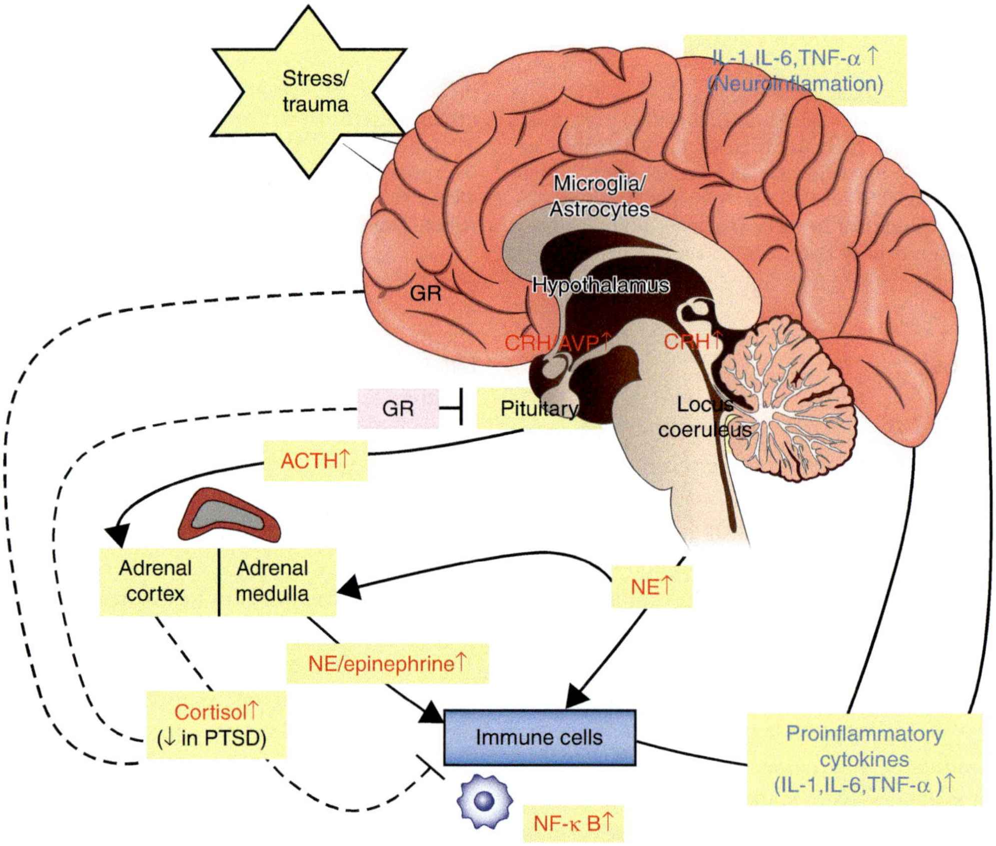

Fig. 19.7 Sensing stress, the amygdala signals the hypothalamus to jumpstart the so-called fight-or-flight response, which releases epinephrine and norephedrine (NE) into the bloodstream and activates the sympathetic nervous system (see Fig. 19.8). Epinephrine is excreted by the adrenal glands, while norephedrine (NE) is released from several nuclei within the brain, primarily the locus coeruleus. Additional excretion of corticotropin-releasing hormone (CRH) and arginine vasopressin (AVP) from the hypothalamus induces the pituitary gland to release adrenocorticotropic hormone (ACTH). ACTH then signals to the adrenal glands to produce cortisol. While glucocorticoid receptors (GR) throughout the limbic system regulate cortisol levels via a negative feedback function, cortisol can also interact with nuclear factor-κB in the peripheral immune system and lead to higher levels of proinflammatory cytokines (IL-1, IL-6, TNF). When in the CNS, these proinflammatory cytokines are associated with neuroinflammation due to overactivation of microglia and astrocytes and the production of additional proinflammatory cytokines. High levels of neuroinflammation re-stimulate HPA axis activity, thereby leading the cycle to begin anew. This should result in a surge in cortisol, but individuals with PTSD appear to not respond to increased ACTH with more cortisol, but with less. Some hypothesize that this cortisol deficiency is key to understanding the neurochemistry of PTSD. Such an abnormality would make it more difficult for the GR-regulated negative feedback mechanism to bring the limbic system back to stasis and mean hypocortisolism is a heritable risk factor for developing PTSD following exposure to trauma [5]

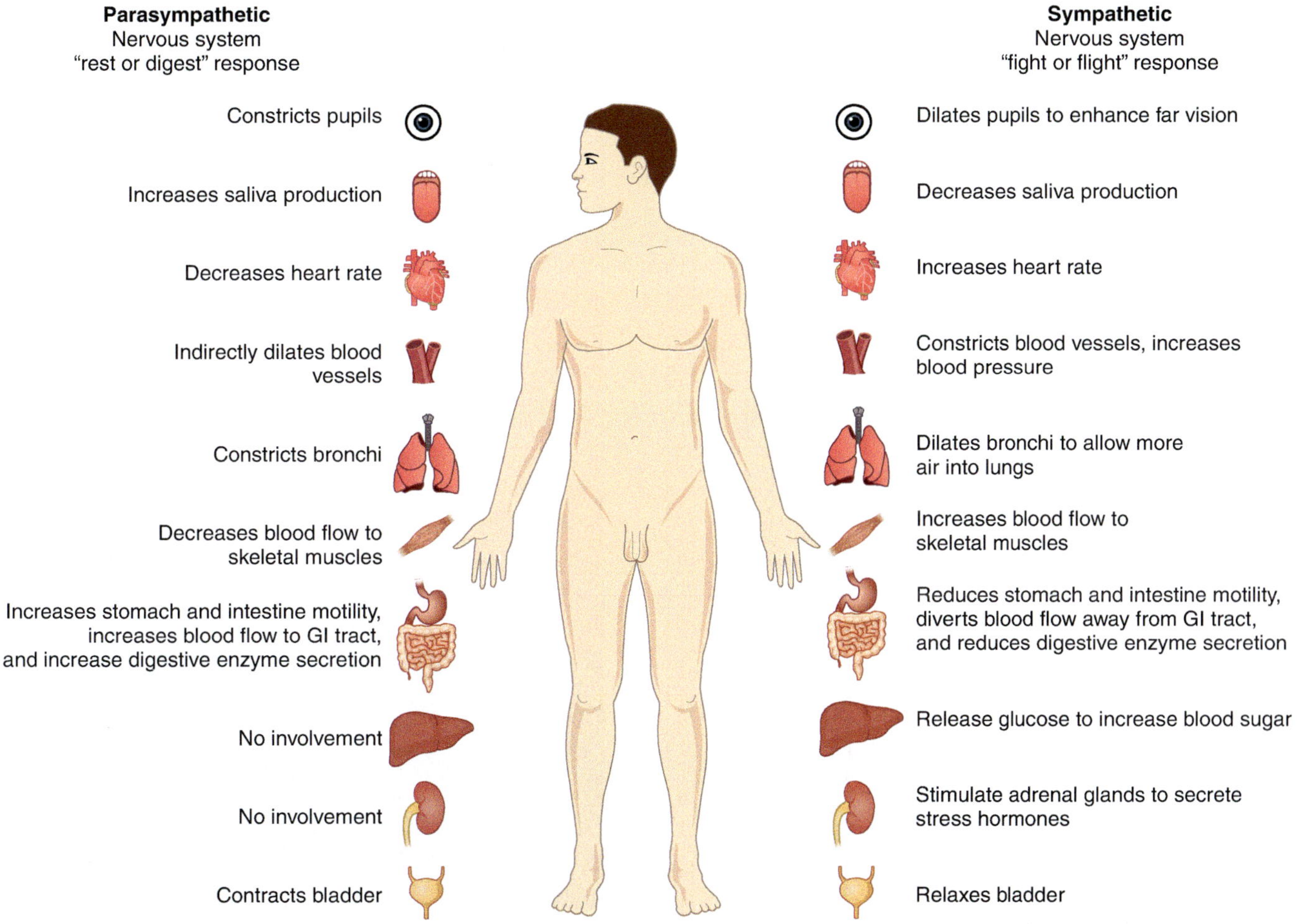

Fig. 19.8 The sympathetic nervous system and the parasympathetic nervous system. Activation of the sympathetic nervous system readies the body for action in the face of danger (fight or flight). The parasympathetic nervous system brings the body back into a state of ease once the threat has passed (rest and digest). The figure below describes specific parts of the body describes specific parts of the body and how they are affected by the two systems

to the high degree of variability among types of trauma [12]. For example, male gender is more commonly associated with traumatic experiences involving unintentional injuries and physical violence, while female gender is more commonly associated with traumatic experiences involving intimate partner violence [11]. Prior exposure to trauma, particularly during childhood, appears to be a strong predictor of future traumatic experiences [7]. Additionally, certain types of trauma are more strongly associated with the risk of ASD and PTSD, particularly assaultive violence [13].

Posttraumatic Stress Disorder

Of the disorders covered in this chapter, posttraumatic stress disorder (PTSD) has been studied the most, largely due to its debilitating nature and relatively high prevalence (3.9% worldwide) [8]. As noted above, as many as 82.7% of adults in the United States may experience trauma severe enough to potentially warrant a diagnosis of PTSD, but rate of incidence in the United States is estimated to be only 6.9% (see Table 19.1) [8]. Rate of incidence can also be influenced by the amount of time since the traumatic event, with one study finding incidence of PTSD at the 3-, 12-, and 24-month marks to be 8.5%, 9.5%, and 6.8%, respectively [14]. PTSD is also estimated to be 2.5 times higher among veterans than the general population in the United States [15].

PTSD is a condition that is characterized by hyperarousal, avoidant behavior, and the re-experiencing of previous traumatic events. DSM-5 acknowledges the additional symptom cluster of negative mood and cognition as a necessary feature, but ICD-11 does not.

History and Nosology

Even though there was no formal nomenclature for the condition until relatively recently, PTSD has been documented throughout history, particularly among soldiers [16]. The first attempt to classify the condition came in the 1688 dis-

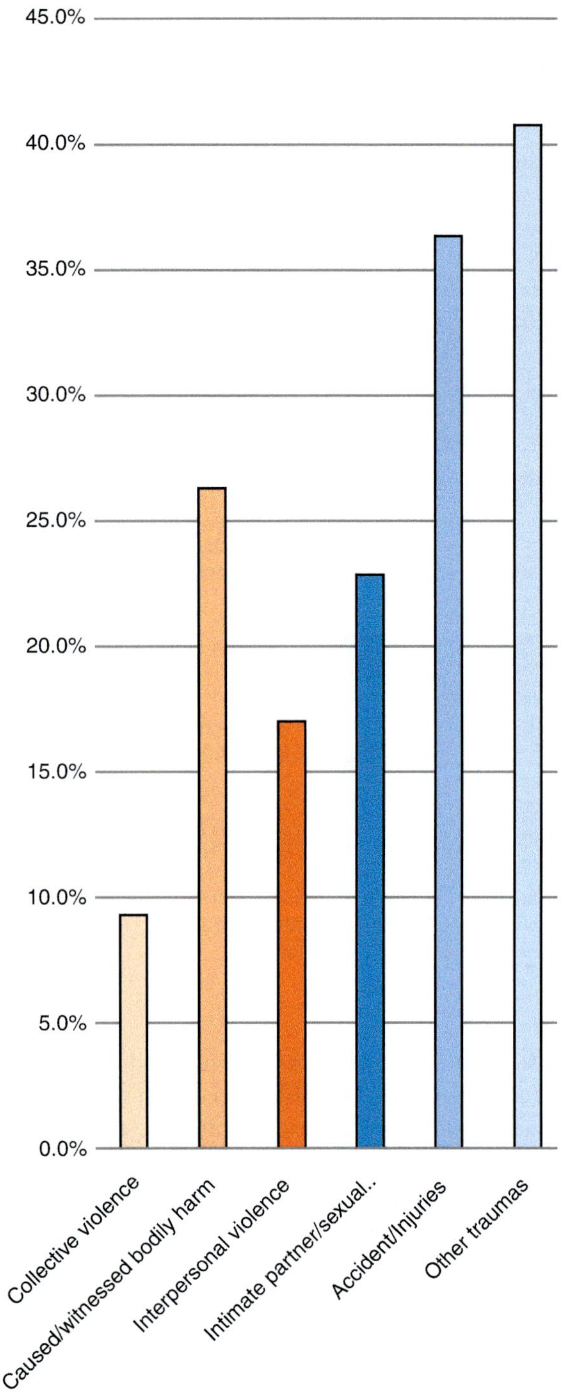

Specific Incident Type	Pct.	S.E.
Civilian in a war zone	5.0%	0.2
Refugee from a war zone	2.3%	0.1
Civilian in a terrorized region	3.9%	0.1
Relief worker in a war zone	1.1%	0.1
Kidnap victim	1.1%	0.1
Purposefully injured/tortured	1.0%	0.1
Combat experience	3.2%	0.1
Accidentally caused injury/death	1.4%	0.1
Saw atrocities	3.7%	0.1
Witnessed death/dead body/injury	23.7%	0.3
Battered by caregiver	7.9%	0.1
Witnessed physical fights at home	12.9%	0.2
Assault by a non-caregiver	5.9%	0.1
Rape	3.2%	0.1
Sexual assault	5.8%	0.1
Battered by spouse/partner	4.5%	0.1
Stalked	5.4%	0.1
Traumatic event to loved one	5.6%	0.1
Private event	4.9%	0.1
Other event	4.2%	0.1
Child with serious illness	7.9%	0.1
Natural disaster	7.7%	0.1
Life-threatening illness	11.8%	0.2
Toxic chemic exposure	4.2%	0.1
Auto accident	14.0%	0.2
Other life-threatening accident	6.2%	0.1
Unexpected death of loved one	31.4%	0.3
Mugged or threatened with a weapon	14.5%	0.2
Man-made disaster	4.0%	0.1

Fig. 19.9 Prevalence of traumatic event by type. Not all stressors are traumatic, though all traumatic events are stressful. A World Health Organization (WHO) survey identified 27 specific types of traumatic events that met Criterion A in DSM-IV, as well as 2 non-specific forms of traumatic events listed under the "intimate partner/sexual violence" trauma cluster as "other events" and "private event" (see Table 19.2) (Some of these traumatic events, such as being diagnosed with a debilitating or life-threatening disease, no longer satisfy Criterion A in DSM-5)

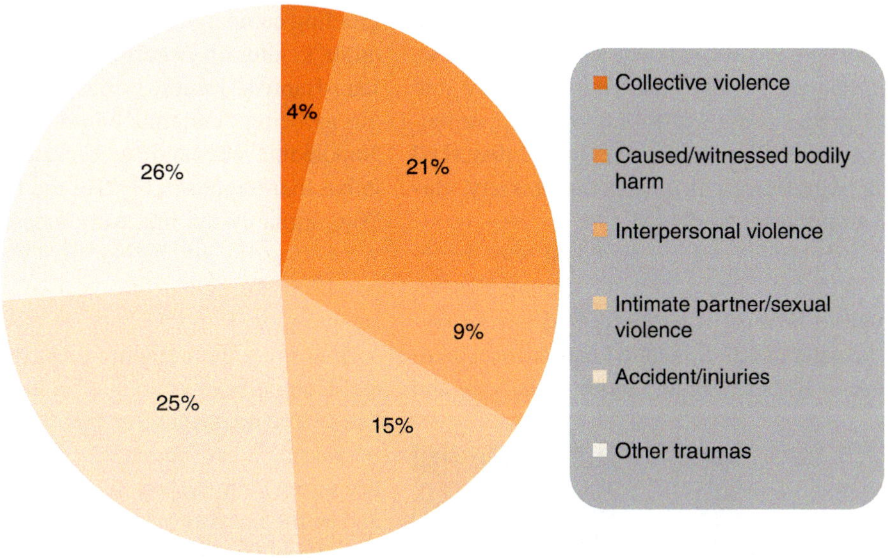

Incident Type	Pct.	S.E.
Incident Type	1.4%	0.0
Refugee from a war zone	0.7%	0.0
Civilian in a terrorized region	1.1%	0.0
Relief worker in a war zone	0.3%	0.0
Kidnap victim	0.4%	0.0
Purposefully injured/tortured	0.7%	0.0
Combat experience	1.0%	0.0
Accidentally caused injury/death	0.7%	0.0
Saw atrocities	2.4%	0.1
Witnessed death/dead body/injury	16.8%	0.2
Battered by caregiver	2.5%	0.0
Witnessed physical fights at home	2.5%	0.0
Assault by a non-caregiver	3.6%	0.1

Incident Type	Pct.	S.E.
Rape	1.8%	0.1
Sexual assault	3.6%	0.1
Battered by spouse/partner	1.4%	0.0
Stalked	3.0%	0.1
Traumatic event to loved one	2.7%	0.1
Private event	1.5%	0.0
Other event	1.3%	0.0
Child with serious illness	3.1%	0.1
Natural disaster	4.1%	0.1
Life-threatening illness	5.1%	0.1
Toxic chemic exposure	3.6%	0.1
Auto accident	6.1%	0.1
Other life-threateing accident	2.9%	0.1
Unexpected death of love one	16.5%	0.2
Mugged or threatened with a weapon	7.4%	0.1
Man-made disaster	2.1%	0.1

Fig. 19.10 Incident type as a percentage of all traumatic events. Not all stressors are traumatic, though all traumatic events are stressful. A World Health Organization (WHO) survey identified 27 specific types of traumatic events that met Criterion A in DSM-IV, as well as 2 non-specific forms of traumatic events listed under the "intimate partner/sexual violence" trauma cluster as "other events" and "private event" (see Table 19.2) (Some of these traumatic events, such as being diagnosed with a debilitating or life-threatening disease, no longer satisfy Criterion A in DSM-5)

sertation of French physician Johannes Hofer, who coined the neologism “nostalgia” (also known as homesickness, *Heimweh*, or *maladie du pays*) to describe a malady that seemed to affect the Swiss more often than others, particularly Swiss mercenaries. Symptoms included “disturbed sleep or insomnia, weakness, loss of appetite, anxiety, cardiac palpitations, stupor and fever” [17].

Over the next roughly 200 years, nostalgia was recognized as a condition that affected people throughout Europe, though it continued to be most widely reported among soldiers. As armies became more regimented and professionalized and the nature of warfare became more about long and grueling campaigns during the late seventeenth century, nostalgia’s rate of occurrence increased. Military physician Jean-Baptiste Joseph Tyrbas de Chamberet described nostalgia as being “endemic” among French soldiers during the Napoleonic Wars and “more frequent than scurvy and no less lethal than typhus” [17]. By the time of the American Civil War, arguably the first truly modern war, cases of nostalgia were occurring among Northern white troops at a rate of 2.34 per 1000 during the first year of the war and 3.3 during its second year (Fig. 19.11) [17].

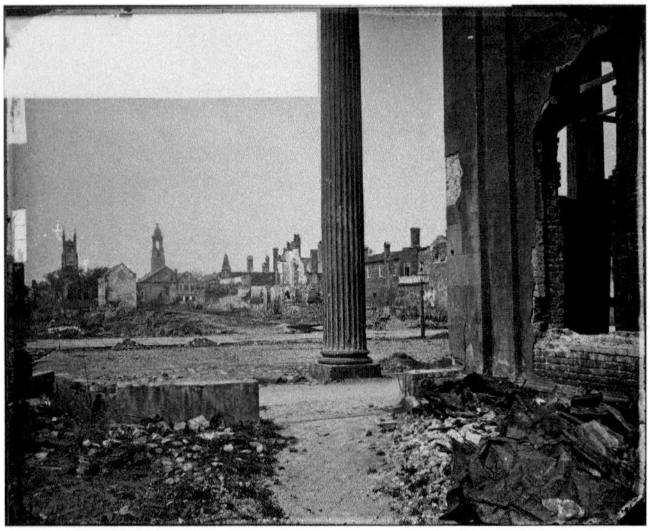

Fig. 19.11 The city of Charleston, SC, in ruins following fighting during the Civil War in the United States. As the scope of warfare became wider during the nineteenth century, this led to more destruction of civilian infrastructure and towns. (From the National Archives [local identifier: 111-B-4667])

Following the war, physicians throughout the United States and Europe began adopting nomenclature such as “soldier’s heart,” “neurasthenia,” or even “hysteria” to denote what was once known as “nostalgia.” Concomitantly, train travel was becoming far more popular throughout industrializing nations, and as the number of commuters rose, so too did the number of rail accidents (Fig. 19.12). Many of those involved in these accidents reported symptoms akin to soldier’s heart. These complaints became so common that the condition was named “railway spine” by British surgeon John Eric Erichsen in 1864 [18]. As industrialization spread and industrial accidents became more common beyond the railway or the battlefield, more physicians became acquainted with patients suffering from these conditions, and the medical community realized that the symptomology shared a common etiological source—i.e., “shock” or trauma—which resulted in the popularization of the term “traumatic neurosis.”

When the First World War broke out, physicians continued to describe patients coming from the frontlines as suffering from “fright neurosis,” “war neurosis,” or neurasthenia. Oftentimes, the symptoms of patients who had been injured due to the concussive force of an exploding shell were indistinguishable from those who had escaped bodily harm in the trenches. Such soldiers were said to suffer from “shell shock”

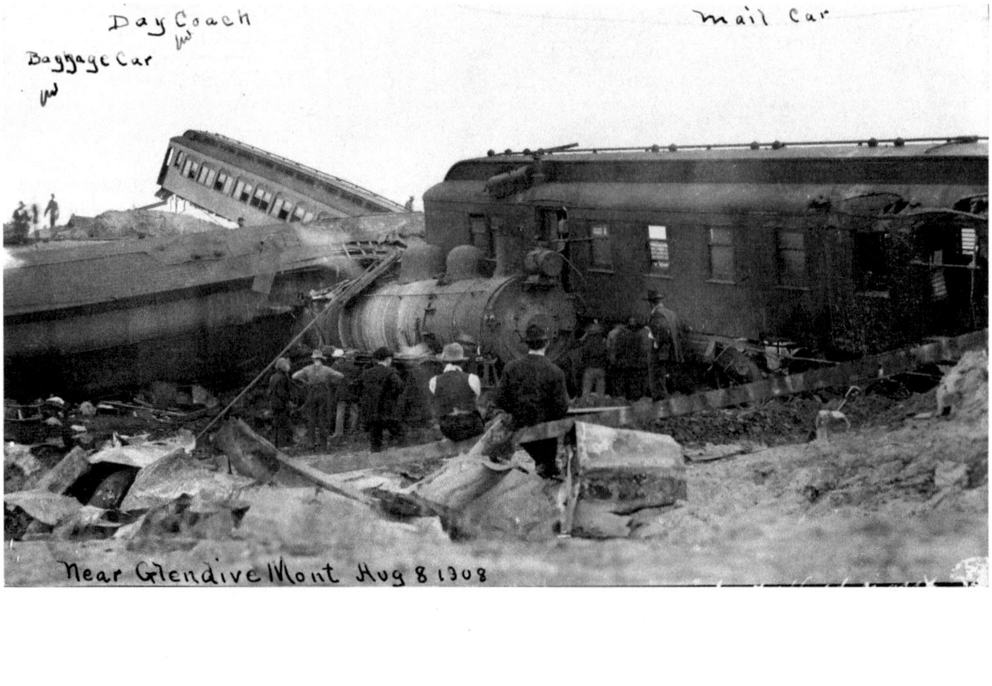

Fig. 19.12 As the nineteenth century progressed and technology produced bigger and faster machines, the violence of the accidents involving these machines became more cataclysmic. Passengers involved in large railway accidents oftentimes walked away unscathed physically but later reported PTSD-like symptoms that became known as “railway spine.” Image, entitled “Near Glendive, Mont.,” is courtesy of the Denver Public Library (call number: Z-5912)

[19]. Figures 19.13, 19.14, and 19.15 reveal some of the horrors of the Great War.

Both the terms "war neurosis" and "shell shock," as well as the broader "traumatic neurosis," would remain in use even after the publication of DSM-I in 1952, which described "Gross Stress Reaction" within the "Transient Situational Personality Disorders" section for patients who had experienced extreme stress either in combat or as civilians (especially Holocaust survivors), but failed to provide detailed criteria. DSM-II, which was released in 1968 at the height of the Vietnam War (see Fig. 19.16), replaced Gross Stress Reaction with "Adjustment Reaction of Adult Life"

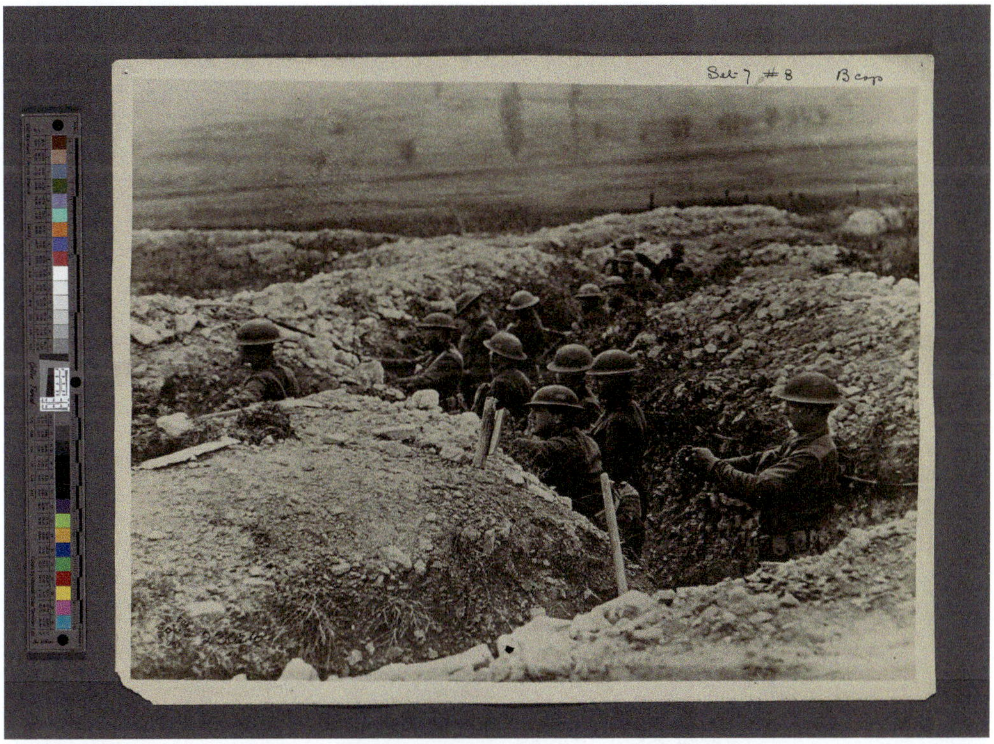

Fig. 19.13 World War I became infamous for its trench warfare. Soldiers were forced to withstand long periods of shelling, gassing, machine gun bursts, sniper fire, disease, infection, and the death of fellow soldiers while confined to narrow, subterranean passageways. Image, entitled "Troops in a trench," is from the New York Public Library's Digital Collection (image ID: 5111995)

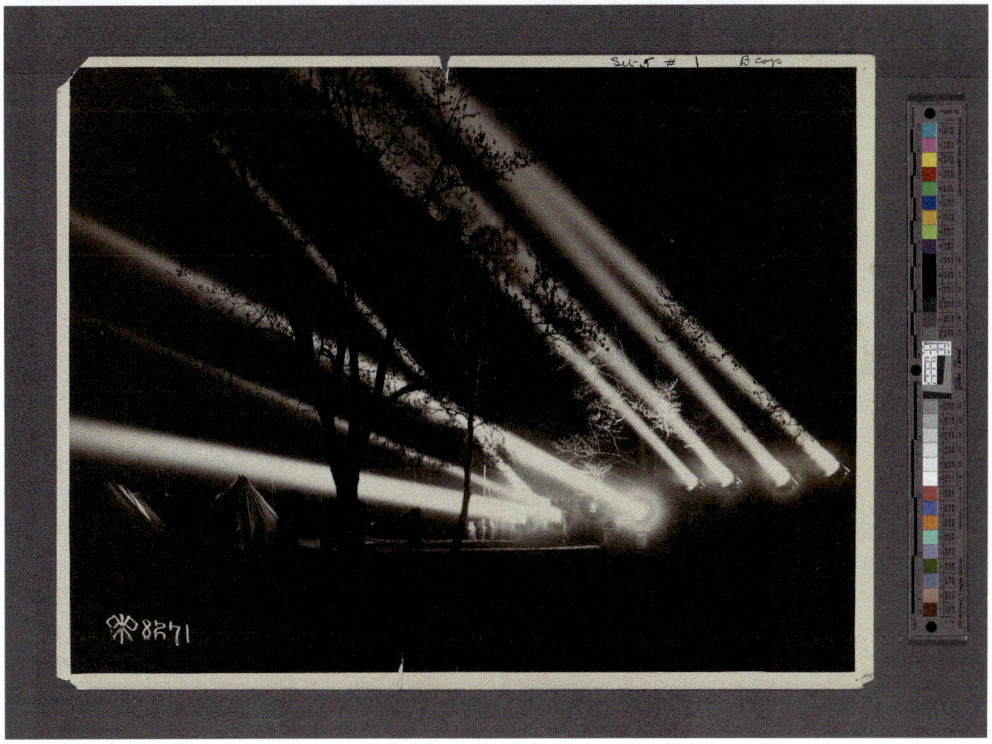

Fig. 19.14 During the Great War, modern technology allowed the fighting to become more all-encompassing than ever before. Air raids begat anti-aircraft searchlights, which only added to the relentless nature of the conflict [17]. Image, entitled "Mobile anti-aircraft searchlights," is from the New York Public Library's Digital Collection (Image ID: 5111981)

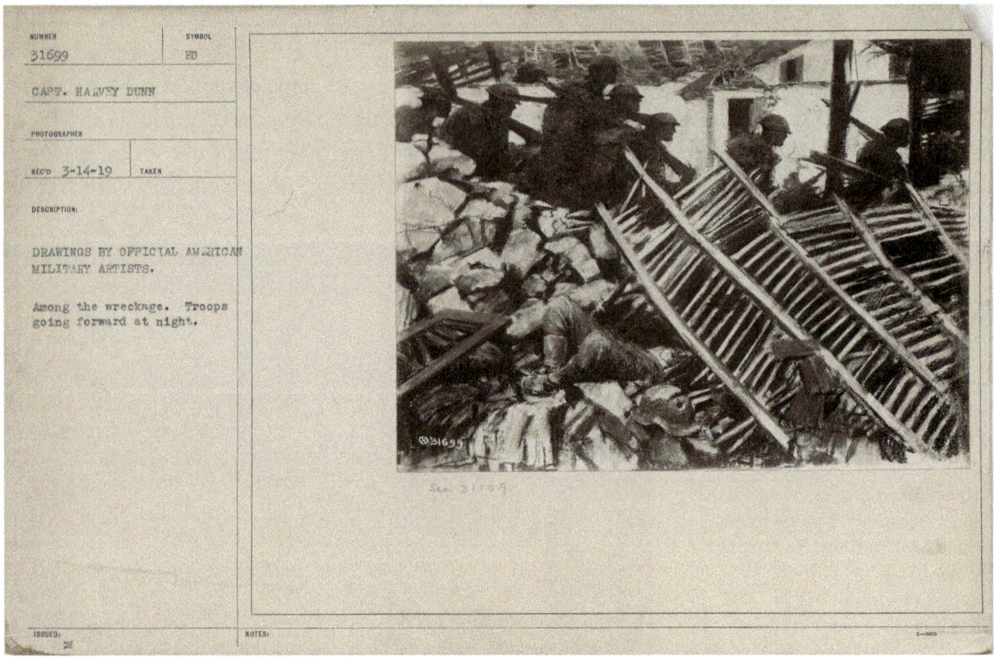

Fig. 19.15 A sketch by Capt. Harvey Dunn gives a terse description of the carnage of the war: "Among the wreckage. Troops going forward at night" (From the National Archives [local identifier: 111-SC-31699])

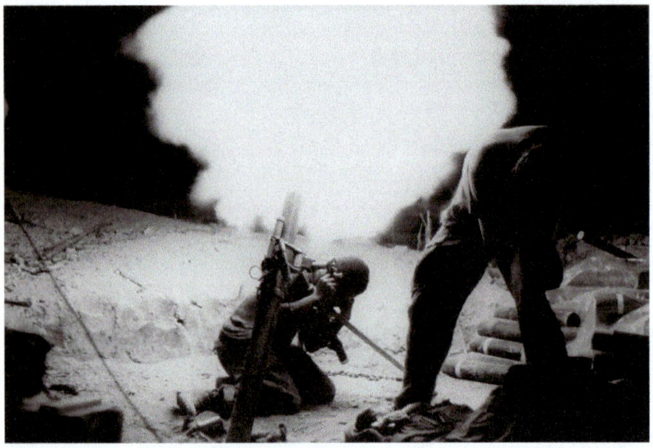

Fig. 19.16 2nd Medallion, 4th Marines firing 81 mm mortars in Quảng Trị province, 1969. (From the Jonathan F. Abel Collection (COLL/3611) at the Marine Corps History Division)

in the section "Transient Situational Disturbances" and once again failed to provide detailed diagnostic criteria for symptoms [20]. Many veterans' rights groups resented the decision. Concurrently, other social movements in the United States began to call attention to the extreme stress responses of civilians who had undergone physical or sexual assaults [21].

Prior to the 1970s, the trauma associated with sexual assault was seldom given proper recognition. For adults (typically women), the trauma was often downplayed. For adolescents and children, the traumatic episodes themselves were considered unrealized fantasies, while any dissociative symptoms related to such episodes were regarded as manifestations of guilt and shame about these repressed fantasies [21]. This response to accusations of molestation or assault was common among Freudian analysts well into the second half of the twentieth century, but Freud himself was not initially in favor of this analysis. As early as 1896, he suggested, instead, that virtually all neuroses could be traced back to childhood sexual trauma [22]. However, this notion, known as "seduction theory," was so toxic that Freud publicly disavowed it because of its truly horrific implications and instead developed some of his more well-known theories, such as the Oedipus complex [23]. More than 30 years later, the Hungarian psychoanalyst Sándor Ferenczi would propose something similar to Freud's seduction theory. Like Freud in 1896, Ferenczi's 1932 paper, *Confusion of the Tongues Between the Adults and the Child*, was met with outrage when he read it to the public [24]. Even American textbooks in 1980 claimed that the rate of incest among women was one in one million and, while rare, was not especially traumatizing [21].

Upon the publication of DSM-III in 1980, all patients who had experienced any form of trauma—soldiers, Holocaust survivors, victims of rape, and others—were pooled together under a single disorder: PTSD [21]. Since then, the conceptualization of PTSD as a disorder and its symptomology in DSM and ICD has evolved. The evolution in DSM can be found in Table 19.3 [20]. ICD has evolved in a similar manner. Like DSM-5, ICD-11 has categorized PTSD as a disorder specifically associated with stress rather than an anxiety disorder but does not include negative thoughts or mood (Criterion D in DSM-5) as a necessary feature of PTSD [25].

Validity

When introduced, PTSD was considered controversial, and it continues to receive criticism to this day. However, relatively few now question the validity of PTSD symptoms or consider it to be a psychosocial construct. There is general consensus that the core symptom clusters include re-experiencing, avoidance, and hyperarousal, but other criteriological disputes remain, particularly with relation to CPTSD [20].

In the past, there was criticism concerning the lack of biological evidence for PTSD, but this has been resolved due to advances in neuroimaging technology over the last 20 years, and there are clear neural correlates between PTSD and the amygdala, hippocampus, and medial prefrontal cortex, as well as other brain regions (Fig. 19.17) [26]. Several studies have found that small hippocampal volumes are associated with PTSD, but the directionality of this correlation remains unclear (Fig. 19.18) [26].

PTSD has also been validated by myriad cross-cultural studies [20, 27].

Risk Factors

Some risk factors associated with PTSD include previous trauma exposure, younger age at time of trauma exposure, female gender, lower socioeconomic status, lower level of education, and lack of social resources either via a strong family or community [27]. For survivors of disasters or catastrophic events, proximity to the epicenter may be another factor [27]. Genetics also plays a role in determining susceptibility to PTSD following trauma [28].

Another indicator that a patient may develop PTSD subsequent to a traumatic experience is a diagnosis of acute stress disorder (ASD). Half of those who develop ASD will go on to develop PTSD, though the converse is not true; a majority of individuals who are eventually diagnosed with PTSD did not meet full ASD criteria [13].

Comorbidities

Comorbid mental disorders such as major depressive disorder, anxiety disorders, and substance use disorders have been found to be 80% more common among individuals with PTSD compared to those without the disorder. Half of individuals with PTSD also meet criteria for depression, and approximately 40% meet criteria for substance use disorder [7]. Traumatic brain injury is also a common concurrent condition among veterans. DSM-5 reports that 48% of veterans of the recent wars in Afghanistan and Iraq who have been diagnosed with PTSD have mild TBI [1].

Risk for suicide attempts and suicidal ideation is estimated to be sixfold higher for individuals with PTSD relative to those without PTSD [7].

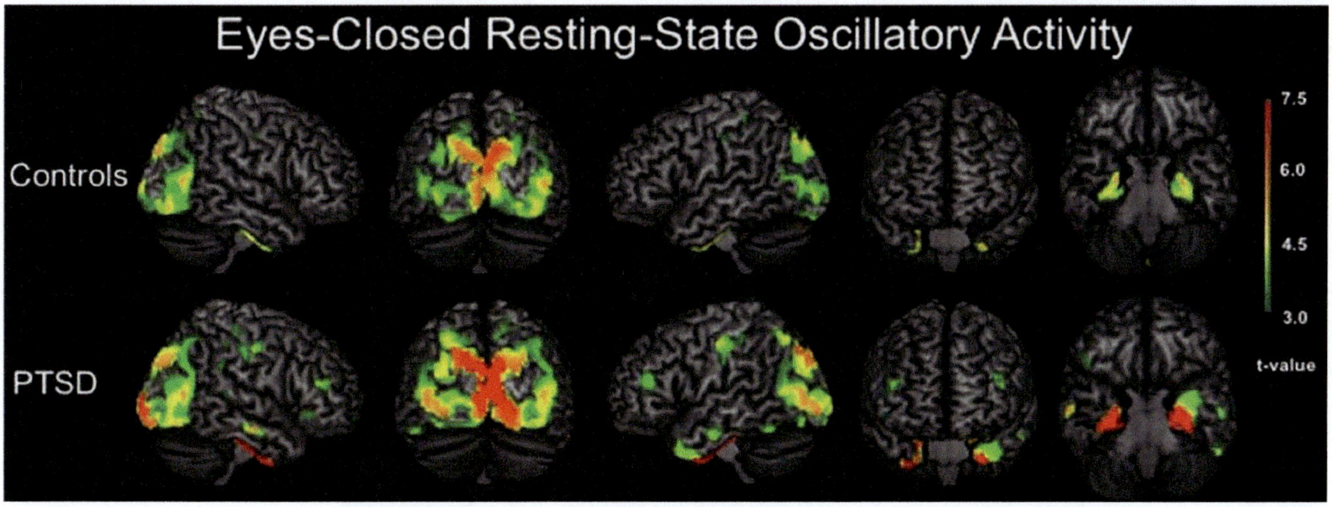

Fig. 19.17 Badura-Brack and colleagues used magnetoencephalography (MEG) to examine the brain activity of veterans diagnosed with PTSD and veterans who had not been diagnosed with PTSD in a resting state. As the figure below indicates, the PTSD group showed stronger activity relative to control in bilateral motor regions, lateral temporal areas, dorsolateral prefrontal cortices, hippocampi, and the amygdala. Respective t-values are indicated by a color scale bar to the right. (*From* Badura-Brack et al. [15]; Creative Commons Attribution License [CC BY 4.0]; https://creativecommons.org/licenses/by/4.0)

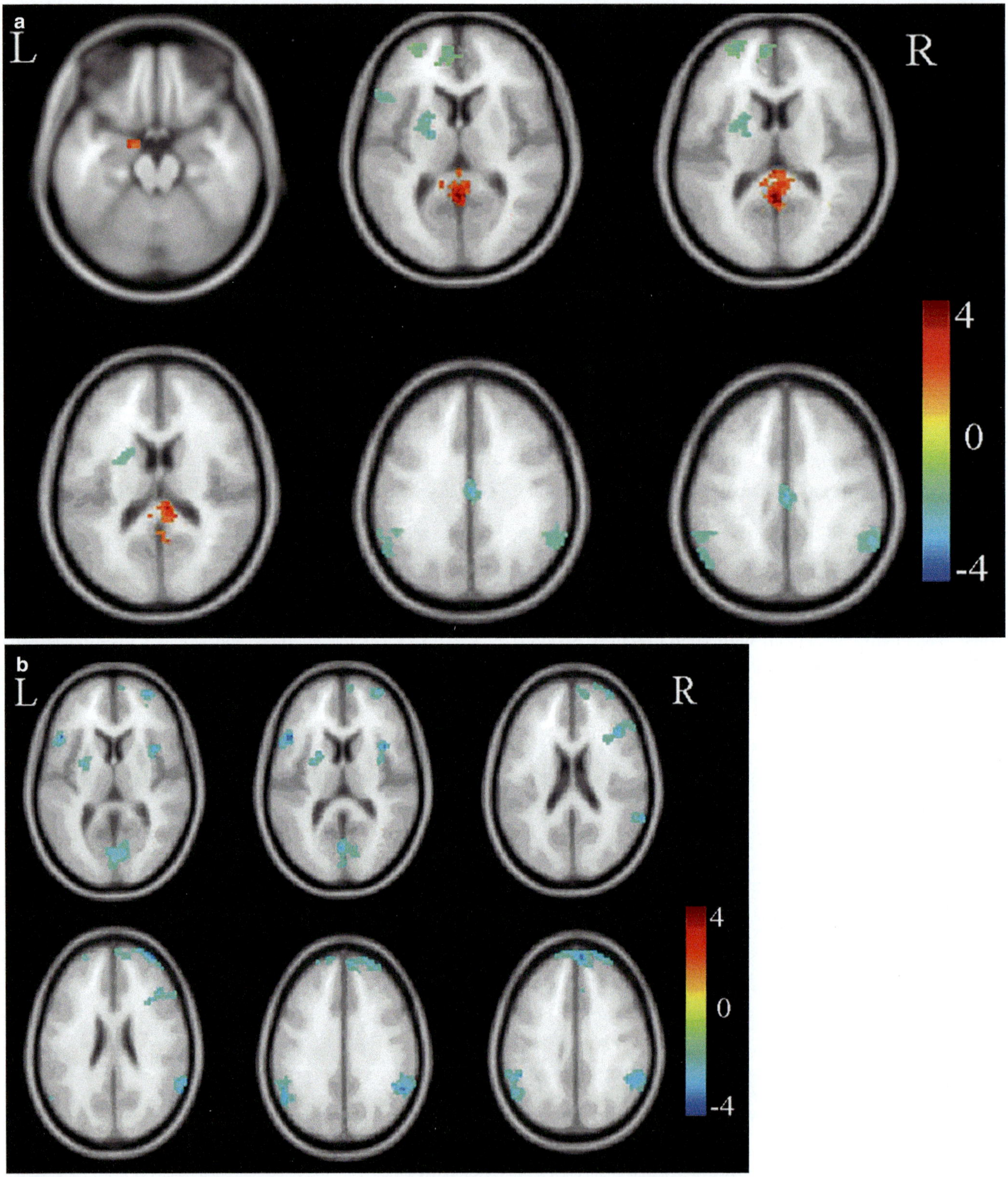

Fig. 19.18 Magnetic resonance imagining of the brains of two patients, one with PTSD (**a**) and one without PTSD (**b**). (**c**) Hippocampal volume is notably smaller in patient on the right. (*From* Bremner et al. [26]; *with permission*)

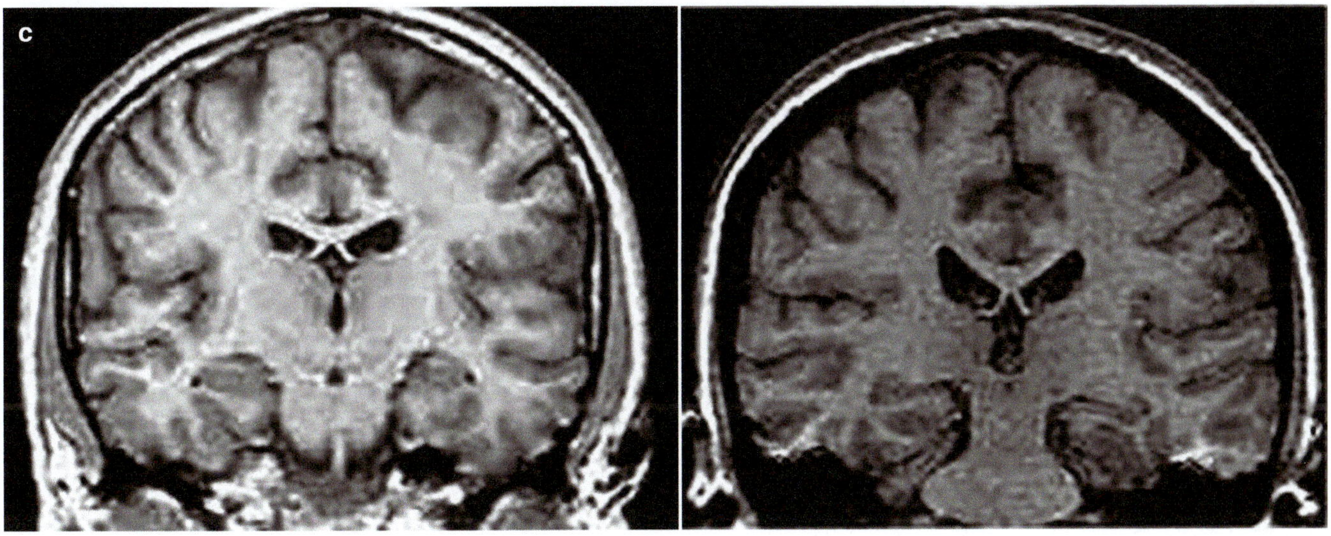

Fig. 19.18 (continued)

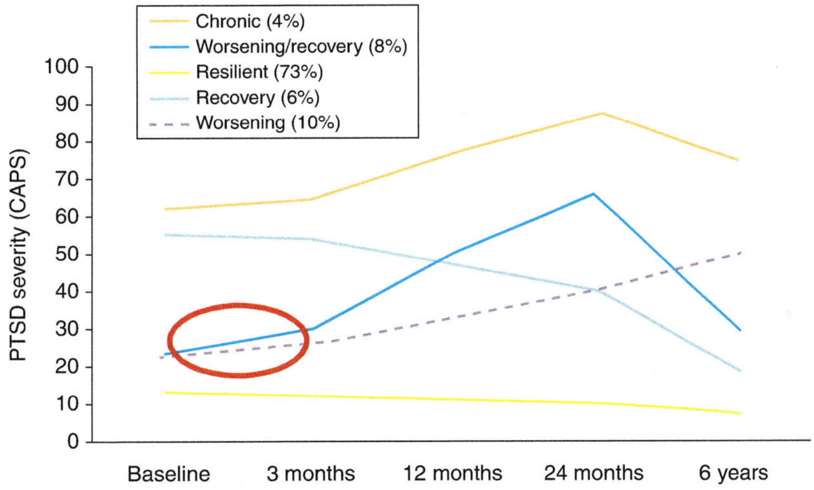

Fig. 19.19 A rough depiction of the data presented by Bryant and colleagues shows that patients tend to follow one of the five trajectories following traumatic injury [29]. The most common is resilient, which occurs when one remains relatively unaffected by the traumatic experience. A patient who follows the recovery trajectory is one who initially shows significant PTSD symptoms that fade with time. The chronic trajectory refers to patients whose severe PTSD symptoms persist for long periods of time. An individual with a delayed trajectory would show moderate symptoms in the months immediately following the experience. These symptoms would only later become more severe. Bryant et al. observed two forms of this trajectory: one where symptoms become far more severe after a delay of a few months and then remit (worsening/recovery) and one where symptoms gradually become worse without remitting (worsening)

Course

As Bryant and colleagues convincingly have argued, the course of PTSD follows one of the five trajectories, resilient, delayed, delayed/recovered, recovered, and chronic, as shown in Fig. 19.19 [29]. These trajectories can also be superimposed over the diagrams originally seen in Figs. 19.4 and 19.5. Frequency of occurrence for each course is far more difficult to discern due to the heterogeneous etiology of PTSD and a multitude of confounding factors influencing an individual patient's symptom trajectory. Research has indicated that delayed onset becomes less likely if patients remain asymptomatic for 12 months or more following the traumatic event [14], while estimates of how many individuals with PTSD develop chronic symptoms range from 17% to 33% and that those who have suffered traumatic interpersonal violence tend to experience symptoms for longer than those who have experienced other forms of traumatic events [2].

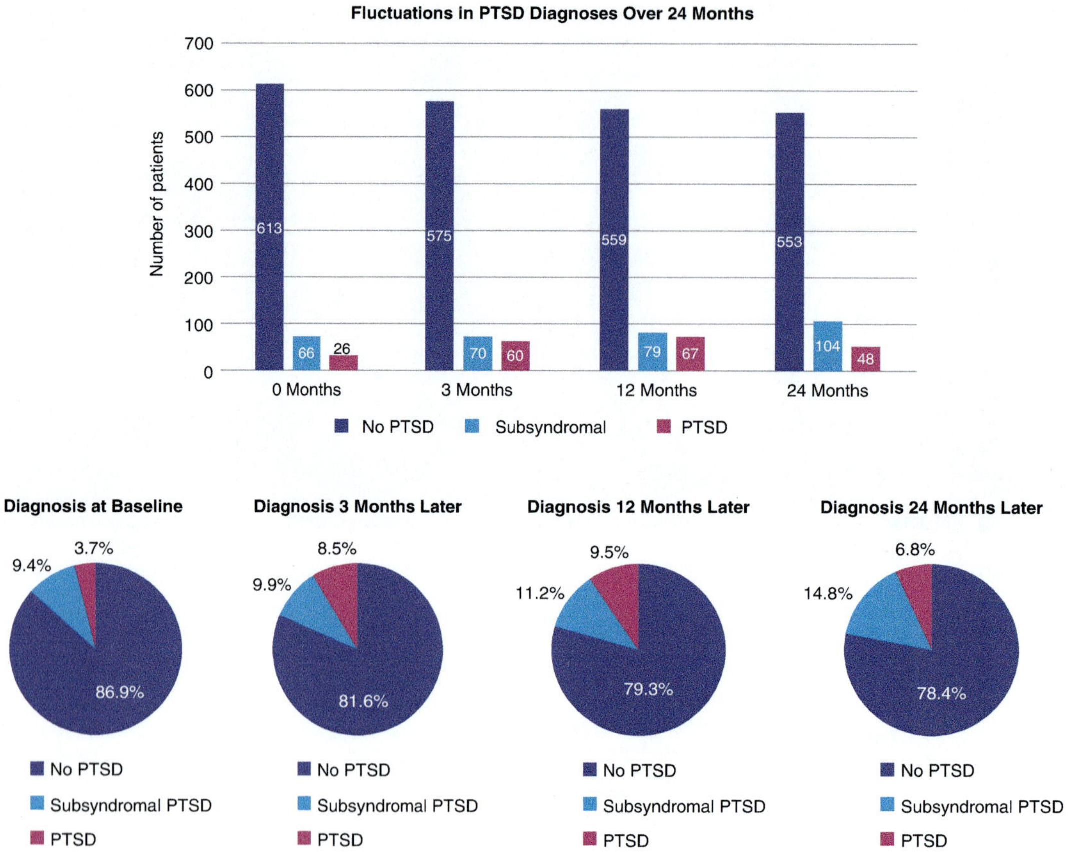

Fig. 19.20 These charts follow the fluctuations in symptoms among a group of 705 patients admitted to one of the four level I trauma centers in Australia between April 1, 2004, and February 28, 2006, who served as the subjects in Bryant and colleagues' 2013 paper [14]. PTSD was assessed using the Clinician-Administered PTSD Scale IV (CAPS). Pink indicates patients who met criteria for PTSD ("PTSD"). Blue indicates patients who did not meet full criteria for PTSD but met criteria for at least two symptom clusters ("subsyndromal PTSD"). Purple indicates patients who did not meet criteria for PTSD but may have met criteria for one symptom cluster ("no PTSD"). (*Top*) The number of individuals who fell into each of the three groups at baseline (0 months) and at 3 months, 12 months, and 24 months after injury. (*Lower*) The percentage of the 705 patients who fell into each of the three groups at baseline and then 3 months, 12 months, and 24 months after injury, respectively

Figures 19.19, 19.20, 19.21, 19.22, and 19.23 explore the data presented in a 2013 paper by Bryant and colleagues about the fluctuation of PTSD symptoms over time among individuals who had been admitted to hospital following a traumatic injury [14]. Of particular note is the greater frequency of patients following the delayed or delayed/recovered course. Most estimates tend to place the figure closer to 25%, but 37.3% of the patients who had PTSD at 12 months had not met criteria for PTSD at 3 months [14].

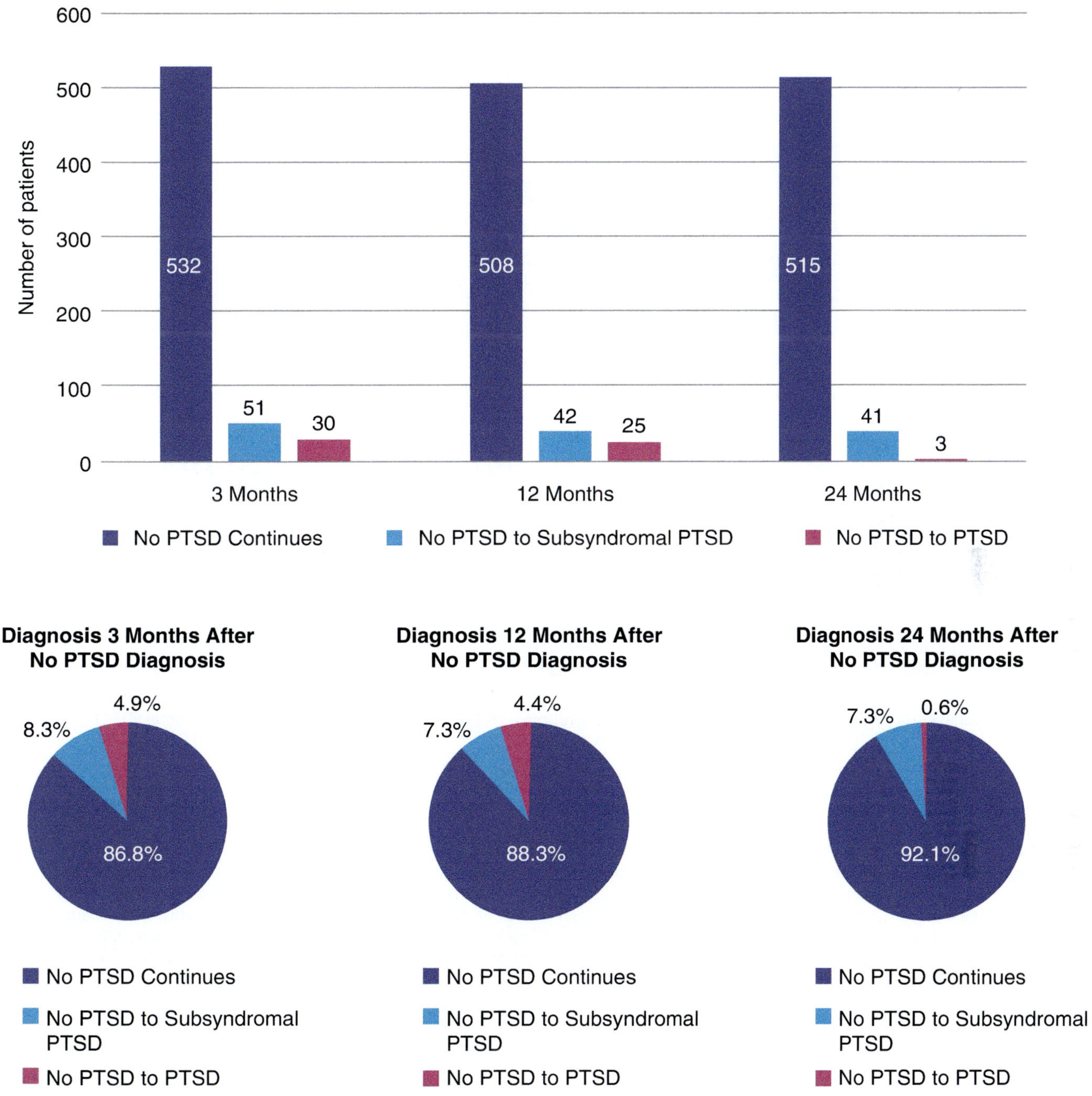

Fig. 19.21 These charts follow the fluctuations in symptoms among the patients from Bryant and colleagues' 2013 paper who presented no PTSD symptoms at baseline [14]. They were assessed 3 months, 12 months, and 24 months following injury. Blue indicates patients who met criteria for PTSD after showing no symptoms of PTSD at baseline ("no PTSD to PTSD"). Pink indicates patients who initially did not meet any criteria for PTSD, but who later met criteria for at least two symptom clusters, but not full PTSD ("no PTSD to subsyndromal PTSD"). Purple indicates patients who continued to not meet criteria for PTSD but may have met criteria for one symptom cluster ("no PTSD continues")
(*Top*) The number of individuals who fell into each of the three groups at 3 months, 12 months, and 24 months after injury. (*Bottom*) The percentages of the patients who fell into each of the three groups at 3 months (total = 613), 12 months (total = 575), and 24 months (total = 559) after injury, respectively

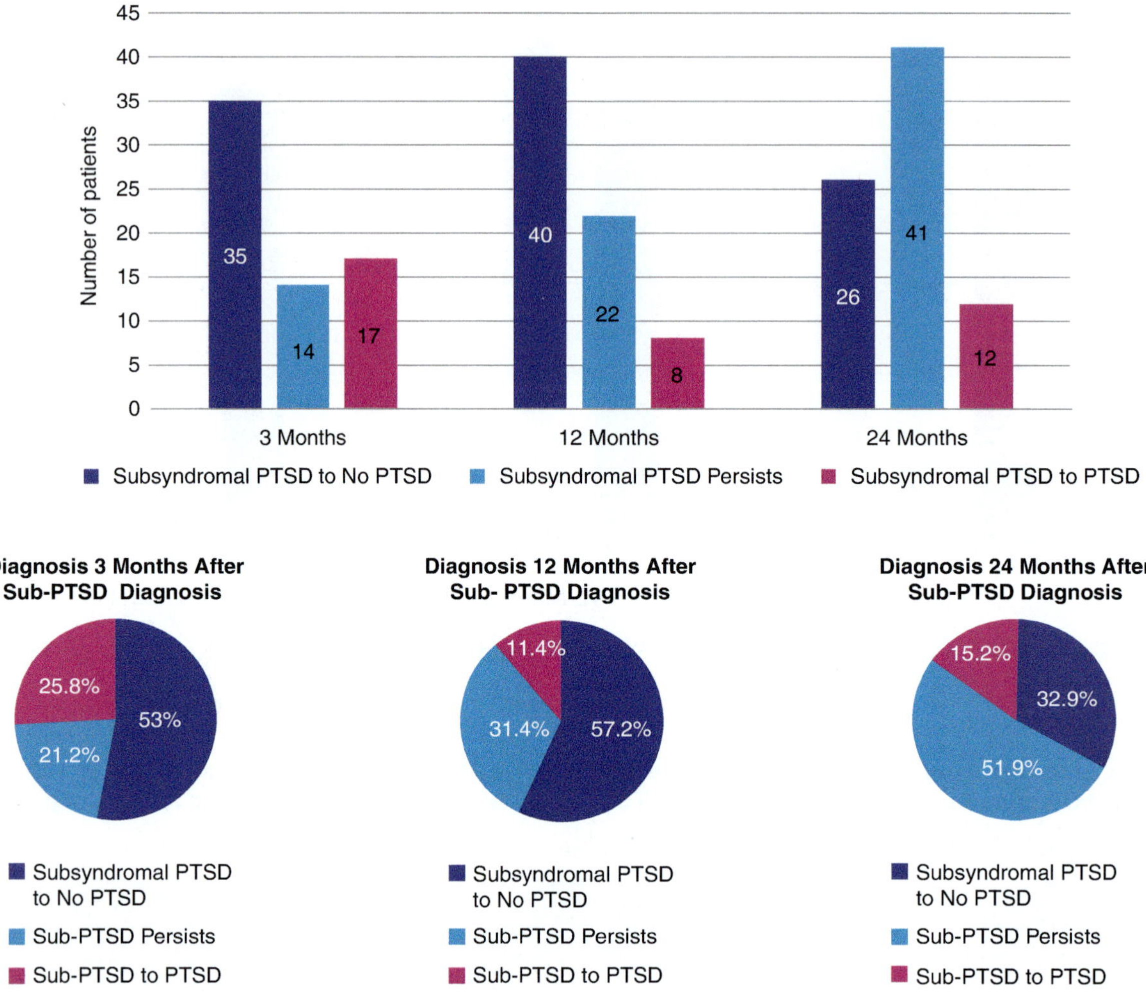

Fig. 19.22 These charts follow the fluctuations in symptoms among the patients from Bryant and colleagues' 2013 paper who did not meet full criteria for PTSD at baseline but did meet criteria for at least two symptom clusters. They were assessed 3 months, 12 months, and 24 months following injury. Blue indicates patients who did not initially meet criteria for PTSD at baseline, but later did ("subsyndromal PTSD to PTSD"). Purple indicates patients whose subsyndromal PTSD continued ("subsyndromal PTSD persists"). Pink indicates patients whose symptoms resolved between baseline and assessment ("subsyndromal PTSD to no PTSD"). (*Top*) The number of individuals who fell into each of the three groups at 3 months, 12 months, and 24 months after injury. (*Bottom*) The percentages of the patients who fell into each of the three groups at 3 months (total = 66), 12 months (total = 70), and 24 months (total = 79) after injury, respectively

Treatment

Worldwide, less than half of those who suffer from PTSD get any form of treatment (see Table 19.4), and only 16.8% of individuals in low-income countries see a healthcare professional of any kind [8]. Even in nations with robust healthcare programs, less than one third of individuals with PTSD ever see a psychiatrist or other specialist to receive treatment [8].

Despite an alarming number of individuals not seeking treatment, there are dozens of treatments that include early interventions, psychological interventions, pharmacological modalities, and more experimental treatment options (see Tables 19.5 and 19.6) [35]. Many of these treatments appear to also be effective at treating other trauma- and stressor-related disorders, and there is strong evidence to indicate that early intervention can attenuate the severity of or potentially even prevent the development of symptoms for many trauma- and stressor-related disorders, not just PTSD.

As for pharmacological treatments, selective serotonin reuptake inhibitors (SSRIs), such as sertraline (Zoloft) and paroxetine (Paxil), are considered first-line treatments due to their efficacy, tolerability, and safety ratings and

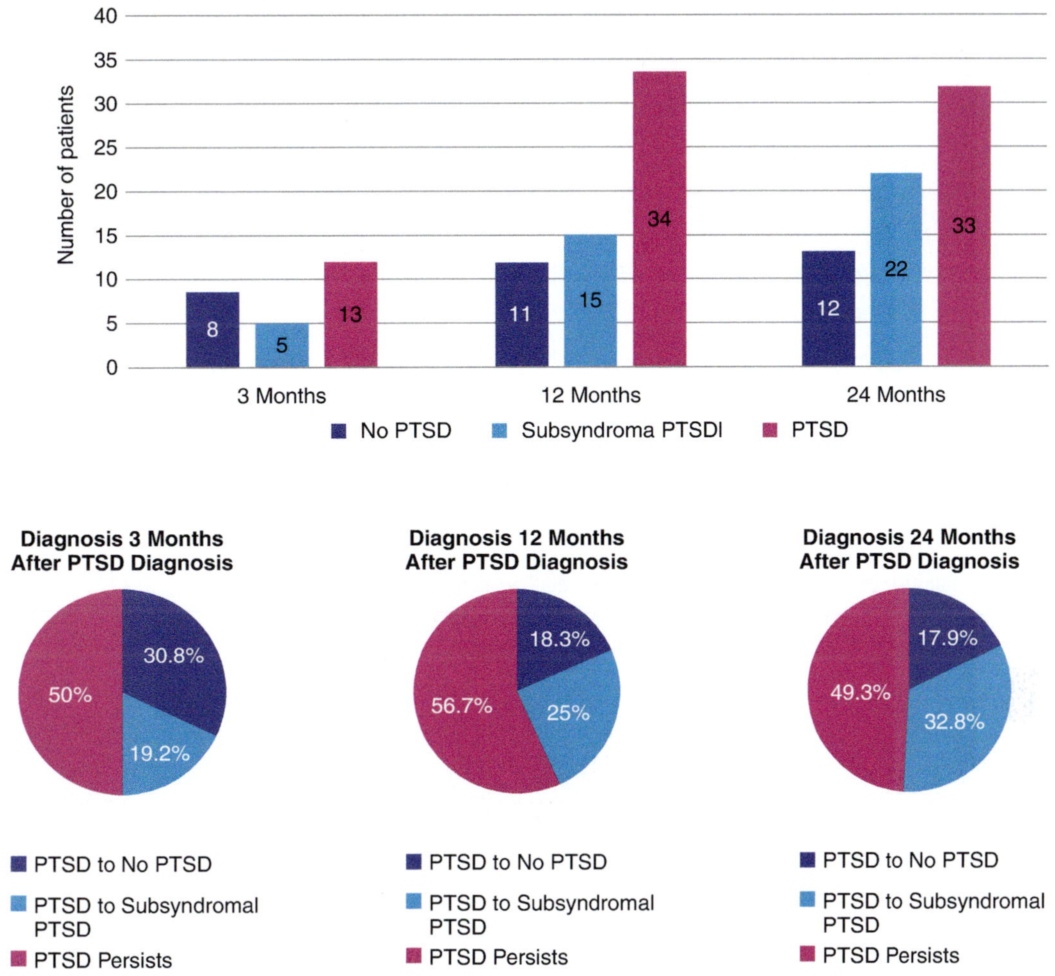

Fig. 19.23 These charts follow the fluctuations in symptoms among the patients from Bryant and colleagues' 2013 paper who met full criteria for PTSD at baseline [14]. They were assessed 3 months, 12 months, and 24 months following injury. Blue indicates patients who continued to meet criteria for PTSD at follow-up assessment ("PTSD persists"). Pink indicates patients whose symptoms improved to the point that they no longer met full criteria for PTSD but continued to meet criteria for at least two symptom clusters ("PTSD to subsyndromal PTSD"). Purple indicates patients whose symptoms resolved between baseline and assessment and no longer met at least two symptom clusters ("PTSD to no PTSD"). (*Top*) The number of individuals who fell into each of the three groups at 3 months, 12 months, and 24 months after injury. (*Bottom*) The percentages of the patients who fell into each of the three groups at 3 months (total = 26), 12 months (total = 60), and 24 months (total = 67) after injury, respectively

are effective in improving symptoms unique to PTSD, as well as PTSD symptom clusters. Buspirone (BuSpar), which also targets the serotonergic system, may also be of use [36].

A number of well-controlled clinical trials have found that the use of imipramine (Tofranil) and amitriptyline (Elavil), two tricyclic drugs, can be beneficial in the treatment of PTSD. Other drugs that may be useful include:

- Monoamine oxidase inhibitors (MAOIs) (e.g., phenelzine [Nardil])
- Trazodone (Desyrel)
- Anticonvulsants (e.g., carbamazepine [Tegretol], valproate [Depakene])
- Reversible monoamine oxidase inhibitors (RIMAs)

Clonidine (Catapres) and propranolol (Inderal), both antiadrenergic agents, may be effective at treating PTSD considering the theories about noradrenergic hyperactivity in the disorder [36]. One of the more novel treatments that has gained a great deal of media attention is the use of 3,4-methylenedioxymethamphetamine (MDMA) in conjunction with more conventional psychotherapy [37]. It appears to be effective, but remains controversial because of MDMA's status as an illicit drug.

Table 19.4 Percentages of individuals with PTSD who receive treatment and treatment from

Region	Mental health specialist	General practitioner	Any healthcare professional	Alternative healer	Religious or non-medical counselor	Alternative healer or non-medical counselor	Any treatment
High-income nations	28.7% (1.6)	36.0% (1.7)	36.0% (1.8)	9.9% (1.0)	7.0% (0.9)	14.7% (1.2)	53.5% (1.8)
Middle-income nations	11.8% (2.7)	16.8% (3.9)	24.6% (4.3)	4.2% (2.1)	2.5% (1.2)	6.6% (2.4)	28.7% (4.6)
Lower-income nations	3.2% (1.9)	14.5% (4.5)	16.8% (4.6)	N/A	7.1% (2.2)	7.6% (2.2)	22.8% (5.5)
Total	25.3% (1.3)	32.4% (1.5)	44.4% (1.6)	8.8% (0.9)	6.4% (0.8)	13.3% (1.0)	48.8% (1.6)

The high-income nations include Australia, Belgium, France, Germany, Israel, Italy, Japan, New Zealand, Northern Ireland, Portugal, Spain, Spain (Murcia), the Netherlands, and the United States. The middle-income nations include Brazil, Bulgaria, Colombia (Medellin), Lebanon, Mexico, Romania, and South Africa. The lower-income nations include Colombia, Iraq, Peru, People's Republic of China, and Ukraine [8]

[a] Figures in parentheses refer to standard error

Table 19.5 ISTSS guidelines for preventative interventions and treating posttraumatic stress disorder

Strong recommendation	• Cognitive behavioral therapy (CBT) with a trauma focus • Cognitive processing therapy (CPT) • Cognitive therapy (CT) • Eye movement desensitization and reprocessing (EMDR) therapy • Prolonged exposure
Standard recommendation	• CBT without a trauma focus • Group CBT with a trauma focus • Guided Internet-based CBT with a trauma focus • Narrative exposure therapy • Present-centered therapy
Intervention with emerging evidence (recommendation)	• Couples CBT with a trauma focus • Group and individual CBT with a trauma focus • Reconsolidation of traumatic memories • Single-session CBT • Virtual reality therapy • Written exposure therapy
Intervention with insufficient evidence to recommend	• Brief eclectic psychotherapy for PTSD • Dialogical exposure therapy • Emotional freedom techniques • Group interpersonal therapy • Group stabilizing treatment • Group supportive counseling • Individual psychoeducation/self-help • Interpersonal psychotherapy • Observed relaxation training • REM desensitization • Supportive counseling • Trauma-focused counseling

CPT presumes a psychological model of PTSD wherein there is a dissonance between the patient's pre-trauma belief structures and post-trauma appraisal of the traumatic event and then seeks to reconcile the two into a singular context and narrative through the practice of Socratic dialogue and other counseling modalities [30]. **Cognitive therapy**, which is derived from **CBT**, presumes a model in which the patient continues to feel a current sense of threat following a traumatic experience and seeks to minimize PTSD symptoms by identifying and then altering negative cognitions and evaluations of the event [31]. **EDMR** presumes that inadequate processing of the traumatic event leads to symptoms of PTSD (particularly avoidance and re-experiencing); that this pathology arises when triggered by the resurfacing of improperly processed memories; and that symptoms can be resolved by reintegrating them into adaptive memory networks through an eight-phase approach [32]. **Prolonged exposure** presumes that PTSD symptoms stem from the erroneous emotional valence attributed to stimuli associated with the traumatic event and then works to resolve these erroneous associations—and therefore avoidant behavior and intrusive memories—by modifying cognitive-emotional networks via interactions with stimuli that are perceived as threatening in a controlled and safe environment [33]. For a more detailed examination of these treatments, see the recently published (2020) *Effective Treatments for PTSD: Practice Guidelines from the International Society for Traumatic Stress Studies* by Forbes et al. [34]

Table 19.6 ISTSS guidelines for early or preventative interventions for posttraumatic stress disorder

	Single preventative session, early interventions	Multiple preventative sessions, early interventions	Early treatment	Early pharmacological interventions
Standard recommendation			• CBT Ten • Cognitive therapy • EMDR therapy	
Intervention with low effect			• Stepped or collaborative care	
Intervention with emerging evidence	• EDMR therapy • Group 512 PM	• Brief dyadic therapy • Self-guided Internet-based intervention	• Internet-based guided self-help • Structured writing intervention	• Hydrocortisone[a]
Intervention with insufficient evidence to recommend	• Computerized visuospatial task • Heart stress counseling • Individual debriefing • Psychoeducation • Reassurance • Trauma-focused counseling • Group debriefing • Group education • Group stress management	• Brief interpersonal psychotherapy • Brief individual trauma processing therapy • Collaborative care • Communication facilitator in an intensive care setting • Guided self-help • Intensive care diaries in an intensive care context • Supported psychoeducational intervention • Telephone-based cognitive behavioral therapy • Brief parenting intervention (following premature birth)	• Behavioral activation • Brief cognitive processing therapy • Internet virtual reality therapy • Nurse-led psychological intervention • Supportive counseling • Telephone-based cognitive behavioral therapy	• Docosahexaenoic acid[a] • Escitalopram[a] • Gabapentin[a] • Oxytocin[a] • Propranolol[a]

For a more detailed examination of these treatments, see the recently published (2020) *Effective Treatments for PTSD: Practice Guidelines from the International Society for Traumatic Stress Studies* by Forbes et al. [34]

[a]Within the first 3 months of the traumatic event

Dissociative Subtype of PTSD

DSM-5 recognizes a subtype of PTSD with dissociative symptoms (PTSD-DS). Dissociative symptoms may present as depersonalization, wherein the patient feels as though they are an outside observer or somehow divorced from the immediate experience of subjective reality, or derealization, wherein one's perception feels dreamlike or otherwise unreal [1]. PTSD-DS has been found to have a range of prevalence between 11% and 30% among those with PTSD [38].

Complex PTSD

The concept of complex posttraumatic stress disorder (CPTSD) was first described in the 1990s but has only recently been included in a formal diagnostic system [39]. Its first appearance was in ICD-11. As it is still a newly recognized disorder, no studies have reported on the efficacy of treatments specifically for CPTSD [40]. Samples have indicated that prevalence of CPTSD is approximately 13% among veterans and 0.6% among the wider community [39].

CPTSD is similar to PTSD but has a significantly different profile that includes a total of six symptom clusters—three that are included within the ICD-11 conceptualization of PTSD (re-experiencing, avoidance, and hyperarousal) and three additional symptom clusters categorized as disturbances of self-organization (DSO) that include difficulties regulating emotion, a diminished sense of self, and interpersonal problems that include avoiding, denigrating, or terminating relationships when inconvenienced (Fig. 19.24a) [25]. These symptom clusters are typically more inhibitive to social or occupational functioning than PTSD and are believed to be more common in individuals who have experienced prolonged mistreatment (prisoners of war, torture victims, refugees, etc.) [41]. Though it is more common among these populations, CPTSD should not be conceptualized as a disorder that is simply a more severe form of PTSD, nor should chronic and repeated traumas be assumed to be a requirement for CPTSD [40]. They certainly increase the risk of developing CPTSD, but these risks can be mitigated by strong social resources and a protective environment. These elements help to prevent the development of a pathology characterized by a profound sense of interpersonal betrayal, which seems to be at the

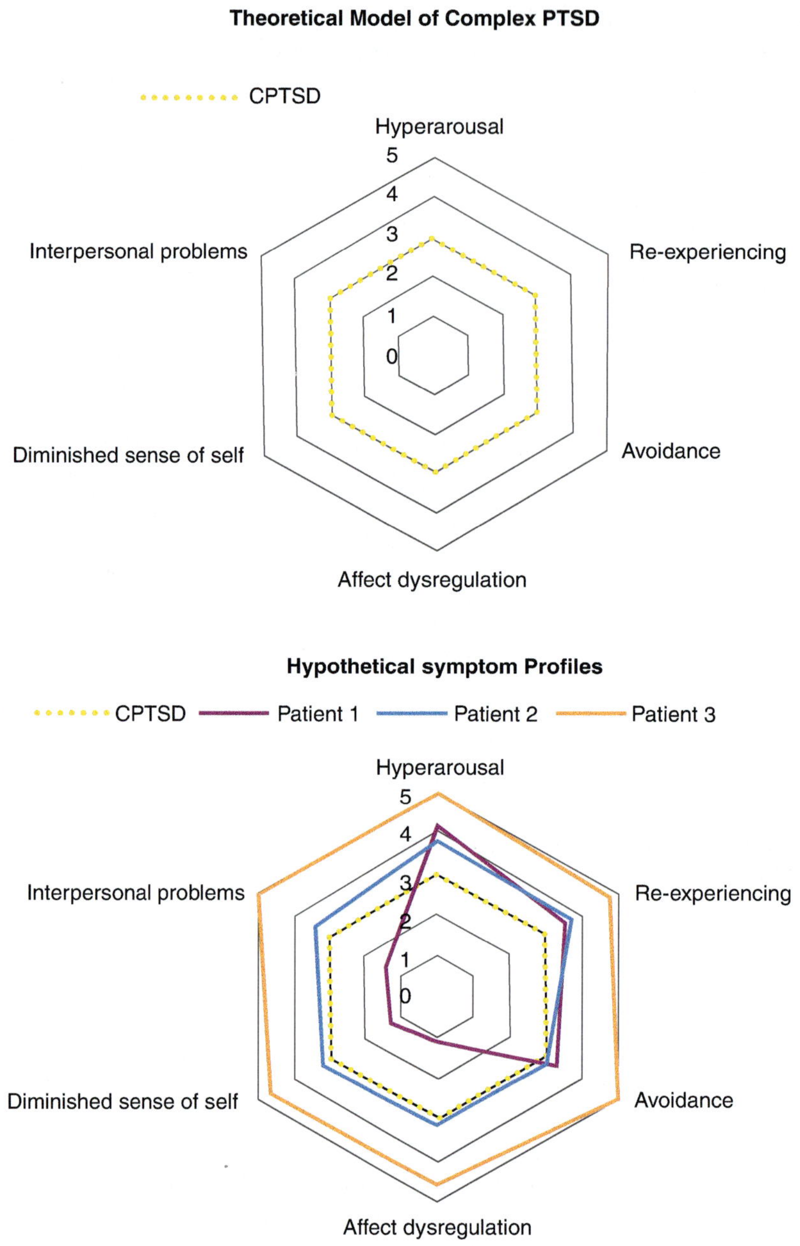

Fig. 19.24 (*Top*) Complex posttraumatic stress disorder is characterized by six symptoms following a traumatic experience: hyperarousal, re-experiencing of the traumatic event, avoidance, affect dysfunction (e.g., inability to manage negative emotions), diminished sense of self (e.g., feelings of worthlessness, shame, or guilt), and interpersonal problems (e.g., feeling alienated from others and avoiding even casual levels of intimacy). In this theoretical model, the yellow dotted line indicates the level of symptom severity that an individual would need to exhibit to meet criteria for the symptom. Points closer to the center of the diagram indicate lower symptom severity. Points further away from the center indicate higher symptom severity. (*Bottom*) This diagram imagines three hypothetical patients who have been assessed following a deeply traumatic event and symptoms that have persisted for several months. Patient 1 scores high on the three core symptoms of PTSD (hyperarousal, re-experiencing of the trauma, and avoidant behavior), but their scores are low enough to not meet criteria for the remaining symptoms collectively known as disturbances of self-organization (DSO). Like Patient 1, Patient 2 scores high on the PTSD. They also score relatively high on the DSO symptoms. Patient 3, meanwhile, scores extremely high on both PTSD symptoms and DSO symptoms. As noted in the text, there is little empirical evidence to support the belief that individuals like Patient 2 are well represented in any population. Most patient symptoms parallel those of Patient 1 (satisfies criteria for PTSD but with subsyndromal DSO symptoms) or Patient 3 (severe symptoms in all six categories)

core of CPTSD [42]. Seen in this light, it becomes conceivable, although perhaps rare, that an individual may suffer a singular traumatic event and develop CPTSD due to a lack of social resources.

There is some controversy about the construct validity of CPTSD. In current models, an individual with PTSD and an individual with CPTSD could conceivably have similar symptom severity with respect to the three core criteria for PTSD, but the individual with CPTSD would meet criteria for DSO criteria, whereas the individual with PTSD would not (Fig. 19.24b). Research, however, has found that individuals with CPTSD do tend to have more severe PTSD symptoms in conjunction with severe DSO symptoms and that between 40% and 80% of individuals with PTSD meet criteria for at least one symptom from the DSO cluster [39, 43]. This suggests that CPTSD only emerges when symptoms of PTSD are severe enough. Additionally, some have argued that a diagnosis of PTSD and borderline personality disorder (BPD) would be indistinguishable from CPTSD, though this seems less accurate upon reflection. BPD is characterized by extreme vicissitudes, volatile interpersonal relationships, and an unstable sense of self, whereas CPTSD is characterized by a constant avoidance of intimacy and a persistently negative view of self [40].

Like PTSD, common comorbidities with CPTSD include substance abuse disorder, anxiety disorders, and major depressive disorders [44].

Acute Stress Disorder

Acute stress disorder (ASD) is intimately related to PTSD. It arises following a traumatic experience as defined by the same diagnostic criteria as Criterion A for PTSD in DSM-5 that causes clinically significant impairment (Criterion D). As noted elsewhere in this chapter, ASD is included in DSM-5, but not ICD-11, because it is believed to represent a normal stress response following a traumatic event. Rates of prevalence vary widely, with some sources claiming that less than 20% of individuals involved in non-violent traumatic events develop ASD, while between 20% and 50% of individuals who experience trauma that involves interpersonal violence develop ASD [1]. Others have found the rate of prevalence following motor vehicle accidents to be as low as 5% and as high as 46% [45]. Most recently, Geoffrion and colleagues found an overall rate of ASD following trauma of 20.4% and a rate of 36% for interpersonal trauma, 15.9% for accident-related trauma, 21.9% for disaster-related trauma, 14.1% for war-related trauma, and 20.7% for life-threatening illnesses [45].

Table 19.7 Potential symptoms of acute stress disorder

Symptoms of intrusion	• Involuntary and distressing memories • Distressing dreams • Flashbacks • Distress from external triggers
Symptoms of mood	• No capacity for positive emotion
Symptoms of dissociation	• Depersonalization/derealization • Dissociative amnesia
Symptoms of avoidance	• Avoidance of feelings or memories about traumatic event • Avoidance of external reminders associated with traumatic event
Symptoms of arousal	• Sleep problems • Aggressive outbursts of emotion • Hypervigilance • Inability to concentrate • Overexcited startle response

Unlike PTSD, patients do not need to exhibit symptoms from each symptom cluster to be diagnosed with acute stress disorder (ASD). DSM-5 states that any combination of nine of the above symptoms warrants a diagnosis of acute stress disorder [1]

Diagnosis of ASD requires the presence of at least nine symptoms from Table 19.7 to be present between 3 days and up to 1 month (Criterion C) following trauma [1]. As noted above, half of those who develop ASD will go on to develop PTSD [13]. Treatment of ASD and early intervention treatments for PTSD are virtually indistinguishable [13].

Adjustment Disorder

Adjustment disorder (AjD) represents an emotional or behavioral response to one or more identifiable stressors that can be considered out of proportion to the severity of antecedent stressors. AjD is also characterized by clinically significant impairment that interferes with one's ability to fulfill their occupational, academic, or social duties, but neither meets the criteria for another mental disorder nor stems from the exacerbation of a preexisting one. An additional criterion (see Table 19.8) is that symptoms arise within either 1 month (ICD-11) or 3 months (DSM-5) of the onset of the stressor and dissipate within 6 months of the elimination of the stressor or its consequences [1, 25]. DSM-5 and ICD-10 recognize various subtypes as illustrated in Table 19.9.

Table 19.8 Adjustment disorder criteria differences in DSM-5 and ICD-11

DSM-5	ICD-11
A. Development of symptoms within 3 months of psychosocial stressor appearance or onset	1. Development of symptoms within 1 month of psychosocial stressor appearance or onset
B. Symptoms can be deemed clinically significant based on one or both of the following: 1. Symptom severity exceeds the expected response to the stressor after accounting for cultural norms and context 2. Symptom severity inhibits the performance of social, occupational, or other duties	2. Preoccupation with stressor or its consequences with at least one of the following: (a) Excessive worry over stressor or its consequences (b) Distressing and frequent thoughts about stressor or its consequences (c) Persistent rumination about stressor or its consequences 3. Failure to adapt to stressor or its consequences, thereby inhibiting the performance of social, occupational, or other duties
C. Symptoms do not meet the criteria for another disorder or represent the exacerbation of an existing disorder	4. Symptoms not severe or specific enough to satisfy criteria for another disorder
D. Symptoms do not constitute normal bereavement	
E. Following the elimination of the stressor or its consequences, symptoms dematerialize within 6 months	5. Following the elimination of the stressor or its consequences, symptoms typically dematerialize within 6 months, but may persist if stressor persists

Though included in the larger category of "disorders specifically associated with stress," ICD-11 conceptualizes adjustment disorder slightly differently than previous editions of ICD or DSM-5 by noting that the disorder stems not only from a failure to adapt to the stressor but preoccupation with either the stressor or its consequences [25]

Table 19.9 Subtypes of adjustment disorder in DSM-5

Subtype	Predominating symptom
With depressed mood	Sense of hopelessness; low mood
With anxiety	Sense of dread or worry; separation anxiety
With mixed anxiety and depressed mood	A combination of the two above subtypes
With disturbance of conduct	Reckless or antisocial behavior
With mixed disturbance of emotions and conduct	Combination of all three
Unspecified	Other maladaptive behaviors or actions

ICD-11 includes no subtypes

AjD was first described in ICD-9 (1978) and the third edition of the DSM (1980) as a standalone disorder [46]. It has been argued that it was included as a pragmatic bridge for symptom constructs that did not meet the criteria for more established disorders (e.g., major depression disorder, persistent bereavement disorder) and that it is simply a reaction to stressors that extends beyond what is considered socially acceptable [46]. This conceptualization of AjD as a subsyndromal catchall has made the disorder somewhat controversial. Likewise, the reliance on non-specific signifiers like "stressor" and "clinically significant" has also been deemed problematic [46]. Vague language and a shifting conceptualization of the disorder, as well as a general skepticism about AjD's standing as a unique affliction, have resulted in limited research [46].

Although a survey of almost 5000 psychiatrists found AjD to be the fifth most problematic mental disorder due to these reasons, the same survey found that AjD is the seventh most frequently diagnosed mental disorder [46]. Prevalence in the general population is estimated to be less than 1% to upward of 2%, with high-risk groups and populations that have experienced similar stressful events being unsurprisingly higher [3]. A study that followed 330 individuals whose jobs were terminated found that core symptom patterns were present in 27.3% of participants within 12 months of being terminated and that 15.5% of participants developed AjD with the same 12-month period [47]. As Fig. 19.25 shows, the study's authors observed multiple risk factors.

Depending on the nature of the stressor, AjD can be either transient or chronic, but it is self-resolving once the stressor or its consequences have been eliminated. Still, the need for intervention is supported by evidence of a link between the disorder and both self-harm and suicide [3]. There is limited evidence about the efficacy of pharmaceuticals in treating AjD with preliminary studies having found the use of anxiolytics and antidepressants to be beneficial [46]. Validated disorder-specific psychosocial treatments are wanting, but ongoing trials suggest that existing treatment modalities for other trauma- and stressor-related disorders can be repurposed to alleviate AjD symptoms.

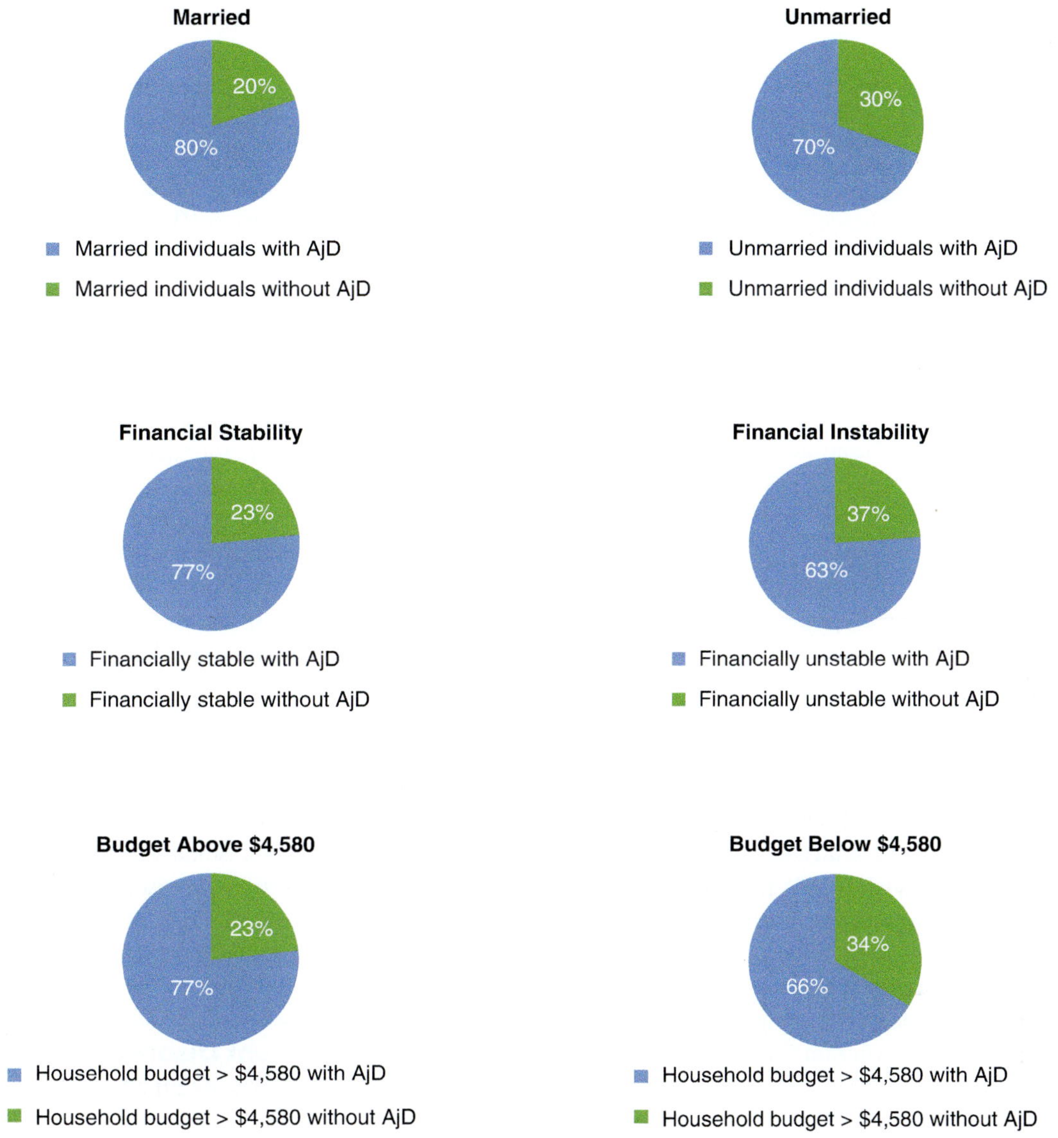

Fig. 19.25 Beyond showing that adjustment disorder (AjD) occurs with relative frequency, these charts indicate the extent to which sociodemographic factors contribute as risk factors to AjD diagnoses. Increased stability, whether due to marriage or financial security, did not eliminate risk for AjD; it merely mitigated it [47]. (*Middle*) The figure given in the study was 4,000 Swiss francs (CHF), which was converted to US dollars (USD). CHF to USD conversion ($1.0512) was based on the average conversion rate for October 15, 2015, as found on poundsterlinglive.com (4,000 SFr = $4204.77). According to the US Bureau of Labor Statistics, $4204.77 in October 2015 had the same buying power of $4580.68 in July 2020 (https://www.bls.gov/data/inflation_calculator.htm)

Prolonged Grief Disorder

Similar to models of resilience already explored above, most individuals experience bereavement as a highly stressful event, but their distress levels eventually decrease and stabilize [48]. Approximately one in ten bereaved individuals, however, will experience disordered or pathological grief following the death of a loved one [49]. At present, there are three distinct variations of pathological grief with their own separate diagnostic criteria: complicated grief (CG), persistent complex bereavement disorder (PCBD), and prolonged grief disorder (PGD) [50]. PGD is the only one to be included in a major diagnostic system (ICD-11). PCBD has only been recognized as a condition for further study in DSM-5 [1].

The disorder is primarily characterized by an extended period of profound bereavement following a death, one that lasts well beyond the timeframe that is considered socially acceptable within the bereaved individual's culture. The diagnostic criteria for PGD in ICD-11 specify that clinical presentation is also defined by at least one of the two key diagnostic features that include preoccupation with the deceased or a persistent yearning to be with the deceased that persist for a minimum of 6 months [51]. Such preoccupation

Table 19.10 Proposed Criteria B and C for persistent complex bereavement disorder in DSM-5

Criterion B (at least one)	Criterion C (at least six)
Persistent yearning for the deceased	Difficulty accepting death of the deceased
Intense emotional pain	Emotional numbness
Preoccupation with the deceased	Trouble reminiscing about deceased positively
Preoccupation with the deceased cause of death	Bitterness over death
	Maladaptive beliefs about relation either with the deceased or to the death
	Avoidance of reminders of decedent
	Desire to die and be with decedent
	Difficulty trusting others
	Feeling alienated from others
	Feeling unable to live without deceased
	Diminished sense of self
	Lack of interest in activities or plans for the future

Under the proposed criteria for persistent complex grief disorder, DSM-5 includes 4 potential symptoms under Criterion B and 12 potential symptoms under Criterion C

is often accompanied by intense emotional pain, disengagement from social activities, and other behaviors associated with grief, as well as impairment in core areas of functioning (occupational, academic, social, etc.) [51]. This diagnostic criterion is far less rigorous than previously proposed criteria for PGD, CG, or PCBD as outlined in DSM-5, which additionally specifies the necessity of distress-related impairment (Criterion D), as well as at least one symptom under Criterion B and six symptoms under Criterion C for at least 12 months in adults and 6 months in children (see Table 19.10) [1].

Common comorbidities of PGD include PTSD (especially if the death is violent or unexpected), depressive disorders, and substance use disorders. Differentiating between PGD and either PTSD or depressive disorders can be difficult. What is key to remember is that the core distinguishing mark of PGD is preoccupation with the deceased themselves or the relationship with the deceased. Depressive disorders and PTSD tend to lack such focus or focus on the manner of the decedent's death—as being unfair. Separation anxiety, meanwhile, fixates on separation from current attachment figures rather than the deceased.

Major risk factors associated with PGD are similar to those associated with other trauma- and stressor-related disorders, though Lundorff and colleagues found that older age was associated with higher rates of PGD [49]. Loss of an only child was also associated with significantly higher rates of PGD [52].

Childhood Trauma

Children may respond to traumatic events differently than adults. As discussed below, attachment disorders may develop when young children experience extreme caregiver negligence or mistreatment. Likewise, children may be more vulnerable to prolonged grief disorder or PTSD after experiencing or witnessing an event that meets the definition of traumatic stress found in Criterion A of DSM-5 [53]. It is estimated that 16% of children and adolescents exposed to traumatic stress will develop PTSD and children from disadvantaged socioeconomic backgrounds appear to be at greater risk of exposure [53]. Difficulties pertaining to family functioning—including drug abuse, marital conflict, or severe mental health issues—may also put a child at a higher risk of exposure [53].

DSM-5 has included a subtype of PTSD for children under the age of 6 with avoidant behaviors and negative cognition appearing as a single symptom cluster, while negative beliefs about the world or self and blaming behavior have been excised [1]. In this subtype of PTSD and in cases of PTSD among children slightly older, the manifestation of symptoms may be slightly different than in adults. For example, children may not be able to fully comprehend or convey the frightening content of distressing dreams or dissociative experiences (flashbacks), and they instead may be expressed as a form of reenactment during play. Studies have also found that children who are exposed to interpersonal violence that satisfies Criterion A are at a greater risk of revictimization both in childhood and once they have become adults [53].

Reactive Attachment Disorder and Disinhibited Social Engagement Disorder

Reactive attachment disorder (RAD) and disinhibited social engagement disorder (DSED) (also known as disinhibited attachment disorder) are childhood disorders that arise when a child experiences significant neglect in the early stages of their development. As the two share a common etiology and both represent abnormalities in attachment behaviors among children over the age of 9 months, they were initially considered a single disorder until being separated in ICD-10 and then in DSM-5 [4]. The two are now grouped in the trauma- and stressor-related disorders sections of ICD-11 and DSM-5 instead of the group dedicated to disorders typically first diagnosed in childhood.

During the earliest stages of development, infants are motivated to seek comfort from and form bonds with a variety of caregivers or adults. As children reach the age of

7–9 months, they begin to show preference for specific caregivers and to direct attachment behaviors toward these individuals. When a child both seeks comfort from and can be soothed by a specific caregiver, this is known as a "secure attachment" [54]. Disorganized attachment, conversely, indicates that the child has not established a means of obtaining comfort from caregivers, something that may or may not be due solely to inadequate caregiving, since children with Williams syndrome, a genetic disorder, may exhibit behavior akin to DSED [4].

Both RAD and DSED represent disorganized forms of attachment, and they can only be diagnosed in instances of extreme neglect or when children are presented with limited opportunities to form stable attachments (e.g., due to being in a poorly staffed institution or frequent caregiver changes) [54]. DSM-5 also specifies that symptoms of RAD must be evident before the child reaches the age of 5 (Criterion F) but does not provide a similar criterion for DSED [1].

RAD is characterized by emotional withdrawal, indifference to caregivers, and a lack of both comfort-seeking behavior and response to attempts to comfort when distressed. DSED is characterized by an "indiscriminate friendliness" and a willingness to be overly familiar when interacting with unknown adults or attachment figs [55]. Children with DSED show a potentially dangerous penchant of wandering off with strangers without hesitation.

Both disorders are more common in institutional settings than in more traditional homes and are believed to be exceptionally rare globally [54]. Even among severely neglected children, DSM-5 estimates prevalence of RAD to be 10% and prevalence of DSED to be 20% [1]. A longitudinal study involving Romanian children who were at least partly raised while in an institution placed these numbers lower—4.1% and 17.6%, respectively [56]. Meanwhile, a study in South Korea by Hong and colleagues reported only 736 cases of either disorder among more than 14 million children under the age of 10 in the years 2010, 2011, and 2012 and an average incidence of 5.25 per 100,000 (5.39 in 2010, 4.90 in 2011, 5.45 in 2012) [57]. Prevalence appears to peak among children aged 3 years before declining (Fig. 19.26) [57]. In some cases, signs may endure into adolescence [55]. Comorbid stereotypies and developmental delays—behavioral, cognitive, and language-based—may persist as well [54].

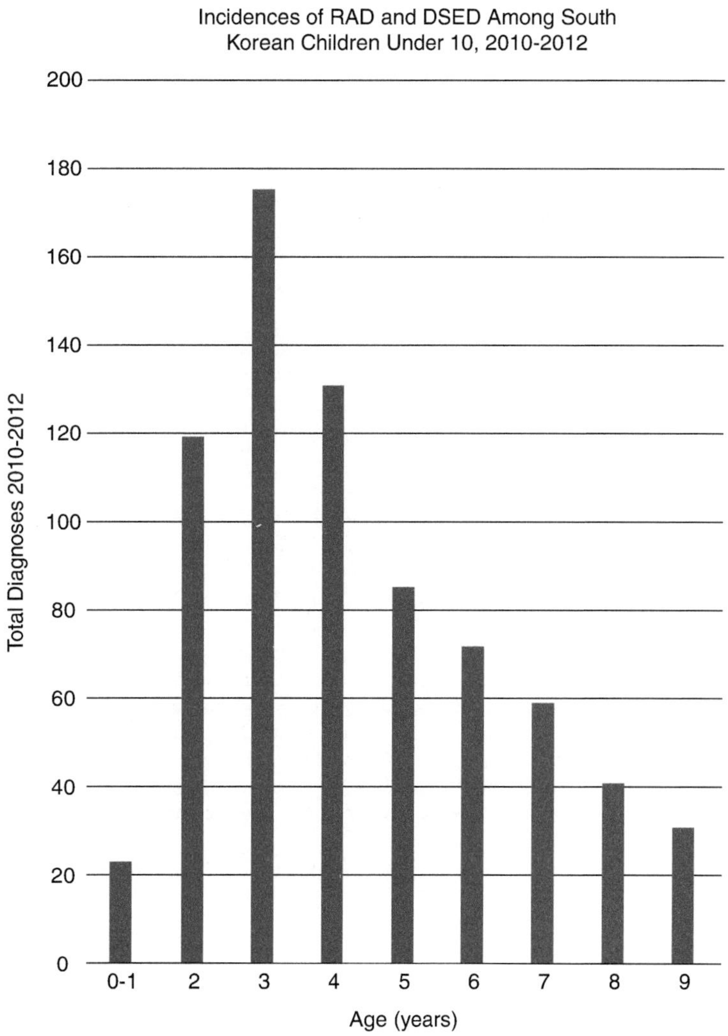

Fig. 19.26 The total number of diagnoses of either reactive attachment disorder (RAD) or disinhibited social engagement disorder (DSED) by age (in years) among South Korean children in the combined years of 2010, 2011, and 2012

The course of RAD is strongly influenced by environmental factors, and children who are deprived of basic levels of comfort and affection from caregivers will continue to exhibit signs of RAD. When placed in a more responsive environment, these signs dissipate [54]. The same is not true for DSED. Even into adolescence and beyond, some will continue to exhibit indiscriminate behavior after being placed in a healthier environment [54].

As Criterion E of DSM-5 implies, RAD and autism spectrum disorder may be difficult to distinguish in some instances, and this same criterion precludes the possibility of concurrent RAD and autism, though this exclusive disjunction is not a feature in other diagnostic systems [57]. Cognitive delays and decreased social reciprocity are associated with both disorders, but the key distinguishing represent disorganized forms of feature is that selective impairment and limited interests are signs of autism and not of RAD. RAD must be distinguished from not just autism but also unrelated intellectual disabilities and depressive disorders, although depression may be a comorbidity. DSED must be distinguished from attention-deficit/hyperactivity disorder (ADHD). Social impulsivity may be a shared feature of DSED and ADHD, but lack of attention and hyperactivity are not characteristic of DSED (Fig. 19.27) [1].

Other Trauma- and Stressor-Related Disorders

DSM-5 acknowledges that clinicians may recognize symptoms indicative of a trauma- and stressor-related disorder that is causing the patient significant distress or functional impairment but may fail to meet specific criteria within either diagnostic system, but ICD-11 does not [1].

Clinicians may choose to designate a disorder as "other specified trauma- and stressor-related disorder" in instances where there is a specific reason why the patient presents a constellation of symptoms beyond the scope of the diagnostic system. For example, a patient may present with adjustment disorder-like symptoms that have arisen several months after the consequences of the traumatic event have dissipated, a patient may meet criteria for persistent complex bereavement disorder, or they may be experiencing a culture-bound syndrome (see Table 19.11).

A clinician may also choose not to provide a specific reason for which criteria have not been met. This is typically because the clinician has yet to amass sufficient information to make a diagnosis [1].

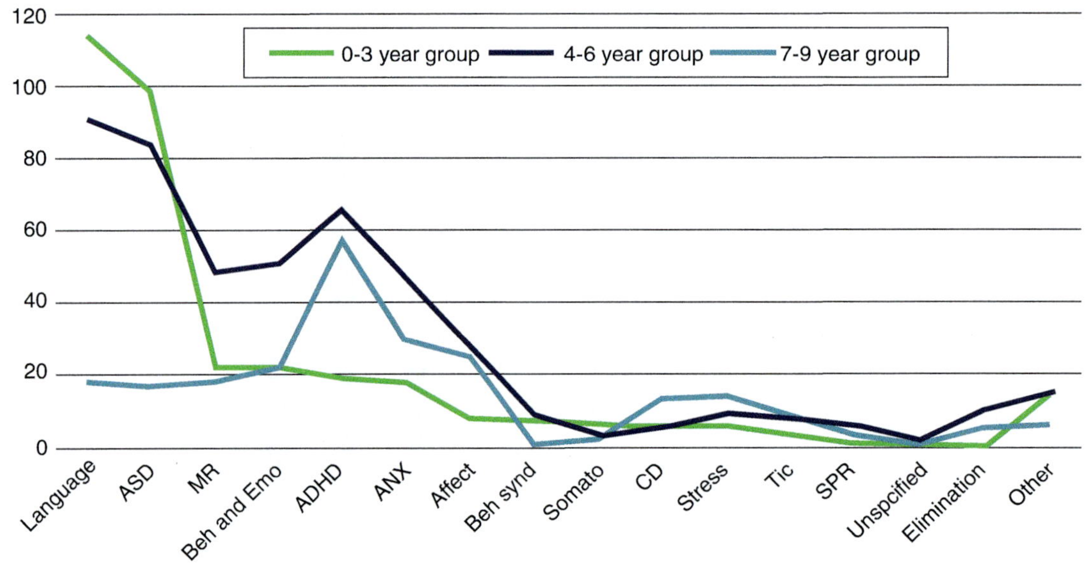

Fig. 19.27 There is limited evidence about comorbid disorders associated with either RAD or DSED, though Hong and colleagues [57] found varying comorbidity rates by age group. *ASD* autism spectrum disorder; *MR* mental retardation; *Beh* and *Emo* behavioral and emotional disorders; *ADHD* attention-deficit/hyperactivity disorder; *ANX* anxiety disorder; *Affect* affective disorder; *Beh synd* behavioral syndromes associated with physiological disturbances and physical factors; *Somato* somatoform disorders; *CD* conduct disorder; *Stress* reaction to severe stress/adjust disorder; *Tic* tic disorder; *SPR* schizophrenia; *Unspecified* unspecified mental disorder; *Elimination* enuresis and encopresis

Table 19.11 Culture-bound trauma- and stressor-related syndromes

Syndrome	Culture/region	Symptoms
Ataque de nervios	Latinx	Translated: "attack of the nerves." May include emotional outbursts, trembling, panic attacks, fainting episodes, and dissociative experiences
Falling out	Afro-Caribbean/ Black	Fainting episodes and dissociative experiences
Ghost sickness	Indigenous North American	Similar to prolonged grief disorder, but often with confusion, anxiety, weakness, troubling dreams, and a pervasive sense of dread
Khyâl cap	Cambodia	Translated: "wind attacks." Similar to panic attacks but with additional symptoms associated with autonomic arousal
Kufungisisa	Zimbabwe	Translated: "thinking too much." Cultural idiom for rumination that may itself be indicative of preoccupation with a distressing event or death
Piblokto	Circumpolar cultures	Aggression and irrational or dangerous behavior, typically with dissociative amnesia
Shin-byung	Korea	Translated: "divine illness." Initial symptoms are anxiety and somatic complaints (fatigue, insomnia, loss of appetite, etc.) followed by dissociative states believed to be caused by spirit possession
Susto	Continental Latinx	Translated: "fright." Despondency, sleep irregularities, troubling dreams, appetite disturbances, low self-worth, and somatic symptoms (headache, fatigue, stomachache, etc.)
Ufufunyane	Southern and Eastern Africa	Spirit possession by malice. Pseudolalia, dissociative states, and severe somatic symptoms like paralysis and temporary blindness
Zār	Africa, Middle East	"Zār" is both the type of spirit (a zār spirit) and the name of an affliction that is associated with zār possession. Symptoms include dissociative experiences, as well as headaches, vocal outbursts, and apathy

The above is a non-comprehensive list of culture-bound syndromes that often arise following trauma or stress or have symptoms that are related to disorders explored in this chapter

Dissociative Disorders

Dissociative disorders (DDs) are characterized by dissociative symptoms. Dissociative symptoms are characterized by disruptions or rifts in the normal integration of the core elements of cognitive functioning, including memory, identity, emotion, and even consciousness itself [1]. As noted above, patients suffering from trauma- and stressor-related disorders or borderline personality disorder (BPD) may have dissociative symptoms, but antecedent trauma is not a necessary criterion for DD in DSM-5 or ICD-11. Still, many of the risk factors associated with trauma- and stressor-related disorders are the same as those associated with DD, and antecedent trauma is so common and that many would contend that the two are casually linked (see Fig. 19.27) [58]. DSM-5 and ICD-11 recognize close relationship between them and have placed the two side by side.

Dissociative symptoms come in many forms and may include intrusive or involuntary altered states, as is the case with depersonalization, derealization, or dissociative identity disorder (DID). They may also refer to the inability to voluntarily access autobiographical information, as is the case with dissociative amnesia (previously known as psychogenic amnesia). According to ICD-11, somatic symptom disorders are also categorized as DDs, but this will be discussed in Chap. 20 [25].

Two schools of thought have arisen to explain dissociative symptoms. The first claims that pathological dissociation is a theoretical defense mechanism that sequesters and divorces traumatic experiences and memories in a manner that makes them less accessible or even inaccessible to the traumatized individual [59]. The trauma is effectively edited out of one's normal narrative or, in the case of dissociative amnesia, excised entirely. The other school believes in an iatrogenic model of dissociation. In this model, DDs are cultural constructs that owe their existence to stories within the media, suggestible patients, and clinicians who overzealously diagnose the disorder. To parallel the earlier discussion about Freud's seduction theory, many who ascribe to the iatrogenic model claim that the previously dissociated memories that are recovered are either false or involuntarily manufactured through clinician suggestion [60].

The iatrogenic model is less popular than it once was. Studies that measure suggestibility using the Gudjonsson Suggestibility Scale found that those with DID scored as less suggestible than individuals with PTSD or BPD or even controls who had experienced trauma [61]. Additionally, recent investigations involving neuroimaging support the traumatic model (see Fig. 19.28) [60, 62]. That individuals with DID typically receive 3–4 incorrect diagnosis and spend 5–12.4 years in institutions before correct diagnosis supports this claim and suggests that DDs may be underdiagnosed [60]. One possible explanation for the underdiagnosis is that clinicians simply do not seriously screen for DDs because they believe them to be exceptionally rare or to not affect the population they are assigned to treat [63]. However, after implementing improved screening techniques, epidemiological studies the world over have evinced that DDs are more common than previously believed, especially in inpatient settings and among patients who have suffered childhood trauma or currently struggle with severe and persistent mental illnesses [64–66]. Lifetime prevalence could be upward of 10% [61].

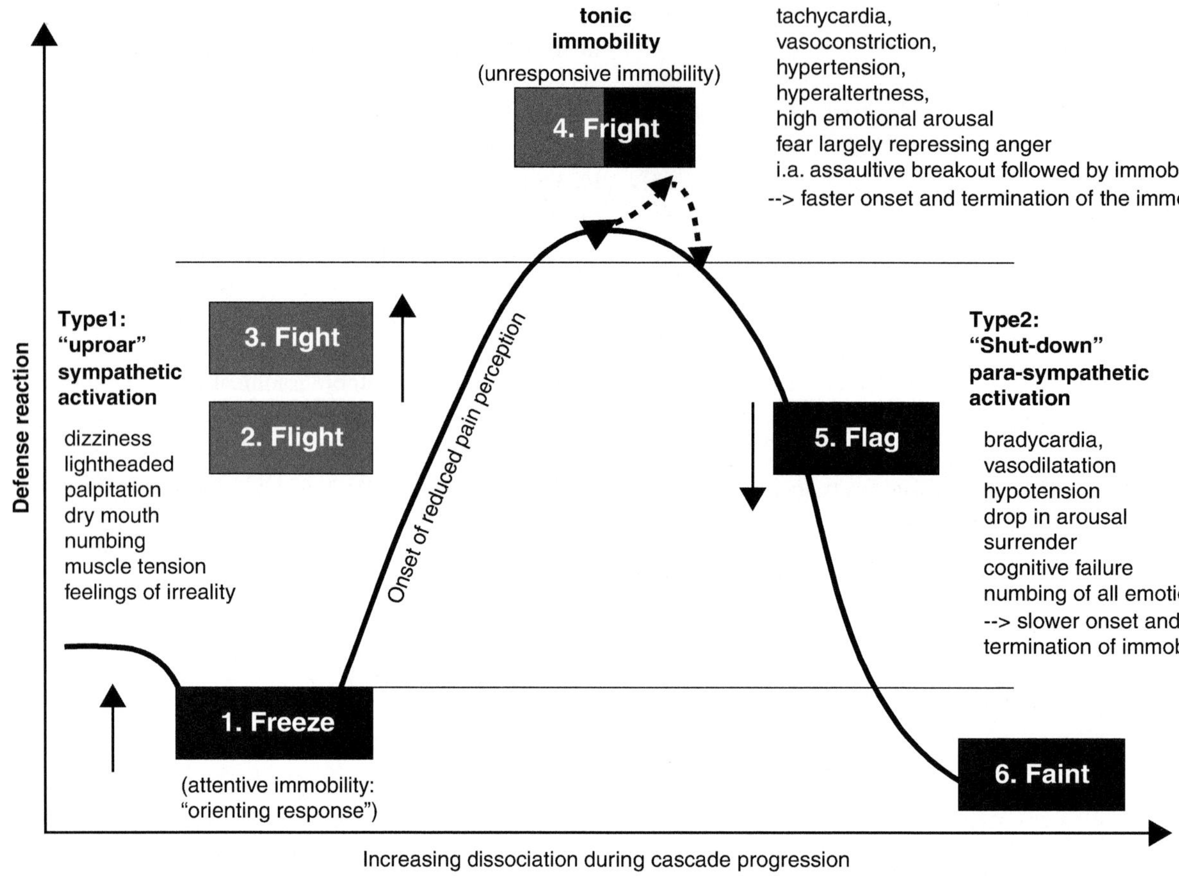

Fig. 19.28 The earlier discussion of stress responses in section "Trauma and Stress" described the limbic system and the sympathetic nervous system (SNS) and parasympathetic nervous system (PNS) (see Figs. 19.6, 19.7 and 19.8). The below model posits a more complex defense response to traumatic stress: (1) freeze, to assess the situation; (2) flee if the threat is far enough away; (3) fight if the threat is near; (4) fright, tense up, go into a state of numbness and effectively "play dead" if trauma is imminent; (5) flag, go into a state of flaccid immobility; and (6) faint, lose consciousness due to hypotension and bradycardia. The initial three stages involve the SNS. At the fourth stage, the SNS has led to a state of tonic immobility and numbing/analgesia with decreased vocalization. Immobility reserves energy to resume flight or fight when opportune, avoids additional tissue damage, and may induce predator disinterest. Throughout, the processing of somatic events becomes less organized. PNS stimulation produces further numbing, cognitive failure, and, eventually, loss of consciousness. This theory posits that pathological posttraumatic symptoms stem from fear conditioning based on the defense mechanisms employed during previous traumatic experiences. Surviving a traumatic experience with only SNS activation may result in PTSD-like symptoms when reminded of trauma by a trigger, while those who experienced the full arc resulting in PNS dominance may exhibit dissociative symptoms when fear responses are triggered

Comorbidities of DDs include PTSD, somatic symptom disorder, conversion disorder, dependent or avoidant personality disorders, and especially BDP [1]. As Fig. 19.29 shows, dissociative symptoms are also commonly found in other psychiatric disorders [67].

Dissociative Amnesia

Dissociative amnesia typically occurs following a traumatic event and can be conceptualized as dissociation of memory from a specific episode (localized), from details within a specific episode (selective), or from one's life history and identity (generalized) [1]. It can also prevent the formation of new memories (continuous amnesia) or recall of categories of information (systemized amnesia) [1]. Prevalence is estimated to be between 1% and 2% in the general population and appears to be more common among women than men [1, 61]. From the perspective of the trauma model, amnesia could either be a mechanism employed to exclude potentially debilitating memories from awareness to either preserve one's sense of self or to maintain concentration on a more vital task [68]. As Fig. 19.30 suggests, tonic immobility is a response to stress and may reduce neural network activity, including connectivity between the hippocampus and neocortical areas resulting in memory fragmentation [70]. Kikuchi and colleagues, meanwhile, used fMRI in two patients with dissociative amnesia and observed reduced hippocampal activity and increased activity in the prefrontal cortex while testing for recall [71]. Suffice to say, dissociative amnesia can lead to significant impairment of memory well beyond the traumatic episode.

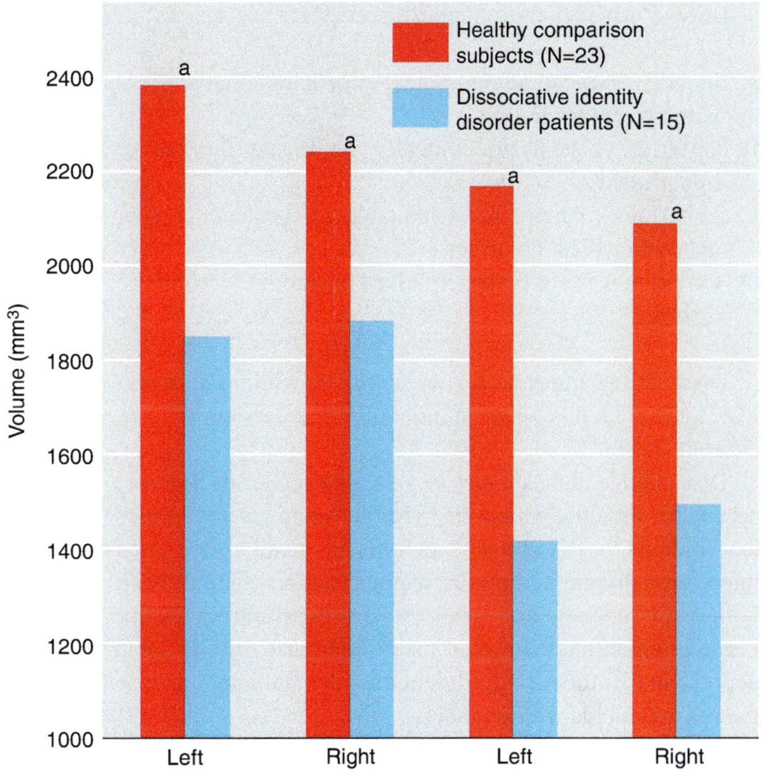

Fig. 19.29 Vermetten and colleagues found left and right hippocampal volumes to be 19.2% smaller in DID patients when compared with healthy controls and that left and right amygdala volumes were 31.6% smaller in DID patients when compared with controls

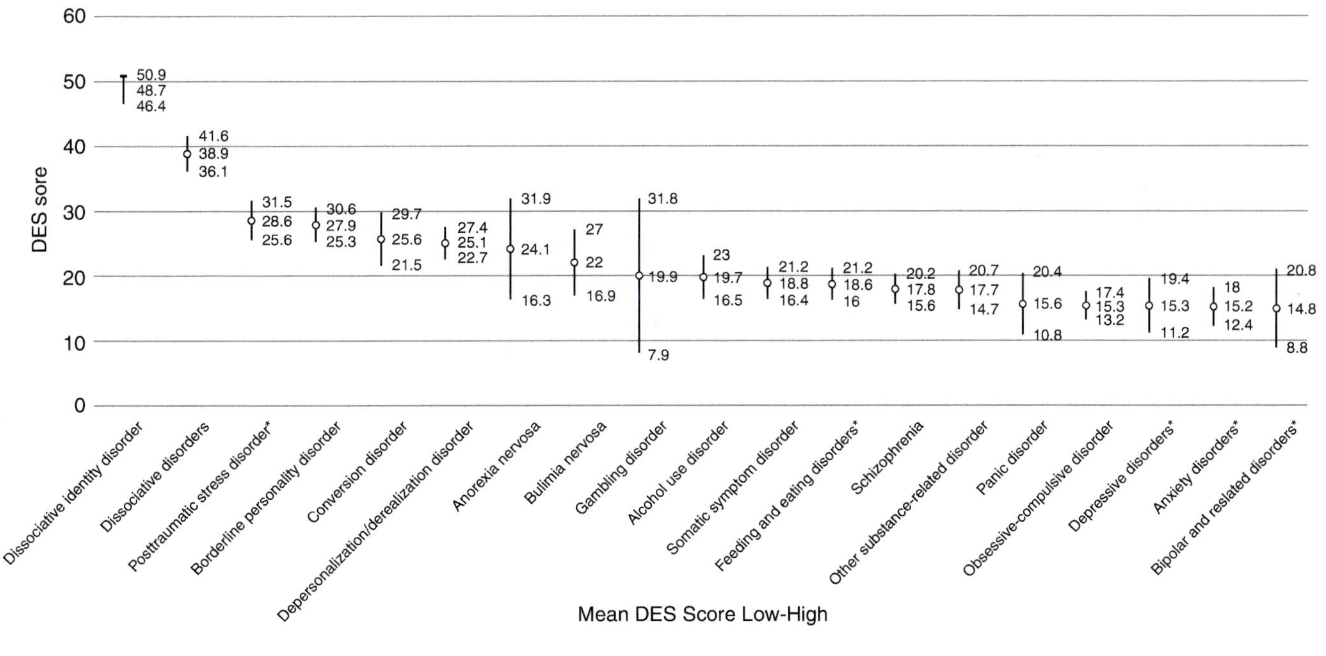

Fig. 19.30 Lyssenko and colleagues performed a meta-analysis on dissociative symptoms in psychiatric disorders and relied on the Dissociative Experiences Scale (DES) or the Dissociative Experiences Scale-II (DES-II) to measure symptom severity. DES is comprised of 28 questions about dissociative experiences that asks patient to self-rate by making slash marks where they fall on a continuum ranging from 0% to 100%. DES-II is similar but asks patients to circle an approximate percentage on the same 0%–100% continuum using an 11-point Likert scale in 10% intervals. For reference, van Ijzendoorn and Schüngel reported a mean DES score among healthy samples and students to be 11.57 and 14.27, respectively [69]. An asterisk (*) indicates entire DSM-5 category

DSM-5 provides four diagnostic criteria:

A. Inability to recall autographical information inconsistent with normal forgetting.
B. Criterion A leads to clinically significant distress or impairment.
C. Criterion A cannot be attributable to substance use or another medical condition.
D. Criterion A is not better explained by another psychiatric disorder.

Dissociative amnesia can occur with or without dissociative fugue, which is when an individual wanders while in an amnesia state [1].

Dissociative amnesia may resolve in a matter of hours or persist for months, which may require treatment modalities that include psychotherapy, pharmacologically facilitated interviews, hypnotherapy, or a combination thereof [61]. Following treatment and recall, patients experience a host of negative emotions that could meet diagnostic criteria for a depressive disorder or adjustment disorder and may increase the risk of suicidal behavior [1].

Depersonalization/Derealization Disorder

In DSM-5, depersonalization/derealization disorder is characterized by frequent experiences of either depersonalization or derealization (Criterion A). Depersonalization is the feeling of observing reality while detached from somatic experience, while derealization occurs when individuals or objects are experienced as unreal or significantly distorted. DSM-5 specifies that reality testing must remain intact throughout the experience (Criterion B) and that the distortion in perception causes significant distress or impairment (Criterion C), cannot be attributable to a substance or alternative medical condition (Criterion D), and cannot be better explained by another psychiatric disorder (Criterion E) [1].

While trauma is commonly reported by individuals with depersonalization/derealization disorder, it is frequently less severe than with other DDs. In many cases, no significant trauma is reported at all, and the disorder arises following acute intoxication caused by the use of either hallucinogen drugs or cannabis. As such, clinicians should be wary of making a diagnosis if patient intoxication is possible. Additionally, the disorder may be symptom associated with another dissociative disorder or another psychiatric disorder (e.g., PTSD, ASD, schizophrenia), or it may be linked to a neurological condition including, but not limited to, a brain tumor, postconcussive syndrome, migraine, or seizure disorders [61].

Depersonalization/derealization disorder has a lifetime prevalence of 2%, affects men and women equally, has a mean age of onset of 16, and can be episodic or chronic, lasting for years or decades [1]. Even transient forms of the disorder can also be extremely debilitating and alienating as patients often feel emotionally divorced from the world. Systematic data on the treatment of the disorder with psychotherapy is wanting, as is clinical evidence to support the use of medications, though limited data suggests that lamotrigine, in combination with serotonin reuptake inhibitors, may reduce depersonalization/derealization symptoms [72]. Medications that treat concurrent anxiety or mood disturbances have been effective at improving quality of life but may also pose the risk of exacerbating the patient's lack of emotional responsiveness [61].

Dissociative Identity Disorder

As described by Criterion A in DSM-5, dissociative identity disorder (DID) is characterized by a discontinuity in identity and the presentation of at least two distinct personality states (often referred to as "alters") that may include a disruption in sense of self, agency, or memory and may be accompanied by symptoms associated with other DDs, including amnesia, trance states, or depersonalization/derealization [1]. ICD-11 specifies that individual alters can and do assume control over executive function of the individual, while ICD-11 and DSM-5 note that this may result in potentially severe episodes of amnesia (Criterion B), that the disruptions lead to distress or impairment (Criterion C), and that the symptoms are not better explained by another condition or due to the use of a substance (Criterion E) [1, 25]. DSM-5 precludes similar disturbances if they are part of a widely accepted cultural practice (Criterion D) [1]. ICD-11, meanwhile, recognizes partial DID as a unique disorder wherein the non-dominant alters only occasionally and transiently assume control of executive functions during moments of extreme stress [25].

DID has been the target of skepticism since well before its inclusion in DSM-III when it was known as multiple personality disorder (MPD), but it is far more common than once thought, with an estimated lifetime prevalence rate of 1.5% [63]. In ten studies on DID patients, between 77 and 100% (median 94%) reported sexual and physical abuse, often beginning before the age of 6 [60].

Symptoms may be covert and rarely resemble the kind of violent switching frequently portrayed in fiction and film, as patients may be unaware of the symptoms or they may attempt to conceal them out of shame or embarrassment. Consequently, failure to detect DID is an extremely common phenomenon, and clinicians must take proactive steps to avoid misdiagnosing patients with BPD, PTSD-DS, schizoaffective disorder (in instances where frequent switches between alters may be confused for rapid cycling), or psychotic disorders [61].

Treatment typically follows a triphasic model, including (1) the creation of a safe environment and the stabilization of symptoms; (2) providing attention to the traumatic material; and (3) integration, wherein the patient begins to eschew patterns of victimization and traumatization [61]. As Loewenstein notes, "DID is more like a never-assembled psychological jigsaw puzzle, not a shattered mirror" [60].

Other Dissociative Disorders

Apart from the disorders described above, ICD-11 recognizes two forms of trance disorder ("trance disorder" and "trance disorder with possession"), as well as a secondary dissociative syndrome, a category to be used by clinicians when dissociative symptoms are present but the presumed underlying condition is not classified as a mental or behavioral disorder [25]. DSM-5 meanwhile includes a category for unspecified dissociative disorder when dissociative symptoms are present and causing distress or impairment, but either the symptoms do not meet full criteria for another DD or the clinician lacks sufficient information to make a diagnosis, as well four DDs categorized under other specified dissociative disorder [1]. Prior to the publication of DSM-5, they were known as dissociative disorder not otherwise specified (DDNOS) (see Fig. 19.31) [61].

Dissociative trance disorder may be an involuntary narrowing of awareness of surroundings or loss of one's sense of personal identity without the emergence of an alter or change in identity. It frequently manifests as an intense unresponsiveness to environmental stimuli, and individuals may find themselves capable of limited and repeated gestures or utterances. Before diagnosis, clinicians should confirm that the state is not part of a broadly accepted religious or cultural practice. Furthermore, clinicians should rule out seizure disorders or movement disorders like Huntington's disease [61].

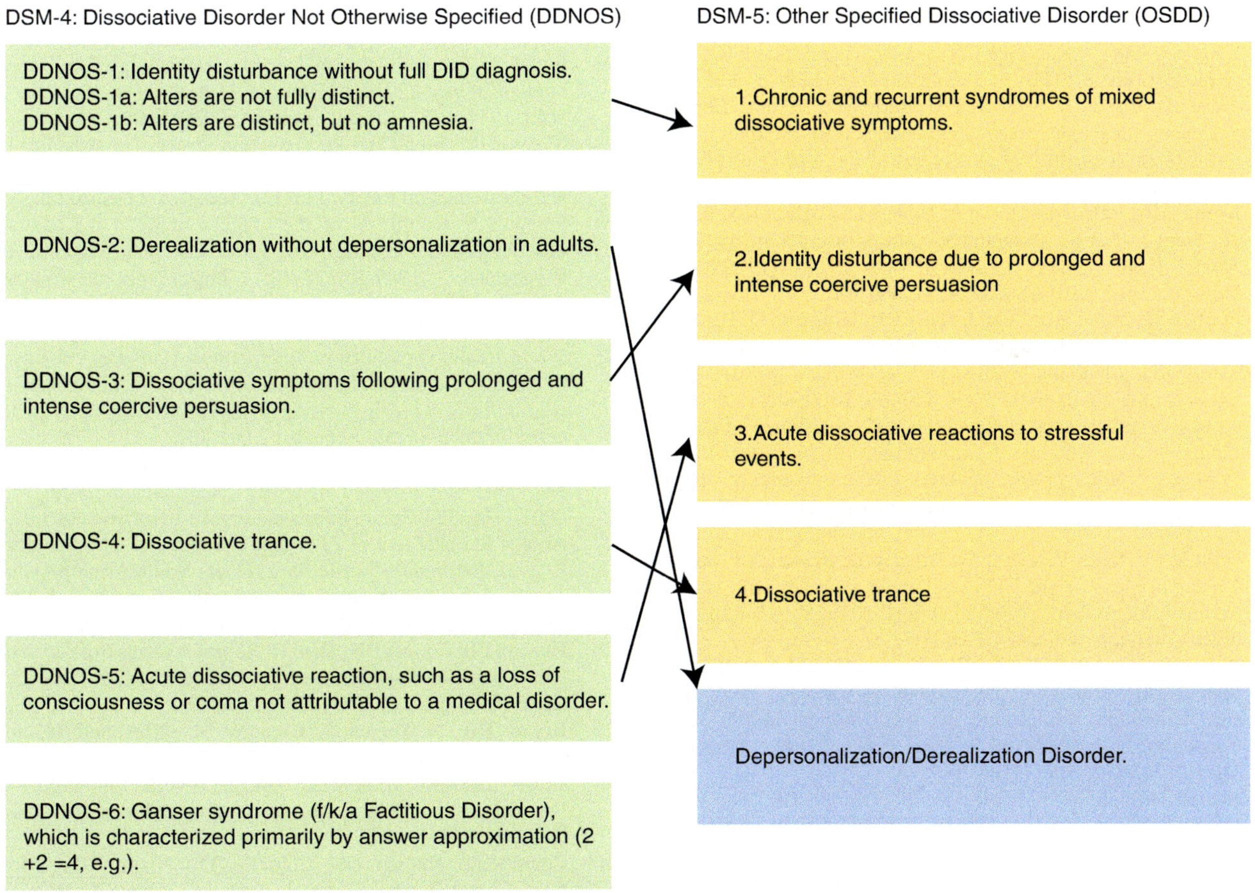

Fig. 19.31 Dissociative disorder not otherwise specified (DDNOS) and other specified dissociative disorder (OSDD) are conceptually similar, as they provide limited diagnostic criteria for DDs that do not meet criteria for DID, DA, or depersonalization/derealization disorder, but there are notable differences. Replacing DDNOS-1a and DDNOS-1b is a single category, which is known as "chronic and recurrent syndromes of mixed dissociative symptoms," which may be often used by clinicians as a placeholder when patients show potential signs of DID or DA or should they fail to meet full criteria for either. DDNOS-2 has been subsumed by depersonalization/derealization disorder. DDNOS-3 is largely the same as OSDD-2 and is conceptually akin to the concept of "brainwashing." Such individuals are susceptible to depersonalization, amnesia, trance-like behavior, and emotional numbing to justify actions previously considered anathema to their values. The state often dissipates upon removal from the source of the coercion. DDNOS-4 and DDNOS-5 are largely the same as OSDD-4 and OSDD-3, respectively. DDNOS-6 is no longer a recognized condition in DSM-5

References

1. American Psychiatric Association. Diagnostic and statistical manual on mental disorders. 5th ed. Washington: The American Psychiatric Association; 2013.
2. Shalev AY, Marmar CR. Posttraumatic stress disorder. In: Sadock BJ, Sadock VA, Ruiz P, editors. Kaplan & Sadock's comprehensive textbook of psychiatry, vol. 1. 10th ed. Philadelphia, PA: Wolters Kluwer; 2017. p. 1812–26.
3. O'Donnell ML, Agathos JA, Metcalf O, Gibson K, Lau W. Adjustment disorder: current developments and future directions. Int J Environ Res Public Health. 2019;16(14):2537. https://doi.org/10.3390/ijerph16142537.
4. Zeanah CH, Gleason MM. Annual research review: attachment disorders in early childhood—clinical presentation, causes, correlates and treatment. J Child Psychol Psychiatry. 2015;56(3):207–22. https://doi.org/10.1111/jcpp.12347.
5. Kim TD, Lee S, Yoon S. Inflammation in post-traumatic stress disorder (PTSD): a review of potential correlates of PTSD with neurological perspective. Antioxidants. 2020;9(2):107. https://doi.org/10.3390/antiox9020107.
6. Ganzel BL, Morris PA, Wethington E. Allostasis and the human brain: integrating models of stress from the social and life sciences. Psychol Rev. 2010;117(1):134–74. https://doi.org/10.1037/a0017773.
7. Korte KJ, Jiang T, Koenen KC, Gradus J. Trauma and PTSD: epidemiology, comorbidity, and clinical presentation in adults. In: Forbes D, Bisson JI, Monson CM, Berliner L, editors. Effective treatments for PTSD: practical guidelines from the International Society for Traumatic Stress Studies. New York: The Guilford Press; 2020. p. 13–29.
8. Koenen KC, Ratanatharathorn A, Ng L, McLaughlin KA, Bromet EJ, Stein DJ, et al. Posttraumatic stress disorder in the World Mental Health Surveys. Psychol Med. 2017;47(13):2260–74. https://doi.org/10.1017/S0033291717000708.
9. Forman-Hoffman VL, Bose J, Batts KR, Glasheen C, Hirsch E, Karg RS, et al. Correlates of lifetime exposure to one or more potentially traumatic events and subsequent posttraumatic stress among adults in the United States: results from the mental health surveillance study, 2008-2012. Substance Abuse and Mental Health Services Administration. 2016. https://www.samhsa.gov/data/report/correlates-lifetime-exposure-one-or-more-potentially-traumatic-events-and-subsequent. Accessed 2 Dec 2022.
10. Gillikin C, Habib L, Evces M, Bradley B, Ressler KJ, Sanders J. Trauma exposure and PTSD symptoms associate with violence in inner city civilians. J Psychiatr Res. 2016;83:1–7. https://doi.org/10.1016/j.jpsychires.2016.07.027.
11. Benjet C, Bromet E, Karam EG, Kessler RC, McLaughlin KA, Ruscio AM, et al. The epidemiology of traumatic event exposure worldwide: results from the World Mental Health Survey Consortium. Psychol Med. 2016;46(2):327–43. https://doi.org/10.1017/S0033291715001981.
12. McCall-Hosenfeld JS, Mukherjee S, Lehman EB. The prevalence and correlates of lifetime psychiatric disorders and trauma exposures in urban and rural settings: results from the National Comorbidity Survey Replication (NCS-R). PLoS One. 2014;9(11):e112416. https://doi.org/10.1371/journal.pone.0112416.
13. Howlett JR, Stein MB. Prevention of trauma and stressor-related disorders: a review. Neuropsychopharmacology. 2016;41(1):357–69. https://doi.org/10.1038/npp.2015.261.
14. Bryant RA, O'Donnell ML, Creamer M, McFarlane AC, Silove D. A multisite analysis of the fluctuating course of posttraumatic stress disorder. JAMA Psychiat. 2013;70(8):839–46. https://doi.org/10.1001/jamapsychiatry.2013.1137.
15. Badura-Brack AS, Heinrichs-Graham E, McDermott TJ, Becker KM, Ryan TJ, Khanna MM, Wilson TW. Resting-state neurophysiological abnormalities in posttraumatic stress disorder: a magnetoencephalography study. Front Neurosci. 2017;11:205. https://doi.org/10.3389/fnhum.2017.00205.
16. Crocq MA, Crocq L. From shell shock and war neurosis to posttraumatic stress disorder: a history of psychotraumatology. Dialogues Clin Neurosci. 2000;2(1):47–55.
17. Ellis PS. The origins of the war neuroses (Part I). J Roy Nav Med Serv. 1984;70:168–77. https://archive.org/details/JRNMSVOL70Images/page/n185/mode/2up. Accessed 2 Dec 2022.
18. Glynn TR. The traumatic neuroses. Lancet. 1910;176(4549):1332–6. https://doi.org/10.1016/S0140-6736(00)52735-4.
19. Ellis PS. The origins of the war neuroses (Part II). J Roy Nav Med Serv. 1985;71:32–44. https://archive.org/details/JRNMSVOL71Images/page/n43/mode/2up. Accessed 2 Dec 2022.
20. North C, Suris AM, Smith RP, King RV. The evolution of PTSD criteria across editions of DSM. Ann Clin Psychiatry. 2016;28(3):197–208.
21. van der Kolk BA. The history of trauma in psychiatry. In: Friedman MJ, Keane TM, Resick PA, editors. Handbook of PTSD: science and practice. New York; The Guilford Press; 2007. p. 19–36.
22. Freud S. The aetiology of hysteria. 1896. https://icpla.edu/wp-content/uploads/2012/10/Freud-S.-Aetiology-of-Hysteria-C.P.-vol.1-1924-p.183-221.pdf. Accessed 2 Dec 2022.
23. Masson JM. Freud and the seduction theory. The Atlantic. 1984. https://www.theatlantic.com/magazine/archive/1984/02/freud-and-the-seduction-theory/376313/. Accessed 2 Dec 2022.
24. Ferenczi S. Confusion of the tongues between the adults and the child—(the language of tenderness and passion). Int J Psychoanal. 1949;30:225–30. https://icpla.edu/wp-content/uploads/2012/11/Ferenczi-S-Confusion-of-Tongues-Intl-J-Psychoa.-vol.30-p.225-1949.pdf. Accessed 2 Dec 2022..
25. World Health Organization. International statistical classification of diseases and related health problems. 11th ed. 2020. https://icd.who.int/browse11/l-m/en#/http%3a%2f%2fid.who.int%2ficd%2fentity%2f991786158. Accessed 2 Dec 2022.
26. Bremner JD. Neuroimaging in posttraumatic stress disorder and other stress-related disorders. Neuroimaging Clin N Am. 2007;17(4):523–38, ix. https://doi.org/10.1016/j.nic.2007.07.003.
27. Ahmad S, Feder A, Lee EJ, Wang Y, Southwick SM, Schlackman E, et al. Earthquake impact in a remote South Asian population: psychosocial factors and posttraumatic symptoms. J Trauma Stress. 2010;23(3):408–12. https://doi.org/10.1002/jts.20535.
28. Duncan LE, Cooper BN, Shen H. Robust findings from 25 years of PTSD genetics research. Curr Psychiatry Rep. 2018;20(12):115. https://doi.org/10.1007/s11920-018-0980-1.
29. Bryant RA, Nickerson A, Creamer M, O'Donnell M, Forbes D, Galatzer-Levy I, et al. Trajectory of post-traumatic stress following traumatic injury: 6-year follow-up. Br J Psychol. 2015;206(5):417–23. https://doi.org/10.1192/bjp.bp.114.145516.
30. Chard KM, Kaysen DL, Galovski TE, Nixon RDV, Monson CM. Cognitive processing therapy. In: Forbes D, Bisson JI, Monson CM, Berliner L, editors. Effective treatments for PTSD: practical guidelines from the International Society for Traumatic Stress Studies. New York: The Guilford Press; 2020. p. 210–33.
31. Ehlers A. Cognitive therapy. In: Forbes D, Bisson JI, Monson CM, Berliner L, editors. Effective treatments for PTSD: practical guidelines from the International Society for Traumatic Stress Studies. New York: The Guilford Press; 2020. p. 255–71.

32. Shapiro F, Russell MC, Lee C, Schubert SJ. Eye movement desensitization and reprocessing therapy. In: Forbes D, Bisson JI, Monson CM, Berliner L, editors. Effective treatments for PTSD: practical guidelines from the International Society for Traumatic Stress Studies. New York: The Guilford Press; 2020. p. 234–54.
33. Riggs DS, Tate L, Chrestman K, Foa EB. Prolonged exposure. In: Forbes D, Bisson JI, Monson CM, Berliner L, editors. Effective treatments for PTSD: practical guidelines from the International Society for Traumatic Stress Studies. New York: The Guilford Press; 2020. p. 188–209.
34. Forbes D, Bisson JI, Monson CM, Berliner L. Effective treatments for PTSD: practical guidelines from the International Society for Traumatic Stress Studies. New York: The Guilford Press; 2020.
35. Bisson JI, Lewis C, Roberts NP. ISTSS PTSD prevention and treatment guidelines: methodology. In: Forbes D, Bisson JI, Monson CM, Berliner L, editors. Effective treatments for PTSD: practical guidelines from the International Society for Traumatic Stress Studies. New York: The Guilford Press; 2020. p. 90–108.
36. Sadock BJ, Ahmad S, Sadock VA. Kaplan & Sadock's pocket handbook of clinical psychiatry. 6th ed. Philadelphia: Wolters Kluwer; 2019.
37. Gorman I, Belser AB, Jerome L, Hennigan C, Shechet B, Hamilton S, et al. Posttraumatic growth after MDMA-assisted psychotherapy for posttraumatic stress disorder. J Trauma Stress. 2020;33(2):161–70. https://doi.org/10.1002/jts.22479.
38. Eidhof MB, June ter Heide FJ, van Der Aa N, Schreckenbach M, Schmidt U, Brand BL, et al. The dissociative subtype of PTSD interview (DSP-I): development and psychometric properties. J Trauma Dissociation. 2019;20(5):564–81. https://doi.org/10.1080/15299732.2019.1597806.
39. Wolf EJ, Miller MW, Kilpatrick D, Resnick HS, Badour CL, Marx BP, et al. ICD-11 complex PTSD in US nationals and veteran samples: prevalence and structural associations with PTSD. Clin Psychol Sci. 2015;3(2):215–29. https://doi.org/10.1177/2167702614545480.
40. Cloitre M, Karatzias T, Ford JD. Treatment of complex PTSD. In: Forbes D, Bisson JI, Monson CM, Berliner L, editors. Effective treatments for PTSD: practical guidelines from the International Society for Traumatic Stress Studies. New York: The Guilford Press; 2020. p. 365–82.
41. Liddell BJ, Nickerson A, Felmingham KL, Malhi GS, Cheung J, Den M, et al. Complex posttraumatic stress disorder symptom profiles in traumatized refugees. J Trauma Stress. 2019;32(6):822–32. https://doi.org/10.1002/jts.22453.
42. Ford JD. New findings questioning the construct validity of complex posttraumatic stress disorder (cPTSD): let's take a closer look. Eur J Psychotramtol. 2020;11(1):1708145. https://doi.org/10.1080/20008198.2019.1708145.
43. Achterhof R, Huntjens RJC, Meewisse ML, Kiers HAL. Assessing the application of latent class and latent profile analysis for evaluating the construct validity of complex posttraumatic stress disorder: cautions and limitations. Eur J Psychotramtol. 2019;10(1):1698223. https://doi.org/10.1080/20008198.2019.169223.
44. Karatzias T, Hyland P, Bradley A, Cloitre M, Roberts NP, Bisson JI, Shevlin M. Risk factors and comorbidity of ICD-11 PTSD and complex PTSD: findings from a trauma-exposed population based sample of adults in the United Kingdom. Depress Anxiety. 2019;36(9):887–94. https://doi.org/10.1002/da.22934.
45. Geoffrion S, Goncalves J, Robichaud I, Sader J, Giguère CE, Fortin M, et al. Systematic review and meta-analysis on acute stress disorder: rates following different types of traumatic events. Trauma Violence Abuse. 2020. https://doi.org/10.1177/1524838020933844.
46. Bachem R, Casey P. Adjustment disorder: a diagnosis whose time has come. J Affect Disord. 2018;227:243–53. https://doi.org/10.1016/j.ad.2017.10.034.
47. Perkonigg A, Lorenz L, Maercker A. Prevalence and correlates of ICD-11 adjustment disorder: findings from the Zurich Adjustment Disorder Study. Int J Clin Health Psychol. 2018;18(3):209–17. https://doi.org/10.1016/j.ijchp.2018.05.001.
48. Lenferink LIM, Nickerson A, de Keijser J, Smid GE, Boelen PA. Trajectories of grief, depression, and posttraumatic stress in disaster-bereaved people. Depress Anxiety. 2020;37(1):35–44. https://doi.org/10.1002/da.22850.
49. Lundorff M, Holmgren H, Zachariae R, Farver-Vestergaard I, O'Connor M. Prevalence of prolonged grief disorder id adult bereavement: a systematic review and meta-analysis. J Affect Disord. 2017;212:138–49. https://doi.org/10.1016/j.jad.2017.01.030.
50. Eisma MC, Lenferink LIM. Response to: prolonged grief disorder for ICD-11: the primacy of clinical utility and international applicability. Eur J Psychotramtol. 2018;9(1):1512249. https://doi.org/10.1080/20008198.2018.1512249.
51. Killikelly C, Maercker A. Prolonged grief disorder for ICD-11: the primacy of clinical utility and international applicability. Eur J Psychotramatol. 2017;8(Suppl 6):1476441. https://doi.org/10.1080/20008198.2018.1476441.
52. Djelantik AAAMJ, Smid GE, Mroz A, Kleber RJ, Boelen PA. The prevalence of prolonged grief disorder in bereaved individuals following unnatural losses: systematic review and meta regression analysis. J Affect Disord. 2020;265:146–56. https://doi.org/10.1016/j.jad.2020.010.34.
53. Alisic E, Conroy R, Thoresen S. Epidemiology, clinical presentation, and development considerations in children and adolescents. In: Forbes D, Bisson JI, Monson CM, Berliner L, editors. Effective treatments for PTSD: practical guidelines from the International Society for Traumatic Stress Studies. New York: The Guilford Press; 2020. p. 30–48.
54. Zeanah CH, Chesher T, Borris NW. American Academy of Child and Adolescent Psychiatry (AACAP) Committee on Quality Issues (CQI). Practice parameter for the assessment and treatment of children and adolescents with reactive attachment disorder and disinhibited social engagement disorder. J Am Acad Child Adolesc Psychiatry. 2016;55(11):990–1003. https://doi.org/10.1016/j.jaac.2016.08.004.
55. Humphreys KL, Nelson CA, Fox NA, Zeanah CH. Signs of reactive attachment disorder and disinhibited social engagement disorder at 12 years: effects of institutional care history and high-quality foster care. Dev Psychopathol. 2017;29(2):675–84. https://doi.org/10.1017/S0954579417000256.
56. Gleason MM, Fox NA, Drury S, et al. Validity of evidence-derived criteria for reactive attachment disorder: indiscriminately social/disinhibited and emotionally withdrawn/inhibited types. J Am Acad Child Adolesc Psychiatry. 2011;50(3):216–31. https://doi.org/10.1016/j.jaac.2010.12.012.
57. Hong M, Moon DS, Chang H, Lee SY, Cho SW, Lee KS, et al. Incidence and comorbidity of reactive attachment disorder: based on national health insurance claims data, 2010-2012 in Korea. Psychiatry Investig. 2018;15(2):118–23. https://doi.org/10.30773/pi.2017.11.01.
58. Schauer M, Elbert T. Dissociation following traumatic stress. Z Psychol. 2010;218(2):109–27. https://doi.org/10.1027/0044-3409/a000018.
59. van der Hart O, Horst R. The dissociation theory of Pierre Janet. J Trauma Stress. 1989;2(4):397–412. https://doi.org/10.1007/BF00974598.

60. Loewenstein RJ. Dissociation debates: everything you know is wrong. Dialogues Clin Neurosci. 2018;20(3):229–42. https://doi.org/10.31887/DCNS.2018.20.3/rloewenstein.
61. Loewenstein RJ, Frewen P, Lewis-Fernández R. Dissociative disorders. In: Sadock BJ, Sadock VA, Ruiz P, editors. Kaplan & Sadock's comprehensive textbook of psychiatry. 10th ed. Philadelphia, PA: Wolters Kluwer; 2017. p. 1866–952.
62. Vermetten E, Schmahl C, Lindner S, Loewenstein RJ, Brener JD. Hippocampal and amygdalar volumes in dissociative identity disorder. Am J Psychiatry. 2006;163(4):630–6. https://doi.org/10.1176/appi.ajp.163.4.630.
63. Reinders AATS, Veltman DJ. Dissociative identity disorder: out of the shadows at last? Br J Psychiatry. 2020;219:413–4. https://doi.org/10.1192/bjp.2020.168.
64. Foote B, Smolin Y, Kaplan M, Legatt ME, Lipschitz D. Prevalence of dissociative disorders in psychiatric outpatients. Am J Psychiatry. 2006;163(4):623–9. https://doi.org/10.1176/appi.ajp.163.4.623.
65. Yu J, Ross CA, Keyes BB, Li Y, Dai Y, Zhang T, et al. Dissociative disorders among Chinese inpatients diagnosed with schizophrenia. J Trauma Dissociation. 2010;11(3):358–72. https://doi.org/10.1080/15299731003793468.
66. Sun P, Alvarez-Jimenez M, Lawrence K, Simpson K, Peach N, Bendall S. Investigating the prevalence of dissociative disorders and severe dissociative symptoms in first episode psychosis. Early Interv Psychiatry. 2019;13(6):1366–72. https://doi.org/10.1111/eip.12773.
67. Lyssenko L, Schmahl C, Bockhacker L, Vonderlin R, Bohus M, Kleindienst N. Dissociation in psychiatric disorders: a meta-analysis of studies using the dissociative experiences scale. Am J Psychiatry. 2018;175:37–46. https://doi.org/10.1176/appi.ajp.2017.17010025.
68. Anderson MC, Hanslmayr S. Neural mechanisms of motivated forgetting. Trends Cogn Sci. 2014;18(4):279–92. https://doi.org/10.1016/j.tics.2014.03.002.
69. van Ijzendoorn MH, Schungel C. The measurement of dissociative experiences in normal and clinical populations: meta-analytic validation of the Dissociative Experiences Scale (DES). Clin Psychol Rev. 1996;16(5):365–82. https://doi.org/10.1016/0272-7358(96)00006-2.
70. Radulovic J, Lee R, Ortony A. State-dependent memory: neurobiological advances and prospects for translation to dissociative amnesia. Front Behav Neurosci. 2018;12:259. https://doi.org/10.3389/fnbeh.2018.00259.
71. Kikuchi H, Fujii T, Abe N, Suzuki M, Takagi M, Mugikura S, Takahashi S, Mori E. Memory repression: brain mechanisms underlying dissociative amnesia. J Cogn Neurosci. 2009;22(3):602–13. https://doi.org/10.1162/jocn.2009.21212.
72. Sierra M, Baker D, Medford N, Lawrence E, Patel M, Phillips ML, David AS. Lamotrigine as an add-on treatment for depersonalized disorder: a retrospective study of 32 cases. Clin Neuropharmacol. 2006;29(5):253–8. https://doi.org/10.1097/01.WNF.0000228368.17970.DA.
73. Wicking M, Steiger F, Nees F, Diener SJ, Grimm O, Ruttorf M, et al. Deficient fear extinction memory in posttraumatic stress disorder. Neurobiol Learn Mem. 2016;136:116–26. https://doi.org/10.1016/j.nlm.2016.09.016.

Somatic Symptom and Related Disorders

20

Maria Kleinstäuber

The diagnostic entities belonging to the group of somatic symptom and related disorders (SSRD) share one common feature: persistent somatic symptoms [1]. *Somatic symptom disorder (SSD)*, *functional neurological symptom disorder (FNSD)*, and *psychological factors affecting other medical conditions (PFAOMC)* focus on distress, interference, and problems in adjusting to somatic symptoms. Although individuals with *illness anxiety disorder (IAD)* do not present with somatic symptoms, their mind is preoccupied with signs of somatic illness. Individuals with *factitious disorder (FD)* falsify somatic or psychological symptoms.

The diagnostic classification of somatic symptom-related psychological distress has gone through a dramatic change over the past decade. With the publication of the fifth revision of the *Diagnostic and Statistical Manual of Mental Disorders* (DSM-5), the group of somatic symptom and related disorders was introduced and replaced its precursor, the somatoform disorders. The previous diagnostic entities of somatization disorder, undifferentiated somatoform disorder, and pain disorder in DSM-IV [2] were replaced with the SSD. FNSD forms the equivalent to the former conversion disorder as does IAD to the former hypochondriasis. PFAOMC and FD were not part of the group of somatoform disorders in DSM-IV [2] but were integrated in other chapters. The category of somatoform disorders in DSM-IV was criticized for reinforcing a body-mind dualistic thinking through requiring somatic symptoms to be not or not sufficiently explained by a medical cause [3]. Physicians worldwide were concerned that the label "somatoform" would not be well accepted by patients. Because of the dominating focus on a lack of a medical explanation, individuals regarded the diagnosis as stigmatizing and implying that their symptoms are made up or "not real." The criteria of SSRD do not distinguish between medically unexplained and explained somatic complaints but shift the focus to the symptom-related psychological distress. In this sense, DSM-5 makes a first serious step of counteracting body-mind dualism by including psychological features as classification criteria and conceptualizing somatic symptoms in a sense of a biopsychosocial model (see Fig. 20.1).

M. Kleinstäuber (✉)
Department of Psychology, Utah State University, Logan, UT, USA
e-mail: maria.kleinstaeuber@usu.edu

W. W. IsHak (ed.), *Atlas of Psychiatry*, https://doi.org/10.1007/978-3-031-15401-0_20

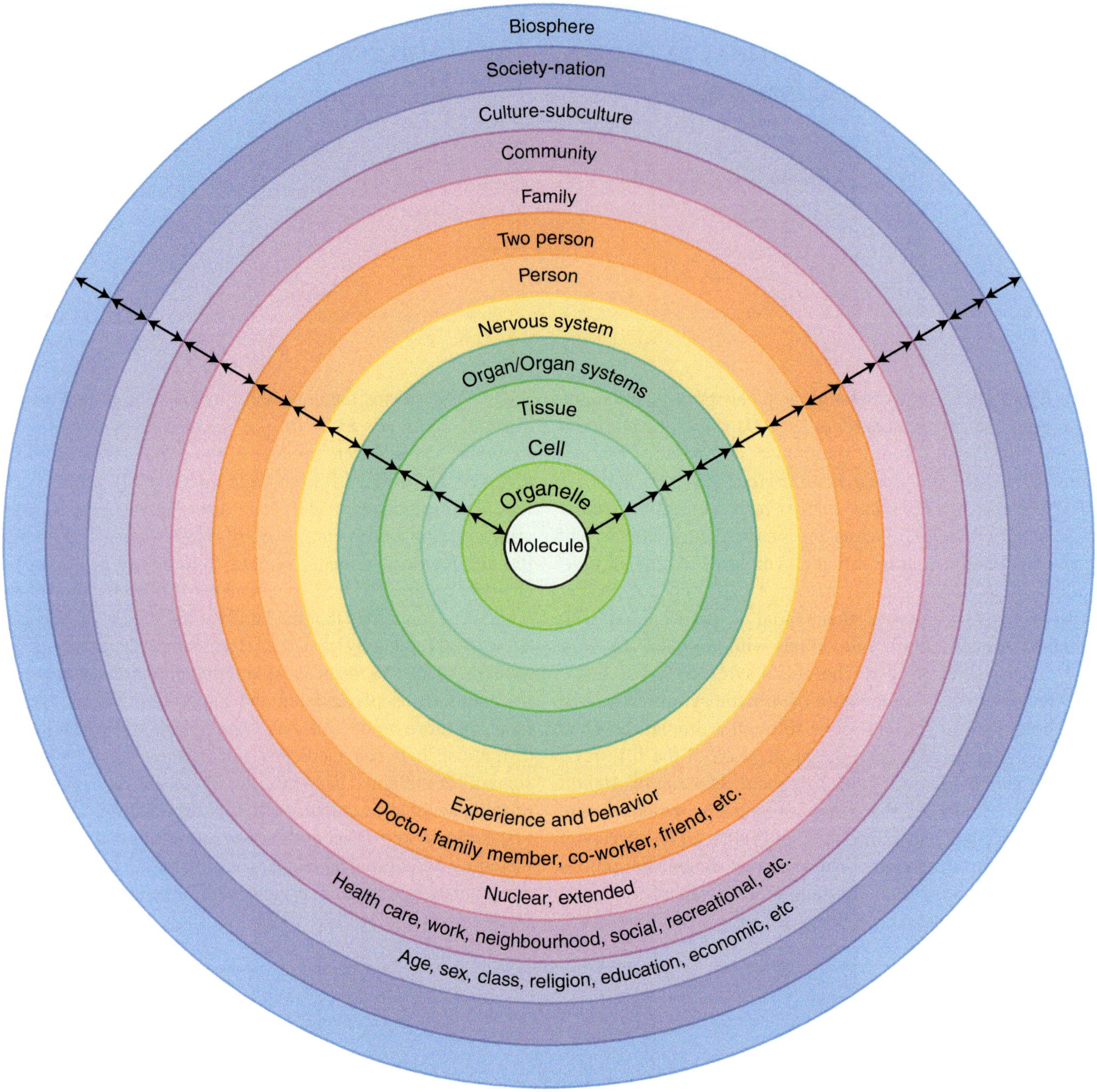

Fig. 20.1 The biopsychosocial model of a human being represents the natural system in a hierarchy and continuum. Each level in the hierarchy is assumed to operate according to a unique system (e.g., tissues and organs at biological level). The integration of these systems is critical in terms of understanding the biopsychosocial nature of the patient's problem. (*Adapted from* Engel et al. [74]; *with permission*)

Somatic Symptom Disorder

Phenomenology and Classification

The core characteristics of somatic symptom disorder (SSD) are described in Table 20.1. This diagnostic entity covers a very heterogeneous group of individuals [4]. SSD can be used to classify individuals with [4]:

(a) Persistent distressing somatic symptoms of monosymptomatic nature that are not or not sufficiently better explained by another medical condition (e.g., gastrointestinal symptoms in irritable bowel syndrome)
(b) Persistent distressing somatic symptoms of polysymptomatic nature that are not or not sufficiently better explained by another medical condition (e.g., former somatization disorder in DSM-IV)

Table 20.1 Checklist of characteristics of somatic symptom disorder according to the classification criteria in DSM-5

	Y	N	?
≥1 somatic symptom(s) that is(are) distressing or result(s) in significant disruption of daily life			
≥1 of the following psychological features:			
(a) Disproportionate and persistent thoughts about the seriousness of one's symptom			
(b) Persistently high level of anxiety about health or symptoms			
(c) Excessive time and energy devoted to these symptoms or health concerns			
Symptomatic state present >6 months (one somatic symptom may not be continuously present)			
Criteria of somatic symptom disorder met?			
Specifier: With dominant pain			
Specifier: Persistent (>6 months)			
Specifier: current severity (a) Mild (1 psychological feature) (b) Moderate (≥2 psychological features) (c) Severe (≥2 psychological features + multiple/one very severe somatic complaint(s))			

(c) Persistent distressing somatic symptoms caused by a known biomedical condition (e.g., fear of recurrence in successfully treated individual with cancer who has side effects from the medical treatment)
(d) Persistent distressing, more or less medically explained, pain symptom(s)
(e) Illness anxieties and present persistent distressing physical symptoms (IAD according to DSM-5 excludes present somatic symptoms)

Common functional somatic syndromes (FSS) are "characterized by patterns of persistent bodily complaints for which adequate examination does not reveal sufficiently explanatory structural or other specified pathology" [5; p. 946]. FSS are usually characterized by a strong interaction of biomedical and psychosocial factors, and individuals with FSS often show psychological features that meet the criteria of a SSD. Therefore, we introduce the characteristics of the three most common and best investigated FSS: irritable bowel syndrome (IBS) [6] (see Table 20.2), chronic fatigue syndrome (CFS) [7] (see Table 20.3), and fibromyalgia (FMS) [8] (see Table 20.4).

Table 20.2 Checklist of characteristics of irritable bowel syndrome (IBS) according to Rome IV criteria [6]

	Y	N	?
Recurrent abdominal pain, on average, ≥1 day per week in the last 3 months			
Abdominal pain associated with ≥2 of the following characteristics: (a) Related to defecation (worsening or improvement with defecation) (b) Associated with a change in frequency of stool (c) Associated with a change in form (appearance) of stool			
Criteria fulfilled for the last 3 months with symptom onset at least 6 months before diagnosis			
Criteria of irritable bowel syndrome met?			
Three subtypes of IBS: (a) IBS with predominant constipation (b) IBS with predominant diarrhea (c) IBS with predominant irregular bowel habits (mixed constipation and diarrhea)			

Table 20.3 Checklist of characteristics of chronic fatigue syndrome (CFS) according to the criteria by the International Chronic Fatigue Syndrome Study Group [7]

	Y	N	?
Clinically evaluated, unexplained, persistent, or relapsing chronic fatigue that meets all of the following criteria:			
(a) New or definite onset			
(b) Not the result of ongoing exertion			
(c) Not substantially alleviated by rest			
(d) Results in substantial reduction in previous levels of occupational, educational, social, or personal activities			
Concurrent occurrence of ≥4 of the following symptoms, all of which must have persisted or recurred during ≥6 consecutive months of illness and must not have predated the fatigue:			
(a) Self-reported impairment in short-term memory or concentration severe enough to cause substantial reduction in previous levels of occupational, educational, social, or personal activities			
(b) Sore throat			
(c) Tender cervical or axillary lymph nodes			
(d) Muscle pain, multi-joint pain without joint swelling or redness			
(e) Headaches of a new type, pattern, or severity			
(f) Unrefreshing sleep			
(g) Post-exertional malaise lasting more than 24 h			
Criteria of chronic fatigue syndrome met?			

Table 20.4 Checklist of characteristics of fibromyalgia (FMS) according to the criteria by the American College of Rheumatology [8]

Symptom severity scale (SSS)				
For each of the following three symptoms, indicate the level of severity over the past week using the following scale: 0 = no problem 1 = slight or mild problems, generally mild or intermittent 2 = moderate, considerable problems, often present and/or at a moderate level 3 = severe: pervasive, continuous, life-disturbing problems				
(a) Fatigue	0	1	2	3
(b) Waking unrefreshed	0	1	2	3
(c) Cognitive symptoms	0	1	2	3
Considering somatic symptoms in general, indicate whether the patient has: 0 = no symptoms 1 = few symptoms 2 = a moderate number of symptoms 3 = a great deal of symptoms				
Somatic symptoms in general[a]	0	1	2	3
SSS score[b]:				
Widespread pain index (WPI)				
Note the number of areas in which the patient has had pain over the last week				
Left shoulder girdle	Y	N		
Right shoulder girdle	Y	N		
Left upper arm	Y	N		
Right upper arm	Y	N		
Left lower arm	Y	N		
Right lower arm	Y	N		
Left hip (buttock, trochanter)	Y	N		
Right hip (buttock, trochanter)	Y	N		
Left upper leg	Y	N		
Right upper leg	Y	N		
Left lower leg	Y	N		
Right lower leg	Y	N		
Left jaw	Y	N		
Right jaw	Y	N		
Chest	Y	N		
Abdomen	Y	N		
Upper back	Y	N		
Lower back	Y	N		
Neck	Y	N		
In how many areas has the patient had pain? Score will be between 0 and 19 **WPI score:**				
	Y	N	?	
Three diagnostic criteria of fibromyalgia according to ACR				
(a) WPI score $\geq$ 7 and symptom severity (SS) scale score $\geq$ 5 OR WPI 3–6 and SS scale score $\geq$ 9				
(b) Criterion (a) met for $\geq$3 months				
(c) Pain cannot be explained better by another disorder				
All of the following three criteria of fibromyalgia by the ACR are met?				

[a]Somatic symptoms that might be considered: muscle pain, irritable bowel syndrome, fatigue/tiredness, thinking or remembering problems, muscle weakness, headache, pain/cramps in the abdomen, numbness/tingling, dizziness, insomnia, depression, constipation, pain in the upper abdomen, nausea, nervousness, chest pain, blurred vision, fever, diarrhea, dry mouth, itching, wheezing, Raynaud's phenomenon, hives/welts, ringing in ears, vomiting, heartburn, oral ulcers, loss of/change in taste, seizures, dry eyes, shortness of breath, loss of appetite, rash, sun sensitivity, hearing difficulties, easy bruising, hair loss, frequent urination, painful urination, and bladder spasms

[b]The SSS score is the sum of the severity of the three symptoms (fatigue, waking unrefreshed, cognitive symptoms) plus the extent (severity) of somatic symptoms in general. The final score is between 0 and 12

Epidemiology

Persistent, psychologically distressing somatic symptoms for which a medical cause cannot or not sufficiently be identified are a common phenomenon in the general population [9]. The prevalence of SSD is not known. The prevalence of an undifferentiated somatoform disorder according to DSM-IV (which requires minimum one symptom) was estimated to be 19.7% [10]. The lifetime prevalence of the Somatization Index-4,6 indicating a minimum of four or six somatoform symptoms in men or women, respectively, is 5.6%, and the 12-month prevalence is 4.3% [11].

Individuals who meet the criteria of a somatization disorder make 1% of the general population [12]. Pain disorder (according to DSM-IV) has a 12-month prevalence of 8.1% [11]. The point-prevalence rate of CFS according to the criteria by Fukuda et al. [7] ranges between 0.2% and 0.4% [13, 14]. The point-prevalence of individuals meeting the criteria of FMS according to the American College of Rheumatology [8] is estimated to be 3.3% [15]. The Rome IV criteria of IBS are met by 3.2% of the general population [16].

Etiology and Pathophysiology

SSD is conceptualized rather as complex interaction of physiological, cognitive, emotional, and behavioral responses [17–19] than as one specific disease process. Most of the etiological models of SSD distinguish between predisposing, precipitating, and perpetuating factors. We provide one example, the cognitive perceptional model of somatoform disorders by Kirmayer and Taillefer in Fig. 20.2. This model describes perceptual, cognitive, emotional, behavioral, and

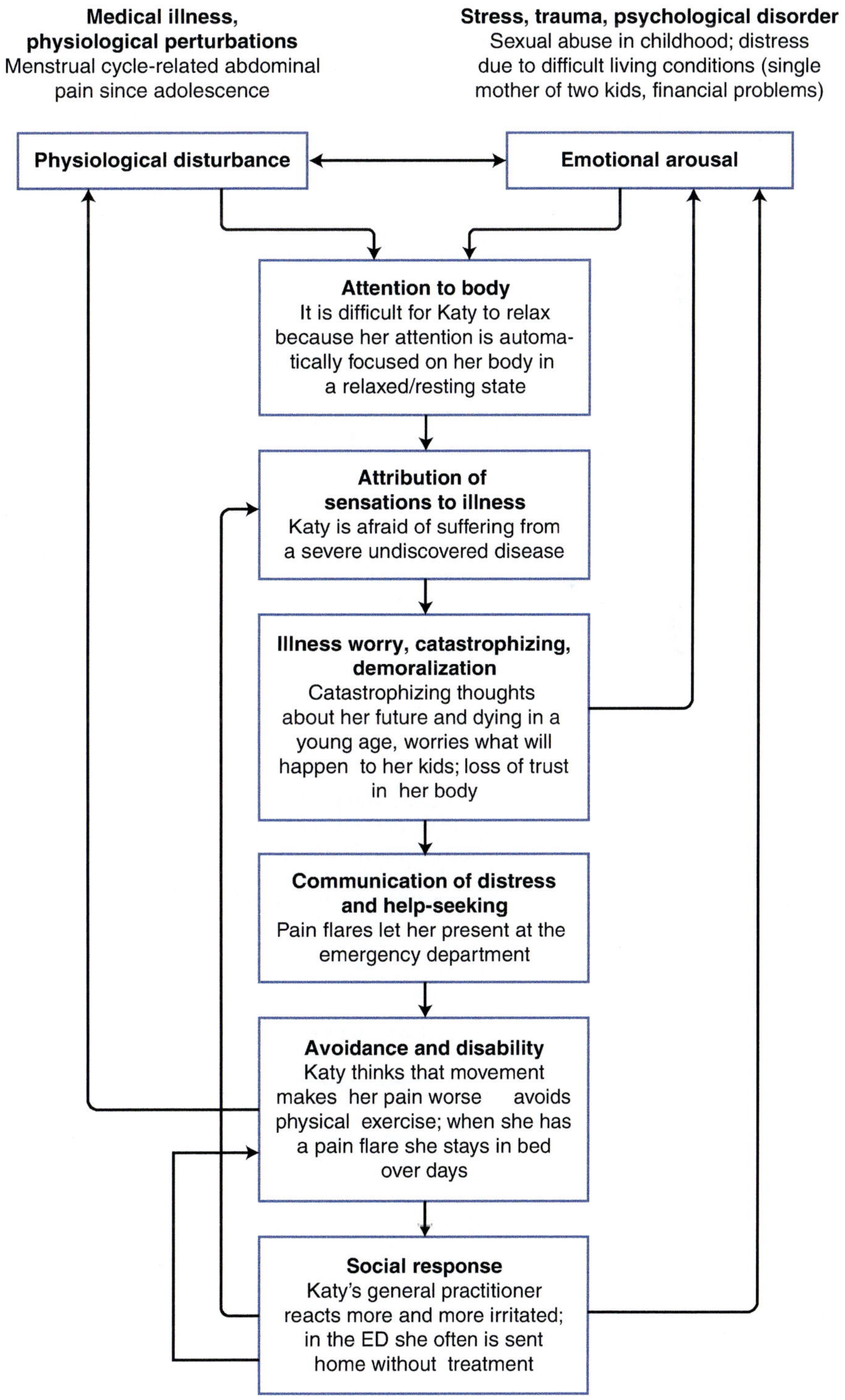

Fig. 20.2 Cognitive perceptional model of somatoform disorders. According to this model, a physical sensation can be caused by different processes (e.g., medical illness or distress). It is interpreted as a sign of illness and triggers help-seeking behavior which becomes a perpetuating factor. Due to negative doctor-patient interactions and the interpretation of their sensations as threatening symptoms, distress develops. This model integrates also the social response of the individual's environment (e.g., negative reactions from health-care providers) which further lowers the motivation to proactively self-manage symptoms. (*Adapted from* Kirmayer and Taillefer [75]; *with permission*)

interactional processes that may contribute to somatic distress.

Predictive coding models of somatic symptom distress focus on our perceptual system [20] (Fig. 20.3). In contrast to previous etiological models, predictive coding models suggest that body perceptions are a result of a continuous process of generating, testing, and refining hypotheses of our perceptual system. Whereas previous etiological model assumed that SSD mostly starts with a peripheral physiological input (e.g., a stress reaction), a predictive coding model can also explain the phenomenon of symptom perceptions that appear without this peripheral physiological input.

Placebo and nocebo mechanisms are another important paradigm to explain SSD. The placebo effect occurs after the administration of a placebo, an inert treatment [21]. Placebo-related effects can also occur in situations where actually no placebo is given; they describe a "biological phenomenon that is due to psychosocial context of the patient and therapy" [21]. By definition, the nocebo effect means "negative health-related changes in the mind-brain body unit" that are initiated and modulated by individuals' expectations [22]. Figure 20.4 summarizes mechanisms of a placebo and nocebo response [21].

Recent research shifts focus on the role of emotions in the chronic manifestation of somatic symptoms. We know from experimental research that negative affectivity has significant impact on physical symptom perception. Figure 20.5 introduces a model of an "emotional shift" explaining potential mechanisms that are involved in the transition from acute to chronic pain [23].

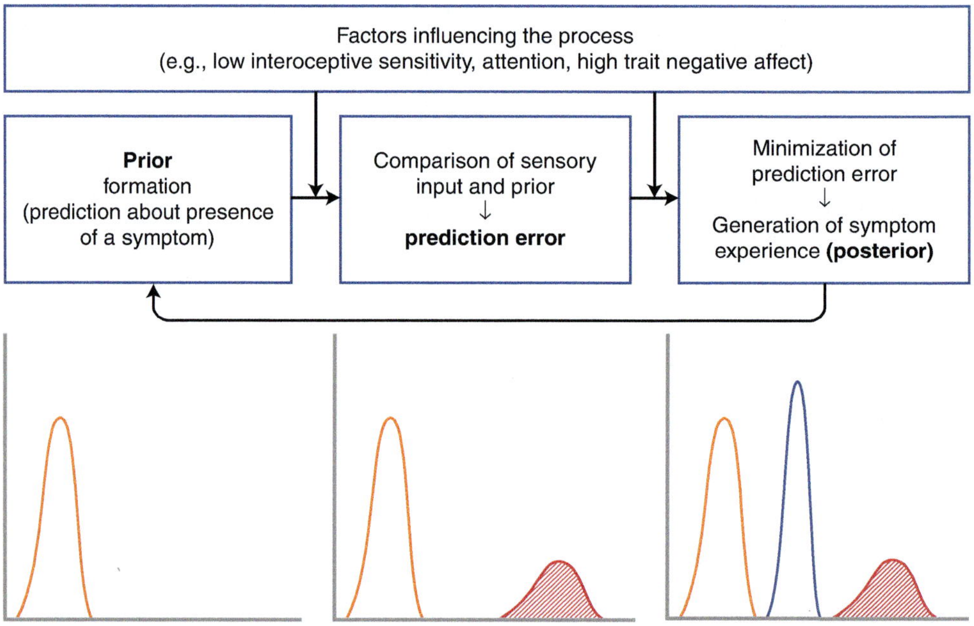

Fig. 20.3 A predictive coding model of somatic symptom disorder proposes that the process of symptom perception starts with the formation of a so-called prior which is a prediction about the presence of symptoms based on expectations and previous experiences with symptoms. Afferent sensory input is compared to this prediction or prior, and when they deviate, a prediction error occurs. Our perceptual system is based on minimizing the prediction error and generates a symptom experience (or posterior) that best matches the prior and prediction error. The posterior functions as input that determines the prior in a next episode of symptom perception. (*Adapted from* van den Bergh [20]; *with permission*)

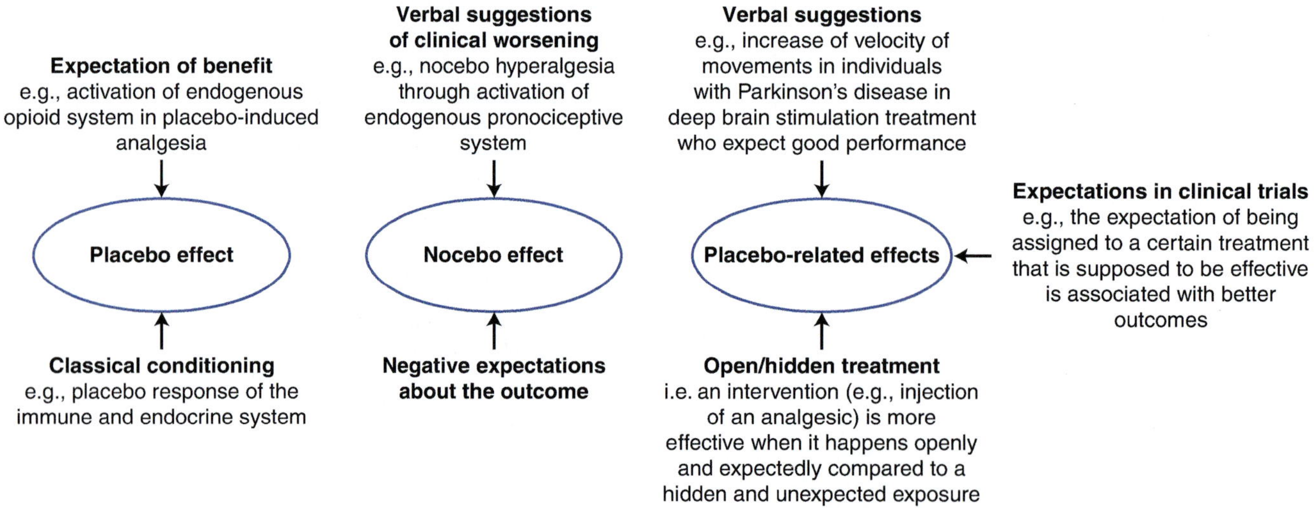

Fig. 20.4 Summary of clinical observations and potential mechanisms of placebo, nocebo, and placebo-related responses

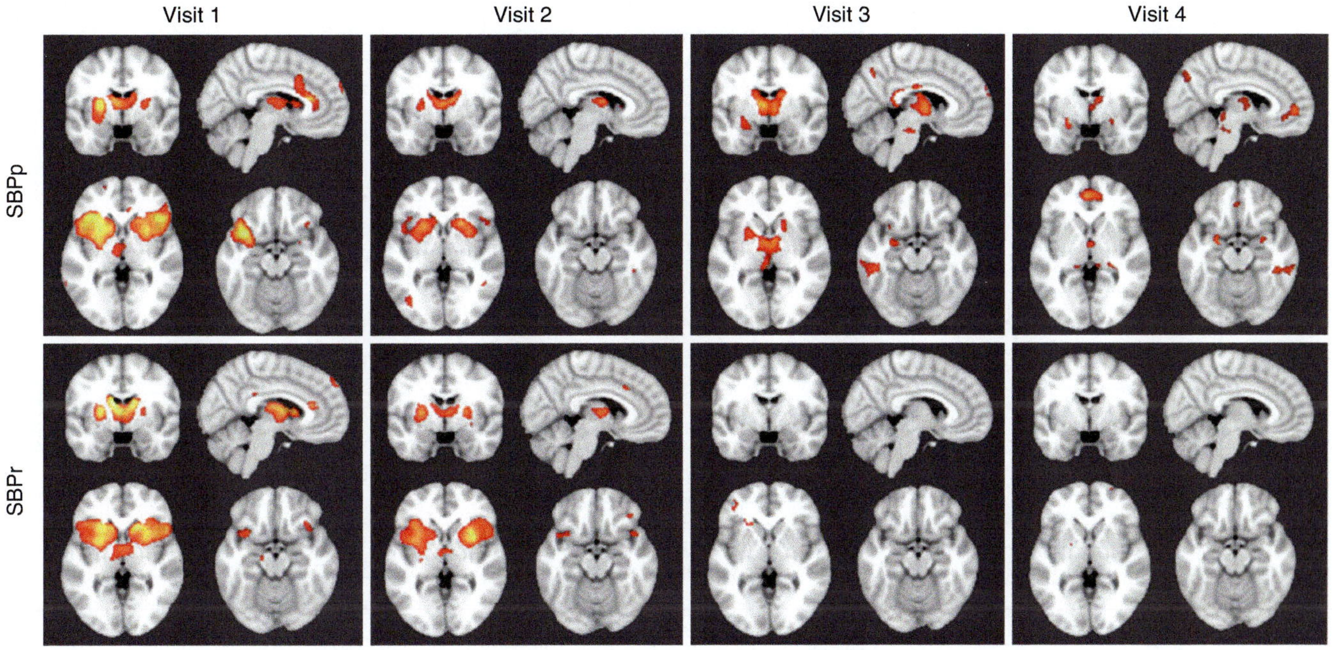

Fig. 20.5 Studies of areas of the brain that are involved in the transition from acute to chronic pain showed that in the context of a chronic manifestation of pain, there is a shift away from classic pain-processing regions in the brain toward emotional networks. This "emotional shift" could explain the fact that pain may persist in patients with emotional distress [23]. The figure shows changes in the activation of brain areas in individuals with persisting and recovering subacute back pain (SBPp and SBPr, respectively) across four visits. At visits 1 and 2 in both groups, similar brain areas are activated (e.g., bilateral thalamus, insula, mid-anterior cingulate cortex, basal ganglia). At visit 4, individuals with persistent SBP show increased activation in the medical prefrontal cortex and the amygdala, whereas recovered individuals showed no significant activity. (*From* Hashmi et al. 2013 [23])

Research on certain FSS, such as IBS, CFS, and FMS, has given increasing insight to the pathophysiology of SSD. In IBS, different underlying mechanisms associated with a dysfunction of the so-called gut-brain axis have been identified [24]. They are summarized in Fig. 20.6. Figures 20.7 and 20.8 show indicators of acute enteric infection and low-grade mucosal inflammation, both potential pathophysiological mechanisms of IBS [24].

Most recent studies show that CFS reflects the activation of biologically ancient, evolutionary responses to injury and a pathological inability of the human body to turn these responses off [25]. Figure 20.9 summarizes a sickness behavior inflammation model of CFS.

Most recent research has demonstrated that FMS is a disorder of pain regulation and central sensitization [26]. Results of different research methods have shown that individuals with FMS show perturbations of their pain processing and regulation that amplify the sensation of pain or decrease pain inhibition (e.g., greater neuronal activity in pain-processing brain regions, exaggerated pain response to experimental stimuli, changes in brain morphology, regulation of peripheral or brain receptors, and altered levels of pain-related neuropeptides). Figure 20.10 shows results of a meta-analysis of functional MRI (fMRI) studies of areas activated by noxious stimulation in individuals with FMS and healthy controls.

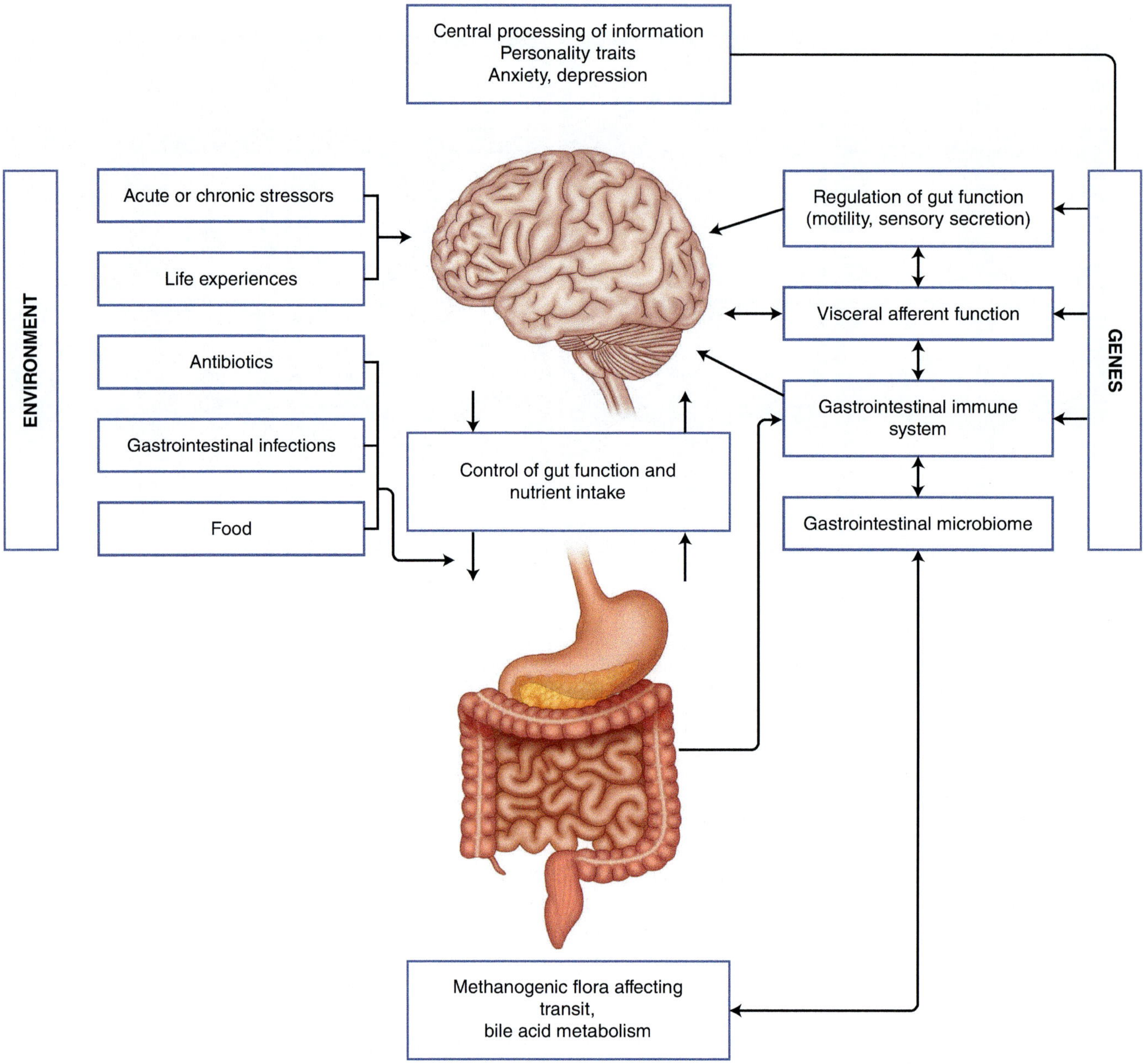

Fig. 20.6 A model of factors that are proposed to be involved in the manifestation of irritable bowel syndrome (IBS). The model assumes that multiple interacting pathways have impact on the manifestation of IBS: genetic factors (e.g., mutation of SCN5A), post-infectious changes (e.g., post-inflammatory neuroplastic changes, visceral hyperalgesia, and muscle hypercontractility), disturbances in the intestinal microbiota (e.g., small intestinal bacterial overgrowth), low-grade mucosal inflammation, immune activation and altered intestinal permeability, disordered bile salt metabolism, abnormalities in serotonin metabolism, and alterations in the brain function (e.g., reduced inhibitory feedback on the emotional arousal network). (*Adapted from* Holtmann et al. [24]; *with permission*)

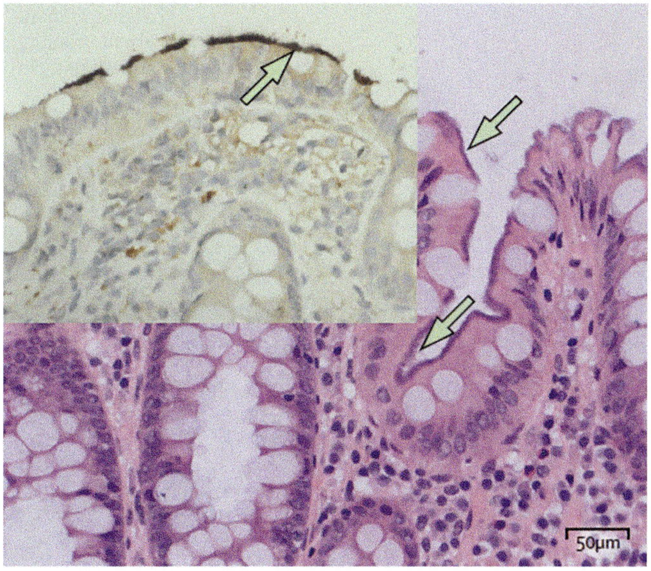

Fig. 20.7 Histological presentation of a colonic spirochetosis in an individual with irritable bowel syndrome (IBS), indicated by blue fringe arrows on hematoxylin and eosin staining and, inset, Warthin-Starry staining. Colonic spirochetosis is an example of a gastrointestinal infection that frequently precedes the onset of IBS. (*Reprinted from* Holtmann et al. [24]; *with permission*)

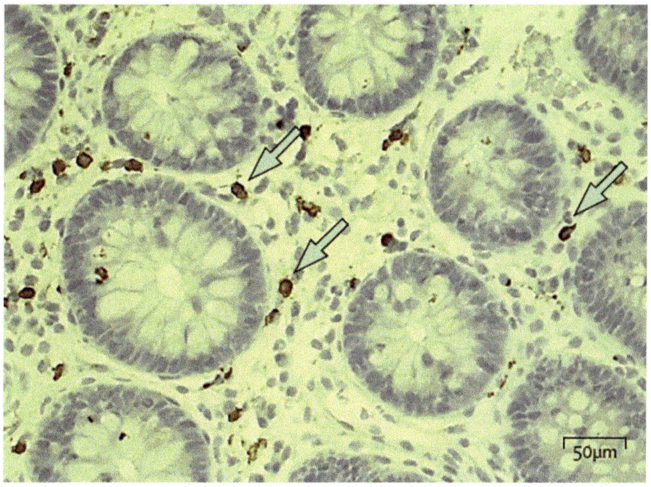

Fig. 20.8 Immunostaining of colonic mucosa shows increased mast cells in colonic mucosa in the lamina propria in a patient with irritable bowel syndrome (IBS) (CD117 immunostaining). Studies have shown indicators of low-grade mucosal inflammation in individuals with IBS, for example, increased concentrations of pro-inflammatory cytokines and mast cells in close proximity to the enteric nerve fibers in the gastrointestinal mucosa. (*Reprinted from* Holtmann et al. [24]; *with permission*)

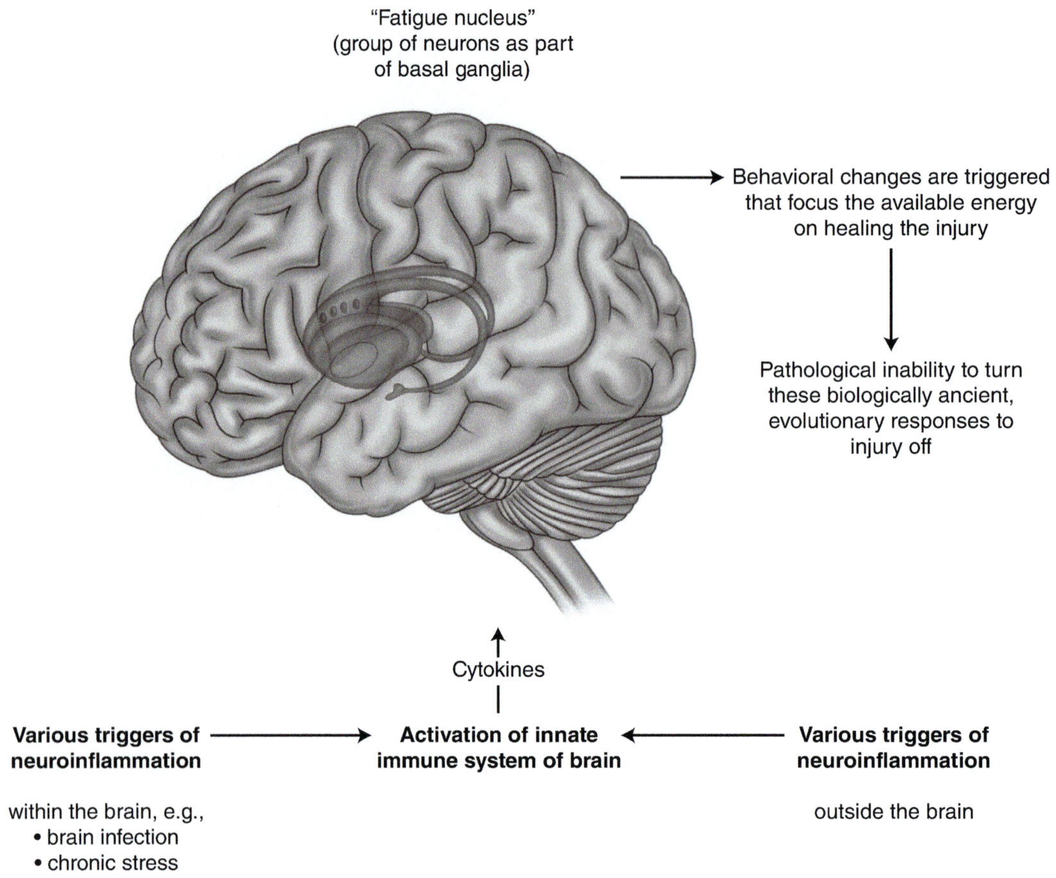

Fig. 20.9 Komaroff (2019) [25] postulates processes of inflammation and sickness behavior as underlying mechanisms of chronic fatigue syndrome (CFS). Results of most recent studies inspired the discussion of CFS reflecting the activation of biologically ancient, evolutionary responses to injury and a pathological inability to turn these responses off. The theory assumes that a neuroinflammation can be induced by numerous different reasons within the brain (e.g., brain infection, chronic stress) or outside the brain. The neuroinflammation produces cytokines that activate an innate immune system inside the brain (a group of neurons called "fatigue nucleus" as part of the basal ganglia). Behavioral changes are triggered that focus the available energy on healing the injury. This theory goes along with evidence of indicators of hypometabolism, high numbers of pro-inflammatory species and low numbers of anti-inflammatory species, and a general downregulation of the hypothalamic-pituitary-adrenal axis

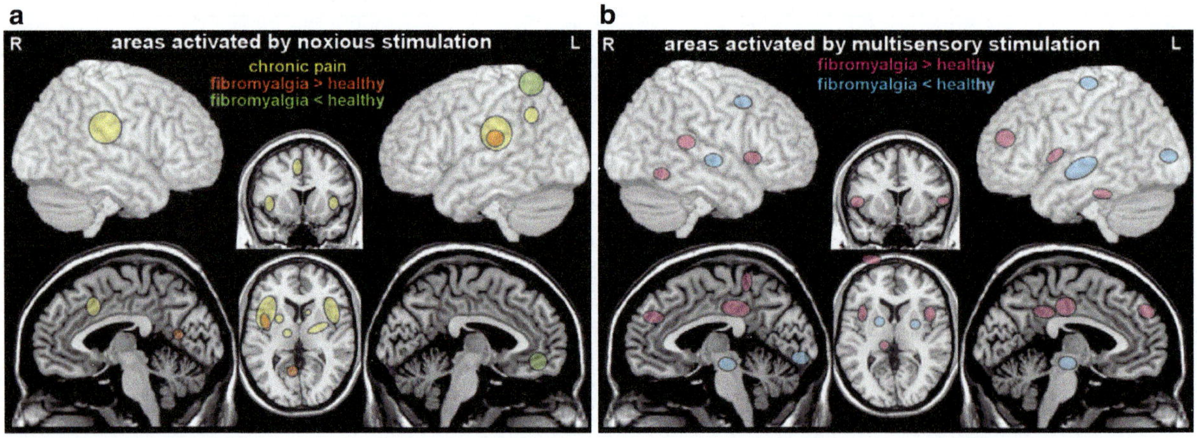

Fig. 20.10 (**a**) A meta-analysis of functional MRI (fMRI) studies of areas activated by *noxious* stimulation reported very similar patterns in healthy individuals (not depicted) and in individuals with chronic pain conditions (highlighted in yellow) [76]. A meta-analysis that combined studies using multiple functional imaging techniques to compare areas activated by *noxious* stimulation identified areas that were more (orange) or less (green) activated in individuals with fibromyalgia compared to healthy subjects [77]. (**b**) Machine learning analyses based on fMRI responses to *sensory* stimuli were applied in a recently published meta-analysis to identify a pattern of activation differences that accurately distinguished subjects with fibromyalgia from healthy individuals [78]. The derived classifier map comprised enhanced activations (highlighted in pink) in heteromodal and self-referential regions and reduced activations (highlighted in blue) in primary and secondary visual and auditory regions, lateral prefrontal cortex, cerebellum, diencephalon, and midbrain. (*Reprinted from* Richard et al. 2019 [79], *with permission*)

Treatment

This subsection refers to the subgroups (a), (b), (d), and (e) of SSD described under the section "Phenomenology and Classification" and excludes persistent distressing somatic symptoms caused by a known biomedical condition because the latter requires specific treatments related to the underlying medical condition. The treatment pathway of individuals suffering from SSD and related disorders is usually initiated with appointments with the general practitioner or medical specialists. Figure 20.11 summarizes general principles of the assessment of individuals with SSD as well as a stepped-care approach to adequately address patients' needs in this early phase of the course of treatment [27].

There are various psychological approaches to treat SSD. They are an important component of a multidisciplinary treatment of moderate to severe forms of SSD (see Fig. 20.11). Figure 20.12 summarizes common psychological approaches for SSD and selected FSS that have demonstrated evidence of efficacy in randomized controlled trials.

Regarding pharmacotherapy for SSD and related FSS, the following recommendations are given [27–29]:

- Different types of antidepressants are recommended for severe forms of SSD that are associated with dominant pain and/or with comorbid mental health problems.
- Peripheral pharmacotherapy to regulate bowel function and antidepressants have low evidence of efficacy in the treatment of IBS.
- Centrally acting agents such as antidepressants and anticonvulsants (e.g., gabapentin, pregabalin) show low to moderate evidence of efficacy in the treatment of FMS. Tricyclic antidepressants show moderate effects, and their efficacy has been more extensively examined than the efficacy of newer antidepressants or other antidepressant agents.

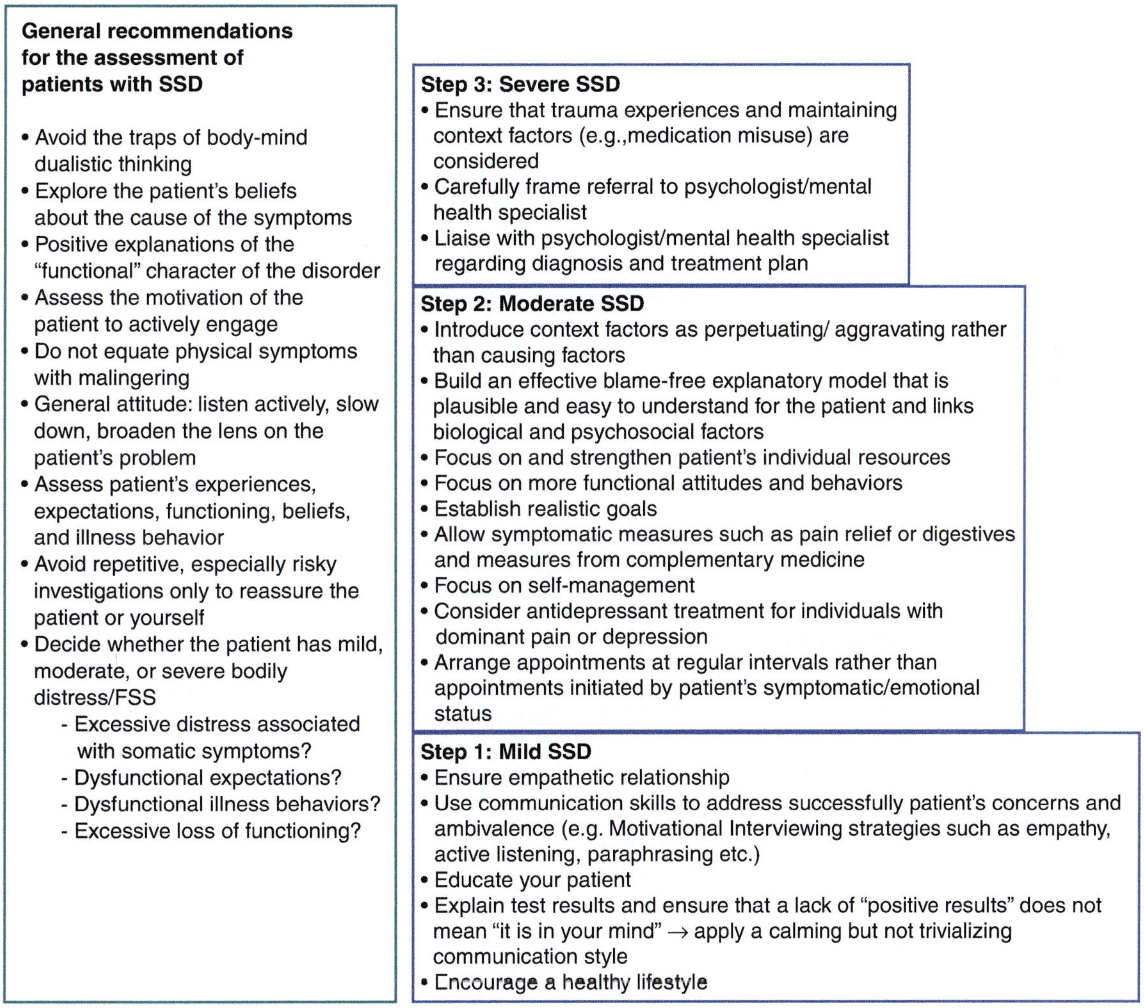

Fig. 20.11 Summary of general principles of the assessment and a stepped-care approach for the management of individuals with somatic symptom disorder (SSD)

Cognitive behavior therapy	Patient education: biopsychosocial model, stress management, reducing body-focused attention, cognitive reappraisal, reduction of illness behaviors
Psychodynamic interpersonal therapy	Clarifying the link between emotions and bodily complaints in the context of patients' actual and early interpersonal relationships. It is assumed that early dysfunctional bodily relationship experiences shape the tendency to experience disabling bodily symptoms that the patient cannot explain or control later in life.
Acceptance and commitment therapy	Patients learn to commit to alternative behaviors than controlling and avoidance behaviors. They learn to focus on living a full and meaningful life. Patients have the choice between controlling their somatic symptoms and related negative emotions/cognitions or living according to chosen values.
Mindfulness-based cognitive behavior therapy	Different kinds of mediation, yoga exercises, and body scans help patients to learn to be mindful towards their body, emotions, mental states, and mind states. Patients are helped to move towards acceptance of their symptoms and increase self-compassion.
Graded exercise therapy (CFS)	Therapeutic approach is based on deconditioning and exercise intolerance theories: Somatic symptoms and distress are perpetuated by reversible physiological changes of deconditioning and avoidance of activity.
Adaptive pacing therapy (CFS)	Therapeutic approach is based on chronic fatigue syndrome as an organic disease process that is not reversible by changes in behavior and which results in a reduced and finite amount (envelope) of available energy. Adaptation is achieved by helping the participant to plan and pace activity to reduce or avoid fatigue, achieve prioritized activities and provide the best conditions for natural recovery.
Gut-directed hypnotherapy (IBS)	Applies certain hypnotherapeutic strategies to induce a deep state of relaxation and to guide patients to learn how to control their gut function. Suggestions and strategies on how to overcome tendencies to anxiety or fear of imminent catastrophe and developing the ability to gain control over other coincidental problems are provided.
Biofeedback	Instruments are applied that provide information on the activity of certain physiological functions (e.g., heart rate, muscle tension) with a goal of being able to manipulate them at will. Biofeedback helps to facilitate relaxation response, to demonstrate links between body and mind, to activate awareness of the own body, and to bring back a sense of control over the body.

Fig. 20.12 Psychological approaches to treat somatic symptom disorder (SSD) and selected functional somatic syndromes [80]

Illness Anxiety Disorder

Phenomenology and Classification

The core symptom of IAD is intense fear about the possibility of having or developing a serious illness (see Table 20.5). The criteria of IAD according to DSM-5 emphasize the *absence* of somatic symptoms and the prominence of worry and reassurance seeking. Individuals who predominantly experience somatic symptoms and develop anxieties about their symptoms and behaviors that aim at symptom relief are classified with SSD (see Table 20.1). The classic presentation of IAD involves frequent visits to physicians to seek reassurance about a feared illness. A substantial subgroup of individuals with IAD avoids physicians due to intense anxiety of receiving a confirmation of a diagnosis they fear [30].

Table 20.5 Checklist of characteristics of illness anxiety disorder according to the classification criteria in DSM-5

	Y	N	?
Preoccupation with having or acquiring a serious illness			
Somatic symptoms are not present (if present, only mild intensity; if medical condition/risk of developing medical condition present, preoccupation is disproportionate)			
High level of anxiety about health			
Excessive health-related behaviors or maladaptive avoidance			
Symptomatic state present ≥6 months			
Psychological factors not better explained by another mental disorder (e.g., somatic symptom disorder, panic disorder, generalized anxiety disorder, body dysmorphic disorder, obsessive-compulsive disorder, delusion disorder [somatic type])			
Criteria of illness anxiety disorder met?			
Specifier: (a) Care-seeking type: frequent health-care utilization (b) Care-avoidant type: rare utilization of health-care services			

Epidemiology

The epidemiology of IAD as defined in DSM-5 is unknown [30]. Most epidemiological studies refer to the precursor diagnosis of IAD in DSM-IV [2], hypochondriasis. In contrast to IAD, hypochondriasis does not exclude the presence of somatic symptoms. In population-based studies, the point prevalence of hypochondriasis is estimated to be 0.04–4.5%. In the clinical context, the prevalence of hypochondriasis is higher (general medical practices, 0.3–8.5%; specialty clinics, 12–20%; psychiatric populations, 1.6–3.5%). Clinically significant health anxieties are much more common in the general population (2.1–13.1%) and in various medical specialty settings (up to 20%) or psychiatric settings (19–31%). Studies show a relatively even distribution between men and women. The onset of the illness seems to be in early to middle adulthood. The disorder is often chronic [31]. IAD is associated with a significant financial burden for health-care systems (e.g., visits to emergency departments), increased numbers of days of sick leave, functional impairment, and rates of use of disability benefits [30]. The frequency of comorbid psychiatric disorders is increased in individuals with hypochondriasis (mainly depressive and anxiety disorder) [32] but varies substantially between studies [30]. Several studies do indicate an increased risk of developing medical illness (e.g., ischemic heart disease) in individuals with health anxiety [33].

Etiology and Pathophysiology

Most models of IAD consider predisposing, precipitating, and perpetuating factors of health anxiety, with an emphasis on cognitive and perceptual factors. The cognitive-behavioral model of hypochondriasis and health anxiety by Salkovskis and Warwick is one of the best examined models and is depicted in Fig. 20.13 [34]. A central concept and key component of this model is the process of somatosensory amplification [35] (see Fig. 20.14).

There are just a few neuroimaging studies that examined functional characteristics of hypochondriasis, reporting hypoactivity of regions involved in planning and executive function (dorsolateral prefrontal cortex, striatum, and left thalamus) and increased activity of regions involving anticipatory fear (amygdala) [36]. A neural circuit framework involving regions such as the anterior cingulate cortex, insula, amygdala, hippocampal formation, and striatum is proposed to be a neural correlate of somatosensory amplification, mentioned above [37] (see Fig. 20.15). Aberrancies in these circuits in addition with the frontal and subcortical regions described above may contribute to health anxiety by increasing negative expectancy, negative attentional bias, and catastrophizing [30]. These findings, however, have to be interpreted with caution. They seem to be not specific for IAS and were similar in individuals with obsessive-compulsive and panic disorder.

Treatment

Psychological interventions, cognitive-behavioral therapy (CBT) and third-wave CBT (e.g., acceptance and commitment therapy, mindfulness-based CBT), in particular, are more extensively investigated regarding their efficacy than pharmacological treatments [30]. They consistently show sustainable improving effects on health anxiety across different treatment settings (e.g., individual, group, and Internet-based therapy) [38]. CBT for IAD focuses on misinterpretation of bodily symptoms, identification and modification of less helpful behavioral and cognitive patterns, and generating alternative explanatory models for symptoms and psychological distress. Cognitive changes seem to act as an important treatment mechanism. Evidence regarding pharmacotherapy is limited but shows promising effects on health anxiety. Selective serotonin reuptake inhibitors (SSRIs) demonstrate an efficacy similar to CBT. The combination of CBT and SSRIs has a significantly higher treatment effect than each treatment on its own [30]. As a general principle in the treatment of IAD, communication with patients should be embedded in an empathetic communication style where the health-care provider listens to the patient's concerns and adopts an active and curious attitude toward the patient's experience [30]. Communication between treatment providers and a treatment plan that all providers agree on are essential for a successful therapy [30].

Fig. 20.13 According to the cognitive-behavioral model of hypochondriasis and health anxiety by Salkovskis and Warwick, dysfunctional beliefs about the prevalence and communicability of serious illnesses, the meaning of bodily symptoms, and the course and treatment of an illnesses are assumed to be risk factors of health anxieties. These beliefs can be triggered by a variety of events. These activated beliefs result in automatic hypochondriacal thoughts and interact with an increased awareness and sensitivity toward somatic sensations, the so-called somatosensory amplification. (*Adapted from* Warwick and Salkovskis [81]; *with permission*)

Previous experience

e.g., oneself or family member affected by illness; medical mismanagement; interpretation of symptoms and reactions in family and peer group

↓

Formation of dysfunctional beliefs

e.g., "Somatic symptoms are always a sign that something is wrong with my body. I have to find an explanation and the problem needs to be fixed."

↓

Incident of symptom which suggests illness
(including also incidents in family or social network, e.g., a friend died of a serious illness)

↓

Activation of dysfunctional beliefs

↓

Automatic thoughts
"I did not tell the doctor that I sometimes felt dizzy. My uncle also had complained about dizziness before he was diagnosed with cancer. My dizziness could be a sign of a brain tumor. I have to monitor if the symptoms get worse…"

↓

Health anxiety
Hypochondriasis
Illness anxiety disorder

Somatosensory amplification

Behavioral reactions
- Avoidance
- Body scanning/self-inspection
- Manipulation of affected area
- Reassurance seeking
- Scanning for information
- Preventative measures

Affective reactions
- Anxiety
- Depressive symptoms
- Anger

Cognitive reactions
- Focus on body
- Enhanced bodily misperception
- Monitoring of body changes
- Attention to negative information
- Helplessness
- Preoccupation, rumination
- Discounting positive information

Physiological reactions
- Increased nervousness and arousal
- Changes in body function
- Sleep disturbance

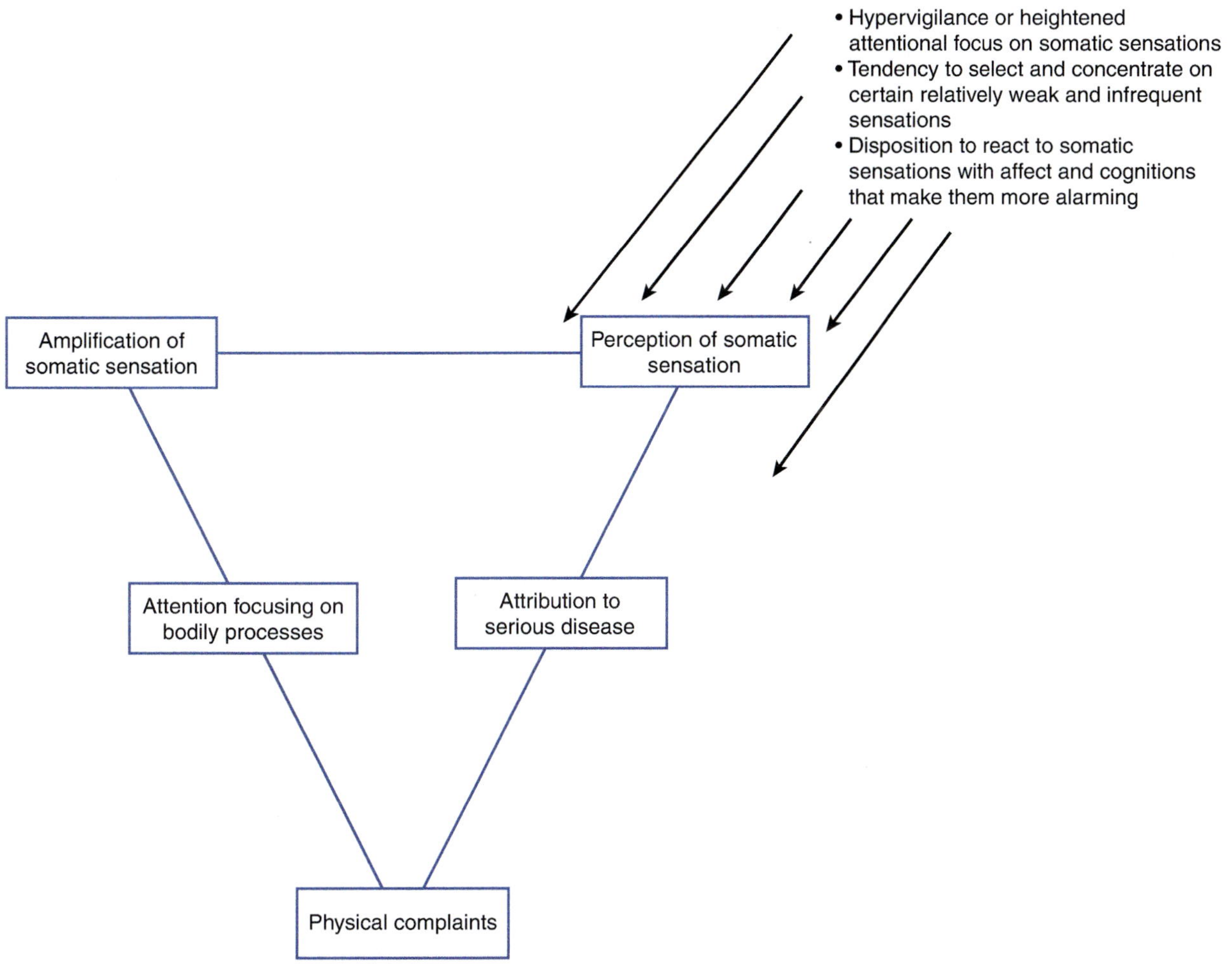

Fig. 20.14 Somatosensory amplification implies that somatic sensations are experienced as more intense, more noxious, more ominous, and more disturbing [35]. Individuals tend to be unusually sensitive to and intolerant of bodily sensations in general. They tend to attribute somatic sensations more frequently to disease than individuals without health anxieties would do

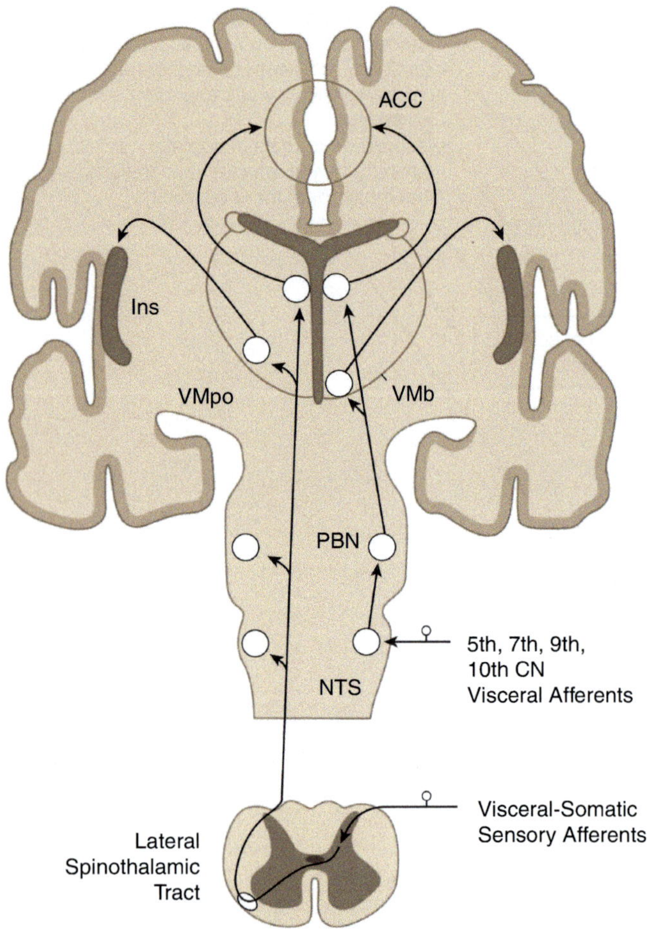

Fig. 20.15 A neural circuit framework involving regions such as the anterior cingulate cortex, insula, amygdala, hippocampal formation, and striatum is proposed to be a neural correlate of somatosensory amplification. This graph depicts the lamina I spinothalamocortical pathway demonstrating convergence of visceral-somatic processing within the brainstem, thalamus, anterior cingulate cortex (ACC), and insula (Ins). (*CN* cranial nerve; *MD* medial dorsal thalamic nuclei; *NTS* nucleus tractus solitarius; *PBN* parabrachial nucleus; *VMb* basal ventral medial thalamic nuclei; *VMpo* ventromedial thalamic nuclei)

Table 20.6 Checklist of characteristics of functional neurological symptom disorder/conversion disorder according to the classification criteria in DSM-5

	Y	N	?
≥1 symptom(s) of altered voluntary motor or sensory function			
Clinical evidence that symptoms are incompatible with recognized medical condition			
Presentation not better explained by another medical condition/mental disorder			
Symptom(s) cause(s) clinically significant distress or impairment (social, occupational, or other area of functioning) or warrants medical evaluation			
Criteria of functional neurological symptom disorder met?			
Specifier: (a) With weakness of paralysis (b) With abnormal movement (c) With swallowing symptoms (d) With speech symptom (e) With attacks or seizures (f) With anesthesia or sensory loss (g) With special sensory symptom (e.g., visual, olfactory, hearing) (h) With mixed symptoms			
Specifier: (a) Acute: <6 months (b) Persistent: ≥6 months			
Specifier: (a) With psychological stressor (b) Without psychological stressor			

Functional Neurological Symptom Disorder

Phenomenology and Classification

The diagnostic criteria of functional neurological symptom disorder (FNSD) according to the DSM-5 are summarized in Table 20.6. The core feature of FNSD is one or more symptoms of altered voluntary motor or sensory function. Symptoms can be various and can be categorized as depicted in Fig. 20.16 [39]. Equivalent terms such as "conversion disorder" or "psychogenic" have become less common. They refer to underlying mechanisms, i.e., unconscious, psychodynamic processes in patients, which are not necessarily present. "Functional symptoms," in contrast, refer to an abnormal functioning of the central nervous system and provide causative neutrality. To make the diagnosis of a FNSD, it is essential that the diagnostic process does not depend on excluding other disorders but on the examination of positive signs (see Figs. 20.17, 20.18, 20.19, and 20.20) [39–41].

Epidemiology

FNSD have an incidence of 4–12 per 100,000 and a prevalence of 50 per 100,000 population per year [39]. FNSD of motor type are the most common subgroup with an incidence of 4–5 per 100,000 population per year [39]. FNSD

Motor symptoms
Poverty of movement
- Leg weakness/paralysis
- Arm weakness/paralysis
- Parkinsonism

Excess of movement
- Tremor, dystonic movements
- Myoclonus
- Dystonia
- Tics

Axial manifestations
- Gait abnormalities
- Abnormal limb posturing
- Balance problems

Speech symptoms
- Dysfluency
- Stuttering
- Articulation deficits
- Dysarthria
- Visible demonstration of speech effort
- Dysphonia
- Aphonia
- Dysprosody

Symptoms with sensory manifestation
- Altered, reduced, or absent skin sensation, sensory loss
- Anesthesia
- Globus (sensation of a lump in the throat and swallowing symptoms)
- Vision-related, e.g., diplopia
- Olfactory
- Hearing disturbance
- Persistent perceptual postural dizziness: persistent disequilibrium or nonspinning dizziness provoked by upright posture, active or passive motion, and exposure to moving visual stimuli

Paroxysmal symptoms
- Paroxysmal akinesia
- Paroxysmal hyperkinesia (e.g., dystonia, tremor, jerks) with no apparent alteration in awareness or convulsive events with falls and variable or complete impairment of consciousness (non-epileptic seizures)

Fig. 20.16 The phenomenology and symptoms of FNSD are various and can be classified within four categories: motor symptoms, speech symptoms, symptoms with sensory manifestation, and paroxysmal symptoms including seizures

is especially common in neurology specialty settings: approximately 5–20% have a primary diagnosis of FNSD [39, 42], and 30% describe neurological symptoms that are somewhat or not at all explained by a medical cause. Incidence rates of FNSD in psychiatric settings are 11–22 per 100,000 [42]. Women are more frequently presented in the population of individuals with FNSD (60–75%) [39]. People with functional motor symptoms usually experience severe distress and disability [43], comparable to those with progressive neurodegenerative conditions [44]. They are at increased risk of developing comorbid mental health disorders (e.g., major depression, anxiety disorders) [45] and of utilizing health-care resources at high rates [43, 46]. FNSD can occur across the lifespan [42]. The onset of non-epileptic seizures peaks in the third decade, and functional motor symptoms have their peak onset in the fourth decade [1]. Symptoms can be transient or persistent. The prognosis may be better in younger children than in adolescents and adults [1].

Etiology and Pathophysiology

The traditional model of FNSD traces back to the concept of "hysteria" from times of ancient Greece and Roman Empire that explains medically unexplained symptoms by abnormalities of the uterus. In the nineteenth century, psychiatrists (e.g., Pierre Briquet, Sigmund Freud) of the psychoanalytic school developed important theories of functional neurological symptoms, among others the concept of "conversion" that describes a process of converting psychological distress into a physical symptom. Contemporary psychodynamic models build up on these precursor concepts and emphasize that symptoms can either suppress emotions or serve to resolve or escape conflicts [39]. Research shows that stressful life events and maltreatment are substantially more common in people with FNSD compared to healthy controls and patient controls; however, they do not have to be necessarily linked to FNSD [47].

Fig. 20.17 Selection of positive signs of functional neurological symptom disorder with motor symptoms

Poverty of movement

General

- Extreme slowness
- Fatigue
- Collapsing weakness (i.e., limb collapses from a normal position with a light touch)
- Give-way weakness (i.e., normal strength is developed and then suddenly collapses)
- Inconsistency in performance

Leg weakness/paralysis

- Hoover sign
- Hip abductor sign (i.e., weakness of fingers abduction that resolves with contralateral finger abduction against resistance)
- Able to stand on toes or ankles despite weak plantarflexion or dorsiflexion on bed
- Spinal injury center test (i.e., patient is unable to lift up knees, legs are passively lifted up in a flexed posture. The paretic leg will not fall in nonorganic weakness.)

Arm weakness/paralysis

- Drift without pronation of the weak arm
- Finger abduction sign (i.e., weakness of fingers abduction that resolves with contralateral finger abduction against resistance)
- Able to remove objects from bag or put on clothes inconsistent with upper limb examination
- Co-contraction sign (i.e., simultaneous contraction of the antagonist muscle [i.e., triceps] when the agonist muscle is being tested [biceps])

Parkinsonism

- Lack of speed or amplitude decrement on repetitive tapping (i.e., sequence effect)
- Variable resistance during passive manipulation

Excess of movement

Tremor

- Variability in frequency
- Entrainment or full suppressibility (i.e., entrainment or ceasing of tremor to externally cued rhythmic movement or an inability to copy movement)
- Tonic co-activation of antagonistic muscles at tremor onset
- Pause during contralateral ballistic movements
- Whack-a-mole sign (i.e., emergence or worsening of an involuntary movement in a separate body part when the initially affected body part is suppressed by someone holding it down)

Myoclonus

- Entrainment or full suppressibility
- Variability in duration and or distribution of jerks or of their latency (if stimulus sensitive)
- Predominance of axial or facial jerks

Dystonia

- Fixed dystonia at onset
- Variable resistance to passive manipulation
- Lack of sensory trick
- Lack of overflow
- Face: tonic pulling of the lips or jaw to one side; closed eyelids resist retraction by examiner

Tics

- Not fully stereotypical
- Interference with speech or voluntary actions
- Lack of premonitory urge
- Inability to voluntarily suppress tics

Axial manifestation

Gait abnormalities

- Knee buckling
- Dragging gait with forefoot in contact with ground
- Excessive slowness or a gait similar to walking on ice
- Chair test (i.e., patients with nonorganic astasia-abasia despite apparently normal power can propel a swivel chair while sitting)

Abnormal limb posturing

- Variability of positions over time
- Inconsistent, uneconomic postures

Balance problems

- No or controlled falls despite excessive swaying when walking
- Swaying and imbalance lessened with dual tasks

Fig. 20.18 Selection of positive signs of functional neurological symptom disorder with sensory symptoms

Midline splitting Test positive if exact splitting of sensory loss of half of the body (does not occur in organic disease, except thalamic lesions)	**Bowlus-Currier test** Patient is asked to place palms together, thumbs down (wrist crossed), fingers interlocked, and then rotate hands to bring them in front of the chest. Examiner performs sensory testing, starting on fifth finger up to the thumb (which is the only uncrossed finger). In functional paresis patient would report that the healthy thumb is anesthetic.
Splitting of vibration Test is positive if difference in the sensation of a tuning fork placed over the left compared to the right side of the sternum or frontal bone	**Non-anatomical sensory loss** i.e., sensory deficits with non-anatomical distribution
Systematic failure Test is positive when the subject fails 100% of the time on a discrimination task (i.e., up going or down going joint)	**Inconsistency/Changing pattern of sensory loss** i.e., findings are not consistent and not reproducible on repeated sensory testing

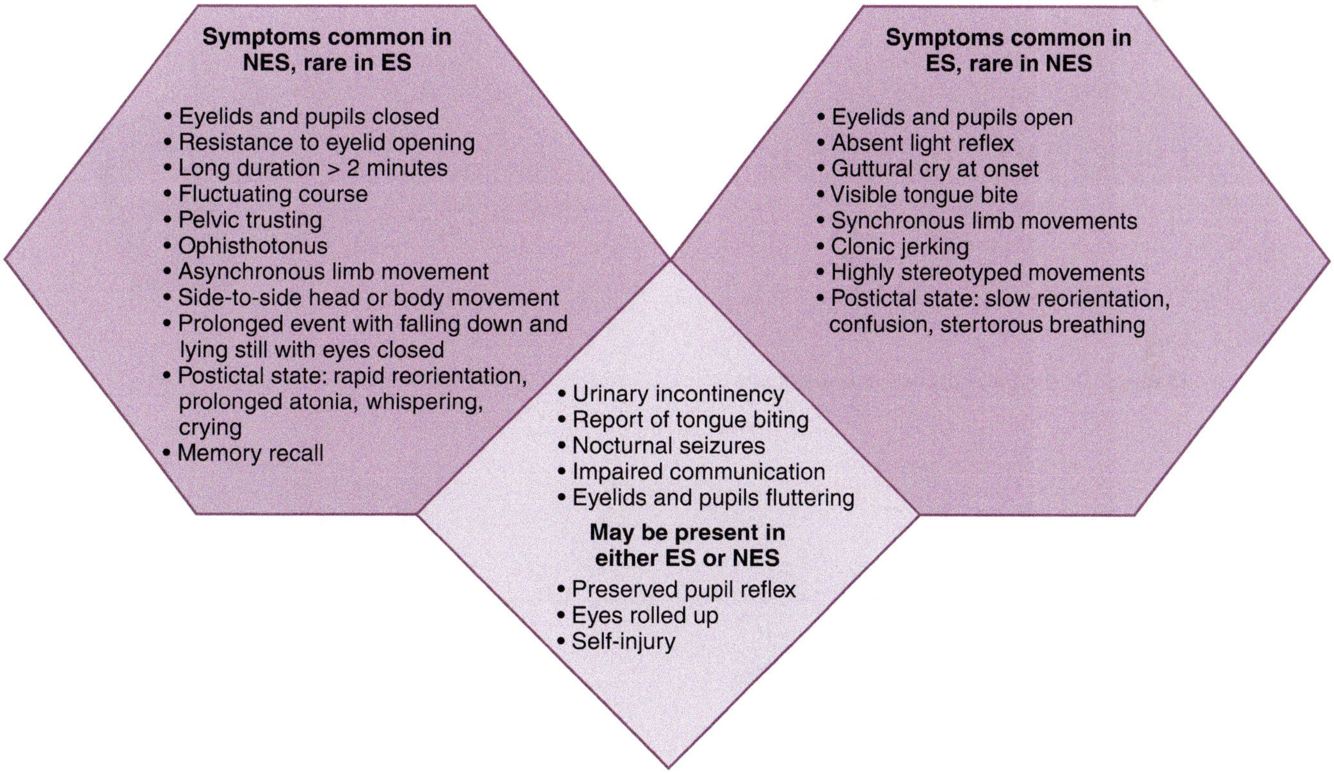

Fig. 20.19 Clinical signs to differentiate between non-epileptic seizures (NES) and epileptic seizures (ES)

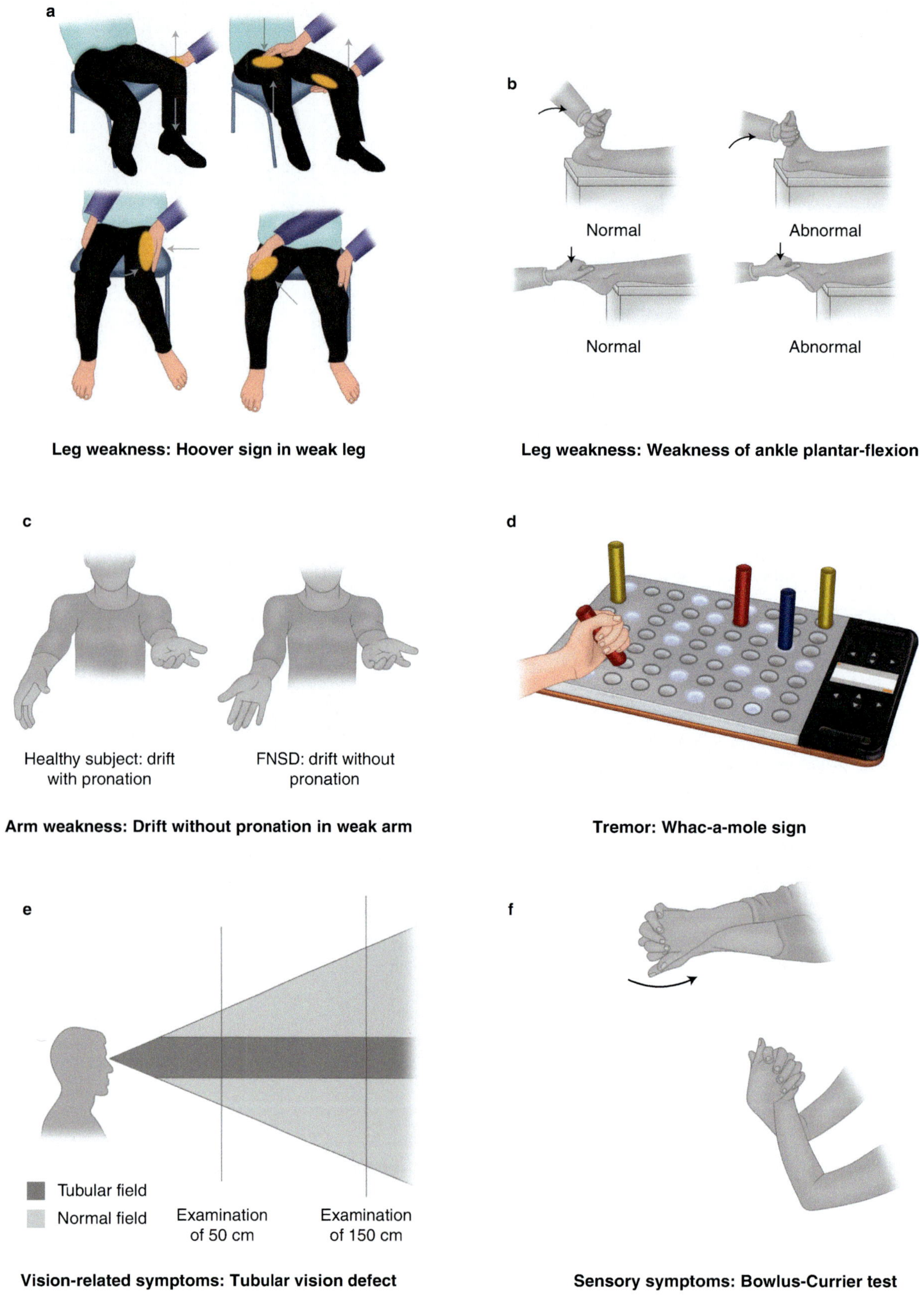

Fig. 20.20 Examples of clinical examinations in selected FNSD

More contemporary psychological theories conceptualize preceding events, such as trauma, medical illness, or physiological events, in the context of hierarchical Bayesian inference in the brain or predictive coding model as described under the section "Etiology and Pathophysiology" [48]. Processes such as attention focused on the body and the emotional state can function as mediating variables.

There are several contemporary psychological theories that focus on more disorder and symptom-specific aspects, for example, non-epileptic seizures (NES) [49]. NES are hypothesized to be based on the breakdown of individuals' ability to synthesize mental contents due to intense stress or emotional states. NES function as an activation of memory fragments dissociated from awareness. Other theories describe NES as an operation of "hard-wired behavioral tendencies" akin to the defensive reflexes seen in animals. Finally, NES can be considered to be a learned behavior that can be positively or negatively reinforced. In this sense, NES can be seen as a consequence of the activation of "learned seizure programs," maintained by factors that increase the activation of seizure programs or undermine the inhibition of them.

Results of neuroimaging and neurophysiological research of individuals suffering from various forms of sensory and motor-type FNSD suggest that higher-order processes (e.g., attention to self and expectations) and bottom-up processes (e.g., trauma, arousal) interact with each other and influence basic motor function (e.g., intention and inhibition of movement) [50]. The brain regions that are assumed to be involved in the pathophysiology across different forms of FNSD are summarized in Figs. 20.21 and 20.22. Research also shows indicators of an altered immune function, inflammation, and neural changes in FNSD [51] (see Table 20.7).

The etiological summary model by Fobian and Elliott [52] (see Fig. 20.23) and the integrative theory of NES by Brown and Reuber [53] (see Fig. 20.24) integrate neurobiological and psychological factors into a biopsychosocial framework of FNSD.

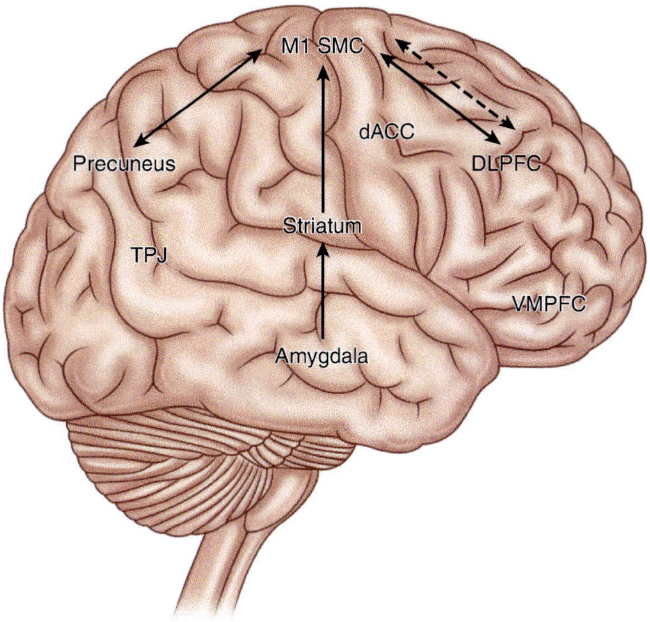

Fig. 20.21 In summary, results of neuroimaging and neurophysiological research of individuals suffering from various forms of sensory and motor-type functional neurological symptom disorder suggest that higher-order processes (e.g., attention to self and expectations) and bottom-up limbic processes (e.g., trauma, arousal) interact with each other and influence basic motor function (e.g., intention and inhibition of movement). Research shows that the activity in the following brain areas is altered: regions mediating emotional processing and regulation and awareness (perigenual anterior cingulate cortex/ventromedial prefrontal cortex [VMPFC], insula, amygdala), cognitive control (dorsolateral prefrontal cortex [DLPFC], dorsal anterior cingulate cortex [dACC], inferior frontal gyrus), self-referential processing (temporoparietal junction [TPJ]/posterior cingulate cortex/precuneus), and motor initiation, intention, and urge and motor inhibitory processes (primary motor cortex [M1], supplementary motor area [SMA]). Since the SMA and amygdala are anatomically not directly connected, the connectivity between motor limbic regions may be mediated by the striatum. Results from neuroimaging studies regarding connectivity are depicted with arrows (solid lines, increased connectivity; dashed lines, decreased connectivity)

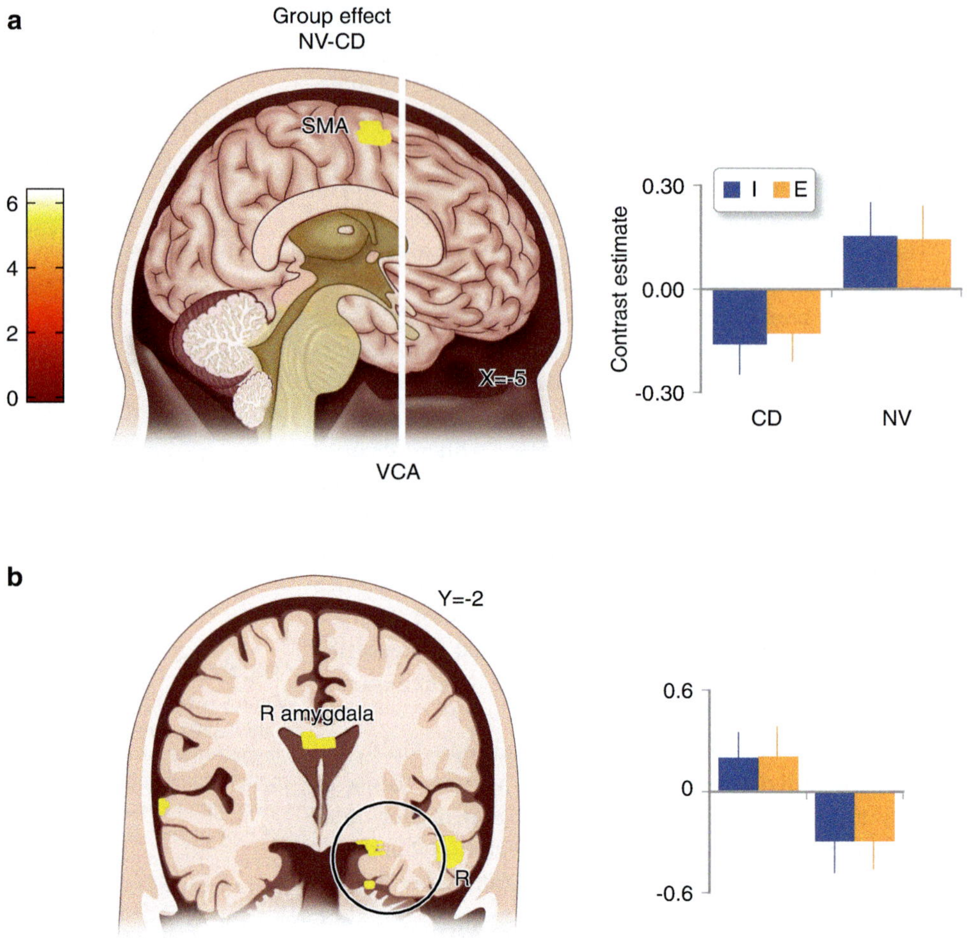

Fig. 20.22 Findings from neuroimaging studies suggest that an interaction between bottom-up limbic processes and higher-order processes has an impact on basic motor function. The supplementary motor area (SMA; involved in motor initiation, intention, and urge and motor inhibitory processes) and the amygdala are areas of the brain that are assumed to play an especially important role. This fMRI study examined individuals with functional motor symptoms and healthy control subjects during a motor preparation task. The fMRI pictures show in individuals with functional motor symptoms (**a**) a decreased activity in the SMA and (**b**) an increased activity in limbic regions (amygdala, anterior insula). (*From* Voon et al. [82]; *with permission*)

Table 20.7 Summary of research of changes in the immune system and neural changes associated with functional neurological symptom disorder (FNSD) [51]

Chronic low-grade inflammation	
High-sensitivity C reactive protein (hsCRP)	• Subgroups of children and adolescents who have experienced maltreatment or who currently suffered from anxiety showed elevated hsCRP values • Raised hsCRP mainly in patients with functional motor symptoms
Tumor necrosis factor-α (TNF-α)	• Changes in TNF-α concentration as the symptoms and disorder progress
Neural changes	
Autonomic nervous system	• Dysregulation of autonomic nervous system with a decreased parasympathetic function and an increase of sympathetic functions resulting in peripheral inflammation that cannot be “switched off” • Children with FNSD showed increased heart rate at baseline and during cognitive/emotional activation
Choroid	• Degenerated and lost mass of choroid
Brain-derived neurotrophic factor (BDNF)	• Decreased levels of BDNF
Hypothalamic-pituitary-adrenal (HPA) axis and immunological changes	• Hyperarousal stress state in FNSD with motor symptoms (altered HPA and ANS biomarker: cortisol and amylase)

Treatment

General treatment principles for FNSD and more specific treatment principles for NES and functional motor symptoms are summarized in Table 20.8 [39]. There are currently two evidence-based treatment approaches: psychological and physical treatments [54]. The *psychological treatments* include disorder-adapted cognitive-behavioral therapy (CBT) for NES and functional motor symptoms, self-management approaches that are based on CBT, and psychodynamic interpersonal approaches. The central goal of CBT is to identify and modify dysfunctional thinking patterns (e.g., ingrained core thoughts about oneself or one’s body, somatic misinterpretations), linked to the functional symptoms, and to promote behavioral changes. Typical CBT strategies include psychoeducation (e.g., understanding mechanisms of symptoms), functional behavioral analysis of symptom triggers, gaining control over movements, and training of assertive communication. *Physical therapy* is especially beneficial for individuals with functional motor symptoms. Mechanisms underlying functional motor symptoms are assumed to be multidimensional and need multidisciplinary interventional approaches. Accordingly, the active ingredients of CBT and physical

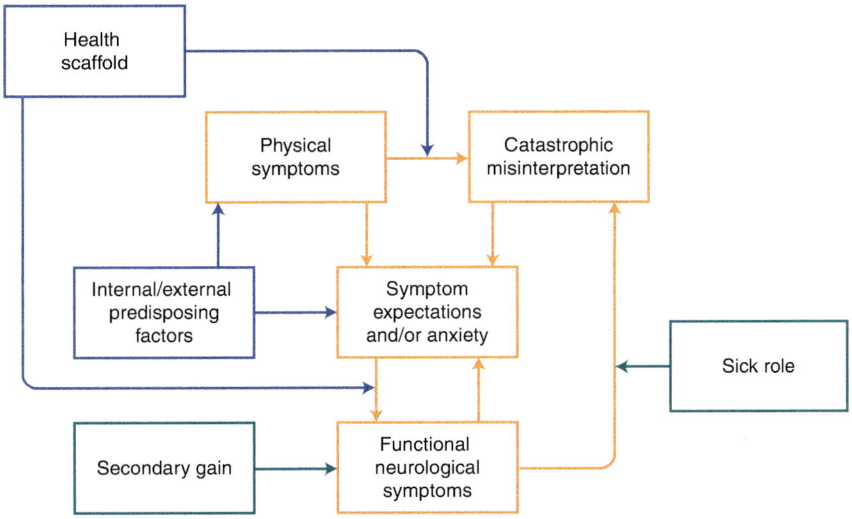

Fig. 20.23 Etiological summary model. This model is based on an interaction between physical symptoms that can be caused by various events or predisposing factors (e.g., trauma, trait anxiety, physical injury; highlighted in white), catastrophic misinterpretations, and the formation of certain symptom expectations. Processes of classical conditioning are proposed to be important mechanisms of this model. Moreover, the model embeds the individual's "health scaffold," a concept that is based on the individual's personal and observed illness experiences and contains classically conditioned neurological behavioral responses to neutral (conditioned) stimuli. Sick role and secondary gain are considered to be reinforcing factors (highlighted in gray) in this model. The model explains common relapse after remission: when a conditioned response is extinguished, the response is not "deleted" but "overwritten" with new learned content. Dotted background represents main model pathway. (*From* Fobian and Elliott [52]; *with permission*)

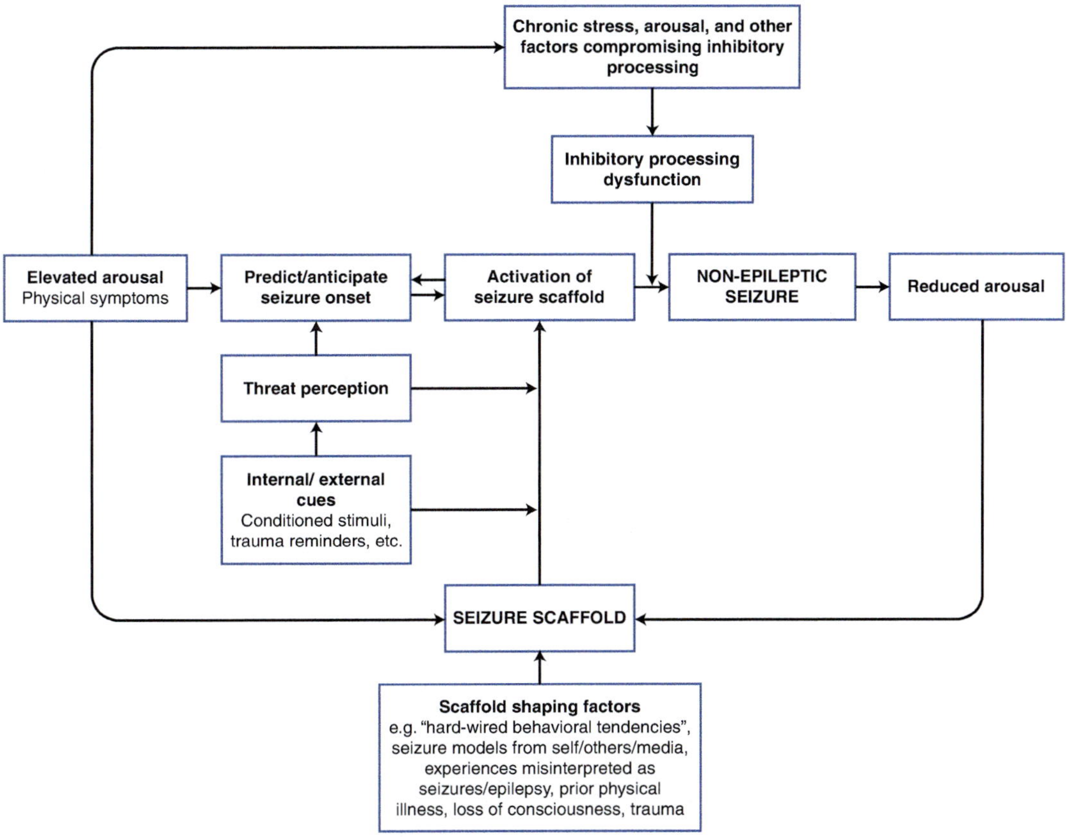

Fig. 20.24 Integrative theory of non-epileptic seizures (NES): the central component of NES in this model is a transient loss in behavioral and cognitive control from the automatic execution of a seizure representation in memory (=seizure scaffold). The model suggests three stages: stage 1 is characterized by an acute increase in sympathetic arousal and autonomic symptoms and the activation of the seizure scaffold, stage 2 means that a cognitive-behavioral component of the seizure scaffold is executed, and in stage 3, the arousal is reduced. (*Adapted from* Brown and Reuber [53]; *with permission*)

Table 20.8 General treatment principles of the therapy of FNSD [39]

General principles
• Diagnosis should be established prior to starting therapy and clearly communicated to the patient within a biopsychosocial framework
• Encourage transparency, especially regarding positive diagnostic features
• Explore and address unhelpful illness beliefs and behaviors
• Ensure that the patient understands potential for reversibility and is motivated to change
• Foster independence and self-management during treatment
• Involve the family and caregivers in treatment
Functional movement disorder-specific principles
• Establish the treatment goal of relearning normal motor control
• Motor retraining begins by establishing elementary movements (e.g., weight-shifting) and consecutively adding more complex movements
• Visual feedback during motor relearning from mirrors and video can be helpful
• Emphasis is placed on the quality of movement instead of the quantity
• Avoid excessive attention to abnormal movements. Treatment adjuncts may enhance movement relearning: treadmill training, electrical stimulation, electromyography biofeedback, and transcranial magnetic stimulation
• Unhelpful cognitions (e.g., "My symptoms indicate a serious disease") should be addressed
• Unhelpful behaviors (e.g., avoidance behaviors) should be addressed
Non-epileptic seizure-specific principles
• Learn techniques to avert episodes if there are warning symptoms
• Foster cognitive awareness of triggers when these are present
• Reduce avoidance using exposure techniques
• Dealing with seizure-related cognitions
• Facilitate the processing of emotions, where appropriate (e.g., history of trauma)
• Make patients more independent and understanding toward the role of significant other in their illness
• Develop a self-management and relapse plan
• Learn to challenge safety or avoidance behaviors around episodes

therapy are combined into an interdisciplinary approach to optimize outcomes. Pharmacotherapy is not indicated to treat FNSD. Pharmacological agents can be helpful to treat comorbid conditions (e.g., anxiety or depressive disorder) or coexisting disease.

Psychological Factors Affecting Other Medical Conditions

Phenomenology and Classification

The category of psychological factors affecting other medical conditions (PFAOMC) describes various psychological factors that add an additional health risk and/or adversely affect the course, the treatment progress and outcome, and the underlying pathology of a medical condition (see Table 20.9) [1]. The effect of psychological factors on the medical condition has to be evident, although it is possible that the direct causal effect underlying the relationship cannot be demonstrated. A selection of psychological factors and common medical conditions that could be classified under PFAOMC is summarized in Table 20.10 and Fig. 20.25. This subsection focuses on a very common type of PFAOMC: psychological factors affecting cardiovascular disease (CVD).

Table 20.9 Checklist of characteristics of psychological factors affecting other medical conditions (PFAOMC) according to the classification criteria in DSM-5

	Y	N	?
Presentation with a medical condition/symptom			
Psychological factor affects medical condition in ≥1 of the following ways:			
(a) Affects course of medical condition: temporal association between psychological factor and development of/exacerbation of/delayed recovery from medical condition			
(b) Interferes with treatment of medical condition			
(c) Constitutes additional health risk			
(d) Affects underlying pathophysiology, precipitating or exacerbating symptoms, or necessitating medical attention			
Psychological factors not better explained by another medical condition/mental disorder (e.g., panic disorder, major depressive disorder, posttraumatic stress disorder)			
Criteria of PFAOMC met?			
Specifier: (a) Mild: increased medical risk (b) Moderate: aggravates underlying medical condition (c) Severe: results in medical hospitalization or emergency room visits (d) Extreme: results in severe, life-threatening risk			

Epidemiology

Profound research evidence shows a strong relationship between CVD and psychological factors, in particular anxiety, depressed mood, and stress [55]. One in five individuals with coronary artery disease (CAD) or heart failure (HF) suffers from *depressive symptoms*. Depressed mood is associated with a 90% increased incidence of coronary heart disease (CHD). A dose-response relationship between depressive symptoms and cardiac events has been demonstrated in individuals with CHD. *Stress*, including chronic exposure to daily hassles and/or traumatic events, increases the risk of developing CVD and is associated with a worse prognosis of an existing CVD. Loneliness and social isolation are associated with a 50% increased risk of incident cardiac events and work-related stress with a 40% increased risk. The increased incidence of CVD events or death in individuals with PTSD ranges between a hazard ratio of 1.46 and 3.28. Results regarding an association between *anxiety* and CVD are more heterogeneous

Table 20.10 Selection of scientific evidence of medical conditions that are affected by psychological factors [72, 73]

Medical conditions (MC) that are demonstrated to be affected by psychological factors	**How do psychological factors and the medical condition interact with each other?**
Cardiovascular disease *For example, coronary heart disease, hypertension, chronic heart failure, arrhythmias*	• Onset and course of MC: e.g., acute and chronic stress, anxiety, depression, anger, hostility • Underlying pathophysiology of MC: various physiological pathways of psychological factors having a damaging effect on cardiovascular system (see Figs. 20.25 and 20.26) • Sequelae of MC: e.g., disability, posttraumatic symptoms after cardiac event or certain treatments, demoralization, irritability, health anxiety • Prognosis of MC: e.g., threat of possible death • Management of MC: e.g., adherence to lifestyle changes
Endocrine disease *For example, Cushing's disease, hyperprolactinemia, Graves' disease, Addison's disease, primary aldosteronism, hyper–/hypothyroidism, hyperparathyroidism*	• Onset and course of MC: e.g., acute and chronic stress, psychiatric comorbidity, irritability • Underlying pathophysiology MC: dysregulation of hypothalamic-pituitary-adrenal (HPA) axis • Sequelae of MC: e.g., disability, sexual dysfunction, fatigue, cognitive dysfunction
Gastrointestinal disorders *For example, functional gastrointestinal disorders*	• Onset and course of MC: e.g., acute and chronic stress, history of sexual and physical abuse, personality traits, somatization, catastrophizing • Underlying pathophysiology of MC: brain-gut axis (see section "Epidemiology") • Sequelae of MC: e.g., disability, stigmatization, somatosensory amplification, health-care seeking
Oncology conditions	• Sequelae of cancer diagnosis and treatment such as surgery, chemotherapy, radiotherapy, or hormone therapy: e.g., changes in the body, impact on relationships/dependency from others, level of functioning, sexuality, loss of certainties, feelings of loneliness, abandonment, anomia, marginalization or stigmatization • Course/prognosis of MC: e.g., threat of possible death, meaning of life/transcendence, fear of recurrence, demoralization
Skin diseases *For example, psoriasis, alopecia areata, atopic dermatitis, acne, urticaria, vitiligo*	• Onset and course of MC: social support, alexithymia, insecure attachment/attachment-related avoidance • Underlying pathophysiology of MC: neuroendocrine-immune network accounting for mind-body connection with the skin through activation of inflammatory process in deeper skin • Sequelae of MC: coping with visible lesions or disfigurement, stigmatization, impaired quality of life and functioning, body image, self-esteem, increased prevalence of suicidal ideation
Metabolic diseases *For example, type 2 diabetes*	• Onset and course of MC: depressive symptomatology • Underlying pathophysiology of MC: multiple pathways involving HPA axis dysregulation, immune and inflammatory mechanisms, brain insulin resistance, or circadian rhythm dysregulation • Sequelae of MC: cognitive decrements, sexual dysfunction, psychiatric comorbidity (e.g., depression, eating disorders), lack of social support • Management of MC: diabetes self-management and glycemic control ("diabetes burnout"), adherence to healthy diet and physical exercise, insulin manipulation
Respiratory diseases *For example, asthma*	• Onset and course of MC: stress • Underlying pathophysiology of MC: multiple pathways between psychological distress and increased risk of respiratory infections, for example, via exacerbated epithelium dysfunction or direct change of bacterial properties • Sequelae of MC: psychiatric comorbidity (e.g., depression, anxiety), emotion regulation, lowered quality of life, anxiety sensitivity toward somatic sensations • Management of MC: lack of self-efficacy, adherence to lifestyle changes (diet, physical activity, obesity), and asthma medication • Course/prognosis of MC: dealing with lifetime diagnosis

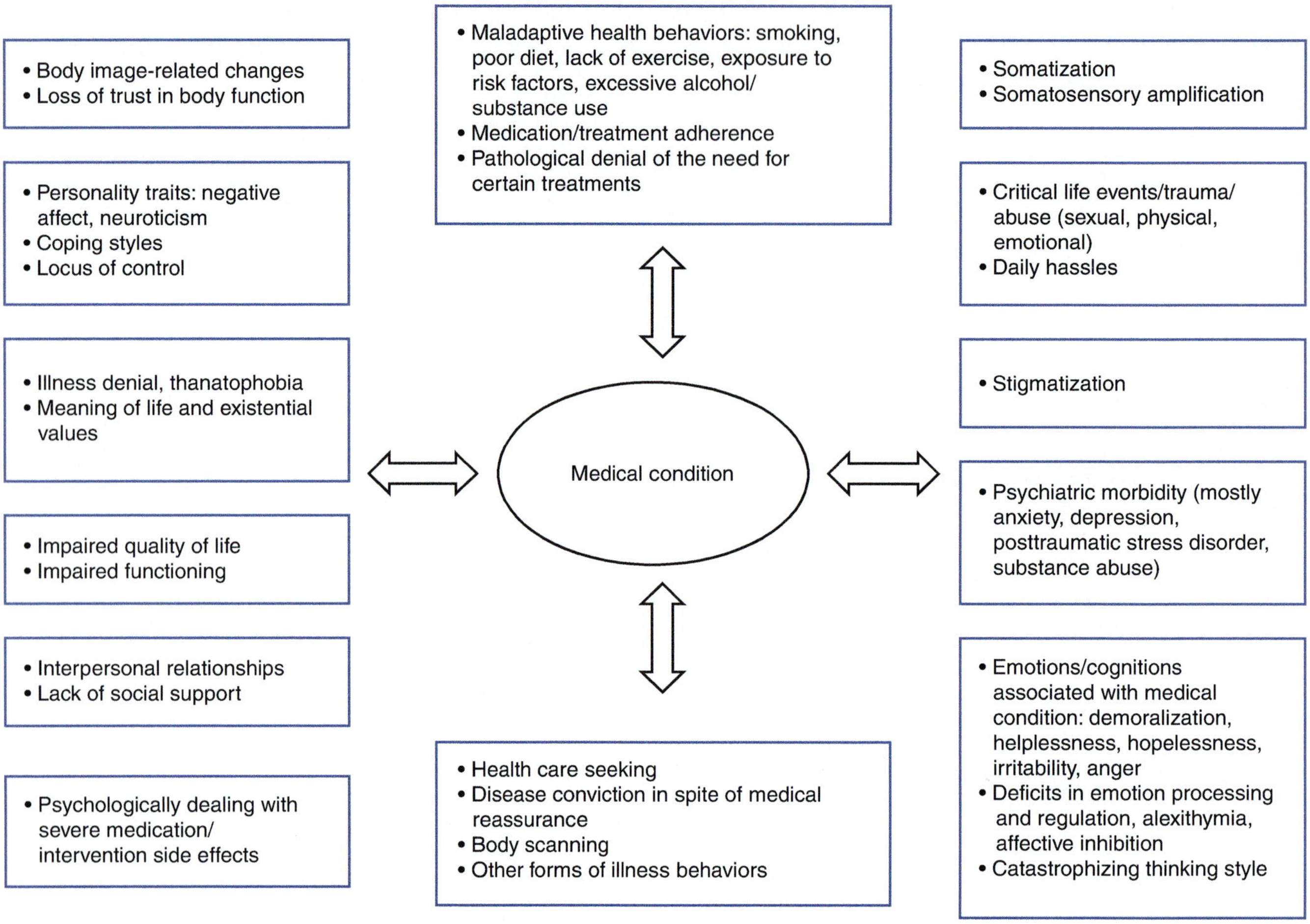

Fig. 20.25 Selection of psychological factors that have been demonstrated to affect medical conditions, in the sense of the DSM-5 diagnosis psychological factors affecting other medical conditions

[56]. Anxiety increases the risk of incidence of CAD by 26%. In individuals with established CAD, anxiety is associated with poor cardiac outcome. However, this relationship seems to be mediated by other medical and psychological factors (e.g., concurrent depression). Anxiety is probably a better predictor of CAD in a period of clinical stability compared to the acute phase after an acute cardiac event.

Etiology and Pathophysiology

Research over the past decades has substantially improved our understanding of the complex mechanisms postulated to mediate the relationship between *anxiety* and CVD (see Fig. 20.26) [56, 57] or *depressed mood* [58–60] and CVD (see Fig. 20.27).

Mechanisms of the relationship between *stress*, *trauma*, and CVD are less well explained [55]. Similar biological and behavioral mechanisms as for anxiety and depressive symptoms are proposed (Figs. 20.26 and 20.27). Animal models emphasize the importance of the individual's response to stress which seems to modulate the activation of neurobiological pathways to cardiovascular damage. A model of mental stress-induced ischemia in individuals with existing CAD explains cardiac events that do not evolve common symptoms such as chest pain and other classic angina symptoms. The model attributes mental stress-induced ischemia to coronary microvascular dysfunction that leads to atypical symptoms such as fatigue and vague discomfort. The damaging impact of psychological stress and trauma on the cardiovascular system may be due to a combination of chronic accumulation of atherosclerotic plaque and acute myocardial ischemia.

Treatment

Screening for depression in individuals with CVD is recommended by professional societies of cardiology worldwide [60]. Brief and validated screening tools such as Patient Health Questionnaire-2 (PHQ-2) are commonly used. Figure 20.28 summarizes a guideline-supported routine depression screen-

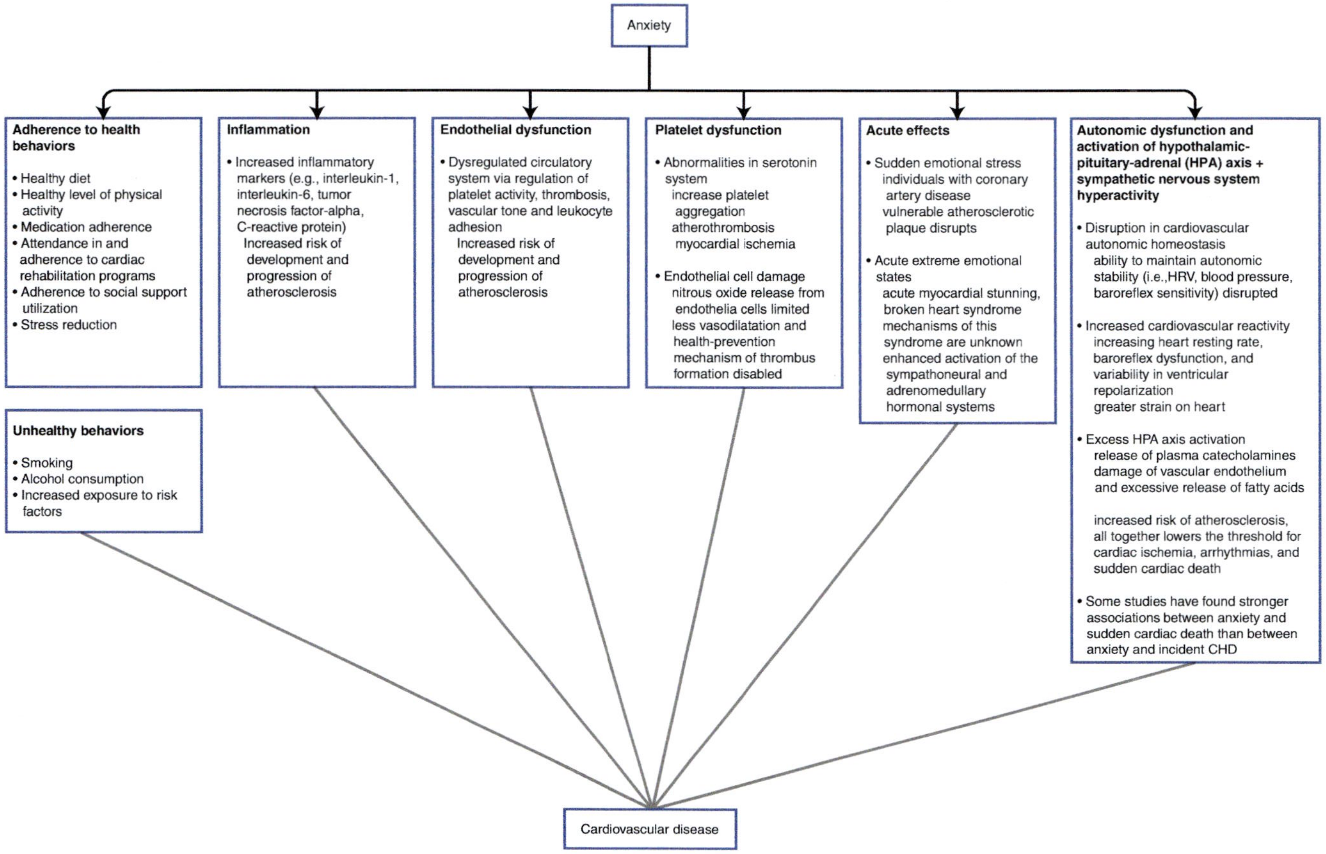

Fig. 20.26 Scientifically examined mechanisms and pathways of anxiety affecting cardiovascular disease [56, 57] mostly based on the assumption that effects of anxiety accumulate over time leading to cardiovascular damage and setting the stage for atherosclerosis and coronary artery disease. Feedback loops linking behavioral and biological factors are proposed

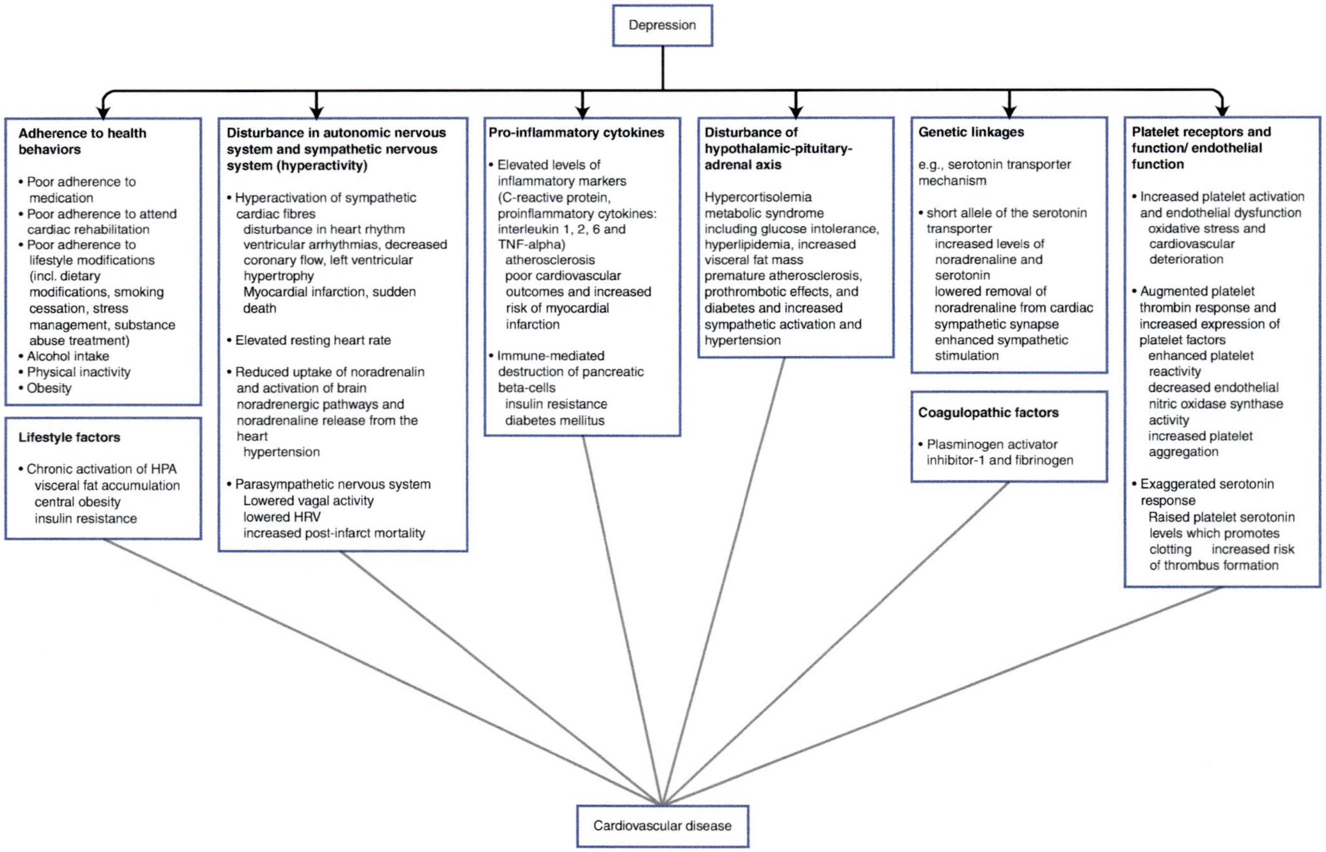

Fig. 20.27 Scientifically examined mechanisms and pathways of depression affecting cardiovascular disease [58–60]. Despite the plausibility of these biological and behavioral mechanisms, inconsistent results have been reported for each of these mechanisms, and there remains a gap in knowledge regarding which mechanisms best account for the association between depression and CVD risk

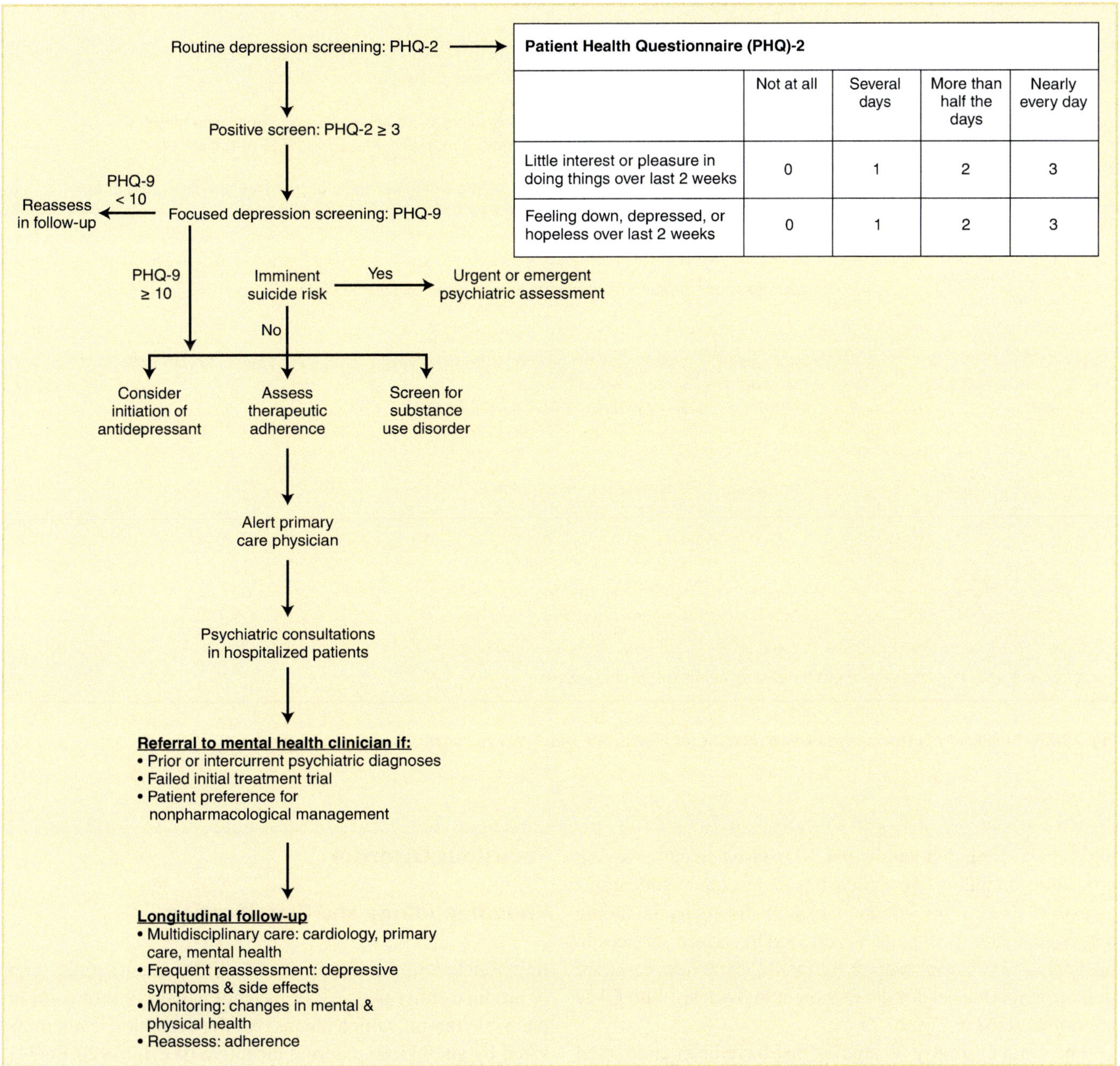

	Not at all	Several days	More than half the days	Nearly every day
Little interest or pleasure in doing things over last 2 weeks	0	1	2	3
Feeling down, depressed, or hopeless over last 2 weeks	0	1	2	3

Fig. 20.28 This guideline-supported routine depression screening pathway in patients with CVD applies a two-step process. This process starts with the two-item Patient Health Questionnaire (PHQ)-2 followed by focused screening with the nine-item PHQ. A multidisciplinary team-based approach (including primary and mental health-care interventions) to manage the symptoms of depression should be used for those who screen positive for depression. (*Adapted from* Jha [60]; *with permission*)

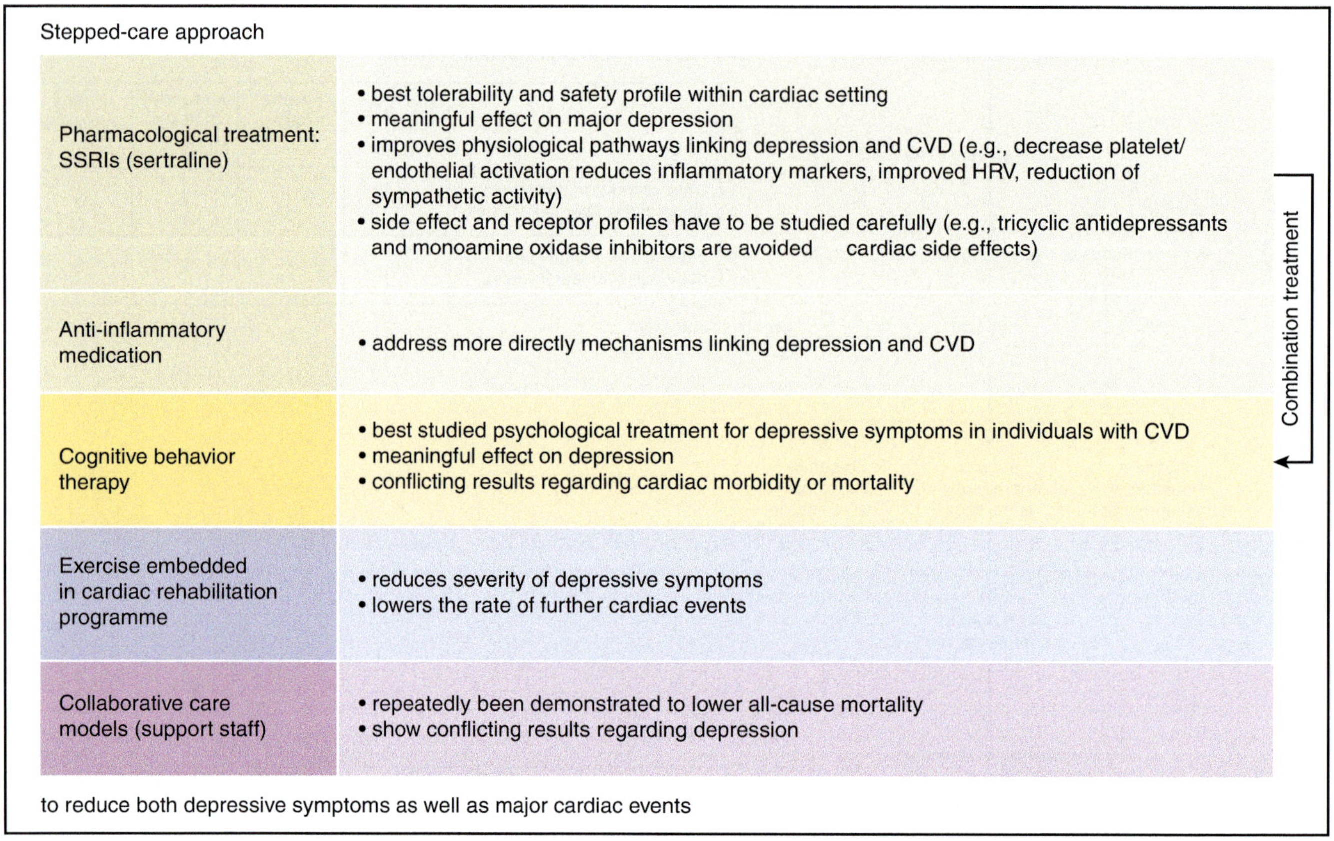

Fig. 20.29 Summary of evidence-based interventions for individuals with CVD and depression

ing pathway for individuals with CVD. Based on the screening procedure, an innovative approach is to develop a clinical service that screens for common mental disorders, including depression, among all patients admitted to cardiac services in hospitals and provides support for them [55]. Evidence-based treatment approaches for depression in individuals with CVD are summarized in Fig. 20.29.

There are currently no studies that have been conducted to examine the efficacy of specific treatments of anxiety problems in individuals with CVD. Antidepressant agents studied in depressed cardiac patients are frequently used in anxious cardiac patients [56, 60]. There are some studies of cognitive-behavioral therapy (CBT) in individuals with acute coronary who have both comorbid anxiety and depressive symptoms. These studies show that CBT substantially lowered the incidence of cardiovascular adverse events and depressive and anxiety symptoms [61]. Specific treatment approaches to help individuals with CVD to improve the way they deal with stress are rare. However, we know from studies of psychosocial interventions (e.g., stress management) that when they are added to traditional cardiovascular rehabilitation programs, they reduce the risk of recurrent CVD events [55].

Factitious Disorder

Phenomenology and Classification

Individuals with factitious disorder (FD) intentionally feign or produce either physical or psychological symptoms for no plausible reason, which means that the deception is not motivated by an obvious external incentive (see Table 20.11) [1]. Historically related is the terminology to the "Münchhausen syndrome" which is a more severe form of chronic fabrication of symptoms [1, 62]. There are two subtypes, FD imposed on self and on another (or "by proxy"). FD imposed on another is an ethically and legally complex condition, in which the perpetrator's behavior might represent criminal behavior [63]. A more modern form of FD is indicated as "by Internet" or "by Google," when stories of illness are disseminated on the Internet [64]. Methods of illness falsification are various (see Fig. 20.30) [1, 65]. The diagnosis of FD does not exclude the presence of a true medical or mental health condition; both can coexist (e.g., diabetes and manipulating blood sugar test results). Malingering has to be differentiated from FD, mainly through the existence of obvious external rewards (see Fig. 20.31).

Table 20.11 Checklist of characteristics of factitious disorder according to the classification criteria in DSM-5

Factitious disorder imposed on self			
	Y	N	?
Associated with identified deception: falsification of physical or psychological symptoms OR induction of injury or disease			
Self-presentation to others as ill/impaired/injured			
Evident deceptive behavior (absence of obvious external rewards)			
Presentation not better explained by another mental disorder (e.g., schizophrenia spectrum or other psychotic disorder)			
Criteria of factitious disorder (imposed on self) met?			
Factitious disorder imposed on another (former factitious disorder by proxy) (the perpetrator but not the victim is diagnosed)			
	Y	N	?
Associated with identified deception: falsification of physical or psychological symptoms OR induction of injury or disease in another			
Presentation of victim individuals to others as ill/impaired/injured			
Evident deceptive behavior (absence of obvious external rewards)			
Presentation not better explained by another mental disorder (e.g., schizophrenia spectrum or other psychotic disorder)			
Criteria of factitious disorder (imposed on another) met?			
Specifier: (a) Single episode (b) Recurrent episodes			

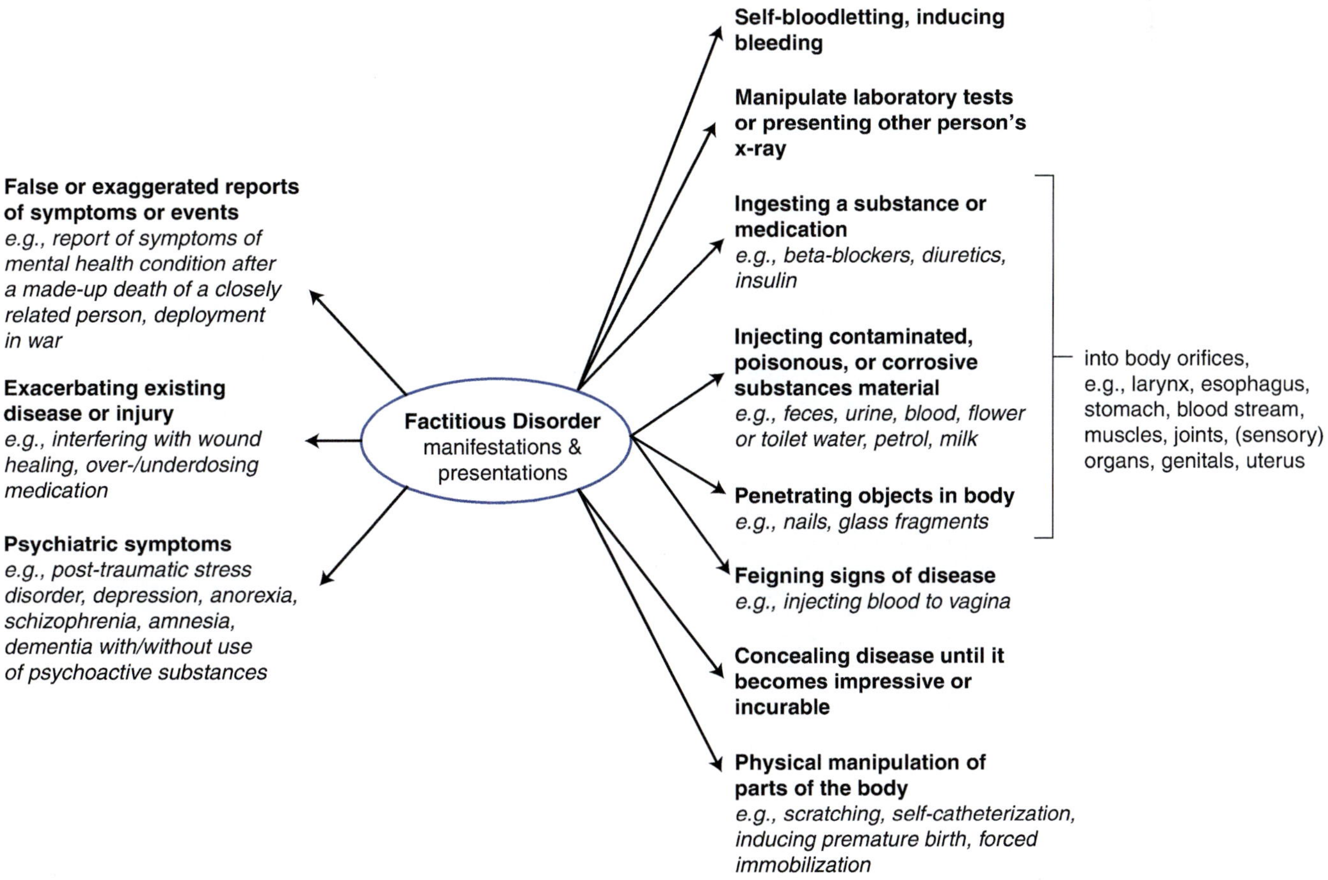

Fig. 20.30 Selection of typical manifestations and presentations of factitious disorder

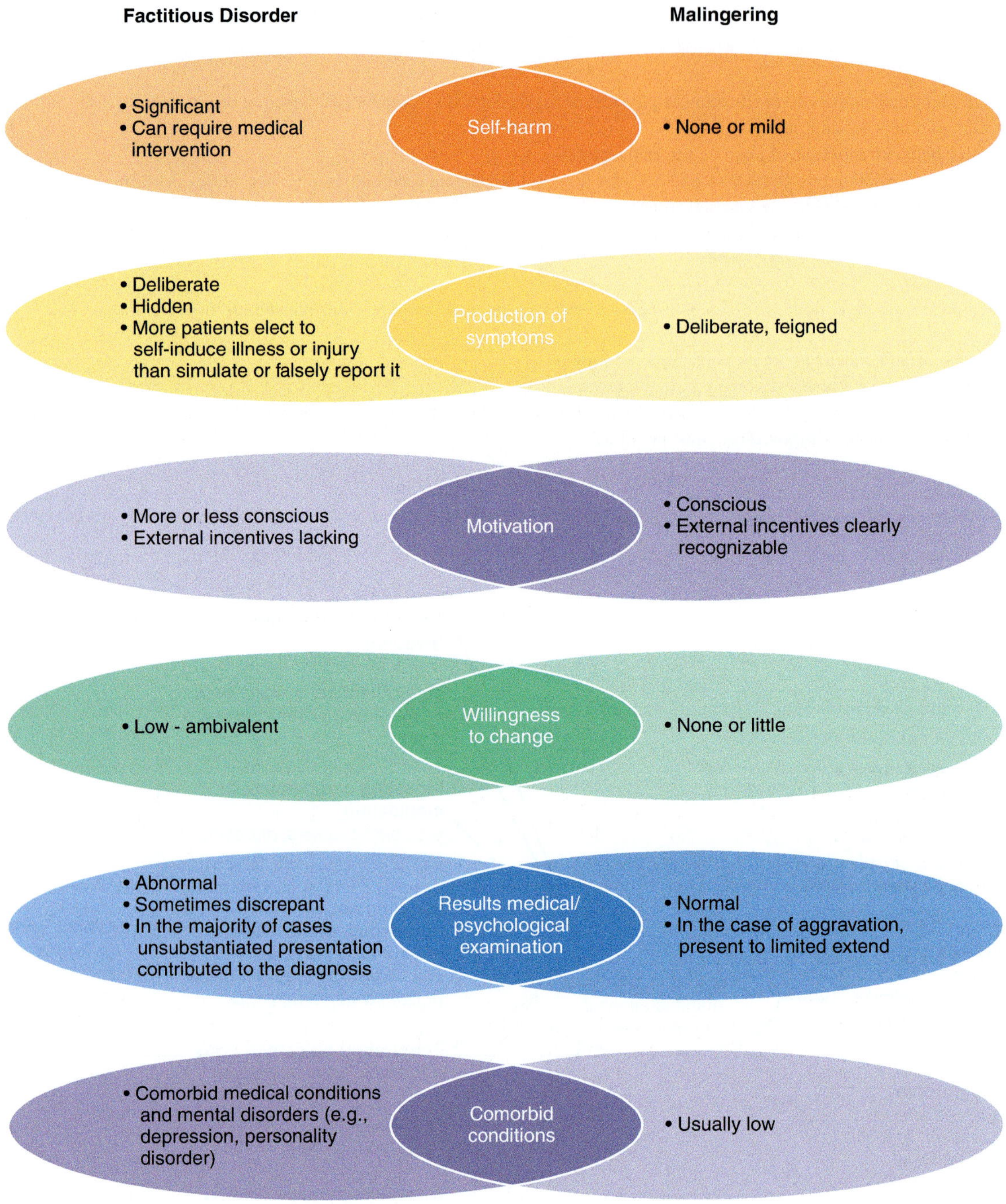

Fig. 20.31 Features that help in distinguishing between factitious disorder and malingering

Epidemiology

FD is assumed to occur in 1–5% in clinical populations [62]. FD by proxy is estimated as 2–2.8/100,000 children less than 1 year of age and 0.4/100,000 children less than 16 years of age [66]. The vast majority of children are younger than 5 years [66]. FD usually appears in intermittent episodes [62]. Onset is usually in early adulthood, often after hospitalization for a medical or mental health condition. A higher prevalence is as twice as high for women compared to men. Individuals with FD are most frequently employed in a healthcare or laboratory profession [67]. More patients elect to self-induce illness or injury than simulate or falsely report symptoms [67]. FD can appear in every medical specialty [67], with particularly high proportions in psychiatry, emergency departments, neurology, infectiology, dermatology, endocrinology, and cardiology [62]. Regarding FD by proxy, most of the abusers are female and the victim's mother [68].

Etiology and Pathophysiology

Knowledge of risk factors and etiological mechanisms of FD are rare. There are risk factors of FD, such as the presence of other mental health problems [67, 68], depressive disorder in particular, health conditions in childhood or adolescence that result in continuous treatments or repeated hospitalizations [69], and the existence of a personality disorder (borderline personality disorder in particular) [68]. Individuals diagnosed with FD have experienced abandonment and/or a history of childhood maltreatment [68].

Treatment

Individuals with FD present a heterogeneous group and there is no single approach to treat them. However, there are central components of the management of FD: the prompt recognition of symptoms and signs and semi-structured basic and consistent documentation. The entire treatment team should be vigilant toward warning signs and indicators. Often patients open up in particular to non-medical staff. Red flags and steps of documentation are summarized in Fig. 20.32 [62]. It is important to avoid developing prejudice toward patients to be saboteurs. At the same time, ongoing denial shared with the patient to avoid conflict should be avoided. Figure 20.33 summarizes the core steps of the management of FD. Supportive confrontation is the basic management tool, embedded in a secure setting and knowledge of the patient to continue to receive active treatment. A good

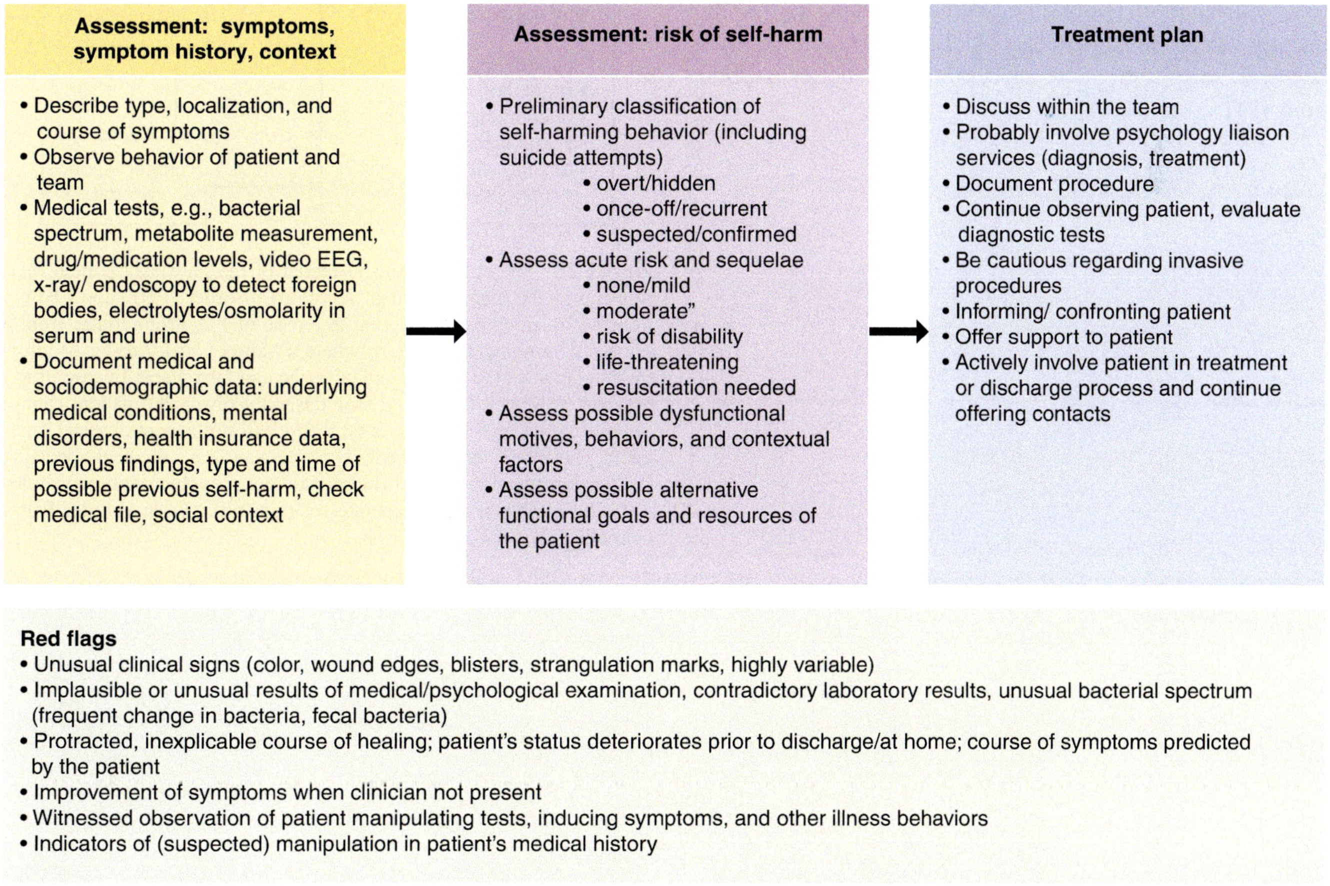

Fig. 20.32 Red flags of and steps of documentation in the management of factitious disorder

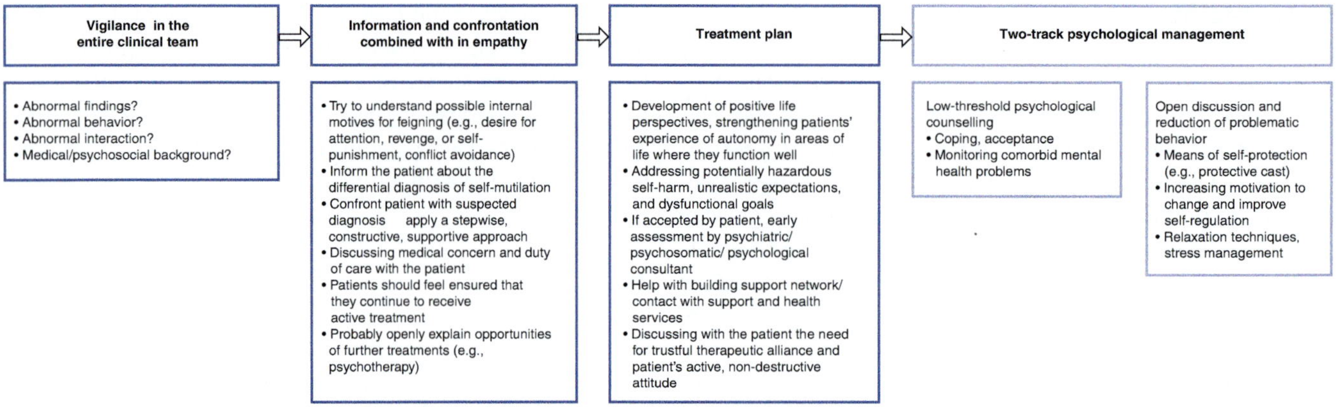

Fig. 20.33 Basic components of the management of factitious disorder: since patients tend to disclose to non-medical staff in particular, the entire team should be vigilant and report and discuss important observed details. As soon as sufficient indicators are given, patients should be informed and confronted in a constructive and supportive approach. Patients should be actively involved in the development of a treatment plan. In the case that patients are willing, engaging them in a psychological treatment can happen in different ways, either as low-threshold counseling or as a more intense approach that directly addresses the patient's problematic behavior

physician-patient relationship that helps in balancing between patient's autonomy and open communication on the one hand and the preservation of the patient's health and the physician's integrity on the other hand is the foundation of a successful confrontation. Figure 20.34 proposes an epistemological model of the physician-patient relationship in the management of FD [70]. Systematic reviews show that neither confrontation, nor psychopharmacotherapy, nor psychotherapy has promising effects [71]. Long-term interventions, however, seem to be more successful than shorter interventions [71].

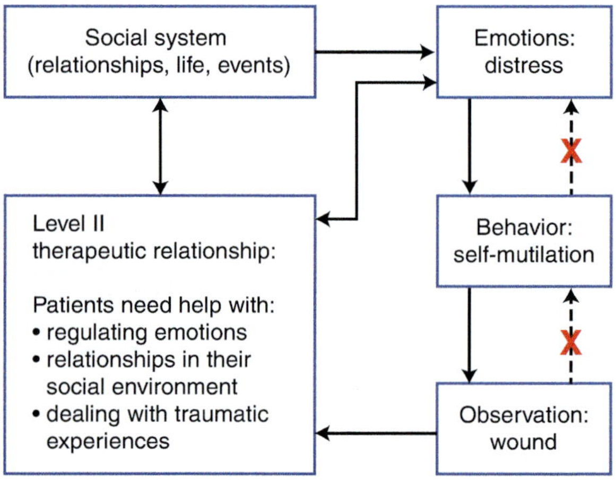

Fig. 20.34 The epistemological model of the physician-patient relationship in the management of factitious disorder (FD) shows how a patient-clinician communication in a case of FD differentiates from a normal communication pattern where a bidirectional transfer of information between the patient and clinician can take place. In case of FD however feedback is blocked (see dashed arrows), the patient cannot accept that he or she harms herself and will not accept external feedback. The model involves a level I clinician (e.g., medical specialist such as a surgeon) and level II clinician (e.g., psychiatrist or psychologist who establishes a therapeutic relationship). (*From* Van der Feltz-Cornelis [70]; *with permission*)

References

1. American Psychiatric Association. Diagnostic and statistical manual of mental disorders. Fifth edition. DSM-5. Washington, DC: APA; 2013.
2. American Psychiatric Association. Diagnostic and statistical manual for mental disorders. Fourth edition, text revision. Washington, DC: American Psychiatric Press; 2000.
3. Sharpe M, Mayou R, Bass C. Concepts, theories and terminology. In: Mayou R, Bass C, Sharpe M, editors. Treatment of functional somatic symptoms. Oxford, UK: Oxford University Press; 1995. p. 3–16.
4. Rief W, Martin A. How to use the new DSM-5 somatic symptom disorder diagnosis in research and practice: a critical evaluation and a proposal for modifications. Annu Rev Clin Psycho. 2014;10:339–67.
5. Henningsen P, Zipfel S, Herzog W. Management of functional somatic syndromes. Lancet. 2007;369(9565):946–55.
6. Lacy BE, Mearin F, Chang L, Chey WD, Lembo AJ, Simren M, et al. Bowel disorders. Gastroenterology. 2016;150(6):1393–407.
7. Fukuda K, Straus SE, Hickie I, Sharpe MC, Dobbins GJ, et al. The chronic fatigue syndrome: a comprehensive approach to its definition and study. Ann Intern Med. 1994;121(12):953–9.
8. Wolfe F, Clauw DJ, Fitzcharles MA, Goldenberg DL, Katz RS, Mease P, et al. The American College of Rheumatology preliminary diagnostic criteria for fibromyalgia and measurement of symptom severity. Arthritis Care Res. 2010;62(5):600–10.
9. Hiller W, Rief W, Brähler E. Somatization in the population: from mild bodily misperceptions to disabling symptoms. Soc Psych Psych Epid. 2006;41(9):704–12.
10. Grabe HJ, Meyer C, Hapke U, Rumpf HJ, Freyberger HJ, Dilling H, et al. Specific somatoform disorder in the general population. Psychosomatics. 2003;44(4):304–11.
11. Jacobi F, Wittchen HU, Holting C, Hofler M, Pfister H, Muller N, et al. Prevalence, co-morbidity and correlates of mental disorders in the general population: results from the German Health Interview and Examination Survey (GHS). Psychol Med. 2004;34(4):597–611.
12. Robins LN, Regier DA, editors. Psychiatric disorders in America: the epidemiological catchment area study. New York: The Free Press; 1991.
13. Jason LA, Richman JA, Rademaker AW, Jordan KM, Plioplys AV, Taylor RR, et al. A community-based study of chronic fatigue syndrome. Arch Intern Med. 1999;159(18):2129–37.
14. Reyes M, Nisenbaum R, Hoaglin DC, Unger ER, Emmons C, Randall C, et al. Prevalence and incidence of chronic fatigue syndrome in Wichita. Kansas Arch Intern Med. 2003;163(13):1530–6.
15. White KP, Speechley M, Harth M, Ostbye T. The London Fibromyalgia Epidemiology Study: comparing the demographic and clinical characteristics in 100 random community cases of fibromyalgia versus controls. J Rheumatol. 1999;26(7):1577–85.
16. Oka P, Parr H, Barberio B, Black CJ, Savarino EV, Ford AC. Global prevalence of irritable bowel syndrome according to Rome III or IV criteria: a systematic review and meta-analysis. Lancet. Gastroenterol Hepatol. 2020;5(10):908–17.
17. Rief W, Broadbent E. Explaining medically unexplained symptoms-models and mechanisms. Clin Psychol Rev. 2007;27(7):821–41.
18. Deary V, Chalder T, Sharpe M. The cognitive behavioural model of medically unexplained symptoms: a theoretical and empirical review. Clin Psychol Rev. 2007;27(7):781–97.
19. Witthöft M, Hiller W. Psychological approaches to origins and treatments of somatoform disorders. Annu Rev Clin Psycho. 2010;6:257–83.
20. Van den Bergh O, Witthöft M, Petersen S, Brown RJ. Symptoms and the body: taking the inferential leap. Neurosci Biobehav Rev. 2017;74:185–203.
21. Benedetti F. Mechanisms of placebo and placebo-related effects across diseases and treatments. Eur Neuropsychopharmacol. 2010;20:S60–S1.
22. Colloca L, Miller FG. Role of expectations in health. Curr Opin Psychiatry. 2011;24(2):149–55.
23. Hashmi JA, Baliki MN, Huang LJ, Baria AT, Torbey S, Hermann KM, et al. Shape shifting pain: chronification of back pain shifts brain representation from nociceptive to emotional circuits. Brain. 2013;136:2751–68.
24. Holtmann GJ, Ford AC, Talley NJ. Pathophysiology of irritable bowel syndrome. Lancet Gastroenterol Hepatol. 2016;1(2):133–46.
25. Komaroff AL. Advances in understanding the pathophysiology of chronic fatigue syndrome. JAMA. 2019;322(6):499–500.
26. O'Brien AT, Deitos A, Pego YT, Fregni F, Carrillo-de-la-Pena MT. Defective endogenous pain modulation in fibromyalgia: a meta-analysis of temporal summation and conditioned pain modulation paradigms. J Pain. 2018;19(8):819–36.
27. Henningsen P, Zipfel S, Sattel H, Creed F. Management of functional somatic syndromes and bodily distress. Psychother Psychosom. 2018;87(1):12–31.
28. Siedentopf F, Hausteiner-Wiehle C. S3 Guideline "Management of Patients with Non-Specific, Functional and Somatoform Physical Complaints" Geburtshilfe Frauenheilkd. 2013;73(3):224–26. https://doi.org/10.1055/s-0032-1328381. https://www.ncbi.nlm.nih.gov/pmc/articles/PMC3964376/. Accessed 2 Dec 2022.
29. Kleinstäuber M, Witthöft M, Steffanowski A, van Marwijk H, Hiller W, Lambert MJ. Pharmacological interventions for somatoform disorders in adults. Cochrane Database Syst Rev. 2014;(11):CD010628. https://doi.org/10.1002/14651858.CD010628.pub2.
30. Scarella TM, Boland RJ, Barsky AJ. Illness Anxiety Disorder: psychopathology, epidemiology, clinical characteristics, and treatment. Psychosom Med. 2019;81(5):398–407.
31. olde Hartman TC, Borghuis MS, Lucassen P, van de Laar FA, Speckens AE, van Weel C. Medically unexplained symptoms, somatisation disorder and hypochondriasis: course and prognosis. A systematic review. J Psychosom Res. 2009;66(5):363–77.
32. Noyes R, Kathol RG, Fisher MM, Phillips BM, Suelzer MT, Woodman CL. Psychiatric comorbidity among patients with hypochondriasis. Gen Hosp Psychiat. 1994;16(2):78–87.
33. Berge LI, Skogen JC, Sulo G, Igland J, Wilhelmsen I, Vollset SE, et al. Health anxiety and risk of ischaemic heart disease: a prospective cohort study linking the Hordaland Health Study (HUSK) with the Cardiovascular Diseases in Norway (CVDNOR) project. BMJ Open. 2016;6(11).
34. Marcus DK, Gurley JR, Marchi MM, Bauer C. Cognitive and perceptual variables in hypochondriasis and health anxiety: a systematic review. Clin Psychol Rev. 2007;27(2):127–39.
35. Barsky AJ, Wyshak G, Klerman GL. The Somatosensory Amplification Scale and its relationship to hypochondriasis. J Psychiatr Res. 1990;24(4):323–34.
36. van den Heuvel OA, Mataix-Cols D, Zwitser G, Cath DC, van der Werf YD, Groenewegen HJ, et al. Common limbic and frontal-striatal disturbances in patients with obsessive compulsive disorder, panic disorder and hypochondriasis. Psychol Med. 2011;41(11):2399–410.
37. Perez DL, Barsky AJ, Vago DR, Baslet G, Silbersweig DA. A neural circuit framework for somatosensory amplification in somatoform disorders. J Neuropsychiatry Clin Neurosci. 2015;27(1):E40–50.
38. Thomson AB, Page LA. Psychotherapies for hypochondriasis. Cochrane Database Syst Rev. 2007;(4):CD006520. https://doi.org/10.1002/14651858.CD006520.pub2.
39. Espay AJ, Aybek S, Carson A, Edwards MJ, Goldstein LH, Hallett M, et al. Current concepts in diagnosis and treatment of functional neurological disorders. JAMA Neurol. 2018;75(9):1132–41.
40. Gasca-Salas C, Lang AE. Neurologic diagnostic criteria for functional neurologic disorders. Handb Clin Neurol. 2016;139:193–212.
41. Daum C, Hubschmid M, Aybek S. The value of 'positive' clinical signs for weakness, sensory and gait disorders in conversion

disorder: a systematic and narrative review. J Neurol Neurosur Ps. 2014;85(2):180–90.
42. Feinstein A. Conversion Disorder. Continuum. 2018;24(3):861–72.
43. Carson A, Stone J, Hibberd C, Murray G, Duncan R, Coleman R, et al. Disability, distress and unemployment in neurology outpatients with symptoms 'unexplained by organic disease'. J Neurol Neurosur Ps. 2011;82(7):810–3.
44. Anderson KE, Gruber-Baldini AL, Vaughan CG, Reich SG, Fishman PS, Weiner WJ, et al. Impact of psychogenic movement disorders versus Parkinson's on disability, quality of life, and psychopathology. Movement Disord. 2007;22(15):2204–9.
45. Feinstein A, Stergiopoulos V, Fine J, Lang AE. Psychiatric outcome in patients with a psychogenic movement disorder. Neuropsychiatr Neuropsychol Behav Neurol. 2001;14(3):169–76.
46. Barsky AJ, Orav EJ, Bates DW. Somatization increases medical utilization and costs independent of psychiatric and medical comorbidity. Arch Gen Psych. 2005;62(8):903–10.
47. Ludwig L, Pasman JA, Nicholson T, Aybek S, David AS, Tuck S, et al. Stressful life events and maltreatment in conversion (functional neurological) disorder: systematic review and meta-analysis of case-control studies. Lancet Psychiat. 2018;5(4):307–20.
48. Edwards MJ, Adams RA, Brown H, Parees I, Friston KJ. A Bayesian account of 'hysteria'. Brain. 2012;135:3495–512.
49. Brown RJ, Reuber M. Psychological and psychiatric aspects of psychogenic non-epileptic seizures (PNES): a systematic review. Clin Psychol Rev. 2016;45:157–82.
50. Voon V, Cavanna AE, Coburn K, Sampson S, Reeve A, LaFrance WC, et al. Functional Neuroanatomy and Neurophysiology of Functional Neurological Disorders (Conversion Disorder). J Neuropsychiatry Clin Neurosci. 2016;28(3):168–90.
51. Ratcliff J, Van der Feltz-Cornelis C. Conversion disorder/functional neurological disorder—a narrative review on current research into its pathological mechanism. Eur J Psychiatry. 2020;34(3):143–52.
52. Fobian AD, Elliott L. A review of functional neurological symptom disorder etiology and the integrated etiological summary model. J Psychiatry Neurosci. 2019;44(1):8–18.
53. Brown RJ, Reuber M. Towards an integrative theory of psychogenic non-epileptic seizures (PNES). Clin Psychol Rev. 2016;47:55–70.
54. Ganslev CA, Storebo OJ, Callesen HE, Ruddy R, Sogaard U. Psychosocial interventions for conversion and dissociative disorders in adults. Cochrane Database Syst Rev. 2020;7(7):CD005331.
55. Cohen BE, Edmondson D, Kronish IM. State of the Art review: depression, stress, anxiety, and cardiovascular disease. Am J Hypertens. 2015;28(11):1295–302.
56. Celano CM, Daunis DJ, Lokko HN, Campbell KA, Huffman JC. Anxiety Disorders and Cardiovascular Disease. Curr Psychiatry Rep. 2016;18(11):101.
57. Thurston RC, Rewak M, Kubzansky LD. An anxious heart: anxiety and the onset of cardiovascular diseases. Prog Cardiovasc Dis. 2013;55(6):524–37.
58. Dhar AK, Barton DA. Depression and the link with cardiovascular disease. Front Psych. 2016;7:33.
59. Hare DL, Toukhsati SR, Johansson P, Jaarsma T. Depression and cardiovascular disease: a clinical review. Eur Heart J. 2014;35(21):1365–72.
60. Jha MK, Qamar A, Vaduganathan M, Charney DS, Murrough JW. Screening and management of depression in patients with cardiovascular disease: JACC state-of-the-art review. J Am Coll Cardiol. 2019;73(14):1827–45.
61. Yu H, Ma YY, Lei R, Xu D. A meta-analysis of clinical efficacy and quality of life of cognitive-behavioral therapy in acute coronary syndrome patients with anxiety and depression. Ann Pallliat Med. 2020;9(4):1886–95.
62. Hausteiner-Wiehle C, Hungerer S. Factitious Disorders in everyday clinical practice. Deutsches Arzteblatt Int. 2020;117(26):452.
63. Hamilton JC, Kouchi KAK. Factitious Disorders and the adjudication of claims of physical and mental injury. Psychol Inj Law. 2018;11(1):9–21.
64. Pulman A, Taylor J. Munchausen by Internet: current research and future directions. J Med Internet Res. 2012;14(4):188–98.
65. Kinns H, Housley D, Freedman DB. Munchausen syndrome and factitious disorder: the role of the laboratory in its detection and diagnosis. Ann Clin Biochem. 2013;50(3):194–203.
66. Galvin HK, Newton AW, Vandeven AM. Update on Munchausen syndrome by proxy. Curr Opin Psychiatry. 2005;17(2):252–7.
67. Yates GP, Feldman MD. Factitious disorder: a systematic review of 455 cases in the professional literature. Gen Hosp Psychiat. 2016;41:20–8.
68. Yates G, Bass C. The perpetrators of medical child abuse (Munchausen Syndrome by Proxy)—a systematic review of 796 cases. Child Abuse Negl. 2017;72:45–53.
69. Mousailidis G, Lazzari C, Bhan-Kotwal S, Papanna B, Shoka A. Factitious disorder: a case report and literature review of treatment. Prog Neurol Psychiatry. 2019;23(2):14–8.
70. Van der Feltz-Cornelis C. The impact of factitious disorder on the physician-patient relationship. An epistemological model. Med Health Care Philos. 2002;5:253–61.
71. Eastwood S, Bisson JI. Management of factitious disorders: a systematic review. Psychother Psychosom. 2008;77(4):209–18.
72. Porcelli P, Sonino N. Psychological factors affecting medical conditions: a new classification for DSM-5. In Fava GA, Fukunishi I, Rosenthal MB, editors. Basel, Switzerland: Karger; 2007.
73. Mukherjee N, Chaturvedi SK. Depressive symptoms and disorders in type 2 diabetes mellitus. Curr Opin Psychiatry. 2019;32(5):416–21.
74. Engel GL. The clinical application of the biopsychosocial model. J Med Philos. 1981;6(2):101–23.
75. Kirmayer LJ, Taillefer S. Somatoform disorders. In: Turner SM, Hersen M, editors. Adult psychopathology and diagnosis. 3rd ed. New York: Wiley; 1997. p. 333–83.
76. Tanasescu R, Cottam WJ, Condon L, Tench CR, Auer DP. Functional reorganisation in chronic pain and neural correlates of pain sensitisation: a coordinate based meta-analysis of 266 cutaneous pain fMRI studies. Neurosci Biobehav Rev. 2016;68:120–33.
77. Dehghan M, Schmidt-Wilcke T, Pfleiderer B, Eickhoff SB, Petzke F, Harris RE, et al. Coordinate-based (ALE) meta-analysis of brain activation in patients with fibromyalgia. Hum Brain Mapp. 2016;37(5):1749–58.
78. López-Solà M, Woo CW, Pujol J, Deus J, Harrison BJ, Monfort J, et al. Towards a neurophysiological signature for fibromyalgia. Pain. 2017;158(1):34–47.
79. Richard JY, Hurley RA, Taber KH. Fibromyalgia: centralized pain processing and neuroimaging. J Neuropsychiatry Clin Neurosci. 2019;31(3):182–7.
80. Kleinstäuber M, Rief W. Somatic symptom disorders. In: Hofmann SG, editor. Clinical psychology: a global perspective. Hoboken, NJ: Wiley-Blackwell; 2017. p. 267–82.
81. Warwick HMC, Salkovskis PM. Hypochondriasis. Behav Res Ther. 1990;28(2):105–17.
82. Voon V, Brezing C, Gallea C, Hallett M. Aberrant supplementary motor complex and limbic activity during motor preparation in motor conversion disorder. Movement Disord. 2011;26(13):2396–403.

Eating Disorders, Feeding, and Elimination Disorders

21

Demetria Pizano, Netasha Pizano, Christopher Martin, Paloma Garcia, and Waguih William IsHak

Anorexia Nervosa

Anorexia nervosa (AN) is an eating disorder that is characterized by disturbances in eating, or eating-related behaviors, that result from altered consumption impairing physical health or psychosocial functioning [1]. With cases of body image distortions observed as early as the twelfth century, it wasn't until 1689 that the first medical account of anorexia nervosa was recorded [2]. Since then, current knowledge has evolved, and there is a deeper understanding of the various components associated with this disorder.

Symptoms, like semi-starvation and purging behaviors, may result in significant or potentially life-threatening medical conditions and can affect major organ systems [1]. Along with behavioral and psychological factors of anorexia, there are several mental disorders highly associated with anorexia. Due to this, there is an increased potential of death due to medical conditions or comorbidity, creating a highly important need for treatment. Through varying levels of intervention, therapeutic approaches, or pharmacological treatments, the goal towards recovery is weight restoration, normalization of eating behaviors, and improvements in body image perceptions [2] (Fig. 21.1).

D. Pizano (✉)
University of Alabama at Birmingham, Birmingham, AL, USA
e-mail: dpizano@uab.edu

N. Pizano
University of California, Santa Barbara, Santa Barbara, CA, USA
e-mail: Nkpizano@ucsb.edu

C. Martin
David Geffen School of Medicine at UCLA, Charles R. Drew University of Medicine and Science, Los Angeles, CA, USA
e-mail: CSMartin@mednet.ucla.edu

P. Garcia
Brown University, Providence, RI, USA
e-mail: paloma_garcia@brown.edu

W. W. IsHak
Cedars Sinai Health System, Department of Psychiatry and Behavioral Neurosciences, University of California Los Angeles, David Geffen School of Medicine, Los Angeles, CA, USA
e-mail: Waguih.IsHak@cshs.org

Epidemiology

Biological Risk Factors

Epidemiological reports of anorexia nervosa identified an average age of onset is between 15 and 19 years old, with an increasing trend of prepubertal children displaying symptoms and mid-to-late life [3]. Approximately between 0.3% and 0.4% of females and 0.1% of males will be diagnosed with AN; nearly 1% of females and 0.3% of males will be diagnosed during their life [4]. Although males make up 25% of people with anorexia, they present a higher risk of dying due to their late diagnoses [5] (Figs. 21.2 and 21.3).

Environmental Risk Factors

With a notable causation from biological risk factors, AN is commonly associated with sociocultural factors, including thin-ideal portrayed in media images and potential exposure of modeled disordered eating behaviors from social structure [8]. Additionally, adverse life events, like sexual or physical abuse, illness, a major move, or pregnancy can also be associated with risk factors commonly experienced prior to onset. Teasing and weight-related comments within a person's environment may act as a contributory factor (Figs. 21.4, 21.5, and 21.6).

Comorbidity

Commonly associated with anorexia nervosa, bipolar, depressive, and anxiety disorders are seen in many people with anorexia nervosa. According to the Diagnostic and Statistical Manual of Mental Disorders, Fifth Edition (DSM-5), individuals tend to report the presence of anxiety symptoms or diagnosed anxiety disorder prior to the onset of their eating disorder [1]. In those with restricting type AN, indi-

W. W. IsHak (ed.), *Atlas of Psychiatry*, https://doi.org/10.1007/978-3-031-15401-0_21

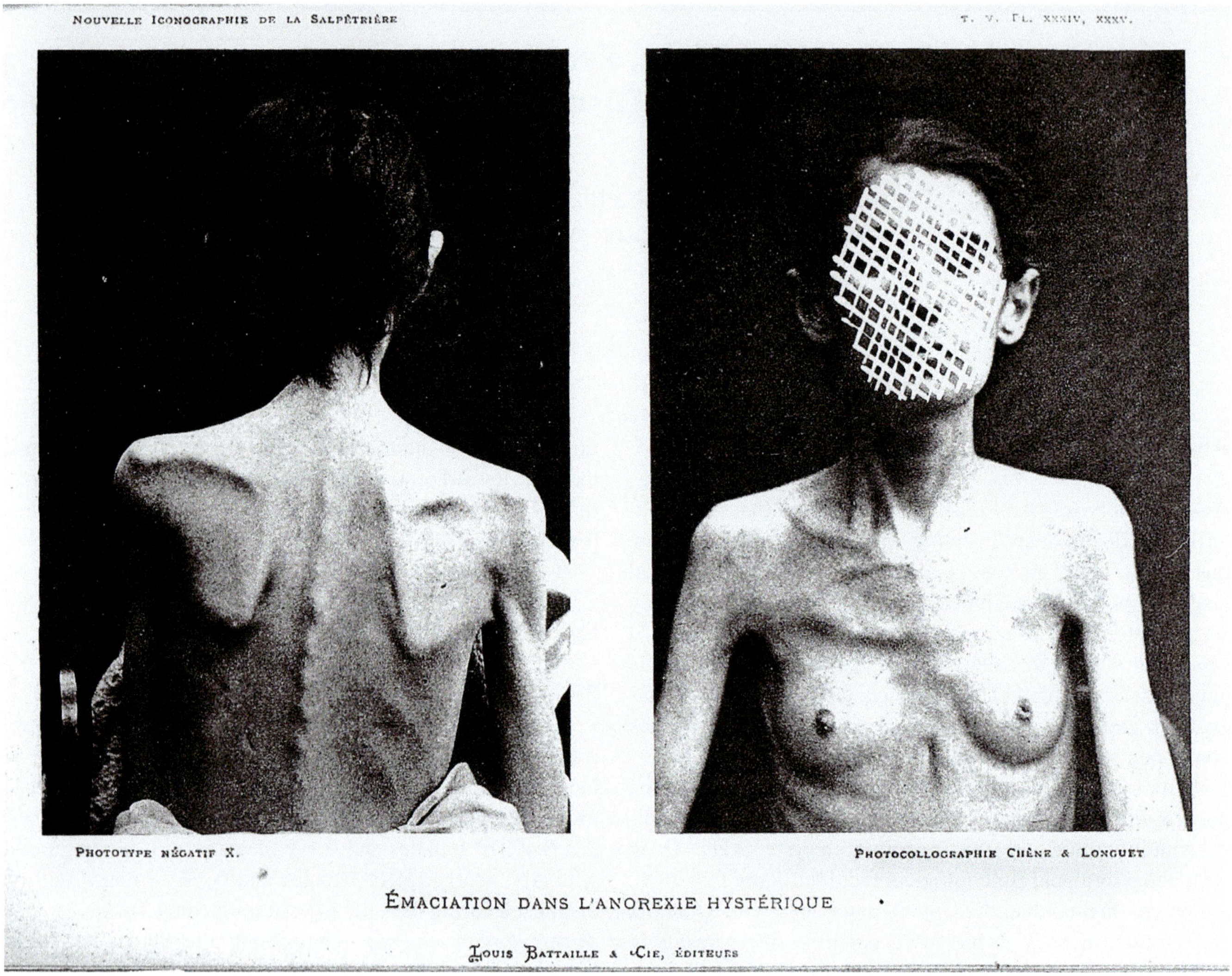

Fig. 21.1 Anorexic emaciation in a "hysteric." Louis Bataille (Welcome Images, L0020548; Creative Commons Attribution 4.0 International; https://creativecommons.org/licenses/by/4.0/). Louis Bataille, 'Deux cas d'anorexie hysterique.' https://commons.wikimedia.org/wiki/File:Louis_Bataille,_%27Deux_cas_d%27anorexie_hysterique%27_Wellcome_L0020548.jpg

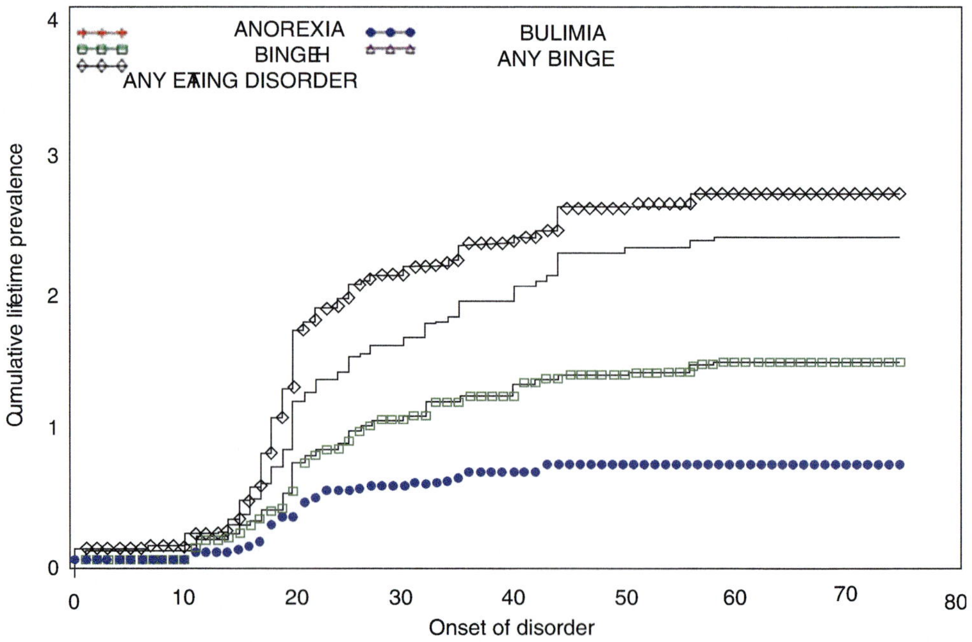

Fig. 21.2 Thomas et al. [6], typical onset begins in adolescence and young adulthood, although many individuals have a period of changed eating behavior prior to full criteria for the disorder being met. (*From* Thomas et al.; *with permission*)

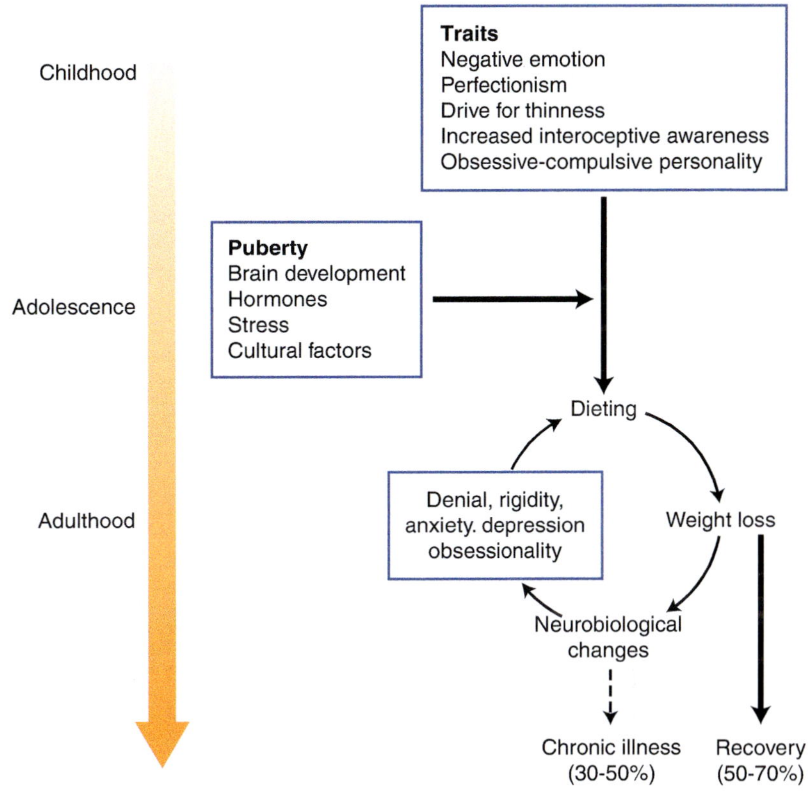

Fig. 21.3 The core characteristics of AN, disturbed appetite and reduced food intake. Identifying premorbid traits in some individuals more susceptible to developing AN, which include personality and temperament. (*From* Kaye et al. [7]; *with permission*)

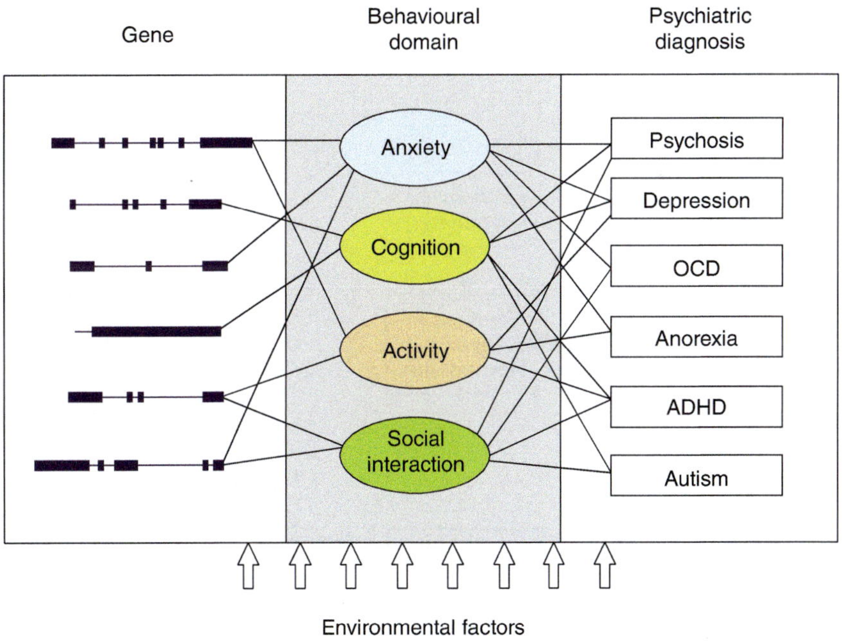

Fig. 21.4 According to Kas and Adan [9], a common genetic variant of the brain-derived neurotrophic factor (BDNF) gene in humans is associated with eating disorders. This also plays a role in the function of neuronal survival, differentiation, and synaptic plasticity. This model outlines certain behavioral domains that are affected in eating disorders that may span across the psychiatric spectrum. (*Reprinted from* Kas et al.; *with permission*)

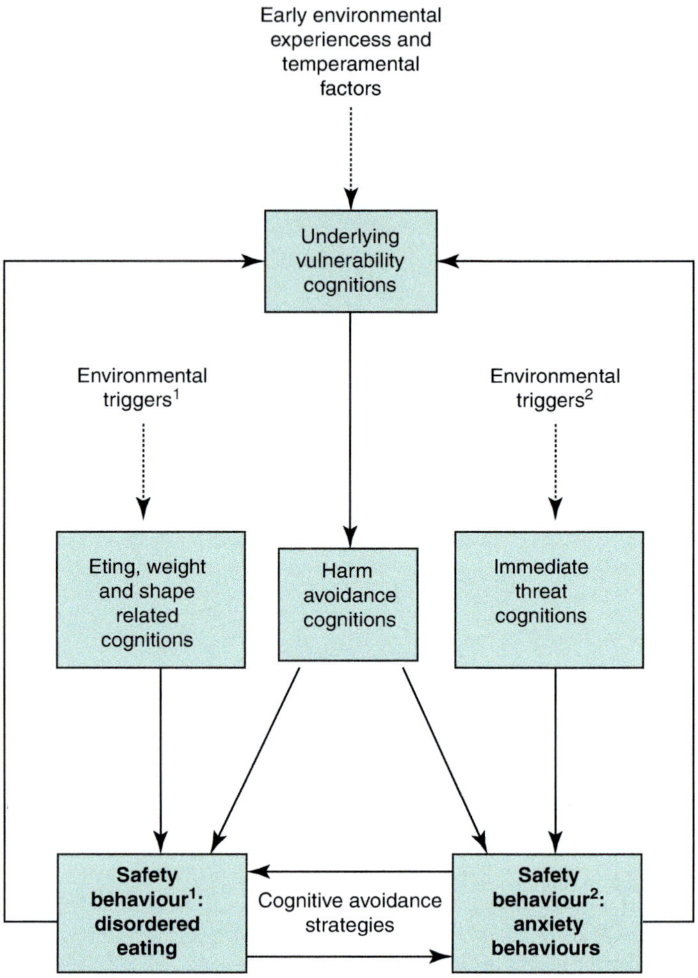

Fig. 21.5 Eating disorders and anxiety are not caused by one another; they stem from the same vulnerability. Rather cognitive avoidance strategy might connect the two disorders, according to Pallister and Waller [10]. (*Reprinted from* Pallister and Waller; *with permission*)

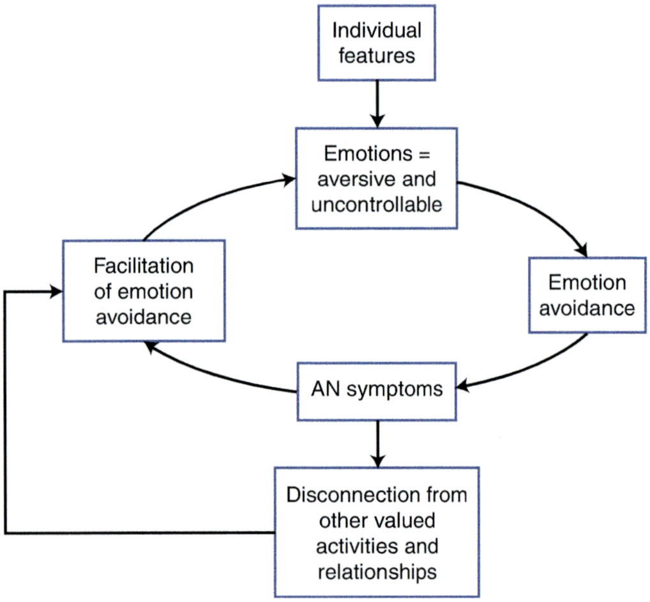

Fig. 21.6 Through emotional acceptance behavioral therapy (EABT), a psychotherapeutic intervention designed for older adolescents and adults, people with AN are often characterized by their harm-avoidant personality trait problems with mood disturbances that shape their experience of uncontrollable and aversive emotions

viduals may experience OCD; alternatively, alcohol and other substance use disorders are more likely seen in those with binge-eating/purging type (Figs. 21.7, 21.8, and 21.9).

Etiology

Genetics and Inheritance

Research suggests that anorexia nervosa is heritable, with estimates ranging from 28 to 74% [11]. Most twin studies have shown higher concordance rates for monozygotic twins than for dizygotic twins. Also, patients with the restrictive subtype tend to have more affected relatives [12]. First-degree relatives are ten times as likely to develop an eating disorder than relatives of individuals without AN [13]. There is also evidence of a positive genetic correlation between AN and schizophrenia [11].

Neurobiology

There are multiple effects on both neurocognition and social cognition, which may persist even after recovery. Neurocognitively, patients with anorexia may show a preference for detail-oriented rather than global process-

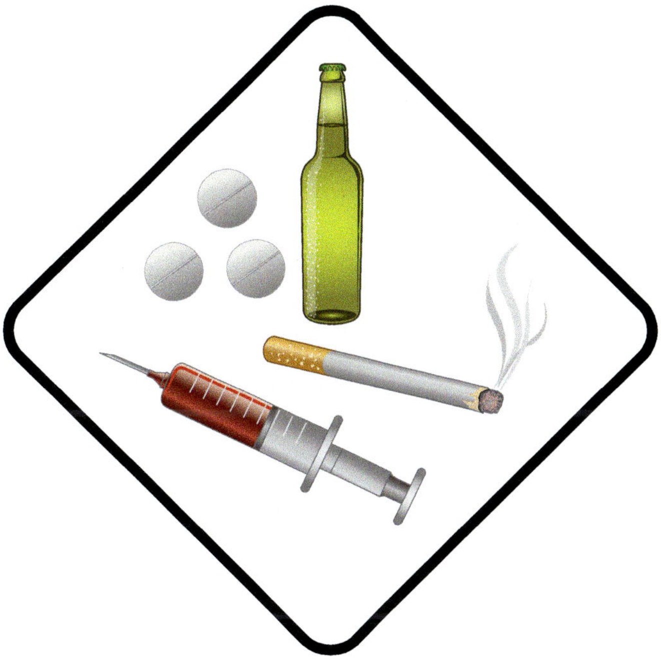

Fig. 21.7 Alcohol use disorder and other substance use disorders may be comorbid with anorexia nervosa, especially among those with binge-eating/purging type. The Noun Project. Substance Abuse Service Icon. https://thenounproject.com/term/substance-abuse-service/41339

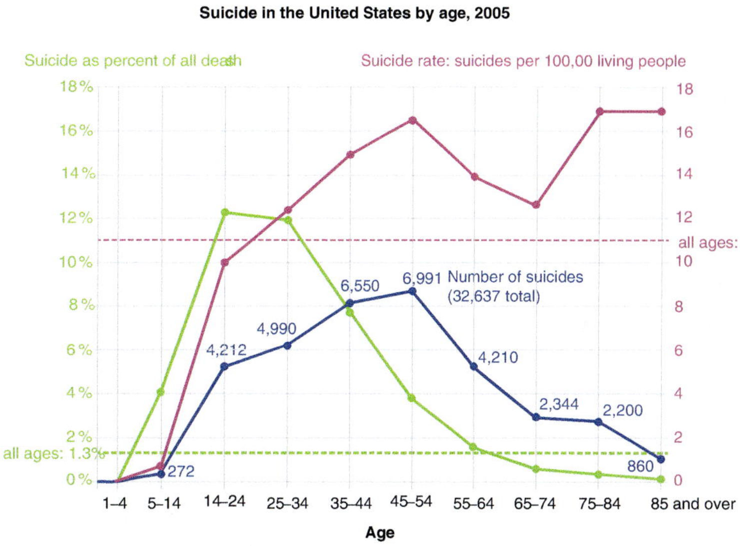

Fig. 21.8 Suicide risk is elevated in anorexia nervosa, with rates reported as 12 per 100,000 per year. Creative Commons Attribution-ShareAlike 3.0 License. WikiMedia. Graph of suicide rates in the United States by age in 2005. Data from the CDC. https://en.wikipedia.org/wiki/File:Suicide_by_age_in_the_US,_2005.png

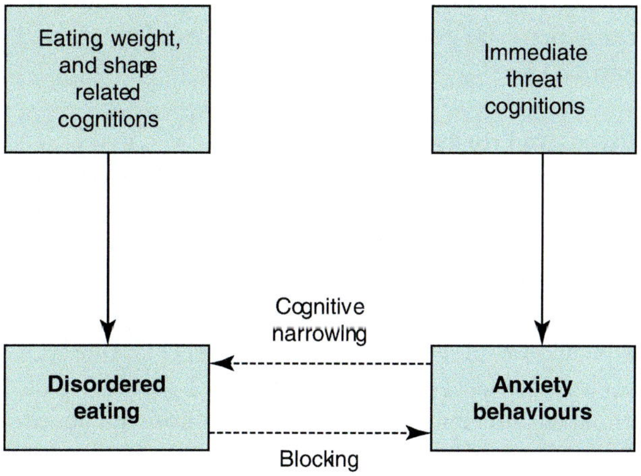

Fig. 21.9 Many individuals with AN report either an anxiety disorder or symptoms prior to the onset of their eating disorder, although Pallister and Waller [10] state one does not cause the other. (*Reprinted from* Pallister and Waller [10]; *with permission*)

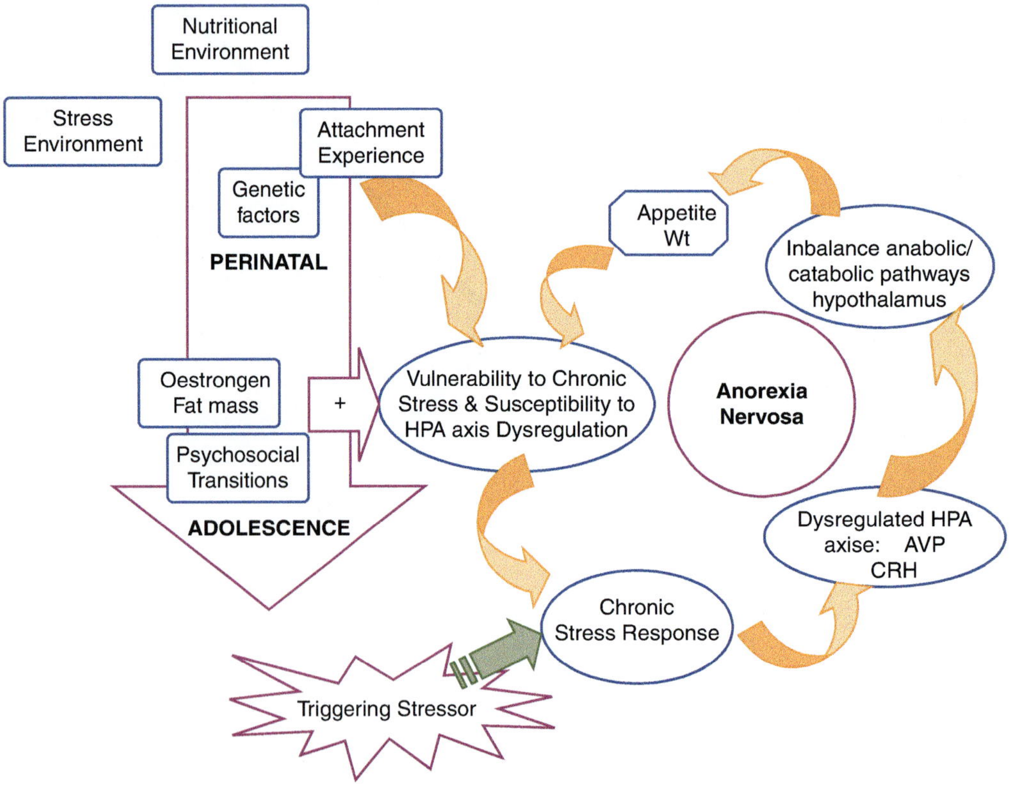

Fig. 21.10 Perinatal exposure and exposures throughout childhood influence vulnerability to chronic stress and Hypothalamic–pituitary–adrenal (HPA) axis dysregulation. Exposure to a "triggering stressor" while vulnerable leads to an impaired HPA axis response that disrupts the hypothalamus. Appetite and weight decrease, and the starvation state sustains the cycle

ing. Set-shifting difficulties, in which patients struggle with switching between tasks, may also occur. Social cognition may also be impaired. Some patients exhibit poor theory of mind, attentional biases, impaired emotional recognition and management [11] (Figs. 21.10, 21.11, and 21.12).

Some evidence suggests that childhood anxiety, obsessions, and perfectionism are risk factors for the development of AN. Restrictive eating may ultimately be a response to imbalances between the serotonergic and dopaminergic systems, with multiple neurobiological models focusing on the relationship between stress, sensations of reward with food restriction, and eventual habitual behavior [11] (Figs. 21.13 and 21.14).

Stressful Life Events

Adverse life events are associated with anorexia nervosa, particularly during times of developmental transition. In infancy, this may include dysmaturity/prematurity, feeding difficulties, and issues with sleeping. Puberty and adolescence represent a uniquely vulnerable and fluid time where typical onset of anorexia nervosa occurs [11]. One well-supported neurodevelopmental model [15] proposes that early childhood attachment experiences combine with genetic factors create susceptibility of HPA axis dysregulation. A stressful event in puberty, especially in females, results in lower AVP levels and elevated levels of CRH, ultimately leading to reduced appetite and weight [16].

Physical, Sexual, and Emotional Abuse

There is some evidence that sexual abuse is associated with increased severity of eating disorder pathology. Sexual abuse has been correlated with binge-eating and purging episodes among patients with anorexia nervosa [17]. Childhood abuse has been hypothesized to relate to AN symptoms, but more research is required. A study on the role of child abuse in patients with AN found that, across subtypes, reports of emotional abuse were most strongly related to emotion dysregulation and AN severity [18]. Data from the National Epidemiologic Survey on Alcohol and Related Conditions found that "the strongest relationships with any eating disorder were sexual abuse and physical neglect among men and sexual abuse and emotional abuse among women" [19].

Substance Abuse

Roughly one in four individuals with anorexia has a comorbid substance use disorder. Individuals with the restricting

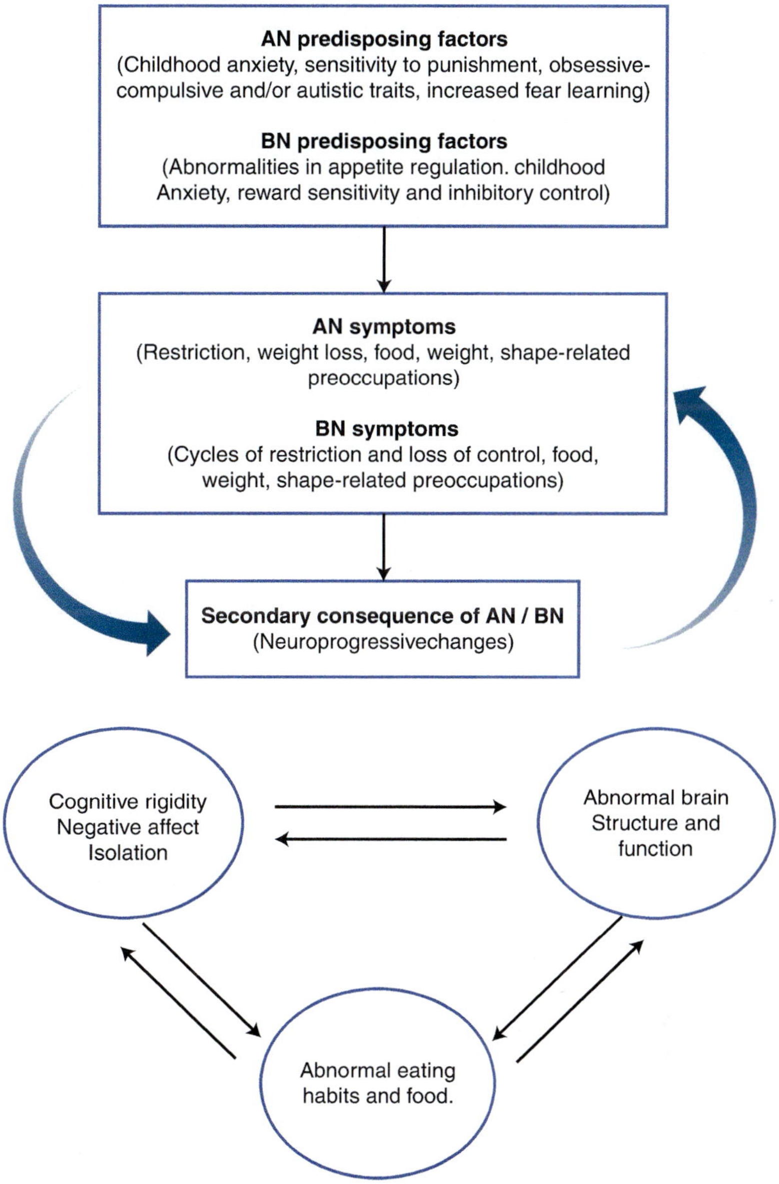

Fig. 21.11 Figure depicts the development of severe AN and BN. Predisposing factors lead to symptoms. Symptoms and neuroprogressive changes reinforce each other

subtype appear to engage in substance abuse less frequently than those with the binge-eating/purging subtype. The severity of caloric restriction is also a predictor of psychostimulant use [20].

Pathophysiology

Physical Signs and Symptoms

The presence of diagnostic markers—such as lowered bone mass, amenorrhea, emaciation, lanugo—is likely observable in people with anorexia nervosa [1]. Bone mass, specifically low bone mineral density in osteopenia or osteoporosis areas, is often seen and may significantly increase the risk of fractures. Amenorrhea, most commonly a consequence of the weight loss, can be observed prior to weight loss. In females, menarche, the first occurrence of menstruation, may be delayed due to severe weight loss. Physical examinations may result in finding emaciation and related heart conditions including hypotension, hypothermia, and bradycardia (Figs. 21.15 and 21.16).

Although not as prevalent, symptoms like lanugo, fine downy body hair, or petechiae which can indicate bleeding diathesis may be seen in people with anorexia nervosa (Figs. 21.17 and 21.18).

Serum Chemistry

In patients diagnosed with an eating disorder, body image distortion includes (1) an inaccurate perception of body size and shape, (2) the level of satisfaction with body silhouette, (3) and the mental image of body structure. Through functional magnetic resonance imaging (fMRI), Gaudio et al.

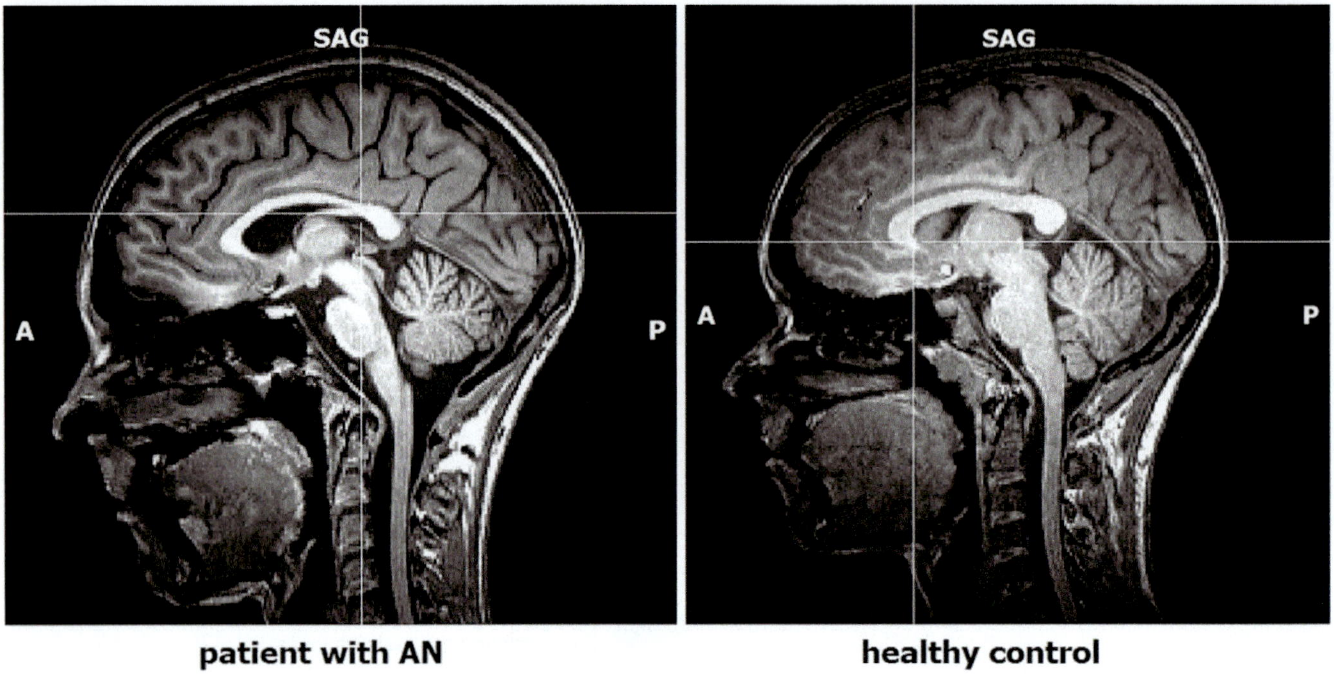

Fig. 21.12 Changes in brain volume can occur as a result of anorexia. Seitz J, Bühren K, von Polier GG, Heussen N, Herpertz-Dahlmann B, Konrad K. Morphological changes in the brain of acutely ill and weight-recovered patients with anorexia nervosa. A meta-analysis and qualitative review. Z Kinder Jugendpsychiatr Psychother. 2014;42(1):7–18. https://doi.org/10.1024/1422-4917/a000265

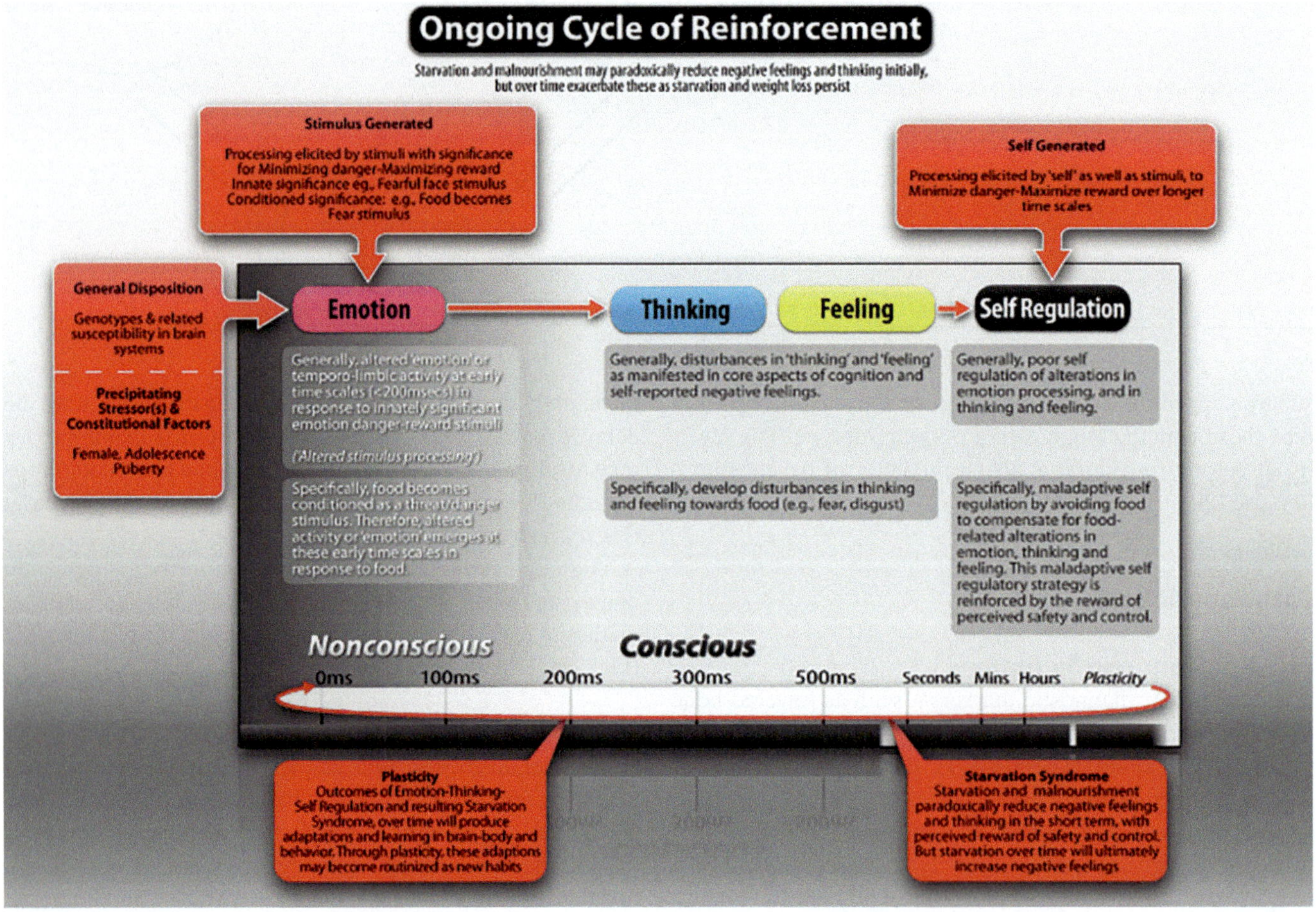

Fig. 21.13 Food becomes a threat/danger stimulus, leading to maladaptive avoidance. (*Reprinted from* Rose and Frampton [14]; *with permission*)

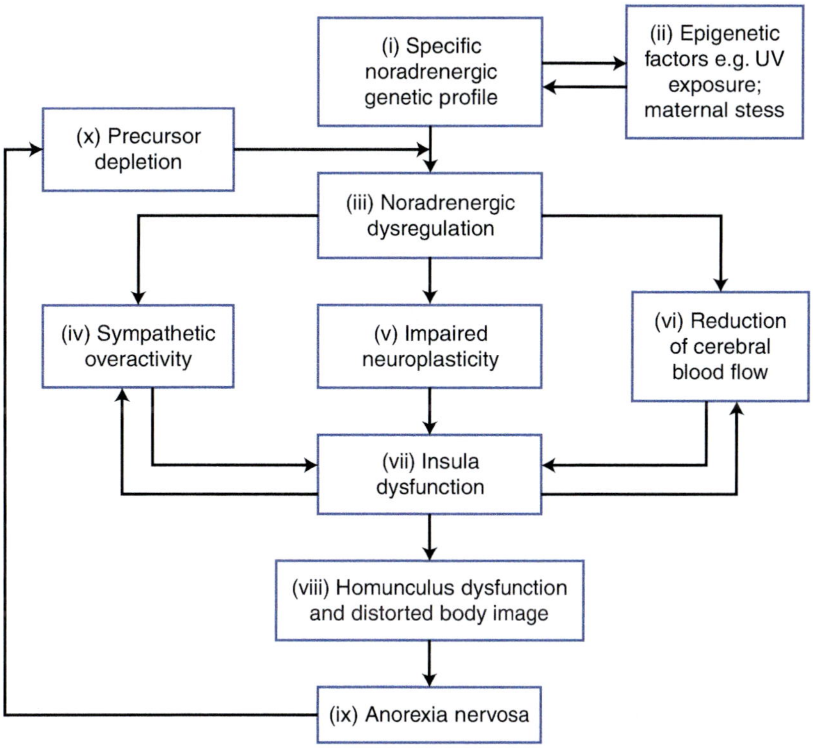

Fig. 21.14 A detailed model of AN that focuses on neurobiology

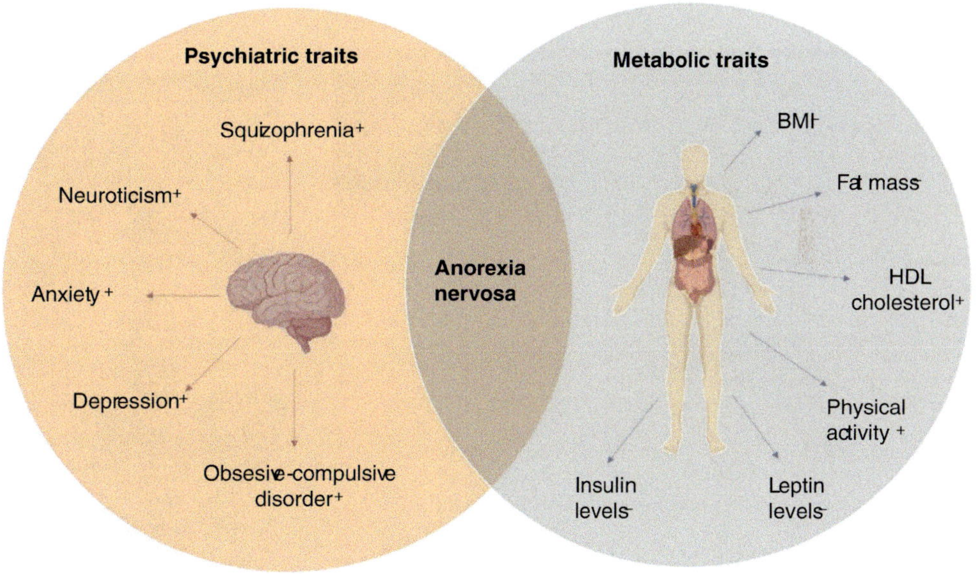

Fig. 21.15 Many of the physical signs and symptoms that are seen in people with AN are attributable to starvation. Wikimedia. [Significant genetic correlations based on the SNP risk loci of Anorexia nervosa with psychiatric and metabolic traits]. 2020

[21] identified the active areas in the brain associated with body image distortion in patients diagnosed with anorexia nervosa. The prefrontal cortex, posterior parietal cortex, extrastriate body area, and insula all play a role in body image distortion. Specifically, the brain's prefrontal area becomes active, while individuals with various eating disorders describe their dissatisfaction with their bodies [22] (Figs. 21.19, 21.20, 21.21, and 21.22).

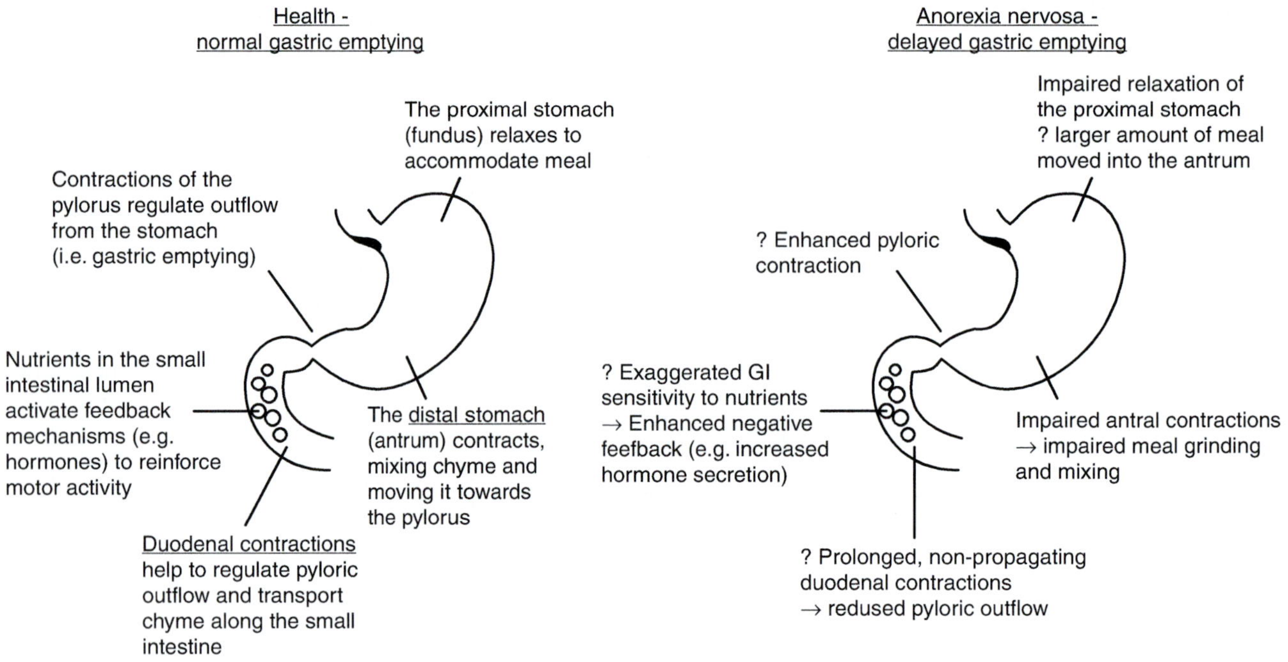

Fig. 21.16 Illustrates the delayed gastric emptying, seen in people with AN, and the reported disturbances in gastrointestinal (GI) motor function. Common disturbances include increased episodes of gastric dysrhythmias, impaired proximal gastric accommodation and antral contractility, and increased postprandial antral distension

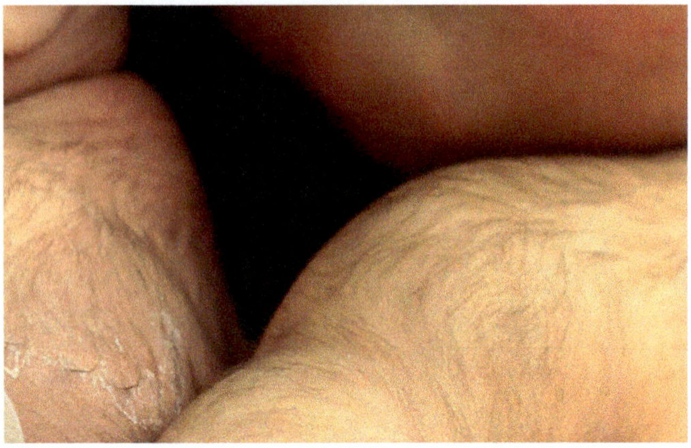

Fig. 21.17 Lanugo can be a diagnostic marker of anorexia

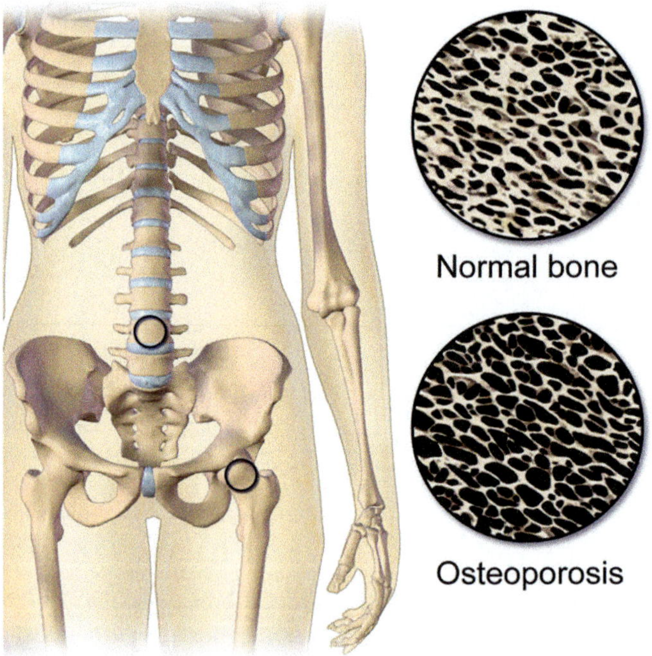

Fig. 21.18 Anorexia can lead to osteoporosis, causing bones to become weak and brittle. Wikimedia. Osteoporosis locations. https://commons.wikimedia.org/wiki/File:Osteoporosis_Locations.png

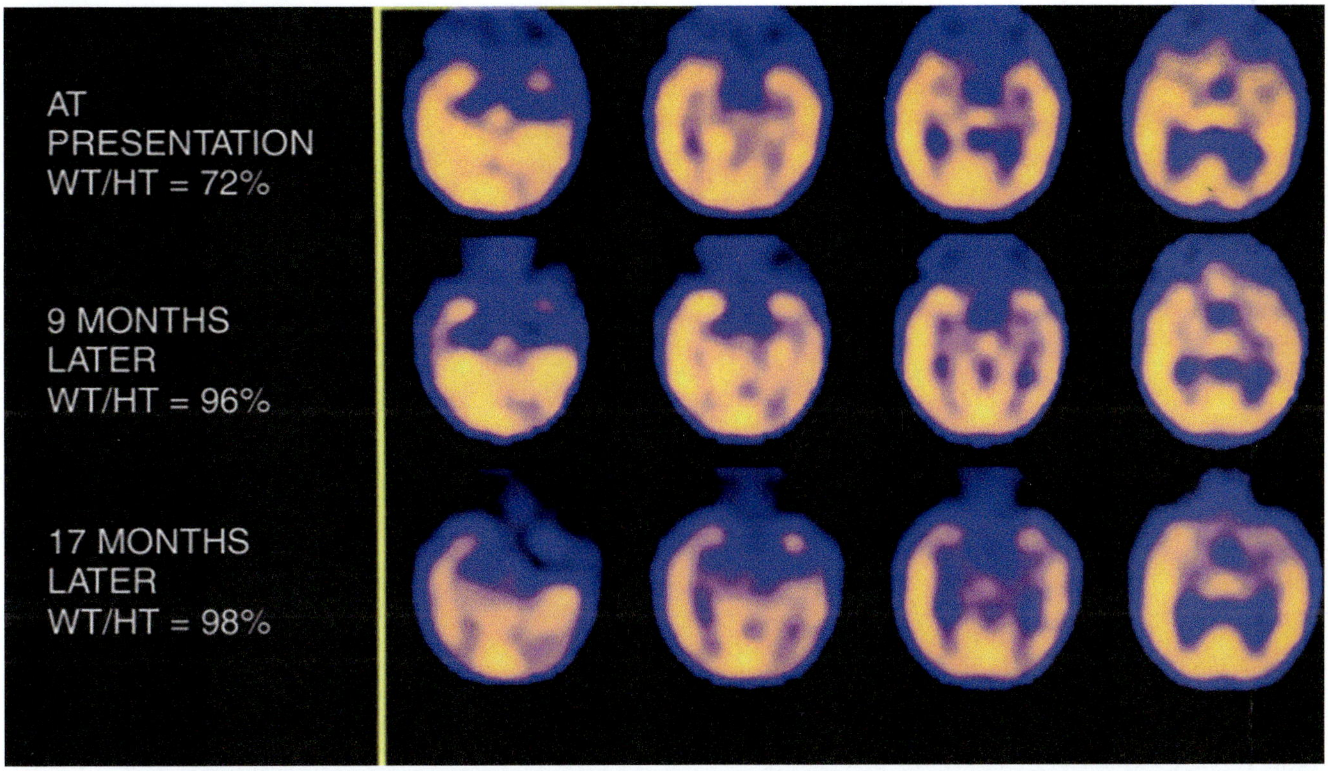

Fig. 21.19 This figure of SPECTS, a tomographic imaging technique using gamma rays, shows brain function by measuring the rate of blood flow in different parts of the brain. Displaying active parts of the brain that require more oxygen and increased perfusion rate that act as fuel to active neurons

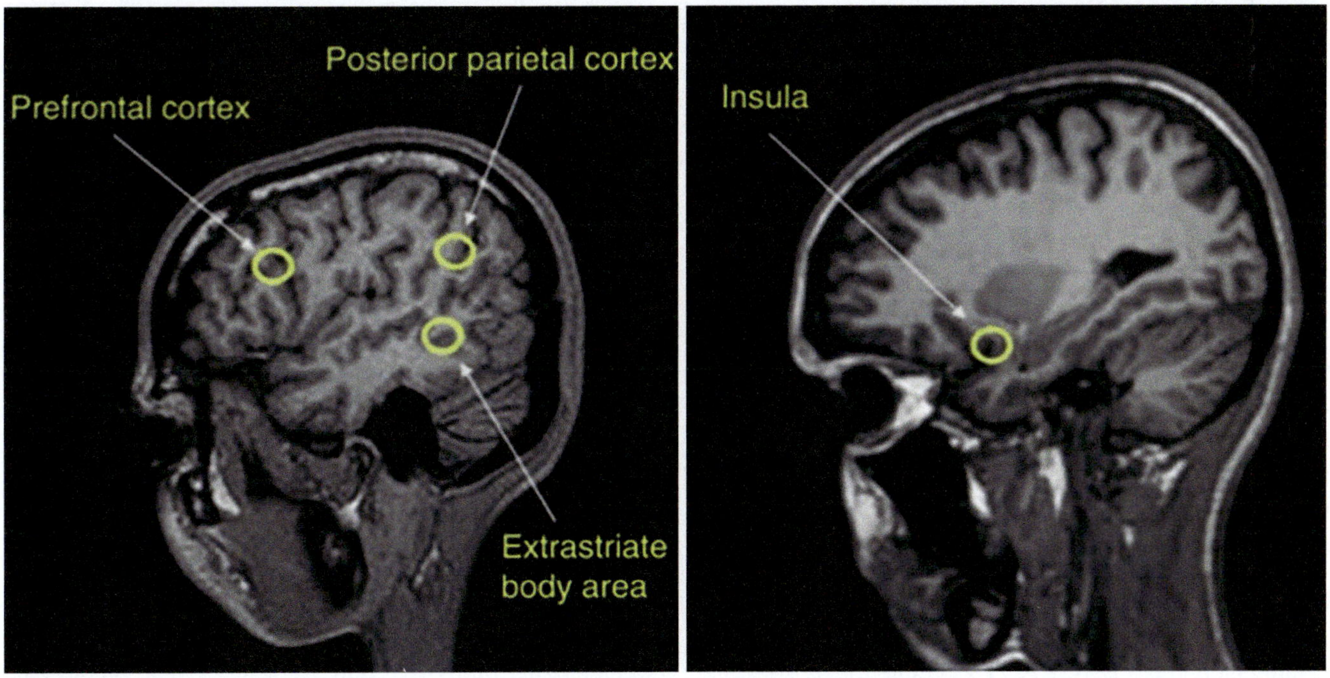

Fig. 21.20 The figure displays and highlights several brain areas associated with body image distortion. The image on the left features the prefrontal cortex, posterior parietal cortex, and extrastriate body area, while the right image focuses on the insula

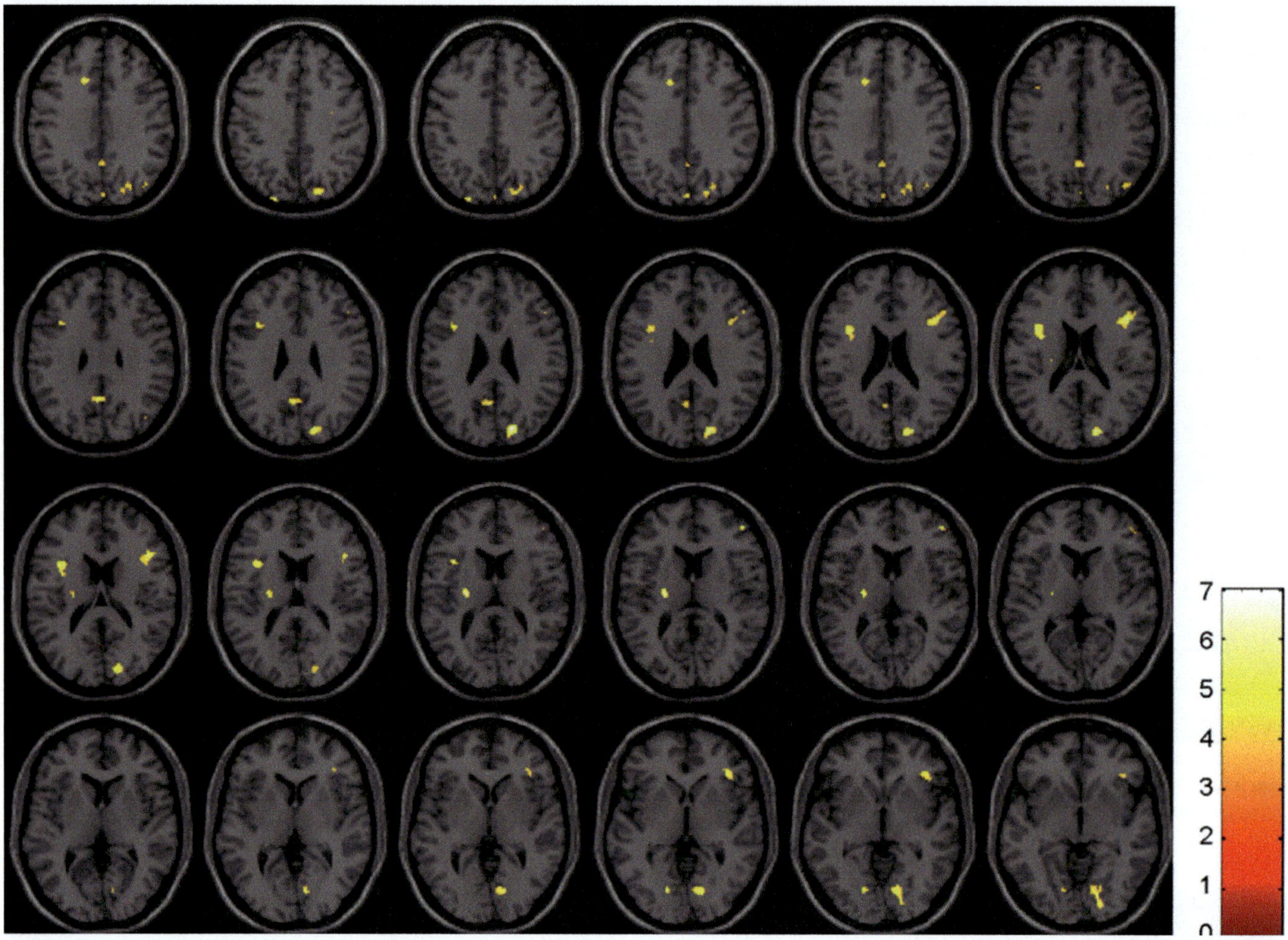

Fig. 21.21 Compared with controls, anorexia patients had reduced activation in the middle frontal gyri, insula, precuneus, and occipital regions when viewing a self-image versus a non-self-image. Sachdev P, Mondatry N, Wen W, Gulliford K. Brains of anorexia nervosa patients process self-images differently from non-self-images: an fMRI study. Neuropsychologia. 2008;46(8):2161–8. https://doi.org/10.1016/j.neuropsychologia.2008.02.031

Phenomenology

Restriction of Energy Intake

According to the American Psychiatric Association [1], caloric intake restriction is one of three required diagnostic symptoms of anorexia nervosa. To further discern the difference in calorie consumption between individuals with anorexic and non-anorexic symptoms, researchers compartmentalized nutrition intake into the number of grams of carbohydrate, fat, and protein consumed. Researchers determined that patients with anorexia nervosa consume significantly fewer grams of carbohydrates, fat, and protein than healthy individuals [23] (Fig. 21.23; Table 21.1).

Fear of Weight Gain or Becoming Fat

Individuals with anorexia nervosa engage in restrictive behavior to control their weight because of the fear of gaining weight or becoming fat [1]. However, in the presence of weight loss, patients will continue to experience high levels of fear. According to the cognitive-behavioral model, while restrictive behaviors play a role, improving cognitions may assist patients with their fears. Therefore, researchers aim to mitigate fears with the use of intensive therapy approaches. For instance, Calugi et al. [24] used intensive cognitive-behavioral therapy to assuage patients' fears. After participating in intensive treatment, patients reported experiencing lower levels of fear of weight gain. Moreover, improvement in fear predicts an increase in body mass index (Figs. 21.24 and 21.25).

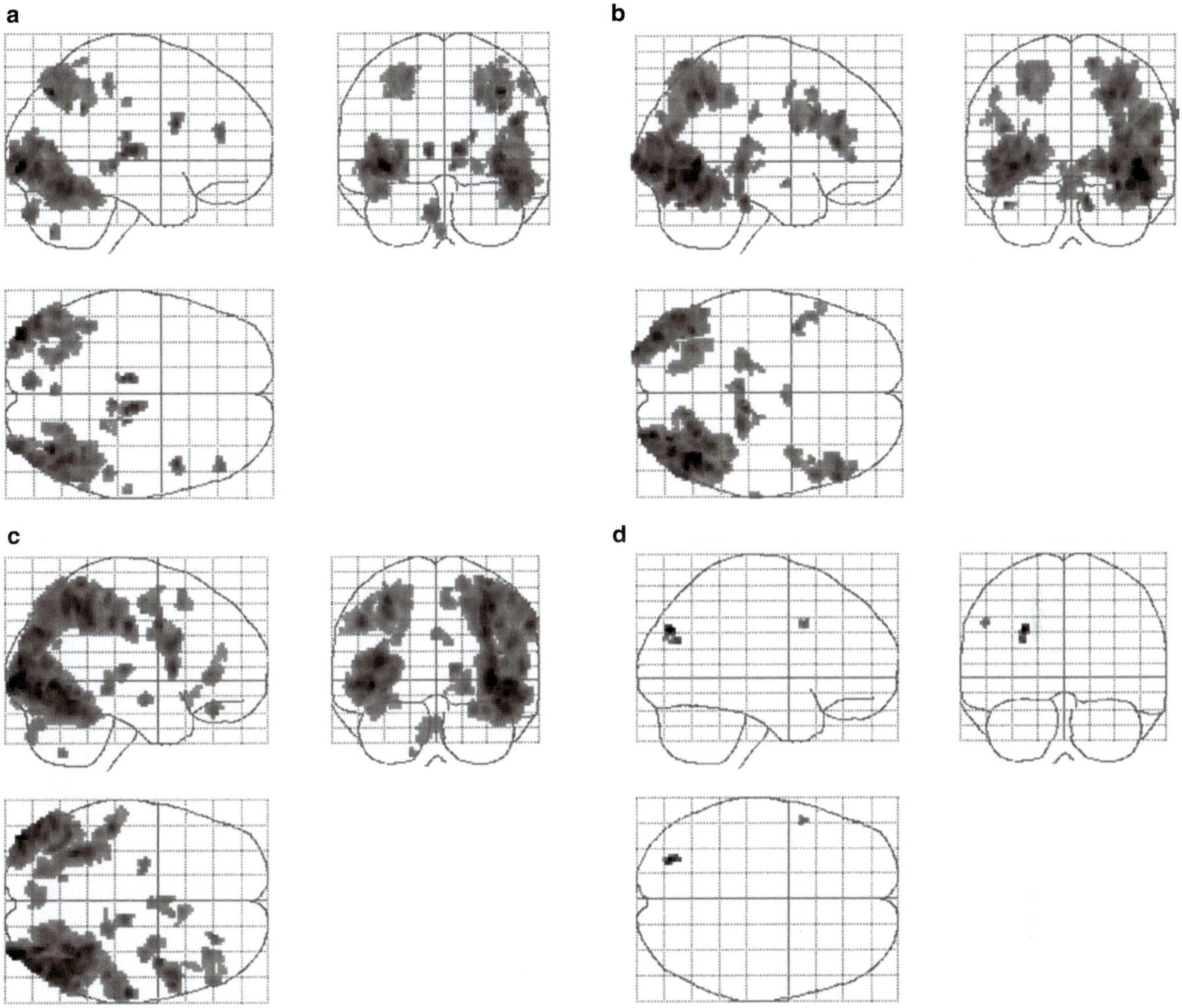

Fig. 21.22 Brain activation patterns observed in controls and patients with anorexia when viewing non-self and self-images compared to baseline. Sachdev P, Mondatry N, Wen W, Gulliford K. Brains of anorexia nervosa patients process self-images differently from non-self-images: an fMRI study. Neuropsychologia. 2008;46(8):2161–8. https://doi.org/10.1016/j.neuropsychologia.2008.02.031

Restrictive vs. Binge-Eating/Purging Type

While all patients with anorexia share three significant symptoms, they may be distinguished into two subtypes of anorexia. The binge-eating/purge subtype of anorexia nervosa, while similar to the restrictive subtype, differs by binge eating followed by purging [1]. Moreover, Gao and Gurd [26] determined that the subtypes significantly differ in energy consumption during meals and snacks. Specifically, patients assigned to binge-eating/purge subtypes report significantly less meal and snack consumption throughout the day than patients with restrictive type anorexia (Fig. 21.26; Table 21.2).

Treatment

Levels of Care

Patients with restrictive and binge-eating/purge subtype symptoms also differ in the type of treatment they are assigned. Since patients with restrictive subtypes engage in dieting, they often are placed in intensive residential treatment programs, such as residential centers and patients. The goal of intensive residential treatment is to prepare patients for less intensive treatment. In lower levels of care, patients still participate in several hours of therapy weekly [28] (Table 21.3).

Fig. 21.23 According to Schebendach et al. [23], when they compared patients, patients diagnosed with AN consumed significantly fewer grams of carbohydrates, proteins, and fats than healthy patients. (*From* Schebendach et al.; *with permission*)

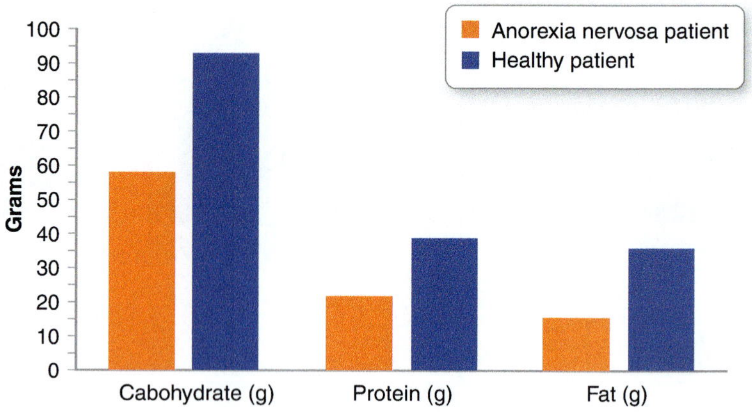

Table 21.1 Comparison of nutrient intake at the multi-item meal study in patients with anorexia nervosa (AN) and healthy control (HC) participants

Multi-item meal intake	AN ($n = 44$)	HC ($n = 48$)	t	df	p [a]	Cohen's d [b]	AN-R ($n = 23$)	AN-BP ($n = 21$)	t	df	p [a]	Cohen's d [b]
Energy (kcal)	469.16 (397.71)	846.40 (346.89)	−4.987	90	<0.001	−1.037	543.22 (477.64)	388.04 (275.51)	1.303	42	0.200	0.397
Carbohydrate (g)[c]	58.40 (45.17)	93.97 (37.10)	−4.115	89	<0.001	−0.86	64.44 (50.36)	51.79 (38.83)	0.926	42	0.360	0.281
Protein (g)[c]	22.06 (17.06)	39.45 (15.18)	−5.141	89	<0.001	−1.076	25.18 (17.59)	18.65 (16.19)	1.278	42	0.208	0.386
Fat (g)	16.45 (20.43)	36.74 (18.90)	−4.949	90	<0.001	−1.031	20.54 (25.97)	11.97 (10.71)	1.452	29.832	0.157	0.431
% kcal carbohydrate[c]	52.09 (20.69)	43.85 (6.60)	2.524	51.162	0.015	0.536	48.22 (16.99)	56.34 (23.81)	−1.310	42	0.197	−0.392
% kcal protein[c]	20.41 (13.46)	19.41 (6.07)	0.451	58.934	0.654	0.095	22.43 (13.52)	18.20 (13.37)	1.042	42	0.303	0.314
% kcal fat	22.95 (13.81)	36.68 (8.03)	−5.757	67.817	<0.001	−1.214	24.99 (13.77)	20.72 (13.85)	1.023	42	0.312	0.308
Diet energy density (DEDS)[d]	0.607 (0.509)	0.978 (0.293)	−4.232	67.433	<0.001	−0.892	0.647 (0.542)	0.563 (0.480)	0.537	42	0.594	0.162
Diet variety (DVS)[e]	5.80 (3.46)	8.96 (2.66)	−4.934	90	<0.001	−1.023	6.39 (3.94)	5.14 (2.79)	1.201	42	0.236	0.365

All values expressed as mean + standard deviation (SD). (*From* Schebendach et al. [23]; *with permission*)
[a]Independent samples t-test
[b]Cohen's d: small effect = 0.2; medium effect = 0.5; large effect = 0.8
[c]Values for carbohydrate (g and %) and protein (g and %) missing for 1 HC participant ($n = 47$)
[d]DEDS: energy intake (kcal) divided by the gram weight of all food/beverage items consumed
[e]DVS: the number of energy-containing food/beverage items consumed divided the number of energy-containing food and beverage items served

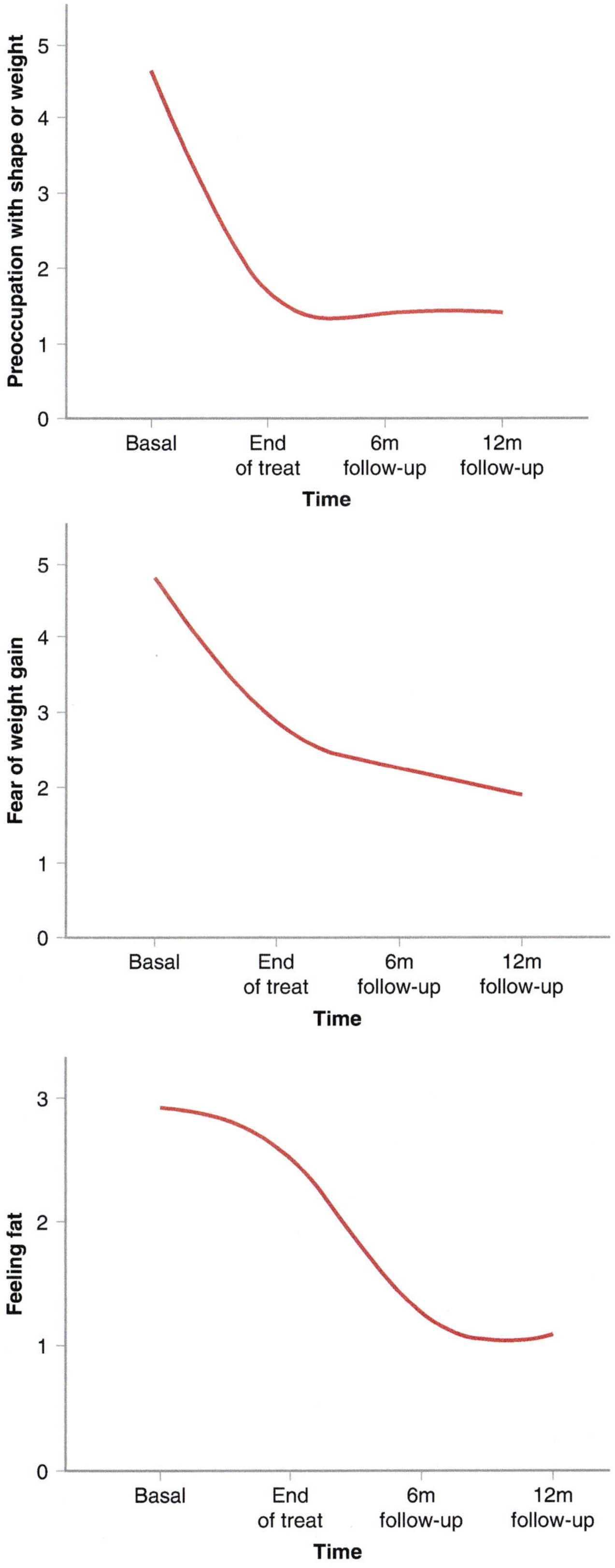

Fig. 21.24 Calugi et al. found estimated means of body image concern components in which estimates were obtained using individual growth curve models. (*From* Calugi et al.; *with permission*)

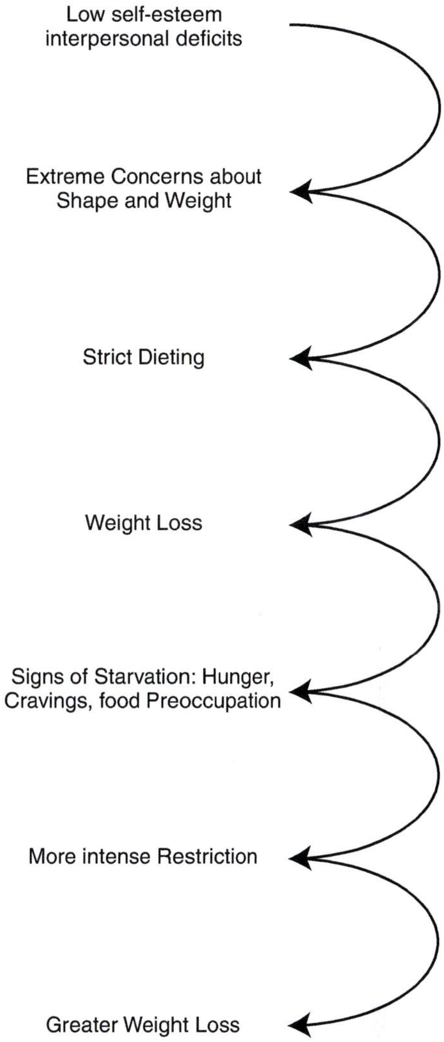

Fig. 21.25 The diagram illustrates the effects of fear of weight gain and the behavioral patterns that lead to weight loss. (*From* Peat [25]; *with permission*)

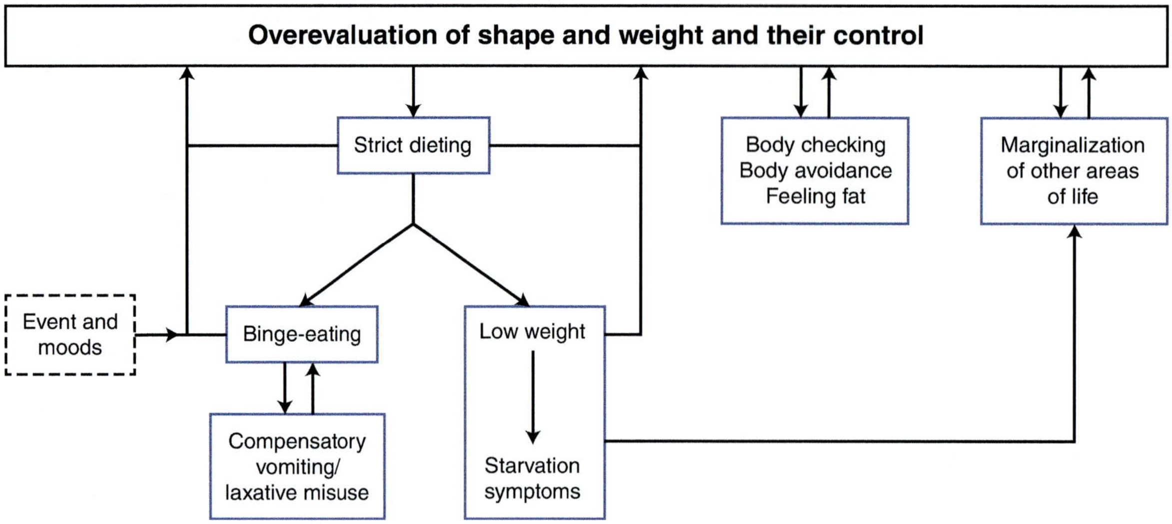

Fig. 21.26 This chart demonstrates the patterns associated with the over-evaluation of shape and weight. (*From* Riva et al. [27]; *with permission*)

Table 21.2 Reported meal and snack consumption on the EDE in the past 28 days with age and BMI as covariates, M (SD)

	Full sample (n = 160)	Restricting AN (n = 120)	Binge purge AN (n = 40)	Test statistic
Breakfast	23.4 (8.1)	24.7 (8.1)	19.8 (10.3)	F(2,158) = 9.25**, partial = 0.56
Mid-morning snack	7.3 (9.2)	8.2 (9.6)	4.4 (7.2)	F(2,158) = 5.59*, partial = 0.035
Lunch	22.9 (7.8)	24.5 (6.6)	18.2 (9.3)	F(2,158) = 18.64***, partial = 0.107
Mid-afternoon snack	14.7 (10.3)	15.6 (10.3)	11.7 (9.5)	F(2,158) = 5.66**, partial = 0.035
Dinner	25.3 (5.7)	26.2 (4.4)	22.5 (7.3)	F(2,158) = 12.12**, partial = 0.072
Evening snack	12.9 (10.1)	13.5 (10.3)	11.5 (9.3)	F(2,158) = 3.74, partial = 0.023
Meals per day	2.55 (0.63)	2.69 (0.51)	2.16 (0.80)	F(2,158) = 19.82***, partial = 0.113
Snack per day	1.24 (0.86)	1.33 (0.89)	0.98 (0.67)	F(2,158) = 7.54**, partial = 0.046

Note. *$p < 0.05$, **$p < 0.01$, ***$p < 0.001$

From Gao and Gurd [26];

Interpersonal Psychotherapy

Interpersonal psychotherapy (IPT) aims to improve eating disorder symptoms, such as binge eating and purging, by addressing social functioning issues [29]. Specifically, individuals may improve their social problems by addressing past personal relationship issues and poor social adjustment. Tanofsky-kraff and Wilfley [29] provide an example of IPT approaches to mitigate a patient's interpersonal problems (Table 21.4).

Cognitive-Behavioral Therapy

With the development of virtual reality (VR) technology, researchers and clinicians may aim to help patients with distorted body image. Experiential cognitive therapy is a cognitive-behavioral therapy treatment that uses virtual reality to ameliorate poor body satisfaction and increase treatment motivation. Through immersive virtual reality, patients view a virtual representation of themselves in a realistic virtual environment. Within the virtual setting, clinicians address the patient's unrealistic body perspectives and affective body dissatisfaction [27] (Figs. 21.27 and 21.28).

Antidepressants

In addition to therapy, clinicians prescribe medication to maintain weight and promote weight gain. McElory et al. [31] review the antidepressants, antipsychotics, appetite stimulants, prokinetics, hormonal agents, and other highly used medications to restore and maintain weight. The following table demonstrates that few medications are effective in restoring the weight of patients with anorexia. Moreover, there are fewer medications that help with the maintenance of weight (Table 21.5).

Table 21.3 Settings for the treatment of individuals with eating disorders

Setting	Description	Indications
Outpatient	Individual or group-based sessions are available, and patients often select or are recommended for several treatment components, often offered by clinicians from different clinical disciplines (e.g., psychology, nutrition, medicine). Outpatient treatment is optimized when providers communicate regularly in order to coordinate care, creating a treatment "team"	An outpatient program is the most commonly used setting for eating disorder treatment. Many patients utilize outpatient treatment as they begin engagement in eating disorder treatment or because they are unable to access higher levels of care because of geographic or other resource limitations. Outpatient treatment is most appropriate for individuals who are achieving or maintaining behavioral goals using this level of care
Intensive outpatient program (IOP)	IOP refers to a routine of outpatient sessions in which visits include several hours of treatment per visit offered at a frequency of several visits (e.g., three) each week. Supervised meals are often available as part of an IOP visit	An IOP is appropriate for individuals who are medically stable and require small amounts of meal instruction or meal supervision without additional daily programmatic structure. An IOP is often used as a step-down from higher levels of care
Partial hospital program (PHP)	Also known as day treatment programs, PHPs offer more hours of weekly treatment than do IOPs. A PHP may serve as a transition from inpatient to outpatient care or may help some individuals avoid the need for hospitalization. PHPs generally include 4–7 days of treatment with two or three supervised meals each treatment day	A PHP is appropriate when meal supervision is needed without requirement for 24-h supervision. PHP admission generally requires that patients be at or above a minimally acceptable weight (e.g., ≥80% ideal body weight) and maintain other evidence of medical stability. A PHP is often used as a step-down from a higher level of care, or as a step-up from a lower level of care
Residential treatment center (RTC)	RTCs offer specialized treatment delivered in a full-time setting; however, they are less structured than hospital programs. They include less medical monitoring and less staffing at night than do hospital-based programs	An RTC is appropriate for patients with low weight (e.g., <85% ideal body weight) and/or evidence of eating disorder behaviors who are in need of close supervision but not in need of daily medical attention. Patients in an RTC must demonstrate motivation needed for voluntary treatment
Inpatient program	Psychiatric hospitalization represents the highest level of care and may be necessary for some individuals with eating disorders, especially those at low weights and those with comorbidities. Specialized inpatient programs include medical personnel, such as psychiatrists and nurses	An inpatient program is appropriate for patients with significantly low weight (e.g., <75% ideal body weight) and/or the presence of other signs of medical or psychiatric instability (e.g., vital sign or electrolyte disturbance; comorbidity, including behavioral dyscontrol and/or suicidality). Inpatient treatment is also appropriate for individuals who have failed to respond to treatment at an RTC

Table 21.4 Interpersonal problem areas

Main problem area	Description	IPT strategies
Grief	Pathological grief stemming from fears of being unable to tolerate the painful affect associated with the loss	Facilitate the mourning process. Help the patient reestablish interest in relationships to substitute for what has been lost
Interpersonal role disputes	Disputes with partner, children, or other family members or coworkers	Identify the dispute. Choose a plan of action. Modify expectations and faulty communication to bring about a satisfactory resolution
Role transitions	Economic or family change: children leaving for college, new job, divorce, retirement, parent's caretaker	Mourn and accept the loss of the old role. Restore self-esteem by developing a sense of mastery regarding the demands of new roles
Interpersonal deficits	A long-standing history of social isolation, low self-esteem, loneliness, and an inability to form or maintain intimate relationships	Reduce the patient's social isolation. Encourage the formation of new relationships

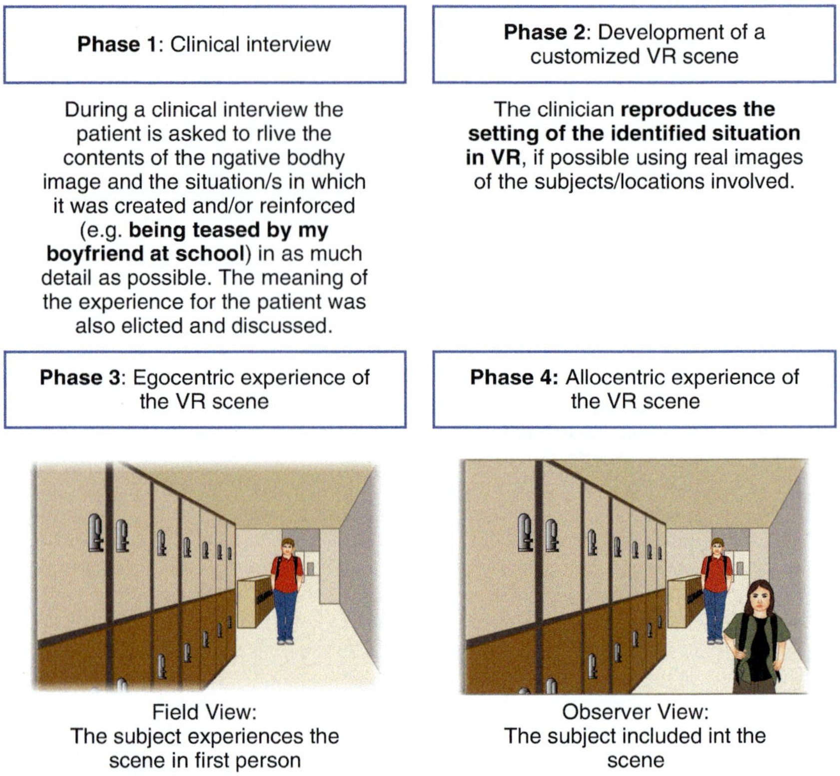

Fig. 21.27 Through the utilization of VR, participants can engage in real-life scenarios that provoke thoughts of negative body image. (*From* Riva et al. [27]; *with permission*)

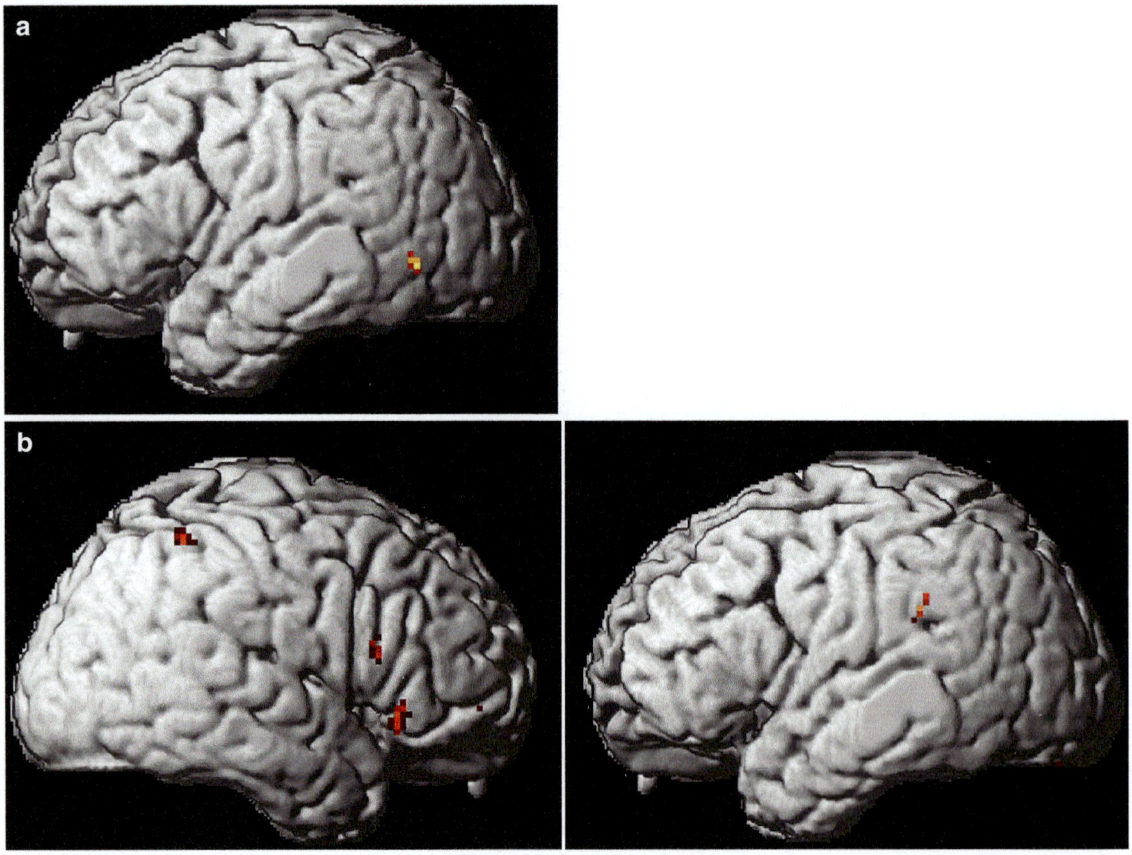

Fig. 21.28 Vocks et al. [30] compared brain activation while viewing one's body for patients with anorexia nervosa before and after body image therapy. Activation in the right middle temporal gyrus (containing the extrastriate body area) was significantly increased post-treatment (Image (**a**) post to pre contrast, (**b**) pre to post contrast). (*From* Vocks et al. [30]; *with permission*)

Table 21.5 Medications studied for anorexia nervosa in randomized, placebo-controlled trials: qualitative results

Medication	Maximum dosage studied (mg/day)	Effect on weight restoration	Effect on weight maintenance
Antidepressants			
Amitriptyline	175	–	NDA
Clomipramine	50	–	NDA
Fluoxetine	60	–	+/–
Antipsychotics			
Olanzapine	15	++	NDA
Pimozide	6	+/–	NDA
Sulpiride	400	–	NDA
Appetite stimulants			
Cyproheptadine	32	+	NDA
Prokinetics			
Cisapride	30	+/–	NDA
Hormonal agents			
rhGH	0.33	+/–	NDA
Testosterone	300 μg	–	NDA
Other agents			
Lithium	NDA [a]	+	NDA
Zinc	100	+	+/–

NDA no data available; *SSRI* selective serotonin reuptake inhibitors; *rhGH* recombinant human growth hormone
[a]Mean plasma lithium level = 1.0 mEq/L

Bulimia Nervosa

Bulimia nervosa—featuring binge-eating and inappropriate compensatory behaviors, feeling ashamed of their eating problems, and attempts to conceal their symptoms—remains as prevalent as anorexia nervosa while highly isolated from one another [1]. Many people with bulimia face similar medical health conditions derived from anorexia nervosa, as well as comorbidities and treatment options. However, several unique factors remain specific to BN, such as weight mass, impacted physical functions caused by abuse of laxatives/diuretics, and disproportionate gender diagnostic issues.

Epidemiology

Biological Risk Factors

Similar to anorexia, bulimia nervosa typically onsets in individuals during their adolescents or young adulthood age [1]. With peak onset in older adolescence, it's uncommon to see individuals with onset before puberty or after the age of 40. Being most prevalent in females than males with a 10:1 ratio, bulimia has a 1–1.5% 12-month prevalence in females (Figs. 21.29 and 21.30).

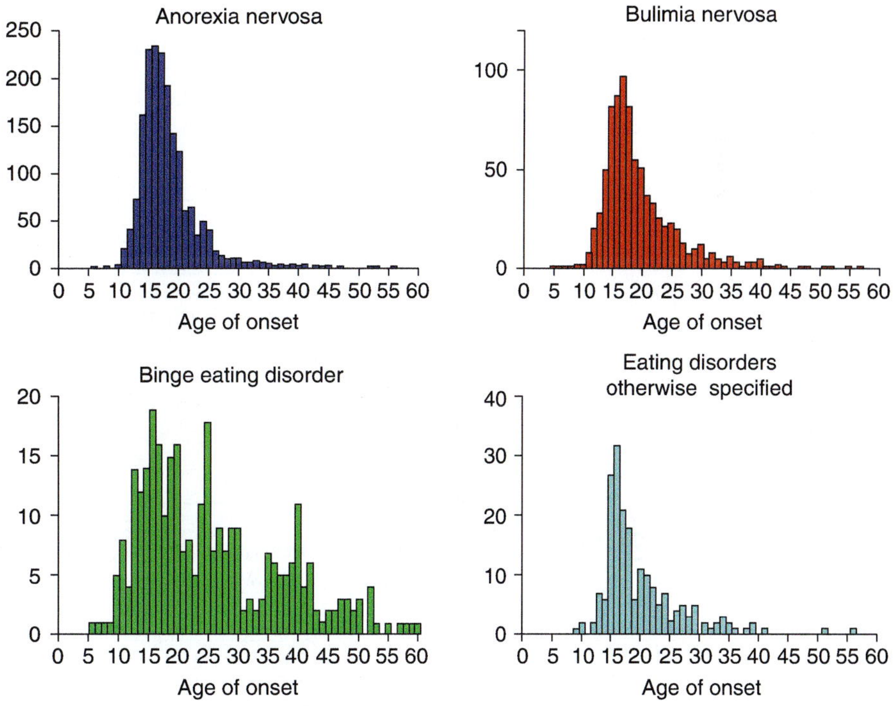

Fig. 21.29 According to Favaro et al. [32], all eating disorders (ED) but binge-eating disorder typically onset during adolescence, with 80% of AN, 69% of BN, and 67% of ED otherwise specified were affected before 20 years old. While BED, onset is typically after 20 years old. (*From* Favaro et al. [32]; *with permission*)

Individuals with BN stereotypically are classified as normal to overweight and are less likely to be obese. The American Psychiatric Association [1] cites that childhood obesity and early pubertal maturation are known to increase the risk of onset, as well as familial transmission and genetic vulnerabilities (Fig. 21.31).

Social Environment

Although there is limited data to support eating disorders are caused by parental expectation or parent-child relationship, social environment is a known factor towards developing disordered eating [33]; within the context of bulimia, a social environment is highly dynamic and significantly influenced by sociocultural model and socialization with parents and peers. Through social interactions, people may engage in body comparison and further internalize the thin ideal [34] (Figs. 21.32 and 21.33).

Through social-environmental exposure, the thin ideal is perpetuated and internalized, thus increasing the risk for developing weight concerns [1]. According to Smahel and friends [34], mass media exposure has been linked to disordered eating, which in turn influences eating patterns (Figs. 21.34 and 21.35).

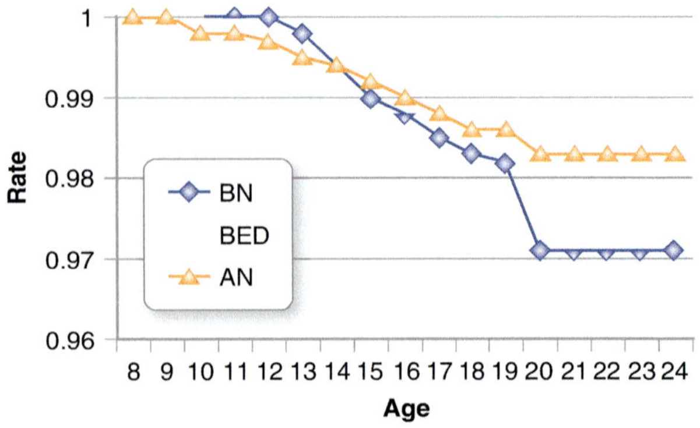

Fig. 21.30 Research has found AN and BN having an average onset of 15 with increasing prevalence throughout the early 20s

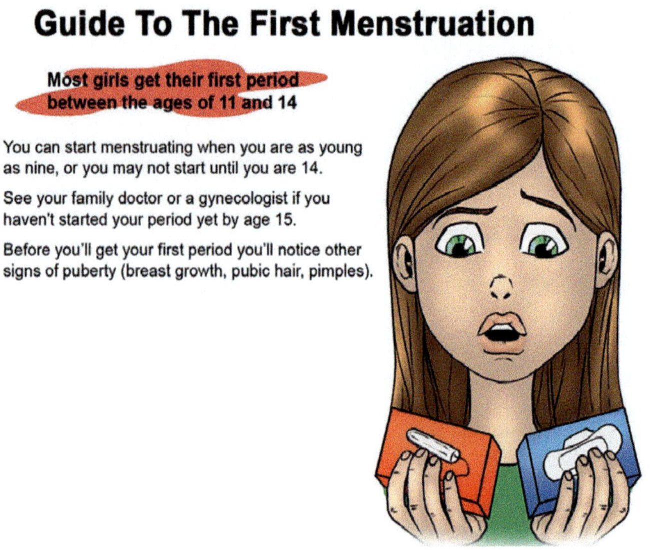

Fig. 21.31 Menstrual irregularity or amenorrhea often occurs among females with BN. SteadyHealth. A girl's guide to the first menstruation. 2020. https://www.steadyhealth.com/articles/a-girls-guide-to-the-first-menstruation

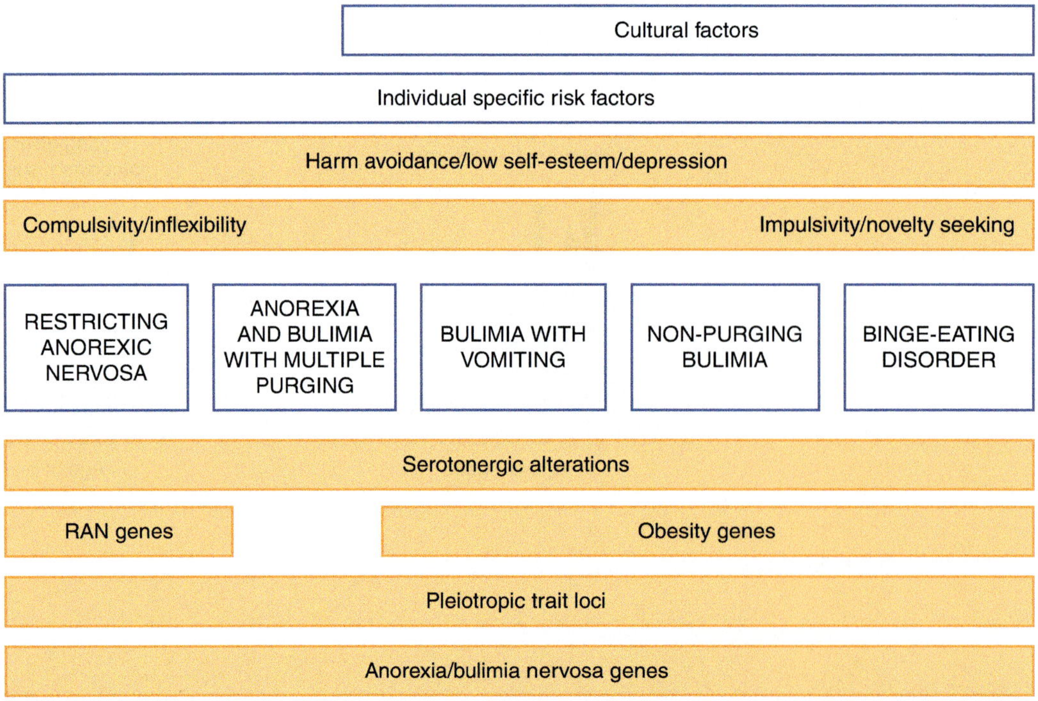

Fig. 21.32 Collier and Treasure [35], like many other researchers, acknowledge the dynamic influences that are regularly associated with eating disorders

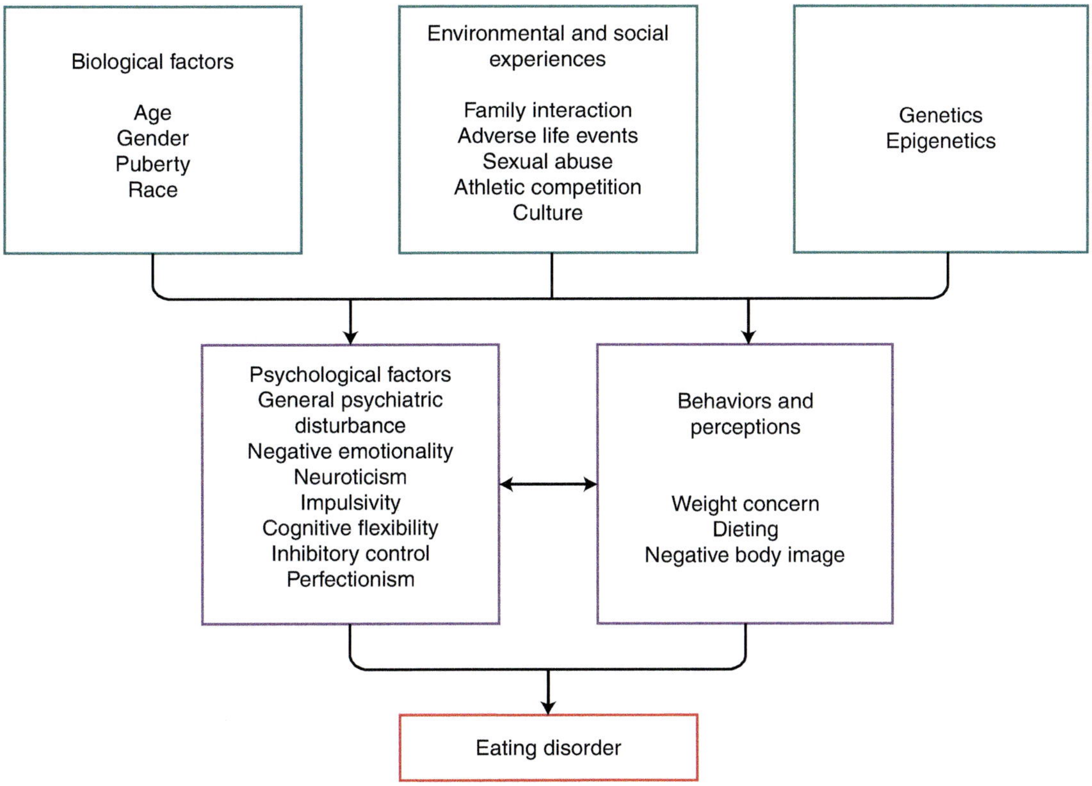

Fig. 21.33 There are various known social, environmental, and biological factors that can be involved in the development of ED. Mayhew AJ, Pigeyre M, Couturier J, Meyre D. An evolutionary genetic perspective of eating disorders. Neuroendocrinology. 2018;106(3):292–306. https://doi.org/10.1159/000484525

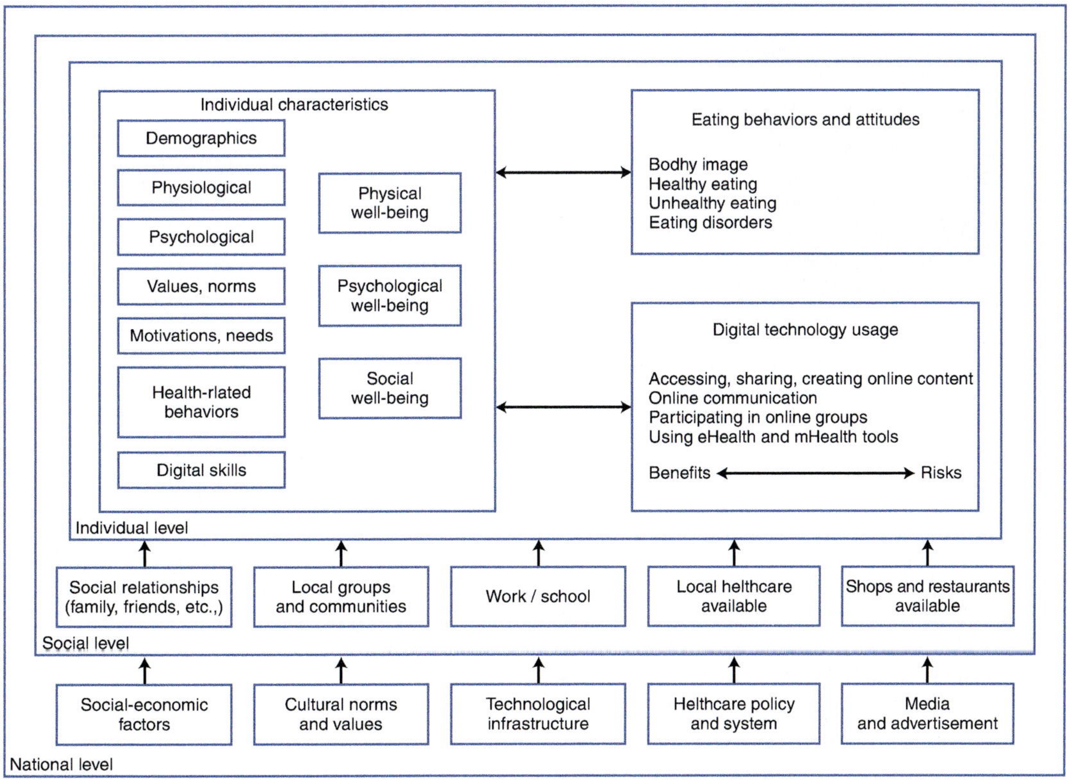

Fig. 21.34 Various factors are associated with ED. Specifically, demonstrating the influence of digital usage

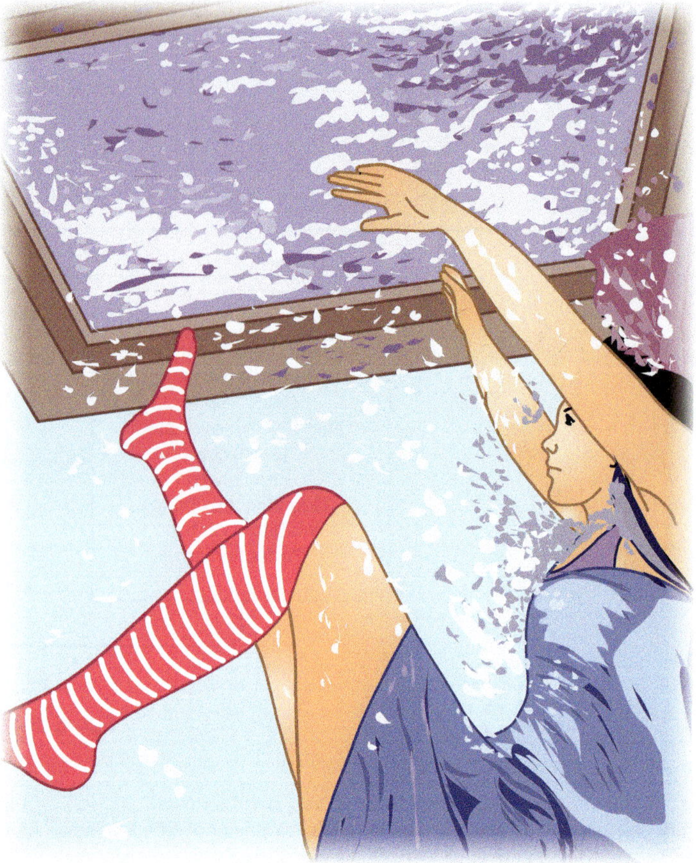

Fig. 21.35 People with BN may be negatively influenced by their body image exposure through social media use. The Eating Disorders Association Inc. Understanding eating disorders. 2014

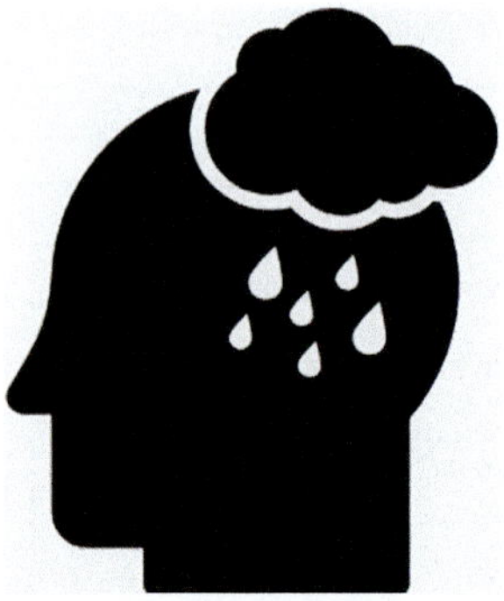

Fig. 21.36 There is an increased frequency of depressive symptoms seen in patients with eating disorders. The Noun Project. Depression Icon. https://thenounproject.com/term/depression/1000159/

Comorbidity

According to Kendler et al. [33], their research found similar comorbidities to those displayed in individuals with bulimia nervosa, such as major depressive disorder. In addition to depressive symptoms, the DSM-5 includes a range of mental disorders that are associated with bulimia, including bipolar disorder, anxiety disorder, and symptoms for personality disorders. A large number of people with bulimia, at least 30% of individuals, have a lifetime prevalence of substance use disorder, specifically alcohol or stimulant use [1] (Figs. 21.36 and 21.37).

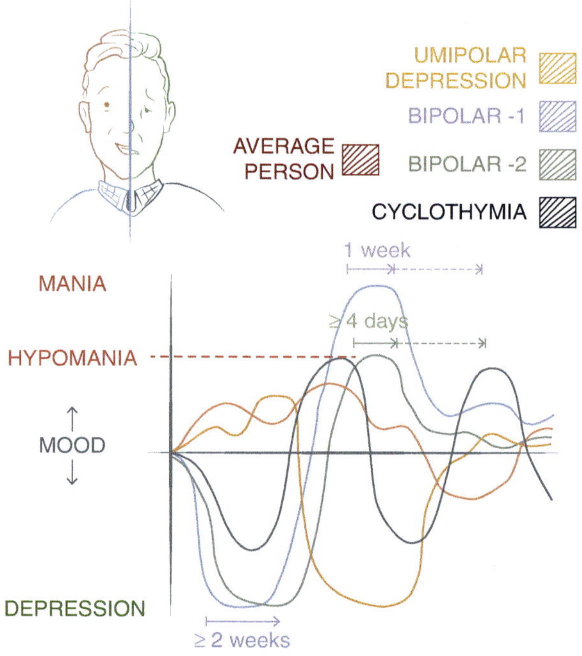

Fig. 21.37 Bipolar disorder is one of several disorders commonly associated with BN. Wikimedia. Graphical representation of Bipolar disorder and Cyclothymia. https://commons.wikimedia.org/wiki/File:Bipolar_mood_shifts.png

Etiology

Inheritance
Twin studies have provided evidence of genetics influencing the incidence of BN (Figs. 21.38, 21.39, and 21.40). For first-degree relatives of patients with BN, the relative risk is 4.4 [13].

Hormones
While the effect of hormones on BN is still poorly understood, multiple studies have suggested estrogen and progesterone are associated with increased binge eating and elevated emotional eating risk. Elevated testosterone levels may also promote binge eating and purging in women [37].

Neurobiology
Serotonin is linked to impulsivity across a range of behavioral disorders. The 5-HT1a receptor likely plays a role, as elevated levels of the receptor have been found in patients with BN [38].

Stressful Life Events
Among monozygotic female twins with lifetime incidence of BN, research has shown an association with frequent comments regarding physicality growing up and high levels of parental expectations [39].

Physical, Sexual, and Emotional Abuse
Childhood physical, sexual, and emotional abuse have shown significant associations with suicide attempts in BN patients [40]. Recent research suggests that emotional abuse may also be associated with greater severity of bulimic symptoms. Also, emotional abuse is associated with higher variability in anger-hostility measurements and increased negative affect among BN patients [41].

Substance Abuse
Many patients with bulimia nervosa also have alcohol use disorder. Estimates of lifetime prevalence of alcohol use disorder have ranged from 9 to 49%, with most studies reporting 20–25% [42]. A nationwide inpatient study of patients with bulimia nervosa (N = 3319) found that drug abuse (21.5%) and alcohol abuse (17.1%) were frequent comorbidities [43].

Pathophysiology

Erosive Soft Palate
Dental lesions have commonly been associated with BN due to vomiting behaviors. As these behaviors persist or increase in frequency, the erosion will worsen. Palatal pain can be a product of self-induced vomiting due to stimulation of the gag reflex using mechanical irritation of fingers or objects used to evoke vomiting [44, 45] (Figs. 21.41 and 21.42).

Cardiovascular and Gastrointestinal
Patients who engage in binge-purge behavior suffer from a cornucopia of physical ailments. Uniquely, patients with bulimia nervosa experience heartburn, blood in regurgitation, upper abdominal pain, and constipation. Notably, the cardiovascular and gastrointestinal symptoms that patients with bulimia experience are similar to anorexia nervosa [46] (Table 21.6; Figs. 21.43, 21.44, and 21.45).

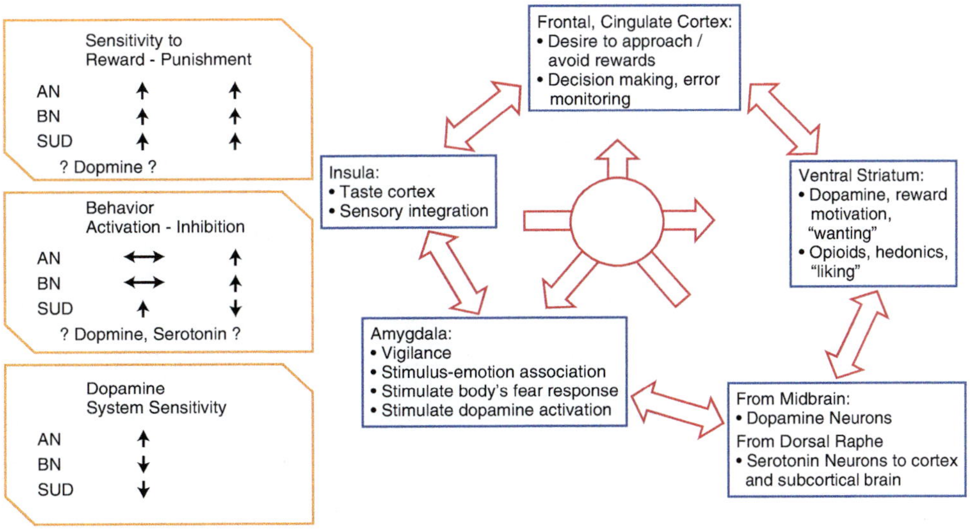

Fig. 21.38 A clear-cut depiction of the brain and multiple pathways that may influence eating disorders. It could be placed in multiple sections

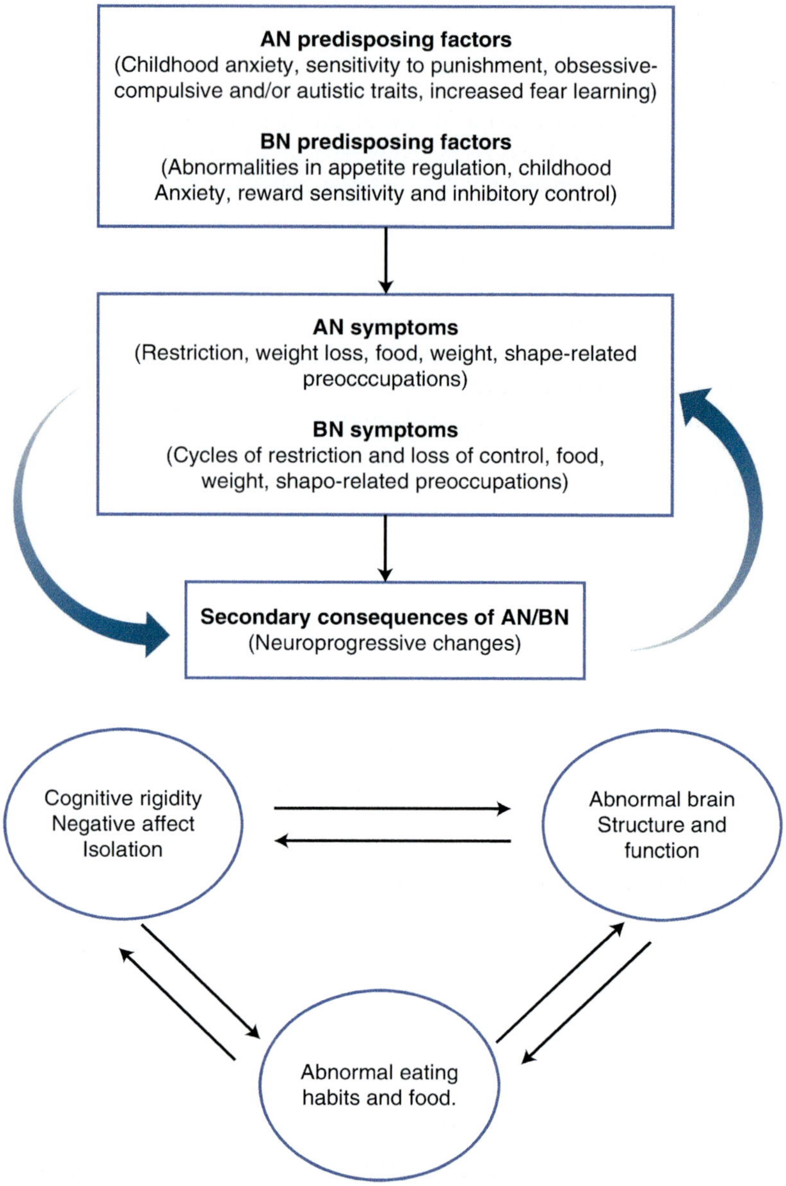

Fig. 21.39 The development of severe AN and BN. Predisposing factors lead to symptoms. Symptoms and neuroprogressive changes reinforce each other

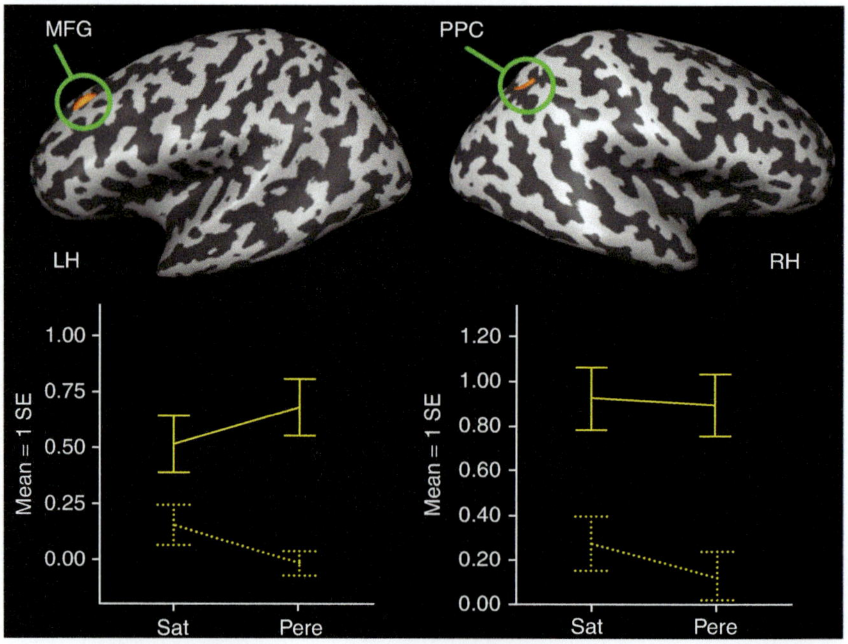

Fig. 21.40 Mohr et al. [36] demonstrated differential brain activation between controls and patients with bulimia in regard to body image processing, specifically in the middle frontal gyrus and posterior parietal cortex

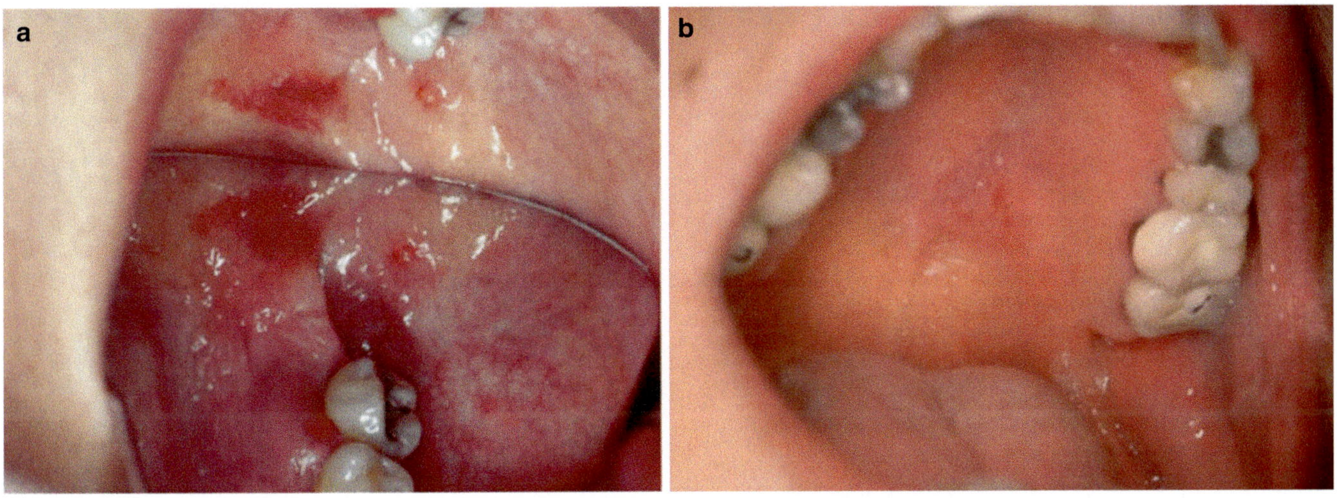

Fig. 21.41 (**a** and **b**) The long-term impact of digital trauma in BN, displaying ulceration of the soft palate

Fig. 21.42 Lesions on the knuckles and the back of the hand can form after many repeated instances of self-induced vomiting. These are known as Russell's sign. Wikimedia. Russell's Sign on the knuckles of the index and ring fingers. https://commons.wikimedia.org/wiki/File:Russell%27s_Sign.png

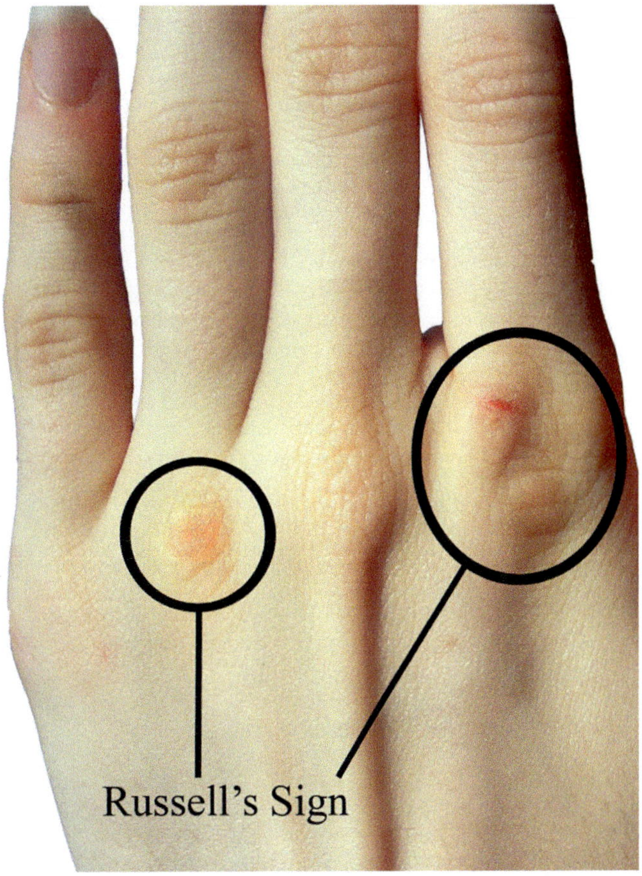

Table 21.6 Physical signs and symptoms associated with eating disorders

System	Anorexia nervosa	Bulimia nervosa
General	– Weight loss – Feeling cold – Dehydration – Fatigue – Irritability/mood changes – Depression – Hypothermia	– Weight fluctuations – Irritability/mood changes – Dehydration – Fatigue
Head, eyes, ears, nose, and throat	– Dry, cracked lips and tongue	– Dry lips and tongue – Palatal scratches – Sore throat – Painful teeth and gums – Dental caries/enamel erosion – Parotid gland swelling
Cardiovascular	– Dizziness – Chest pain – Palpitations – Orthostatic blood pressure or heart rate changes – Cold and/or blue hands and feet – Delayed capillary refill – Ankle swelling	– Dizziness – Chest pain – Palpitations – Arrhythmias – Orthostatic blood pressure or heart rate changes – Ankle swelling
Gastrointestinal	– Early satiety – Episodes of abdominal pain and discomfort – Constipation – Bloating after meals	– Heartburn – Blood in vomitus – Epigastric tenderness – Diarrhea or constipation
Endocrine	– Absent or irregular menses – Fractures – Delay puberty	– Absent or irregular menses
Dermatologic	– Dry skin – Pallor – Lanugo – Brittle nails – Carotenoderma (yellow or orange discoloration of skin) – Thin, dry hair	– Calluses on the dorsum of hand (Russell's sign) – Dry mouth
Musculoskeletal	– Fatigue, muscle weakness, and cramps	– Fatigue, muscle weakness, and cramps
Neurological	– Decreased concentration, memory, thinking ability	– Decreased concentration, memory, thinking ability

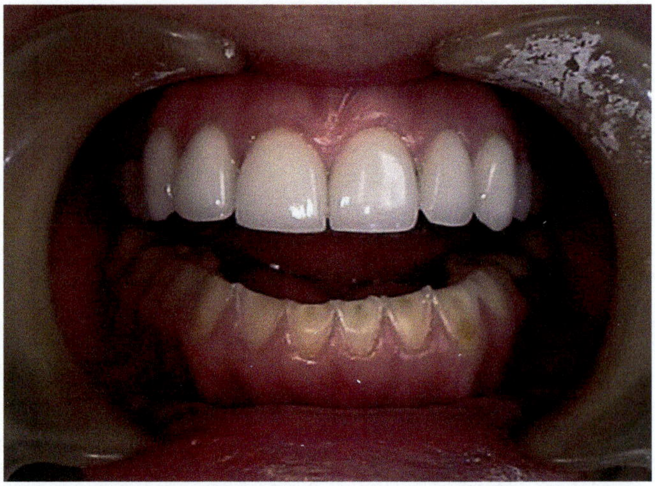

Fig. 21.43 Frequent exposure to gastric acid damages tooth enamel and can cause premature decay

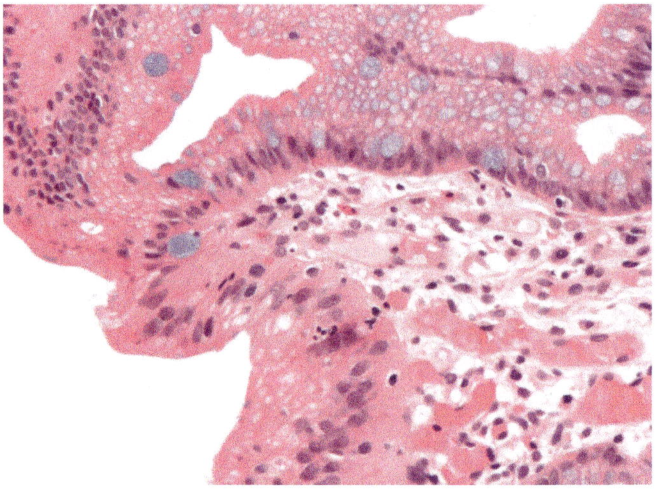

Fig. 21.44 Barrett's esophagus can occur as a result of repeated exposure to stomach acid, characterized by the presence of goblet cells (stained blue) lining the esophagus rather than squamous cells

Phenomenology

Body Dissatisfaction

Grilo et al. [47] determined that body dissatisfaction and over-evaluation in bulimia nervosa patients did not relate to purge frequency, restraint, eating concerns, and binge-eating frequency (Figs. 21.46 and 21.47).

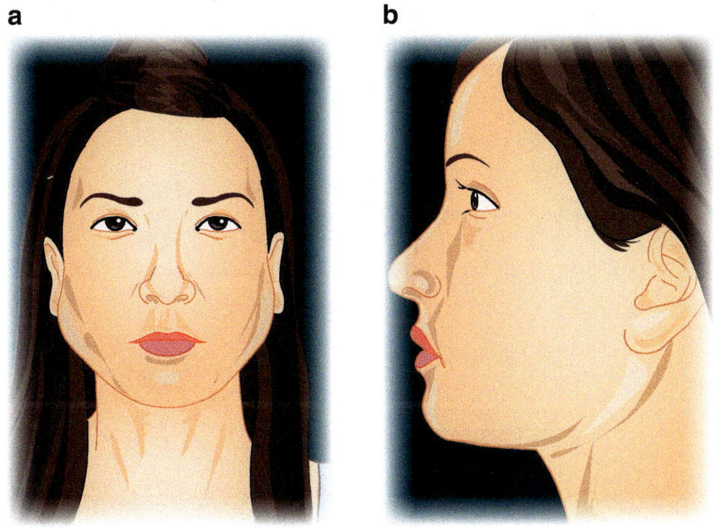

Fig. 21.45 Long-term bulimia can cause salivary gland hypertrophy (sialadenosis) (**a**) Anterior, (**b**) Lateral

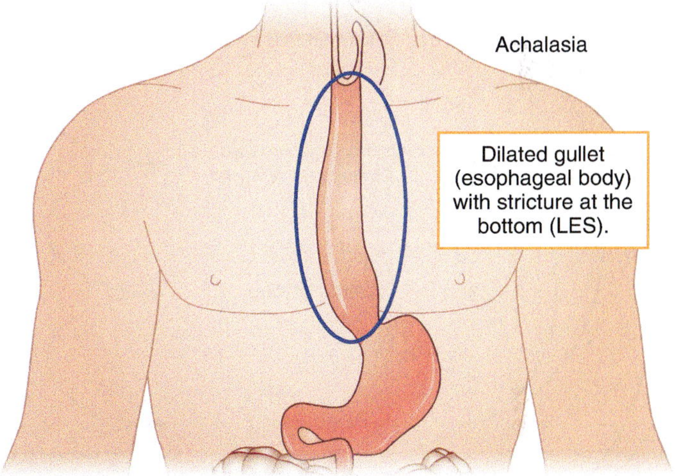

Fig. 21.46 Achalasia, a condition that makes it difficult for food and liquid to reach the stomach, can occur as a complication of bulimia. Pixabay. Achalasia. https://pixabay.com/photos/achalasia-what-is-achalasia-5208564/

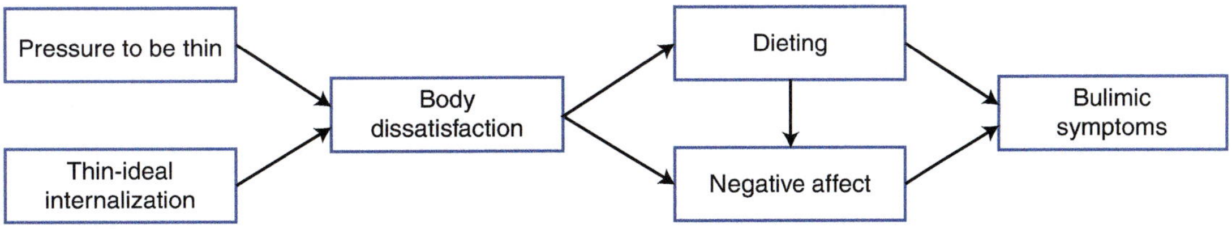

Fig. 21.47 The tripartite influence model of body image and eating patterns

Treatment

Cognitive-Behavioral Therapy

While using the cognitive-behavioral therapeutic approach, clinicians focus on addressing maladaptive thoughts about food, body image, and weight in patients with bulimia. According to the cognitive-behavioral model, negative thoughts and feelings of low self-esteem are factors that lead patients to engage in deleterious eating disorder behaviors, such as binge eating and purging [25]. Cognitive-behavioral therapy is highly efficacious for patients diagnosed with BN. As seen in Figs. 21.55 and 21.56, patients report engaging in fewer bulimia nervosa behaviors and depressive feelings [48]. Moreover, the efficacy of cognitive-behavioral therapy remains consistent across time (Figs. 21.48 and 21.49).

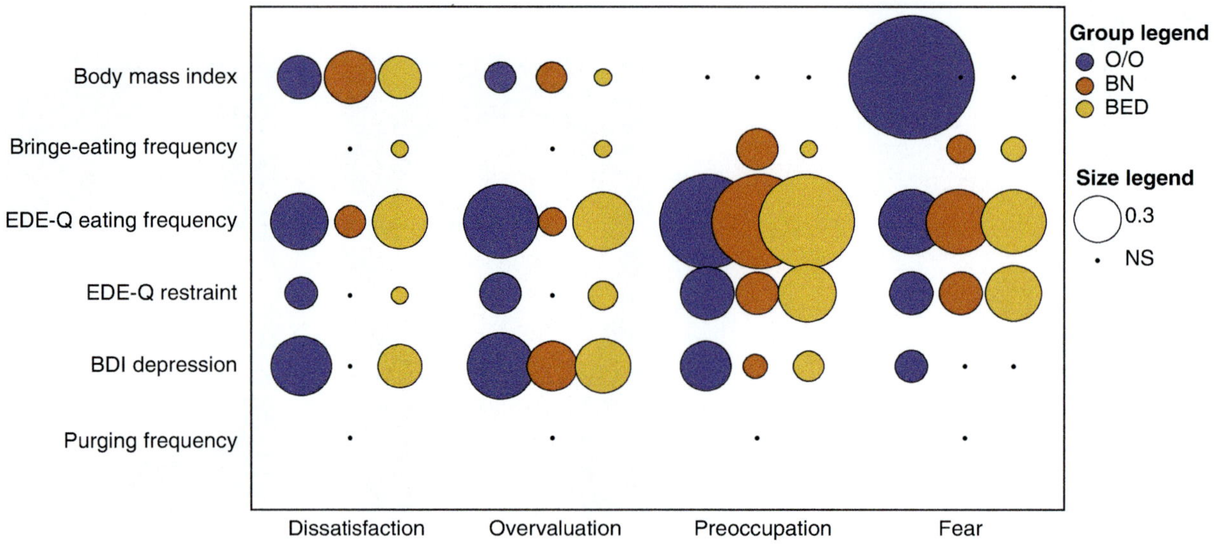

Fig. 21.48 With over 9000 surveys, Hudson et al. [49] found a lifetime prevalence of 3.5% BED in females and 2.0% in males

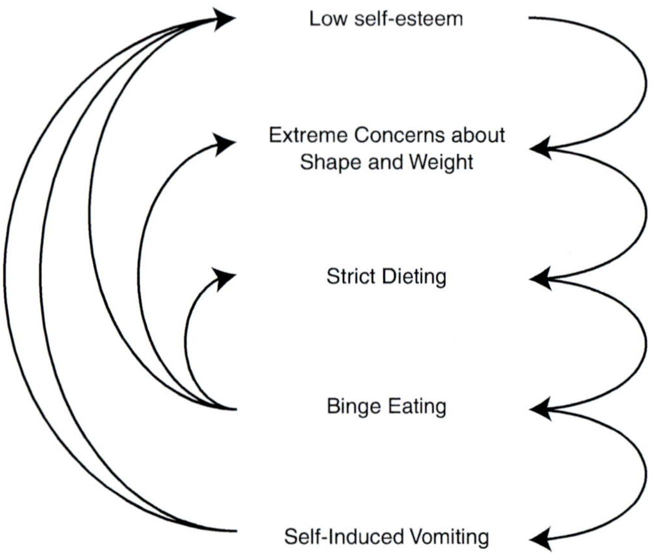

Fig. 21.49 Cognitive-behavioral model of BN maintenance

Family-Focused Therapy

Uniquely, family-focused therapy is a therapeutic approach for adolescent patients and their families. Unlike cognitive-behavioral therapy, family-focused therapy only focuses on correcting harmful eating behaviors. This therapy can be especially helpful working with adolescents and their families collaborating to assuage deleterious eating behaviors. Le Grange and Lock [50] evaluated differences in purging behaviors across patients who receive family-based therapy and supportive psychotherapy. Across time, patients in the supportive psychotherapy condition report engaging in fewer purging behaviors than patients in the family-based therapy condition. While there are differences in purging behaviors, patients' purging behaviors in the family-based therapy condition are not significantly higher later (Fig. 21.50).

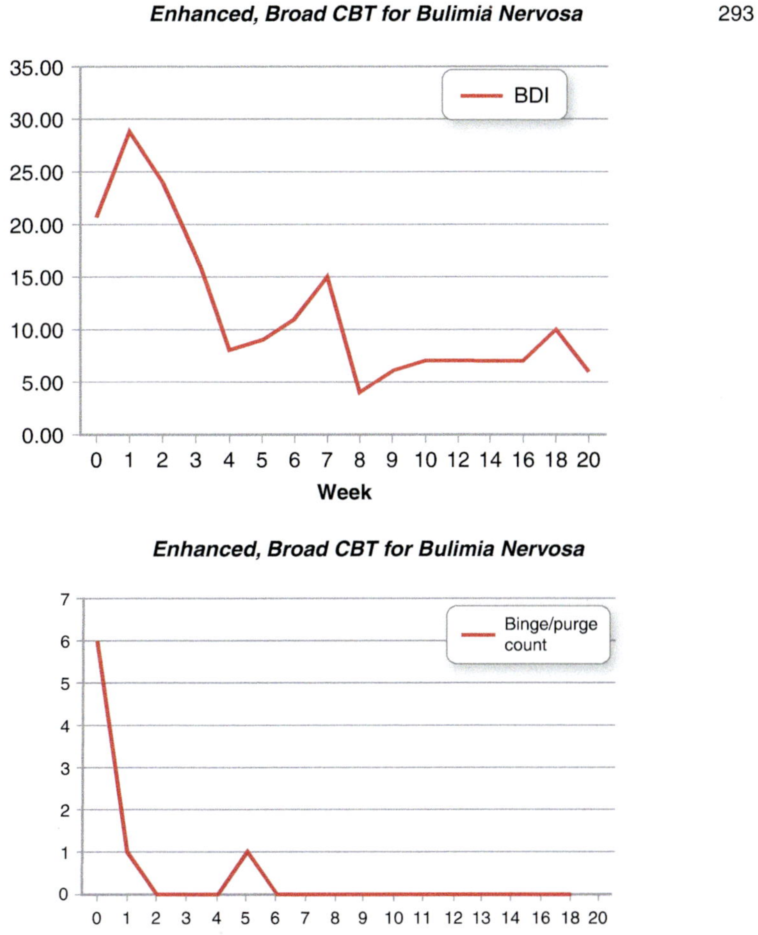

Fig. 21.50 *Top*: Beck Depression Inventory (DBI) scores over treatment course. *Bottom*: Binge-purge count over treatment course

Other Interventions

In addition to cognitive therapy, clinicians use pharmacology interventions to treat patients who suffer from bulimic symptoms. Across medication trials, patients mostly report a significant decrease in binge-eating frequency compared to patients in control groups. Specifically, fluoxetine, desipramine, trazodone, topiramate, and ondansetron effectively reduce binge-eating behavior [51]. Another highly efficacious alternative intervention to CBT is integrative cognitive-affect therapy (ICAT). ICAT, an extension of CBT, addresses the flaws identified with the intervention. Unlike cognitive-behavioral, ICAT focuses on emotions and interpersonal behavior. Moreover, ICAT emphasizes the importance of motivation and healthy meal planning [52] (Fig. 21.51; Table 21.7).

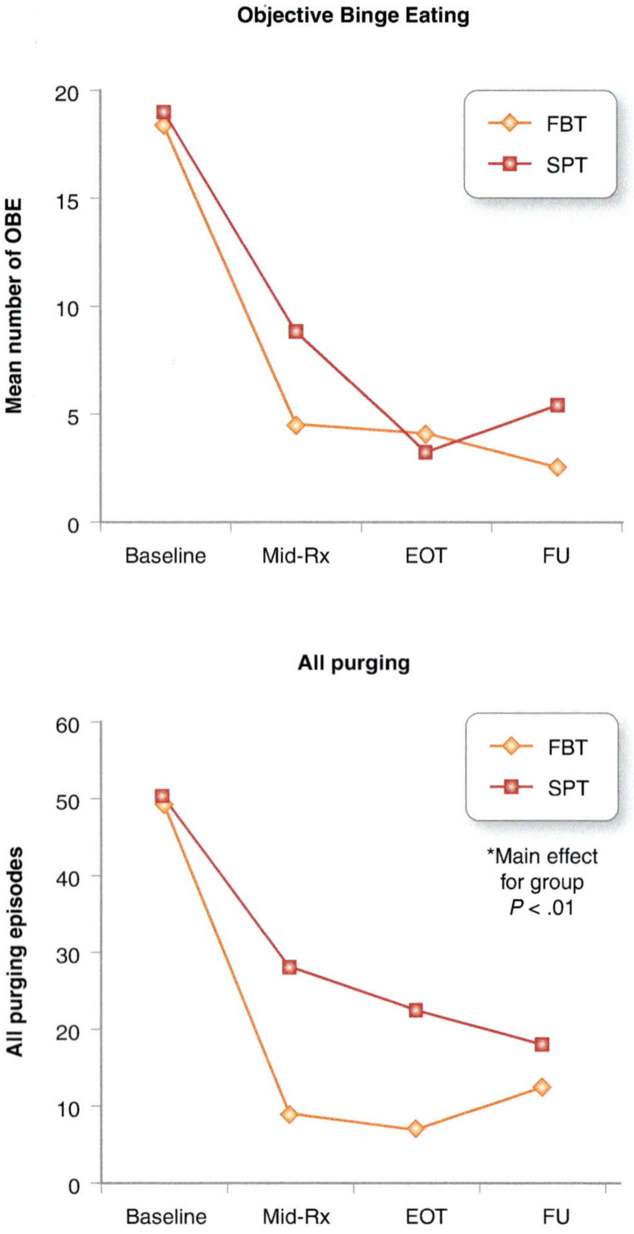

Fig. 21.51 Objective binge eating and purging for family-based treatment (FBT)-BN and supportive psychotherapy (SPT). *OBE* objective binge eating; *Mid-Rs* midtreatment; *EOT* end of treatment; *FU* follow-up

Table 21.7 Summary of ICAT phases

Phases of ICAT	Treatment strategies	Specific interventions
Phase I: Introduction and motivation	1. Conduct motivational enhancement 2. Present psychoeducational material 3. Engage in emotion identification	1. Discuss current behavior vs. broader goals and emotional significance 2. Self-monitor food intake and context 3. Introduce FEEL skill
Phase II: Nutritional rehabilitation	1. Begin meal planning 2. Continue food logs 3. Identify emotions associated with eating	1. Encourage meal plan and regular consumption of meals/snacks (CARE skill) 2. Activity teach coping skills for purpose of assisting meal planning (PDA) 3. Monitor context of symptoms 4. Monitor and elicit affect regarding meal plan, especially monitoring emotional avoidance
Phase III: Interpersonal patterns and self-directed styles	1. Conduct interpersonal pattern and self-directed style analysis 2. Conduct historical analysis of patterns (optional) 3. Focus on changing interpersonal patterns and self-directed styles 4. Focus on reducing self-discrepancy 5. Continue food logs	1. Identify interpersonal patterns of patient and specific others as well as self-directed style 2. Attempt to identify historical factors associated with underlying beliefs and interpersonal rules that inform and direct the interpersonal pattern (optional) 3. Carefully elicit and clarify affect in interpersonal situations 4. Focus on assertiveness training and increasing self-accepting self-regulatory style (SAID, SPA, WAIT skills) 5. Address and modify maladaptive evaluative standards; heavy emphasis on workbook 6. Elicit and monitor affect
Phase IV: Relapse prevention	1. Discuss components of a healthy lifestyle 2. Develop written relapse prevention plan 3. Address feelings related to termination	1. Review progress in treatment 2. Formalize relapse prevention plan 3. Elicit and monitor affect

Binge-Eating Disorder

Binge-eating disorder (BED) was first included as its own entity in DSM-5, the latest edition of the American Psychiatric Association's diagnostic manual [2]. In the previous DSM edition, BED was added provisionally under Eating Disorders Not Otherwise Specified, requiring further studies on specific diagnostic criteria and an outlined distinction from bulimia nervosa. Updated knowledge now identifies BED differing from bulimia nervosa in terms of clinical presentation, recurrent inappropriate compensatory behavior, and lack of sustained dietary restrictions. With this new diagnostic code, clinicians are able to provide appropriate treatments, acknowledging the overlapping and individualistic features of this disorder (Fig. 21.51).

Epidemiology

Biological Risk Factors

It is unclear whether the age of onset has been decreasing over time or if cases of BED are being detected more effectively. The age of onset for BED is often earlier than the age of onset for AN and BN [53] (Fig. 21.52).

Binge-eating disorder is more commonly diagnosed in women than men, and the lifetime prevalence of this disorder is 2.6% within the United States [54].

Comorbidity

Nearly half of patients with BED have a lifetime history of two or more comorbidities. The most prevalent in descending order is specific phobia (37%), social phobia (32%), PTSD (26%), and alcohol use disorder (21%) [55].

Etiology

Inheritance

Twin studies of BED have reported heritability estimates between 41% to 57% [13].

Substance Abuse

Substance abuse, physical abuse, and sexual abuse are known risk factors for the development of BED [56] (Fig. 21.53).

Pathophysiology

The prominent affect regulation model proposes that binge-eating episodes are triggered by negative effects and relieved by binging. Many patients endorse challenges with emotional regulation and emotional awareness. Neuroimaging studies have shown hyperactivity of the medial orbitofrontal cortex and hypoactivity in the prefrontal network [56] (Figs. 21.54 and 21.55).

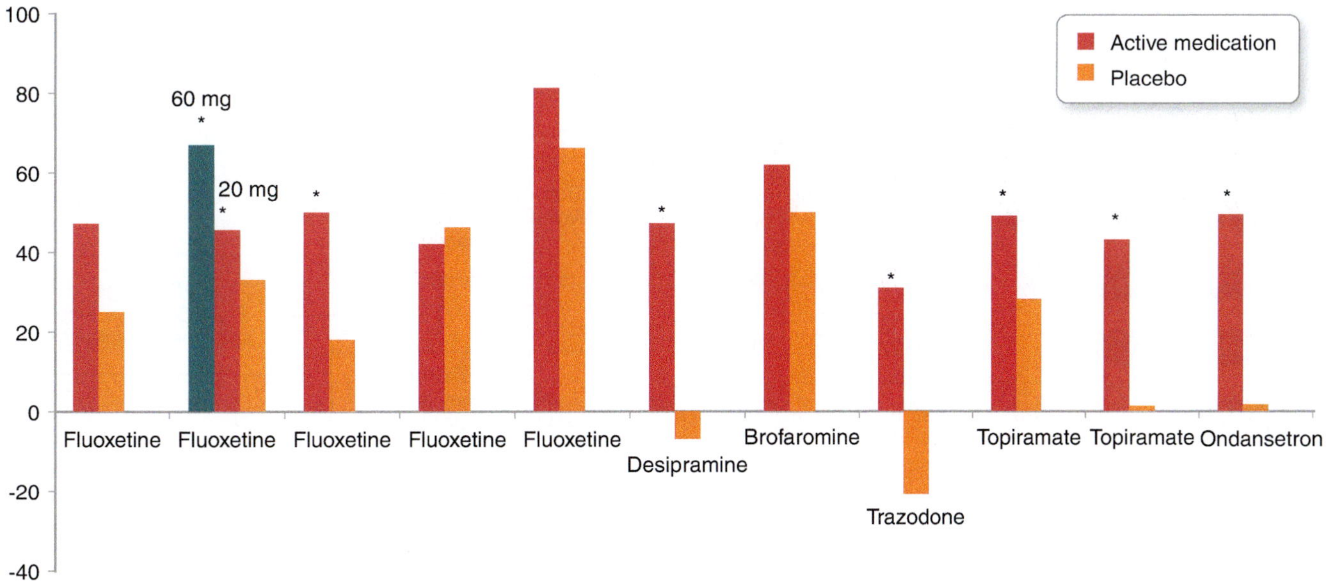

Fig. 21.52 Binge-eating frequency reduction

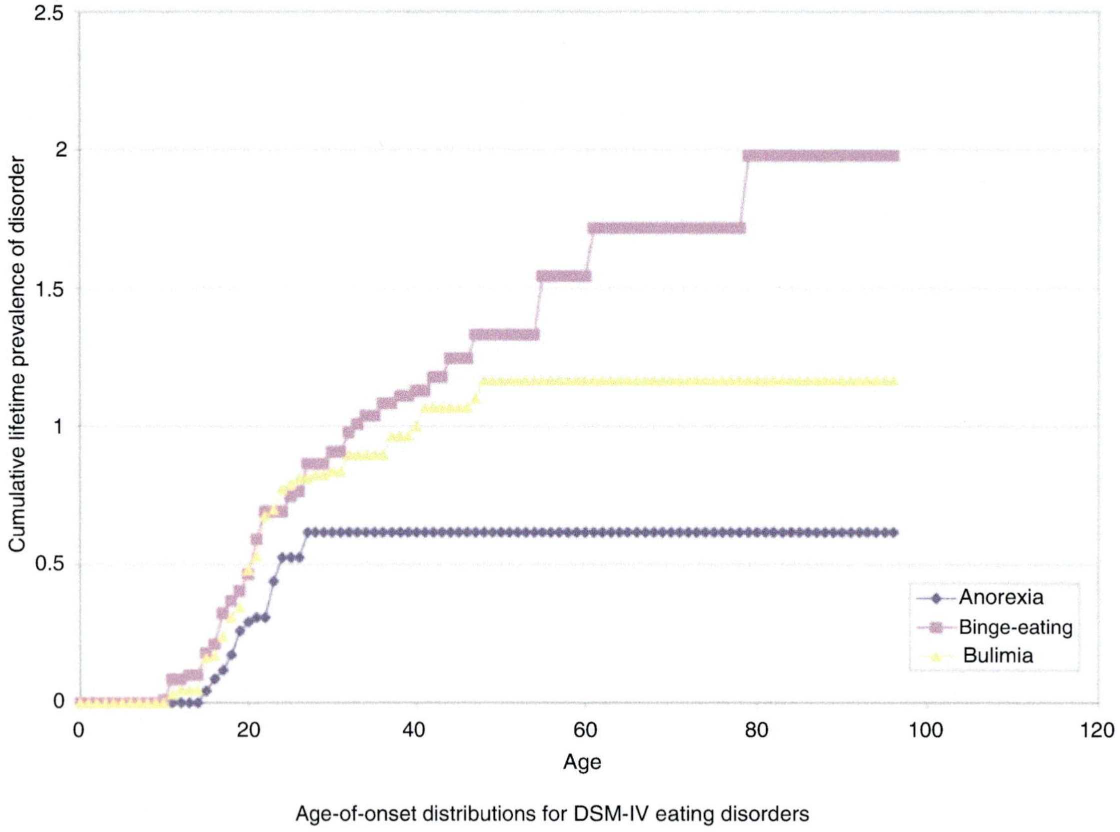

Fig. 21.53 Age of onset distributions of DSM-IV eating disorders

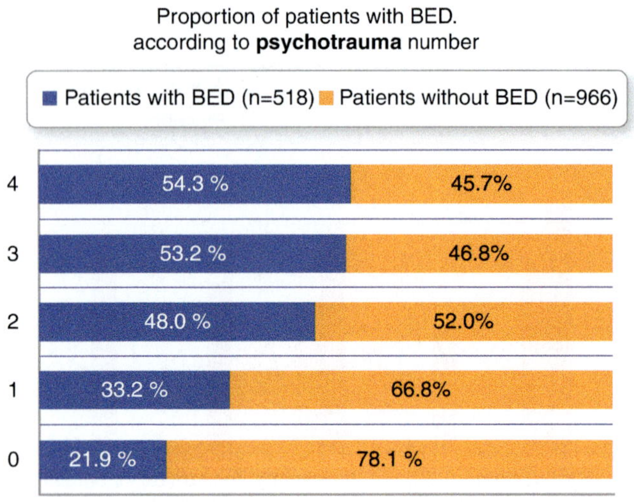

Fig. 21.54 Early traumatic experiences are a significant predictor of binge-eating disorder. Quilliot D, Brunaud L, Mathieu J, Quenot C, Sirveaux MA, Kahn JP, Ziegler O, Witkowski P. Links between traumatic experiences in childhood or early adulthood and lifetime binge eating disorder. Psychiatry Res. 2019;276:134–41. https://doi.org/10.1016/j.psychres.2019.05.008

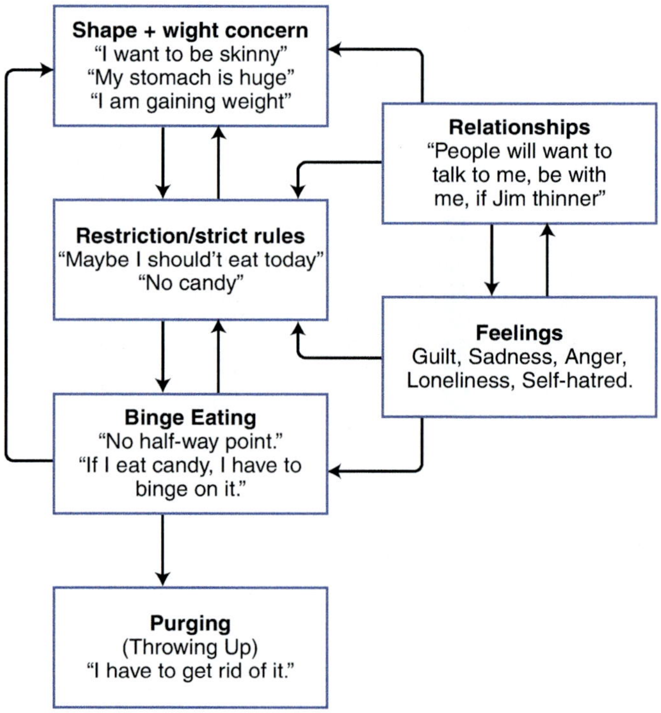

Fig. 21.55 Personalized formulations

Phenomenology

Binge-Eating Episode

According to the American Psychiatric Association [1], individuals diagnosed with binge-eating disorder experience uncontrollable eating episodes. In a short amount of time, BED patients consume a large amount of food (Fig. 21.56).

Marked Distress Regarding Binge Eating

Marked distress about binge eating, diagnosis criteria of BED, plays a significant role. Grilo and White [58] determined that patients with all criteria of BED had significantly higher depression levels and BED psychopathologies than individuals who did not meet full criteria of BED. Marked distress further distinguishes between individuals who experience symptoms without marked distress in comparison to who do (Fig. 21.57).

Severity

According to the American Psychiatric Association [1], patients with BED vary in severity across binge-eating episodes. Unsurprisingly, patients with higher levels of BED severity differ in body mass index, eating disorder symptoms, and mood from patients with all other BED levels of severity [59] (Table 21.8; Fig. 21.58).

Treatment

Level of Care

Treatment of binge-eating disorder is typically conducted in outpatient settings. Partial hospital, residential, and inpatient are required in circumstances that require greater observation [1].

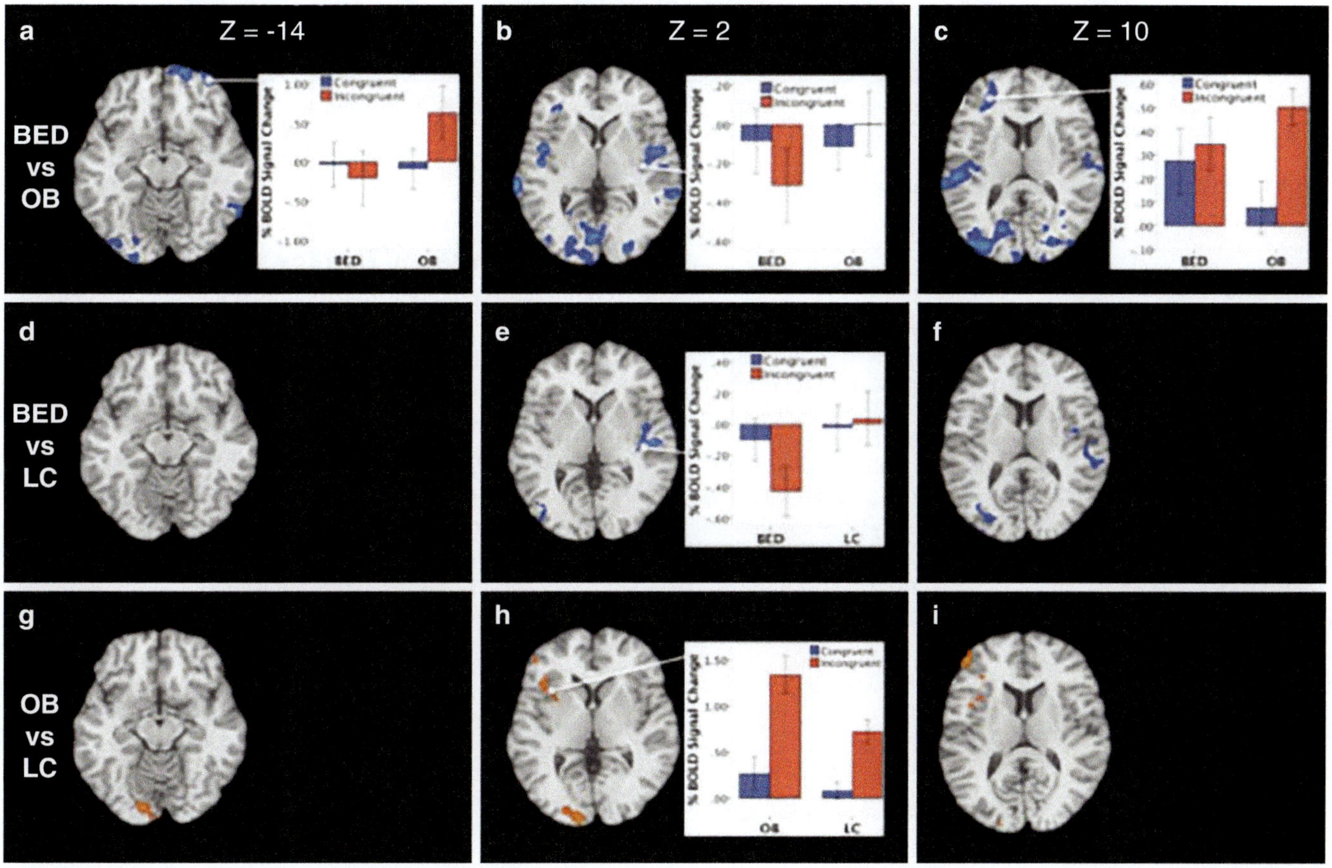

Fig. 21.56 Compared with obese individuals without binge-eating disorder, obese individuals with binge-eating disorder had decreased activity in areas including the vmPFC, IFG, and insula during an inhibitory control task. Blue areas represent areas of decreased activity between groups for images (**a–i**) [57]

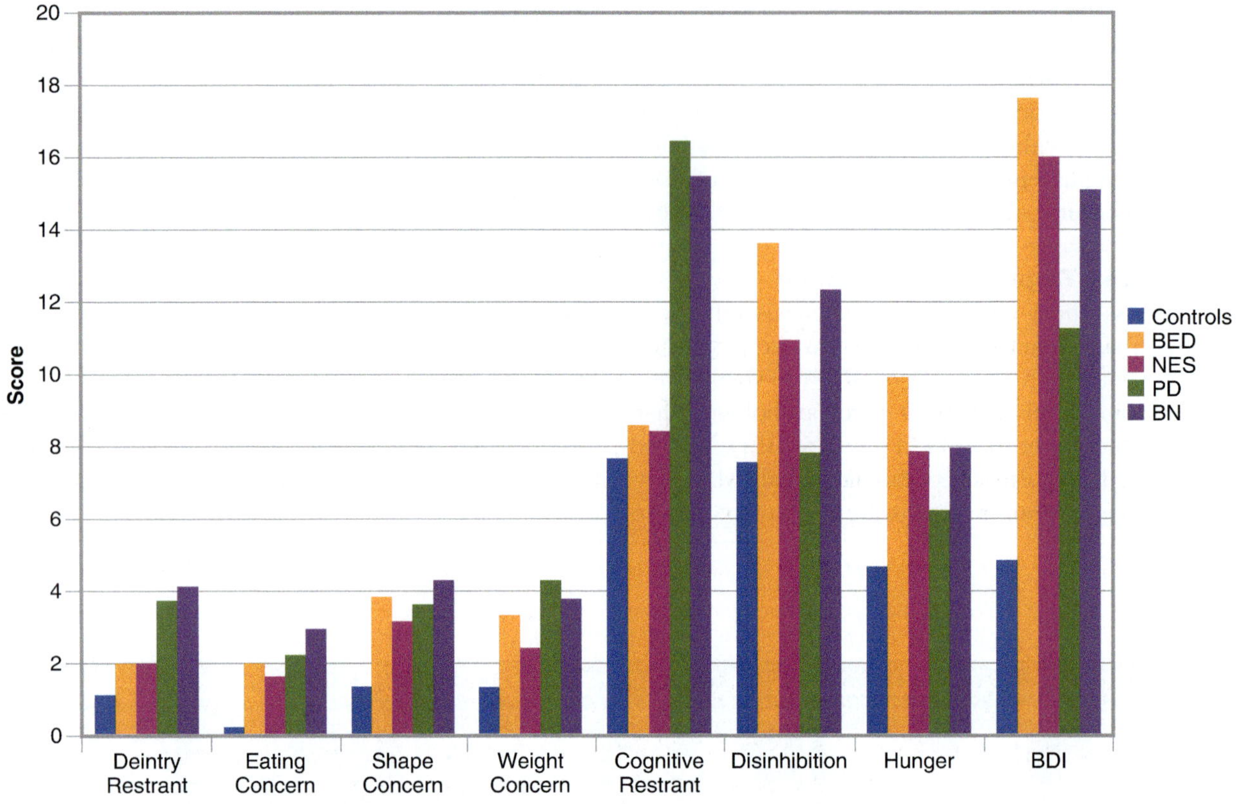

Fig. 21.57 Multiple symptoms that commonly occur in BED

Table 21.8 Binge-eating disorder diagnostic criteria

1. Recurrent binge-eating episodes are denoted by short periods of time when large amounts of food are uncontrollably consumed
2. Binge-eating episodes associated symptoms with eating rapidly, eating until uncomfortable, eating when not physically hungry, feeling of embarrassment, disgust, and depression
3. Binge-eating episodes are associated with feelings of distress
4. Binge-eating occurs at least once a week across 3 months, on average
5. Binge-eating is not followed by compensatory behaviors that are present in bulimia and does not occur exclusively with anorexia nervosa or bulimia nervosa

Cognitive-Behavioral Therapy

Psychotherapy is the first-line treatment and appears to have a more significant clinical effect than pharmacological therapy. CBT appears to be the most commonly form of therapy [56].

Antidepressants

Pharmacotherapy can be an effective initial treatment for those unable or unwilling to receive therapy. SSRIs, epileptic drugs, ADHD medications, and armodafinil have proven effective [56] (Fig. 21.59).

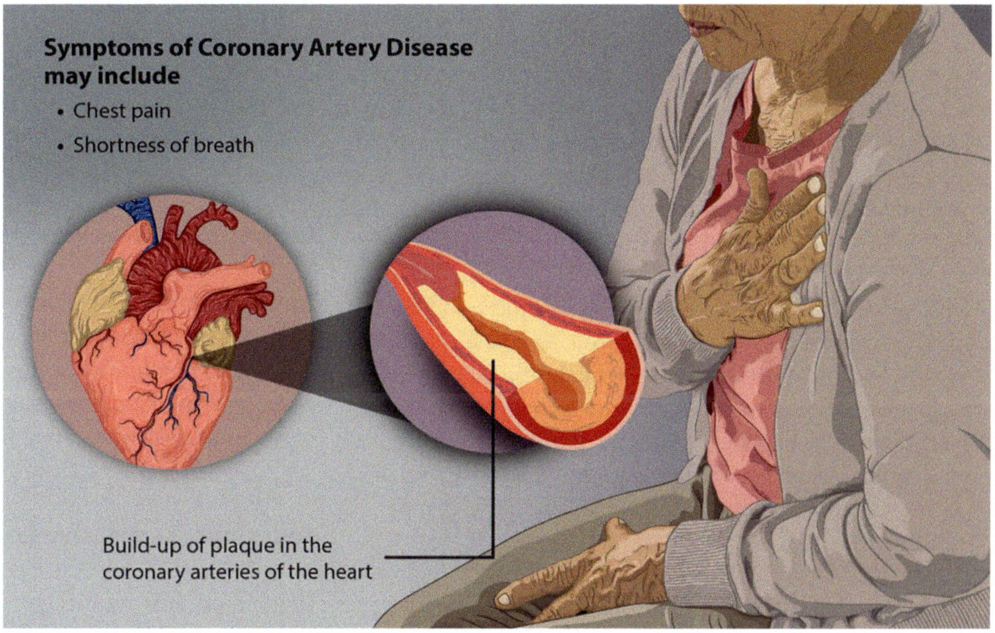

Fig. 21.58 Binge-eating disorder often co-occurs with obesity and can lead to significant complications such as coronary artery disease, heart failure, and high cholesterol. Wikimedia. Depiction of a person suffering from coronary artery disease. https://commons.wikimedia.org/wiki/File:Depiction_of_a_person_suffering_from_Coronary_Artery_Disease.png

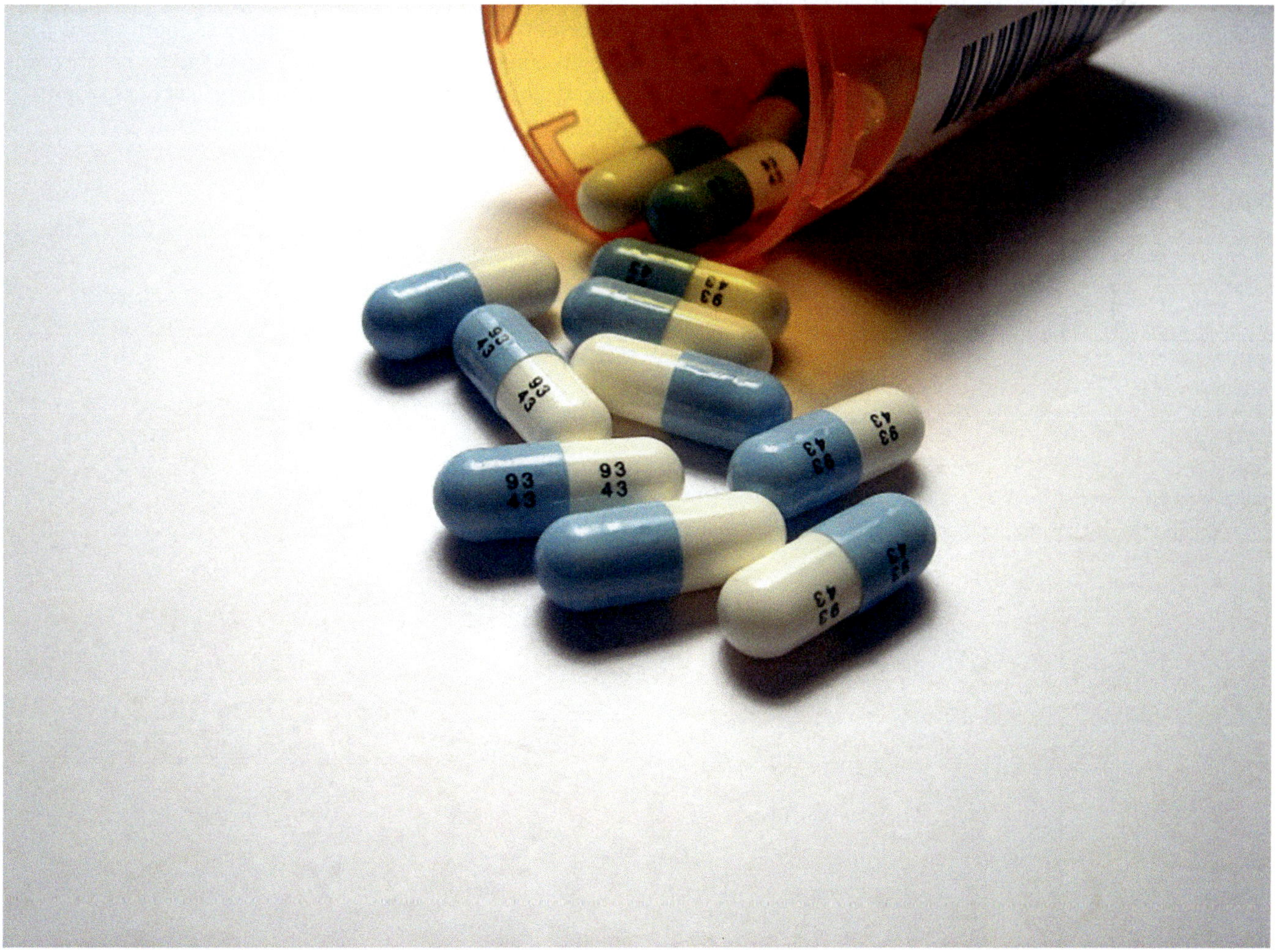

Fig. 21.59 SSRIs and other medications can be used to treat binge-eating disorder. Wikimedia. Prozac pills. https://commons.wikimedia.org/wiki/File:Prozac_pills.jpg

Other Eating Disorders

Diagnostic criteria for rumination, avoidant/restrictive food intake disorder, and other eating disorders differentiate themselves by the classification schemes that are mutually exclusive [1]. However, there are multiple behavioral and psychological components in the clinical course of their disorder and their outcomes/treatment that highly differ. Uniquely, pica and rumination disorders may be diagnosed in the presence of any of the other eating disorders and are not exclusive to anorexia or bulimia nervosa. As a new addition to the DSM-5, avoidant/restrictive food intake disorder (ARFID) was acknowledged by the American Psychiatric Association [1] as a means to capture individuals that fail to meet nutritional and/or energy needs while addressing differentiating pathological limits to food variety and the development of food selectivity [2].

Pica

Pica is the consumption of non-food substances without nutritional value for at least 1 month. Ingested items may include but are not limited to ice, earth, raw starch, and chalk. It is frequently seen in young children and in patients with intellectual impairment. In women, it is most often seen during pregnancy. Pica can lead to ingestion of materials that are harmful to the fetus, such as long-term neurological disability (lead poisoning) and delays in childhood motor function (geophagy). No definitive cause of this condition has been established [60] (Table 21.9).

Rumination Disorder

Rumination disorder is a poorly understood condition with unclear prevalence. Patients repeatedly regurgitate food for at least 1 month. This regurgitation is not due to a medical condition and cannot be solely attributed to AN, BN, BED, or avoidant/restrictive food intake disorder [1].

Avoidant/Restrictive Food Intake Disorder

It is important to clearly distinguish this disorder from BN and AN. While significant weight loss and nutritional deficiency may occur, there is no preoccupation with body image. Patients with ARFID do not intentionally engage in weight loss but have a disinterest in food, avoid food due to uncomfortable sensory experiences, or are concerned about consequences of eating, such as vomiting [62] (Fig. 21.60).

Table 21.9 Description of the substances consumed by the 52 pregnant women who reported pica practice

Pica					
	Reason for ingestion				
	Did not specify the crave reason	Sensorial	Physical	Anxiety	Cultural
Substances consumed	*n* = 37	*n* = 14	*n* = 2	*n* = 4	*n* = 1
Earth/sand/brick	21 (36,2)	8 (13,8)	–	–	1 (1,7)
Ice	1 (1,7)	–	1 (1,7)	1 (1,7)	–
Raw rice	1 (1,7)	2 (3,5)	–	–	–
Flower/leaf	2 (3,5)	–	–	–	–
Feces	1 (1,7)	–	–	–	–
Others	11 (19,0)	4 (6,9)	1 (1,7)	3 (5,2)	–

From Santos et al. [61]; *with permission*

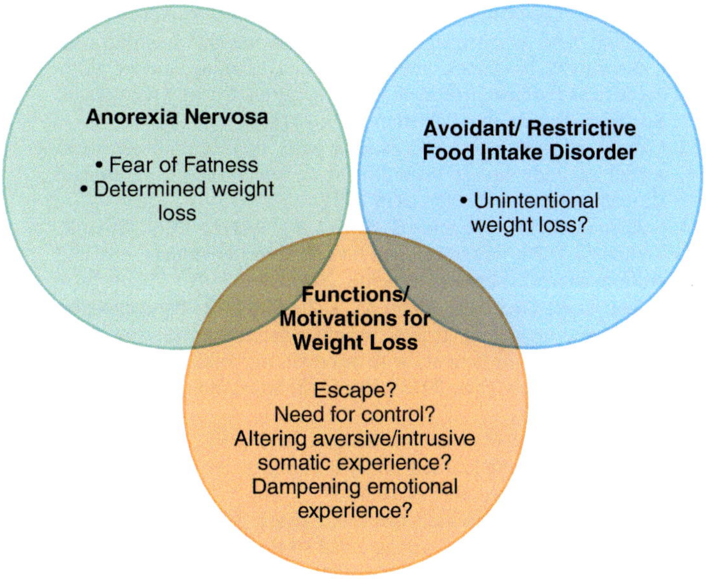

Fig. 21.60 The distinct features of each ARFID vs. anorexia nervosa vs. weight loss

Unspecified Feeding or Eating Disorder

This diagnosis applies to patients with an eating disorder that causes significant distress or functional impairment but does not fit the criteria of other eating disorders [1]. This diagnosis may be given when there is not enough available information to make a more definitive diagnosis (acute care, nonverbal patient, etc.).

References

1. American Psychiatric Association. Diagnostic and statistical manual of mental disorders. 5th ed. 2013. https://doi.org/10.1176/appi.books.9780890425596
2. Wade E. Encyclopedia of feeding and eating disorders. Springer; 2017. https://doi.org/10.1007/978-981-287-104-6.
3. Bulik CM, Reba L, Siega-Riz AM, Reichborn-Kjenneurd T. Anorexia nervosa: definition, epidemiology, and cycle of risk. Int J Eat Disord. 2005;37(S2–9):52–9. https://doi.org/10.1002/eat.20107.
4. Keski-Rhkonen A, Hoek HW, Susser ES, Linna MS, Sihvola E, Raevuori A, Bulik CM, Kaprio J, Rissanen A. Epidemiology and course of anorexia nervosa in the community. Am J Psychiatr. 2007;164(8):1259–65. https://doi.org/10.1176/appi.ajp.2007.06081388.
5. Mond JM, Mitchison D, Hay P. Prevalence and implications of eating disordered behavior in men. In: Cohn L, Lemberg R, editors. Current findings on males with eating disorders. Philadelphia, PA: Routledge; 2014.
6. Thomas JJ, Lee S, Becker AE. Updates in the epidemiology of eating disorders in Asia and the Pacific. Curr Opin Psychiatry. 2016;29(6):354–62. https://doi.org/10.1097/YCO.0000000000000288.
7. Kaye W, Fudge J, Paulus M. New insights into symptoms and neurocircuit function of anorexia nervosa. Nat Rev Neurosci. 2009;10:573–84. https://doi.org/10.1038/nrn2682.
8. Mazzeo SE, Bulik CM. Environmental and genetic risk factors for eating disorders: what the clinician needs to know. Child Adolesc Psychiatr Clin N Am. 2009;18(1):67–82. https://doi.org/10.1016/j.chc.2008.07.003.
9. Kas MJH, Adan RAH. Animal models of eating disorder traits. In: Adan R, Kaye W, editors. Behavioral neurobiology of eating disorders. Current topics in behavioral neurosciences, vol. 6. Berlin/Heidelberg: Springer; 2011. https://doi.org/10.1007/7854_2010_84.
10. Pallister E, Waller G. Anxiety in the eating disorders: understanding the overlap. Clin Psychol Rev. 2008;28(3):366–86. https://doi.org/10.1016/j.cpr.2007.07.001.
11. Zipfel S, et al. Anorexia nervosa: aetiology, assessment, and treatment. Lancet Psychiatry. 2015;2(12):1099–111. https://doi.org/10.1016/s2215-0366(15)00356-9.
12. Lombardi L, et al. Anorexia nervosa is associated with neuronatin variants. Psychiatr Genet. 2019;29:103–10. https://doi.org/10.1097/ypg.0000000000000224.
13. Himmerich H, Bentley J, Kan C, Treasure J. Genetic risk factors for eating disorders: an update and insights into pathophysiology. Ther Adv Psychopharmacol. 2019;9:2045125318814734. https://doi.org/10.1177/2045125318814734.
14. Rose M, Frampton. Conceptual models. In: Eating disorders and the brain. Lask B, Frampton I, editors. Hoboken, NJ: Wiley; 2011. Pg. 159,
15. Connan F, Campbell IC, Katzman D, et al. A neurodevelopmental model for anorexia nervosa. Physiol Behav. 2003;79:13–24.
16. Lask B, Frampton I. Eating disorders and the brain. Wiley-Blackwell: A John Wiley & Sons, Ltd; 2011.
17. Calugi S, et al. Anorexia nervosa and childhood sexual abuse: treatment outcomes of intensive enhanced cognitive behavioural therapy. Psychiatry Res. 2018a;262:477–81. https://doi.org/10.1016/j.psychres.2017.09.027.
18. Racine SE, Wildes JE. Emotion dysregulation and anorexia nervosa: an exploration of the role of childhood abuse. Int J Eat Disord. 2015;48(1):55–8. https://doi.org/10.1002/eat.22364.
19. Afifi TO, Sareen J, Fortier J, Taillieu T, Turner S, Cheung K, Henriksen CA. Child maltreatment and eating disorders among men and women in adulthood: results from a nationally representative United States sample. Int J Eat Disord. 2017;50(11):1281–96. https://doi.org/10.1002/eat.22783. Epub 2017 Oct 9
20. Barbarich-Marsteller NC, Foltin RW, Walsh BT. Does anorexia nervosa resemble an addiction? Curr Drug Abuse Rev. 2011;4(3):197–200. https://doi.org/10.2174/1874473711104030197.

21. Gaudio S, Dakanalis A, Fariello G, Riva G. Neuroscience, brain imaging, and body image in eating and weight disorders. In: Cuzzolaro M, Fassino S, editors. Body image, eating, and weight: a guide to assessment, treatment, and prevention. Cham, Switzerland: Springer International Publishing AG; 2018. p. 97–111.
22. Gaudio S, Quattrocchi CC. Neural basis of a multidimensional model of body image distortion in anorexia nervosa. Neurosci Biobehav Rev. 2012;36(8):1839–47.
23. Schebendach JE, Uniacke B, Walsh BT, Mayer LES, Attia E, Steinglass J. Fat preference and fat intake in individuals with and without anorexia nervosa. Appetite. 2019;139:35–41.
24. Calugi S, El Ghoch M, Conti M, Dalle Grave R. Preoccupation with shape or weight, fear of weight gain, feeling fat and treatment outcomes in patients with anorexia nervosa: a longitudinal study. Behav Res Ther. 2018b;105:63–8. https://doi.org/10.1016/j.brat.2018.04.001.
25. Peat CM. Cognitive behavioral therapy. In: Claes L, Muehlenkamp JJ, editors. Non-suicidal self-injury in eating disorders. Heidelberg, Germany: Springer; 2014. p. 105–25.
26. Gao T, Gurd B. Reported meal and snack consumption on the EDE in the past 28 days with age and BMI as covariates, M (SD). BMC Health Serv Res. 2019;19(1):6. https://doi.org/10.1186/s12913-019-3907-6.
27. Riva G, Gaudio S, Serino S, Dakanalis A, Ferrer-García M, Gutiérrez-Maldonado J. Virtual reality for the treatment of body image disturbances in eating and weight disorders. In: Cuzzolaro M, Fassino S, editors. Body image, eating, and weight: a guide to assessment, treatment, and prevention. Cham, Switzerland: Springer International Publishing AG; 2018. p. 333–51.
28. Steinglass J, Mayer L, Attia E. Treatment of restrictive eating and low-weight conditions, including anorexia nervosa and avoidant/restrictive food intake disorder. In: Walsh BT, Attia E, Glasofer DR, Sysko R, editors. Handbook of assessment and treatment of eating disorders. Arlington, VA: American Psychiatric Association Publishing; 2016. p. 259–78.
29. Tanofsky-Kraff M and Wilfley DE. Interpersonal psychotherapy for the treatment of eating disorder. In Agras WS (Ed.), The Oxford Handbook of Eating Disorders. New York, NY: Oxford University Press, Inc. 2010;348–72.
30. Vocks S, Busch M, Schulte D, Grönermeyer D, Herpertz S, Suchan B. Effects of body image therapy on the activation of the extrastriate body area in anorexia nervosa: an fMRI study. Psychiatry Res. 2010;183(2):114–8. https://doi.org/10.1016/j.pscychresns.2010.05.011.
31. McElory SL, Guerdjikova AI, O'Melia AM, Mori N, Keck PE. Pharmacotherapy of eating disorders. In: Agras WS, editor. The Oxford handbook of eating disorders. New York, NY: Oxford University Press, Inc.; 2010. p. 417–51.
32. Favaro A, Busetto P, Collantoni E, Santonastaso P. The age of onset of eating disorders. In: de Girolamo G, McGorry P, Sartorius N, editors. Age of onset of mental disorders. Cham: Springer; 2019. https://doi.org/10.1007/978-3-319-72619-9_11.
33. Kendler KS, MacLean C, Neale M, Kessler R, Heath D, Eaces L. The genetic epidemiology of bulimia nervosa. Am J Psychiatry. 1991;148(12):1627–37.
34. Smahel D, Machackova H, Smahelova M, Cevelicek M, Almenara CA, Holubcikova J, editors. Digital technology, eating behaviors, and eating disorders. Springer; 2018. https://doi.org/10.1007/978-3-319-93221-7.
35. Collier D, Treasure J. The aetiology of eating disorders. Br J Psychiatry. 2004;185(5):363–5. https://doi.org/10.1192/bjp.185.5.363.
36. Mohr HM, Röder C, Zimmermann J, Hummel D, Negele A, Grabhorn R. Body image distortions in bulimia nervosa: investigating body size overestimation and body size satisfaction by fMRI. NeuroImage. 2011;56(3):1822–31. https://doi.org/10.1016/j.neuroimage.2011.02.069.
37. Berner LA, Brown TA, Lavender JM, Lopez E, Wierenga CE, Kaye WH. Neuroendocrinology of reward in anorexia nervosa and bulimia nervosa: beyond leptin and ghrelin. Mol Cell Endocrinol. 2019;497:110320. https://doi.org/10.1016/j.mce.2018.10.018.
38. Hildebrandt T, Alfano L, Tricamo M, Pfaff DW. Conceptualizing the role of estrogens and serotonin in the development and maintenance of bulimia nervosa. Clin Psychol Rev. 2010;30(6):655–68. https://doi.org/10.1016/j.cpr.2010.04.011.
39. Wade TD, Gillespie N, Martin NG. A comparison of early family life events amongst monozygotic twin women with lifetime anorexia nervosa, bulimia nervosa, or major depression. Int J Eat Disord. 2007;40(8):679–86. https://doi.org/10.1002/eat.20461.
40. Smith CE, Pisetsky EM, Wonderlich SA, Crosby RD, Mitchell JE, Joiner TE, Bardone-Cone A, Le Grange D, Klein MH, Crow SJ, Peterson CB. Is childhood trauma associated with lifetime suicide attempts in women with bulimia nervosa? Eat Weight Disord. 2016;21(2):199–204. https://doi.org/10.1007/s40519-015-0226-8. Epub 2015 Oct 13.
41. Wonderlich SA, Rosenfeldt S, Crosby RD, Mitchell JE, Engel SG, Smyth J, Miltenberger R. The effects of childhood trauma on daily mood lability and comorbid psychopathology in bulimia nervosa. J Trauma Stress. 2007;20(1):77–87. https://doi.org/10.1002/jts.20184.
42. Trace SE, Thornton LM, Baker JH, et al. A behavioral-genetic investigation of bulimia nervosa and its relationship with alcohol use disorder. Psychiatry Res. 2013;208(3):232–7. https://doi.org/10.1016/j.psychres.2013.04.030.
43. Patel RS, Olten B, Patel P, Shah K, Mansuri Z. Hospitalization outcomes and comorbidities of bulimia nervosa: a nationwide inpatient study. Cureus. 2018;10(5):e2583. https://doi.org/10.7759/cureus.2583.
44. Panico R, Piemonte E, Lazos J, Gilligan G, Zampini A, Lanfranchi H. Oral mucosal lesions in Anorexia Nervosa, Bulimia Nervosa and EDNOS. J Psychiatr Res. 2018;96:178–82. https://doi.org/10.1016/j.jpsychires.2017.09.022.
45. Strumia R. Eating disorders and the skin. Clin Dermatol. 2013;31(1):80–5. https://doi.org/10.1016/j.clindermatol.2011.11.011.
46. Katzman DK, Kanbur NO, Steinegger CM. Medical screening and management of eating disorders in adolescents. In Agras WS (Ed.), The Oxford handbook of eating disorders. New York, NY: Oxford University Press, Inc. 2010;267–91.
47. Grilo CM, Ivezaj V, Lydecker JA, White MA. Toward an understanding of the distinctiveness of body-image constructs in persons categorized with overweight/obesity, bulimia nervosa, and binge-eating disorder. J Psychosom Res. 2019;126:109757. https://doi.org/10.1016/j.jpsychores.2019.109757.
48. Thompson-Brenner H. Casebook of evidence-based therapy for eating disorders. 2015.
49. Hudson JI, Hiripi E, Pope HG, Kessler R. The prevalence and correlates of eating disorders in the National Comorbidity Survey Replication. Biol Psychiatry. 2007;61(3):348–58. https://doi.org/10.1016/j.biopsych.2006.03.040.
50. le Grange D, Lock J. Family-based treatment for adolescent with BM. In: Grilo CM, Mitchell JE, editors. The treatment of eating disorders: a clinical handbook. New York, NY: The Guilford Press; 2010. p. 372–87.
51. Broft A, Berner L, Walsh BT. Pharmacotherapy for bulimia nervosa. In book: The Treatment of Eating Disorders: A Clinical Handbook (Editors: Carlos M. Grilo, James E. Mitchell). The Guilford Press, 2010.
52. Wonderlich SA, Peterson CB, Smith TL, Klein M, Mitchell JE, Crow SJ, Engel SG. Integrative cognitive-affective therapy for bulimia nervosa. In: Grilo CM, Mitchell JE, editors. The treatment of eating disorders: a clinical handbook. New York, NY: The Guilford Press; 2010. p. 317–38.

53. Smink FRE, van Hoeken D, Hoek HW. Epidemiology of eating disorders: incidence, prevalence and mortality rates. Curr Psychiatry Rep. 2012;14:406–14. https://doi.org/10.1007/s11920-012-0282-y.
54. Kessler RC, Berglund PA, Chiu WT, Deitz AC, Hudson JI, Shahly V, Aguilar-Gaxiola S, Alonso J, Angermeyer MC, Benjet C, Bruffaerts R, de Girolamo G, de Graaf R, Maria Haro J, Kovess-Masfety V, O'Neill S, Posada-Villa J, Sasu C, Scott K, Viana MC, Xavier M. The prevalence and correlates of binge eating disorder in the World Health Organization World Mental Health Surveys. Biol Psychiatry. 2013;73(9):904–14.
55. Wilson GT, Wilfley DE, Agras WS, Bryson SW. Psychological treatments of binge eating disorder. Arch Gen Psychiatry. 2010;67(1):94–101.
56. Iqbal A, Rehman A. Binge eating disorder. In: StatPearls. Treasure Island, FL: StatPearls Publishing; 2020. https://www.ncbi.nlm.nih.gov/books/NBK551700/.
57. Balodis IM, Molina ND, Kober H, Worhunsky PD, White MA, Sinha R, Grilo CM, Potenza MN. Divergent neural substrates of inhibitory control in binge eating disorder relative to other manifestations of obesity. Obesity (Silver Spring, Md.). 2013:21(2);367–77. https://doi.org/10.1002/oby.20068.
58. Grilo CM, White MA. A controlled evaluation of the distress criterion for binge eating disorder. J Consult Clin Psychol. 2011;79:509–14. https://doi.org/10.1037/a0024259.
59. Dakanalis A, Riva G, Serino S, Colmegna F, Clerici M. Classifying adults with binge eating disorder based on severity levels. Eur Eat Disord Rev. 2017;25:268–74.
60. Al Nasser Y, Muco E, Alsaad AJ. Pica. In: StatPearls. Treasure Island, FL: StatPearls Publishing; 2020. https://www.ncbi.nlm.nih.gov/books/NBK532242/.
61. Santos AM, Benute GR, Nomura RM, Santos NO, De Lucia MC, Francisco RP. Pica and eating attitudes: a study of high-risk pregnancies. Matern Child Health J. 2016;20(3):577–82. https://doi.org/10.1007/s10995-015-1856-1.
62. Norris ML, Robinson A, Obeid N, Harrison M, Spettigue W, Henderson K. Exploring avoidant/restrictive food intake disorder in eating disordered patients: a descriptive study. Int J Eat Disord. 2014;47:495–9. https://doi.org/10.1002/eat.22217.

Further Reading

American Psychiatric Association. Treatment of patients with eating disorders, third edition. American Psychiatric Association. Am J Psychiatry 2006;163(7 Suppl):4–54.

Balodis IM, Molina ND, Kober H, Worhunsky PD, White MA, Sinha R, Grilo CM, Potenza MN. Divergent neural substrates of inhibitory control in binge eating disorder relative to other manifestations of obesity. Obesity (Silver Spring, MD). 2013;21(2):367–77. https://doi.org/10.1002/oby.20068.

Grave RD, Calugi S. Transdiagnostic cognitive behavioral theory and treatment of body image disturbance in eating disorders. In: Cuzzolaro M, Fassino S, editors. Body image, eating, and weight: a guide to assessment, treatment, and prevention. Cham, Switzerland: Springer International Publishing AG; 2018. p. 309–21.

Haines J, Neumark-Sztainer D. Prevention of obesity and eating disorders: a consideration of shared risk factors. Health Educ Res. 2006;21(6):770–82. https://doi.org/10.1093/her/cyl094.

Javaras KN, et al. Familiality and heritability of binge eating disorder: results of a case–control family study and a twin study. Int J Eat Disord. 2008;41(2):174–9.

Preti A, de Girolamo G, Vilagut G, Alonso J, de Graaf R, Bruffaerts R, Demyttenaere K, Pinto-Meza A, Haro JA, Morosini P. The epidemiology of eating disorders in six European countries: results of the ESEMeD-WMH project. J Psychiatr Res. 2009;43(14):1125–32. https://doi.org/10.1016/j.jpsychires.2009.04.003.

Robinson P, Skarderud F, Sommerfeldt B. Hunger: mentalization-based treatments for eating disorders. Springer. 2019; https://doi.org/10.1007/978-3-319-95121-8.

Smolak L, Levine MP. The Wiley handbook of eating disorders: basic concepts and foundational research, vol. 1. Wiley; 2015.

Stewart Agras W. The oxford handbook of eating disorders. Oxford University Press; 2010.

Wikimedia. Lanugo on the shoulder and back of twin girls. https://commons.wikimedia.org/wiki/File:Lanugo.png

Wikimedia. Micrograph of Barrett's esophagus (high magnification). https://commons.wikimedia.org/wiki/File:Barretts_esophagus_alcian_blue_high_mag.jpg.

Wikimedia. Oral manifestation of bulimia. https://commons.wikimedia.org/wiki/File:Oral_manifestation_of_Bulimia.jpg.

Wildes JE, Marcus MD. Diagnosis, assessment, and treatment planning for binge-eating disorder and eating disorder not other specified. In: Grilo CM, Mitchell JE, editors. The treatment of eating disorders: a clinical handbook. New York, NY: The Guilford Press; 2010. p. 44–65.

Yeomans M. Eating, body shape and health. In: Adler B, Abraham C, van Teijlingen E, Porter M, editors. Psychology and sociology applied to medicine. Kidlington, United Kingdom: Churchill Livingstone; 2009. p. 86–7.

Sexual Dysfunctions, Gender Dysphoria, and Paraphilic Disorders

22

Sam Nishanth Gnanapragasam, Fraser Scott, and Dinesh Bhugra

Introduction

All healthcare professionals are likely to manage patients who have sexual dysfunctions, gender dysphoria, and/or paraphilic disorders. These encounters may be directly related to the assessment and management of these disorders themselves, or while treating other conditions. At the same time, individuals who have these disorders are often stigmatized, face significant barriers to care, and may have associated mental health comorbidities. As such, it is necessary that care provided is respectful, compassionate, nonjudgmental, evidence-based, and culturally relevant. In this chapter, we provide an overview of these disorders based upon the Diagnostic and Statistical Manual of Mental Disorders Fifth Edition (DSM-5). We outline the epidemiology, etiology, pathophysiology, phenomenology, and treatment of these disorders.

Sexual Dysfunctions

Introductory Text

The DSM-5 defines sexual dysfunction as "a clinically significant disturbance in a person's ability to respond sexually or to experience sexual pleasure" [1]. For each specified disorder, the morbidity criteria required for a diagnosis include the following: symptoms are experienced on almost all or all occasions (approx. 75–100% or are "persistent or recurrent" in the case of Male Hypoactive Sexual Desire Disorder), symptoms have been present for at least 6 months, and the symptoms result in clinically significant distress [1]. The one exception is for substance- or medication-induced sexual dysfunction, where the duration criterion is not applied. This represents a significant change from the Diagnostic and Statistical Manual of Mental Disorders, Fourth Edition, Text Revision (DSM-IV-TR), which only stipulated the criterion of causing significant distress. The full diagnostic categories in DSM-5 are presented in Table 22.1.

The impact of sexual dysfunction on an individual's physical and psychological health can be striking. The psychological effects can take the form of depression, anxiety disorders, and subjective feelings of inadequacy and distress in the patient or even their partner [2]. It has also been demonstrated that quality of life is lower among those with sexual dysfunction (between 1.2 and 19.1% lower than the population mean) [3]. Therefore, it is vital that healthcare professionals have a reasonable understanding of the many potential causes, presentations, and treatment(s) of sexual disorders.

S. N. Gnanapragasam (✉) · F. Scott
South London and Maudsley NHS Foundation Trust, London, UK
e-mail: Sam.Gnanapragasam@slam.nhs.uk; fraser.scott@slam.nhs.uk

D. Bhugra
Institute of Psychiatry, Psychology & Neuroscience, King's College London, London, UK
e-mail: Dinesh.Bhugra@kcl.ac.uk

W. W. IsHak (ed.), *Atlas of Psychiatry*, https://doi.org/10.1007/978-3-031-15401-0_22

Table 22.1 Classification of sexual dysfunctions as recorded in DSM-5. The morbidity criteria are outlined in section "Phenomenology" diagnosis (above) and are the same for all disorders, unless otherwise specified

DSM-5 Sexual dysfunction categorization
Female problems
Female orgasmic disorder: either of the following must be present: 1. Marked delay in, marked infrequency of, or absence of orgasm 2. Markedly reduced intensity of orgasmic sensation
Female sexual interest/arousal disorder (FSIAD): diagnosis requires the presence of three or more of: 1. Absent/reduced interest in sexual activity 2. Absent/reduced sexual/erotic thoughts or fantasies 3. No/reduced initiation of sexual activity and typically unreceptive to a partner's attempts to initiate 4. Absent/reduced sexual excitement/pleasure during sexual activity on all/almost all sexual encounters 5. Absent/reduced sexual interest/arousal in response to any internal or external sexual/erotic cues (written, verbal, or visual) 6. Absent/reduced genital or nongenital sensations during sexual activity on almost all or all sexual encounters
Genito-pelvic pain/penetration disorder: persistent/recurrent difficulty with one or more of: 1. Having vaginal intercourse/penetration 2. Marked pelvic or vulvovaginal pain during vaginal intercourse 3. Marked fear or anxiety about either vulvovaginal or pelvic pain in anticipation of, during, or as a result of vaginal penetration 4. Marked tensing or tightening of the pelvic floor musculature during attempts at vaginal penetration
Male problems
Delayed ejaculation: either of the following symptoms: 1. Marked delay in ejaculation 2. Marked infrequency or the absence of ejaculation
Erectile disorder: at least of the following three symptoms must be present: 1. Marked difficulty in obtaining an erection during sexual activity 2. Marked difficulty in maintaining an erection until the completion of sexual activity 3. Marked decrease in rigidity of erections
Male hyposexual desire disorder: persistently deficient or absent sexual/erotic thoughts or fantasies and desire for sexual activity
Premature (early) ejaculation: a persistent/recurrent pattern of ejaculation occurring during sexual activity with a partner within approximately 1 min following vaginal penetration and before the individual wishes it

Epidemiology

The changes in morbidity criteria from DSM-IV-TR to DSM-5 have limited comparative epidemiological studies of sexual dysfunction, as they themselves likely resulted in a marked impact on the population prevalence of these disorders. The third National Survey of Sexual Attitudes and Lifestyles (Natsal-3) was a stratified probability sample survey of over 15,000 men and women in Britain aged 16–74 years and used very similar morbidity criteria to DSM-5 [4, 5]. In this study, overall 4.2% of sexually active men reported one or more of the following: lack of interest in having sex (0.8%), trouble getting or maintaining an erection (1.8%), difficulty in reaching climax (0.5%), or reaching climax more rapidly than they would like (1.7%) in the last year, which met all three DSM-5 morbidity criteria [4]. Of the above difficulties, getting or maintaining an erection was the only one to significantly increase in prevalence with age.

For sexually active women in Natsal-3, 3.6% reported one or more of the following problems, which met DSM-5 criteria for morbidity in the last year: lacked interest or arousal (0.6%), difficulty in reaching climax (1.9%), or feeling physical pain as a result of sex (1.9%). In this survey, there did not appear to be a clear linear association with age, although this is not consistent with findings reported from others [6].

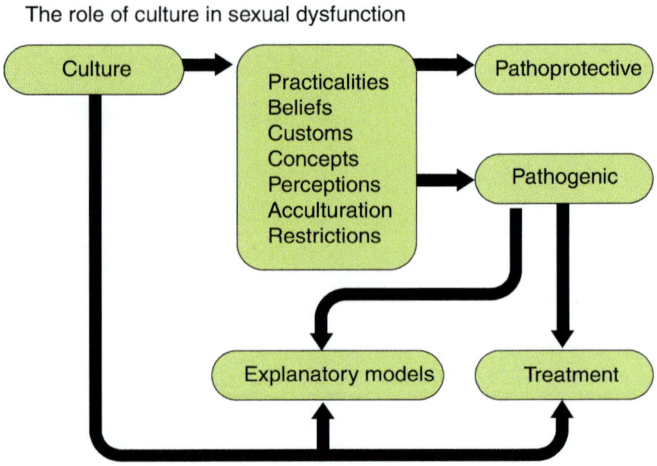

Fig. 22.1 The role of culture in sexual dysfunction

Etiology

Unsurprisingly, for such a varied group of disorders, there are numerous etiological factors which are implicated in sexual dysfunction. DSM-5 has included a wider range of associated features than DSM-IV-TR. These include partner factors, relationship factors, individual vulnerability factors, psychiatric comorbidity or stressors, cultural or religious factors, and medical factors [1]. See Fig. 22.1 for the role of culture in sexual dysfunction. Both physical and psychological factors can play a role, including mood or anxiety disorders, stress or performance anxiety, and past trauma (outlined in Fig. 22.2). Various etiological factors of male and female sexual disorders are outlined in Table 22.2.

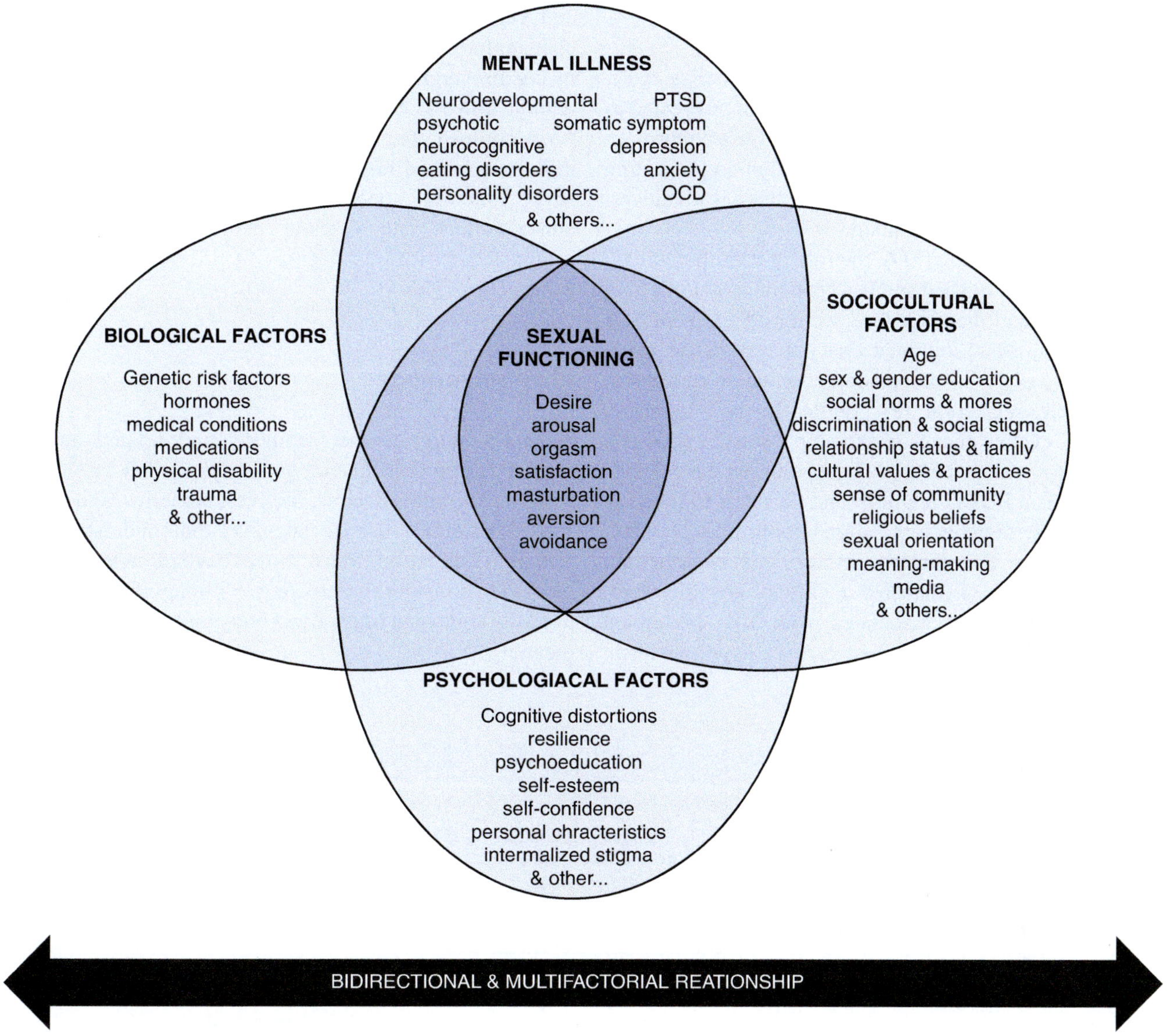

Fig. 22.2 The relationship between mental illness and sexual functioning is bidirectional and multifactorial. (*From* Klimowicz et al. [36]; *with permission*)

Table 22.2 Summary of the major physical and psychological factors that are implicated in the etiology of sexual dysfunction. This list is not exhaustive and merely serves to illustrate the diversity of possible causes of sexual dysfunction, which is to be expected of such a heterogeneous collection of disorders

Physical	
Normal age-related	**Men:** decreased testosterone, decreased penile rigidity and blood flow, increased refractory period, increased difficulty sustaining erections
	Women: decreased testosterone, vaginal atrophy, decreased vaginal lubrication
Cardiovascular	Atherosclerosis, heart failure, peripheral arterial disease, hyperlipidemia
Metabolic and endocrine:	Diabetes mellitus, pituitary dysfunction, Addison's disease, hypo-/hyperthyroidism, obesity
Neurological	Spinal cord injury, multiple sclerosis, Parkinson's disease, peripheral neuropathy
Genitourinary	Prostate disease and surgery, Peyronie's disease, renal failure, genital or urological cancer, pelvic radiation, urinary tract infection
Musculoskeletal	Pelvic fracture or injury
Pharmacological	Alcohol, recreational drugs (opiates, amphetamines, cocaine, benzodiazepines, and barbiturates), antidepressants (selective serotonin reuptake inhibitors (SSRIs), serotonin and norepinephrine reuptake inhibitors (SNRIs), tricyclic antidepressants (TCAs) and monoamine oxidase inhibitors (MAOIs)), antipsychotics, antihypertensive drugs (angiotensin-converting enzyme inhibitors, beta-blockers, alpha-adrenergic blockers, diuretics), estrogen, and anti-androgens
Psychological	
Stressors	General stress, guilt, anger, performance anxiety, previous trauma or abuse
Psychiatric	Depression, anxiety disorders, psychosis, mania, obsessive compulsive disorder (OCD)

Pathophysiology

Normal sexual response is divided into a four stage cycle, which is outlined in Fig. 22.3. Desire was later suggested as a fifth stage [7]. Sexual disorders can occur from abnormalities in one or more stages. Given the variation in presenting features of the different sexual disorders, there is no universal pathophysiological mechanism.

In erectile dysfunction (ED), the role of endothelial dysfunction is well established and has been the target of effective pharmaceutical therapies (see section "Treatment"). A review by Kaminetsky outlined that impaired nitric oxide (NO) activity results in decreased endothelium-dependent smooth-muscle relaxation [8]. Indirectly, NO increases intracellular cyclic guanosine monophosphate (cGMP), which is in turn broken down by phosphodiesterase-5 (PDE-5). Sildenafil is a PDE-5 inhibitor and thus acts to increase levels of cGMP, thereby increasing smooth muscle relaxation. Conditions that directly damage the endothelium (e.g., hypertension or diabetes mellitus) are therefore, unsurprisingly, strongly associated with ED. Hormonal abnormalities, such as low testosterone or hypogonadism, and central nervous system (CNS) and neurotransmitter changes have additionally been implicated in ED. Alterations in dopaminergic and serotonergic activity have both been demonstrated in ED.

In contrast, female sexual dysfunction has been much more overlooked historically. Disturbances in genital sensory function, pelvic floor musculature, hormonal abnormalities, and vascular pathologies have all been implicated to various degrees in different female sexual dysfunctions [9].

Phenomenology

Aanstoos suggests that sexuality and related acts have deep meaning for a person and are the result of one's own unique biography, desires, motives, anxieties, and relationship dynamics [10]. He suggests that understanding of sexual dysfunction must move beyond neurobiological models to consider the loss (e.g., of imagination and intentionality) between one's lived body and the wider world of meaning.

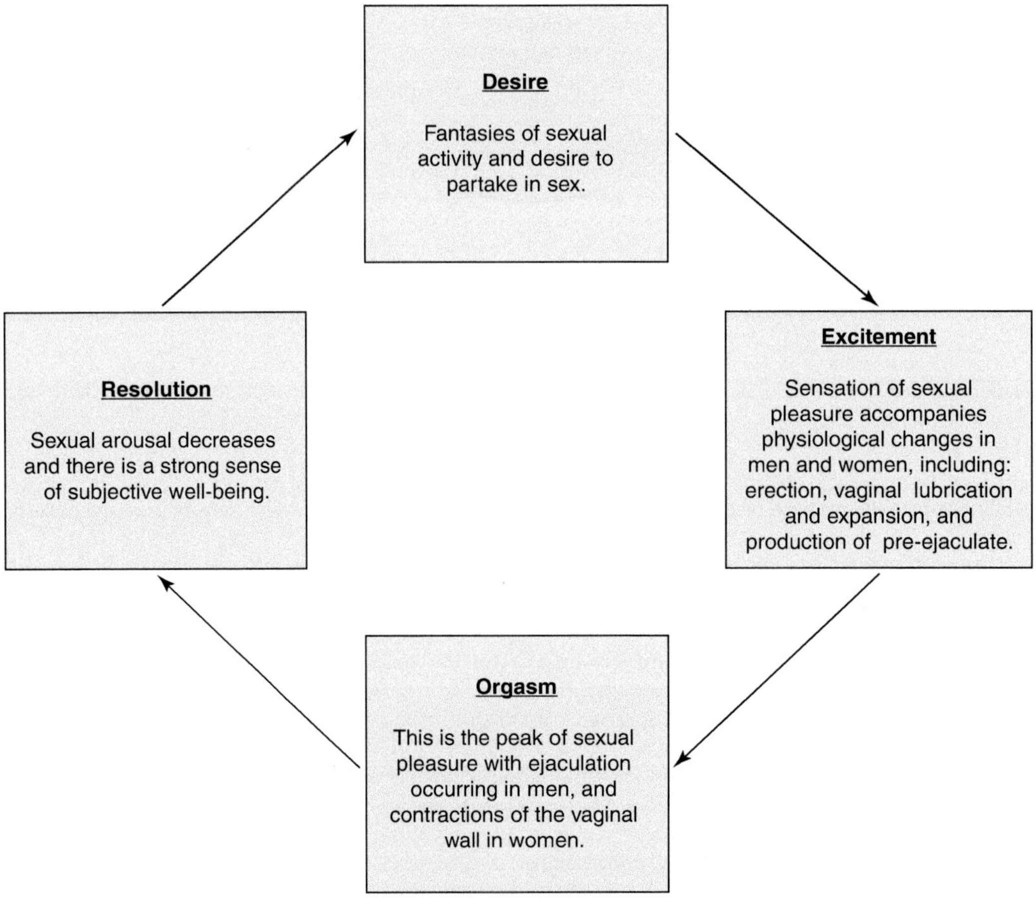

Fig. 22.3 An overview of the normal human sexual response cycle. Some sources include Plateau as a distinct stage between excitement and orgasm

Treatment

The first step in assessment and management of a patient presenting with sexual difficulties is a comprehensive history of the presenting complaint, in addition to a full medical, psychiatric, social, and sexual history, including current and past medications (and any recent dose alterations). For female patients, this should include a full gynecological history and information on birth control and hormone therapy. It is of paramount importance that a trusting patient–doctor relationship is formed, as patients can feel uncomfortable disclosing more private aspects of their sexual difficulties. A five-step "ALLOW" algorithm to facilitate this process is outlined in Fig. 22.4.

A detailed physical examination is required, which may include the abdomen, thyroid, general appearance (e.g., hair distribution, body habitus), peripheral vascular examination, examination of testes, penis, digital rectal examination, and internal examination (where appropriate).

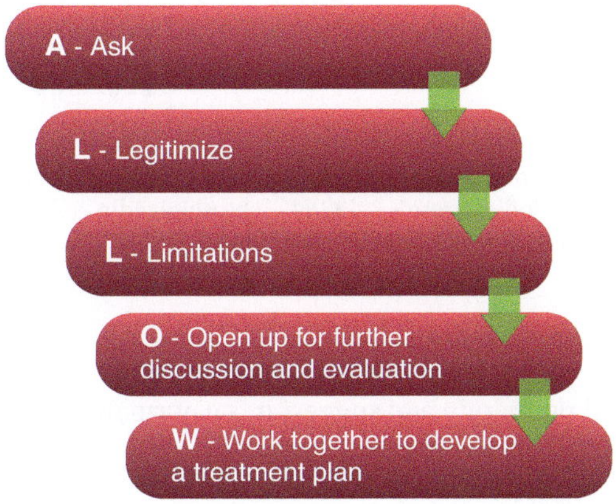

Fig. 22.4 The five-step "allow" algorithm for managing sexual dysfunction

In terms of investigations, a detailed workup may include full blood count, thyroid function tests, serum prolactin, serum testosterone, luteinizing hormone (LH) and follicle-stimulating hormone (DSH) levels, sex hormone-binding globulin, and estradiol. More specialized investigations are available including penile duplex ultrasonography and nocturnal penile tumescence and rigidity testing for use where appropriate [11].

In general terms, the treatment of sexual dysfunctions can be divided into pharmacological and psychological. However, it is important to acknowledge the myriad different etiologies that can produce sexual symptoms and dysfunction. Therefore for a number of patients, treatment of underlying disorders may improve sexual function.

Pharmacological strategies have been found to be most useful for ED. The most commonly used agents are PDE-5 inhibitors and include: sildenafil, tadalafil, and vardenafil. These drugs have also shown themselves to be of use in antidepressant-induced sexual dysfunction [12]. The mechanism of action of PDE-5 inhibitors is shown in Fig. 22.5. In this condition, other options include switching to a different antidepressant with a lower risk of sexual side effects, reducing the dose, a drug holiday, or waiting for spontaneous remission [13]. Conversely, in premature ejaculation, using this side effect of SSRIs is a treatment option [12].

Psychological treatments of sexual dysfunction have some evidence for efficacy in a variety of disorders. Sex therapy uses cognitive behavioral techniques to help a couple overcome sexual problems in their relationship. Psychological approaches have been used with varying degrees of success in the treatment of: impaired sexual desire, ED, premature ejaculation, and vaginismus [12].

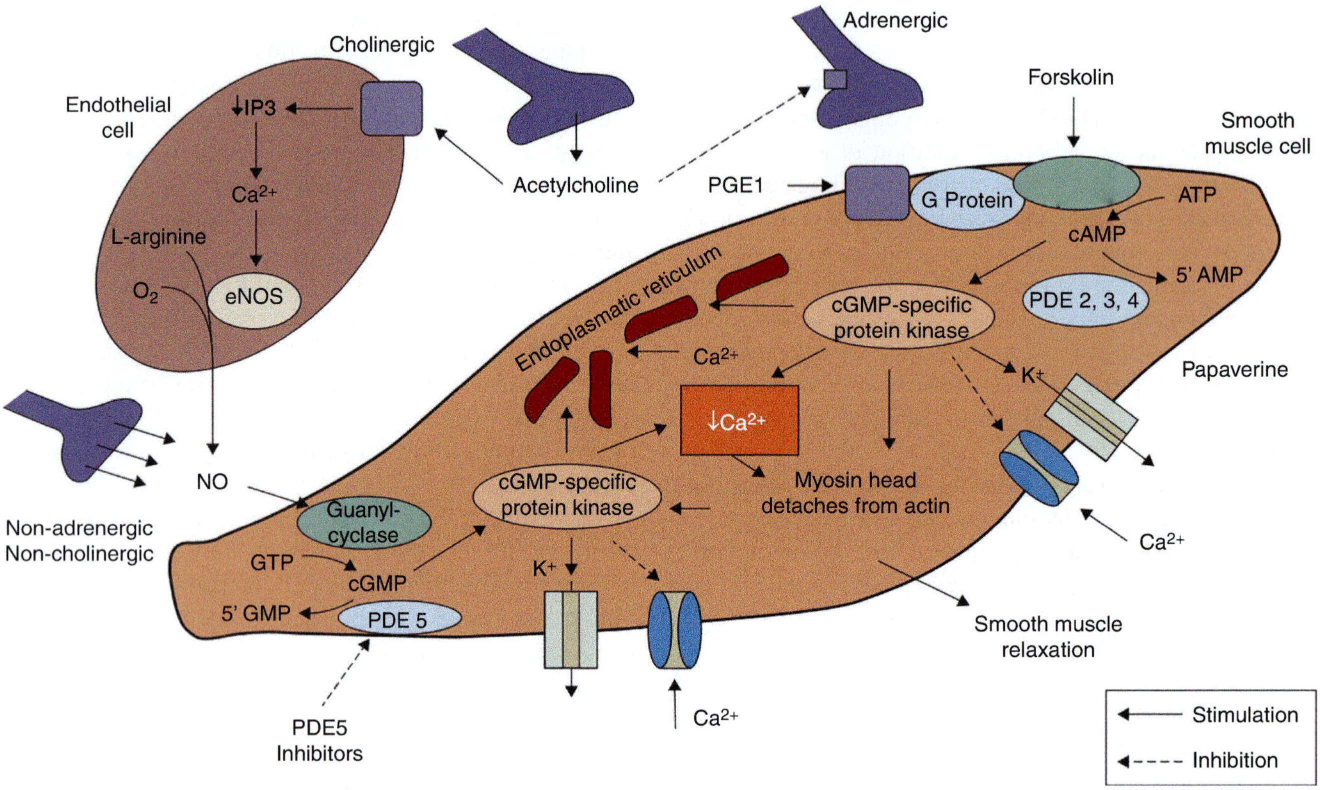

Fig. 22.5 Regulation of penile corpus cavernosum smooth muscle relaxation and effect of PDE5 inhibitors. *ATP* adenosine triphosphate; *cAMP* cyclic adenosine monophosphate; *cGMP* cyclic guanosine monophosphate; *eNOS* endothelial nitric oxide synthase; *GTP* guanosine-5′-triphosphate; *IP3* inositol trisphosphate; *NO* nitric oxide; *PDE* phosphodiesterase; *PGE1* prostaglandin E1. (*From* Hatzimouratidis et al. [35]; *with permission*)

Gender Dysphoria

Introductory Text

Gender dysphoria (GD) is the marked incongruence between one's gender identity and assigned sex at birth. The DSM-5 provides diagnostic criteria for this and outlines the diagnostic differences in children and adolescents/adults (Table 22.3). Crucially, the DSM-5 clarifies that gender nonconformity is not in itself a mental health disorder and that the key element to consider is the presence of clinically significant distress or impairment in social, occupational, or other areas of functioning [1]. Further, not all individuals are identified as transgender or gender diverse experience dysphoria. GD is not linked to sexual orientation, and people with GD may identify as straight, gay, lesbian, bisexual, or other self-identifications.

The GD definitions and criteria are not without debate. Indeed, there has been and continues to be an evolution in gender terminology across different parts of the world and time periods. This has been reflected in varied diagnostic definitions throughout iterations of the DSM, as well as in management and treatment guidelines/practices. It is also noted that some scholars and activists contest whether GD is a medical pathology and suggest it is a normal variant in gender identity and expression.

Epidemiology

There are varied estimates, and these relate to different research methods used (Fig. 22.6). Notably, national epidemiological surveys that look at mental disorder do not typically include GD.

DSM-5 estimates prevalence of 0.005–0.014% in birth assigned adult males and 0.002–0.003% in birth assigned adult females [1]. This estimate is based on clinical populations of those who received either a diagnosis of GD or the ICD-10 criteria of transsexualism and had sought binary transition (e.g., female to male or male to female). Studies in the Netherlands showed varied gender trends, with 0.008% of transgender women and 0.003% of transgender men seeking treatment at specialist clinics for GD [14]. Similarly, a Swedish study found rates of 0.013% among transgender women and 0.008% among transgender men [15].

Self-estimates show vastly higher prevalence numbers. A study of adults in the United States of America (USA) found

Table 22.3 DSM-5 criteria for gender dysphoria

Children	Adolescents and adults
Marked incongruence between one's experienced/expressed gender and their assigned gender, lasting at least 6 months	
As manifested by **at least six** of the following (one of which must be the first criterion): – Strong desire to be of the other gender or an insistence that one is the other gender (or some alternative gender different from one's assigned gender) – In boys (assigned gender), a strong preference for cross-dressing or simulating female attire or in girls (assigned gender), a strong preference for wearing only typical masculine clothing and a strong resistance to the wearing of typical feminine clothing – A strong preference for cross-gender roles in make-believe play or fantasy play – A strong preference for the toys, games, or activities stereotypically used or engaged in by the other gender – A strong preference for playmates of the other gender – In boys (assigned gender), a strong rejection of typically masculine toys, games, and activities and a strong avoidance of rough-and-tumble play or in girls (assigned gender), a strong rejection of typically feminine toys, games, and activities – A strong dislike of one's sexual anatomy – A strong desire for the physical sex characteristics that match one's experienced gender	As manifested by **at least two** of the following: – Marked incongruence between one's experienced/expressed gender and primary and/or secondary sex characteristics (or in young adolescents, the anticipated secondary sex characteristics) – A strong desire to be rid of one's primary and/or secondary sex characteristics because of a marked incongruence with one's experienced/expressed gender (or in young adolescents, a desire to prevent the development of the anticipated secondary sex characteristics) – A strong desire for the primary and/or secondary sex characteristics of the other gender – A strong desire to be of the other gender (or some alternative gender different from one's assigned gender) – A strong desire to be treated as the other gender (or some alternative gender different from one's assigned gender) – A strong conviction that one has the typical feelings and reactions of the other gender (or some alternative gender different from one's assigned gender)
And associated with clinically significant distress or impairment in social, school, or other important areas of functioning	

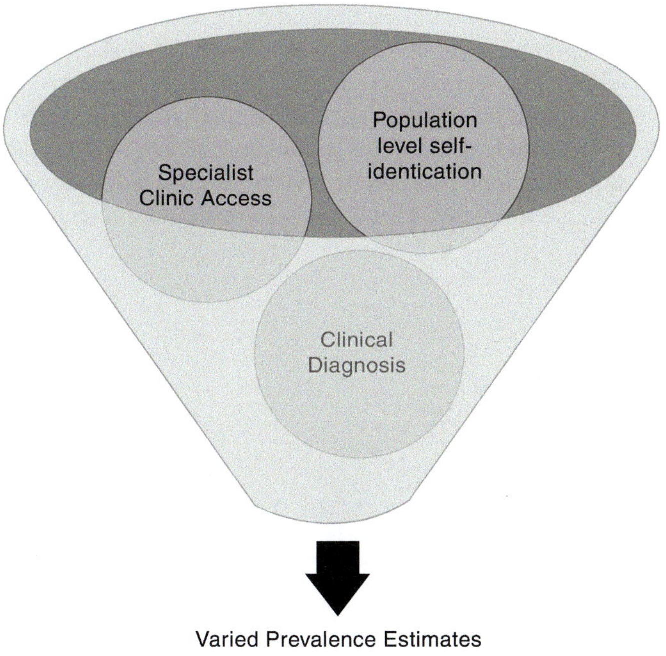

Fig. 22.6 Sources of prevalence estimates in gender dysphoria that account for varied prevalence. Some studies measure the proportion of people who have received a clinical diagnosis in health institutions, while others report the number of individuals accessing specialist clinic support and a few population level studies identify the number of people who self-identify with the disorder

0.6% identified as being transgender [16] and a different study of Dutch adults found incongruent gender identify rate of 1.1% among those assigned male sex at birth and 0.8% among those assigned female sex at birth [17].

The same is true among younger people, with prevalence numbers even greater in this group—for example, a study of middle school students in the United States found 1.3% identified as transgender [18]. Similarly, 1.2% of high school students in New Zealand are identified as transgender [19].

These findings suggest that estimates gained through clinical diagnosis or access to services may underestimate the prevalence. This is likely owing to individuals not seeking transition care or receiving hormones by self-administration/outside of specialist clinics, as well as the wider stigma/barriers to care that are associated with gender variation. It is also possible however, as noted by the DSM-5 GD definition, that some of the individuals who self-identify as transgender do not meet the diagnostic threshold as they do not suffer with clinically significant distress or impairment in functioning.

Finally, it is hard to fully ascertain the changes in prevalence over time, on account of varying diagnostic criteria. While some evidence suggests an increase over the last 50 years, it remains unclear whether increased rates may instead reflect greater comfort among those identified as GD, owing to wider societal decrease in stigma, depathologization, and more available specialist support.

Etiology

The exact cause of GD is unclear; however, it is thought to be multifactorial with biopsychosocial influencers. Biological factors, including genetic makeup, determine gender identity. It is suggested that there may be a heritable component, with studies showing higher concordance rates among monozygotic twins compared with dizygotic twins [20]. Further, it is thought that hormonal exposure (e.g., progesterone or other estrogenic drugs) may also impact gender identity, although firm evidence is lacking. In addition, developmental and social factors including emotional bond and relationship with parents and socialization in gendered behavior from birth also influence gender role and identity. There is evidence that childhood emotional, sexual, and physical abuses are neglected and maltreatment may be associated with GD.

DSM-5 also recognizes as a specifier that GD can present in congenital adrenal hyperplasia or partial androgen insensitivity syndrome (Fig. 22.7).

Pathophysiology

GD is found to be higher in patients with other psychiatric comorbidities such as schizophrenia and autism spectrum disorder. The link between these conditions and GD appears to be related to neuroanatomy, and further research is necessary to investigate this. Neuroanatomical links found in studies include hypothalamic link differentials [21] and variations in hemispheric ratios and amygdala connectivity [22]. In addition, a magnetic resonance imaging study of male-to-female conversion also found that the transgender putamen was within the normal range for women and larger than that of men [23]. It has also been suggested that changes in the third interstitial nucleus of the anterior hypothalamus (INAH3) (subnucleus of the hypothalamic uncinate nucleus) and the bed nucleus of the stria terminalis may be related to variation [24].

Phenomenology

A systematic review and meta-synthesis that included 20 papers (1606 participants) considered the lived experience of individuals with GD [25]. The study identified four key overarching themes (see Fig. 22.8).

The findings suggested a reciprocal relationship between the societal response and an individual's feeling about their own gender. Further, it underlined that an individual's distress was due to both gender identification incongruence and social factors.

Treatment

Healthcare assessments occur in a range of primary, inpatient, and specialist care settings. During these interactions, it is important to be mindful of the societal stigma, barriers to access, and related pressures individuals may have had to contend with in seeking support. As such, it is crucial that healthcare professionals are nonjudgmental and empathetic, as well as conscious of different terms used by individuals in their self-identification as this may be reflective of rapid evo-

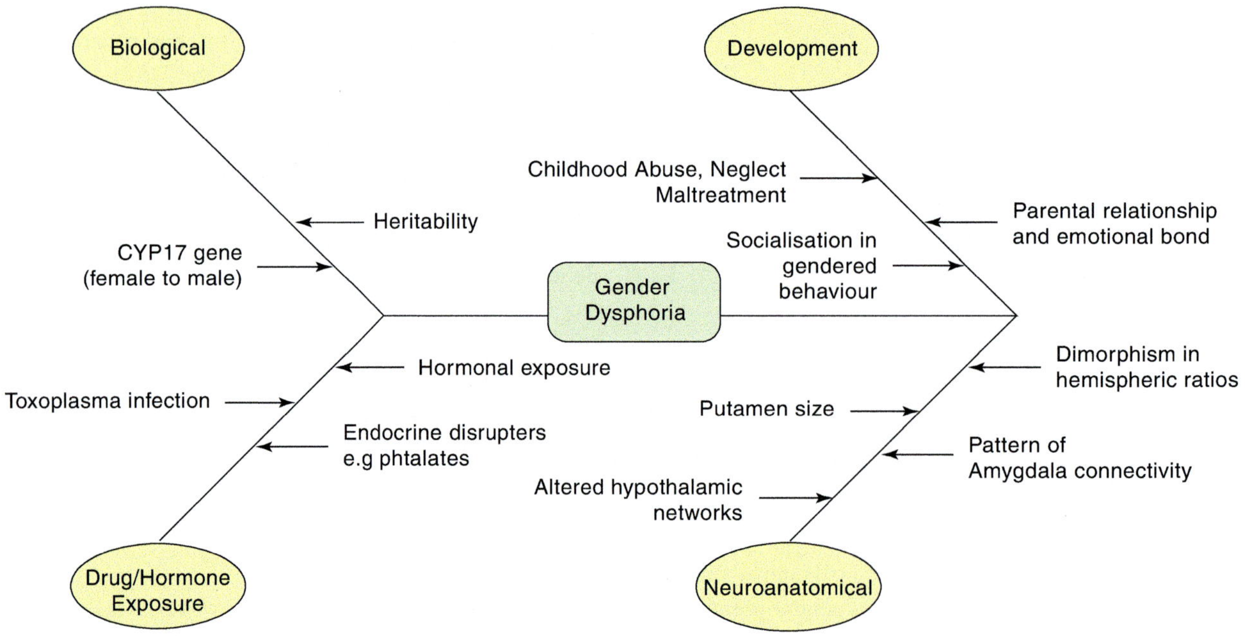

Fig. 22.7 Etiology of gender dysphoria

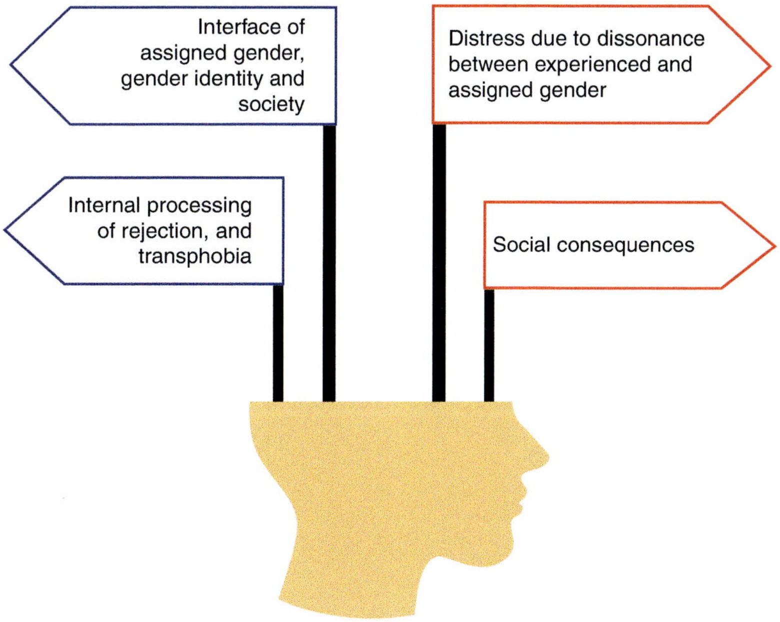

Fig. 22.8 Lived experience of gender dysphoria. Four key themes that emerged from systematic review and meta-synthesis

lution in gender terminology. Healthcare assessments are strengthened by undertaking a thorough history that covers psychiatric, medical, substance, social, family, and developmental domains. A particularly important aspect to consider is previous trauma and abuse.

Treatment options for the patients include social affirmation (using pronouns/names to match their gender identity), legal affirmation (changing name/gender markers on official legal and governmental identifiers), psychological support (such as individual and group psychotherapy), medical management (such as pubertal suppression for adolescents, or the use of hormones such as estrogen/testosterone for adults), and surgical management (such as sex reassignment and other gender-affirming surgery).

It is to be noted that medical and surgical treatment can be divided into fully reversible therapy (such as puberty blockers), partially reversible therapy (such as estrogen or androgen hormones) or irreversible (such as surgical procedures like mastectomy and vaginoplasty). Decision to undertake medical and surgical therapies are often done with a multidisciplinary team, which often includes endocrinologist, surgeons, and mental health professionals. The approach is varied dependent on age (see Figs. 22.9 and 22.10) and clinical presentation.

In management, it is necessary to take a collaborative decision making approach with adequate counseling. This is particularly important to help individuals have realistic expectations of treatment options (e.g., including of limitations), evaluate risks/benefits of therapy (e.g., related to bone mineral density and pubertal suppression), understand fertility preservation (e.g., the patient may lose the ability to reproduce), and wider sexual health education. Patients also benefit from help in establishing a supportive network of peers, friends, and family, as this network is often predictive of adverse mental health outcomes. Further, individuals may need ongoing support with comorbid mental health conditions and substance use problems. This is particularly important given these patients show higher rates of depression, anxiety, and suicidal acts.

It is to be noted that historical and current practices of psychological attempts to "convert" individuals to be cisgender, also known as "gender identity conversion therapy," are considered as unethical and in some countries illegal.

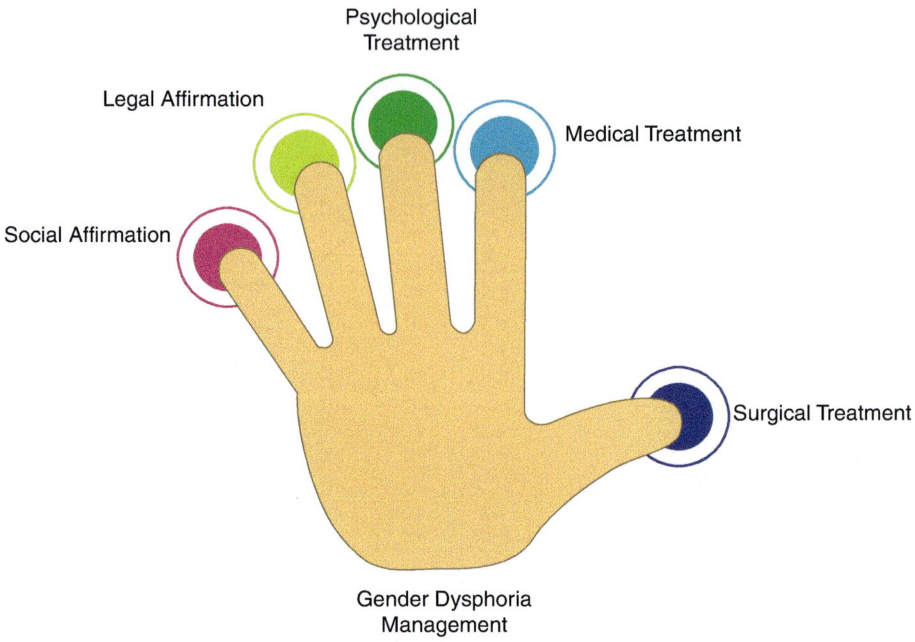

Fig. 22.9 Gender dysphoria management domains

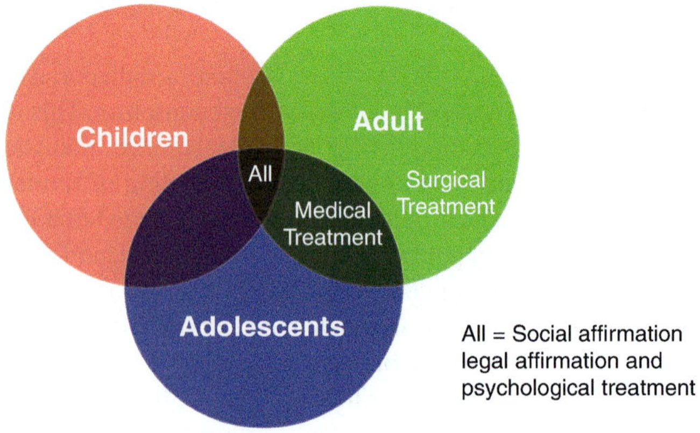

Fig. 22.10 Gender dysphoria treatment offered by age groups. For children, individual, family, and group, therapy is of benefit to explore and support gender identity. The World Professional Association for Transgender Health published Standards of Care that recommend against irreversible interventions such as surgery until someone is of a legal age and has lived has lived in the gender role congruent with their gender identify for at least one year [25]. For adolescents, hormonal treatment and psychotherapy is to be considered concurrently. In management of adults, psychotherapy, hormonal, and surgical management options are considered

Paraphilic Disorders

Introductory Text

Paraphilic disorders refer to a set of disorders in which sexual urges, interests, and excitement are dependent on objects, situations, or behaviors that are considered atypical or unusual. This broad definition and what is considered as unusual remains highly controversial within clinical, social, and political spheres. The definition and societal interpretation are often dependent on the cultural context, and there has been significant variation over time related to malleability of sexual norms (Figs. 22.11, 22.12, and 22.13).

These nuances and challenges are reflected in the evolution of psychiatric classification of disorders. Prior to DSM-III, paraphilic disorders were not distinct entities, and behaviors were instead classified under personality and other nonpsychotic mental disorder domains. Further, acts that are now accepted as sexual norms were pathologized (e.g., homosexuality).

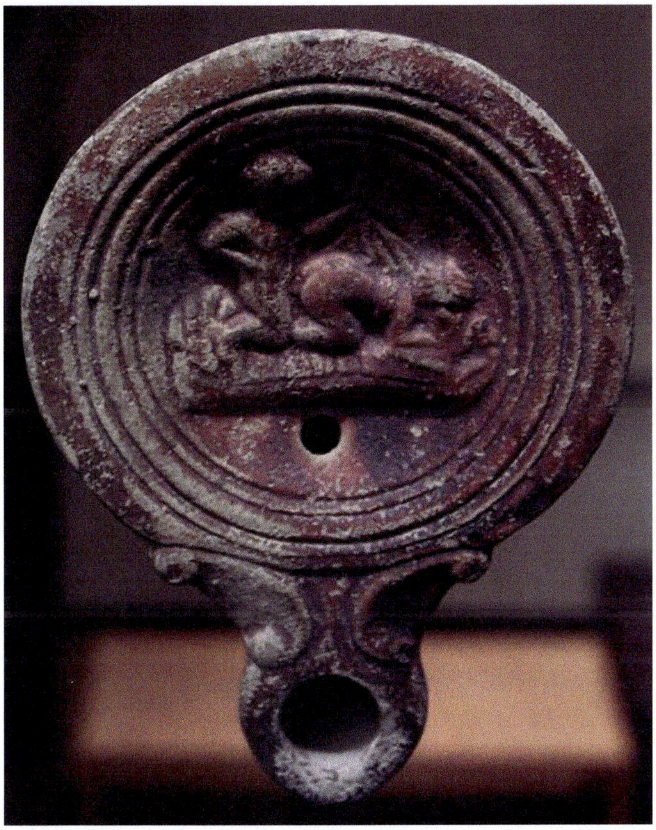

Fig. 22.11 Roman oil lamp depicting erotic art

The DSM-5 has clarified that most people with atypical sexual interest do not have a mental disorder and diagnostic threshold is only met if the interest(s) either cause mental distress to the individual and the well-being of others (including psychological, physical or death) or involves someone who is unable or unwilling to give consent [1]. This is reflected in the change in DSM-5 nomenclature from "paraphilia" to "paraphilic disorder."

The current working definition in DSM-5 remains broadly unchanged from the DSM-IV-TR:

> *recurrent, intense sexually arousing fantasies, sexual urges, or behaviors generally involving i) non-human objects, ii) the suffering or humiliation of oneself or one's partner, or iii) children or other non-consenting persons that occur over a period of at least 6 months* [26].

In total, there are eight listed paraphilic disorders in the DSM-5 (see Table 22.4).

Epidemiology

There are limited reliable population level incidence and prevalence estimates, particularly outside of nonclinical samples. This is owing to the cultural variation, change across time periods, and due to the reluctance of individuals to disclose atypical sexual interest to researchers, particularly given some activities have legal implications. Further, these disorders are often not included in national epidemiological surveys of mental disorders.

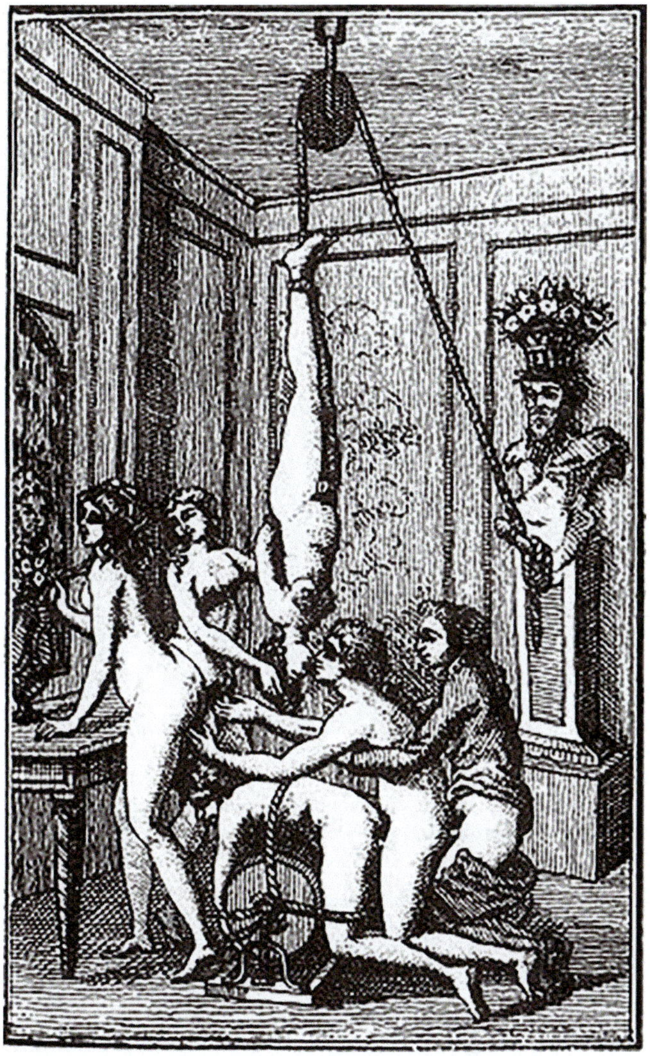

Fig. 22.12 Erotic illustration from the 1917 novel Juliette by Marquis de Sade

Population estimates, such as the Australian Study of Health and Relationships, found 2.2% and 1.3% of sexually active men and women, respectively, were involved in masochism activities in the prior year [27]. A recent study that had a demographically representative sample from Canada found almost half of the participants expressed an interest in one or more paraphilic behaviors, with approximately a third of participants acting on the interest [28]. While this is not the same as having a disorder, it does show that the paraphilic behaviors may be much more common than previously estimated. The exact prevalence of individual disorders within this group is also understood to be varied, and it is

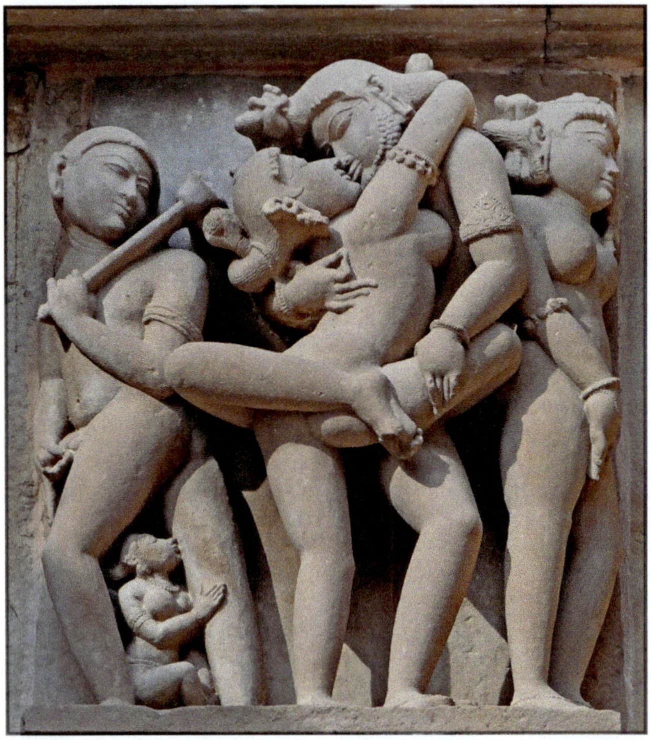

Fig. 22.13 Khajuraho temples, Madhya Pradesh, India, and a UNESCO world heritage site famous for erotic figures. The erotic art constitute for approximately 10% of total monumental art at the site

Table 22.4 DSM-5 paraphilic disorder

Disorder	Atypical sexual interest
Voyeuristic disorder	Watch a person while naked, undressing, performing sexual acts or activities without their knowledge
Exhibitionistic disorder	Exposing one's genitalia or performing sexual acts unsuspecting strangers
Frotteuristic disorder	Touching/rubbing against non-consenting other
Sexual masochism disorder	Being humiliated, beaten, tied-up, or other suffering
Sexual sadism disorder	Inflicted pain or humiliation (physical or psychological suffering) of another person
Pedophilic disorder	Prepubescent children
Fetishistic disorder	Inanimate objects or nongenital body parts
Transvestic disorder	Clothing and accessories associated with the opposite sex

thought that paraphilic disorders largely impact men more than women with the notable possible exceptions of masochism and fetishism.

Etiology

Paraphilic disorders typically emerge during an individual's adolescence and once established tend to be chronic. The etiology of paraphilic disorders remains unknown, and it is likely multifactorial. There are a number of psychoanalytic, developmental, biological, and imaging/structural models that seek to explain the etiology.

Money sought to explain these behaviors through the concept of "lovemaps." He suggested that paraphilic "lovemaps" may emerge rather than heterosexual or homosexual ones during a process of "vandalizing" that results from abuse (e.g., sexual) or nonsexual genitally stimulating childhood experiences [29]. Freund suggested that certain paraphilias can be considered as expressions of a disturbance in a common regulatory development system, particularly the normal "courtship" process for men [30]. Biological studies have found that there may be genetic associations with sexual behavior, including paraphilic behaviors such as pedophilia [31]. Interestingly, paraphilic disorders are also frequently comorbid with other paraphilic disorders, substance misuse disorders, and other mental health disorders (e.g., personality disorders).

Pathophysiology

Paraphilic behaviors have been associated with neurological disorders such as traumatic brain injury, stroke, dementia, and Parkinson's disease. These comorbidities provide valuable data points in investigating causative links. Solla and colleagues suggest that intensity of paraphilic urges in Parkinson's may be attenuated by the dopamine pathways [32]. Further studies suggest that central dopamine may play a key role in the pathogenesis of paraphilic disorders and in regulation of behavior. One study found that urine samples showed increased levels of serotonin and norepinephrine and decreased levels of DOPAC (3,4-dihydroxyphenylacetic acid) [33].

Phenomenology

The distinctive phenomenological feature of paraphilic disorders is the intense urge or craving to engage in behaviors that most people would not find sexually arousing. Among those that do, it is often difficult, sometimes even impossible, to control these impulses. This distinction is important—when we take the example of pedophilia, not all related sex offenders are individuals with paraphilic disorders and similarly not all those with a pedophilia paraphilic disorder are sex offenders.

Treatment

A thorough psychiatric and sexual history and mental state and neurological examination are needed as part of the assessment. An empathetic and nonjudgmental approach is

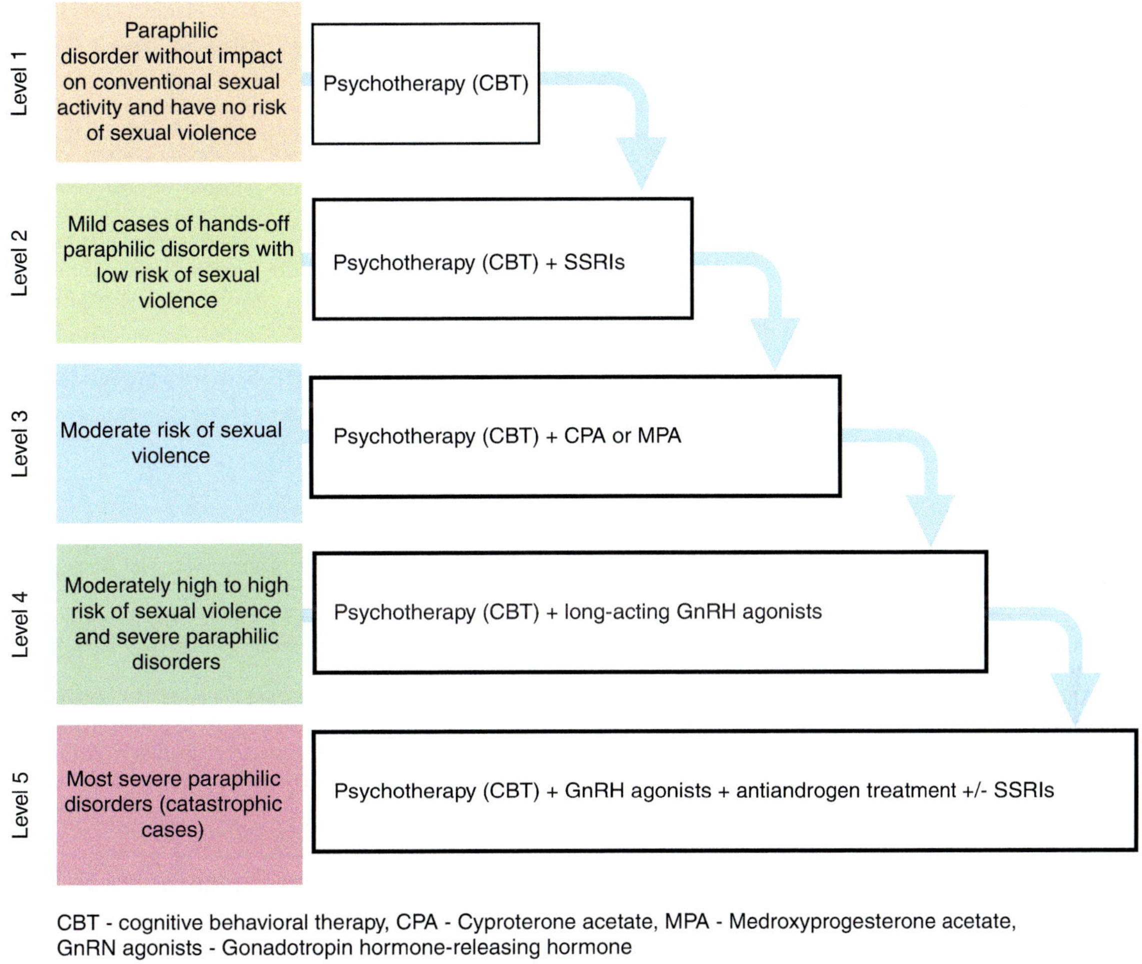

Fig. 22.14 Overview of World Federation of Societies of Biological Psychiatry 2020 guidelines for the pharmacological treatment of paraphilic disorders [34]. Initiation of medication must be balanced with prior medical history, comorbid psychiatric history, ongoing medication, and allergy history. It is also important to recognize that these medications do not cure paraphilic disorders and should often be combined with therapy such as CBT

crucial during this process, as these disorders have often been stigmatized and may have legal ramifications. Clinical assessments should also screen for any evidence of emotional, physical, or sexual abuse. There is benefit in complementing this with investigations such as blood tests (particularly endocrinological markers), phallometric tests, and EEG, to aid the diagnostic process.

Treatment itself poses a number of challenges—firstly, the context in which treatment is accessed is significant. Most people who seek support for paraphilic disorders are either convinced by family or friends, or are legally mandated to do so as part of a forensic assessment. This is owing to the ego-syntonic/ego-dystonic dual nature of paraphilic disorders, in which most individuals feel ashamed or guilty, while at the same time continue to engage in activities due to sexual pleasure/satisfaction. Secondly, there may be legal implications that may serve as a barrier to access.

Management options include psychological and medical treatments, and current evidence suggests that comprehensive treatment plans encompassing both components offer the best clinical outcomes for those with most severe cases. The decision to combine both treatment options is dependent on nature and intensity of sexual interest/activity and the related risk of violence to self/others (Fig. 22.14).

Psychological approaches, in particular cognitive behavioral therapy (CBT), have been shown to be efficacious in managing a range of paraphilic disorders. While the evidence base for specific pharmacological approaches is more varied, they offer helpful approaches and are part of treatment algorithms for varying severity. Pharmacological options include selective serotonin reuptake inhibitors, steroidal antiandrogens, and gonadotropin-releasing hormone analogs (Table 22.5).

Table 22.5 Pharmacological treatments of paraphilic disorders

Medication class	Medication examples	Primary mechanism of action	Treatment effect
Serotonin selective reuptake inhibitors	Fluoxetine, sertraline, fluvoxamine	Inhibition of serotonin reuptake via serotonin transporter, thereby increasing extracellular level of serotonin	Impaired libido including with orgasm and arousal Helpful for those with prominent obsessive paraphilic thoughts and compulsive-related behaviors Management of comorbid mental health conditions such as depression and anxiety
Gonadotropin-releasing hormone analogs	Triptorelin acetate, leuprolide acetate	Suppression of luteinizing hormone release, thereby reduced stimulation of testes to produce testosterone	Reduced sex drive and urges
Steroidal antiandrogens	Medroxyprogesterone acetate, cyproterone acetate	Increased catabolism of testosterone, increased testosterone protein binding, suppression of the hypothalamic-pituitary-gonadal axis	Reduced paraphilic interests and behaviors

References

1. Association AP. Diagnostic and statistical manual of mental disorders (DSM-5®). American Psychiatric Pub; 2013.
2. Rosen RC, Althof S. Impact of premature ejaculation: the psychological, quality of life, and sexual relationship consequences. J Sex Med. 2008;5(6):1296–307.
3. Ventegodt S. Sex and the quality of life in Denmark. Arch Sex Behav. 1998;27(3):295–307.
4. Mitchell SJ, Madrigal-Matute J, Scheibye-Knudsen M, Fang E, Aon M, González-Reyes JA, et al. Effects of sex, strain, and energy intake on hallmarks of aging in mice. Cell Metab. 2016;23(6):1093–112.
5. Mercer CH, Tanton C, Prah P, Erens B, Sonnenberg P, Clifton S, et al. Changes in sexual attitudes and lifestyles in Britain through the life course and over time: findings from the National Surveys of Sexual Attitudes and Lifestyles (Natsal). Lancet. 2013;382(9907):1781–94.
6. Laumann EO, Waite LJ. Sexual dysfunction among older adults: prevalence and risk factors from a nationally representative US probability sample of men and women 57–85 years of age. J Sex Med. 2008;5(10):2300–11.
7. Archer J, Lloyd B. Sex and gender. Cambridge University Press; 2002.
8. Kaminetsky J. Epidemiology and pathophysiology of male sexual dysfunction. Int J Impot Res. 2008;20(1):S3–S10.
9. Levin RJ, Both S, Georgiadis J, Kukkonen T, Park K, Yang CC. The physiology of female sexual function and the pathophysiology of female sexual dysfunction (Committee 13A). J Sex Med. 2016;13(5):733–59.
10. Aanstoos C. A phenomenology of sexual experiencing. In New directions in sex therapy: Innovations and alternatives. New York: Routledge; 2012. p. 51–68.
11. Krakowsky Y, Grober ED. A practical guide to female sexual dysfunction: an evidence-based review for physicians in Canada. Can Urol Assoc J. 2018;12(6):211.
12. Nagaraj AK, Pai NB, Nanjegowda RB, Rajagopal R, Shivarudrappa NK, Siddika N. Etiology and management of sexual dysfunction. Online J Health Allied Sci. 2009;8(2):1.
13. Taylor DM, Barnes TR, Young AH. The Maudsley prescribing guidelines in psychiatry. Wiley; 2018.
14. Bakker A, van Kesteren PJ, Gooren LJ, Bezemer PD. The prevalence of transsexualism in the Netherlands. Acta Psychiatr Scand. 1993;87(4):237–8.
15. Dhejne C, Öberg K, Arver S, Landén M. An analysis of all applications for sex reassignment surgery in Sweden, 1960–2010: prevalence, incidence, and regrets. Arch Sex Behav. 2014;43(8):1535–45.
16. Flores AR, Brown TN, Herman J. Race and ethnicity of adults who identify as transgender in the United States: Williams Institute, UCLA School of Law, Los Angeles, CA; 2016.
17. Kuyper L, Wijsen C. Gender identities and gender dysphoria in the Netherlands. Arch Sex Behav. 2014;43(2):377–85.
18. Shields JP, Cohen R, Glassman JR, Whitaker K, Franks H, Bertolini I. Estimating population size and demographic characteristics of lesbian, gay, bisexual, and transgender youth in middle school. J Adolesc Health. 2013;52(2):248–50.
19. Clark TC, Lucassen MF, Bullen P, Denny SJ, Fleming TM, Robinson EM, et al. The health and well-being of transgender high school students: results from the New Zealand adolescent health survey (Youth'12). J Adolesc Health. 2014;55(1):93–9.
20. Heylens G, De Cuypere G, Zucker KJ, Schelfaut C, Elaut E, Bossche HV, et al. Gender identity disorder in twins: a review of the case report literature. J Sex Med. 2012;9(3):751–7.
21. Berglund H, Lindström P, Dhejne-Helmy C, Savic I. Male-to-female transsexuals show sex-atypical hypothalamus activation when smelling odorous steroids. Cereb Cortex. 2008;18(8):1900–8.
22. Savic I, Lindström P. PET and MRI show differences in cerebral asymmetry and functional connectivity between homo-and heterosexual subjects. Proc Natl Acad Sci. 2008;105(27):9403–8.
23. Luders E, Sánchez FJ, Gaser C, Toga AW, Narr KL, Hamilton LS, et al. Regional gray matter variation in male-to-female transsexualism. NeuroImage. 2009;46(4):904–7.
24. Garcia-Falgueras A, Swaab DF. A sex difference in the hypothalamic uncinate nucleus: relationship to gender identity. Brain. 2008;131(12):3132–46.
25. Cooper K, Russell A, Mandy W, Butler C. The phenomenology of gender dysphoria in adults: a systematic review and meta-synthesis. Clin Psychol Rev. 2020:101875.

26. Association AP. Diagnostic and statistical manual of mental disorders, 4th Edition. DSM-1V-TR. Washington, DC: American Psychiatric Association; 2000.
27. Richters J, Grulich AE, de Visser RO, Smith AM, Rissel CE. Sex in Australia: autoerotic, esoteric and other sexual practices engaged in by a representative sample of adults. Aust N Z J Public Health. 2003;27(2):180–90.
28. Joyal CC, Carpentier J. The prevalence of paraphilic interests and behaviors in the general population: a provincial survey. J Sex Res. 2017;54(2):161–71.
29. Money J. Paraphilias: phenomenology and classification. Am J Psychother. 1984;38(2):164–79.
30. Freund K, Watson R. Mapping the boundaries of courtship disorder. J Sex Res. 1990;27(4):589–606.
31. Cengiz M, Cezayirli E, Bayoglu B, Asliyuksek H, Kocabasoglu N. Catechol-O-Methyltransferase Val158Met and brain-derived neurotrophic factor Val66Met gene polymorphisms in paraphilic sexual offenders. Indian J Psychiatry. 2019;61(3):253.
32. Solla P, Bortolato M, Cannas A, Mulas CS, Marrosu F. Paraphilias and paraphilic disorders in Parkinson's disease: a systematic review of the literature. Mov Disord. 2015;30(5):604–13.
33. Kamenskov MY, Gurina O. Neurotransmitter mechanisms of paraphilic disorders. Zh Nevrol Psikhiatr Im S S Korsakova. 2019;119(8):61.
34. Thibaut F, Cosyns P, Fedoroff JP, Briken P, Goethals K, Bradford JM, et al. The World Federation of Societies of Biological Psychiatry (WFSBP) 2020 guidelines for the pharmacological treatment of paraphilic disorders. World J Biol Psychiatry. 2020:1–79.
35. Hatzimouratidis K, Salonia A, Adaikan G, Buvat J, Carrier S, El-Meliegy A, McCullough A, Torres LO, Khera M. Pharmacotherapy for erectile dysfunction: recommendations from the Fourth International Consultation for Sexual Medicine (ICSM 2015). J Sex Med. 2016;13(4):465–88.
36. Klimowicz A, Janicic A, IsHak WW. Sex and chronic psychiatric illness. In: IsHak W, editor. The textbook of clinical sexual medicine. Cham: Springer; 2017. https://doi.org/10.1007/978-3-319-52539-6_32.

Sleep-Wake Disorders

23

Luigi Ferini-Strambi, Andrea Galbiati, Marco Sforza, Francesca Casoni, and Maria Salsone

The issue of sleep need and duration is highly heterogeneous across individuals and during aging and represents only a small part of a healthy sleep. Indeed, according to the most recent classification of sleep disorders (International Classification of Sleep Disorders 3rd edition, ICSD-3), sleep disturbances are more than 60, ranging from abnormal behaviors during sleep to hypersomnias, from insomnia to sleep-related movement disorders. The aim of this chapter is to provide a schematic and essential overview of the most prevalent sleep disorders encountered in clinical practice. The DSM-5 Sleep-Wake Disorders Work Group worked closely with ICSD-3 nosology system, and a lot of effort was undertaken to achieve the greatest degree of concordance between these two classifications. We chose to follow ICSD-3 since it represents the most widely used classification system for sleep disorders.

L. Ferini-Strambi (✉) · A. Galbiati · M. Sforza
Università Vita-Salute San Raffaele,
Milan, Italy

Department of Clinical Neurosciences, Neurology,
Sleep Disorders Center, IRCCS San Raffaele
Scientific Institute, Vita-Salute San Raffaele University,
Milan, Italy
e-mail: ferinistrambi.luigi@hsr.it

F. Casoni
Department of Clinical Neurosciences, Neurology,
Sleep Disorders Center, IRCCS San Raffaele Scientific Institute,
Milan, Italy
e-mail: Casoni.francesca@hsr.it

M. Salsone
Department of Clinical Neurosciences, Neurology,
Institute of Molecular Bioimaging and Physiology,
National Research Council, Sleep Disorders Center,
IRCCS San Raffaele Scientific Institute,
Milan, Italy

Introduction

Sleep is a dynamic state. The sleeping brain, in fact, continues its own internal physiological and psychological activity during sleep with an alternation of state that is unlikely reducible to a simple restoration function.

Based on electroencephalography (EEG), electrooculography (EOG), and electromyography (EMG), that constitutes polysomnography (PSG), it is possible to identify two different sleep phases, rapid eye movement sleep (REM), and non-REM (NREM) sleep.

During NREM sleep, EEG pattern is synchronous, and characteristic waveforms such as sleep spindles, K-complexes, and high-voltage slow waves are present. We can identify three different NREM stages N1, N2, and N3 that gradually reflect a sleep deepening.

Vice versa, REM sleep is defined by an incremented EEG activation, muscle atonia, and sudden rapid eye movements.

Healthy human enters sleep throughout NREM sleep, with the first occurrence of REM sleep 80 min after sleep onset. Then, during the night, NREM and REM sleep alternate within a 90 min cycle. During eye-closed relaxed wakefulness, trains of sinusoidal 8–13 Hz activity, namely alpha rhythm, are recorded over occipital derivations (Fig. 23.1).

The first sleep cycle starts with stage 1, which represents wake-to-sleep transition, and it is characterized by the disappearance of alpha rhythm and the presence of low amplitude and mixed frequency EEG activity, predominantly at 4–7 Hz (theta activity). Commonly, an increased amount of this stage during the night is a sign of disrupted sleep.

The most predominant sleep stage during an overnight PSG recording is stage 2 (N2). N2 is primarily defined by the presence of sleep spindle, a group of rhythmic waves characterized by a progressively increasing, then gradually decreasing, amplitude, generally in the range of 12–14 Hz, and K-complexes, a sharp wave that is maximum at the vertex and has a duration of at least 0.5 s. The presence of delta activity (<2 Hz, 75 microvolts) has to be less than 20% of the epoch (Fig. 23.2).

W. W. IsHak (ed.), *Atlas of Psychiatry*, https://doi.org/10.1007/978-3-031-15401-0_23

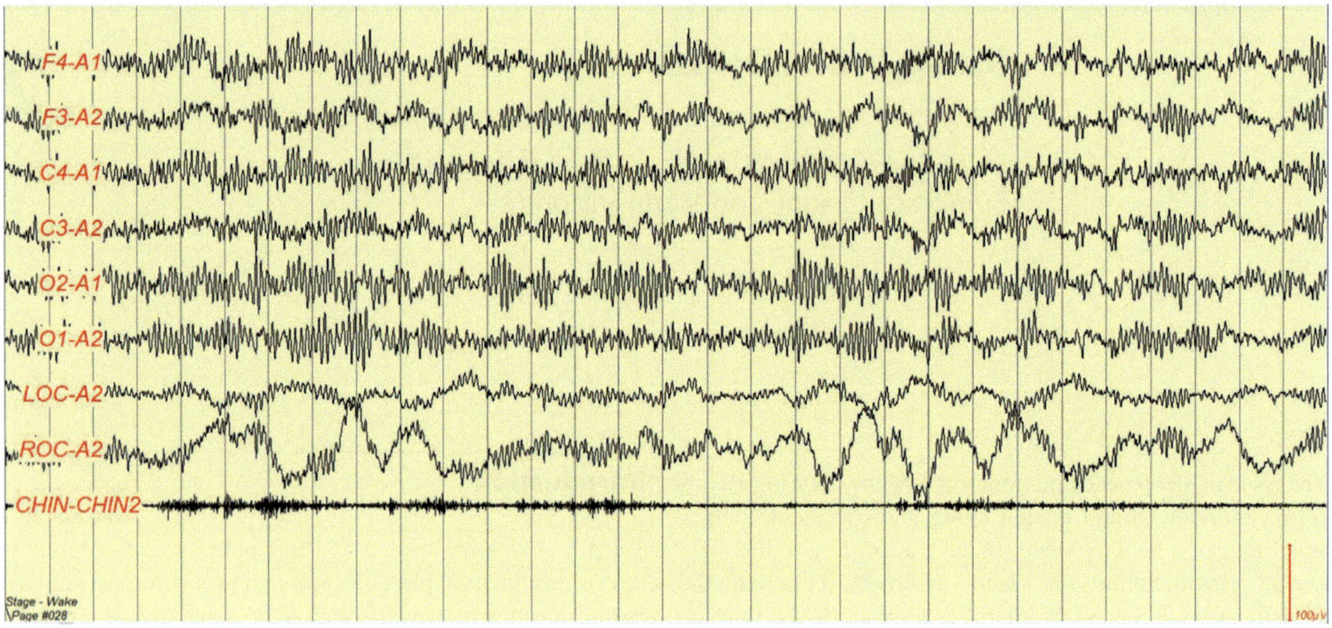

Fig. 23.1 Alpha rhythm is observed predominantly on occipital derivations

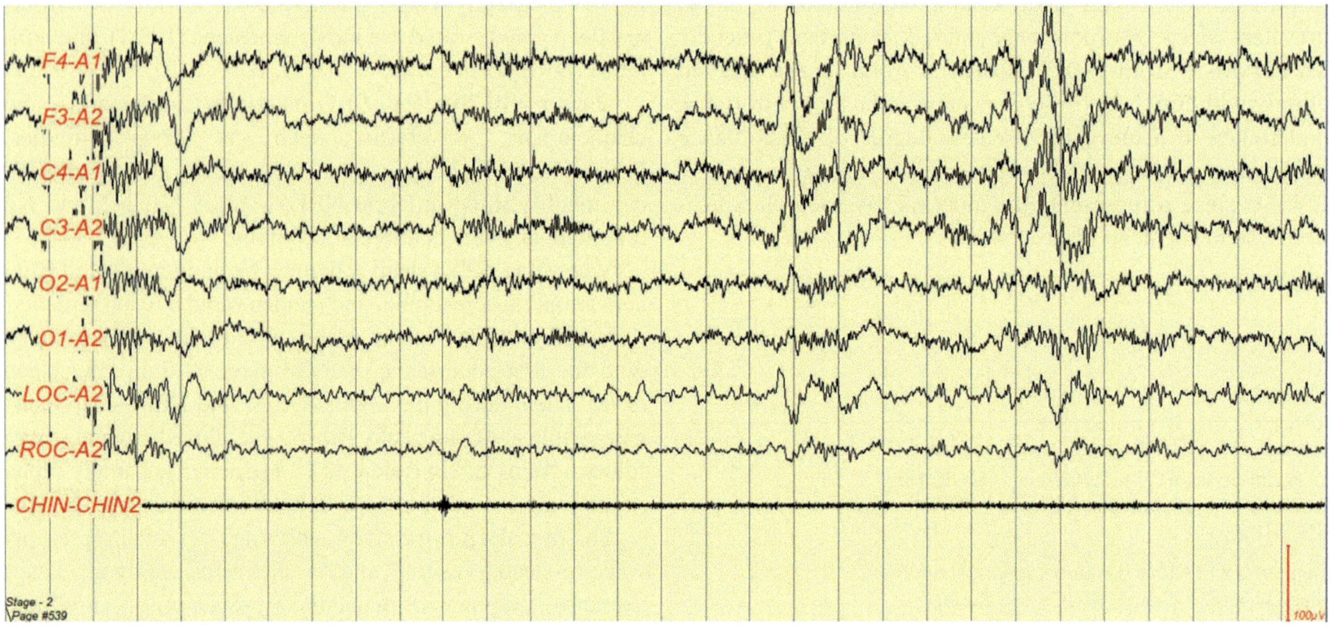

Fig. 23.2 Non-REM sleep Stage 2

The deepest stage of sleep is N3 (or slow wave sleep, SWS) that is determined by an increased delta activity measured mainly over the frontal derivation; in particular, its presence has to be more than 20% of an epoch (Fig. 23.3).

REM sleep is defined by the presence of conjugate, irregular, sharply peaked eye movement with an initial deflection usually lasting <500 ms, the presence of muscular atonia or low EMG tone, and the presence of low amplitude with mixed frequency EEG activity (Fig. 23.4).

The alternation between NREM and REM sleep is cyclical throughout the night. After a short period of N1, N2 continues for 10–25 min. An episode of N3 might then occur, followed again by 5–10 min of N2, preceding the first REM episode (usually not until 80 min or longer). During the first cycle of the night, REM sleep is usually short-lived and then becomes longer across the night. Vice versa, N3 is particularly represented in the first cycle of the night and diminishes from later cycles, with N2 that occupies the NREM sleep portion of the cycle. Throughout the night, the average

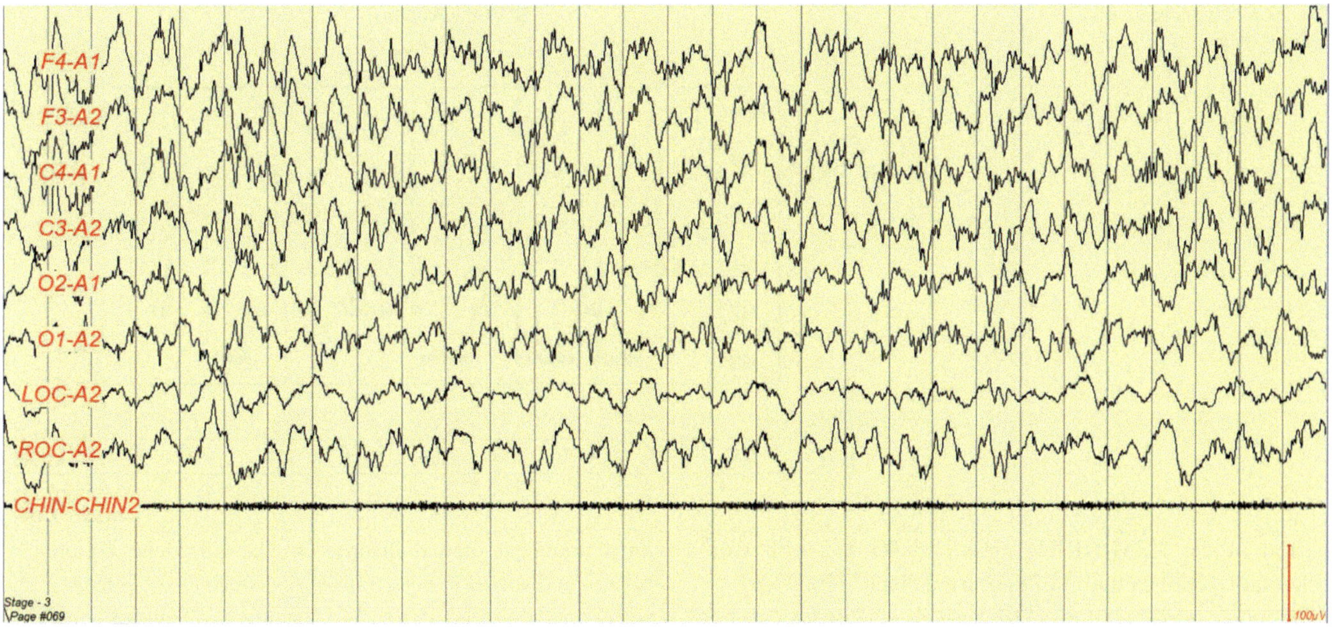

Fig. 23.3 Slow wave sleep

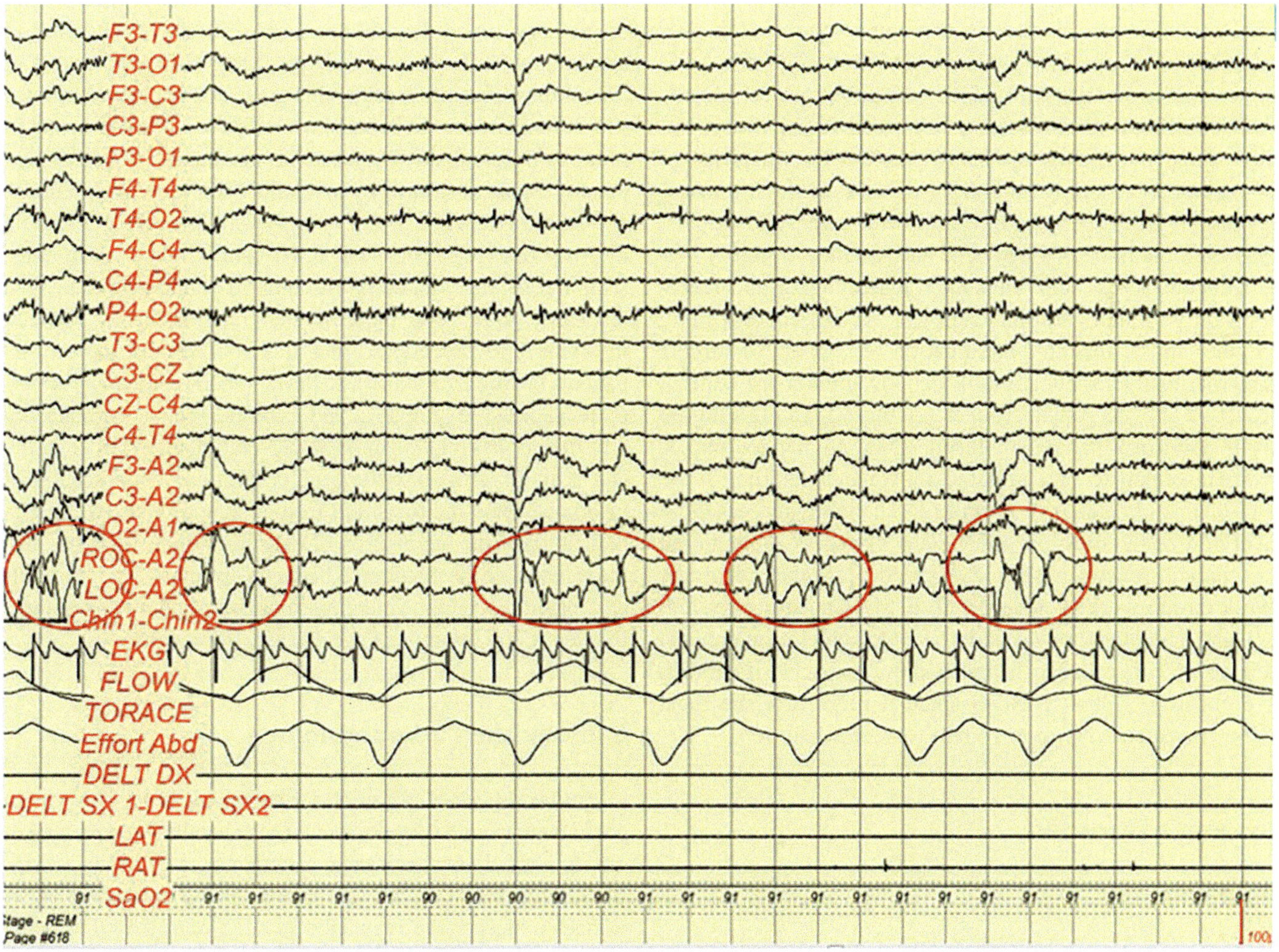

Fig. 23.4 REM sleep. Example of REMs in red circles

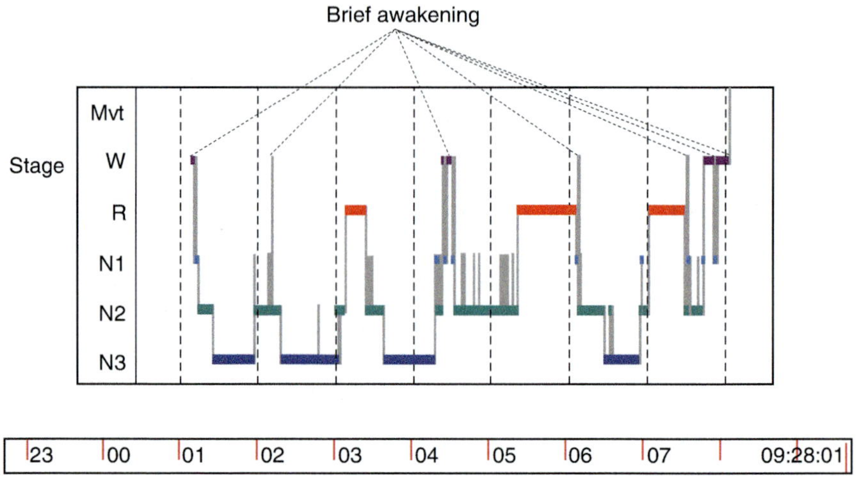

Fig. 23.5 Hypnogram of a healthy sleeper

period of the REM-NREM cycle is ~90–110 min (for a schematic representation of nocturnal sleep, Fig. 23.5).

Another important tool to objectively quantify sleep periods is actigraphy. This is a non-invasive method used to evaluate human rest/activity cycles with a wristwatch-like motion-sensing device. The advantage in comparison with PSG is that it can be used in the home environment over extended time periods. However, by the actigraphy, it is impossible to identify and quantify the different sleep stages.

It is difficult to characterize a normal length sleep pattern, since it depends on many factors. The majority of young adults report 7.5 h a night on weekday, with longer nocturnal sleep period, 8.5 h, during weekend nights. However, the issue of sleep need and duration is highly heterogeneous across individuals and during aging and represents only a small part of a healthy sleep. Indeed, according to the most recent classification of sleep disorders (International Classification of Sleep Disorders 3rd edition, ICSD-3) [1], sleep disturbances are more than 60, ranging from abnormal behaviors during sleep to hypersomnias, from insomnia to sleep-related movement disorders. The aim of this chapter is to provide a schematic and essential overview of the most prevalent sleep disorders encountered in clinical practice. The DSM-5 Sleep-Wake Disorders Work Group worked closely with ICSD-3 nosology system [2], and a lot of effort was undertaken to achieve the greatest degree of concordance between these two classifications. We chose to follow ICSD-3 since it represents the most widely used classification system for sleep disorders.

Insomnia Disorder

Epidemiology

Insomnia disorders (ID) is a common health problem, about 10% of the population meets the diagnostic criteria, and a third of the population reports sleep complaints. ID is the second most prevalent mental disorder in the European Union [3]. Insomnia disorder is determined by disturbance of sleep onset, sleep maintenance, and early morning awakenings with dissatisfaction with sleep quantity or quality. Moreover, the disease is characterized by impaired daytime functioning, i.e., fatigue and reduced energy, impaired attention, concentration or memory, mood disturbances, and difficulty functioning in academic or occupational settings. Sleep difficulty occurs at least three nights per week and is present for at least 3 months [2]. Time specifiers in diagnostic criteria result fundamental in order to differentiate ID and acute insomnia, i.e., a transient phenomenon constituted by insomnia symptoms that naturally go into remission in a few days or weeks. Conversely, insomnia disorder tends to be persistent and became chronic in 3 months. ID is frequently associated with other psychiatric and medical disorders [4–6]. The most studied relationship is between insomnia and depression, and literature results showed ID patients having twofold risk to develop depression [7]; furthermore, depressive symptoms and insomnia seem to be linked by a bi-directional relationship [8]. Several changes occur in the last years in terms of diagnostic criteria and classification of insomnia. First, the transition from a symptom-based conceptualization to the recognition of a disorder on its own; but also the removal of the distinction between "primary" and "secondary" insomnia; and the integration of a minimum of symptoms frequency and duration of the disease [9] was applied.

Etiology and Pathophysiology

Literature suggested a partial attribution by genetic factors in predicting insomnia development. Some results showed an association not only between sleep disturbance and circadian clock genes alterations [10] but also neurotransmitter function genes related to sleep-wake regulation [11, 12]. On the other hand, recent genetic studies displayed risk genes overlap between insomnia and depression and stress and anxiety disorders, rather than with other sleep disorders or clock-related genes [13, 14].

ID pathophysiology suggests hyperarousal during both sleep and wakefulness (Fig. 23.6) [15].

Results in the literature suggested increased levels of cortisol, indicating a fundamental role of stress circuit activity of the hypothalamic-pituitary-adrenal axis [16]. Furthermore, elevated body temperature, metabolic rate, resting heart rate, and altered heart rate variability parameters in insomnia patients compared with controls demonstrated a modified activity of the autonomic nervous system [17–20]. If macrostructural polysomnographic indices failed to characterize a consistent pattern of insomnia patient [21], EEG quantitative analyses seem to be more informative. Insomnia patients showed an increase in fast frequencies in nocturnal EEG (Fig. 23.7) [22, 23], which seems to be linked with the known phenomenon of sleep misperception in insomnia (overestimation of sleep latency and wake after sleep onset and underestimation of sleep time), interpreted as an increase in sensorimotor and cognitive activity (Fig. 23.8) [24].

On the other hand, insomnia patients present a reduced low-frequency activity (slow-wave activity <4 Hz) [25–27], specifically in slow-oscillation (0.5–1 Hz) [28]. In line with previous findings and therefore with the hypothesis of an insomnia deficit of sleep homeostatic drive, a research group revealed a relative deficit in initial sleep drive, as manifested in lower initial NREM EEG delta power and less rapid decline of delta power over the night [29]. Furthermore, rapid eye movement (REM) sleep features seem to characterize insomnia objective sleep. Specifically, "restless REM sleep" indices, REM sleep with a high number of phasic events, including arousals and eye movements, seem to interfere with the overnight resolution of emotional distress, and it could contribute to its accumulation, leading to a chronically hyperarousal state (Fig. 23.9) [30, 31].

Also imaging studies corroborated hyperarousal insomnia theory, suggesting overactivation of the arousal system, the emotion-regulating system, and parts of the cognitive system accompanied by reduced activation of the prefrontal cortex (PFC) and the caudate head [9]. Furthermore, a brain imaging study using FDG (18F-fluorodeoxyglucose)-PET showed ID patients with increased brain metabolism in brain networks, such as the arousal, emotion-regulating, and the cognitive system [32].

The Psycho-Biosocial Point of View

Consistently with the previous approach, Spielman and colleagues in 1987 [33] elaborated the three factor model, by integrating perpetuating, precipitating, and predisposing factors. The genetic and hyperarousal characteristics, described previously, psychological factors (e.g., worry and rumination) and social factors (such as incompatible work or partner schedule) in insomnia patients constitute the predisposing factors and the premorbid condition of the subjects. At this point, if the subject will undergo a stressful event (e.g., related to work, school, family, or health), insomnia symptoms could exceed the threshold and became clinically significant. On the other hand, precipitating factors are acute occurrences that interact with the patient's predisposition for insomnia to produce a transient phenomenon that naturally go into remission in a few days or weeks. Nevertheless, chronic insomnia occurs with the presence of perpetuating factors, interacting with the two previous factors and consequently leading to chronicization of the disorder. The maintenance factors refer to cognitive and behavioral strategies aimed at responding to stress; such as arousal conditioned (e.g., negative state of arousal rather than state of relaxation associated at the bedroom), sleep effort (e.g., extended time in bed and avoid evening or morning activities in order to straining to sleep), and worry about sleep, daytime, and health consequences (Fig. 23.10). These cognitive and behavioral dysfunctional strategies will be targets of the non-pharmacological intervention.

Diagnosis and Treatments

The European and US guidelines suggest a clinical evaluation of ID patients, just through subjective assessment [34, 35]. Indeed, sleep objective evaluation is not mandatory for the diagnosis of insomnia disorders. However, objective evaluation could provide fundamental information regarding nocturnal sleep and for evaluating other pathologic disease secondary to the disorder.

According with the main treatment guidelines, cognitive-behavioral therapy for insomnia (CBT-I) is the first-choice treatment for chronic insomnia. Its effectiveness has been proved to be greater in the long term with fewer side effects in comparison with pharmacotherapy [34–37]. CBT-I [38–40] is a multicomponent approach encompassing psycho-education on sleep hygiene [39], behavioral interventions (e.g., stimulus control [41] and sleep restriction [33]), and relaxation [42], as well as cognitive techniques [40]. Most studies used subjective indices in order to evaluate CBT-I efficacy. Nevertheless, it seems that also objective CBT-I efficacy has been proven, not through traditional EEG or polysomnography-derived sleep macro-structural indices [43, 44], but rather specific microstructural sleep features (sleep spindles) [45], and quantitative EEG indices [28, 29, 46], that resulted very informative in evaluating CBT-I efficacy.

The literature concerning pharmacotherapy in ID patients suggests that if the first-line treatment is not effective or not available, in short term, benzodiazepines and benzodiazepine receptor agonists should be used, with high-quality evidence. In addition, in short-term, antidepressants could be used with moderate-quality evidence in literature. On the

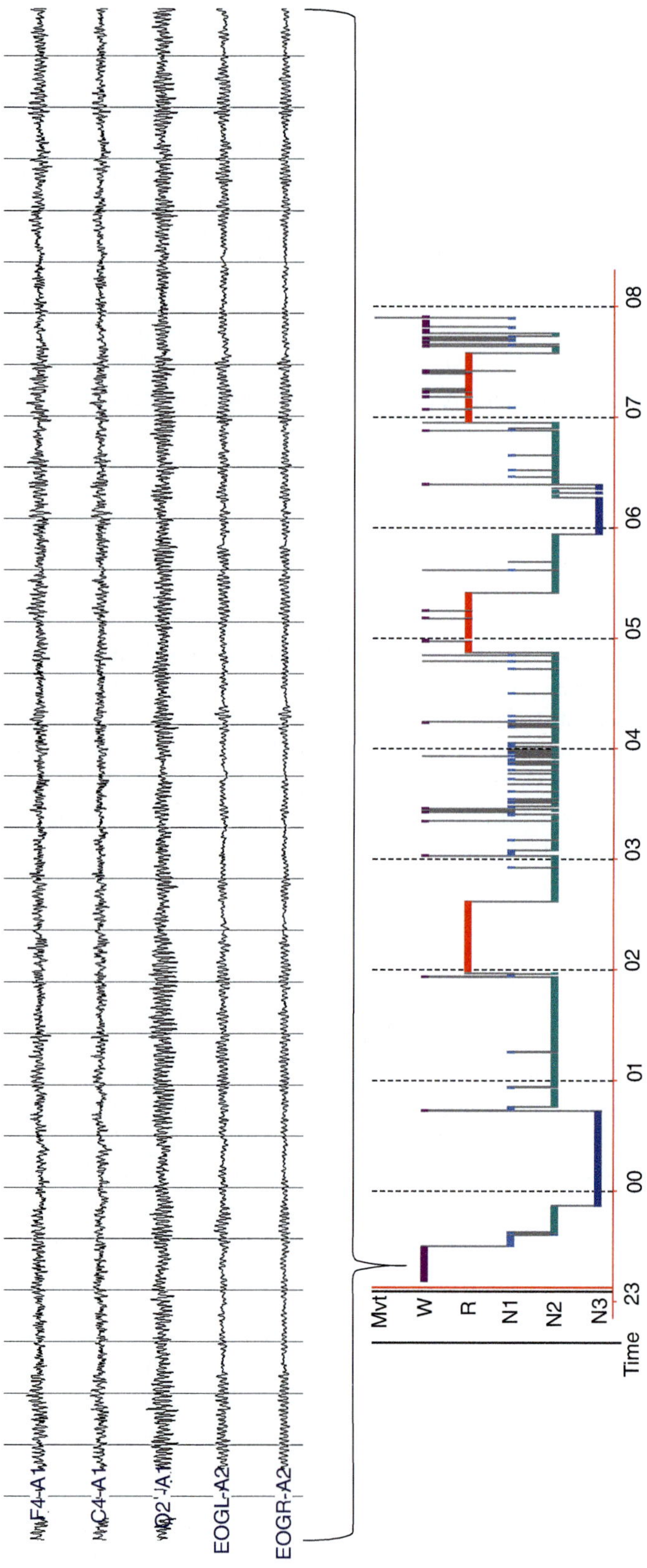

Fig. 23.6 Prolonged periods of alpha rhythm during sleep onset in a patient with insomnia with difficulties initiating and maintaining sleep

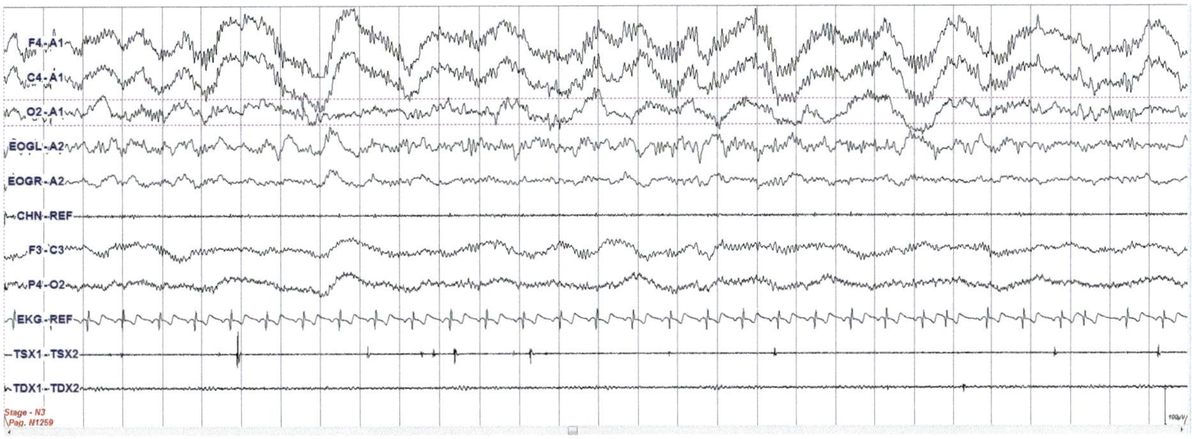

Fig. 23.7 Alpha-delta sleep. High EEG frequencies during slow wave sleep, i.e., insomnia hyperarousal during sleep

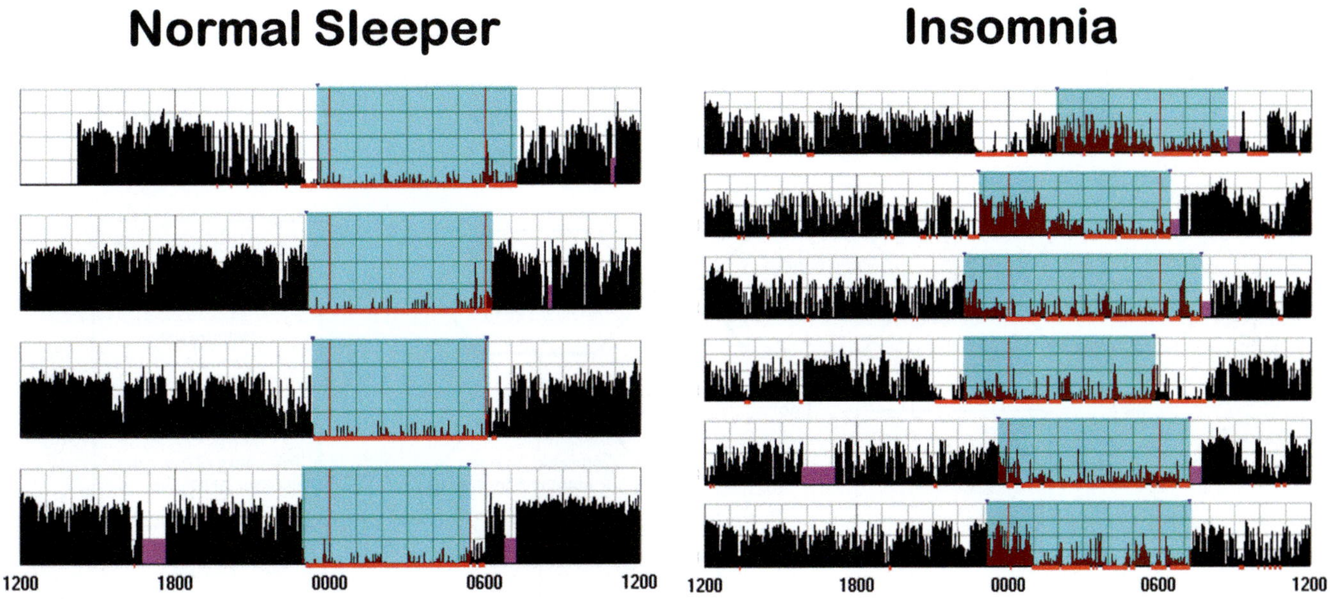

Fig. 23.8 Actigraphy recording of a normal sleeper and an insomnia patient

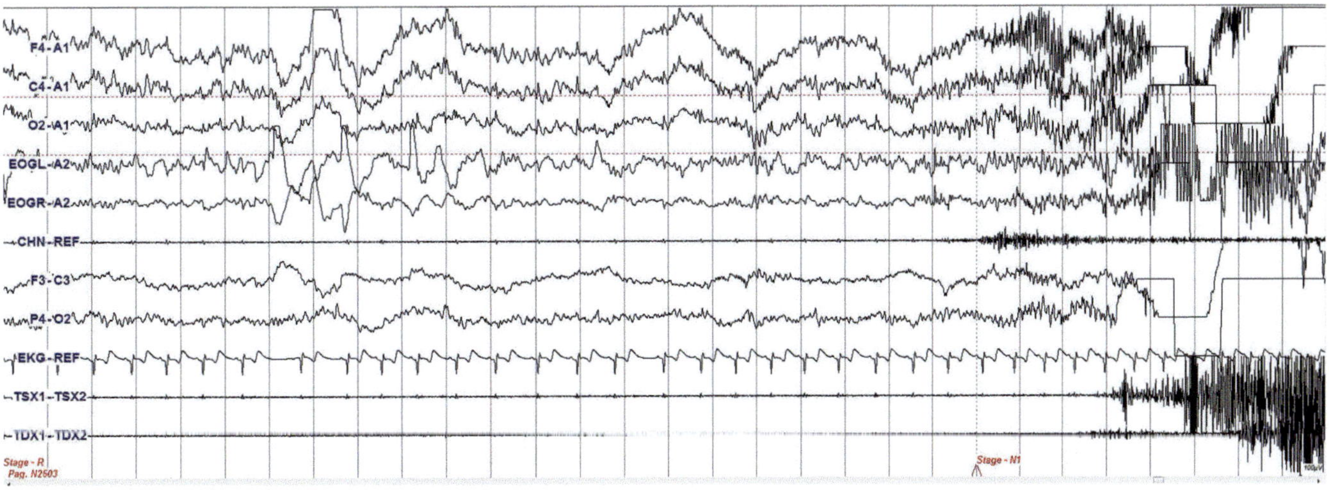

Fig. 23.9 Arousal during REM sleep. A REM epoch with an arousal that can be classified as a "restless REM sleep" epoch

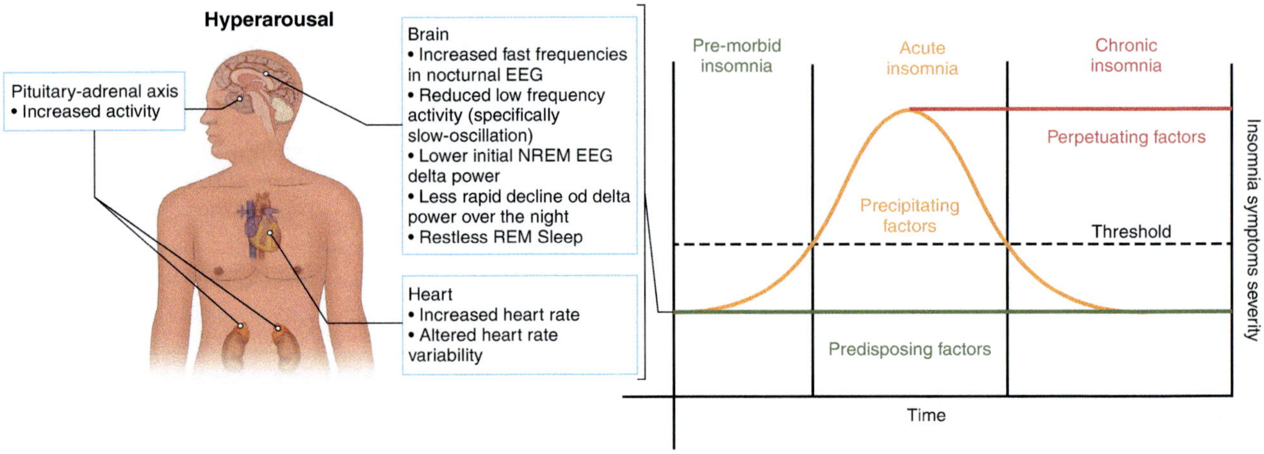

Fig. 23.10 Hyperarousal and three factor model along time. (*Adapted from* Spielman et al. [33] and Morin et al. [9]; *with permission*)

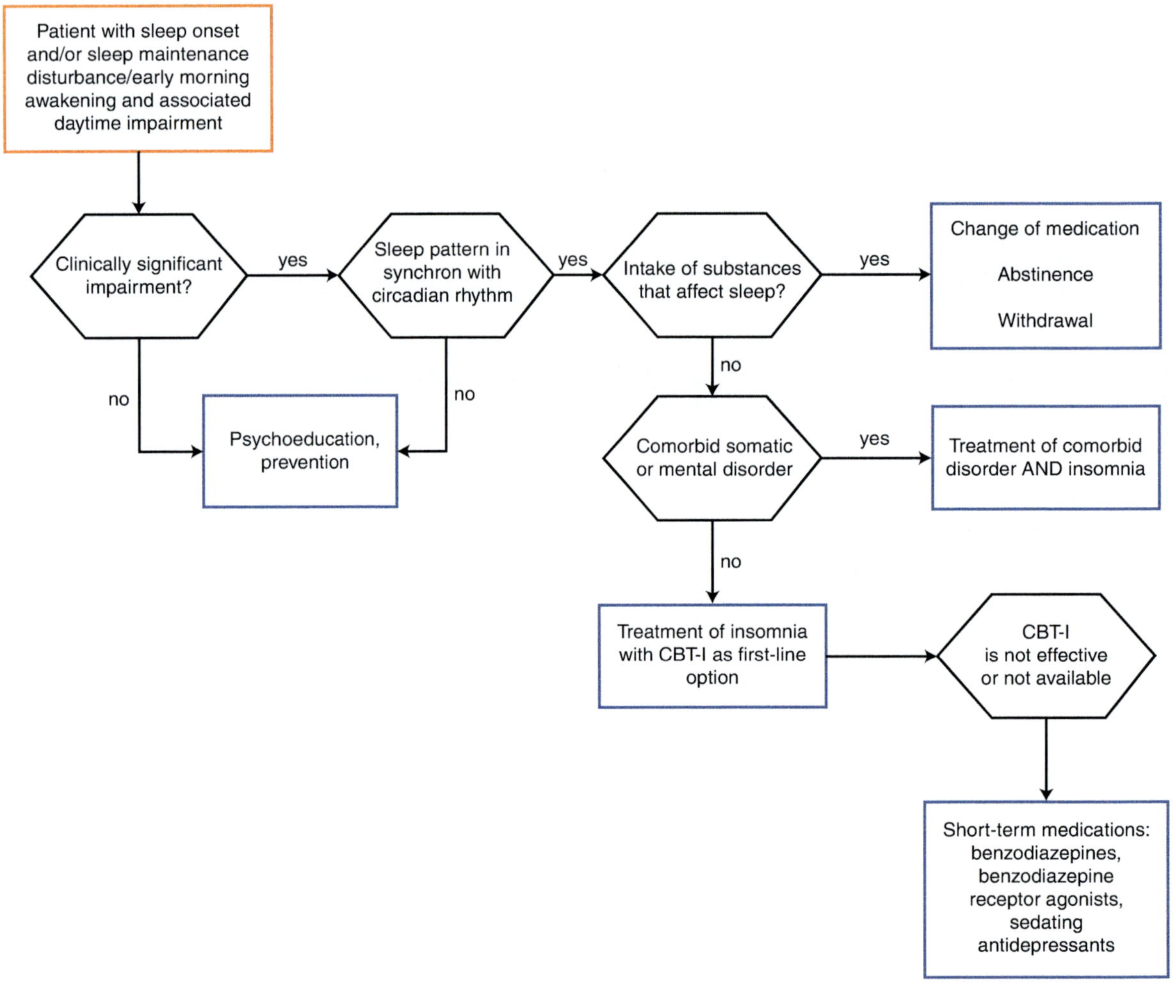

Fig. 23.11 Clinical algorithm for the diagnosis and treatment of insomnia. (*Adapted from* Riemann et al. [34]; *with permission*)

other hand, antipsychotics, antihistamines, melatonin, and phytotherapeutics are not recommended, due to low to very low quality of efficacy evidence literature. Light therapy and/or exercise could be used as ancillary therapies [34] (Fig. 23.11).

Central Disorders of Hypersomnolence

Excessive daytime sleepiness (EDS) is the core complaint of hypersomnias. EDS is characterized by failure in staying awake and alerted during the major waking periods of the day, culminating in episodes of unquenchable need of sleep. In some cases, despite large amount of daily sleep, patient does not report feeling of restoration; in other cases, naps during the day could alleviate hypersomnolence symptom [47]. Sleepiness is directly related to sleep drive modulated by the physiological processes of homeostasis and circadian drives, which regulate sleep across the 24-h cycle [48].

In order to quantify the severity of EDS, the clinician has two options, the subjective and the objective evaluation, which usually does not correlate with each other. On the other hand, both are useful for the diagnostic purpose. The subjectively EDS report can be quantified using Epworth Sleepiness Scale (ESS), a self-report scale investigating, during the preceding months, sleep propensity in real-life situations. It is composed of eight items with 0–3 points each, and the total score ranges from 0 to 24 [49]. The objective EDS evaluation can be quantified using the multiple sleep latency test (MSLT), i.e., an objective test that measures the tendency to fall asleep under controlled conditions. Specifically, even if insufficient sleep, drugs, activity, and arousal level could bias MSLT outcome, the test showed validity and reliability in diagnostic evaluation of narcolepsy and idiopathic hypersomnia. It consists of four to five naps given 2 h apart during the day, following a standardized procedure. The mean sleep latency from all naps is used as the measure of sleepiness [50]. However, the EDS instrumental assessment must be used accordingly with an appropriate clinical judgment, in order to pursue the diagnostic purpose.

Narcolepsy

Narcolepsy is a chronic sleep disorder characterized by EDS and, in most patients, cataplexy; i.e., brief (<2 min) episode of sudden loss of muscle tone with retained consciousness usually bilaterally symmetrical is triggered by strong emotions. A diagnosis of narcolepsy requires a reduction in the mean sleep latency (to ≤8 min), with two or more SOREMPs (occurrence of REM sleep within 15 min of sleep onset) observed on the MSLT when performed after a minimum of 6 h of sleep (documented by nocturnal polysomnography). Furthermore, patients might present sleep paralysis, hypnagogic (falling sleep) or hypnopompic (waking up) hallucinations, and disturbed sleep (i.e., objectively and subjectively reported frequent brief awakenings and a high level of N1 sleep, which is also associated with poor quality of sleep at night) [47, 51, 52].

Epidemiology

The world prevalence is 25–50 cases per 100.000 subjects [53–57]. Literature reported two peaks in the age-of-onset profile with one peak in adolescence and one peak at 30–39 years of age [58, 59].

Etiology and Pathophysiology

Two subtypes of narcolepsy have been described, Type 1 and Type 2. Even if both types showed similar clinical profiles, these differ on the basis of the presence of cataplexy. In more detail, patients with Type 1 narcolepsy have cataplexy and/or low levels of hypocretin 1 in the cerebrospinal fluid (CSF). Conversely, patients with Type 2 narcolepsy do not have cataplexy and show normal levels of hypocretin 1. The most reliable pathogenic hypothesis of Type 1 pathogenesis, even if the lack of direct evidences, is the autoimmune destruction of hypothalamic neurons that produce hypocretin, supported by immune-related genetic and environmental factors findings in Type 1 patients (Fig. 23.12) [60].

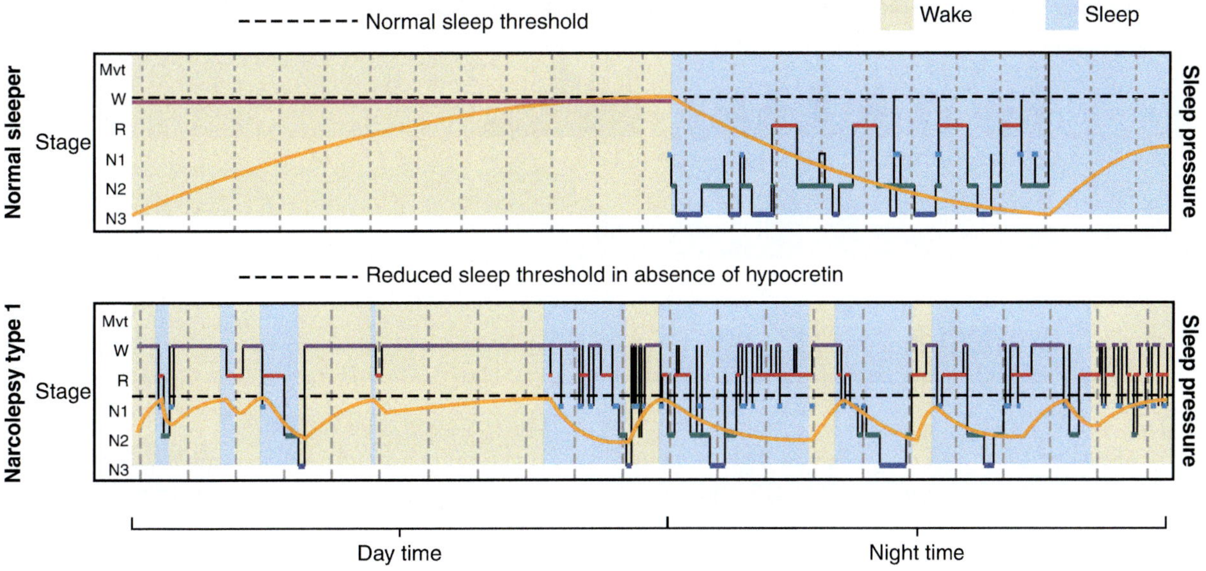

Fig. 23.12 Hypocretin wake-promoting role in normal sleeper and in narcolepsy type 1. In patients with narcolepsy, a loss of hypocretin neurons activity could lead to a lower threshold of sleep pressure and, consequently hypersomnia. (*Adapted from* Kornum et al. [59]; *with permission*)

Diagnosis and Treatment

Most frequently, wrong diagnoses, including psychiatric conditions and attention deficit hyperactivity disorder (ADHD), may contribute to diagnostic delay [58, 61]. Despite new scientific discoveries about its pathophysiology, treatments remain scarce and only symptomatic (moreover, mainly pharmacological interventions for children are still "off-label" prescribed). Several classes of drugs are used for the management of narcolepsy, including stimulants and antidepressants. The first-line treatment for excessive daytime sleepiness in patients with narcolepsy is modafinil. However, modafinil has no direct effect on cataplexy or on the other core symptoms of narcolepsy [62, 63]. Methylphenidate, due to side effects [64] and the potential for abuse, is now considered a second-line treatment for EDS. It could be considered an add-on treatment before monotonous circumstances (driving, meeting, or studying) [60]. In order to intervene on hallucinations, sodium oxybate and venlafaxine seem to be effective [64]. Moreover, sodium oxybate seems to be an effective treatment not only for cataplexy but also in reducing disturbed sleep and consolidating nocturnal sleep. In addition, pitolisant, a small molecule acting as an antagonist/inverse agonist at the H3 receptor subtype, showed promising results in order to treat EDS and cataplexy in narcolepsy [65]. Solriamfetol, a dopamine/norepinephrine reuptake inhibitor, resulted effective for EDS in narcoleptic patients [66]. Furthermore, behavioral and psychosocial interventions are useful in helping patients and their family in improving patients' quality of life [67].

Idiopathic Hypersomnia

The identification of the idiopathic hypersomnia (IH) is much more recent than the other central disorders of hypersomnolence [68]. IH is a chronic neurologic disorder characterized by EDS present for at least 3 months, occurring in the absence of cataplexy, and not explained by another disorder or substance. Moreover, differently than Type 1 narcolepsy, hypocretin deficiency is not present; even if enhancement of GABAergic transmission was found in IH patients and in other central disorders of hypersomnolence. The objective evaluation of this disease should suggest no more than one SOREMP (sleep-onset REM) on MSLT, but with mean sleep latency of at least 8 min and at least 11 h of sleep per 24 h documented. In addition, these patients are characterized by long sleep duration, prolonged and unrefreshing naps, and difficulty in awakening in the morning or at the end of daytime naps (Fig. 23.13) [47].

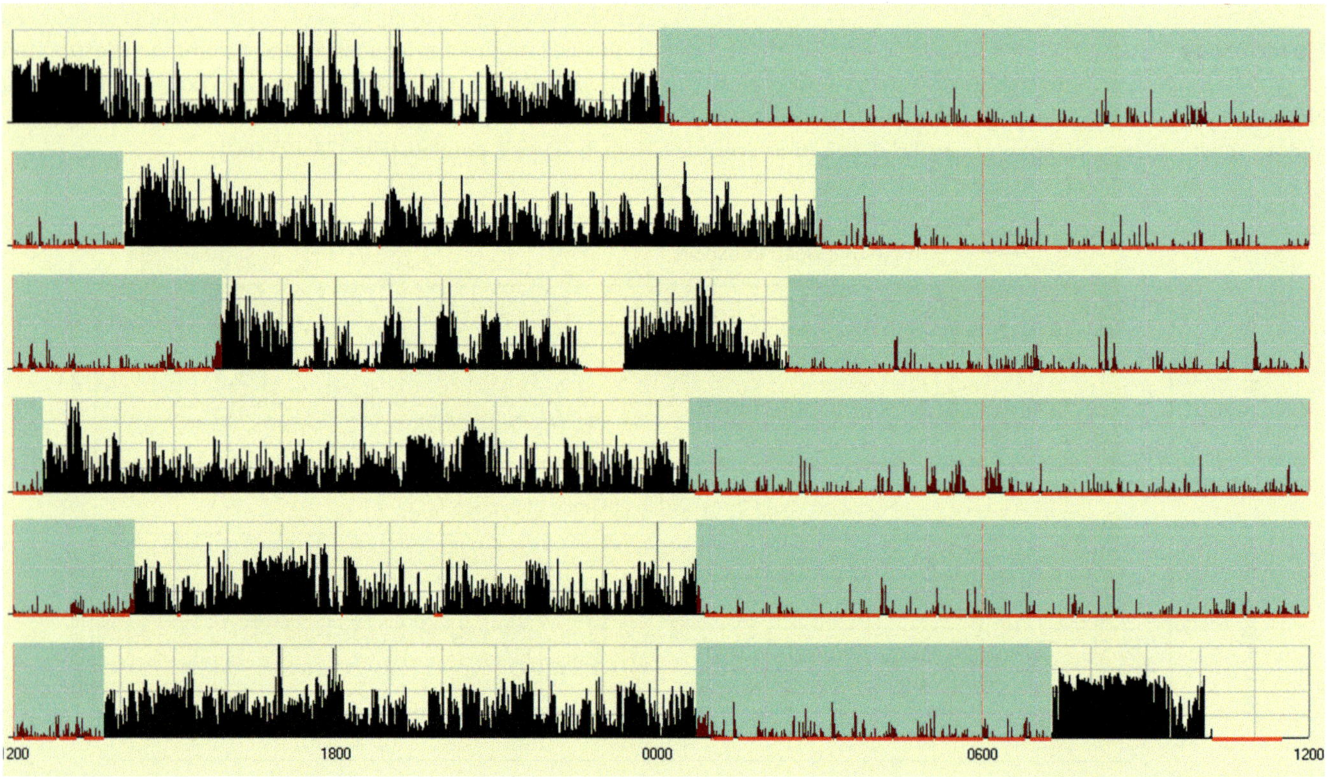

Fig. 23.13 Actigraphy recording highlighting prolonged sleep duration in idiopathic hypersomnia

Etiology and Pathophysiology

A familial predisposition to IH has been reported, although more rigorous studies with clinical interviews and sleep studies in relatives are warranted. Furthermore, viral illness, head trauma, and general anesthesia have been proposed as precipitating factors but no definitive link has been proven [69].

Treatment

Unfortunately, behavioral treatments of idiopathic hypersomnia are not as successful as in narcolepsy. In addition, no medications are currently approved by the US Food and Drug Administration, specifically for the treatment of IH. and there are no published, randomized, controlled trials of any treatment for IH. Nevertheless, current pharmacological treatments of idiopathic hypersomnia still mirror those of hypersomnolence in narcolepsy types 1 and 2, and, even if not effective in all patients, modafinil appears beneficial in a modest majority of patient [69, 70].

Kleine-Levin Syndrome

Epidemiology

Kleine-Levin syndrome (KLS) is a rare disorder with an estimated prevalence of one to five cases per million population and that mainly affected adolescent men (about 3:1) [71]. KLS is characterized by recurrent episodes of hypersomnia (at least two recurrent episodes of excessive sleepiness and sleep duration, each persisting for 2 days to 5 weeks), usually including various behavioral and cognitive disturbances, eating disorder, signs of dysautonomia, and disinhibited behavior [47, 72–75].

Etiology and Pathophysiology

There is currently no biomarker for KLS, and diagnosis relies on clinical evaluation.

Treatment

Due to KLS insufficiency in general population, few systematic studies have been conducted to evaluate treatments, and no medication has been consistently demonstrated as efficacious in the treatment of the disease. Treatment is for the most part supportive, with stimulant medications such as modafinil, which may be considered if prescribed at onset of the disorder [76, 77].

Sleep-Related Breathing Disorders

The sleep-related breathing disorders are characterized by abnormalities of respiration during sleep. The disorder are grouped into obstructive sleep apnea (OSA) disorders, central sleep apnea disorder, sleep relate hypoventilation disorder, and sleep related hypoxemia disorder [1].

The central sleep apnea syndromes are characterized by reduction or cessation of airflow due to absent o reduced respiratory effort. In primary central sleep apnea, the cause of the disorder is unknown (idiopathic), but often, patients with this disorder have congestive heart failure or neurological conditions like stroke.

Obstructive Sleep Apnea

Obstructive sleep apnea (OSA) is the most common sleep-related breathing disorder, characterized by repetitive collapse of the upper airway during sleep resulting in increased microarousals, sleep fragmentation, and decreased oxygenation [1]. To date, OSA diagnosis comprises a clinical assessment supported by an objective demonstration on full-night polysomnography (PSG) of impaired breathing during sleep [78]. (See Table 23.1 for diagnostic criteria and Fig. 23.14 for an example of episodes of obstructive apnea).

Epidemiology

The prevalence of OSA is strictly related on its gravity, ranging from 6% to 17% in the general population at ≥15 events/h apnea-hypopnea index (AHI) and shows a higher rate in men and increases with age [79].

Etiology

Excessive body weight represents the main predisposing factor for OSA. Indeed, a high morbidity with obesity has been

Table 23.1 Diagnostic Criteria for OSA according to the International Classification of Sleep Disorders-3rd edition

Diagnostic criteria
(**A** and **B**) or **C** satisfy the criteria
A. The presence of one or more of the following:
1. The patient complains of sleepiness, nonrestorative sleep, fatigue, or insomnia symptoms
2. The patient wakes with breath holding, gasping, or choking
3. The bed partner or the observer reports habitual snoring, breathing interruptions, or both during the patient's sleep
4. The patient has been diagnosed with hypertension, a mood disorder, cognitive dysfunction, coronary heart disease, stroke, congestive heart failure, atrial fibrillation, or type 2 diabetes mellitus
B. Polysomnography (PSG) or out-of-center sleep testing (OCST) demonstrates:
1. Five or more predominantly obstructive respiratory events (obstructive and mixed apneas, hypopneas, or respiratory effort related arousal [RERAs]) per hour of sleep during a PSG or per hour of monitoring (OCST)
Or
C. PSG or OCST demonstrates:
1. Fifteen or more predominantly obstructive respiratory events (apneas, hypopneas, or RERAs) per hour of sleep during a PSG or per hour of monitoring (OCST)

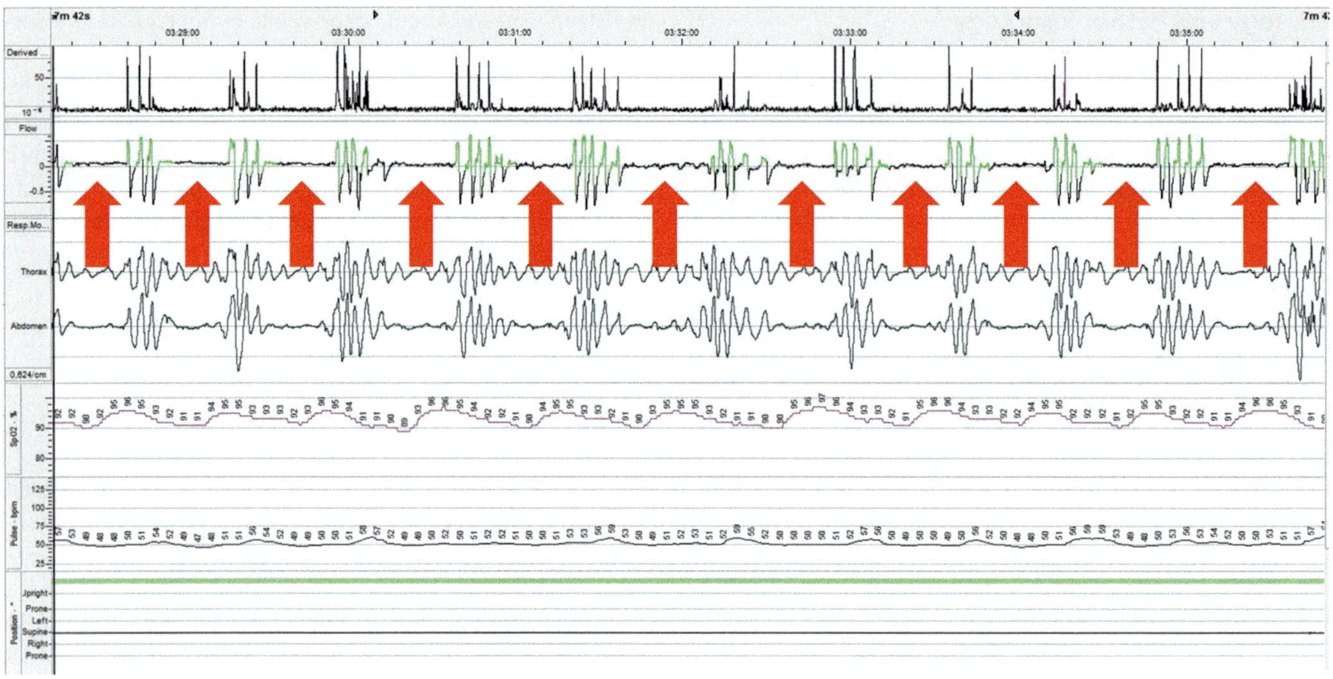

Fig. 23.14 Episodes of obstructive apnea in a patient with OSA

reported. In subjects with normal body weight, OSA might be ascribable to maxillomandibular malformation or adeno-tonsillar enlargement that leads to upper way obstruction. Moreover, also increased neck circumference can predict OSA severity [1]. In woman, menopause is a risk factor for OSA.

Pathophysiology

OSA pathophysiology is multifactorial. In general, it is the result of a combination of abnormal neuromuscular control and anatomical narrowing of upper airway. During REM sleep, there is an exacerbation of the neuromuscular failure, which contributes to longer and more pronounced obstructive events. The end of these events may depend on chemical and mechanical stimuli causing augmentation of upper airway muscle tone or on change of sleep state, causing sleep fragmentation. Decreased ventilator drive facilitates upper airway collapse leading to hypoxemia, hypercapnia, and sleep disruption that may result in neurobehavioral and medical deficits. Neuroimaging evidence suggests that OSA may accelerate the neurodegenerative processes in the brain [80]. A consistent number of neuroimaging studies have well documented that human OSA brain may be characterized by several tissue damages including alterations of white matter integrity, free water content, brain metabolites, and regional gray matter volume changes. To question how OSA affects the brains is of importance not only for the perspective of the OSA pathology it-self but also especially for an emerging hypothesis as OSA is considered a bridge versus the neurodegeneration. Consistent evidence links neurodegenerative disorders, in particular Alzheimer's disease (AD) [81]. The neurobiological link between OSA and AD is probably mediated to an increase of ß-amyloid deposition in the brain, hallmark of AD neuropathology (Fig. 23.15).

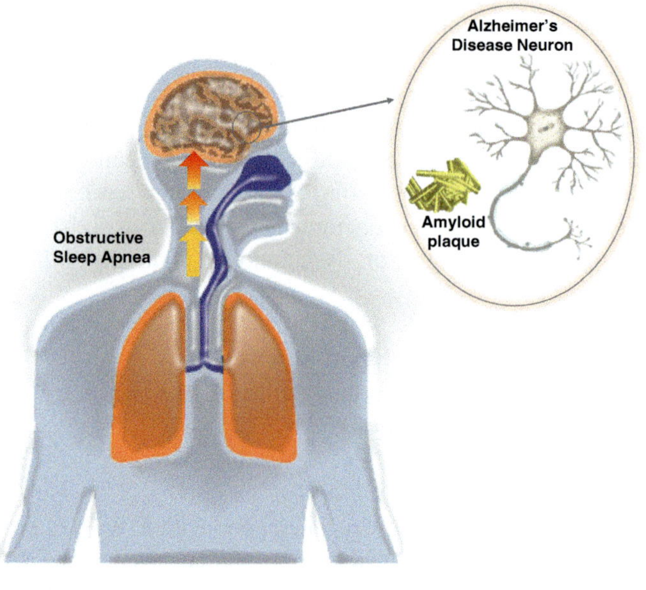

Fig. 23.15 OSA might increase ß-amyloid deposition in the brain, an hallmark of AD neuropathology

Phenomenology

OSA is characterized by repetitive episodes of complete (apnea) or partial (hypopnea) upper airway obstruction occurring during sleep. These events often results in reduction of blood oxygen saturation. By definition, apneic or hypopneic events not only last a minimum of 10 s, commonly lasting from 10 to 30 s, but also may persist for more than 1 min [1]. Events can occur at any stage of sleep. Snoring between apneas, episodes of gasping, or choking and body movements are typically reported by bed partners. Nocturnal disruption of sleep by repetitive arousals due to obstructive events result in the typical features of this disorder, including excessive daytime sleepiness (EDS), stress-related disorder fatigue, and mood problems. OSA is also associated with several severe conditions such as medical, neurocognitive, and cardiovascular. In addition, OSA patients may exhibit neurocognitive dysfunctions with impairment in attention, episodic memory, and executive functions [82].

Treatment

The first-choice treatment of this disorder is continuous positive airway pressure (CPAP), which provides continuous air pressure to the upper airways during the sleep. This therapy is the most efficacious treatment in the complete resolution of sleep apnea, reducing the frequency of respiratory events during sleep, sleep fragmentation, sleepiness, and improve daytime functioning [83]. Based on the severity and characteristics of the disorder, other treatment can be tailored like oral appliance (OA) therapy, positional therapy, or surgical intervention.

Sleep-Related Movement Disorders

Sleep-related movement disorders include restless legs syndrome (RLS), periodic limb movement disorder (PLMD), sleep-related leg cramps, sleep-related bruxism, sleep-related rhythmic movement disorder, benign sleep myoclonus of infancy, and propriospinal myoclonus at sleep onset (Table 23.2). These movements can manifest at the onset or during sleep.

Table 23.2 Sleep-related movement according to the ICSD-3

Sleep-related movement disorders
Restless legs syndrome
Periodic limb movement disorder
Sleep-related leg cramps
Sleep-related bruxism
Sleep-related rhythmic movement disorder
Benign sleep myoclonus at sleep onset
Propriospinal myoclonus at sleep onset
Sleep-related movement disorder due to a medical disorder
Sleep-related movement disorder due to a medication or substance
Sleep-related movement disorder, unspecified

Restless Legs Syndrome (RLS/WED)

Restless legs syndrome (RLS/WED), also known as Willis-Ekbom disease (RLS/WED/WED), is a sleep related movement disorder that affects predominantly the legs, characterized by an urge to move, frequently associated or triggered by unpleasant sensations in the limbs, with a specific circadian rhythm.

Typically, RLS/WED symptoms occur during periods of rest and inactivity, can be partially or totally relieved by activity, and worsens in the evening or at night, resulting in severe sleep disruption and consequent impairs quality of life [84]. Treatments can improve quality of life [85], although management of the disease shows different problems developing overtime [86].

RLS/WED can occur associated with other clinical conditions such as cardiovascular disease, diabetes, renal failure, arterial hypertension, multiple sclerosis, Parkinson disease, pregnancy, and peripheral neuropathy or as an isolated disease [87].

Epidemiology

RLS/WED prevalence has a regional variation, with a higher estimated prevalence in Caucasian populations (5–12%), intermediate in Asian population (1–8%), and lowest in African countries, in which few studies have been performed (less than 1%) [88]. The prevalence in moderate-severe RLS/WED is lower (2–3%). RLS/WED is more common in women, especially with a history of pregnancies, than in men and prevalence increase with advancing age.

RLS/WED is strongly associated with other clinical condition, mainly iron deficiency (prevalence up to 35%) and end-stage renal disease [89].

Pathophysiology

Pathophysiology of RLS/WED is not fully understood. Epidemiological studies founded a strong familial clustering, and some genome-wide association studies have identified single-nucleotide polymorphisms within the genes BTBD9, MEIS1, PTPRD, MAP 2K5, SKOR1, and TOX3 and on an intergenic region on chromosome 2 (rs6747972) with higher risk for RLS [90]. Dopamine metabolism and iron deficiency are the two main pathophysiological mechanisms studied in RLS/WED physiology. A hyperdopaminergic state superimposed upon the circadian changes in dopamine availability has been involved in the pathophysiology of RLS/WED.

Phenomenology

Clinical diagnosis of RLS/WED is based on the criteria of the International RLS Study Group [91], the ICSD-3 [47], and the Diagnostic and Statistical Manual of Mental Disorders, Fifth Edition (DSM-5) [2] (see Table 23.2).

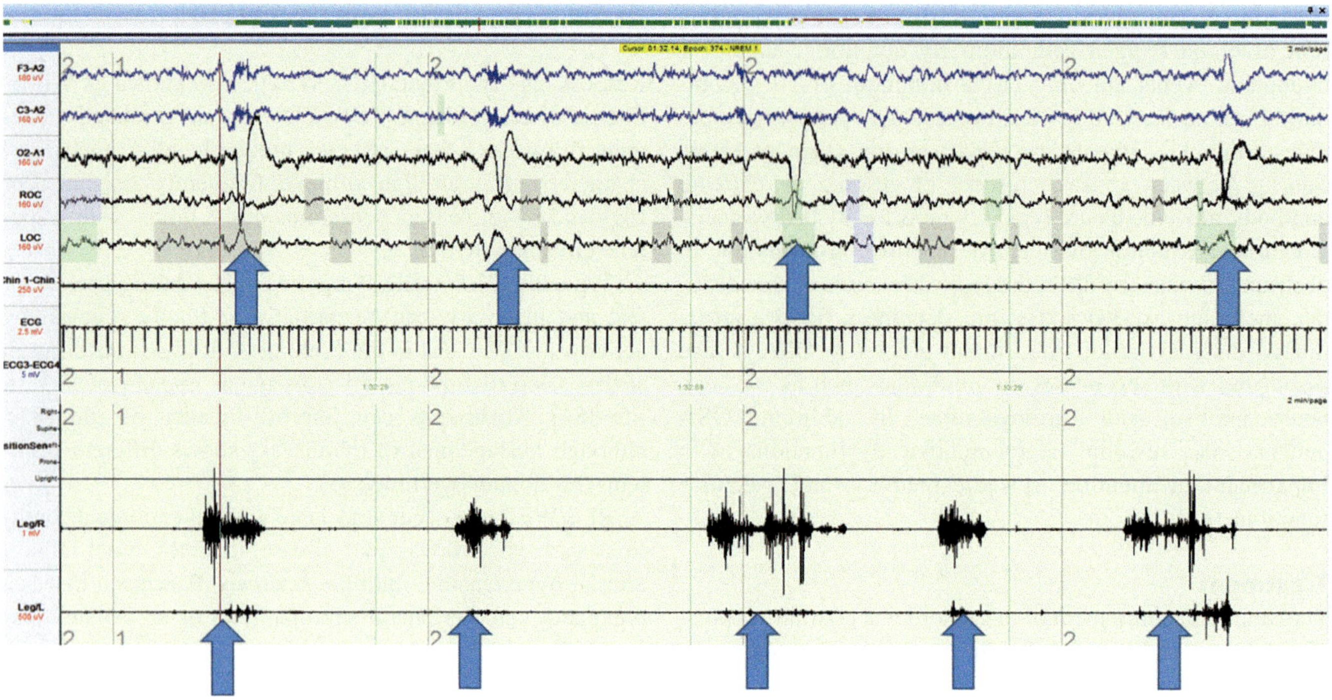

Fig. 23.16 PLMs associated with arousals in a patient with RLS

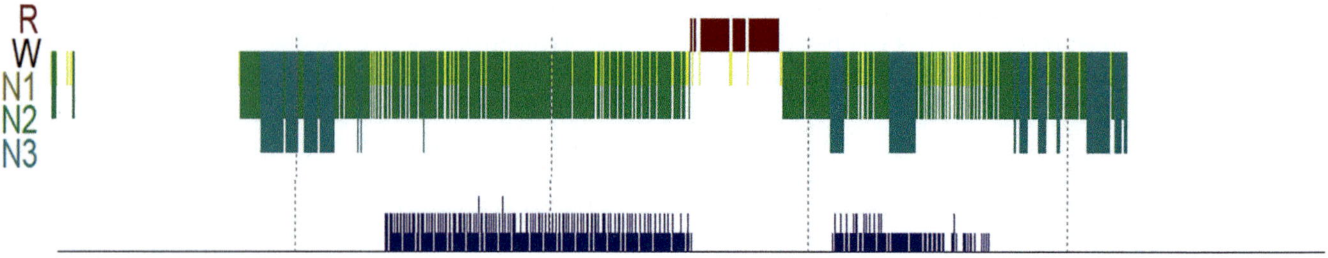

Fig. 23.17 In this hypnogram, an example of sleep fragmentation induced by PLMs (in blue) in a patient with RLS

To confirm the diagnosis, instrumental examination (e.g., polysomnography) is not strictly required. However, polysomnography can be useful to detect the periodic leg movements of sleep (PLMS) (Fig. 23.16).

These movements are stereotyped leg movements, occurring in about 90% of RLS patients. They can cause instability and fragmentation of the micro- and macrostructure of sleep (Fig. 23.17).

Some drugs can provoke or aggravate RLS/WED disease. Use of antihistamines, neuroleptics/dopamine-receptor blockers (e.g., olanzapine, risperidone, or quetiapine), serotonergic and noradrenergic antidepressants (e.g., amitriptyline, fluoxetine, sertraline, venlafaxine, and mirtazapine), or anti-emetics (e.g., metoclopramide) can worse symptoms. Antidepressants with dopaminergic activity, as trazodone or bupropion, should be preferred [92] (see Table 23.3 for diagnostic criteria).

Other disorder affecting the legs must be taken into consideration in the diagnosis of RLS. Peripheral neuropathy, radiculopathy, arthritis, leg cramps, venous stasis, myalgia, or sleep related leg cramps can mimic RLS/WED symptoms and confound the clinicians. Usually, these conditions are characterized by the absence of a circadian pattern. Common mimics are listed in Table 23.4.

Treatment

The treatment of RLS/WED includes pharmacological and non-pharmacological therapies. Dopamine agonists (such as pramipexole, ropinirole, and rotigotine) and calcium channel alpha-2-delta ligands are recognized as the first-line treatment. Iron, benzodiazepines, and opioids are considered second-line treatment options, however. Management of RLS/WED requires long-term interventions, since the typical manifestation of this disorder is chronic.

Table 23.3 Diagnostic criteria for RLS/WED according to International Restless Legs Syndrome Study Group (IRLSSG) consensus diagnostic criteria

Essential diagnostic criteria (all must be met):
1. An urge to move the legs usually but not always accompanied by, or felt to be caused by uncomfortable and unpleasant sensations in the legs [a,b]
2. The urge to move the legs and unpleasant sensations begin or worsen during periods of rest or inactivity such us lying down or sitting
3. The urge to move the legs and unpleasant sensations are partially or totally relieved by movement, such as walking or stretching, at least as long as the activity continues [c]
4. The urge to move the legs and any accompanying unpleasant sensations during rest or inactivity only occur or are worse in the evening or night than during the day [d]
5. The occurrence of the above features is not solely accounted for as symptoms primary to another medical or a behavioral condition (e.g., myalgia, venous stasis, leg edema, arthritis, leg cramps, positional discomfort, and habitual foot tapping) [e]
Specifiers for clinical course of RLS/WED [f]
A. Chronic-persistent RLS/WED: symptoms when not treated would occur on average at least twice weekly for the past year
Specifier for clinical significance of RLS/WED:
The symptoms of RLS/WED cause significant distress or impairment in social, occupational, educational, or other important areas of functioning by their impact on sleep, energy/vitality, daily activities, behavior, cognition, or mood
Supportive criteria:
Family history of RLS/WED/WED among first-degree relatives
Dopaminergic treatment response
Periodic leg movements during wakefulness or sleep
Lack of profound daytime sleepiness

From Allen et al. [90]; *with permission*

[a] Sometimes the urge to move the legs is present without the uncomfortable sensations and sometimes the arms or other parts of the body are involved in addition to the legs

[b] For children, the description of these symptoms should be in the child's own words

[c] When symptoms are very severe, relief by activity may not be noticeable but must have been previously present

[d] When symptoms are very severe, the worsening in the evening or night may not be noticeable but must have been previously present

[e] These conditions, often referred to as "RLS/WED mimics," have been commonly confused with RLS/WED particularly in surveys because they produce symptoms that meet or at least come very close to meeting criteria 1–4. The list here gives some examples that have been noted as particularly significant in epidemiological studies and clinical practice. RLS/WED may also occur with any of these conditions, but the RLS/WED symptoms will then be more in degree, conditions of expression or character than those usually occurring as part of the other condition

[f] The clinical course criteria do not apply for pediatric cases nor for some special cases of provoked RLS/WED such as pregnancy or drug-induced RLS/WED where the frequency may be high but limited to duration of the provocative condition

Periodic Limb Movement Disorder

Periodic limb movement disorder (PLMD) is a sleep disorder characterized by the presence of PLMS on PSG, without the typical symptoms of RLS. PLMD cause sleep fragmentation and is associated with symptoms of either insomnia or excessive daytime sleepiness. PLMS are associated to RLS, narcolepsy (about 75%), RBD (up to 70%), and sleep-related breathing disorder, so an accurate clinical interview is necessary in order to exclude the presence of other sleep disorder [93]. The diagnostic criteria are listed in Table 23.5.

The exact prevalence of this disorder is not known. PLMD prevalence tends to increase with advancing age, occurring in over 45% of the elderly.

Presence of PLMS on PSG recording has been associated with RLS risk genes, suggesting common underlying pathogenetic mechanisms in these two conditions.

It is still debated the correct treatment of PLMD. A positive effect of clonazepam and valproate on sleep quality but not on PLMS index is reported by some studies, whereas melatonin reduced PLMS index [94].

Table 23.4 Differential diagnosis of RLS/WED (RLS/WED mimics)

Common conditions
Leg cramps [a]
Positional discomfort [a]
Local leg injury
Arthritis
Leg edema
Venous stasis
Peripheral neuropathy [a]
Radiculopathy [a]
Habitual foot tapping/leg rocking
Anxiety
Myalgia
Drug-induced akathisia
Less common
Myelopathy
Myopathy
Vascular or neurogenic claudication
Hypotensive akathisia
Orthostatic tremor
Painful legs and moving toes

From Allen et al. [90]; *with permission*

[a] More likely to fulfill all of criteria 1–4. Any of these conditions can coexist with RLS/WED

Propriospinal Myoclonus at Sleep Onset

Propriospinal myoclonus (PSM) is a rare condition characterized by sudden myoclonic jerks occurring at the relaxed wakefulness preceding sleep onset and during transition from wake to sleep, provoking a rapid reappraisal of wake state; therefore, it prevents the sleep onset and determining a sleep onset insomnia [95]. Diagnostic criteria for PSM are listed in Table 23.6.

The jerks arise mainly form a thoracic or abdominal spinal source (myoclonic generator) (Fig. 23.18) and spread rostrally and caudally along a propriospinal pathway intrinsic the spinal cord with a slow conduction velocity through a multisynaptic slow-conduction pathways.

PSM can be idiopathic, secondary to a wide range of medical conditions or functional [95].

It is not age related but is typical of middle age subjects, more frequent in men (symptomatic forms more frequent in women) and rare in children.

Polymyography is essential for the diagnosis of PSM although formal criteria do not exist.

No guidelines are available regarding the treatment of true PSM at sleep onset. For secondary PSM, the treatment of the underlying condition is indicated. Functional PSM can benefit from non-pharmacological therapy.

Table 23.5 Diagnostic criteria for PLMD

Diagnostic criteria
Criteria A–D must be met:
A. Polysomnography demonstrates PLMS as defines in the America Academy of Sleep Medicine (AASM) Manual for the scoring of Sleep and Associated Events
B. The frequency is >5/h in children or >5/h in adults
C. The PLMS cause clinically significant sleep disturbance or impairment in mental, physical, social, occupational, educational, behavioral, or other important areas of functioning
D. The PLMS and the symptoms are not better explained by another sleep disorder, medical or neurological disorder, or mental disorder (e.g., PLSM occurring with apneas or hypopneas should not be scored)

Table 23.6 Diagnostic criteria for propriospinal myoclonus at sleep onset

Diagnostic criteria
Criteria A–E must be met:
A. The patient complains of sudden jerks, mainly of the abdomen, trunk, and neck
B. The jerks appear during relaxed wakefulness and drowsiness, as the patient attempt to fall asleep
C. The jerks disappear upon mental activation and with onset of a stable sleep stage
D. The jerks result in difficulty initiating sleep
E. The disorder is not better explained by another sleep disorder, medical, or neurological disorder, mental disorder, medication use, or substance use disorder

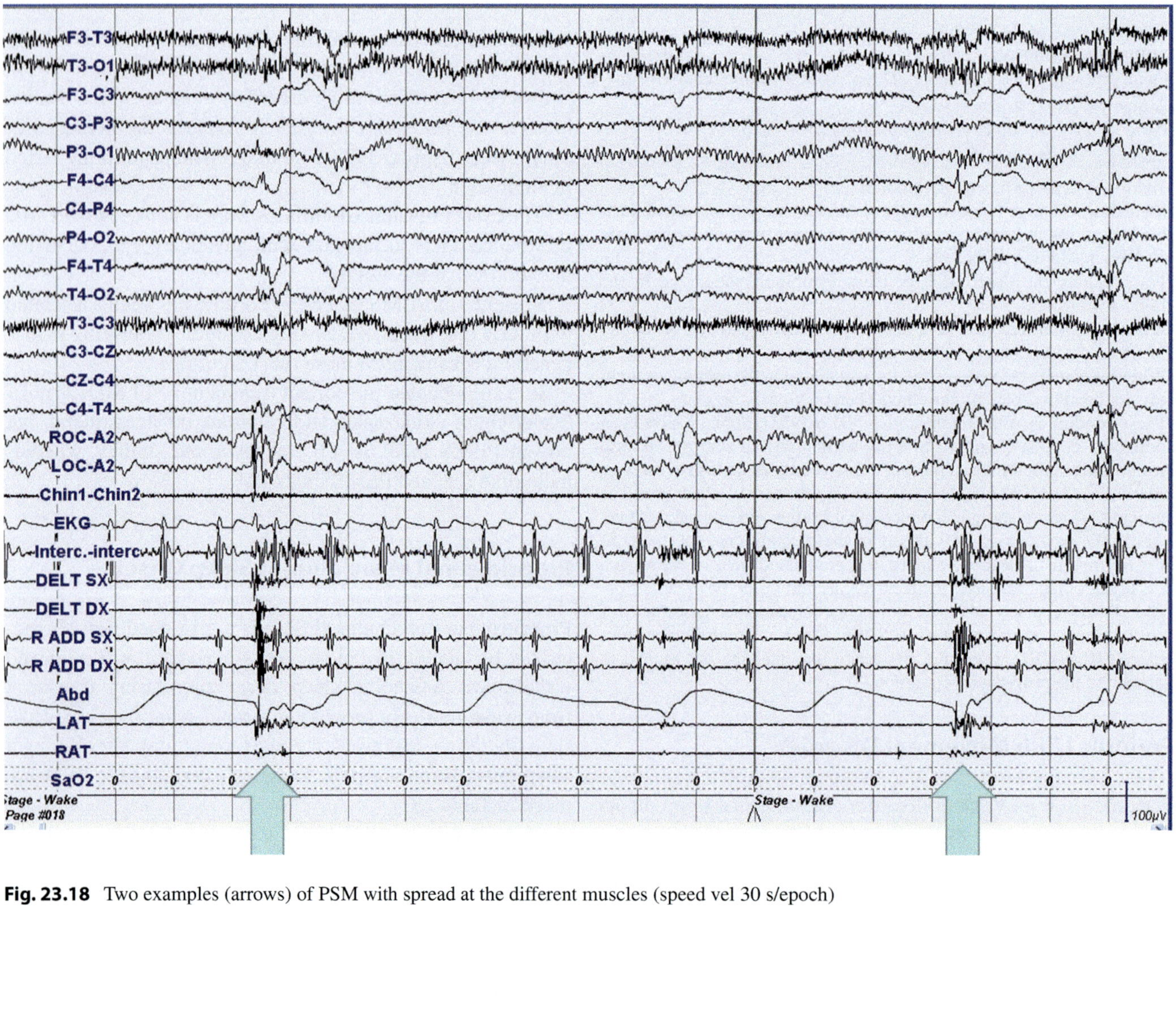

Fig. 23.18 Two examples (arrows) of PSM with spread at the different muscles (speed vel 30 s/epoch)

Parasomnias

Parasomnias are defined as unpleasant or undesirable experiences or behaviors that occur mainly during a sleep period, the transition from wake to sleep or vice versa. According to ICSD-3, parasomnias are categorized according to the sleep phase of origin: NREM sleep parasomnias, REM sleep parasomnias, or other parasomnias [96].

Disorder of Arousal (DOA)

Parasomnias that manifest themselves during NREM sleep are commonly listed as disorders of arousal (DOA). This group includes confusional arousals, sleepwalking, and sleep terrors that result from incomplete arousals from deep sleep. Another disorder, sleep-related eating syndrome (SRED) is included among NREM parasomnias but not under the category of DOA (for DOA diagnostic criteria see Table 23.7).

Table 23.7 Diagnostic criteria for confusional arousal, sleepwalking, and sleep terrors

General diagnostic criteria for DOA (criteria A-E must be met):		
A. Recurrent episodes of incomplete awakening from sleep **B.** Inappropriate or absent responsiveness to efforts of others to intervene or redirect the person during the episode **C.** Limited (e.g., a single visual scene) or no associated cognition or dream imagery **D.** Partial or complete amnesia for the episode **E.** The disturbance is not better explained by another sleep disorder, mental disorder, medical condition, medication, or substance use		
Confusional arousals	**Sleepwalking**	**Sleep terrors**
A. The disorder meets general criteria for NREM disorders of arousal **B.** The episodes are characterized by mental confusion or confused behavior that occurs while the patient is in bed **C.** There is an absence of terror or ambulation outside of the bed	**A.** The disorder meets general criteria for NREM disorders of arousal **B.** The arousals are associated with ambulation and other complex behaviors out of bed	**A.** The disorder meets general criteria for NREM disorders of arousal **B.** The arousals are characterized by episodes of abrupt terror, typically beginning with an alarming vocalization such as a frightening scream **C.** There is intense fear and signs of autonomic arousal, including mydriasis, tachycardia tachypnea, and diaphoresis during an episode

For Confusional arousal, criteria A–C must be met; for sleepwalking, A–B; and for sleep terrors, A–C. All these disorders share common clinical diagnostic criteria

Epidemiology

DOA are especially prevalent during childhood and also in adults younger than 35 years, with a similar prevalence of sleepwalking and confusional arousals. There is no sex difference.

Sleep terror is present in up to 34% of children at 1.5 years of age and sleepwalking in up to 13% of children at 10 years of age. DOA often resolve by puberty; however, they are far more common in adults than is generally acknowledged, with a 2–4% prevalence of sleepwalking or sleep terror in both men and women [97, 98]. The lifetime prevalence of DOAs is around 29%, with two or more episodes per month reported by 1% of adults. In clinical cohorts, adult onset DOA account for 17–27% of cases [99, 100].

Pathophysiology

Even if overall sleep architecture is generally preserved in DOA, dysfunction of slow-wave sleep can be found. The occurrence of slow-wave sleep instability is supported by a consistent number of findings [101], and recent focus was given to slow-wave activity dynamics in DOA, in terms of organization of sleep [102, 103] and specifically in relation to DOA episodes [104].

In these patients, EEG frequently shows features of both typical sleep- like and wake-like activity, and in contrast to what reported in diagnostic criteria, they occasionally report dreaming. From a research standpoint, DOA provide a unique natural model to investigate the coexistence of local sleep and wake brain activity and the dissociation between behavior and various aspects of consciousness [105].

Etiology

DOA are the result of a combination of predisposing and precipitating factors. Genetic contribution might represent the main predisposing factor, in particular in those patients where episodes persist beyond adulthood. Precipitating factors are several and generally, ranges from conditions that increase deep sleep (such as sleep deprivation and several drugs) to those that induce sleep fragmentation (obstructive sleep apneas, periodic leg movements, chronic pain, stress, and anxiety).

Phenomenology

Patients exhibit a variety of behaviors with consciousness that is not preserved; therefore, no dream imagery and complete amnesia for the episodes are frequent.

Confusional arousals occur with the patient in bed. They generally start with the subject sitting up in the bed and looking around in a confused manner. They may precede an episode of sleepwalking that initiates when the patients leave the bed (Fig. 23.19).

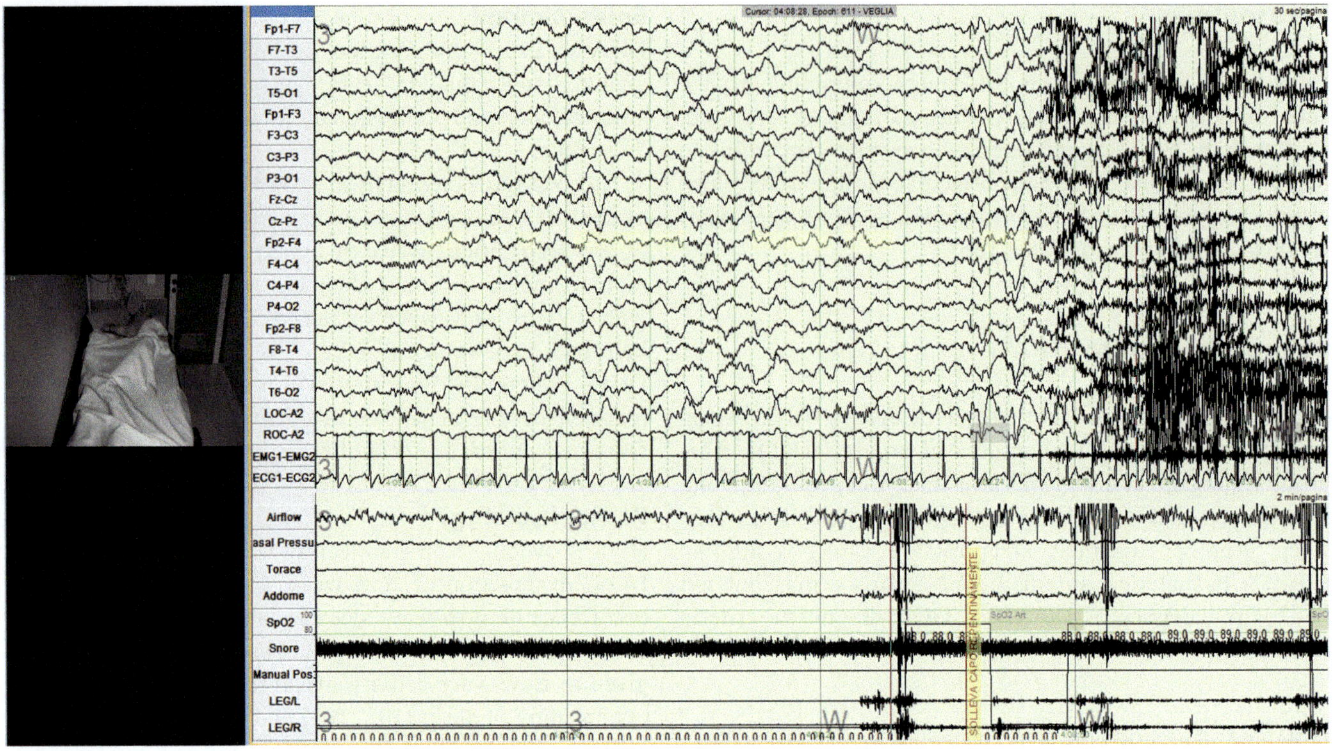

Fig. 23.19 Arousal from deep sleep in a patient with DOA

Sleepwalking episodes can begin as confusional arousal or with the patient that leaves the bed and walk from the bed and can last from seconds to more than 30 min. Behaviors may be simple and non-goal-directed, or complex. Misperception and unresponsiveness to external stimuli, mental confusion, perceived threat, and variable retrograde amnesia are very frequent among patients after the episodes. The subject is generally disoriented in time and place, with slow speech, diminished mentation, and blunted response to questions or requests. Blockade of sensory input results in a diminished external perception; however, the patient may appear to be awake during an episode but with reduced vigilance and impaired cognition.

Sleep terrors differ from the other DOA since the episodes are characterized by a cry or scream, associated by behavioral manifestation of intense fear and activation of the autonomic nervous system. The patient usually sits up in the bed, is not responsive to external stimuli, and is confused and disoriented when awakened. In the adults, jumping out of the bed, running, and violent behaviors may occur. Prolonged inconsolability after the episode is frequent, especially in children.

Treatment

The primary therapy for all parasomnias is adequate patient and bed partner education. In fact, the disease course is usually benign and tends to resolve spontaneously with time. Both the patient and bed partner should be educated about safety precautions for the bedroom environment, aimed at reducing potential sources of the injury. The partner should avoid waking up the patient during an episode, as this can possibly trigger violent behavior.

Confusional Arousals

There is no specific pharmacological management for confusional arousals (CA). However, when symptoms become persistent and severe, benzodiazepine (clonazepam) or antidepressants (imipramine and clomipramine) have been suggested to be effective. Scheduled or anticipatory awakening has been suggested as a behavioral technique to prevent these events. This consists in awakening the child 15–20 min before the usual time of occurrence of CA, in order to alter the sleep state and therefore to abort the event [106].

Sleepwalking

The first-line treatment is supportive and includes avoiding precipitants factors such as sleep deprivation and alcohol ingestion, creating a safe environment, giving the sleepwalker quiet guidance back to bed if necessary. It can be also noteworthy to reassure the patient that sleepwalking is not linked with underlying psychiatric illness. A number of nonpharmacologic treatments, including anticipatory awakening, psychotherapy, and hypnotherapy, have been proposed [106]. The pharmacological treatment of sleepwalking, relying mainly on benzodiazepines, antidepressants such as tricyclic antidepressants or serotonin-selective reuptake inhibitors, remains largely anecdotal.

Sleep Terrors

In this case, the first approach, especially in children with infrequent episodes of sleep terror, is still reassured, since they often resolve spontaneously with time. Patients should avoid trigger factors such as alcohol or sleep deprivation. Behavioral methods such as psychotherapy, relaxation therapy, autogenic training, and hypnosis can be used. Anticipatory or scheduled awakening have also been proposed [106]. When the episodes become more frequent, self-injurious, or persistent into adulthood, pharmacological treatment might be considered. Proposed pharmacological treatment includes benzodiazepines (diazepam and clonazepam) and antidepressants (imipramine, trazodone, clomipramine, and paroxetine) in adults and melatonin and L-5-hydroxytryptophan in children.

Sleep-Related Eating Disorder

Sleep-related eating disorder (SRED) is a non-REM sleep parasomnia that is not listed under the category of DOA. SRED is characterized by recurrent episodes of involuntary eating and drinking during an arousal from sleep. Typically, the diminished level of consciousness does not allow the recall of the event.

Epidemiology

Different rates of SRED have been reported according to the studied population. SRED was reported by 16.7% of subjects in an inpatient eating disorders group, while 8.7% of those in an outpatient eating disorders program and 4.6% of college students reported behavior consistent with SRED [107]. It is more frequent in women; accordingly, females comprise 60–83%, with a mean age of 22–39 years.

Pathophysiology

The pathophysiology of SRED remains unclear. SRED shares features with both eating and sleep disorders, in particular DOA; however, its peculiar presentation supports the classification as a separate entity. In accordance, the presence of another parasomnia is a risk factor. The most common PSG finding is the presence of confusional arousals from SWS, with chewing and swallowing movements that are frequently associated with EEG arousals [107].

Etiology

Predisposing and precipitating factors are similar to those observed in DOA.

Phenomenology

Patients generally arouse and eat 2–3 h after sleep onset. The episodes are characterized by a rapid ingestion of food, reported by subjects as "out of control" or compulsive. Level of consciousness is heterogeneous ranging from full awareness to unawareness typical of a DOA episode. Next day, amnesia is usually in line with the self-reported level of consciousness during the episodes, with confusional arousals associated with more impairment of recollection. Diurnal consequences comprise daytime fatigue that results from frequent nocturnal awakenings and weight gain due to the large number of calories consumed during episodes. Morning anorexia, due to overeating throughout the night, might be present in SRED patients.

Diagnosis is based on clinical criteria with PSG that might be useful to investigate the presence of other pathological condition (for SRED diagnostic criteria see Table 23.8).

Treatment

Both pharmacological and non-pharmacological treatments are used for SRED. The treatment of sleep pathologies that cause fragmentation of sleep, such as, PLMD or OSA, can reduce the number of arousals from sleep, which may drive nocturnal eating episodes. For example, dopaminergic agents (carbidopa/L-dopa; bromocriptine), benzodiazepine, and selective serotonin reuptake inhibitors are efficacious in those patients with concomitant RLS, sleepwalking, and daytime eating disorders, respectively. Furthermore, also topiramate is useful in reducing nighttime eating behaviors [107].

REM-Related Parasomnias

REM-related parasomnias comprise the abnormal behaviors that arise during REM sleep. This group includes REM sleep behavior disorder (RBD), recurrent-isolated sleep paralysis and nightmare disorder. Usually, these parasomnias are most common in the second half of the night when the body spends

Table 23.8 Diagnostic criteria for SRED according to ICSD-3

Diagnostic criteria
Criteria A–D must be met:
A. Recurrent episodes of dysfunctional eating that occur after an arousal during the main sleep period
B. The presence of at least one of the following in association with the recurrent episodes of involuntary eating:
1. Consumption of peculiar forms or combinations of food or inedible or toxic substances
2. Sleep-related injurious or potentially injurious behaviors performed while in pursuit of food or while cooking food
3. Adverse health consequences from recurrent nocturnal eating
C. There is partial or complete loss of conscious awareness during the eating episode, with subsequent impaired recall
D. The disturbance is not better explained by another sleep disorder, mental disorder, medical disorder, or substance abuse

more time in REM sleep. Notably, according to ICSD-3, PSG recording is mandatory only in the RBD diagnosis.

REM Sleep Behavior Disorder

REM sleep behavior disorder (RBD) is a parasomnia described for the first time by Schenck and colleagues in 1986 [108]. It is characterized by the loss of normal atony during the REM sleep phase, associated with abnormal and often violent behavior and movements, usually in relation to an unpleasant or terrifying dream.

According to the ICSD-3, the diagnosis is based on the history of repeated episodes of vocalizations and/or complex motor behaviors, usually in the second part of the night, and a video-polysomnographic (VPSG) documentation of such behavior or increase muscle tone during REM sleep (for diagnostic criteria see Table 23.9).

Epidemiology

Using specific questionnaires, the prevalence in elderly people is estimated around 4.6–7.7% [109]. But when the PSG is performed, the prevalence seems to be lower (0.3–1.15%) [110].

This disorder seems to predominantly affect male subjects. The reason for male prevalence is unclear: circulating sex hormones are normal in patients with RBD [111]. It is more probable, an under estimation in women due to a less violent behaviors. RBD is usually diagnosed in individuals over 50 years old [112].

Etiology

This pathology can be the result of other primary disease and can be associated with other neurological disorders. In these cases, RBD can be classified as "secondary." However, in its isolated or idiopathic form, it can precede insurgence of α-synucleinopathies (in particular Parkinson's disease (PD) and dementia with Lewy bodies (DLB)) by many years, thus representing a prodromal form of neurodegeneration.

Pathophysiology

The correlation between RBD and neurodegeneration in the forms initially identified as "idiopathic" is of utmost importance. The majority of RBD patients will convert to PD (43%), followed by DLB (25%) over the years [113]. It is also interesting that RBD patients may show abnormalities typical of PD such as hyposmia, depression, constipation, and orthostatic hypotension.

Table 23.9 Diagnostic criteria for REM sleep behavior disorder (RBD) according to ICSD-3

Diagnostic criteria
Criteria A–D must be met:
A. Repeated episodes of sleep related vocalization and/or complex motor behaviors
B. These behaviors are documented by polysomnography to occur during REM sleep or, based on clinical history of dream enactment, are presumed to occur during REM sleep
C. Polysomnographic recording demonstrates REM sleep without atonia (RSWA)
D. The disturbance is not better explained by another sleep disorder, mental disorder, and medication or substance use

In patients with RBD, several biomarkers of neurodegeneration have been identified, including imaging data, impaired color vision and olfactory function, EEG slowing, and neurocognitive impairments. The evidence that the degenerative process underlying the RBD involves also structures such as the olfactory system, the nigrostriatal system, and the autonomic system, with deposits of α-synuclein led to the hypothesis that this parasomnia should be considered part of the neurodegenerative process rather than a predisposing risk factor [114].

Phenomenology

Sleep- and dream-related behaviors include both violent and, less commonly, nonviolent behaviors. Most patients experience terrifying dreams, characterized by the presence of people, insects, or animals, which attack, chase, or bite the patient himself or people close to him. If awakened during an episode, patients are usually oriented and can detail the dream content in detail, remembering vivid details of the dream. In addition to the motor behavior, patients show various types of vocalization, which usually reflect the unpleasant content of the dream, like screams, curses, and insults. Violent movements can also cause injuries to the patient himself or, more frequently, to the bed-partner, in some cases even leading to lethal consequences.

The current diagnostic criteria for RBD published in 2014 [1] require a PSG confirmation of increased muscle tone during REM sleep on the polysomnogram (REM sleep without atonia-RSWA) (Fig. 23.20).

Treatment

Protection measures are recommended to improve the safety of the sleep environment, such as removing dangerous objects from the bedroom, installing bed rails, placing cushions on the floor next to the bed, or sleeping in separate beds or bedrooms. It is also important to avoid drugs like antidepressant or some beta-blockers that can induce or worsen RBD symptoms. First-line drug treatments are clonazepam and melatonin at bedtime [115].

Recurrent-Isolated Sleep Paralysis

Recurrent isolated sleep paralysis (RISP) is characterized by an inability to perform voluntary movements at sleep onset (hypnagogic form) or on waking from sleep (hypnopompic), in the absence of a diagnosis of narcolepsy (Table 23.10).

Epidemiology

Sleep paralysis (SP) is surprisingly common, but the exact prevalence of this disorder varies widely due to the specific measurements used for assessment (i.e., questionnaires or clinical interviews), the age, cultural, and ethnic factors. At least one SP episode over the course of their life is experi-

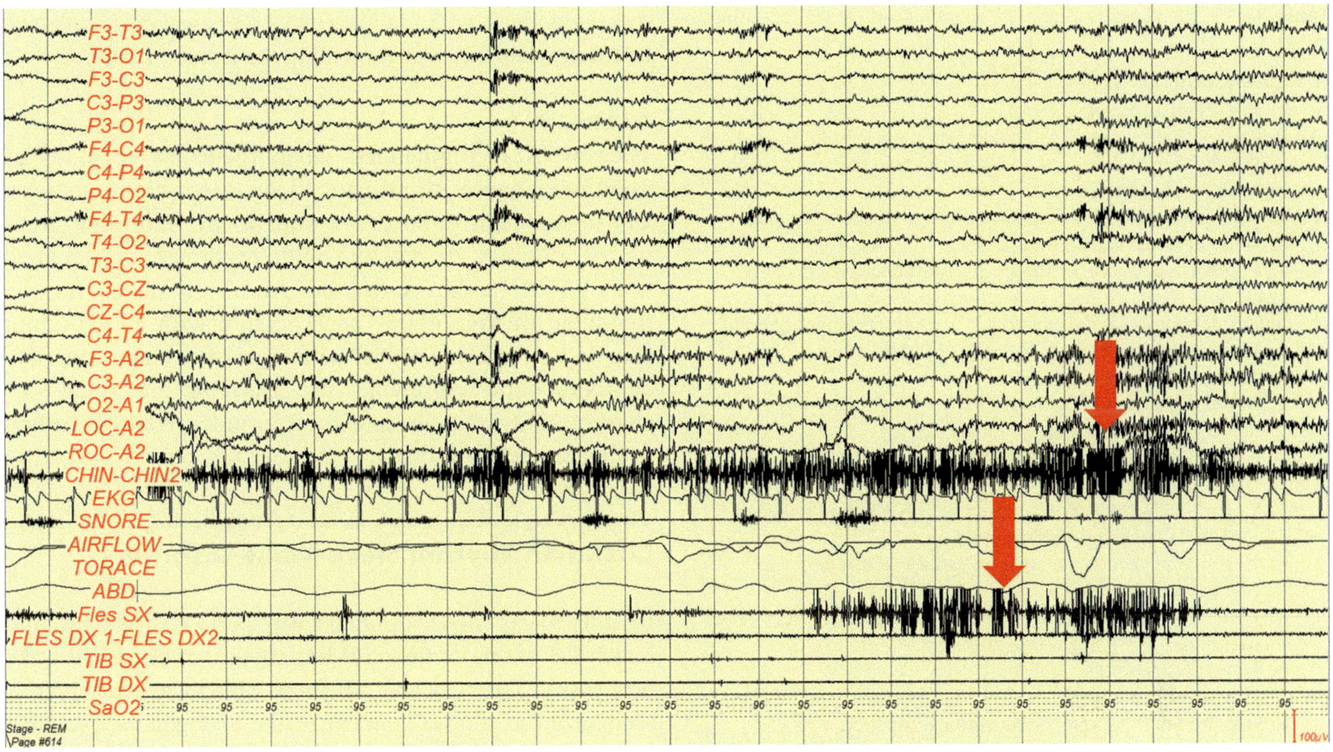

Fig. 23.20 Thirty-second PSG epoch of an RBD patient. RSWA is observable on both chin and flexor digitorum superficialis EMG

Table 23.10 Diagnostic criteria for recurrent isolated sleep paralysis according to ICSD-3

Diagnostic criteria
Criteria A–D must be met:
A. A recurrent inability to move the trunk and all of the limbs at sleep onset or upon awakening from sleep
B. Each episode lasts seconds to a few minutes
C. The episodes cause clinically significant distress including bedtime anxiety or fear of sleep
D. The disturbance is not better explained by another sleep disorder, mental disorder, medical disorder, or substance abuse

enced by 7.6% of the general population, though individual study estimates greatly vary from 2 to 60% [116].

Etiology

SP is frequently associated with narcolepsy and psychiatric dissociative phenomena; however, this condition is frequently described in the context of anxiety disorders in general, panic disorder, and post-traumatic stress disorder. Indeed, evidence reported that stress, chronic fear, and anxiety may act as predisposing factors for the occurrence of SP [116].

Pathophysiology

Only a few studies investigated the underlying neurophysiology of sleep paralysis. It does appear, however, that episodes are linked with sleep disruption and are particularly associated with sleep onset REM Period. SP is an example of state dissociation with elements of REM sleep persisting into wakefulness [117].

Phenomenology

Isolated SP episodes are characterized by muscle atonia upon sleep onset or offset. During an episode, patients are disabled to move the limbs, trunk, and head, but the ocular and respiratory movements remain unaltered, and perception of the immediate environment is clear. Fear, distress, and felling of suffocation may be associated with episodes. An episode can last from seconds to few minutes, and usually it resolves spontaneously. A sensory stimulation can end the episode early [117].

Treatment

Pharmacological agents often used in the context of narcolepsy have been utilized to treat SP. The most commonly used agents are tricyclic antidepressants and selective serotonin reuptake inhibitors. Their hypothesized mechanism of action is the suppression of REM sleep.

SP episodes can be increased by sleep deprivation; therefore, a correct sleep hygiene is highly recommended, such as, daytime naps that should be discouraged as they trigger SP [106].

Nightmare Disorder

Nightmare is defined by the repeated occurrence of nightmares that cause clinically significant distress or impairment in social, occupational, or other important areas of functioning (see Table 23.11). Generally, these dreams occur during REM sleep and often result in awakening.

Table 23.11 Diagnostic criteria for nightmare disorder according to ICSD-3

Diagnostic criteria
Criteria A–C must be met:
A. Repeated occurrences of extended, extremely dysphoric, and well-remembered dreams that usually involve threats to survival, security, or physical integrity
B. On awakening from the dysphoric dreams, the person rapidly becomes oriented and alert
C. The dream experience, or the sleep disturbance produced by awakening from it, causes clinically significant distress or impairment in social, occupational, or other important areas of functioning as indicated by the report of at least one of the following:
1. Mood disturbance (e.g., persistence of nightmare affect, anxiety, and dysphoria)
2. Sleep resistance (e.g., bedtime anxiety and fear of sleep/subsequent nightmares)
3. Cognitive impairments (e.g., intrusive nightmare imagery, impaired concentration, or memory)
4. Negative impact on caregiver or family functioning (e.g., nighttime disruption)
5. Behavioral problems (e.g., bedtime avoidance and fear of the dark)
6. Daytime sleepiness
7. Fatigue or low energy
8. Impaired occupational or educational function
9. Impaired interpersonal/social function

Epidemiology
Occasional nightmares are very common in children (60–75%), but the diagnosis of nightmare disorder, with recurrent episodes, is uncommon. Overall, 3.5–8.3% of the general adult population [118], 6.7–11.3% of children [119], and 15.6–66.7% of adult psychiatric patients (anxiety disorders and post-traumatic stress disorder (PTSD), respectively) [120] report recurrent nightmares. Nightmares occur more frequently in women than in men.

Etiology
Nightmare disorder is frequently associated with psychopathology. Drugs affecting norepinephrine, serotonin, dopamine, and GABA systems and REM sleep suppressive agents are related to nightmares' complaints [1].

Pathophysiology
Not known.

Phenomenology
Patients with nightmare disorder complain about recurrence of extremely dysphoric dream, with typical content of imminent physical danger or other distressing themes. Emotions are characteristically negative and involve anxiety, fear, terror, anger, and embarrassment. Nightmares usually occur during REM sleep and are associated with symptoms of physical arousal such as sweating and shortness of breath, often resulting in awakening. Post-awakening anxiety and difficulty returning to sleep may be present. Contrary to night terrors, individuals with nightmare disorder awaken completely, orient immediately, and remember the dream vividly.

Treatment
Therapy is recommended when recurrent episodes of nightmare cause significant sleep disruption, distress, and impairment in social, occupational, and other areas of functioning. In patients with nightmares associated with PTSD, prazosin can be useful. Evidence for the treatment of nightmares unassociated with PTSD is not established [121]. Several behavioral and cognitive psychotherapeutic approaches are available, but their efficacy remains unclear, and future randomized controlled trials are needed [106].

Circadian Rhythm Sleep-Wake Disorders

In order to experience optimal sleep, periods of sleep should match the timing of the circadian rhythm of sleep and wake propensity. Delayed and advanced sleep-wake disorder is recognized as a misalignment of the endogenous circadian timekeeping system with the desired sleep-wake schedule. Indeed, as reported by the ICSD-3rd edition, a circadian rhythm sleep-wake disorder is "caused by alterations of the circadian time-keeping system, its entrainment mechanisms, or a misalignment of the endogenous circadian rhythm and the external environment" [1].

Delayed Sleep-Wake Phase Disorder

Diagnostic criteria defined by ICSD-3 are reported in Table 23.12.

An example of actigraphy evaluation of a patient with delayed sleep-wake phase disorder is shown in Fig. 23.21.

Table 23.12 Diagnostic criteria for delayed sleep-wake phase disorder according to ICSD-3

Diagnostic criteria
Criteria A–E must be met:
A. There is a significant delay in the phase of the major sleep episode in relation to the desired or required sleep time and wake-up time, as evidenced by a chronic or recurrent complaint by the patient or a caregiver of inability to fall asleep and difficulty awakening at a desired or required clock time
B. The symptoms are present for at least 3 months
C. When patients are allowed to choose their ad libitum schedule, they will exhibit improved sleep quality and duration for age and maintain a delayed phase of the 24-h sleep-wake pattern
D. Sleep log and, whenever possible, actigraphy monitoring for at least 7 days (preferably 14 days) demonstrate a delay in the timing of the habitual sleep period. Both work/school days and free days must be included within this monitoring
E. The sleep disturbance is not better explained by another current sleep disorder, medical or neurological disorder, mental disorder, medication use, or substance use disorder

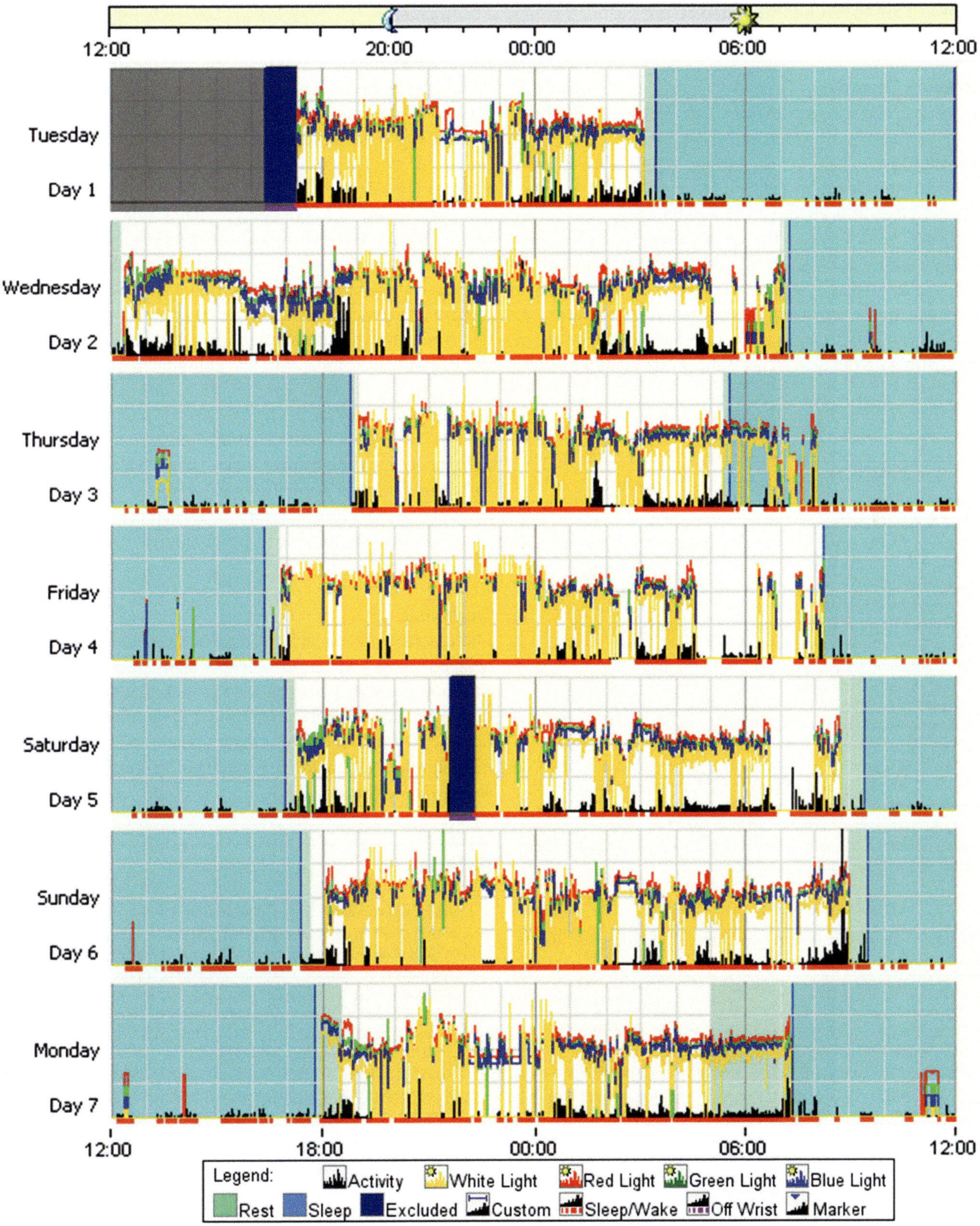

Fig. 23.21 Actigraphy recording of a patient with a delayed sleep-wake phase disorder

Advanced Sleep-Wake Phase Disorder

Diagnostic criteria are reported in Table 23.13.

Shift Work Disorder

Diagnostic criteria are reported in Table 23.14.

Epidemiology

The actual prevalence of delayed sleep-wake phase disorder is not clear. It is reported predominantly in preadolescence and adolescence, but it remains an infrequent condition with a prevalence around 0.17% in population-based studies. Also, the actual prevalence of advanced sleep-wake phase disorder in the general population is unknown, but it is thought to be rare and less frequent in comparison with delayed sleep-wake phase disorder [122].

Table 23.13 Diagnostic criteria for advanced sleep wake disorder according to ICSD-3

Diagnostic criteria Criteria A–E must be met:
A. There is an advance in the phase of the major sleep episode in relation to the desired or required sleep time and wake-up time, as evidenced by a chronic or recurrent complaint of difficulty staying awake until the required or desired conventional bedtime, together with an inability to remain asleep until the required or desired time for awakening
B. The symptoms are present for at least 3 months
C. When patients are allowed to sleep in accordance with their internal biological clock, sleep quality and duration are improved with a consistent but advanced timing of the major sleep episode
D. Sleep log and, whenever possible, actigraphy monitoring for at least 7 days (preferably 14 days) demonstrate advance in the timing of the habitual sleep period. Both work/school days and free days must be included within this monitoring
E. The sleep disturbance is not better explained by another current sleep disorder, medical or neurological disorder, mental disorder, medication use, or substance use disorder

Table 23.14 Diagnostic criteria for shift work disorder according to ICSD-3

Diagnostic criteria Criteria A–D must be met:
A. There is a report of insomnia and/or excessive sleepiness, accompanied by a reduction of total sleep time, which is associated with a recurring work schedule that overlaps the usual time for sleep
B. The symptoms have been present and associated with the shift work schedule for at least 3 months
C. Sleep log and actigraphy monitoring (whenever possible and preferably with concurrent light exposure measurement) for at least 14 days (work and free days) demonstrate a disturbed sleep and wake pattern
D. The sleep and/or wake disturbance are not better explained by another current sleep disorder, medical or neurological disorder, mental disorder, medication use, poor sleep hygiene, or substance use disorder

Etiology

Delayed and advance sleep-wake phase disorders are caused by a desynchronization between endogenous biological clock and desired sleep-wake schedule. Shift work disorder is closely related to work schedules and remits when conventional sleep-wake pattern is restored [1].

Pathophysiology

The pathogenesis of both delayed and advanced sleep-wake phase disorder is the disruption of the circadian timing system. However, although there is evidence for alteration in the circadian clock of these patients, future research is needed to confirm this model [122]. On the contrary, shift work disorder is situational, and alterations of the circadian systems might be induced shift work and consequent behavior.

Phenomenology

Patients with sleep-wake phase disorder experience a habitual and in some case involuntary, sleep wake time that is earlier or later than normal societal average. This frequently causes to daytime impairment, social, and occupational dysfunctions that might lead to psychological and psychiatric consequences [122].

Treatment

Phototherapy and melatonin administration are used for both delayed and advanced sleep-wake phase disorders. Chronotherapy may also be used in these patients; however, up to now, no randomized controlled trials support this practice. Some components of cognitive-behavioral therapy for insomnia are useful for the treatment of circadian rhythm sleep-wake disorder [123].

References

1. American Academy of Sleep Medicine. The international classification of sleep disorders (ICSD-3). 2014.
2. Association AP. American Psychiatric Association. Diagnostic and statistical manual of mental disorders. 5th ed; 2013.
3. Wittchen HU, et al. The size and burden of mental disorders and other disorders of the brain in Europe 2010. Eur Neuropsychopharmacol. 2011;21(9):655–79. https://doi.org/10.1016/j.euroneuro.2011.07.018.
4. Roth T, Jaeger S, Jin R, Kalsekar A, Stang PE, Kessler RC. Sleep problems, comorbid mental disorders, and role functioning in the national comorbidity survey replication. Biol Psychiatry. 2006;60(12):1364–71. https://doi.org/10.1016/j.biopsych.2006.05.039.
5. Sarsour K, Morin CM, Foley K, Kalsekar A, Walsh JK. Association of insomnia severity and comorbid medical and psychiatric disorders in a health plan-based sample: insomnia severity and comorbidities. Sleep Med. 2010;11(1):69–74. https://doi.org/10.1016/j.sleep.2009.02.008.
6. Budhiraja R, Roth T, Hudgel DW, Budhiraja P, Drake CL. Prevalence and polysomnographic correlates of insomnia

comorbid with medical disorders. Sleep. 2011;34(7):859–67. https://doi.org/10.5665/SLEEP.1114.
7. Baglioni C, et al. Insomnia as a predictor of depression: a meta-analytic evaluation of longitudinal epidemiological studies. J Affect Disord. 2011;135(1–3):10–9. https://doi.org/10.1016/j.jad.2011.01.011.
8. Sivertsen B, et al. The Bidirectional Association Between Depression and Insomnia. Psychosom Med. 2012;74(7):758–65. https://doi.org/10.1097/PSY.0b013e3182648619.
9. Morin CM, et al. Insomnia disorder. Nat Rev Dis Prim. 2015;1:15026. https://doi.org/10.1038/nrdp.2015.26.
10. Viola AU, et al. PER3 Polymorphism Predicts Sleep Structure and Waking Performance. Curr Biol. 2007;17(7):613–8. https://doi.org/10.1016/j.cub.2007.01.073.
11. Deuschle M, et al. Association between a serotonin transporter length polymorphism and primary insomnia. Sleep. 2010;33(3):343–7. https://doi.org/10.1093/sleep/33.3.343.
12. Buhr A, et al. Functional characterization of the new GABAA receptor mutation β(R192H). Hum Genet. 2002;111(2):154–60. https://doi.org/10.1007/s00439-002-0766-7.
13. Hammerschlag AR, et al. Genome-wide association analysis of insomnia complaints identifies risk genes and genetic overlap with psychiatric and metabolic traits. Nat Genet. 2017;49(11):1584–92. https://doi.org/10.1038/ng.3888.
14. Jansen PR, et al. Genome-wide analysis of insomnia in 1,331,010 individuals identifies new risk loci and functional pathways. Nat Genet. 2019;51(3):394–403. https://doi.org/10.1038/s41588-018-0333-3.
15. Riemann D, et al. The hyperarousal model of insomnia: a review of the concept and its evidence. Sleep Med Rev. 2010;14(1):19–31. https://doi.org/10.1016/j.smrv.2009.04.002.
16. Zhang J, et al. A community-based study on the association between insomnia and hypothalamic-pituitary-adrenal axis: sex and pubertal influences. J Clin Endocrinol Metab. 2014;99(6):2277–87. https://doi.org/10.1210/jc.2013-3728.
17. Farina B, et al. Heart rate and heart rate variability modification in chronic insomnia patients. Behav Sleep Med. 2014;12(4):290–306. https://doi.org/10.1080/15402002.2013.801346.
18. Spiegelhalder K, et al. Heart rate and heart rate variability in subjectively reported insomnia. J Sleep Res. 2011;20(1 Pt 2):137–45. https://doi.org/10.1111/j.1365-2869.2010.00863.x.
19. Bonnet MH, Arand DL. 24-hour metabolic rate in insomniacs and matched normal sleepers. Sleep. 1995;18(7):581–8. https://doi.org/10.1093/sleep/18.7.581.
20. Lack LC, Gradisar M, Van Someren EJW, Wright HR, Lushington K. The relationship between insomnia and body temperatures. Sleep Med Rev. 2008;12(4):307–17. https://doi.org/10.1016/j.smrv.2008.02.003.
21. Kalmbach DA, et al. Hyperarousal and sleep reactivity in insomnia: current insights. Nat Sci Sleep. 2018;10:193–201. https://doi.org/10.2147/NSS.S138823.
22. Spiegelhalder K, et al. Increased EEG sigma and beta power during NREM sleep in primary insomnia. Biol Psychol. 2012;91(3):329–33. https://doi.org/10.1016/j.biopsycho.2012.08.009.
23. Israel B, Buysse DJ, Krafty RT, Begley A, Miewald J, Hall M. Short-term stability of sleep and heart rate variability in good sleepers and patients with insomnia: for some measures, one night is enough. Sleep. 2012;35(9):1285–91. https://doi.org/10.5665/sleep.2088.
24. Perlis ML, Merica H, Smith MT, Giles DE. Beta EEG activity and insomnia. Sleep Med Rev. 2001;5(5):363–74. https://doi.org/10.1053/smrv.2001.0151.
25. Lamarche CH, Ogilvie RD. Electrophysiological changes during the sleep onset period of psychophysiological insomniacs, psychiatric insomniacs, and normal sleepers. Sleep. 1997;20(9):724–33. https://doi.org/10.1093/sleep/20.9.726.
26. Merica H. Spectral characteristics of sleep EEG in chronic insomnia. Eur J Neurosci. 1998;10(5):1826–34. https://doi.org/10.1046/j.1460-9568.1998.00189.x.
27. Bastien CH, LeBlanc M, Carrier J, Morin CM. Sleep EEG power spectra, insomnia, and chronic use of benzodiazepines. Sleep. 2003;26(3):313–7. https://doi.org/10.1093/sleep/26.3.313.
28. Hogan SE, et al. Slow-oscillation activity is reduced and high frequency activity is elevated in older adults with insomnia. J Clin Sleep Med. 2020;16(9):1445–54. https://doi.org/10.5664/jcsm.8568.
29. Krystal AD, Edinger JD. Sleep EEG predictors and correlates of the response to cognitive behavioral therapy for insomnia. Sleep. 2010;33(5):669–77. https://doi.org/10.1093/sleep/33.5.669.
30. Wassing R, et al. Slow dissolving of emotional distress contributes to hyperarousal. Proc Natl Acad Sci U S A. 2016;113(9):2538–43. https://doi.org/10.1073/pnas.1522520113.
31. Wassing R, Lakbila-Kamal O, Ramautar JR, Stoffers D, Schalkwijk F, Van Someren EJW. Restless REM Sleep Impedes Overnight Amygdala Adaptation. Curr Biol. 2019;29(14):2351–2358.e4. https://doi.org/10.1016/j.cub.2019.06.034.
32. Nofzinger EA, Boysse DJ, Germain A, Price JC, Miewald JM, Kopfer DJ. Functional neuroimaging evidence for hyperarousal in insomnia. Am J Psychiatry. 2004;161(11):2126–8. https://doi.org/10.1176/appi.ajp.161.11.2126.
33. Spielman AJ, Saskin P, Thorpy MJ. Treatment of chronic insomnia by restriction of time in bed. Sleep. 1987;10(1):45–56. https://doi.org/10.1093/sleep/10.1.45.
34. Riemann D, et al. European guideline for the diagnosis and treatment of insomnia. J Sleep Res. 2017;26(6):675–700. https://doi.org/10.1111/jsr.12594.
35. Qaseem A, Kansagara D, Forciea MA, Cooke M, Denberg TD. Management of chronic insomnia disorder in adults: a clinical practice guideline from the American College of Physicians. Ann Intern Med. 2016;165(2):125. https://doi.org/10.7326/M15-2175.
36. Sateia MJ, Buysse DJ, Krystal AD, Neubauer DN, Heald JL. Clinical practice guideline for the pharmacologic treatment of chronic insomnia in adults: an American Academy of Sleep Medicine Clinical Practice Guideline. J Clin Sleep Med. 2017;13(02):307–49. https://doi.org/10.5664/jcsm.6470.
37. Castronovo V, et al. Long-term clinical effect of group cognitive behavioral therapy for insomnia: a case series study. Sleep Med. 2018;47:54–9. https://doi.org/10.1016/j.sleep.2018.03.017.
38. Espie CA. The psychological treatment of insomnia. Chichester: Wiley; 1991.
39. Hauri PJ. Sleep hygiene, relaxation therapy, and cognitive interventions. In Case studies in insomnia. Boston, MA: Springer US; 1991. p. 65–84.
40. Morin CM. Insomnia: psychological assessment and management. Guilford Press; 1993.
41. Bootzin RR, Epstein D, Wood JM. Stimulus Control Instructions. In Case studies in insomnia. Boston, MA: Springer US; 1991. p. 19–28.
42. Lichstein KL. Clinical relaxation strategies. New York: Wiley; 1988.
43. Mitchell LJ, Bisdounis L, Ballesio A, Omlin X, Kyle SD. The impact of cognitive behavioural therapy for insomnia on objective sleep parameters: a meta-analysis and systematic review. Sleep Med Rev. 2019;47:90–102. https://doi.org/10.1016/j.smrv.2019.06.002.
44. Galbiati A, et al. Insomnia patients with subjective short total sleep time have a boosted response to cognitive behavioral therapy for insomnia despite residual symptoms. Behav Sleep Med. 2020;18(1):58–67. https://doi.org/10.1080/15402002.2018.1545650.
45. Dang-Vu TT, et al. Sleep spindles may predict response to cognitive-behavioral therapy for chronic insomnia. Sleep

Med. 2017;39(2017):54–61. https://doi.org/10.1016/j.sleep.2017.08.012.
46. Cervena K, et al. Effect of cognitive behavioural therapy for insomnia on sleep architecture and sleep EEG power spectra in psychophysiological insomnia. J Sleep Res. 2004;13(4):385–93. https://doi.org/10.1111/j.1365-2869.2004.00431.x.
47. Sateia MJ. International classification of sleep disorders-third edition. Chest. 2014;146(5):1387–94. https://doi.org/10.1378/chest.14-0970.
48. Borbely AA. A two process model of sleep regulation. Hum Neurobiol. 1982;1(3):195–204.
49. Johns MW. A new method for measuring daytime sleepiness: the Epworth sleepiness scale. Sleep. 1991;14(6):540–5. https://doi.org/10.1093/sleep/14.6.540.
50. Arand DL, Bonnet MH. The multiple sleep latency test. In Handbook of clinical neurology. 2019.
51. Yoss RE, Daly DD. Narcolepsy. Med Clin North Am. 1960;44:953–68. https://doi.org/10.1016/S0025-7125(16)33982-7.
52. Roth T, et al. Disrupted nighttime sleep in narcolepsy. J Clin Sleep Med. 2013;9(9):955–65. https://doi.org/10.5664/jcsm.3004.
53. Silber MH, Krahn LE, Olson EJ, Pankratz VS. The epidemiology of narcolepsy in Olmsted County, Minnesota: a population-based study. Sleep. 2002;25(2):197–202. https://doi.org/10.1093/sleep/25.2.197.
54. Heier MS, Evsiukova T, Wilson J, Abdelnoor M, Hublin C, Ervik S. Prevalence of narcolepsy with cataplexy in Norway. Acta Neurol Scand. 2009;120(4):276–80. https://doi.org/10.1111/j.1600-0404.2009.01166.x.
55. Hublin C, Partinen M, Kaprio J, Koskenvuo M, Guillerminault C. Epidemiology of narcolepsy. Sleep. 1994;17:S7–S12. https://doi.org/10.1093/sleep/17.suppl_8.s7.
56. Hublin C, et al. The prevalence of narcolepsy: an epidemiological study of the Finnish Twin Cohort. Ann Neurol. 1994;35(6):709–16. https://doi.org/10.1002/ana.410350612.
57. Ohayon MM, Priest RG, Zulley J, Smirne S, Paiva T. Prevalence of narcolepsy symptomatology and diagnosis in the European general population. Neurology. 2002;58(12):1826–33. https://doi.org/10.1212/WNL.58.12.1826.
58. Thorpy MJ, Krieger AC. Delayed diagnosis of narcolepsy: characterization and impact. Sleep Med. 2014;15(5):502–7. https://doi.org/10.1016/j.sleep.2014.01.015.
59. Dauvilliers Y, et al. Age at onset of narcolepsy in two large populations of patients in France and Quebec. Neurology. 2001;57(11):2029–33. https://doi.org/10.1212/WNL.57.11.2029.
60. Kornum BR, et al. Narcolepsy. Nat Rev Dis Primers. 2017;3:16100. https://doi.org/10.1038/nrdp.2016.100.
61. Plazzi G, et al. Complex movement disorders at disease onset in childhood narcolepsy with cataplexy. Brain. 2011;134(Pt 12):3477–89. https://doi.org/10.1093/brain/awr244.
62. Billiard M, et al. Modafinil: a double-blind multicentric study. Sleep. 1994;17(8 Suppl):S107–12. https://doi.org/10.1093/sleep/17.suppl_8.s107.
63. Broughton RJ, et al. Randomized, double-blind, placebo-controlled crossover trial of modafinil in the treatment of excessive daytime sleepiness in narcolepsy. Neurology. 1997;49(2):444–51. https://doi.org/10.1212/WNL.49.2.444.
64. Auger RR, Goodman SH, Silber MH, Krahn LE, Pankratz VS, Slocumb NL. Risks of high-dose stimulants in the treatment of disorders of excessive somnolence: a case-control study. Sleep. 2005;28(6):667–72. https://doi.org/10.1093/sleep/28.6.667.
65. Calik MW. Update on the treatment of narcolepsy: clinical efficacy of pitolisant. Nat Sci Sleep. 2017;9:127–33. https://doi.org/10.2147/NSS.S103462.
66. Dauvilliers Y, et al. Solriamfetol for the treatment of excessive daytime sleepiness in participants with narcolepsy with and without cataplexy: subgroup analysis of efficacy and safety data by cataplexy status in a randomized controlled trial. CNS Drugs. 2020;34(7):773–84. https://doi.org/10.1007/s40263-020-00744-2.
67. Franceschini C, Pizza F, Antelmi E, Folli MC, Plazzi G. Narcolepsy treatment: pharmacological and behavioral strategies in adults and children. Sleep Breath. 2020;24(2):615–27. https://doi.org/10.1007/s11325-019-01894-4.
68. Roth B. Narcolepsy and hypersomnia: review and classification of 642 personally observed cases. Schweiz Arch Neurol Neurochir und Psychiatr. 1976;119(1):31–41.
69. Billiard M, Sonka K. Idiopathic hypersomnia. Sleep Med Rev. 2016;29:23–33. https://doi.org/10.1016/j.smrv.2015.08.007.
70. Trotti LM. Idiopathic Hypersomnia. Sleep Med Clin. 2017;12(3):331–44. https://doi.org/10.1016/j.jsmc.2017.03.009.
71. Arnulf I, Zeitzer JM, File J, Farber N, Mignot E. Kleine-Levin syndrome: a systematic review of 186 cases in the literature. Brain. 2005;128(Pt 12):2763–76. https://doi.org/10.1093/brain/awh620.
72. Kleine W. Periodische Schlafsucht. pp. 285–304. Eur Neurol. 1925;57:285–304. https://doi.org/10.1159/000190426.
73. Levin M. Periodic somnolence and morbid hunger: a new syndrome. Brain. 1936;59:494–504. https://doi.org/10.1093/brain/59.4.494.
74. de Oliveira MM, Conti C, Prado GF. Pharmacological treatment for Kleine-Levin syndrome. Cochrane Database Syst Rev. 2016;2016(5):CD006685. https://doi.org/10.1002/14651858.CD006685.pub4.
75. Afolabi-Brown O, Mason TBA. Kleine-Levin Syndrome. Paediatr Respir Rev. 2018;25:9–13. https://doi.org/10.1016/j.prrv.2016.12.004.
76. Miglis MG, Guilleminault C. Kleine-Levin syndrome: a review. Nat Sci Sleep. 2014;6:19–26. https://doi.org/10.2147/NSS.S44750.
77. Sum-Ping O, Guilleminault C. Kleine-Levin Syndrome. Curr Treat Options Neurol. 2016;18(6):24. https://doi.org/10.1007/s11940-016-0409-2.
78. Kapur VK, et al. Clinical practice guideline for diagnostic testing for adult obstructive sleep apnea: an American academy of sleep medicine clinical practice guideline. J Clin Sleep Med. 2017;13(3):479–504. https://doi.org/10.5664/jcsm.6506.
79. Senaratna CV, et al. Prevalence of obstructive sleep apnea in the general population: a systematic review. Sleep Med Rev. 2017;34:70–81. https://doi.org/10.1016/j.smrv.2016.07.002.
80. Liguori C, et al. Obstructive sleep apnea is associated with early but possibly modifiable Alzheimer's disease biomarkers changes. Sleep. 2017;40(5). https://doi.org/10.1093/sleep/zsx011.
81. Emamian F, et al. The association between obstructive sleep apnea and Alzheimer's disease: a meta-analysis perspective. Front Aging Neurosci. 2016;7:78. https://doi.org/10.3389/fnagi.2016.00078.
82. Ferini-Strambi L, Marelli S, Galbiati A, Castronovo C. Effects of continuous positive airway pressure on cognitition and neuroimaging data in sleep apnea. Int J Psychophysiol. 2013;89(2):203–12. https://doi.org/10.1016/j.ijpsycho.2013.03.022.
83. Bosi M, Incerti Parenti S, Sanna A, Plazzi G, De Vito A, Alessandri-Bonetti G. Non-continuous positive airway pressure treatment options in obstructive sleep apnoea: a pathophysiological perspective. Sleep Med Rev. 2021;60:101521. https://doi.org/10.1016/j.smrv.2021.101521.
84. Stevens MS. Restless legs syndrome/Willis-Ekbom disease morbidity burden, quality of life, cardiovascular aspects, and sleep.

Sleep Med Clin. 2015;10(3):369–73. https://doi.org/10.1016/j.jsmc.2015.05.017.
85. Hornyak M, Scholz H, Kohnen R, Bengel J, Kassubek J, Trenkwalder C. What treatment works best for restless legs syndrome? Meta-analyses of dopaminergic and non-dopaminergic medications. Sleep Med Rev. 2014;18(2):153–64. https://doi.org/10.1016/j.smrv.2013.03.004.
86. Winkelmann J, et al. Treatment of restless legs syndrome: evidence-based review and implications for clinical practice (Revised 2017)§. Mov Disord. 2018;33(7):1077–91.
87. Trenkwalder C, Allen R, Högl B, Paulus W, Winkelmann J. Restless legs syndrome associated with major diseases: a systematic review and new concept. Neurology. 2016;86(14):1336–43. https://doi.org/10.1212/WNL.0000000000002542.
88. Koo BB. Restless leg syndrome across the globe: epidemiology of the restless legs syndrome/Willis-Ekbom disease. Sleep Med Clin. 2015;10(3):189–205. https://doi.org/10.1016/j.jsmc.2015.05.004.
89. Kambampati S, Wasim S, Kukkar V, Awad VM, Malik BH. Restless leg syndrome in the setting of patients with end-stage renal disease on hemodialysis: a literature review. Cureus. 2020;12(8):e9965. https://doi.org/10.7759/cureus.9965.
90. Didato G, Di Giacomo R, Rosa GJ, Dominese A, de Curtis M, Lanteri P. Restless legs syndrome across the lifespan: symptoms, pathophysiology, management and daily life impact of the different patterns of disease presentation. Int J Environ Res Public Health. 2020;17(10):3658. https://doi.org/10.3390/ijerph17103658.
91. Allen RP, et al. Restless legs syndrome/Willis-Ekbom disease diagnostic criteria: updated International Restless Legs Syndrome Study Group (IRLSSG) consensus criteria—history, rationale, description, and significance. Sleep Med. 2014;15(8):860–73. https://doi.org/10.1016/j.sleep.2014.03.025.
92. Kolla BP, Mansukhani MP, Bostwick JM. The influence of antidepressants on restless legs syndrome and periodic limb movements: a systematic review. Sleep Med Rev. 2018;38:131–40. https://doi.org/10.1016/j.smrv.2017.06.002.
93. Stefani A, Högl B. Diagnostic criteria, differential diagnosis, and treatment of minor motor activity and less well-known movement disorders of sleep. Curr Treat Options Neurol. 2019;21(1):1. https://doi.org/10.1007/s11940-019-0543-8.
94. Aurora RN, et al. The treatment of restless legs syndrome and periodic limb movement disorder in adults—an update for 2012: practice parameters with an evidence-based systematic review and meta-analyses. Sleep. 2012;35(8):1039–62. https://doi.org/10.5665/sleep.1988.
95. Antelmi E, Provini F. Propriospinal myoclonus: the spectrum of clinical and neurophysiological phenotypes. Sleep Med Rev. 2015;22:54–63. https://doi.org/10.1016/j.smrv.2014.10.007.
96. Sateia MJ. International classification of sleep disorders-third edition highlights and modifications. Chest. 2014;146(5):1387–94. https://doi.org/10.1378/chest.14-0970.
97. Ohayon MM, Mahowald MW, Dauvilliers Y, Krystal AD, Léger D. Prevalence and comorbidity of nocturnal wandering in the US adult general population. Neurology. 2012;78(20):1583–9. https://doi.org/10.1212/WNL.0b013e3182563be5.
98. Stallman HM, Kohler M. Prevalence of sleepwalking: a systematic review and meta-analysis. PLoS One. 2016;11(11):e0164769. https://doi.org/10.1371/journal.pone.0164769.
99. Lopez R, Jaussent I, Scholz S, Bayard S, Montplaisir J, Dauvilliers Y. Functional impairment in adult sleepwalkers: a case-control study. Sleep. 2013;36(3):345–51. https://doi.org/10.5665/sleep.2446.
100. Bargiotas P, Arnet I, Frei M, Baumann CR, Schindler K, Bassetti CL. Demographic, clinical and polysomnographic characteristics of childhood- and adult-onset sleepwalking in adults. Eur Neurol. 2017;78(5–6):307–11. https://doi.org/10.1159/000481685.
101. Zadra A, et al. Somnambulism: clinical aspects and pathophysiological hypotheses. Lancet Neurol. 2013;12(3):285–94.
102. Jaar O, Pilon M, Carrier J, Montplaisir J, Zadra A. Analysis of slow-wave activity and slow-wave oscillations prior to somnambulism. Sleep. 2010;33(11):1511–6. https://doi.org/10.1093/sleep/33.11.1511.
103. Perrault R, Carrier J, Desautels A, Montplaisir J, Zadra A. Electroencephalographic slow waves prior to sleepwalking episodes. Sleep Med. 2014;15(12):1468–72. https://doi.org/10.1016/j.sleep.2014.07.020.
104. Januszko P, et al. Sleepwalking episodes are preceded by arousal-related activation in the cingulate motor area: EEG current density imaging. Clin Neurophysiol. 2016;127(1):530–6. https://doi.org/10.1016/j.clinph.2015.01.014.
105. Castelnovo A, Lopez R, Proserpio P, Nobili L, Dauvilliers Y. NREM sleep parasomnias as disorders of sleep-state dissociation. Nat Rev Neurol. 2018;14:1–12. https://doi.org/10.1038/s41582-018-0030-y.
106. Galbiati A, Rinaldi F, Giora E, Ferini-Strambi L, Marelli S. Behavioural and cognitive-behavioural treatments of parasomnias. Behav Neurol. 2015;2015:786928. https://doi.org/10.1155/2015/786928.
107. Winkelman JW, Johnson EA, Richards LM. Sleep-related eating disorder. Handb Clin Neurol. 2011;98:577–85.
108. Schenck CH, Bundlie SR, Ettinger MG, Mahowald MW. Chronic behavioral disorders of human REM sleep: a new category of parasomnia. Sleep. 1986;9(2):293–308. https://doi.org/10.1093/sleep/9.2.293.
109. Mahlknecht P, et al. Probable RBD and association with neurodegenerative disease markers: a population-based study. Mov Disord. 2015;30(10):1417–21. https://doi.org/10.1002/mds.26350.
110. Haba-Rubio J, et al. Prevalence and determinants of rapid eye movement sleep behavior disorder in the general population. Sleep. 2018;41(2):1–8. https://doi.org/10.1093/sleep/zsx197.
111. Iranzo A, Santamaría J, Vilaseca I, De Osaba MJM. Absence of alterations in serum sex hormone levels in idiopathic REM sleep behavior disorder. Sleep. 2007;30(6):803–6. https://doi.org/10.1093/sleep/30.6.803.
112. Fernández-Arcos A, Iranzo A, Serradell M, Gaig C, Santamaria J. The clinical phenotype of idiopathic rapid eye movement sleep behavior disorder at presentation: a study in 203 consecutive patients. Sleep. 2016;39(1):121–32. https://doi.org/10.5665/sleep.5332.
113. Galbiati A, Verga L, Giora E, Zucconi M, Ferini-Strambi L. The risk of neurodegeneration in REM sleep behavior disorder: a systematic review and meta-analysis of longitudinal studies. Sleep Med Rev. 2019;43:37–46. https://doi.org/10.1016/j.smrv.2018.09.008.
114. Ferini-Strambi L, Fasiello E, Sforza M, Salsone M, Galbiati A. Neuropsychological, electrophysiological, and neuroimaging biomarkers for REM behavior disorder. Expert Rev Neurother. 2019;19(11):1069–87. https://doi.org/10.1080/14737175.2019.1640603.
115. Högl B, Stefani A, Videnovic A. Idiopathic REM sleep behaviour disorder and neurodegeneration—an update. Nat Rev Neurol. 2018;14(1):40–55. https://doi.org/10.1038/nrneurol.2017.157.
116. Sharpless BA, Barber JP. Lifetime prevalence rates of sleep paralysis: a systematic review. Sleep Med Rev. 2011;15(5):311–5. https://doi.org/10.1016/j.smrv.2011.01.007.
117. Sharpless BA, Denis D. Recurrent isolated sleep paralysis. In The curated reference collection in neuroscience and biobehavioral psychology. 2016.

118. Li SX, Zhang B, Li AM, Wing YK. Prevalence and correlates of frequent nightmares: a community-based 2-phase study. Sleep. 2010;33(6):774–80. https://doi.org/10.1093/sleep/33.6.774.
119. Wiechers S, Schlarb AA, Urschitz MS, Eggebrecht E, Schlaud M, Poets CF. Sleep problems and poor academic performance in primary school children. Somnologie. 2011;15:243–8. https://doi.org/10.1007/s11818-011-0535-8.
120. Swart ML, Van Schagen AM, Lancee J, Van Den Bout J. Prevalence of nightmare disorder in psychiatric outpatients. Psychother Psychosom. 2013;82(4):267–8. https://doi.org/10.1159/000343590.
121. Högl B, Iranzo A. Rapid eye movement sleep behavior disorder and other rapid eye movement sleep parasomnias. Continuum (Minneap Minn). 2017;23(4):1017–34. https://doi.org/10.1212/CON.0000000000000489.
122. Abbott SM, Reid KJ, Zee PC. Circadian rhythm sleep-wake disorders. Psychiatr Clin N Am. 2015;38(4):805–23. https://doi.org/10.1016/j.psc.2015.07.012.
123. Culnan E, McCullough LM, Wyatt JK. Circadian rhythm sleep-wake phase disorders. Neurol Clin. 2019;37(3):527–43. https://doi.org/10.1016/j.ncl.2019.04.003.

Personality Disorders

24

Paul S. Links, James Ross,
and Philippe-Edouard Boursiquot

Historical Background and Current Approaches to Diagnosis

Conceptualizations of personality are long-standing and can be found in ancient Chinese and Greek philosophical traditions [1]. They have continued to change in nature, and their scope has been focused with the use of empirical approaches for the study of personality (Figs. 24.1 and 24.2) and personality disorders (PDs). Additionally, strides in neuroscience have provided neuroanatomical substrates for aspects of personality (Fig. 24.3). Although PDs are now found in the main classification systems (Diagnostic and Statistical Manual of Mental Disorders, 5th edition [DSM-5] and International Classification of Diseases for Mortality and Morbidity Statistics 11th edition [ICD-11]), there is an ongoing debate regarding the preferable approach to diagnosing these conditions, namely whether the use of a categorical system (presence or absence of a specific PD), of a dimensional system (degree of personality traits), or of a hybrid system is more appropriate [2]. In psychology, the self-report five-factor (agreeableness, conscientiousness, extraversion, openness, and neuroticism) model has become a reference for normal and abnormal personality dimensions; its use for clinician-based measurements and the assessment of psychopathology has been difficult due to, in part, its heterogeneity in clinical populations [3]. The DSM-5's alternative model for PDs proposes a hybrid approach while remaining oriented toward the categorical system of the prior edition, DSM-IV-Text Revision, given its more practical nature. In

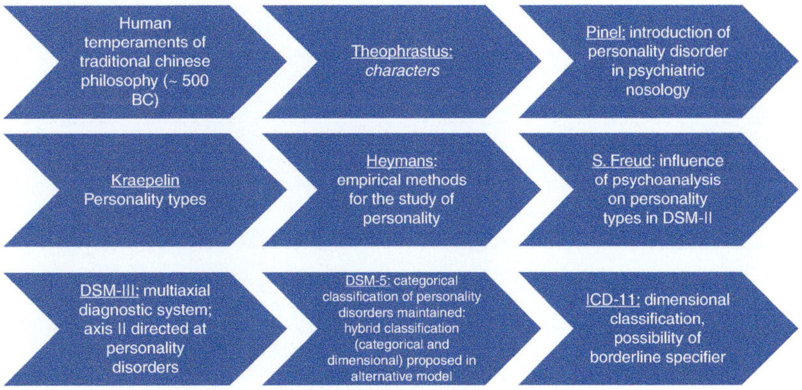

Fig. 24.1 Timeline of classification of personality disorders

P. S. Links (✉) · P.-E. Boursiquot
Department of Psychiatry and Behavioural Neurosciences, McMaster University, Dundas, ON, Canada
e-mail: paul.links@lhsc.on.ca; linksp@mcmaster.ca; boursipe@mcmaster.ca

J. Ross
Department of Psychiatry, Schulich School of Medicine and Dentistry, University of Western Ontario, Parkwood Mental Health Institute, London, ON, Canada
e-mail: james.ross@lhsc.on.ca

W. W. IsHak (ed.), *Atlas of Psychiatry*, https://doi.org/10.1007/978-3-031-15401-0_24

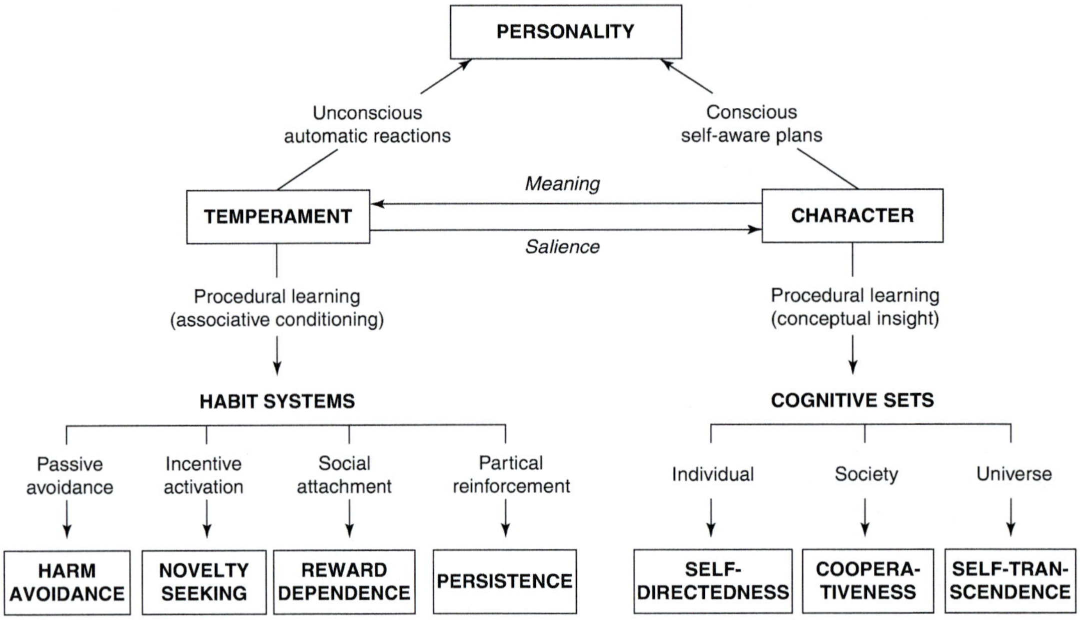

Fig. 24.2 Personality: an integrated psychobiological schema

Fig. 24.3 Personality markers in the brain

PERSONALITY MARKERS IN THE BRAIN		
Extroversion	Extrovents have reduced activity, in response to stimuli, in the neural circuit that keeps the brain aroused (showen here). As aresult, they need more environmental stimuli to keep them feeling energized.	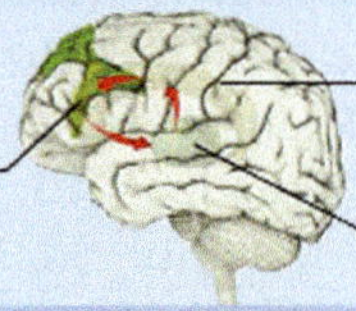
Aggression	People with a version of a gene previously linked to impulsive violence show abnormally redused volume and unusually low activity in the cingulate cortex-an area concernrd with monitoring and guiding behavior.	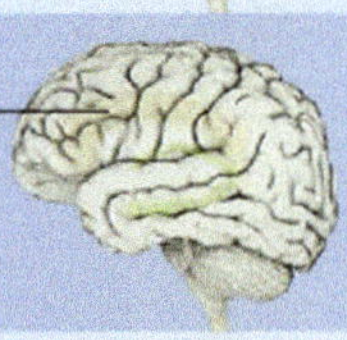
Social behaviour	Socially secure people have a stromger response to friendly looking people in the striatum—tan area concerned with reward—than shy people. Avoidant types shoe a stronger reaction in the amygdala to unfriendly looking people.	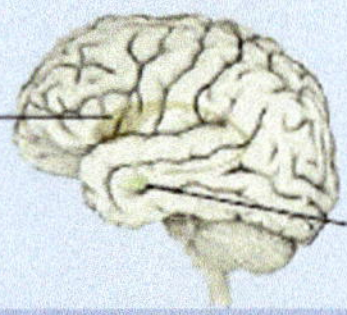
Novelty seeking	People who like novelty may have better connections between areas shown here. The hippocampus sends signals to the striatum—which registers pleasure—when it identifies an experience as new	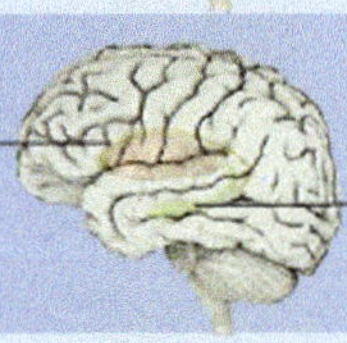
Coorperation	Coorperative people shoe increased activity in the insula if they think their treatment is unfair. Uncooparative people do not register unfairness to the same extent, suggesting an underdeveloped sense of trust.	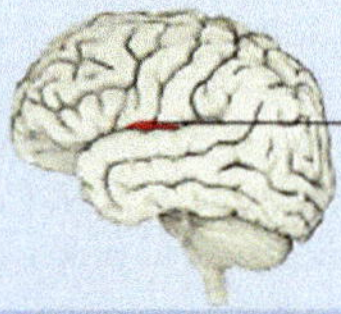
Optimism	Optimism is linked to enhanced activation in the amygdala and in the anrtior cingulate cortex when imagining positive future events relative to negative ones.	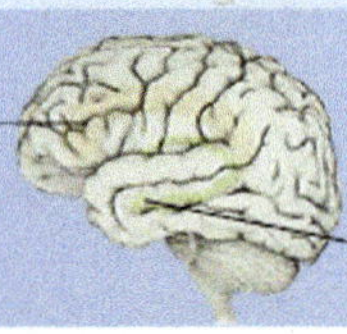

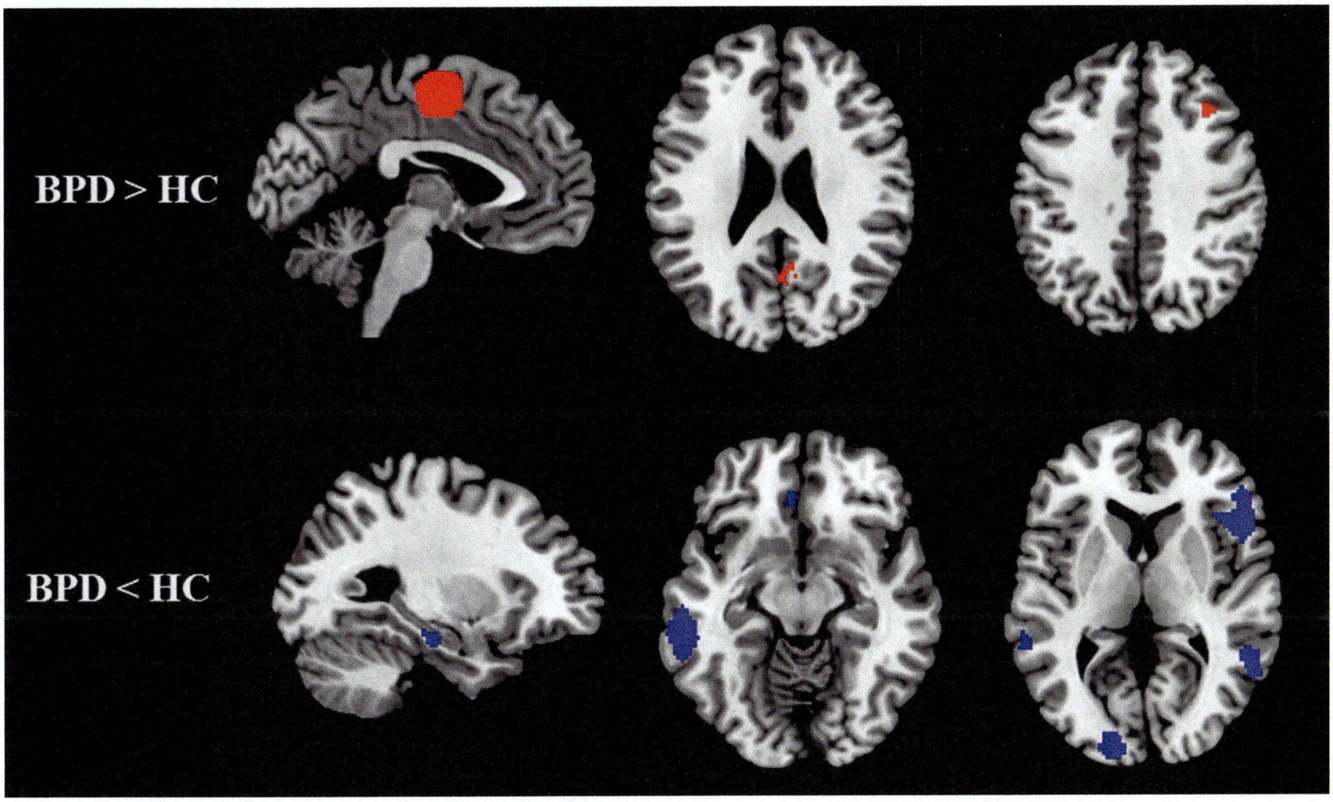

Fig. 24.4 Regions showing gray matter alteration in BPD patients compared with health controls. (From Yang et al. [49] Creative Commons Attribution 4.0 International License; Creative Commons Attribution 4.0 International License; http://creativecommons.org/licenses/by/4.0/)

the DSM-5 alternative model, which is not currently used in practice, self and interpersonal dysfunction is required for the diagnosis, and traits subsumed under five domains (negative affectivity, detachment, antagonism, disinhibition, and psychoticism) provide a dimensional lens to this diagnosis. The following categorical diagnoses (antisocial, avoidant, borderline, obsessive-compulsive, narcissistic, and schizotypal) can be made using this approach; additionally, a personality disorder—trait specified diagnosis— can also be made [4]. There is a departure from the categorical approach in ICD-11 by adopting a fully dimensional model, with the exception of a borderline specifier, in reference to BPD [5].

Researchers are investigating the existence of a general factor of personality impairment—or of general psychopathology—(*g* factor, *p* factor), which may enhance the coherence of PD assessment [6, 7]. There is nevertheless value in specific ("s") factors to identify distinct aspects of personality pathology [6] (Fig. 24.4).

Table 24.1 summarizes the advantages and disadvantages of categorical versus dimensional classifications for PDs.

Table 24.1 Advantages and disadvantages of categorical and dimensional approaches to PD classification

Categorical approach	Dimensional approach
Advantages: – Facilitates communication with other health care professionals and agencies – Allows to expand existing body of research	**Advantages**: – Possibly increased validity of PD diagnoses – Facilitates universality of PD diagnosis [3]
Disadvantages: – Half of patients meeting criteria for a PD do not fall in a specific category [2]	**Disadvantages**: – Potential threat to reliability of PD diagnoses – Difficult to maintain existing PD constructs

Importance of Personality Disorder Diagnoses

Clinicians should recognize the importance of making personality disorder diagnoses as these diagnoses have important implications for understanding and managing patients with complex presentations. A personality diagnosis can be related to the risk of suicidal behavior and suicide, impact patients' general functioning, and lead to comorbid psychiatric and medical problems. The next section of the chapter will also briefly discuss how the clinician can approach making the diagnosis of a personality disorder during a clinical assessment.

Clinicians should recognize that personality disorders are common in making up about 10% of the general population and are much more common in clinical psychiatric settings. For example, 25% of outpatients in psychiatric services and up to 50% of psychiatric inpatients may meet criteria for personality disorders. A diagnosis of a personality disorder also places the patient at increased risk for suicide. Estimates suggested patients with borderline personality disorder have a 3–10% lifetime risk of suicide while patients with antisocial personality disorder have a 5% lifetime risk of suicide [8]. Other personality disorder diagnoses from the so-called cluster A and cluster C diagnoses also are associated with increased risk of suicide but perhaps less so than borderline and antisocial personality disorder.

Establishing a personality disorder diagnosis increases the risk that the patient may have a coexisting clinical disorder (also referred to as "symptom disorders"). In the next sections of this chapter, we discuss the likely comorbidities that are found with the more prevalent personality disorders. The coexistence of clinical disorders with personality disorders in general diminishes patients' response to standard treatments for these clinical disorders. For example, the coexistence of major depression with a personality disorder likely doubles the risk of a poor outcome from treatment and increases the risk of recurrence for depression and many of the symptom disorders [9].

Although the etiology of personality disorders is not well understood, 40–50% of the total prototypic variance in personality function and characteristics in general is related to genetic factors. Research evidence suggests that parental pathology, family breakdown, and traumatic life events are risk factors for developing personality disorders in vulnerable people. Therefore, personality disorders are excellent examples of the interplay between genetic vulnerability plus developmental psychological and social adversity that led to the expression of adult personality disorders. Figure 24.5 depicts the relationship between childhood traumatic experience and personality disorder traits.

Although personality disorders were originally thought to be lifetime diagnoses, important research has clarified that remission from personality disorder diagnoses is quite common; for example, with borderline personality disorder more than 80% of patients will no longer meet criteria for borderline personality disorder over 10 years follow-up [10]. In general, a remission from the diagnosis of borderline personality disorder is relatively stable; however, approximately 10–15% of patients have a relapse to meeting full criteria for borderline personality disorder over the period of 10 years follow-up [10]. Research indicates remission rates are generally similar for avoidant, obsessive-compulsive, and schizotypal personality disorder.

Personality disorders tend to wax and wane over the years, although elements of their difficulties with interpersonal functioning and self-image may be persistent. Personality disordered individuals are more likely to be separated, divorced, and never married [11]. In terms of work performance, personality disordered patients may be more educated but demonstrate poor job performance in relationship to their academic achievements. They have difficulties with interpersonal relationships, and of course, these difficulties can affect their work performance. One aspect that is unclear from previous research is whether this dysfunction is mainly attributable to the personality disorder diagnosis or to the frequent comorbid clinical syndromes that are found in these patients.

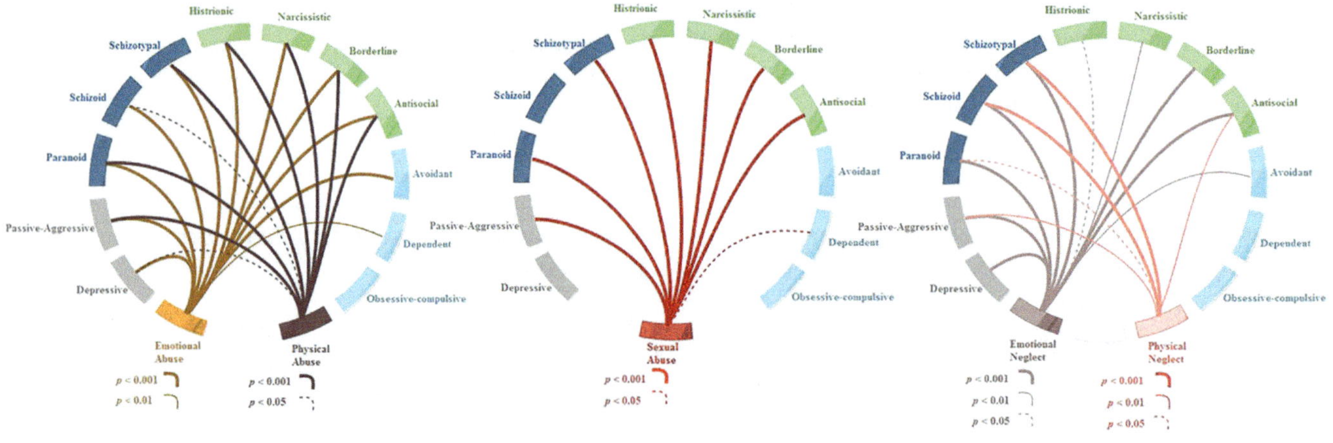

Fig. 24.5 Spearman correlation between childhood traumatic experience and personality disorder traits. (From Yang et al. [49] Creative Commons Attribution 4.0 International License; Creative Commons Attribution 4.0 International License; http://creativecommons.org/licenses/by/4.0/)

Recognizing Patients with Personality Disorders

When assessing patients, one of the primary questions is whether patients are suffering from a clinical disorder or a personality disorder. Besides carefully reviewing the patients' symptoms, it will be important to examine the course of symptoms over time. Clinical disorders tend to remit and recur while personality disorder features tend to wax and wane but some residual problems particularly with self-image and interpersonal functioning may persist. Are the symptoms ego-dystonic or ego-syntonic? Personality disorder characteristics are more likely to be ego-syntonic, and persons may be presenting because of the difficulties they have created for others. When dealing with such patients, recognize how the patients make you feel and observe and reflect on your initial encounters with the patients. You may experience a feeling of being coerced by the patients' interactions, you may have a strong emotional reaction to these patients, and such responses may lead you to consider the possibility of a personality disorder diagnosis. However, remember if you are left frustrated by the encounter, be cautious, many patients can provoke these feelings and they may not necessarily have a personality disorder.

The clinicians should pay attention to the factors that raised their suspicion about the presence of a personality disorder and then see how these factors converge with the essential features of a personality disorder as outlined in the DSM-5 text [4]. For example, if patients present with a pattern of grandiosity and seek admiration, then the clinician should be suspicious of a narcissistic personality disorder. If patients appear anxious and inhibited and present a story of general social inhibition, then the clinician should be on the lookout for avoidant personality disorder. Once the clinician has in mind a particular personality disorder, then seek further evidence for this disorder by examining the patients' interpersonal functioning over time and from their interactions in the clinical interview. Subsequently, the clinician can try to confirm the diagnosis by referring to the full DSM criteria for the specific personality disorder. It is also helpful for clinicians to think about the setting in which they are working because some personality disorders are more common in certain settings. For example, borderline personality disorder is known to be a common diagnosis among patients presenting to emergency departments with suicidality. As discussed below, certain symptom disorders are more common with certain personality disorder diagnoses, and this can be helpful on deciding the personality disorder diagnosis. Personality disorders tend to run in families so the family history of psychiatric illness can also be useful. In addition, the clinicians need to review patients' developmental history for a history of adversity, trauma, or neglect, look for recurrent patterns of interpersonal difficulties, and assess the patients overall functioning.

Although working with personality disorder patients can be challenging, it can also be very rewarding. These patients provoke emotional responses in clinicians, but they often have experienced significant rejection and stigma during interactions with mental health workers. Sharing with the patient your impressions about the diagnosis and the possible management approaches can instill hope in patients and their families.

Antisocial Personality Disorder

ASPD, after BPD, is the second most studied personality disorder in the literature. Similar to BPD, emotion dysregulation and trait impulsivity are key constructs in ASPD. In DSM-5, ASPD has been defined behaviorally in contrast to psychopathy (there is debate as to whether psychopathy is distinct from or a more severe form of ASPD—Fig. 24.6), whose hallmarks include affective features (shallow affect) and interpersonal components (manipulativeness and callousness) in addition to behavioral disturbances [12] (Fig. 24.7). The etiology, pathophysiology, and comorbid disorders of ASPD are presented in Table 24.2.

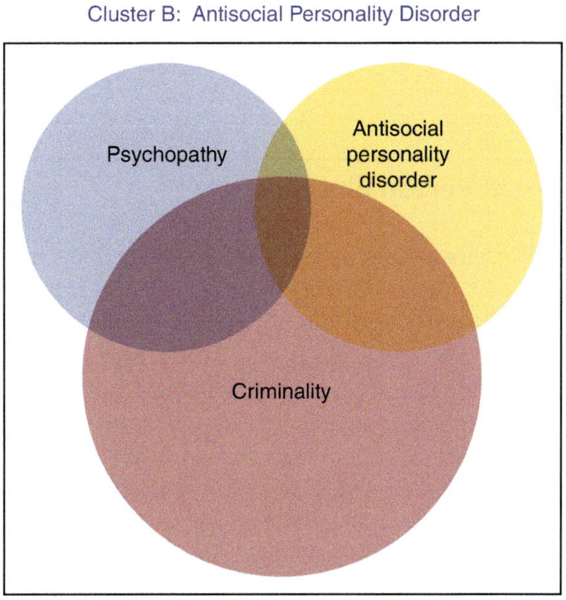

Fig. 24.6 Distinction and overlap between antisocial personality disorder, psychopathy, and criminality

Fig. 24.7 Factor structure of psychopathy

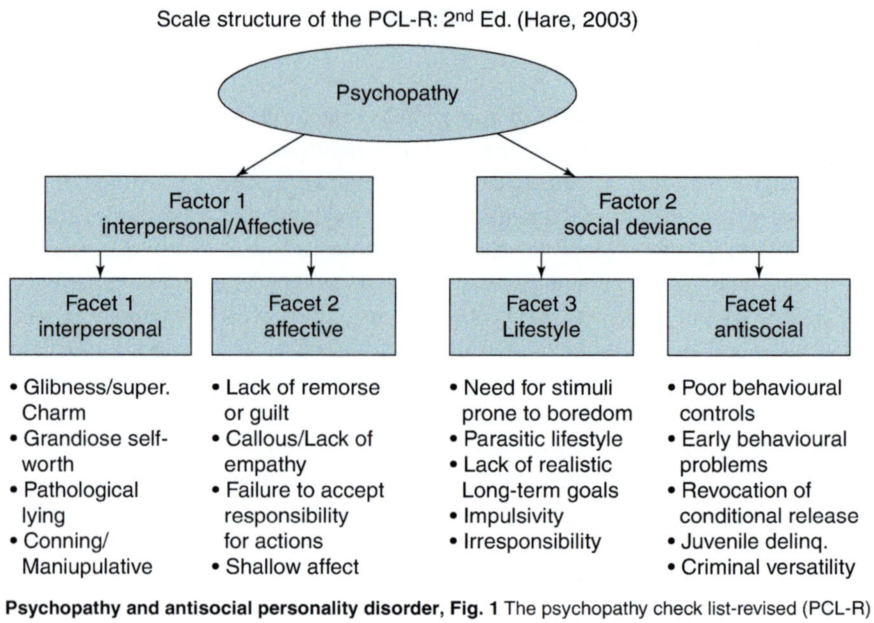

Table 24.2 Antisocial personality disorder: etiology, pathophysiology, and comorbid disorders

Antisocial personality disorder		
Epidemiology	Prevalence: 2–3% of population 3% in men, 1% in women In prison samples, 47% in men, 21% in women	Stability of diagnosis: – Conduct disorder before age 15
Etiology and pathophysiology	Psychosocial: – Low quality of early care – Confounding with genetic factors	Genetic: – Role of genetics more extensive in relatives of females with ASPD – Genetic factors more important in explaining life course in offenders
Comorbid disorders	– Psychopathy – Mood disorders – Substance use disorders – Somatic symptom disorder – Borderline personality disorder	

Avoidant Personality Disorder

AVPD is characterized by social inhibition, feelings of inadequacy, and hypersensitivity to negative evaluation [13]. Those with AVPD tend to have a sense of inferiority when comparing themselves with others and expect rejection. Their sense of identity involves "malignant self-regard," in which poor interpersonal relationships are attributed to oneself, which in turn leads to worse negative self-concept [14]. Unrealistic, perfectionistic standards and expectations of rejection or criticism often lead to behavioral inhibition and avoidance, meaning that individuals with AVPD have limited self-direction and can be significantly psychosocially impaired and may have limitations in their ability to work and make friendships [14]. Deficits in mentalization (thinking about one's own and others' actions in terms of thoughts and feelings and using this knowledge to guide action and reflection in day to day life) [15] or avoidance of mentalization can result from the pervasive need to avoid emotions in an attempt to avoid rejection. Alexithymia, difficulty identifying or articulating emotional states, is often present. Intimacy is impaired as the individual is caught in an "approach-avoidance" conflict or "fearful attachment style" where a desire for intimacy is undermined by interpersonal distrust and fear of rejection. In established relationships, the individual with AVPD will be restrained, often with an anxious/avoidant attachment style [14]. (In an anxious/avoidant attachment style, individuals have developed a tendency, through innate temperament and developmental experiences, to feel insecure in relationships, which leads them to deny their interpersonal emotions or avoid intimacy in relationships [Tables 24.3 and 24.4; Figs. 24.8 and 24.9]).

Table 24.3 Avoidant personality disorder: epidemiology, etiology, and comorbid disorders

Avoidant personality disorder		
Epidemiology	Incidence: – 1.5–2.5% of population – 14.7% of psychiatric outpatients – F > M in some studies	Stability of diagnosis (CLPS, 2004): – 12 months remission rate of 31% – 50% still met criteria at 2 years after initial Dx
Etiology and pathophysiology	Psychosocial: – Millon: early interactions with parents as an important factor – Those with AVPD report fewer positive relationships with older adults with less sexual abuse or physical neglect than other PDs	Genetic: Heritability of 0.64. Temperament characterized by personality rigidity, hypersensitivity, high harm avoidance, low novelty seeking, and overactive behavioral inhibition – Genetic influences on AVPD found to be stable over time (Norwegian twin study)
Comorbid disorders	– Co-occurrence estimates with Social Anxiety Disorder estimated to be 40%, with some studies estimating 88–100% – Large community studies have found that 2/3 of those in this setting meeting criteria for AVPD do not meet additional criteria for SAD – 59% of those with dependent PD also found to meet criteria for AVPD (Stuart)	

From Weinbrecht et al. [13]; *with permission*)

Table 24.4 Social anxiety disorder vs. AVPD phenomenology

Area of pathology	Social anxiety	Avoidant PD	May present in both
Key features	Anxiety about social situations in which the individual is exposed to scrutiny by others and may exhibit anxiety symptoms that will be negatively evaluated	Social inhibition, feelings of inadequacy and hypersensitivity to negative evaluation Fear of relationships with others	Avoidance of social situations (AVPD may involve more avoidance of relationships in general)
Reaction to perceived scrutiny or judgment	Anxiety, avoidance of situations	Self-criticism, worse self-esteem, "malignant self-regard"	
Impairment	Mainly in situations involving new people or social gatherings	Impairment in family relationships and other situations involving intimacy	
Cognitive aspects	Avoidance of social situations, use of safety behaviors that limit evidence that others are scrutinizing them or any signs of anxiety from the patient	Avoidance or deficits in self-reflexive functioning, emotions and mentalization	
Affective	Global anhedonia or alexithymia not characteristic	Anhedonia and/or alexithymia often present	

From Weinbrecht et al. [13]; *with permission*

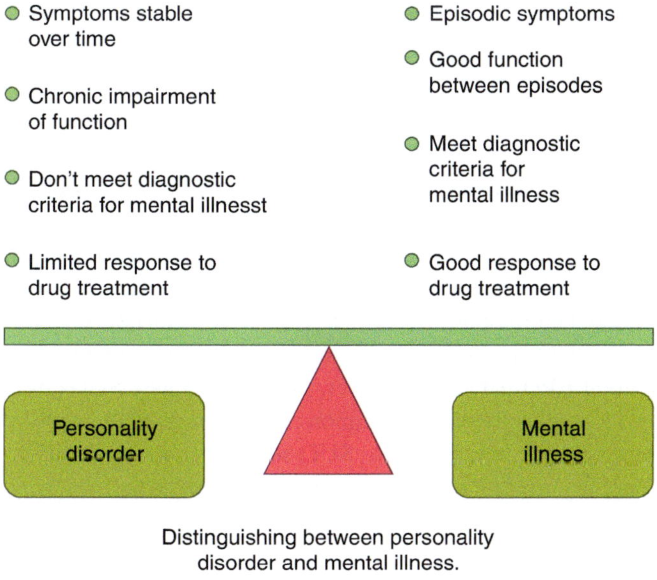

Fig. 24.8 Distinguishing between personality disorders and mental illness

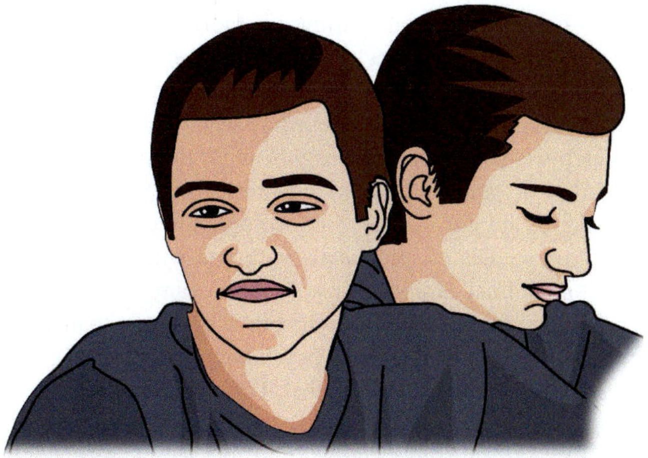

Fig. 24.9 Avoidant personality disorder (AVPD)

Borderline Personality Disorder

BPD is characterized by dysregulation of behaviors, interpersonal dysfunction, dysregulation of emotion, and instability of identity, which contribute to marked impairment in personal, social, and occupational functioning. As shown in Table 24.5, the disorder is prevalent in the community [16] and is associated with considerable morbidity and mortality, leading to substantial societal costs through premature death and the high utilization of health care services [17, 18].

The diagnosis of borderline personality disorder was first introduced into the psychiatric diagnostic classification with the publication of DSM-III (the overall history of personality diagnoses is discussed above). There are now three different approaches to diagnosing BPD:

- Categorical: DSM-5—No changes were made to the BPD diagnosis from the DSM-IVTR version.
- Hybrid—The new alternative model that appears in the Section 3 in DSM 5 is included to encourage further study. In this model, BPD is included as one of six types of personality disorder.
- Dimensional—ICD11 classification of personality disorders only refers to a single **dimension** of severity for all personality dysfunction, ranging from normal (non-disordered) personality to severe personality disorder. However, a Borderline pattern qualifier was included, and the description of the features of this pattern qualifier is adapted from DSM-5 criteria for the categorical diagnosis for BPD.

Since the introduction of DSM-III in 1980 and criteria for BPD, an extensive body of research has flourished over the last four decades. The first two decades of studies, mainly studying clinical samples, demonstrated the frequent occurrence of clinical psychiatric (Axis I; symptom disorders) disorders both current and lifetime, in individuals with BPD [16]. In the last two decades, the research has advanced to include community samples that avoid the bias created by researching only individuals who seek treatment. This research has provided new insights about the occurrence of comorbid disorders in community residents [9]. The other advance in the last decade is the completion of prospective follow-up studies of individuals with and without PDs [9]. The longitudinal designs allow for the examination of the temporal relationship between disorders and begin to characterize how BPD and clinical psychiatric disorders may be etiologically related to one another. The central findings from prospective longitudinal research of the associations between BPD and Axis I disorders leads to the following conclusions. Although many Axis I disorders are found to be comorbid with BPD, mood and anxiety disorders appear most interrelated. For example, remissions of BPD predict the remission of comorbid major depressive disorder and lessen the risk of future major depressive episodes in patients with BPD; thus, treatment interventions for BPD psychopathology must be undertaken to address this comorbidity. Substance use disorders (SUD) represent a recurrent and intermittent problem among BPD patients; however, the onset of new SUDs over the course of BPD is uncommon. The absence of SUD or the remission from a comorbid SUD seems to positively impact the early course of BPD, perhaps over the first 5–7 years. However, over the longer term, the course of BPD is less

Table 24.5 Borderline personality disorder: epidemiology, etiology, and comorbid disorders

Borderline personality disorder		
Epidemiology	Prevalence—general population Mean 1.6% Prevalence—Clinical samples 28% of all patients in outpatients or hospitals 6% of primary care visits 10–15% of all emergency department visits	Stability of diagnosis More than 80% of patients will no longer meet criteria for borderline personality disorder over 10 years follow-up Remission is relatively stable 10–15% of patients relapse to meeting full criteria over the period of 10 years follow-up
Etiology and pathophysiology	Psychosocial evidence supports a **gene X environment interaction**, with adversity throughout childhood and adolescence increasing the risk of BPD in individuals with sensitive genotypes	Genetic Heritability of BPD is ~55% Twin studies suggest a single factor model for liability to BPD rather than a collection of separate traits
Comorbid disorders	Many clinical disorders are found to be comorbid with BPD, mood and anxiety disorders most common Three or more comorbid disorders characteristic of individuals with BPD Remissions of BPD predict the remission of comorbid major depressive disorder Absence of substance abuse disorders or the remission from a comorbid substance abuse disorder seems to improve the early course of BPD	

From Gunderson et al. [47]; *with permission*

Table 24.6 Three different approaches to diagnosing BPD

Diagnostic and statistical manual (DSM)-5 criteria adapted	DSM-5 alternative model—adapted	International classification of disease (ICD) 11 adapted
Categorical	Hybrid -A and B must be met	Dimensional
Five or more of nine criteria	Criterion A—impairment in personality functioning—difficulties in two or more of the following four areas: Identity Self-direction Empathy Intimacy	Classification of personality disorders only refers to a single dimension of severity for all personality dysfunction, ranging from normal (non-disordered) personality to severe personality disorder.
No changes made to the BPD diagnosis from the DSM-IVTR version Abandonment fears Unstable/intense relationships Unstable self-image Impulsivity Recurrent suicidality Affective instability Chronic emptiness Inappropriate anger Paranoid ideation, dissociative symptoms	Criterion B—four or more of the following seven pathological personality traits, at least one of which is impulsivity, risk-taking, or hostility: Emotional liability Anxiousness Separation insecurity Depressivity Impulsivity Risk-taking Hostility	Borderline pattern qualifier was included and the description of the features of this pattern qualifier is adapted from DSM-5 criteria for the categorical diagnosis for BPD

Table 24.7 BPD comorbidity: which disorder is primary? (inserted below)

Disorder	BPD primary disorder	Rationale
Depression	Yes	Will remit if BPD does
Bipolar—mania	No	Unable to use BPD therapy
Bipolar—not manic	Both	Independent courses
Bipolar II	?	More research needed
Generalized and/or social anxiety disorder	Yes	Will remit if BPD does
PTSD—early onset (complex)	No	Too vigilant to attach/be challenged
PTSD—adult onset	Yes	BPD predisposes; will remit if BPD does
Substance use disorder—dependency	No	2–6 months sobriety makes BPD therapy feasible
Substance use disorder—abuse	Probable	Concurrent treatment required
Antisocial personality disorder	?	Are there secondary gains?
Narcissistic personality disorder (NPD)	Yes	Regulate with BPD therapy then individual work for NPD
Eating disorder—anorexia	No	Unable to use BPD therapy
Eating disorder—bulimia	?	Concurrent treatment if physically stable; independent courses

Table 24.8 Borderline personality disorder (BPD) and risk of suicide (inserted below)

Lifetime risk for suicide estimated to be 3–10.3%
Represent 9–33% of all suicides
Half of the chronically suicidal patients seen in the Emergency Department meet criteria for BPD
History of suicidal behavior in 60–78% of individuals with BPD

determined by the presence or absence of Axis I pathology and is more related to temperament and childhood antecedents. Finally, eating disorders are found to be comorbid with BPD; however, the nature of the relationship between these two disorders is less clear, and they appear more independent of each other than say mood disorders, anxiety disorders, and BPD (Tables 24.5, 24.6, and 24.7).

Suicide Risk

The rate of suicide in BPD has been estimated to range as high as 10% and as low as 0%, depending on the setting, patient characteristics, and method of study. In their 27-year follow-up study of patients previously hospitalized with a diagnosis of BPD, Paris and Zweig-Frank reported a suicide rate of 10% [17, 19]. Several recent prospective studies, however, have found a lower rate of suicide. In a 10-year prospective study by Zanarini and colleagues, the rate of death by suicide was only 4% [20]. This same cohort at 24 years of prospective follow-up demonstrated a 5.9% rate of death by suicide [21]. Among patients with BPD recruited at the Austen Riggs voluntary residential treatment center and followed in treatment for 7 years, Perry et al. found no deaths by suicides [22]. Links, Kolla, Guimond, and McMain [23] in a prospective follow-up study of BPD patients who received 1 year of BPD-indicated treatment found that none died by suicide over 1 year of treatment and 2 years of follow-up. These results suggest that patients receiving regular outpatient treatment may be at significantly lower risk compared with an untreated or undertreated population of patients with BPD. The rate of attempted suicide in BPD is much higher than the rate of suicide in these patients, and it is estimated that around 85% of patients have a history of such behavior (Table 24.8) [17].

A review of risk factors within BPD samples [24] summarized statistically significant characteristics related to the

Table 24.9 Risk factors for suicide attempts within BPD (inserted below)

Risk factors	Strength of association
Older age	+
Female	+
Living alone	+
Major depressive disorder	+
Substance abuse	+
Psychosis	+
Low Global Adjustment Scale score	+
Previous attempts	++
Impulsivity	+
Antisocial traits	+
Childhood sexual abuse	++
Low Social Adjustment Scale score	++
Psychiatric hospitalizations	++

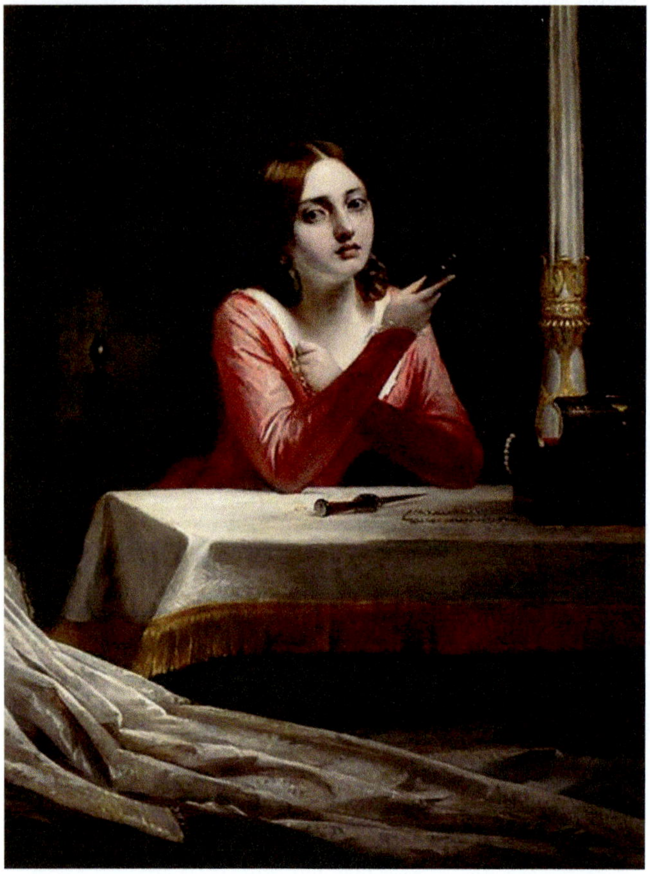

Fig. 24.10 Managing suicide risk in patients with BPD

outcome of suicide and attempted suicide found in more than one study. Major risk factors for suicide were older age, a family history of substance abuse, comorbid substance abuse disorder, comorbid PDs, any Cluster B PD, and Antisocial PD comorbidity. Major depressive disorder comorbidity, previous suicide attempts, a low social adjustment, and psychiatric hospitalization predicted most strongly suicide attempts (Table 24.9; Fig. 24.10).

Narcissistic Personality Disorder

The concept of narcissistic personality disorder has a rich tradition going back to the myth of Narcissus, a young man who fell in love with his own reflection in the fountain. The primary concept of exaggerated states of self-love still seems to be a central element of this disorder. In DSM-5, narcissistic personality disorder is characterized by the identifying features of the person being "arrogant, grandiose, assertive, and aggressive," and this has been described as narcissistic grandiosity [25, 26]. In terms of pathological narcissism, many have argued that two clinical phenotypes of the disorder may present themselves: narcissistic grandiosity and narcissistic vulnerability [27]. Patients with narcissistic vulnerability are "shy, vulnerable, insecure, and shame-ridden" [25, 26]. In terms of interpersonal style, grandiose narcissistic patients demonstrate domineering, vindictive, and intrusive interpersonal behaviors [28]. The vulnerable narcissistic patient interpersonally is cold and aloof and socially avoidant and often senses being taken advantage in their relationships [28]. Although the presentation of narcissistic pathology can be varied, the clinical presentations of narcissistic patients are felt to arise from self-esteem dysregulation, affect dysregulation, and difficulties in interpersonal relationships that characterize pathological narcissism [25]. Overall, the clinical and empirical literature supports the existence of at least two distinct types of narcissistic presentations (Fig. 24.11; Table 24.10) [25].

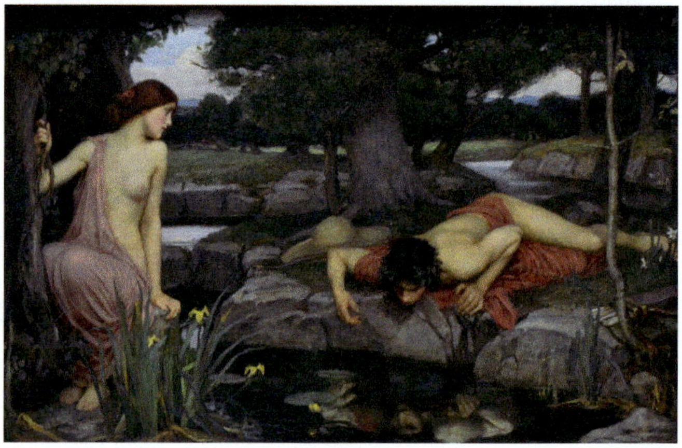

Fig. 24.11 Narcissistic psychopathology

Table 24.10 Narcissistic personality disorder: characteristics (inserted below)

May present as narcissistic grandiosity and/or narcissistic vulnerability
Grandiose—arrogance, assertiveness, and aggressive
Vulnerable—shyness, insecurity, and shame
Lesser impairment in quality of life; can be adaptive
Stable course—improvements can occur related to achievements, relationships or disillusionments

Table 24.11 Narcissistic personality disorder: epidemiology, etiology, and comorbid disorders

Etiology and pathophysiology	Psychosocial Kernberg (1975)—"conflict model" where early childhood experiences of cold, indifferent, or aggressive parenting lead to the child developing feelings of specialness as a retreat Kohut (1971)—"deficit model" of narcissistic personality that arose because parents failure to empathize with their child and the grandiose self emerges to defend the child Core feature dysregulated self-esteem	Genetic Limited research—one study heritability of 24%
Comorbid disorders	Comorbid bipolar affective disorder and/or alcohol use disorders Comorbid with anxiety disorders, anorexia nervosa and post-traumatic stress disorder	

From Yakeley et al. [34]; with permission

In spite of the limited research on NPD, several authors have argued based on clinical experience or studies of trait narcissism that the consequences of narcissism for clinical practice are very significant. Ronningstan [29] and Links [30] have argued that narcissism has a unique association to the risk of suicide over and above the existence of comorbid depression. In addition, the risk of suicide can onset in very dramatic fashion so that narcissistic pathology is important to recognize in patients at risk for suicide. Miller et al. [31] were able to relate narcissistic pathology to aggression in provoked and non-provoked interactions. Narcissistic traits make the person vulnerable to a "self-serving bias" or taking credit for success but blaming others for failure. Narcissistic pathology is related to interpersonal dysfunction and is related to causing distress in others [32]. Miller et al. [32] found that narcissistic pathology was related to various maladaptive behaviors such as pathological gambling, alcohol abuse, compulsive spending, and antisocial behavior. Psychological distress appears less directly related to narcissistic pathology but may arise because of the person's impaired functioning. Finally, the narcissistic person will lack insight into their difficulties. Overall, these authors have argued that a body of related research suggests that understanding narcissistic personality disorder (or patients with significant narcissistic pathology) has considerable clinical utility and these understandings can assist in delivering effect psychotherapy interventions.

Table 24.11 provides a summary of the epidemiology, etiology, and pathophysiology and comorbid disorders related to NPD [33, 34].

Suicide Risk

Data on narcissistic PD and suicide risk are limited but growing. Narcissistic PD may have a very unique relationship to suicide; an individual demonstrating grandiose characteristics may be protected against suicidality versus those with vulnerable characteristics that increase the person's risk. Narcissistic PD also may confer a risk more related to death by suicide than suicide attempts as patients with narcissistic PD may carry out very lethal attempts and hold various motives for their actions, e.g., wanting death before dishonor, but no conscious intention to die (Table 24.12; Fig. 24.11) [35].

Table 24.12 Managing suicidal patients with pathological narcissism (inserted below)

Monitor for evidence of coexisting major depression
Watch for an acute episode of lowered self-esteem resulting from a narcissistic injury
Directly inquire about suicidal thoughts, planning, and intent
Educate significant others about the likely acute onset of suicidality, how to seek emergency help and reduce access to means of suicide (e.g. guns in the home)
Seek permission to communicate patient's safety plan to others as part of the therapeutic contract
Stable therapeutic relationship may lessen suicide risk
Threatened intimate relationship often leads to a suicidal crisis; couple interventions may be helpful

Obsessive Compulsive Personality Disorder

In DSM-5, OCPD is described as "preoccupation with orderliness, perfectionism, and mental and interpersonal control at the expense of flexibility, openness, and efficiency" [4]. Those with OCPD take roles very seriously and often favor doing things themselves rather than delegate to someone else. Their sense of identity is often caught between an outward sense of duty and an inner shame or self-doubt [36]. While often rigid in their opinions and routines, those with OCPD may have difficulty with self-direction since ambivalence and pathological doubt in decision-making can be paralyzing [36]. Future planning will usually be favored over enjoyment in the present, and minute details will be seen rather than a broader picture [37]. Intellectualization, isolation of affect, and a preoccupation with the rational over the emotional make empathizing with others a challenge for many with OCPD. Intimacy is difficult in OCPD, since control and rationality are valued highly and interpersonal, emotional situations and the complexity they bring could lead to a loss of control or loss of face, particularly with regard to emotionality or libidinal drives (Tables 24.13, 24.14, and 24.15; Fig. 24.12) [38].

Table 24.13 Obsessive compulsive personality disorder: epidemiology, etiology, and comorbid Disorders

Obsessive-compulsive personality disorder		
Epidemiology	– Lifetime prevalence 3–8% in community samples – Increased incidence in older, less educated – The most common PD in the general population – Third most common PD in general outpatients, with point prevalence of 8.7% – Second most common PD in inpatients with a rate of 23.3% – Conflicting evidence M = F vs. M > F prevalence	Stability of diagnosis: – In one study (Shea), 58% no longer met diagnostic criteria at 12 months – Grilo et al. found remission rate of 38% within 24 months F/U (<2 criteria for >12 months) – Some OCPD criteria are more stable and may in fact worsen over time
Etiology and Pathophysiology	Psychosocial: Two studies provide evidence of relationship between OCPD and insecure attachment, with having received less care and overprotection in childhood, leading to limited emotional and empathetic development	Genetic: empirical evidence supports heritability of OCPD but inconsistent findings, with heritability between 0.27 and 0.78 in different studies
Comorbid Disorders	Anxiety disorders: Lifetime Dx OCPD present in 23–38% with panic disorder, 34% with GAD, 33% with social anxiety disorder Affective disorders: Lifetime Dx OCPD present in 23–28% with MDD (unipolar) and 26–39% with bipolar disorder OCPD has been found to be present in 22.9–34.7% of those with OCD Increasing evidence of high co-occurrence with Cluster A personalities	

From Diedrich and Voderholzer [37]; *with permission*

Table 24.14 Pathology in obsessive-compulsive disorder (OCD) vs. in obsessive-compulsive personality disorder (OCPD)

Area of pathology	OCD	OCPD	May present in both
Experience of obsessive and compulsive thinking	Usually ego-dystonic	Usually ego-syntonic	
Types of compulsivity	Contamination, cleaning, pure obsessions/ intrusive thoughts	Rigidity, excessive self-control	Symmetry, ordering, hoarding
Key features	*Obsessions*—intrusive thoughts and *compulsions*—actions taken to counteract or address obsessions	Preoccupation with orderliness, perfectionism and mental and interpersonal control	Pathological doubt, especially about actions taken or mistakes Perfectionism, inflexibility
Duration	Waxing and waning course, often with distinct episodes and shifting symptoms	Lifelong, may worsen at times of stress	
Thought process	"Magical thinking"—belief in illogical connections between actions and outcomes that is amenable to evaluation with reason but nonetheless makes compulsions feel necessary	Rigid adherence to rules or principles, loss of larger picture for minute details, avoidance of emotionality	

From Diedrich and Voderholzer [37]; *with permission*, and Starcevic et al. [48]; *with permission*

Table 24.15 Domains of schizotypy

Domains of schizotypy
Interpersonal distress
Cognitive-perceptual disturbances
Disorganization

From Debbané et al. [41]; *with permission*

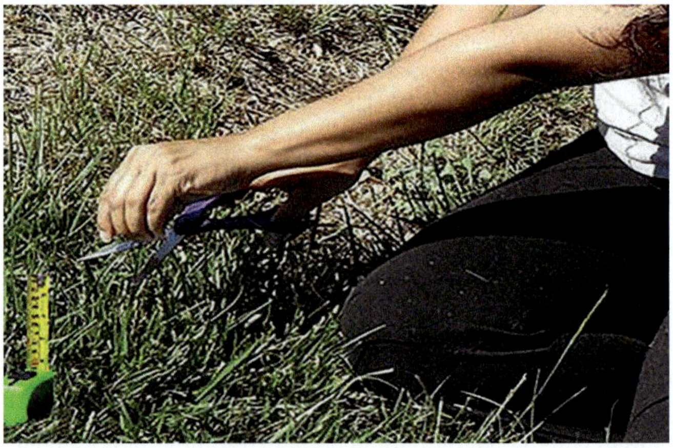

Fig. 24.12 Obsessive compulsive personality disorder (OCPD)

Schizotypal Personality Disorder

Schizotypal personality disorder (STPD) is linked to schizophrenia but sufficiently distinct to stand alone as a separate diagnosis. This is supported by studies of the genetic basis of each condition. STPD rests on the construct of schizotypy [39, 40], which is based on three areas: interpersonal distress, disorganization, and cognitive-perceptual disturbances (Table 24.3) [41]. There can be features of schizotypy in individuals in the general population and in persons with STPD; schizophrenia can be seen as an extreme of this continuum. The individual affected by STPD has acute discomfort in interpersonal settings. There can be disorganization of thought and/or behavior, particularly at times of stress. Unusual thoughts or perceptions can occur. The course of STPD is variable: most individuals have an attenuation of symptoms over time, while a low number progress to schizophrenia. Interpersonal deficits may be more predictive of this poor prognosis. The etiology, pathophysiology, and comorbid disorders of STPD are included in Table 24.16. These, along with the clinical features of STPD, are captured in Fig. 24.13.

Table 24.16 Schizotypal personality disorder: etiology, pathophysiology, and comorbid disorders

Schizotypal personality disorder		
Epidemiology	0.6–4.6% M > F	Stability of diagnosis: – Mainly decreases over time; childhood-onset presentation may be more sustained and severe
Etiology and pathophysiology	Psychosocial: – Child maltreatment	Genetic: – Variable heritability (0.15–0.67)
Comorbid disorders	– Avoidant personality disorder – Obsessive-compulsive disorder – Borderline personality disorder – Major depressive disorder	

From Kirchner et al. [39]; Creative Commons Attribution 4.0 International License; http://creativecommons.org/licenses/by/4.0/

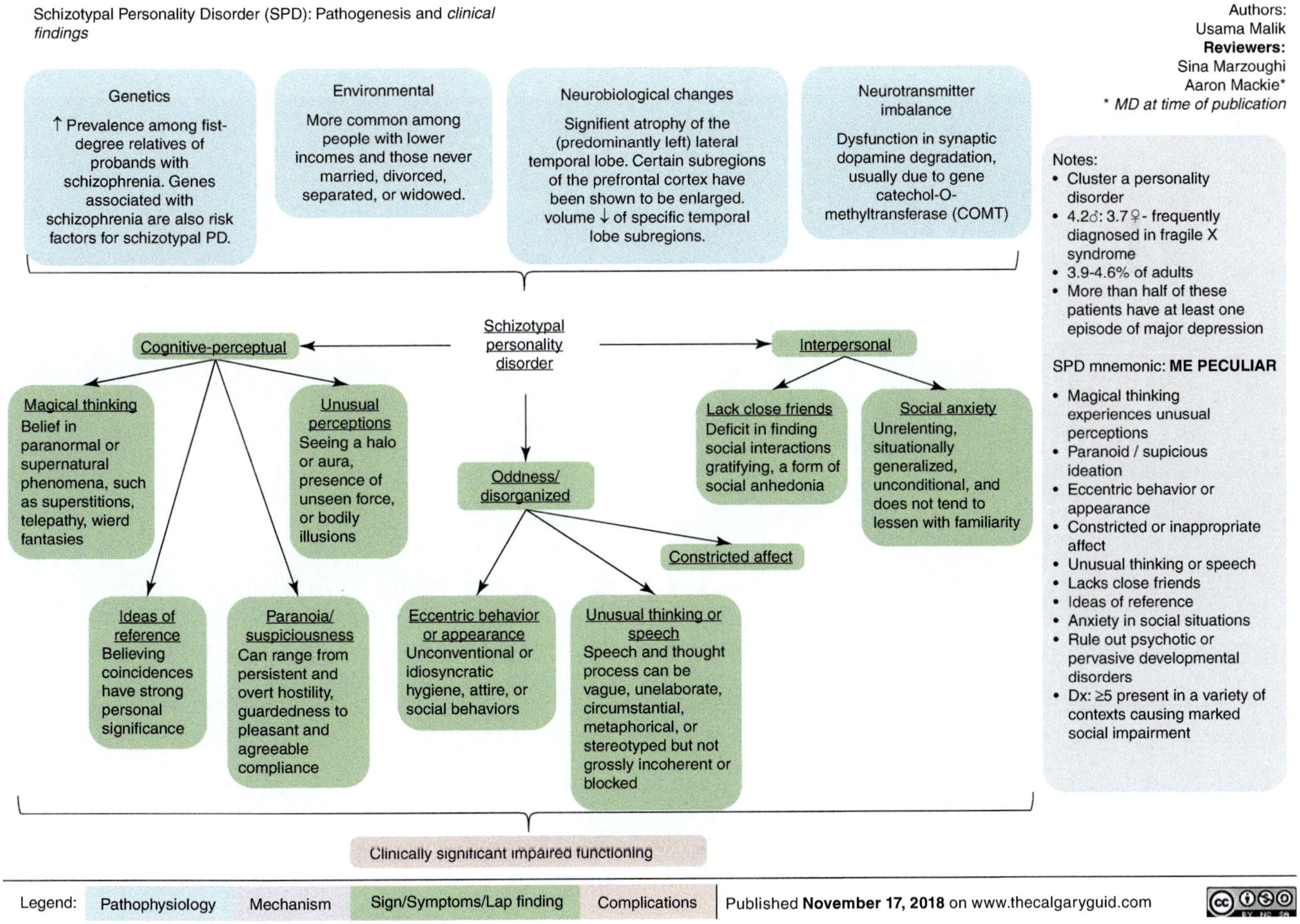

Fig. 24.13 Origins and features of schizotypal personality disorder (public domain)

Other Personality Disorders (Histrionic, Paranoid, Schizoid, and Dependent)

Very little research has been done on other personality disorders such as histrionic, paranoid, schizoid, or dependent personality disorder. Histrionic personality disorder has not been included in the proposed types in DSM-5 alternate model [4]. Sex-biased criteria, significant overlap with other personality disorders such as borderline personality disorder and the lack of empirical literature over the last 35 years, have deterred interest in the Histrionic personality disorder diagnosis. Paranoid personality disorder is one of the more common personality disorders in the community with a reported prevalence of 1.7%; however, these patients seldom seek out mental health services. Patients with paranoid personality disorder have reduced quality of life and live socially isolated lives. However again, there is very little research about this diagnosis. Schizoid personality disorder is a less common personality disorder and with a prevalence rate 0.9% in the community. Dependent personality disorder is even less common with a prevalence of 0.7%. Dependent personality traits can be important to consider particularly in patients with chronic medical concerns that restricts their independence (Fig. 24.14).

Management of Patients with Personality Disorders

Psychopharmacology

Patients with BPD and other PDs will request and are often prescribed multiple medications over the course of their disorder. However, the use of medication in the management of PDs is highly controversial, and no medications have been approved as treatments for PDs. The United Kingdom National Institute for Health and Care Excellence [42] stated that medications are "not to be used" in the management of borderline personality disorder. The NICE treatment guidelines are known to be stringent and directly contrast with the American Psychiatric Association guidelines that recommend a symptom-targeted approach to the pharmacologic management of patients with BPD [43]. In spite of the controversy and the need for further research, medication can play an adjunctive role to psychotherapy in the management of symptoms and in improving the functioning of patients with PDs. Unfortunately, the bulk of the research has been carried out with patients with BPD, and very little research has been done related to the pharmacotherapy of patients with other PDs (Figs. 24.15 and 24.16). Table 24.17 provides

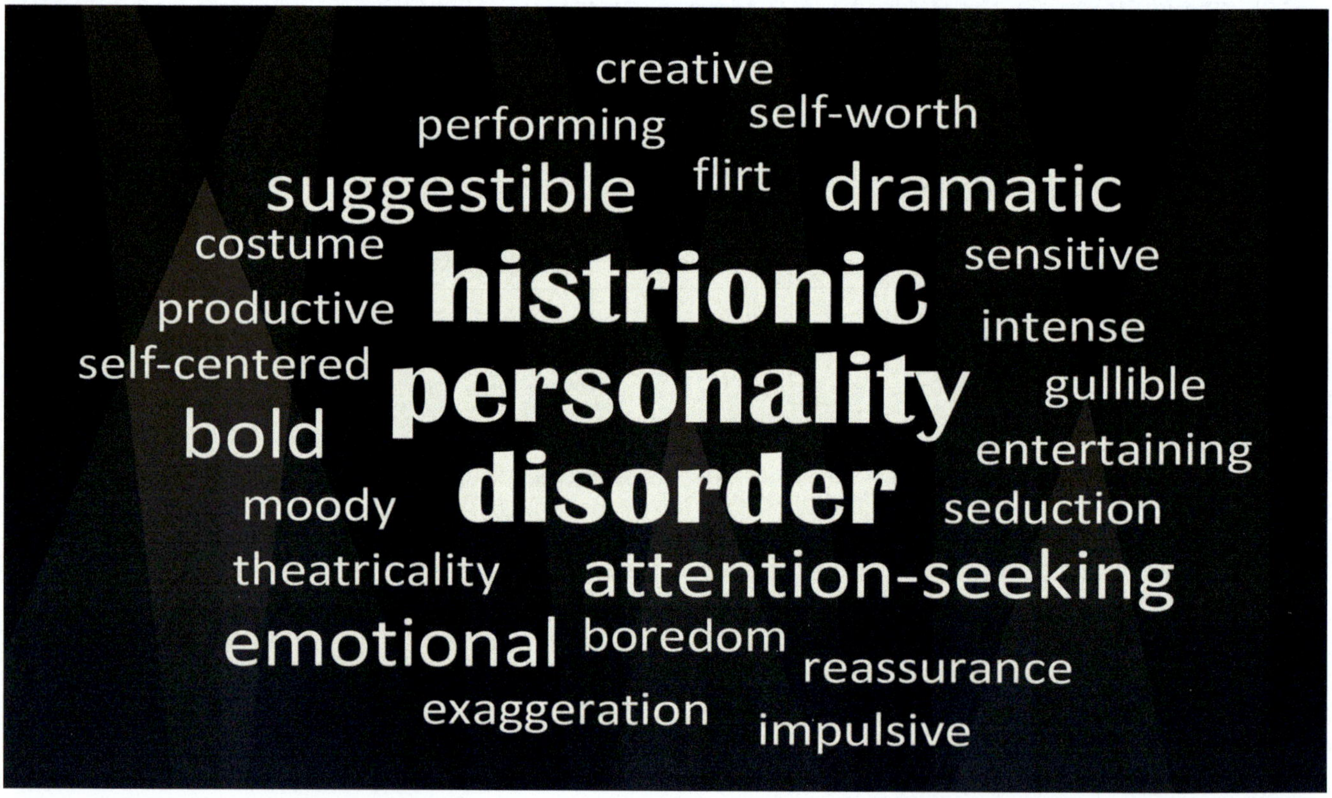

Fig. 24.14 Histrionic personality disorder features

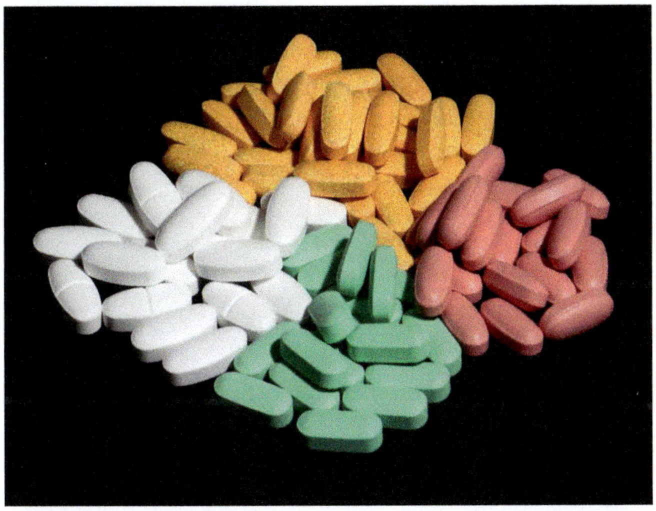

Fig. 24.15 Medication management

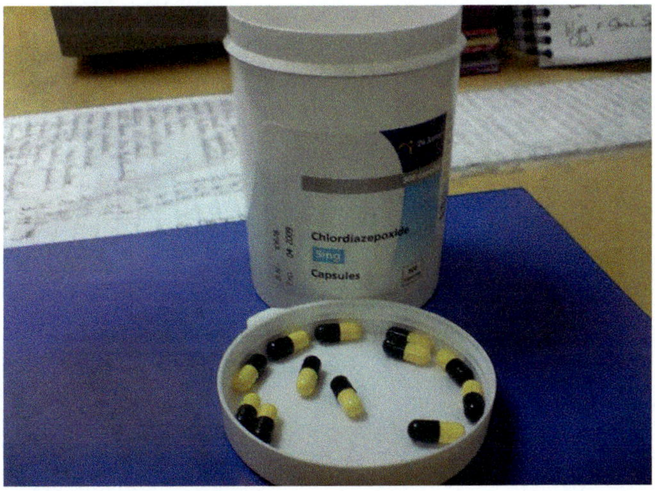

Fig. 24.16 Benzodiazepines for patients with BPD

a summary of the drug types and their role in pharmacotherapy of PDs.

The use of medication for specific symptoms and targeting certain outcomes in patients with BPD and other PDs can be fostered by taking a careful clinical approach [44]. The outcomes for pharmacotherapy should be measurable and be related to the patients' functioning. When medications are to be considered, the clinician should create a partnership with the patient in choosing the medication, in discussing the options, and then in monitoring and evaluating the outcome. Often, patients can be directly engaged in deciding on how best to measure the outcomes of interest. In addition, symptoms that might be possible side effects of the medication should be monitored at baseline and over the course of the medication trial. Some other useful principles to follow when managing patients with PDs are avoiding polypharmacy, treating comorbid Axis I disorders as a priority especially if they interfere with functioning or participation in psychosocial treatment, and eschewing medication changes during crisis episodes. Whenever medications are to be considered, the patient and clinician must evaluate and monitor the risks versus the benefits (Table 24.18).

Psychotherapy

Recognizing and diagnosing personality disorder diagnoses is important because there is a growing evidence that psychotherapy treatment is effective for many of these patients. Particularly for borderline personality disorder, there are at least six individual psychotherapies with proven benefits. For patients with borderline personality disorder, evidence-based treatments are effective in targeting suicidal behaviors and in psychiatry; these therapies are among the most proven

Table 24.17 Pharmacotherapy of personality disorders: summary

Mood stabilizers	Broadest effectiveness, but only modest effectiveness for depression/mood stabilization. More useful for anger/impulsivity Recent negative study of lamotrigine (Crawford et al., 2018)	Lamotrigine Dose: 150–200 mg per day Major side effect: Stevens-Johnson syndrome
Antipsychotics	Second broadest effectiveness. Side effects encourage time-limited trials	Quetiapine Dose: 150–300 mg per day Major side effects: somnolence, fatigue, and increased appetite and weight
Antidepressants	uncertain value, used for comorbid disorders especially for depression/anxiety	Fluoxetine Dose: 20–40 mg per day Major side effect: increased agitation/suicidality
Antianxiety	Benzodiazepines: habit forming, sometimes disinhibiting. Relatively contraindicated; trauma-related arousal/nightmares—clonidine; prazosin	Prazosin Dose: 3–10 mg per day Major side effect: hypotension

Note: No medication FDA approved

Table 24.18 Clinical approach to pharmacotherapy

Psychotherapy primary treatment
Drug management—choose specific outcomes that are measurable and relate to functioning
Create a partnership in choosing and monitoring the treatment
Evaluate symptoms at baseline
Symptom disorders are a priority
Try to avoid polypharmacy
Discuss and monitor risks versus benefits

effective interventions to reduce the risk of recurrent suicidal behavior. Table 24.19 provides a review of the evidence for psychotherapy treatment for patients with BPD [45]. Table 24.20 summarizes the common psychotherapy factors that are found across the evidence-based therapies for patients with BPD [46].

Table 24.19 Psychotherapies for BPD with strong evidence base

Modality	Level of evidence	Key mechanisms of change	Outcomes
Dialectical behavior therapy (DBT)	Multiple RCTs (>10 RCTs, of varying quality) Multiple other non-RCT studies of aspects of DBT in different populations and settings	Conceptualizes BPD as result of high emotional sensitivity and invalidating environments in development Acquisition of skills using mindfulness to tolerate distress, regulate emotions, and manage relationships Individual therapy, group therapy, telephone consultation for patent with therapist and consultation team for the therapist	Decrease in suicidal ideation and non-suicidal self-injury (NSSI) Increased retention in 1:1 treatment in one study Better scores on anger and social adjustment in one study
Mentalization-based treatment (MBT)	Multiple RCTs with differing results and varying quality, most demonstrate advantage for MBT over TAU Multiple other uncontrolled and retrospective studies	Conceptualizes BPD as resulting from deficits in *mentalization* or ability to reflect on one's own and others' mental states while emotionally dysregulated Therapist uses "not knowing stance" to encourage patients to reflect on their own emotional states and those of others in interactions. Change occurs through becoming able to think through hyperactivated emotional states through the process of therapy Individual therapy, group therapy, and team meeting for reflection on process with patients	Reduced suicidality, NSSI, service use, medication use, and "Global Assessment of Functioning" (GAF) score, with increasing benefits over time after completion of the therapy
Transference-focused therapy (TFP)	One major RCT comparing with DBT and supportive therapy	1:1 therapy	Improvements in reflective functioning and attachment style
Schema-focused therapy (SFT)	One major RCT comparing with TFP	1:1 therapy Behavioral, cognitive, and experiential techniques that focus on the therapeutic relationship, daily life outside of therapy and past traumatic experiences Use of four "schema modes"—"detached protector, punitive parent, abandoned/abused child and angry/impulsive child"	More in SFT recovered with reliable clinical improvement SFT patients showed greater increase in quality of life
STEPPS	One major RCT vs. treatment as usual	Group therapy only, meant to compliment other modalities of treatment Psychoeducation, emotion management skills training, behavior management skills	Greater improvement on Zanarini BPD rating scale Improvements in impulsivity, negative affectivity, mood and global functioning
Good psychiatric management of BPD (GPM)	One major RCT demonstrating no difference from DBT in most outcomes	1:1 therapy, often in combination with other treatments Less structure than other approaches, adapted to the needs of the patient and available resources Active therapist, validation, "not-knowing stance," connections made between emotions and events in patient's life with focus on "interpersonal hypersensitivity" Focus on improving functioning through goals in work and relationships. Patient is accountable and change is expected	Vs. baseline, fewer ER visits, fewer suicide episodes, lower number of NSSI behaviors, fewer days in hospital, fewer admissions, lower number of psychotropic medications. Improvement in symptoms of anger, depression. Better interpersonal functioning Results sustained at 2 years follow-up and further improvement in suicidal and NSSI behaviors, anger, interpersonal functioning, anger, symptom distress GPM had better outcome than DBT for depression at 2y F/U
Structured clinical management (SCM)	One major RCT demonstrating similar results to MBT on many outcomes	Use of guidelines for management of BPD based on principles of MBT with less structure	Decreased suicidal behaviors, NSSI, and hospitalizations Increases in Global Assessment of Functioning (GAF) score, self-rated symptom severity, interpersonal functioning and social adjustment (but less than in MBT group)

From Choi-Kain et al. [45]

Table 24.20 Common factors in effective psychotherapies for BPD

Coherent/stable treatment framework
Identification of adverse effects of self-injurious behavior, monitoring for risk or "lethality" of suicidal ideation
Therapist is active, responsive, and validating
Treatment focuses on establishing connections between actions and feelings
Patients are encouraged to assume control of themselves, facilitated through balance of validation and change and fostering a sense of self-agency
Here and now focus—emphasis on current function and relationships
All therapies address core deficits: • Affective Instability—Teach emotion regulation • Impulsivity—Teaching patients to observe, rather than act on feelings • Relationships—Awareness of one's own feeling and feelings of others (mentalization)
Manage and pay careful attention to countertransference
Therapist has ongoing discussion with colleagues/easy access to consultation as part of a team
Contractual alliance as first step—identification of goals, roles, consequences for missed appointments, vacation, therapist limits

Summary

Although patients with PD diagnoses are often considered as challenging and their care can be associated with the risk for suicide and suicide behavior, psychotherapeutic interventions and outpatient psychiatric care appear to be very effective in reducing the short- and long-term risk of recurrent suicidal behavior and assisting these patients to have good clinical outcomes. With the appropriate knowledge, skills, and patient collaboration with treatment, the clinician's work with patients with PDs can be effective and clinically rewarding.

References

1. Crocq MA. Milestones in the history of personality disorders. Dialogues Clin Neurosci. 2013;15:147–53.
2. Paris J. Controversies in the classification and diagnosis of personality disorders. In: Lejuez CW, Gratz KL, editors. The Cambridge handbook of personality disorders. Cambridge University Press; 2020.
3. Trull TJ, Widiger TA. Dimensional models of personality: the five-factor model and the DSM-5. Dialogues Clin Neurosci. 2013;15:135–46.
4. American Psychiatric Association, editor. Diagnostic and statistical manual of mental disorders. 5th ed. Arlington, VA: American Psychiatric Association; 2013.
5. World Health Organization. International classification of diseases for mortality and morbidity statistics (11th Revision); 2018.
6. Sharp C, Wright AGC, Fowler JC, et al. The structure of personality pathology: both general ('g') and specific ('s') factors? J Abnorm Psychol. 2015;124:387–98.
7. Caspi A, Moffitt T. All for one and one for all: mental disorders in one dimension. Am J Psychiatry. 2018;175:831–44.
8. Links PS, Boursiquot P, Links M. Assessing and managing suicide risk. In: Skodol OJ, editor. Textbook of personality disorders. 3rd ed. American Psychiatric Association; in press.
9. Links PS, Eynan R, Shah R. Comorbidity of personality disorders with clinical disorders: current status and future directions. In: Widiger T, editor. Handbook of personality. Oxford Press; in press.
10. Zanarini MC, Frankenburg FR, Reich DB, Fitzmaurice G. Time to attainment of recovery from borderline personality disorder and stability of recovery: a 10-year prospective follow-up study. Am J Psychiatry. 2010;167:663–7.
11. Skodol AE. Impact of personality pathology on psychosocial functioning. Curr Opin Psychol. 2018;21:33–8.
12. Glenn AL, Johnson AK, Raine A. Antisocial personality disorder: a current review. Curr Psychiatry Rep. 2013;15:1–8.
13. Weinbrecht A, Schulze L, Boettcher J, Renneberg B. Avoidant personality disorder: a current review. Curr Psych Rep. 2016;18:29.
14. Lampe L, Malhi G. Avoidant personality disorder: current insights. Psychol Res Behav Manag. 2018;11:55–66.
15. Bateman A, Fonagy P. Mentalization-based treatment for personality disorders: a practical guide. Oxford: Oxford University Press; 2016.
16. Lieb K, Zanarini MC, Schmahl C, et al. Borderline personality disorder. Lancet. 2004;364:453–61.
17. Paris J. Half in love with easeful death: the meaning of chronic suicidality in borderline personality disorder. Harv Rev Psychiatry. 2004;12:42–8.
18. Bender D, Dolan R, Skodol A, et al. Treatment utilization by patients with personality disorders. Am J Psychiatry. 2001;158:295–302.
19. Paris J, Zweig-Frank H. A 27-year follow-up of patients with borderline personality disorder. Compr Psychiatry. 2001;42:482–7.
20. Zanarini MC, Frankenburg FR, Hennen J, et al. Prediction of the 10-year course of borderline personality disorder. Am J Psychiatry. 2006;163(5):827–32.
21. Temes CM, Frankenburg FR, Fitzmaurice GM, Zanarini MC. Deaths by suicide and other causes among patients with borderline personality disorder and personality-disordered comparison subjects over 24 years of prospective follow-up. J Clin Psychiatry. 2019;80(1):30–6.
22. Perry JC, Fowler JC, Bailey A, et al. Improvement and recovery from suicidal and self-destructive phenomena in treatment-refractory disorders. J Nerv Ment Dis. 2009;197(1):28–34. https://doi.org/10.1097/NMD.0b013e3181927598.
23. Links PS, Kolla NJ, Guimond T, McMain S. Prospective risk factors for suicide attempts in a treated sample of patients with borderline personality disorder. Can J Psychiatr. 2013;58(2):99–106.
24. Geissbuhler M, Links P. Prospective risk factors for suicide attempts in borderline personality disorder. Curr Psychiatry Rep. 2009;11(1):53–4.
25. Ronningstam E. Narcissistic personality disorder: facing DSM-V. Psychiatr Ann. 2009;39:111–21.
26. Pincus AL, Lukowitsky MR. Pathological narcissism and narcissistic personality disorder. Annu Rev Clin Psychol. 2010;6:421–46.
27. Gabbard GO. Transference and countertransference: developments in the treatment of narcissistic personality disorder. Psychiatr Ann. 2009;39:129–36.
28. Ogrodniczuk JS, Kealy D. Interpersonal problems of narcissistic patients. In: Ogrodniczuk JS, editor. Understanding and treating pathological narcissism. Washington, DC: American Psychological Association; 2013. p. 113–28.
29. Ronningstam E. Narcissistic Personality disorder in DSM V- in support of retaining a significant diagnosis. J Personal Disord. 2011;25:248–59.
30. Links PS. Pathological narcissism and the risk of suicide. In: Ogrodniczuk JS, editor. Understanding and treating pathological narcissism. Washington, DC: American Psychological Association; 2013. p. 167–82.

31. Miller JD, Widiger TA, Campbell WK. Narcissistic personality disorder and the DSM-V. J Abnorm Psychol. 2010;119:640–9.
32. Miller JD, Campbell WK, Pilkonis PA. Narcissistic personality disorder: relations with distress and functional impairment. Compr Psychiatry. 2007;48:170–7.
33. Dhawan N, Kunik ME, Oldham J, Coverdale J. Prevalence and treatment of narcissistic personality disorder in the community: a systematic review. Compr Psychiatry. 2010;51:333–9.
34. Yakeley J. Current understanding of narcissism and narcissistic personality disorder. Br J Psychiatry Advances. 2018;24:305–15. https://doi.org/10.1192/bja.2018.20.
35. Ronningstam EF, Maltsberger JT. Pathological narcissism and sudden suicide-related collapse. Suicide Life Threat Behav. 1998;28:261–71.
36. Shapiro D. Neurotic styles. New York: Basic Books; 1999.
37. Diedrich A, Voderholzer U. Obsessive-compulsive personality disorder: a current review. Curr Psych Rep. 2015;17:2.
38. McWilliams N. Psychoanalytic diagnosis. New York: The Guilford Press; 2011.
39. Kirchner SK, Roeh A, Nolden J, Hasan A. Diagnosis and treatment of schizotypal personality disorder: evidence from a systematic review. NPJ Schizophr. 2018;4:1–18.
40. Raine A. Schizotypal personality: neurodevelopmental and psychosocial trajectories. Annu Rev Clin Psychol. 2006;2:291–326.
41. Debbané M, Eliez S, Badoud D, et al. Developing psychosis and its risk states through the lens of schizotypy. Schizophr Bull. 2015;41:S396–407.
42. National Institute for Health and Clinical Excellence. Borderline personality disorder: recognition and management. 2015. https://www.nice.org.uk/guidance/cg78/resources/borderline-personality-disorder-recognition-and-management-pdf-975635141317.
43. American Psychiatric Association. Practice guideline for the treatment of patients with borderline personality disorder. Am J Psychiatry. 2001;158:1–52.
44. Gunderson JG, Links PS. Handbook of good psychiatric management for borderline personality disorder. Washington, DC: American Psychiatric Publishing; 2014.
45. Choi-Kain LW, Finch EF, Masland SR, Jenkins JA, Unruh BT. What works in the treatment of borderline personality disorder. Curr Behav Neurosci Rep. 2017;4:21–30.
46. Schiavone FL, Links P. Common elements for the psychotherapeutic management of patients with self-injurious behaviour. Child Abuse Negl. 2013;37:233–8.
47. Gunderson JG, Herpertz SC, Skodol AE, et al. Borderline personality disorder. Nat Rev Dis Primers. 2018;4:18029. https://doi.org/10.1038/nrdp.2018.29.
48. Starcevic V, Brakoulias V. New diagnostic perspectives on obsessive-compulsive personality disorder and its links with other conditions. Curr Opin Psych. 2014;27:62–7.
49. Yang X, Hu L, Zeng J, et al. Default mode network and frontolimbic gray matter abnormalities in patients with borderline personality disorder: a voxel-based meta-analysis. Sci Rep. 2016;6:34247. https://doi.org/10.1038/srep34247.

The Future of Psychiatry

25

Waguih William IsHak, Naira Magakian, William W. Ishak,
Asbasia A. Mikhail, and Russell Lim

Introduction

Psychiatry has a promising future at this point of time as we are getting close to starting the second quarter of the twenty-first century. Expansions in different dimensions of the field are exponential. This chapter is an attempt at capturing some of the most significant future directions in the field including biological, psychological, social, technological, financial, educational, and legal aspects of the field spanning across etiological, diagnostic, therapeutic, and preventative future directions. The World Psychiatric Association (WPA)-Lancet Psychiatry Commission on the Future of Psychiatry was published in 2017, and it is a crucial framework for the future of the field. The Commission addressed six priority areas or parts as shown in Table 25.1 [1].

WPA-LPC Report Part 1: The Future of the Patient and Treatment

Data show that psychiatry will be involved in caring for older, more urban, and migrant populations. Biomarkers will potentially change the way psychiatrists diagnose and treat psychiatric disorders, and digital technology will provide

W. W. IsHak
Cedars-Sinai Health System, Department of Psychiatry and Behavioral Neurosciences, University of California Los Angeles, David Geffen School of Medicine, Los Angeles, CA, USA
e-mail: Waguih.IsHak@cshs.org

N. Magakian
Cedars-Sinai Medical Center, Los Angeles, CA, USA

W. W. Ishak
Brown University, Providence, RI, USA
e-mail: william_ishak@brown.edu

A. A. Mikhail
Department of Emergency Medicine, Huntington Hospital, Pasadena, CA, USA

R. Lim (✉)
Department of Psychiatry, University of California, Davis, Davis, CA, USA

W. W. IsHak (ed.), *Atlas of Psychiatry*, https://doi.org/10.1007/978-3-031-15401-0_25

Table 25.1 The World Psychiatric Association (WPA)-Lancet Psychiatry Commission (LPC) on the future of psychiatry report

Part 1: The patient and treatment
Who will psychiatrists help? The patient population of the future will reflect general demographic shifts toward older, more urban, and migrant populations. While technical advances such as the development of biomarkers will potentially alter diagnosis and treatment and digital technology will facilitate assessment of remote populations, the human elements of practice such as cultural sensitivity and the ability to form a strong therapeutic alliance with the patient will remain central
Part 2: Psychiatry and healthcare systems
Delivering mental health services to those who need them will require reform of the traditional structure of services. Few existing models have evidence of clinical effectiveness and acceptability to service users. Services of the future should consider stepped care, increased the use of multidisciplinary teamwork, more of a public health approach, and the integration of mental and physical health care. These services will need to fit into the cultural and economic framework of a diverse range of settings in high income, low income, and middle income countries
Part 3: Psychiatry and society
Increased emphasis on social interventions and engagement with societal expectations might be an important area for psychiatry's development. This could encompass advocacy for the rights of individuals living with mental illnesses, political involvement concerning the social risk factors for mental illness, and, on a smaller scale, work with families and local social networks and communities. Psychiatrists should therefore possess communication skills and knowledge of the social sciences as well as the basic biological sciences
Part 4: The future of mental health law
Mental health law worldwide tends to be based on concerns about risk rather than the protection of the rights of individuals experiencing mental illness. The United Nations Convention on the Rights of Persons with Disabilities, which states that compulsion based in whole or in part on mental disability is discriminatory and is a landmark document that should inform the future formulation and reform of mental health laws. An evidence-based approach needs to be taken: mental health legislation should mandate mental health training for all health professionals, ensure access to good quality care, and cover wider societal issues, particularly access to housing, resources, and employment. All governments should include a mental health impact assessment when drafting relevant legislation
Part 5: Digital psychiatry—enhancing the future of mental health
Digital technology might offer psychiatry the potential for radical change in terms of service delivery and the development of new treatments. However, it also carries the risk of commercialized and unproven treatments entering the medical marketplace with detrimental effect. Novel research methods, transparency standards, clinical evidence, and care delivery models must be created in collaboration with a wide range of stakeholders. Psychiatrists need to remain up to date and educated in the evolving digital world
Part 6: Training the psychiatrist of the future
Rapid scientific advance and evolving models of health care delivery have broad implications for future psychiatry training. The psychiatrist of the future must not only be armed with the latest medical knowledge and clinical skills but also be prepared to adapt to a changing landscape. Training programs in an age in which knowledge of facts is less important than how new knowledge is accessed and deployed must refocus from the simple delivery of information toward acquisition of skills in lifelong learning and quality improvement

From Bhugra et al. [1]; *with permission*

access for remote populations without compromising the central human elements of psychiatry such as building therapeutic alliance and cultural sensitivity (see Fig. 25.1) [2].

WPA-LPC Report Part 2: The Future of Psychiatry and Healthcare Systems

Reforming traditional mental health services delivery models will be needed including the incorporation of stepped care, multidisciplinary teams, public health approaches, and integrating psychiatric with medical care with diverse cultural and economic considerations (see Fig. 25.2) [1, 3].

WPA-LPC Report Part 3: The Future of Psychiatry and Society

Psychiatrists will be involved in social engagement regarding advocacy for psychiatric patient rights and addressing the social factors that influence psychiatric disorders at the local, regional, national, and international levels, including educational, occupational, residential, financial, health care access factors, and crime, discrimination, and inequality. Given the example of the presence of these problems in local European neighborhoods seen below [4], one could imagine their prevalence in the rest of the world (see Fig. 25.3).

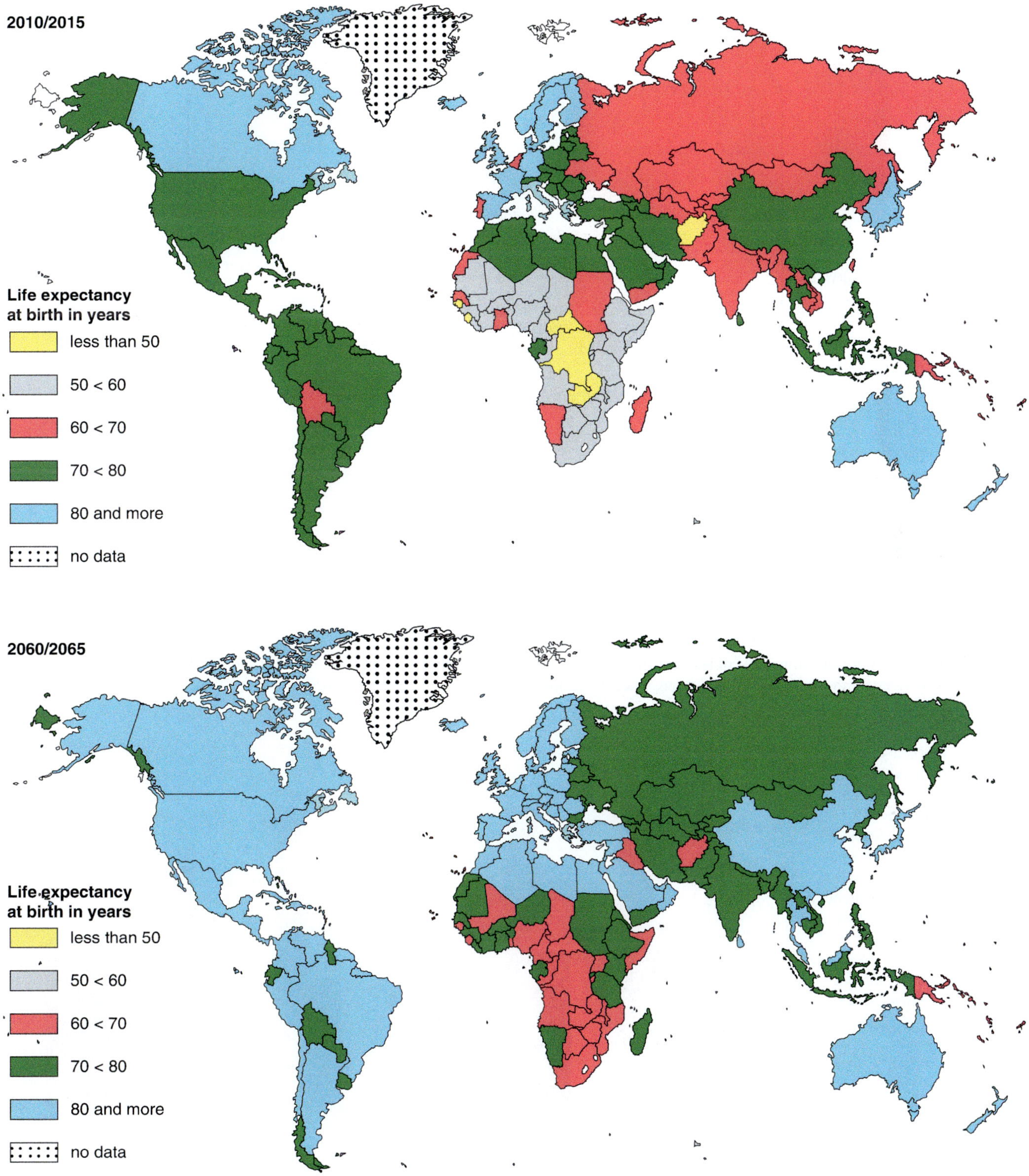

Fig. 25.1 Life expectancy at birth, both sexes 2010–2015 and 2060–2065. (*From* Swiaczny [2]; *with permission*)

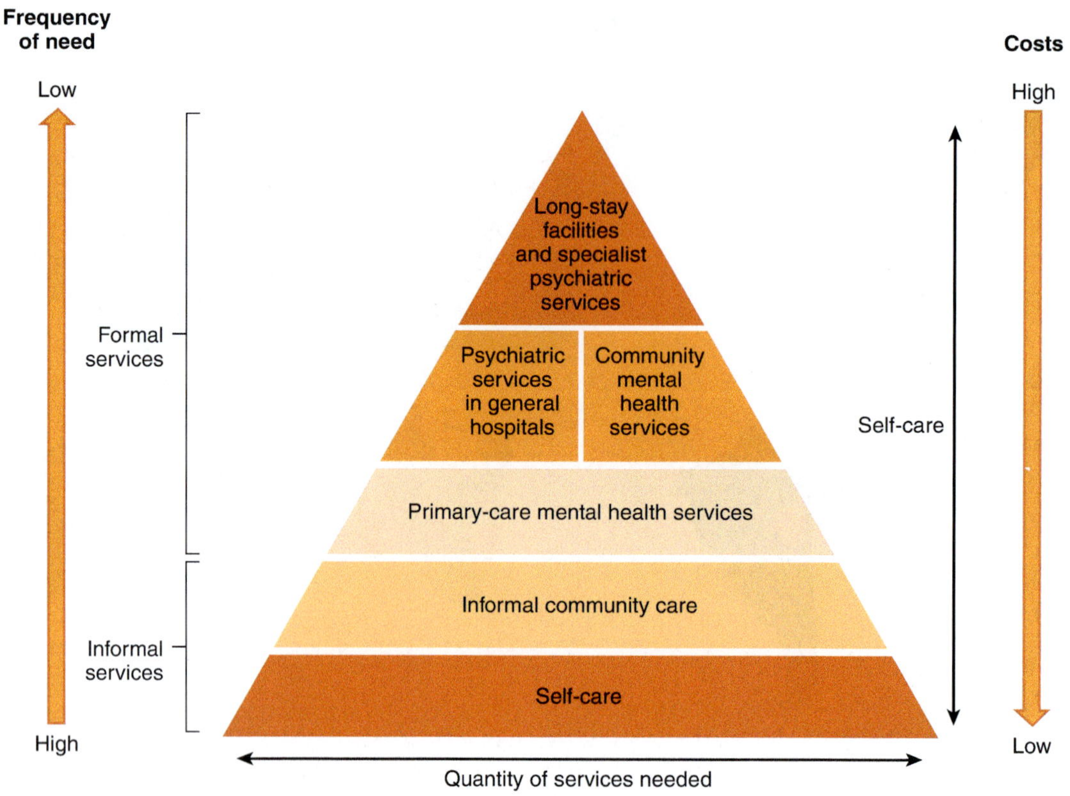

Fig. 25.2 WHO pyramid model. The WHO model is a service organization pyramid describing an optimal mix of services for mental health. The costliest services are the least frequently needed, whereas the most needed services can be provided at a relatively low cost. Self-care features through all services and all levels of the pyramid. (*From* Bhugra et al. [1]; *with permission*)

Fig. 25.3 Problems in the local neighborhood in the European Union. From the European Quality of Life Surveys (EQLS) question#50: "Please think about the area where you live now—I mean the immediate neighborhood of your home. Do you have major, moderate or no problems with the following?" (*From* Ahrendt et al. [4]; *with permission*)

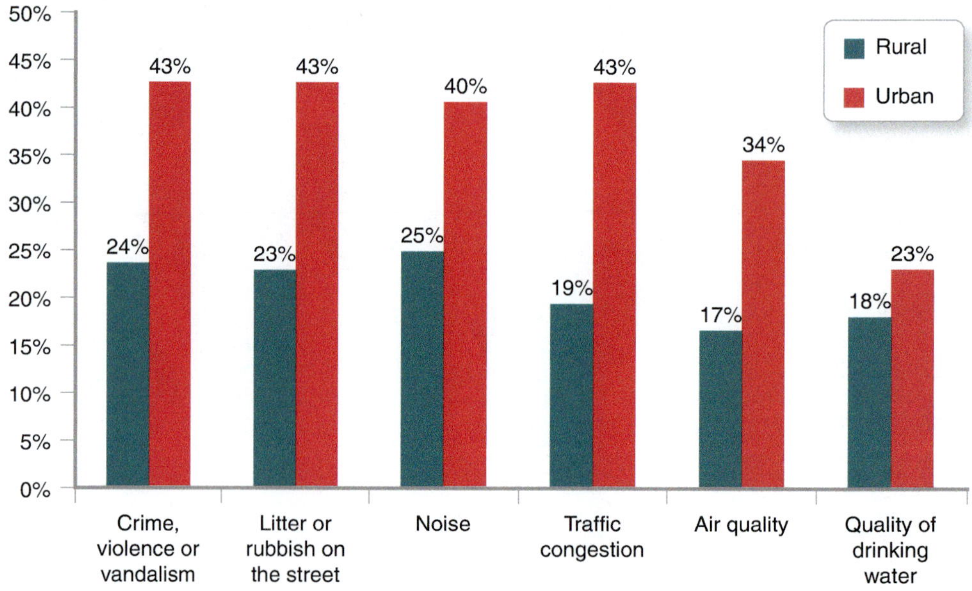

WPA-LPC Report Part 4: The Future of Mental Health Law

The United Nations Convention on the Rights of Persons with Disabilities (CRDP), which had its tenth anniversary this year, is a historic advance in the protection of the rights of psychiatric patients and is expected to drive the reform of mental health laws worldwide. Laws should require access to quality care, health professional behavioral health training, and addressing social factors contributing to psychiatric disorders (see Fig. 25.4) [5].

WPA-LPC Report Part 5: Digital Psychiatry and Enhancing the Future of Mental Health

Digital technology in psychiatry is a promising field in introducing innovative treatments and enhancing treatment delivery as well as collecting real-time research data and optimizing collaboration (see Fig. 25.5) [1, 6].

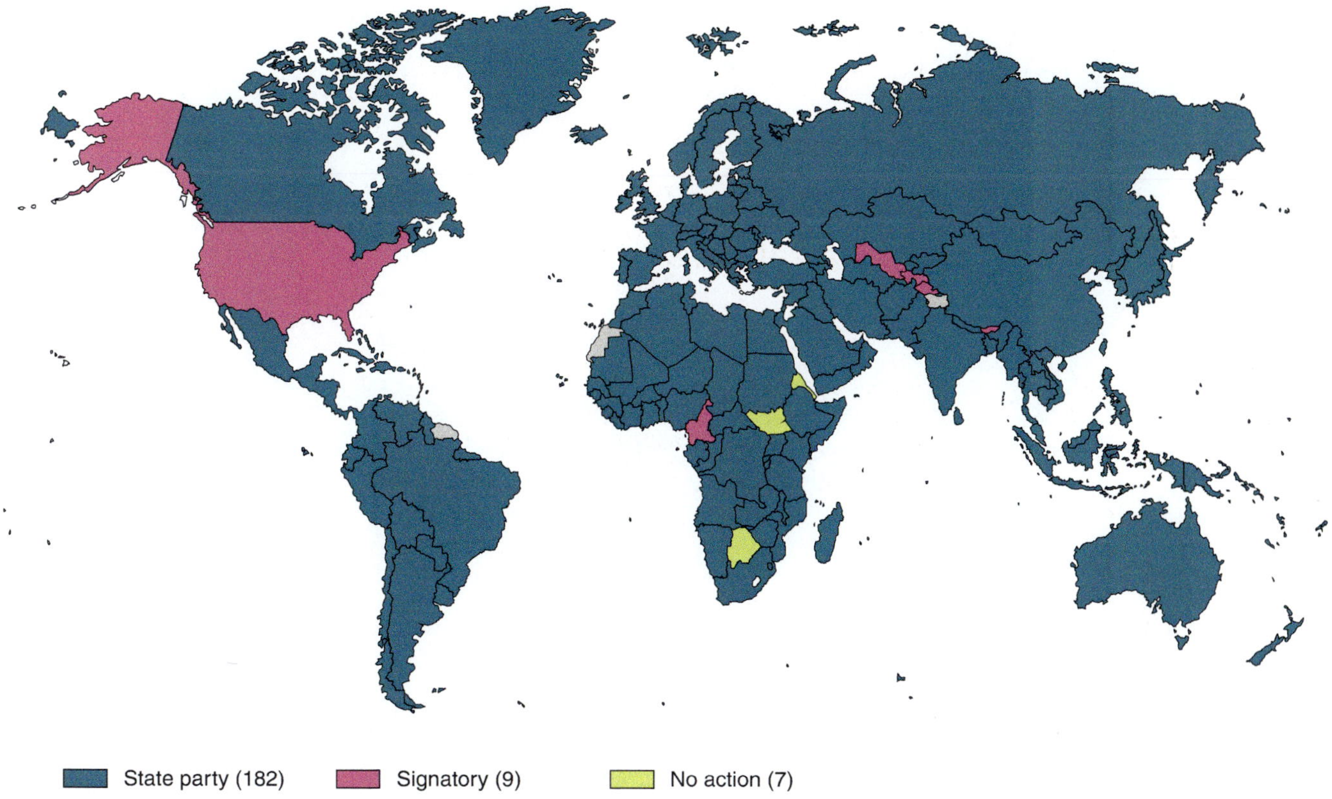

Fig. 25.4 Ratification of the convention on the rights of persons with disabilities. Note: The boundaries and the names shown and the designations used on these maps do not imply official endorsement or acceptance by the United Nations. Final boundary between the Republic of Sudan and the Republic of South Sudan has not yet been determined dotted line represents approximately the Line of Control in Jammu and Kashmir agreed upon by India and Pakistan. The final status of Jammu and Kashmir has not yet been agreed upon by the parties

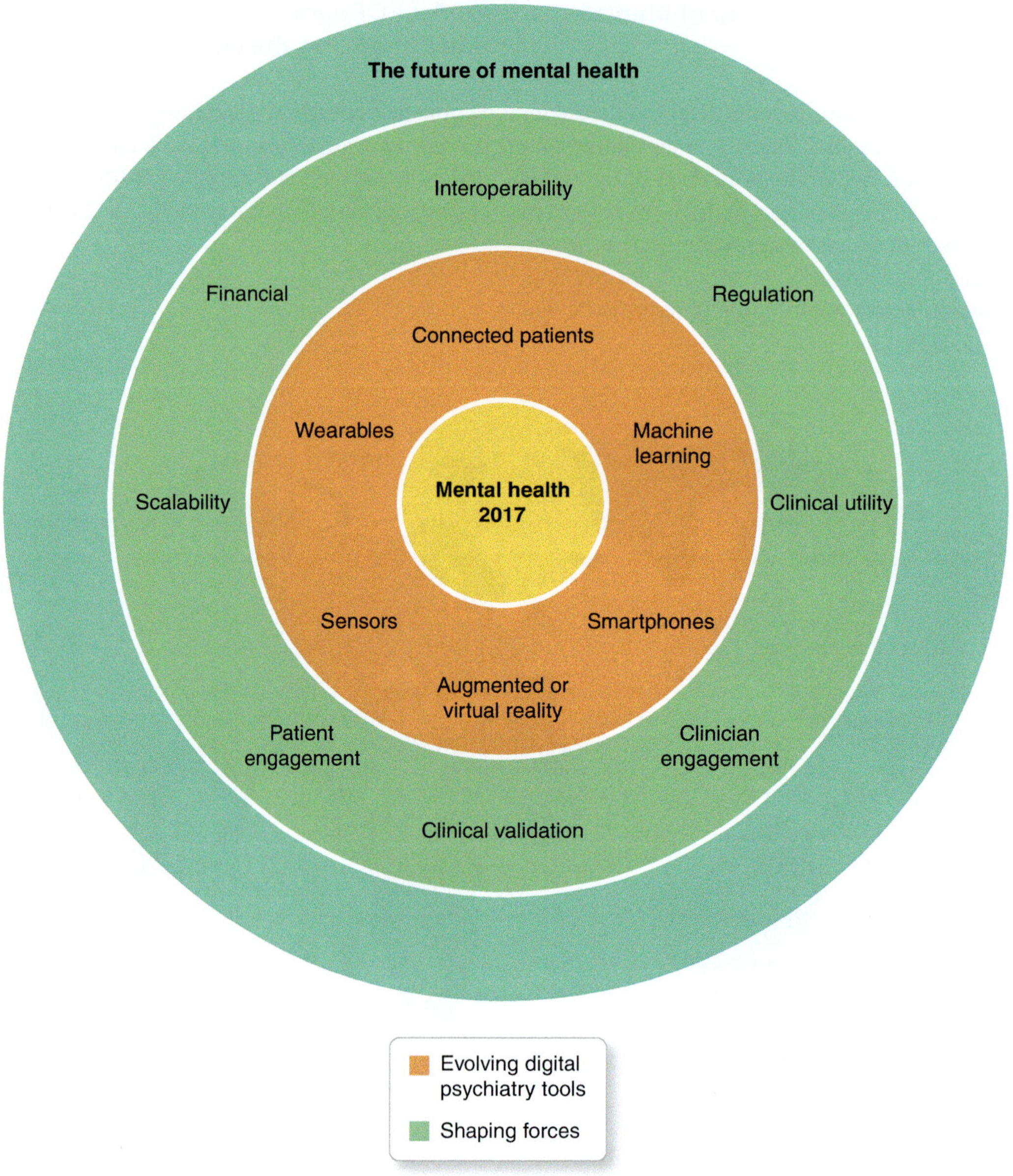

Fig. 25.5 Driving forces for progress in digital psychiatry in the next 10 years. Progress will be driven not only by new technologies but also by numerous shaping forces. (*From* Bhugra et al. [1]; *with permission*)

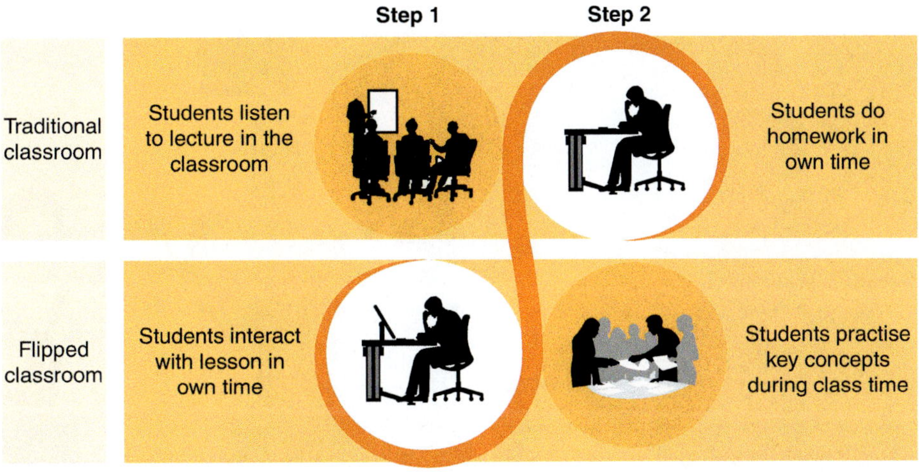

Fig. 25.6 Flipped classroom. Psychiatry trainees are engaged in self-directed learning before attending class by watching a video or reading selected text. Interactive learning techniques using role-play or group discussion take place in the classroom. (*From* Bhugra et al. [1]; *with permission*)

WPA-LPC Report Part 6: Training the Psychiatrist of the Future

Future psychiatrists will master lifelong learning and quality improvement skills as well as building therapeutic relationship and working with key stakeholders, policy makers, and patient advocacy groups (see Fig. 25.6) [1, 7].

The Future of Identification of the Causes of Psychiatric Disorders

The causes of psychiatric disorders have been identified along the lines of predisposing, precipitating, and perpetuating factors, including biological such as genetics and psychosocial such as early trauma.

Genetics

There are clear (yet complex) links between genetics and psychiatric disorders. For instance, suicide was noted in certain families such as Hemingway's as seen in Fig. 25.7 [8].

Using IBM Watson for Drug Discovery, a powerful machine learning text-mining application, Lüscher Dias et al. built the networks below depicting the connections between Psychiatric and Neurological Disorders and genes and drugs from scientific publications in the last 50 years (see Fig. 25.8) [9].

The Future of Genetic and Genomic Research in Psychiatric Disorders

Despite identification of hundreds of genetic variants associated with psychiatric disorders, the potential of genomics to identify genetic risk and link to specific disorders have not been yet achieved. Potential approaches include transcriptome-wide association studies (TWAS) (Fig. 25.9a) [10] and endophenotypes (Fig. 25.9b) [11].

Transcriptome-Wide Association Studies (TWAS)

Hernandez et al. pinpointed in 2021: "Successful next steps require identification of "causal" genetic variants and their proximal biological consequences; placing variants within biologically defined functional contexts, reflecting specific molecular pathways, cell types, circuits, and developmental windows; and characterizing the downstream, convergent neurobiological impact of polygenicity within an individual." Focusing on the transcriptome, the collection of RNAs expressed in a cell/tissue, using transcriptome-wide association studies (TWAS) to prioritize risk genes within genome-wide association studies (GWAS), could help the integration of distinct genetic, genomic, and phenotypic levels, as seen in Fig. 25.9a [10].

Endophenotypes

The potential of identifying the genetic and genomic factors in psychiatric disorders might be in endophenotypes, which are heritable neurobehavioral traits in psychiatric disorders, as described below [11] using suicide as an example (see Fig. 25.9b).

The Effects of Early Trauma

Early trauma has been indirectly linked to inflammation due to hypothalamic-pituitary-adrenal (HPA) axis activation (see Fig. 25.10) [12].

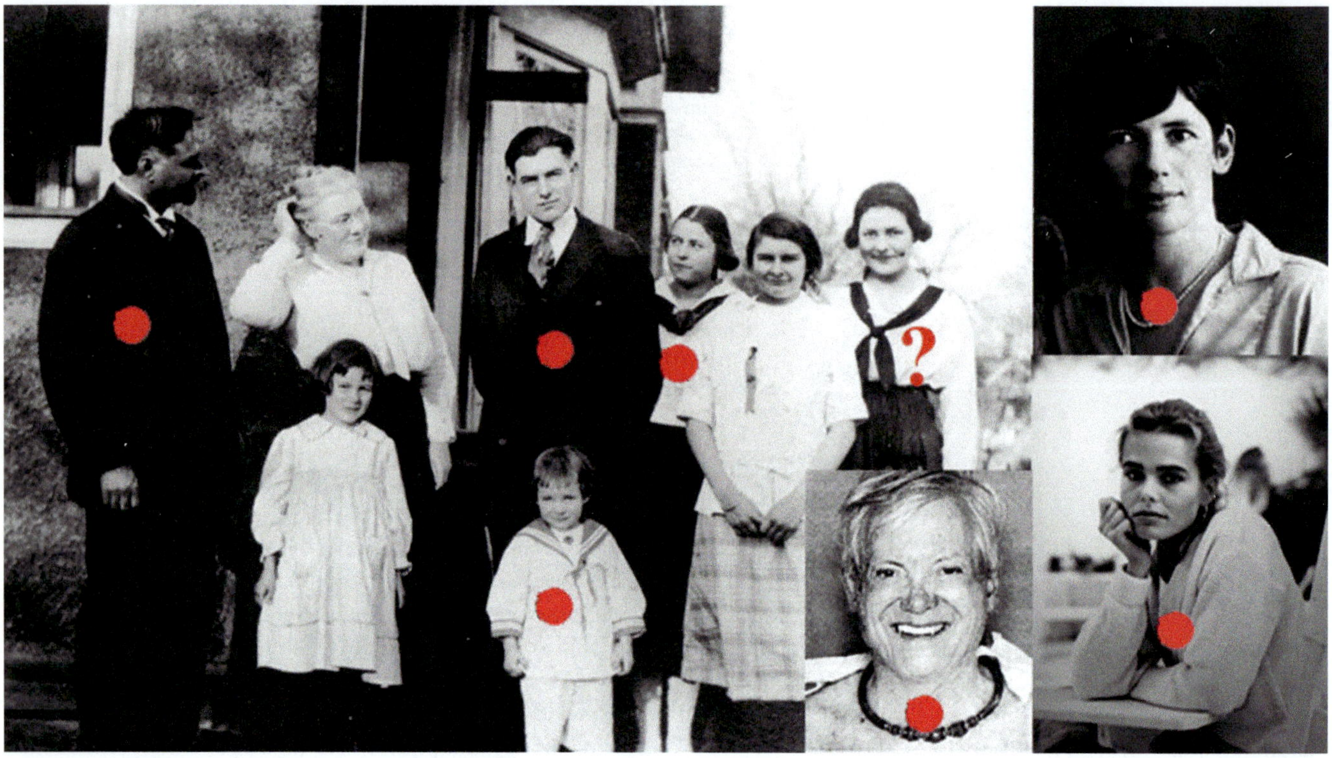

Fig. 25.7 Members of the Hemingway family c. 1917. Red dots mark those who died by suicide. Main photo: Clarence (father), Grace (mother), and offspring (Carol, Ernest, Leicester, Ursula, Madelaine "Sunny," and Marceline). Right top: Pauline Pfeiffer (wife). Right bottom: Gregory (son). Left bottom: Margaux (granddaughter). The question mark stands for a possible suicide for Marceline. (*From* Fountoulakis and Nimatoudis [8]; *with permission*)

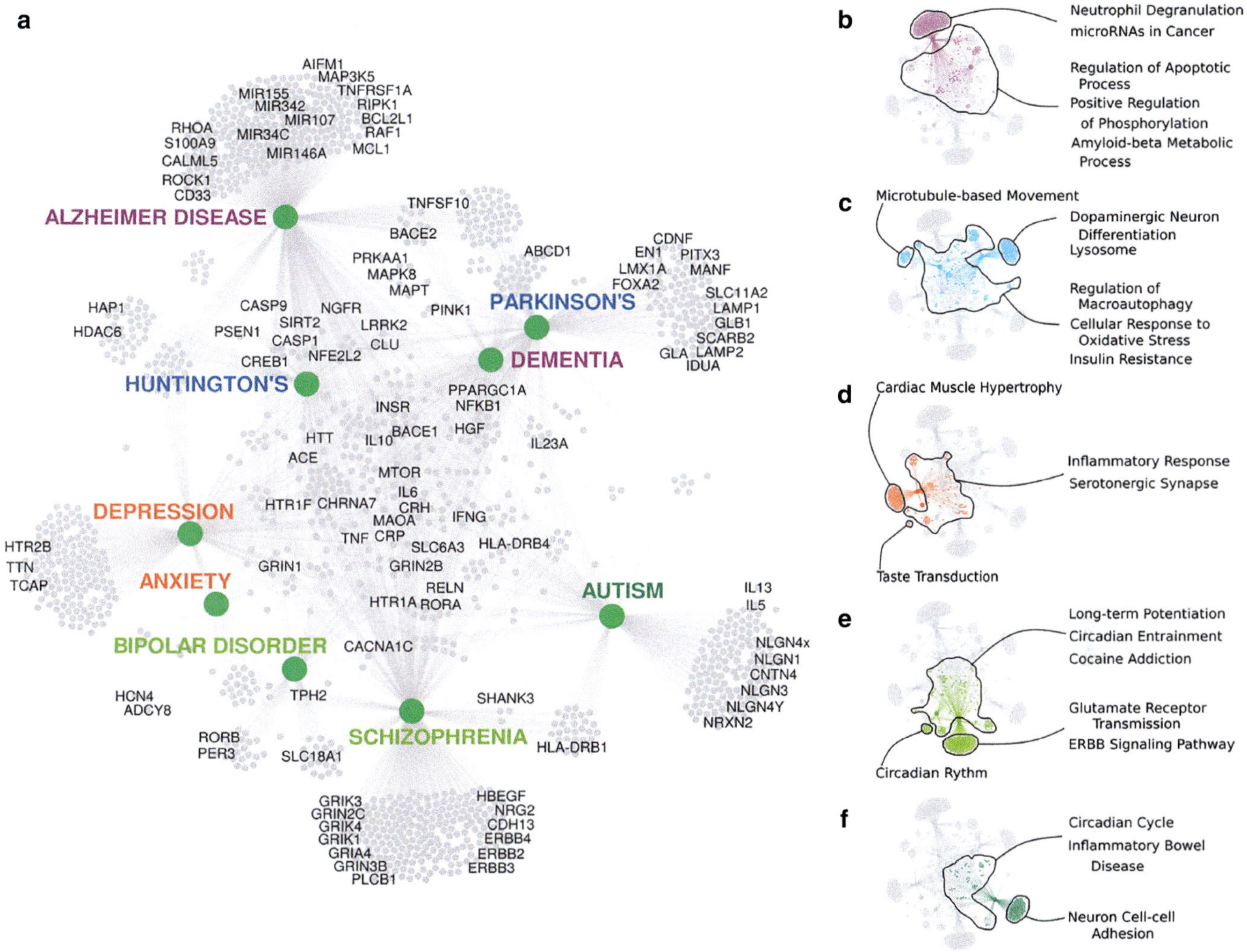

Fig. 25.8 Functional analysis of genes unique to each psychiatric and neurological disorders and network modules. (**a**) A summary of genes connected to PNDs enriched for relevant biological processes (GO) and pathways (KEGG). (**b–f**) The most significant gene enrichment categories for genes in the modules: Alzheimer's and dementia (**b**), Huntington's disease and Parkinson's disease (**c**), depression and anxiety (**d**), schizophrenia and bipolar disorder (**e**), and autism (**f**). (*From* Lüscher Dias et al. [9]; with permission)

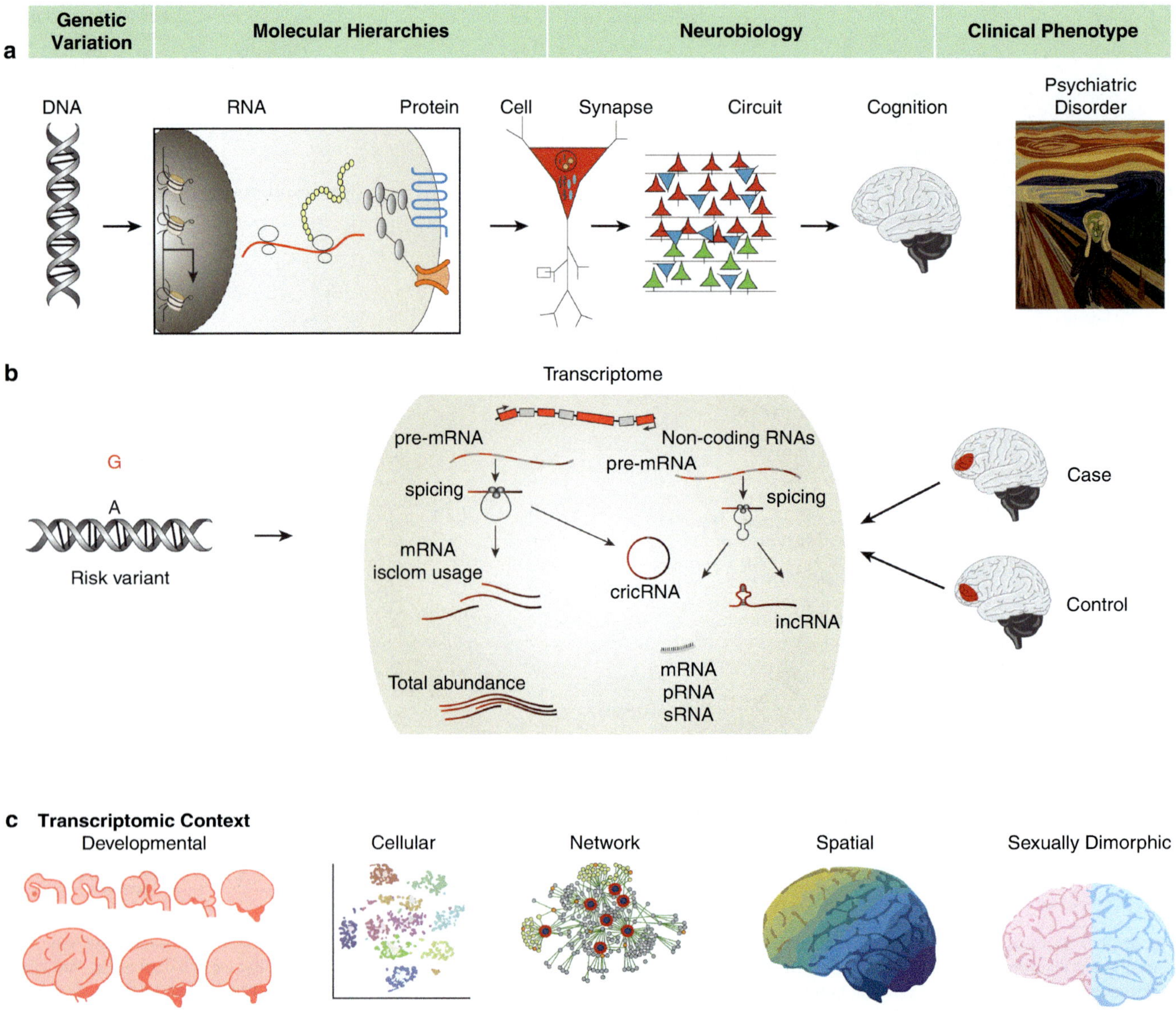

Fig. 25.9 (**a**) A transcriptomic framework for mechanistic dissection of complex psychiatric traits. (A) A hierarchical neurobiological organization linking genotype to phenotype. (B) Two main approaches are highlighted. (Left) Disease-associated genetic risk variants can be integrated with gene expression measures through transcriptome-wide association studies and related approaches to prioritize proximal biological mechanisms, particularly for noncoding variants. (Right) Differential gene expression analyses of brain tissue from subjects with psychiatric disorders (case) compared with controls can be used to identify a reactive, brain-level molecular pathology of disease. (C) Gene expression patterns are highly dynamic and interpretation requires understanding the relevant biological context. *circRNA* circular RNA; *lncRNA* long noncoding RNA; *miRNA* microRNA; *mRNA* messenger RNA; *piRNA* PIWI-interacting RNA; *siRNA* small interfering RNA. (*From* Hernandez et al. [10]; with permission.) (**b**) Candidate gene regions, genes, and endophenotypes implicated in suicide research. The upper portion of the figure indicates the dynamic interplay among genetic, epigenetic, and environmental factors that produce cumulative liability to suicidal behaviors. Although attempted suicide does not always predate a completed suicide as suggested on the reaction surface, it is a significant risk factor. None of the sections of this figure can be definitive; many more gene loci, genes, candidate endophenotypes, and links among the three remain to be discovered. Environment, protective and harmful, includes a substantial number of environmental events (e.g., drug exposure) unmentioned here because of our focus on genetic and neurobiological correlates. Similarly, there are many gene loci, genes, and candidate endophenotypes that were not included because of the conceptual limitations of this figure. (From Courtet et al. [11]; with permission)

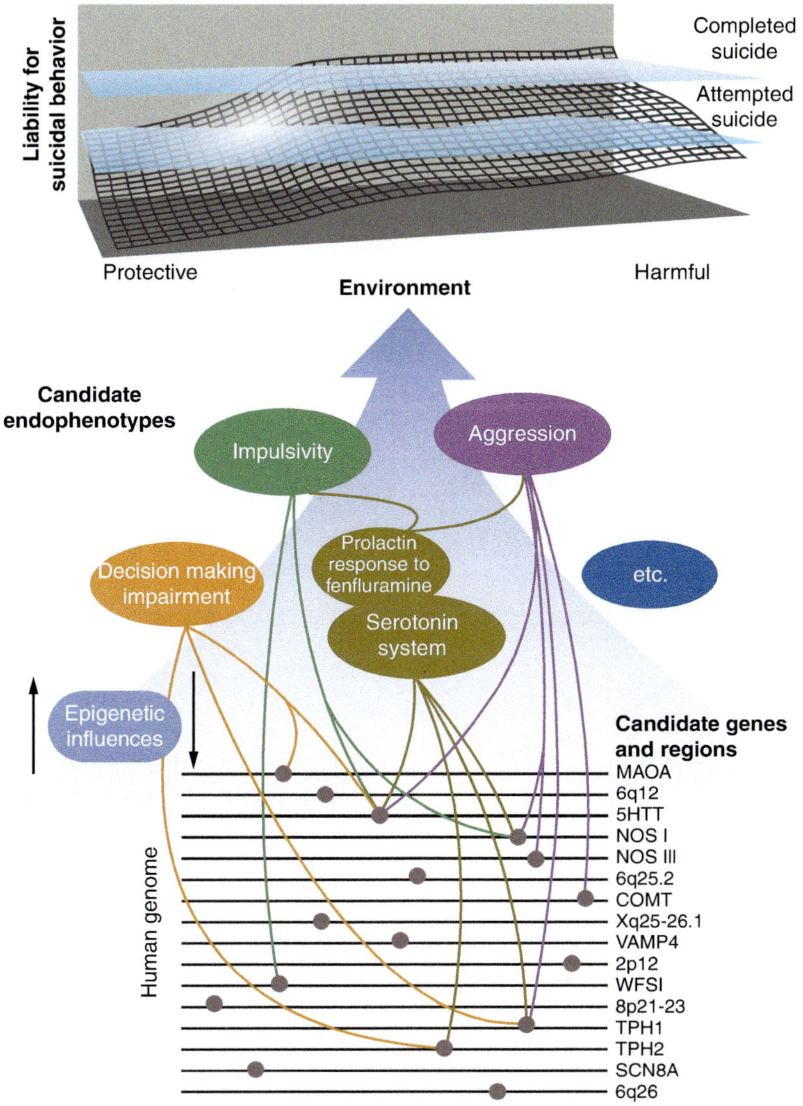

Fig. 25.9 (continued)

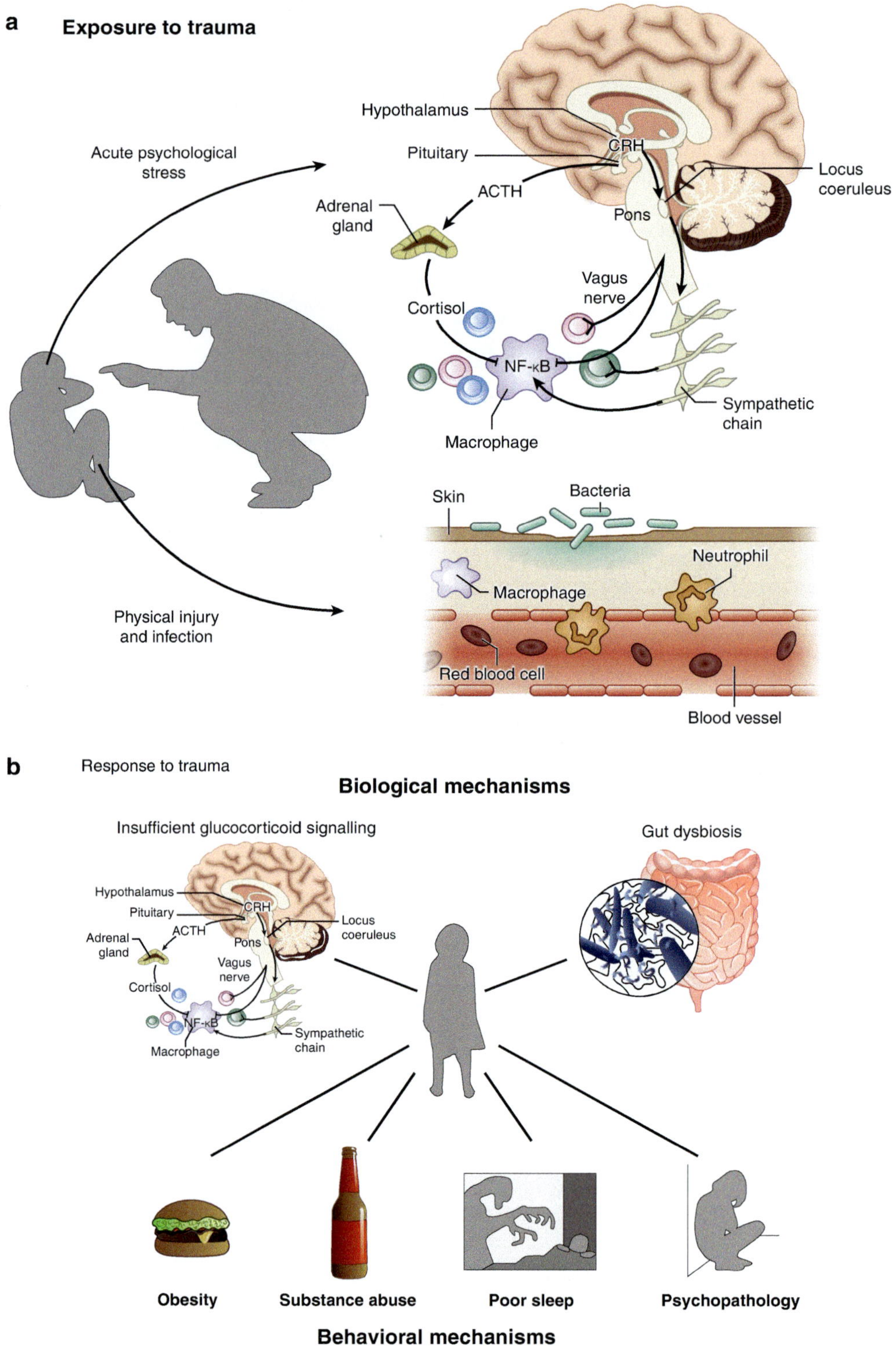

Fig. 25.10 Potential mechanisms linking childhood trauma and inflammation. Panel (**a**) portrays potential mechanisms through which exposure to childhood trauma could elicit an acute inflammatory response. On the one hand, exposure to acute psychological stress can elicit an acute inflammatory response by stimulation of the sympathetic nervous system. On the other hand, psychological trauma may occur in the context of physical trauma. In this case, physical injury and pathogen infection can induce inflammation by triggering innate immunity. Short-term activation of the inflammatory response during sensitive periods in early life may affect the brain development and later microglia and neuroendocrine reactivity. Panel (**b**) portrays potential biological and behavioral mechanisms through which response to childhood trauma could lead to a chronic inflammatory state. (*From* Danese and Lewis [12]; with permission)

The Future of Diagnostics in Psychiatry

The current diagnostic system in psychiatry remains symptom and syndrome based as shown below. New research is mining major psychiatric disorders using different supervised and nature-inspired computing techniques (see Fig. 25.11) [13].

The Future of Classification

Classification of psychiatric disorders is going through a major transformation. Symptom-based classification of mental disorders using the ICD/DSM diagnoses is not mapping well to neurobiological findings. The Biological Classification of Mental Disorders (BeCOME) study will recruit 1000 individuals with affective, anxiety, and stress-related psychiatric disorders and 500 healthy individuals for a control group in order to identify biologically based classes of psychiatric disorders using NIMH Research Domain Criteria (RDoC) through an in-depth collection and examination of clinical laboratory parameters, extraction of blood and plasma DNA, RNA, and peripheral blood mononuclear for the generation of induced pluripotent stem cells, and body measurement, vital signs, heart rate variability, and EKG in addition to tests of psychophysiology, neuropsychology, and neuroimaging as detailed below (see Fig. 25.12) [14].

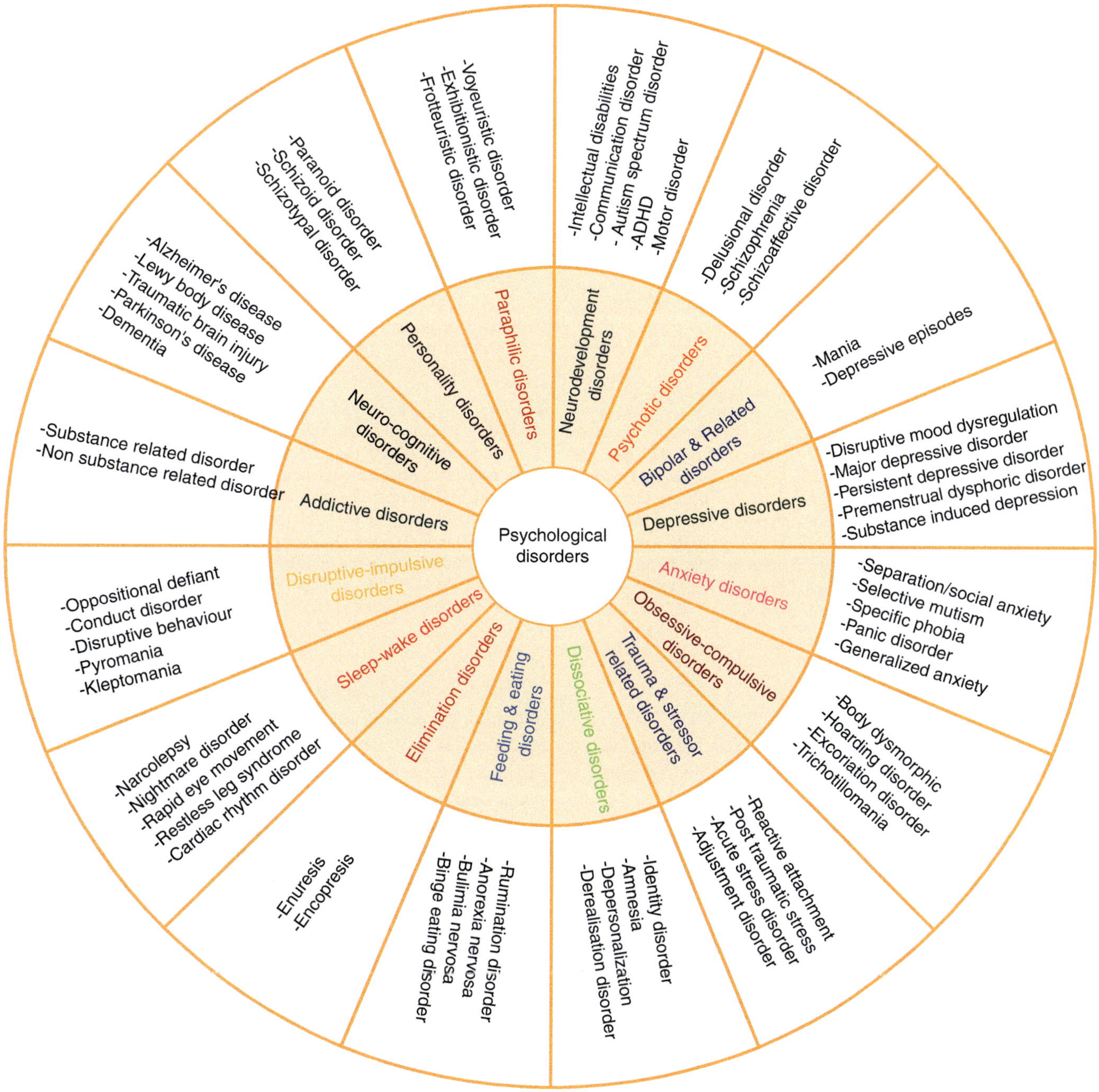

Fig. 25.11 Classification of psychiatric disorders according to the DSM-5. (*From* Kaur and Sharma [13]; with permission)

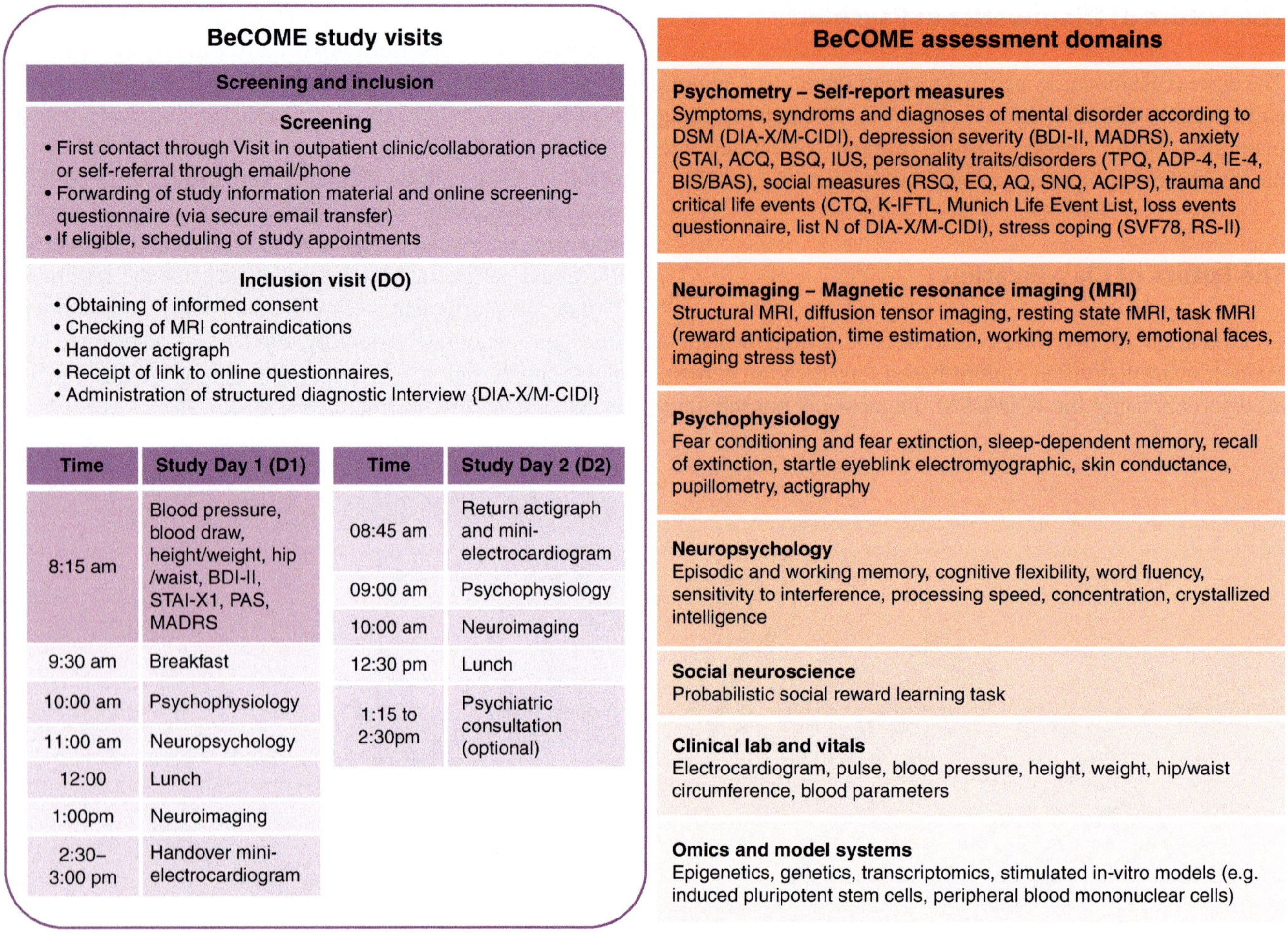

Fig. 25.12 The biological classification of mental disorders (BeCOME) schedule and assessment domains. *DIA-X/M-CIDI* lifetime, and 12-month version of the computer-assisted Munich-Composite International Diagnostic Interview; *BDI-II* Beck Depression Inventory Second Edition; *MADRS* Montgomery-Asberg Depression Rating Scale; *STAI* State-Trait-Anxiety Inventory; *ACQ* Agoraphobic Cognitions Questionnaire; *BSQ* Body Sensations Questionnaire; *IUS* Intolerance-of-Uncertainty Scale; *PAS* Panic and Agoraphobia Scale; *TPQ* Tridimensional Personality Questionnaire; *ADP-IV* Assessment of DSM-IV Personality Disorders; *IE-4* Internal-External Locus of Control Scale; *BIS/BAS* Behavioral Inhibition and Behavioral Approach System Scales; *RSQ* Relationship Scales Questionnaire; *EQ* Empathy Quotient; *AQ* Autism Quotient; *SNQ* Social Network Questionnaire; *ACIPS* Anticipatory and Consummatory Interpersonal Pleasure Scale; *CTQ* Childhood Trauma Questionnaire; *KIFTL* short inventory for the assessment of early traumatic life events; *SVF78* German stress coping questionnaire—78 items version; *RS-11* resilience scale 11 items version. (From Brückl et al. [14]; Creative Commons CC BY)

Noninvasive Tests

Sweat analysis for cortisol is now utilized for noninvasive stress monitoring through the use of wearable and portable electrochemical sensing (see Fig. 25.13) [15].

Biomarkers

Biomarkers are becoming essential tools for the assessment of diagnosis, disease progression, intervention/prevention, patient stratification, therapeutic response, and clinical outcome. The framework for the development of biomarkers in psychiatry is detailed below (see Fig. 25.14) [16].

Biomarkers are highly needed in psychiatric disorders to complement self-report and clinician-rated measures, to predict the risk, confirm the diagnosis, assess the outcome, and estimate the prognosis, paving the road for precision and personalized psychiatry (see Fig. 25.15) [17].

Neuroimmune biomarkers especially in depression have been identified as depicted in Table 25.2 [18].

Central and peripheral immunological markers were also identified throughout the lifetime course of schizophrenia (see Fig. 25.16) [19].

Neuropathology markers and biobanks are now becoming a fundamental aspect of future psychiatric research using the Stanley Neuropathology Consortium as an example as shown in Fig. 25.17 [20].

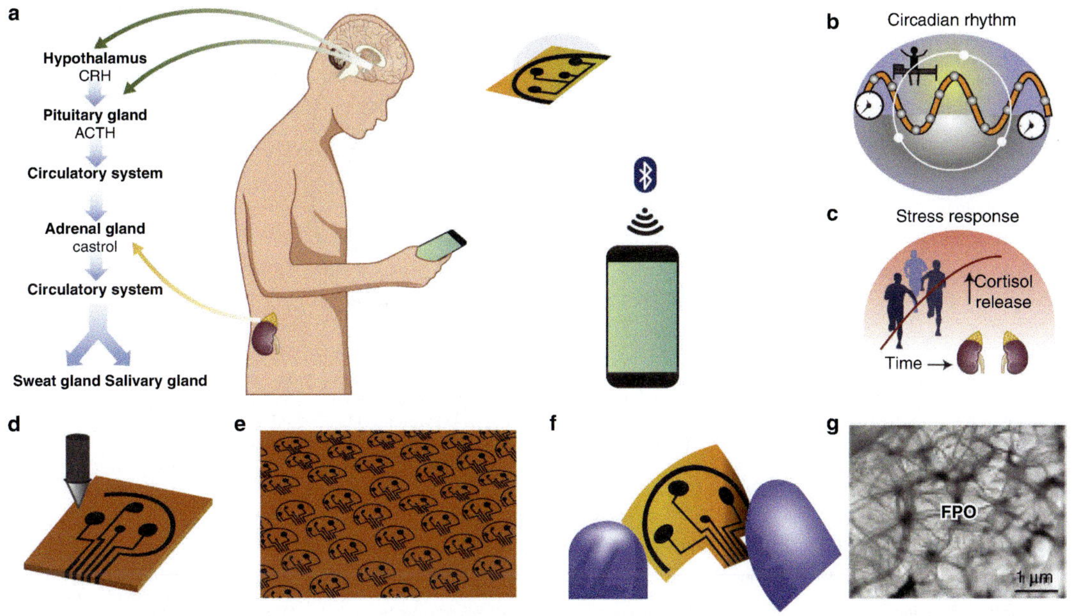

Fig. 25.13 An integrated wireless graphene-based sweat stress sensing system (GS) for dynamic and noninvasive stress hormone analysis. (**a**) Schematic illustration of the origin of cortisol in sweat and saliva and the use of the GS to track the circulating cortisol level. *CRH* corticotropin-releasing hormone; *ACTH* adrenocorticotropic hormone. (**b** and **c**) Conceptual illustration of cortisol dynamics regulated by circadian rhythm (**b**) and triggered by physiological and psychological stress (**c**). (**d**) Illustration of the laser-engraving process of a graphene platform. (**e**) Graphene sensor arrays mass-produced on a polyimide substrate. (**f**) Image of a disposable flexible graphene sensor array. (**g**) TEM image of the graphene electrode surface. (From Torrente-Rodríguez et al. [15]; with permission)

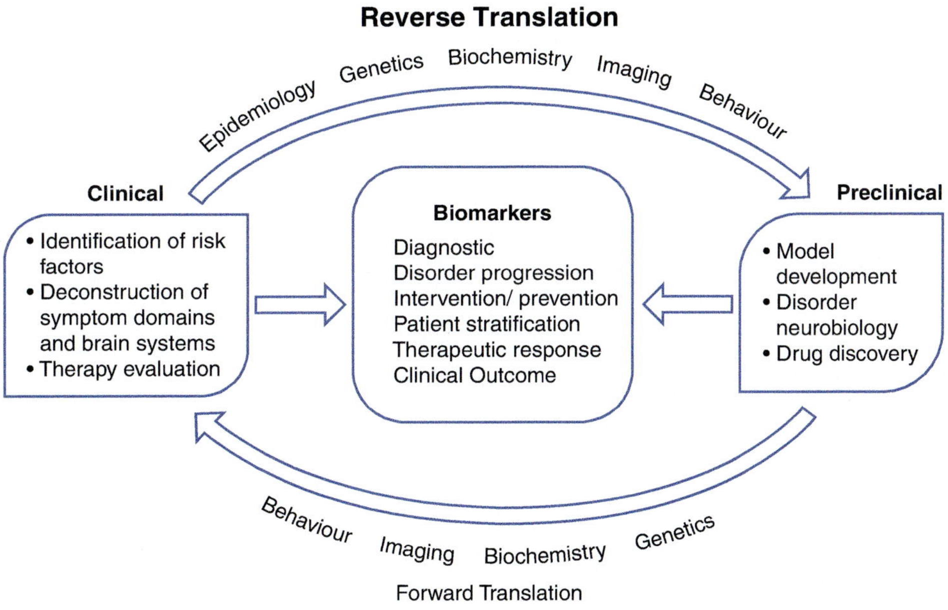

Fig. 25.14 Framework for biomarker development through the adoption of forward and reverse translation approaches. The importance of adopting a reciprocal forward and reverse translation approach that is iteratively updated when additional new information is gained, either preclinically or clinically, offers the greatest opportunity for discovering panels of biomarkers for the diagnosis, prognosis, and treatment of schizophrenia. Note that biomarkers are objective biological measures that can broadly be divided into several categories: (1) diagnostic, where they can aid in predicting risk and diagnosis; (2) prognostic, where they can provide a signpost for clinical course; and (3) predictive of drug response/therapeutic intervention, whether beneficial or adverse and thereby provide a potential means of patient stratification. (From Pratt et al. [16]; with permission)

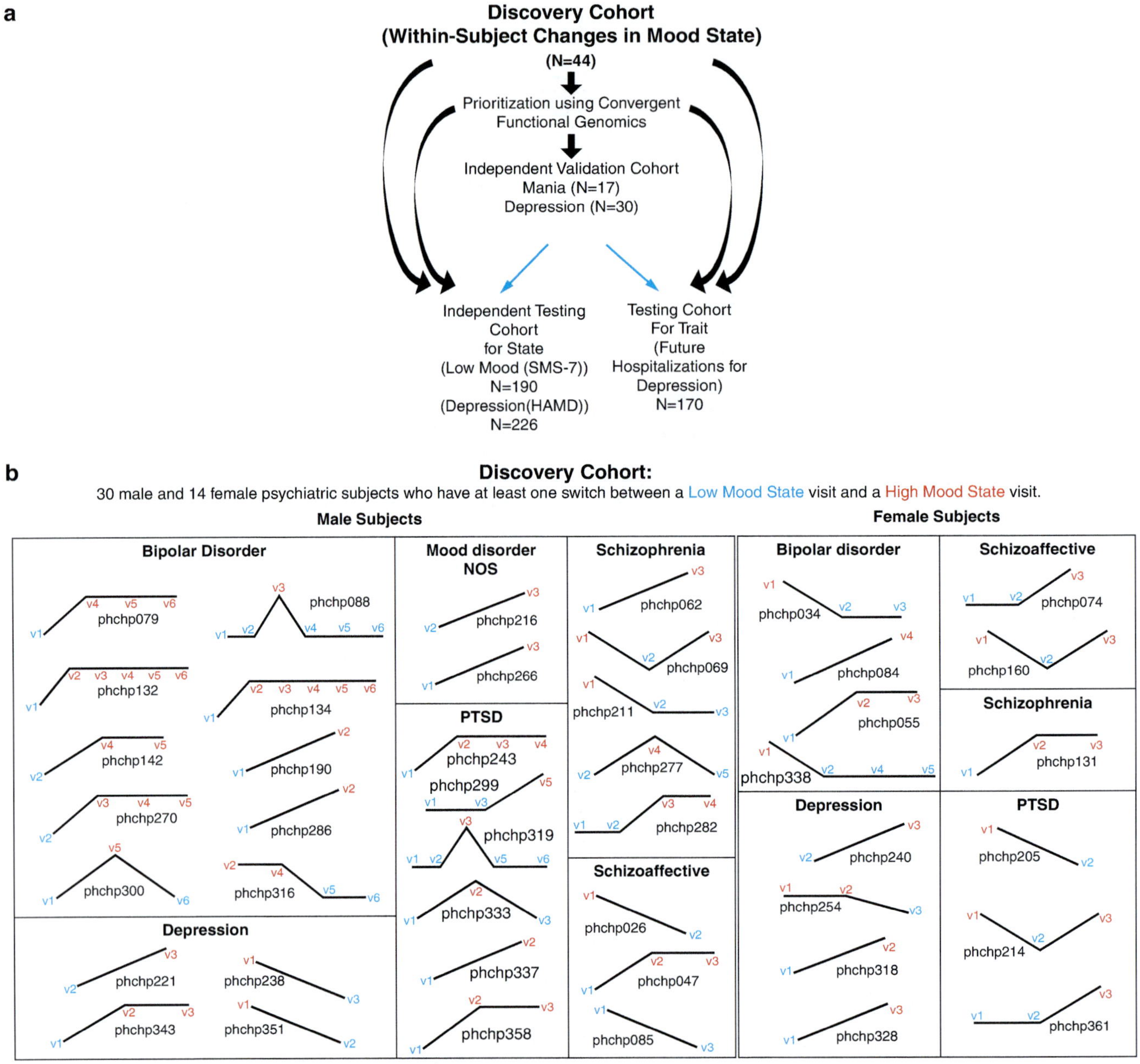

Fig. 25.15 Steps 1–3: Discovery, prioritization, and validation of biomarkers for mood. (**a**) Cohorts used in study, depicting flow of discovery, prioritization, and validation of biomarkers from each step. (**b**) Discovery cohort longitudinal within-subject analysis. Phchp### is study ID for each subject. V# denotes visit number. (**c**) Differential gene expression in the discovery cohort, number of genes identified with differential expression (DE), and absent–present (AP) methods with an internal score of 2 and above. Red increased in expression in high mood; blue decreased in expression in high mood. At the discovery step, probesets are identified based on their score for tracking mood with a maximum of internal points of 6 (33% (2 pt), 50% (4 pt), and 80% (6 pt)). (**d**) Prioritization with CFG for prior evidence of involvement in mood disorders. In the prioritization step, probesets are converted to their associated genes using Affymetrix annotation and GeneCards. Genes are prioritized and scored using CFG for mood evidence with a maximum of 12 points. Genes scoring at least 6 points out of a maximum possible of 18 total discovery and prioritization points are carried to the validation step. (**e**) Validation in two independent cohorts of psychiatric patients with clinically severe depression (HAMD ≥22) and clinically severe mania (YMRS ≥20). In the validation step, biomarkers are assessed for stepwise change from the validation group with mania, to the discovery groups of subjects with high mood, low mood, to the validation group with depression, using ANOVA. *N* is the number of testing visits. Two hundred ninety-one biomarkers were nominally significant, and 1446 biomarkers were stepwise changed. PRPS1 and SLC6A4 are examples of significantly increased, respectively, decreased, biomarkers in validation. There were 26 markers that had an overall Convergent Functional Evidence (CFE) score from Steps 1–3 that was at least as good as SLC6A4, which serves as a de facto positive control and that we decided to use as a cutoff. The markers in red are increased in high mood; the markers in blue are decreased in high mood/increased in depression (color figure online). (From Le-Niculescu et al. [17]; Creative Commons CC BY)

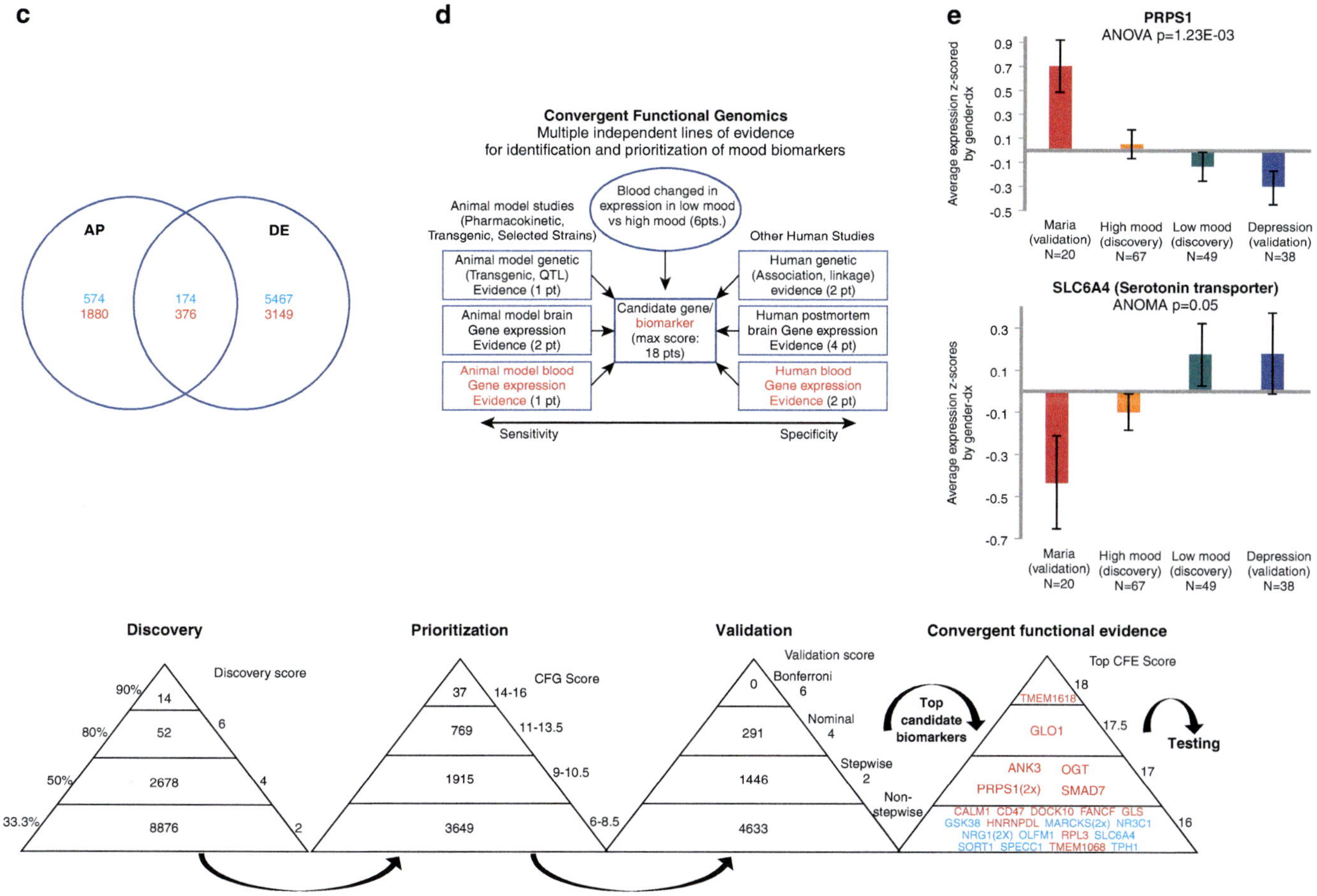

Fig. 25.15 (continued)

Table 25.2 Selected potential neuroimmune biomarkers for depression

Biomarker	Strength of association	Translation potential
IL-6	Supported by meta-analysis	Part of diagnostic array or stratification marker; treatment response indicator
CRP	Supported by meta-analysis	Stratification marker
TNF-α	Supported by meta-analysis	Stratification marker; treatment response indicator
IL-1β	Meta-analytical data variable	Stratification marker; treatment response indicator
MCP-1/CCL2	Supported by meta-analysis	Part of diagnostic array; stratification marker
IL-8/CXCL8	Meta-analytical data uncertain	Part of diagnostic array; stratification marker
IFN-γ	Meta-analytical data uncertain	Stratification marker
IFN-α, IL-4, IL-5, IL-7, IL-10, IL-12, etc.	Data uncertain/ inconclusive	More investigation required to establish relationships more fully

From Herron et al. [18]; with permission

Neuroimaging

The future of diagnostic methods in psychiatry includes advances in structural and functional neuroimaging given the expansion of databases of neuroimaging studies and advances of meta-analysis techniques as seen in Fig. 25.18 [21].

Neuroimaging has been also used to further our understanding of psychological phenomena (see Fig. 25.19) [22].

Brain imaging could be used in future of treatment selection. For the treatment of depression, antidepressant medication and cognitive therapy are effective interventions that share similar neural mechanisms, and each distinguish themselves by distinct ones. Neuroimaging techniques using resting-state PET imaging and task-related fMRI could have value in the future to predict and select best matched patients to each intervention (see Fig. 25.20) [23].

Large brain mapping databases with thousands of functional and structural neuroimaging such as BrainMap and NeuroVault among many others are creating new understandings and classifications in neuroscience and psychiatry (see Fig. 25.21) [24].

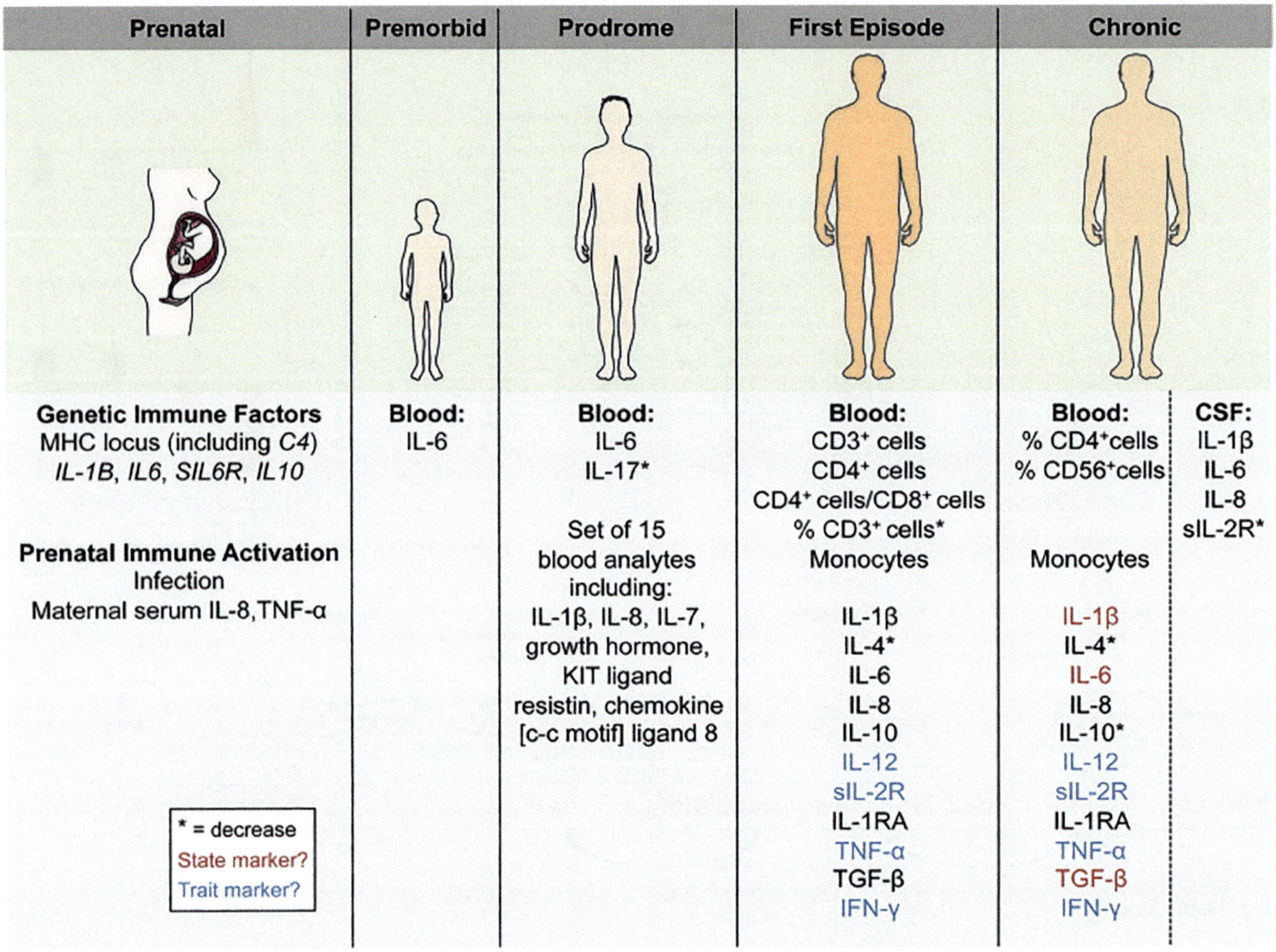

Fig. 25.16 Peripheral and central immune alterations along the clinical course of schizophrenia and their potential as immune-related biomarkers. Relevant immune-related markers are summarized against the background of developmental stages (potential predictive biomarkers) and the clinical course of schizophrenia. All immune markers listed signify increased levels detected in at-risk individuals or patients relative to healthy controls, except when denoted by the symbol (*) (= decrease). Putative state and trait markers are depicted in red and blue color, respectively. Abbreviations: *MHC* major histocompatibility complex; *C4* complement component 4; *IL* interleukin; *TNF* tumor necrosis factor; *CD* cluster of differentiation; *sIL-2R* soluble interleukin 2 receptor; *IL-1RA* interleukin 1 receptor antagonist; *TGF* transforming growth factor; *IFN* interferon. (From Notter [19]; with permission)

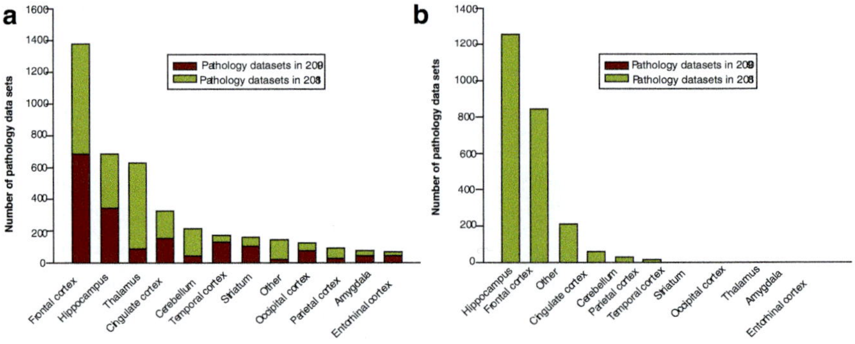

Fig. 25.17 Total numbers of neuropathology markers in the Stanley Neuropathology Consortium Integrative Database. The number of markers from each brain region from the Stanley Neuropathology Consortium (**a**) and the Array Collection (**b**). (From Kim and Webster [20]; with permission)

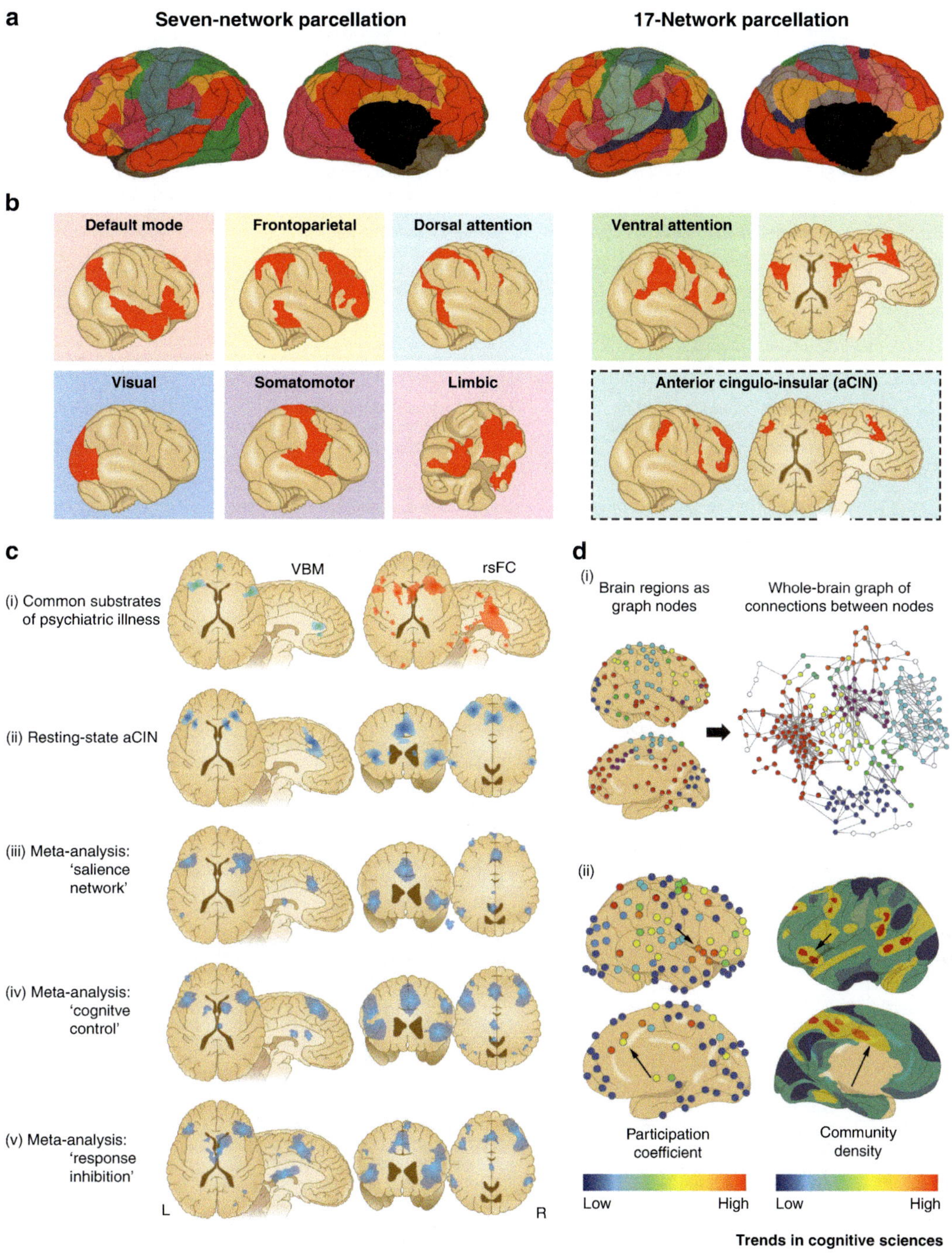

Fig. 25.18 Psychiatric common core regions in the context of the functional architecture of the human brain. (**a**) Consistent networks can be identified within the activity of the resting brain. 7- and 17-network parcellations have been reported as being particularly stable across individuals in data sets of 1000 subjects. (**b**) Replicable networks include visual, somatomotor, and limbic networks, as well as a default-mode network (DMN) active during rest or introspection, two to three frontoparietal networks (FPN) active during cognitive tasks or extrospection, and an anterior cingulo-insular network (aCIN) or salience network (SN), which closely overlaps the common core areas of structural abnormality across psychiatric disorders. (**c**) The common neural substrates across multiple psychiatric illnesses on voxel-based morphometry (VBM) studies comprise a coherent functional network on resting-state functional connectivity (rsFC) mapping (i), corresponding closely to the aCIN (ii), which in turn corresponds closely to the set of regions emerging from Neurosynth meta-analyses of activations in neuroimaging studies of the salience network (iii), and more specifically of the Research Domain Criteria construct "cognitive control" (iv) and response inhibition (v). (**d**) (i) In graph theoretical analyses of the functional architecture of the brain, the aCIN regions (shown in purple) stand in a "crossroads" position, connecting to many other subcommunities. By contrast, other communities, such as low-level visual networks (blue), low-level sensorimotor networks (cyan), or even the DMN itself (red), are relatively self-contained, tightly integrated within themselves but not widely connected to other communities. (ii) Quantitative measures of network centrality, such as the participation coefficient (left) and community density (right), are high in the nodes of the aCIN (dorsal anterior cingulate cortex and anterior insula), supporting the premise that these regions serve as "hubs" or "crossroad" regions within the functional architecture of the brain as a whole. (From Downar et al. [21]; with permission)

Module	Secure Attachment (balanced de- and hyper-activation)	Avoidant Attachment (de-activation)	Anxious Attachment (hyper-activation)
Aversion Module 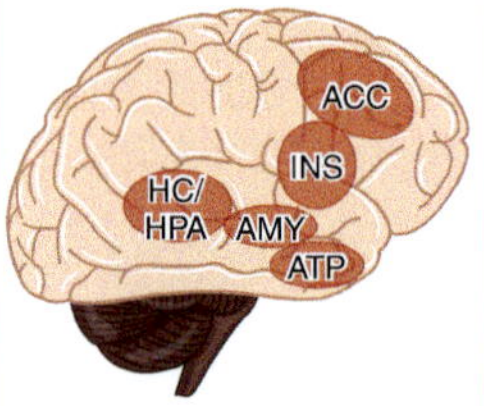	• Beneficial stress-reducing influence of secure-based social interactions, priming, and mental representations (anatomy, function, and connectivity) • Short- and long-term effects • Protective effect of readily available social (co-) regulation during stress & generally lower likelihood of early adversity ↓	• Lower activation during social exclusion due to expectation of rejection by others • Increased activation during negative social information processing when inhibition/suppression as emotion regulation strategy cannot be employed • Indication of long-term elevated stress HPA axis modification • Limited efficiency of deactivating strategies ↑↓	• Higher activation during the processing of negative social information • Anatomical alteration pointing to long-term Elevated Stress/HPA axis modification • This pattern is consistent with hyper-activating strategies that increase the saliency of social cues pointing towards social rejection / the unavailability of others during stressful situations ↑
Approach Module 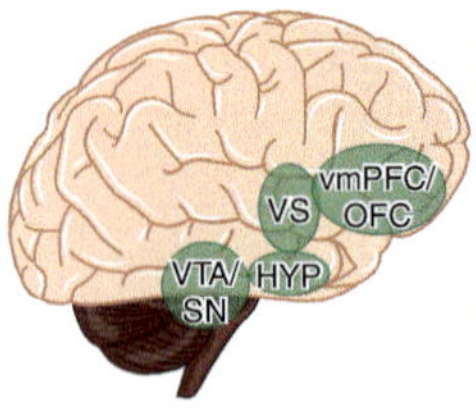	• Activation generally reflecting positive motivational attributes towards, and affective representations of others – especially under conditions of threat and stress, i.e. when others are needed to (co-)regulate negative states • This pattern accords with a positive model of others characteristic for attachment security ↑	• Generally decreased approach module activation (both across close and more distant social contexts) • Role of oxytocin and/or endogenous opioids, apart from dopamine, in such processes • Pattern reflects negative other-model associated with attachment avoidance ↓	• Only limited evidence of altered approach module functionality • Some findings point to increased (automatic) processing of positive social cues, particularly when they occur unexpectedly, i.e, when social rejection is anticipated but does not occur • Patten agrees with a partially positive other-model / wish for closeness and care ↑
Emotion (Self-) Regulation Module 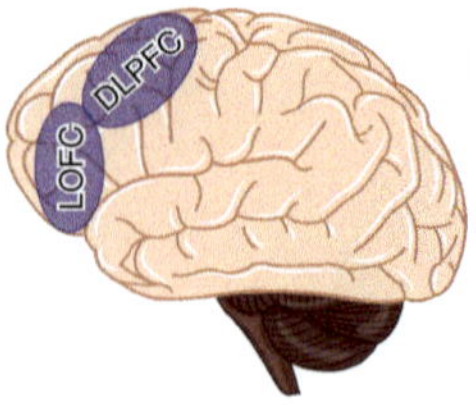	• Emotion (self-)regulation appears functional and efficient (successful aversion module down-regulation through physical contact as well as by positive mental representation of significant others) • Indication of better between the emotion regulation and aversion modules • Mental state representation ↑	• Preferential use of inhibition/suppression when dealing with (social) emotions, both positive and negative • Emotion regulation appears ineffective when inhibition / suppression cannot be employed – e.g. cognitive re-appraisal fails in down-regulating aversion module activity during negative social information processing • Social (co-)regulation appears ineffective and may even exacerbate aversion module activity during stressful situations ↓	• Increased activation during natural processing of (social) negative information • No consistent indication of emotion dawn-regulation difficulties • Both cognitive re-appraisal and suppression / inhibition appear functional when properly instructed • Social (co-)regulation under stress also seems effective • Pattern points to dependence on external contribution towards emotion regulation associated with a negative self-model ↓
Mental State Representation Module 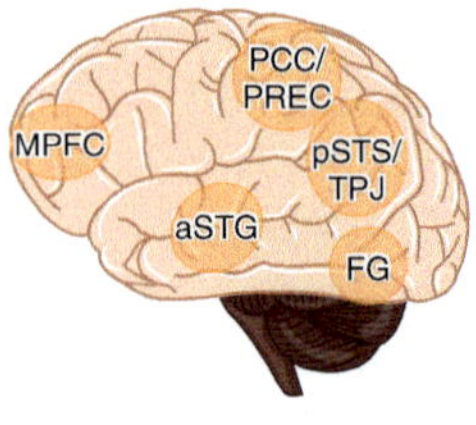	• Seems to develop early • Predominantly positive representation of others • More extensive (functional) connectivity with the other modules ↑	• Only very limited evidence • One Study implies less mentalizing (RMET) • Possible tendency for hyper-mentalizatian due to the need for an early assessment of social situations so that inhibition/suppression can be employed if deemed necessary • More data is still needed ↓	• Only very limited evidence • One study in adolescents indicates both activation in- and decreases as a function of both mentalization content valence (positive versus negative) and focus (self versus close other) • More data is still needed ↓↑

Fig. 25.19 Summary of the most consistent effects regarding attachment security, avoidance, and anxiety on the functioning of affective evaluation (approach and aversion) and cognitive control (emotion regulation and mental state representation). Extended and refined summary of associations between approach, aversion, emotion regulation, and mental state representation module functionality and interindividual differences in attachment security, avoidance, and anxiety, as disclosed by first-person social neuroscience data. Abbreviations: *HPA* hypothalamus-pituitary adrenal; *aversion module*; *ACC* anterior cingulate cortex; *INS* insula; *HC/HPA* hippocampus/HPA-axis; *AMY* amygdala; *ATP* anterior temporal pole; *approach module*; *vmMPF/OFC* ventromedial prefrontal/orbitofrontal cortex; *VS* ventral striatum; *HYP* hypothalamus; *VTA/SN* ventral tegmental area/substantia nigra; *emotion regulation module*; *DLPFC* dorsolateral prefrontal cortex; *LOFC* lateral orbitofrontal cortex; *mental state representation module*; *MPFC* medial prefrontal cortex; *PCC/PREC* posterior cingulate cortex/precuneus; *pSTS/TPJ* posterior superior temporal sulcus/temporo-parietal junction; *aSTG* anterior superior temporal gyrus; *FG* fusiform gyrus. (From Long et al. [22]; Creative Commons CC BY)

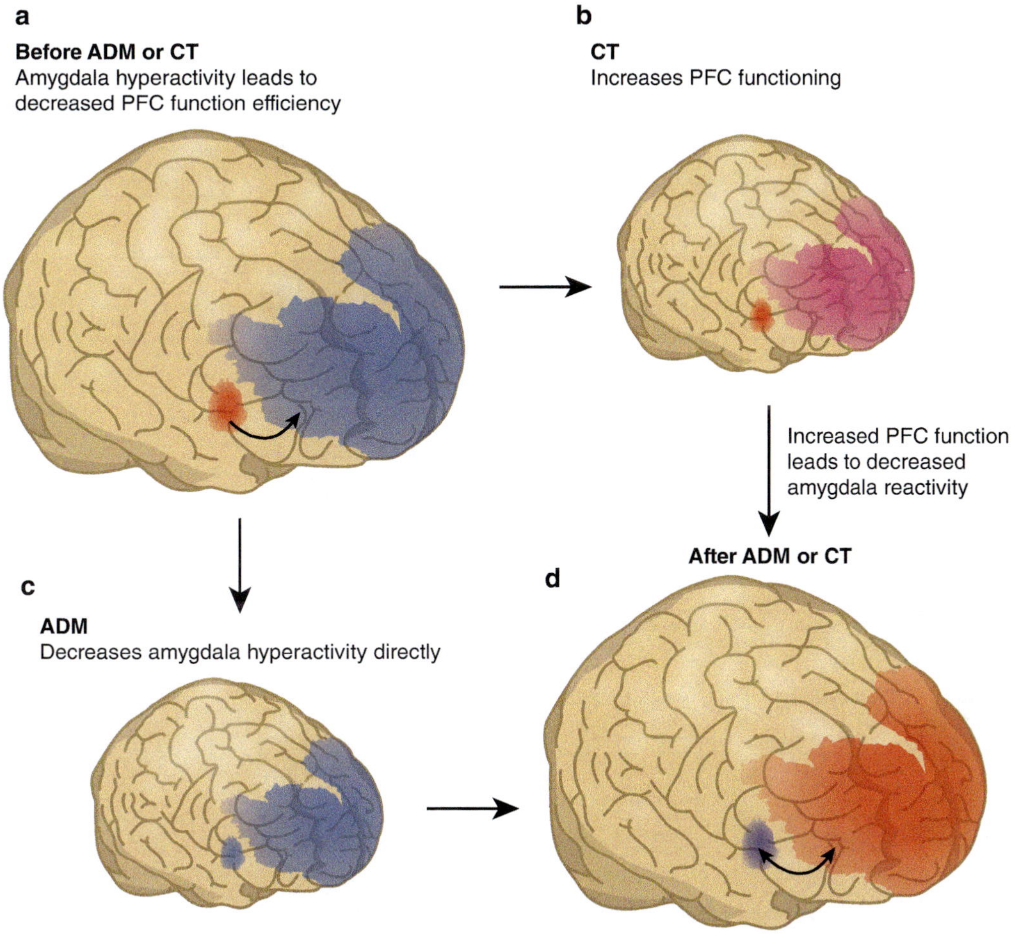

Fig. 25.20 Hypothetical time course of the changes to amygdala and prefrontal function that are associated with antidepressant medication and cognitive therapy based on available evidence. (**a**) During acute depression, amygdala activity is increased (red), and prefrontal activity is decreased (blue) relative to activity in these regions in healthy individuals. (**b**) Cognitive therapy (CT) effectively exercises the prefrontal cortex (PFC), yielding increased inhibitory function of this region. (**c**) Antidepressant medication (ADM) targets amygdala function more directly, decreasing its activity. (**d**) After ADM or CT, amygdala function is decreased, and prefrontal function is increased. The double-headed arrow between the amygdala and the PFC represents the bidirectional homeostatic influences that are believed to operate in healthy individuals. (From DeRubeis et al. [23]; with permission)

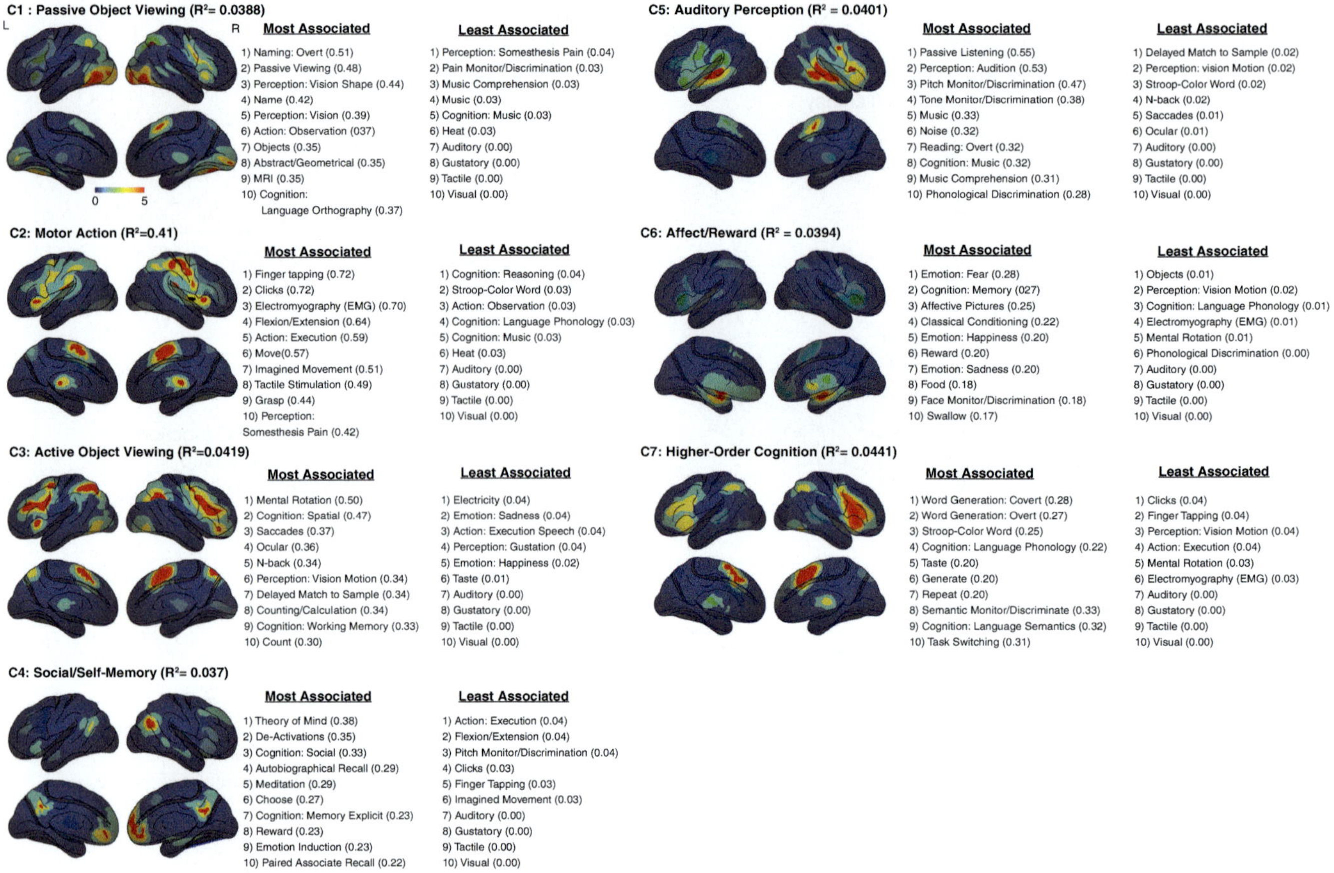

Fig. 25.21 Centroid activation maps and behavioral decoding for seven-cluster solution. (*BD* behavioral domain; *PC* paradigm class; *ExtVariable* external variable; *Stim* stimulus; *Resp* response). Centroid activation maps with preliminary interpretative descriptions for the seven-cluster solution. (From Bolt et al. [24]; with permission)

The Future of Psychiatric Treatment

The future of psychiatric treatment will involve advances in precision psychiatry, psychotherapy, psychopharmacology, and brain-modulation, as well as advanced treatments at the molecular, cascade, cellular, network, person, and population levels.

The Future of Precision Psychiatry

Precision psychiatry, which evolved from precision medicine, uses a treatment and prevention approach that "takes each person's variability in genes, environment, and lifestyle" into account [25]. The future of precision psychiatry will involve the domains and components described in Fig. 25.22 [26].

Psychotherapy

Advanced psychotherapy involves addressing with the psychodynamic and cognitive steps with their neurobiological impact (see Fig. 25.23) [27].

The recent decade has witnessed the growth of online psychotherapy and digital therapeutics delivered through apps culminating in FDA clearance of new psychotherapeutic treatments (see Fig. 25.24) [28].

Psychopharmacology

Psychopharmacology is one of the main stays of psychiatric treatment in the last five decades. More innovative mechanisms of action are still evolving as detailed in the next sections.

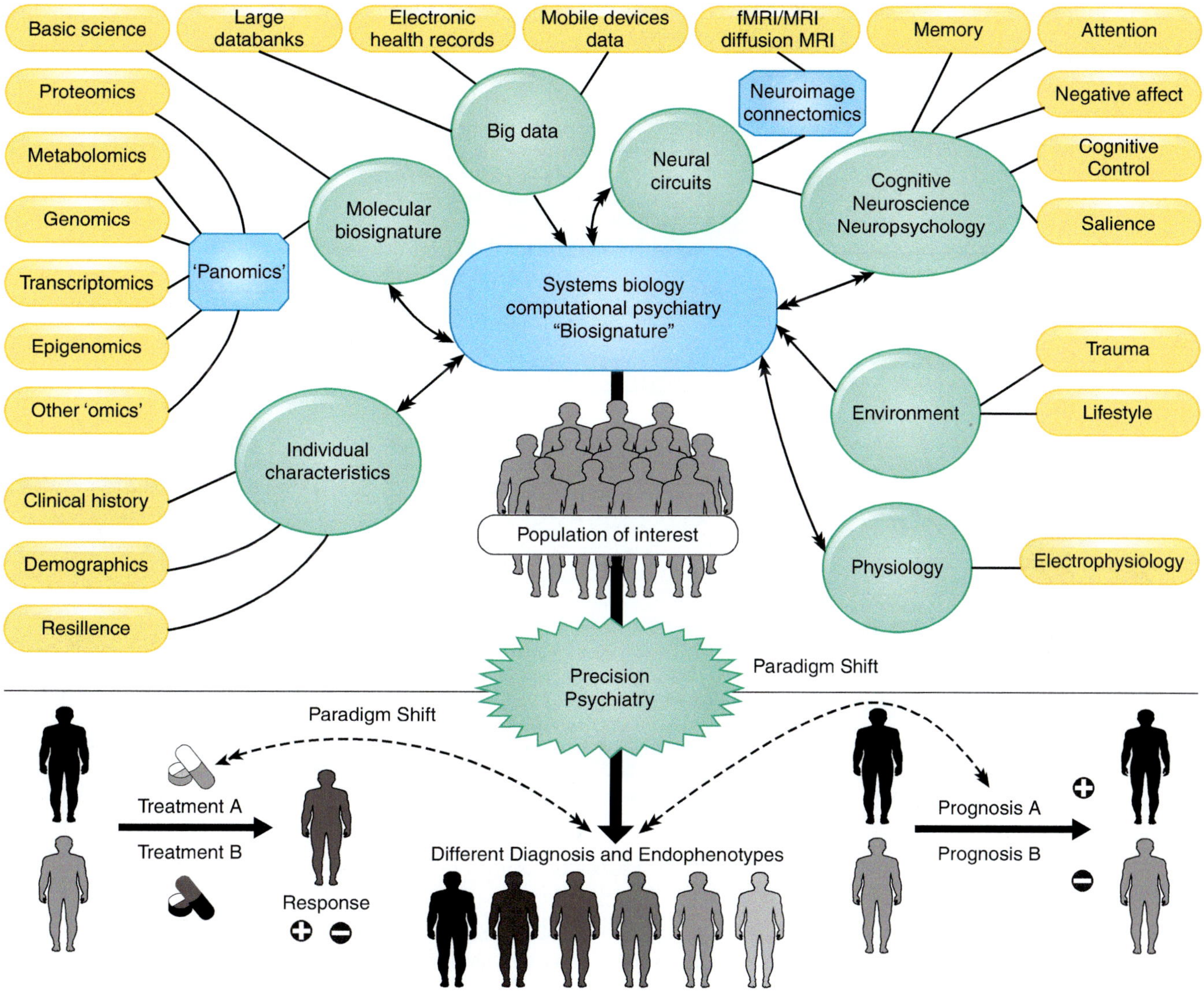

Fig. 25.22 Domains related to "precision psychiatry". Diverse approaches and techniques, such as "omics," neuroimaging, cognition, and clinical characteristics, converge to several domains. These domains can be analyzed using systems biology and computational psychiatry tools to produce a biosignature—a set of biomarkers—that, when applied to individuals and populations, will produce better diagnosis, endophenotypes (measurable components unseen by the unaided eye along the pathway between disease and distal genotype), classifications and prognosis, and tailored interventions for better outcomes. The bottom-up approach from specific areas (such as metabolomics) to domains (such as molecular biosignature), to systems biology and computational psychiatry, and to a resultant biosignature can also be reverted to a top-down approach, with specific biosignatures being analyzed to better understand domains and its specific components. Components and domains are not mutually exclusive, and a subject can belong to more than one component or domain; for instance, "large databanks" can belong to data from "neuroimaging," "mobile devices," and "panomics," all of which are put as different domains. After the establishment of precision psychiatry, persons considered to belong to the same group (agglomerate of persons in grey) will be reclassified into different diagnosis and endophenotypes. Further, after accomplishing precision psychiatry, it will be possible to more accurately predict response or nonresponse to treatment, as well as better prognosis. (From Fernandes et al. [26]; Creative Commons CC BY)

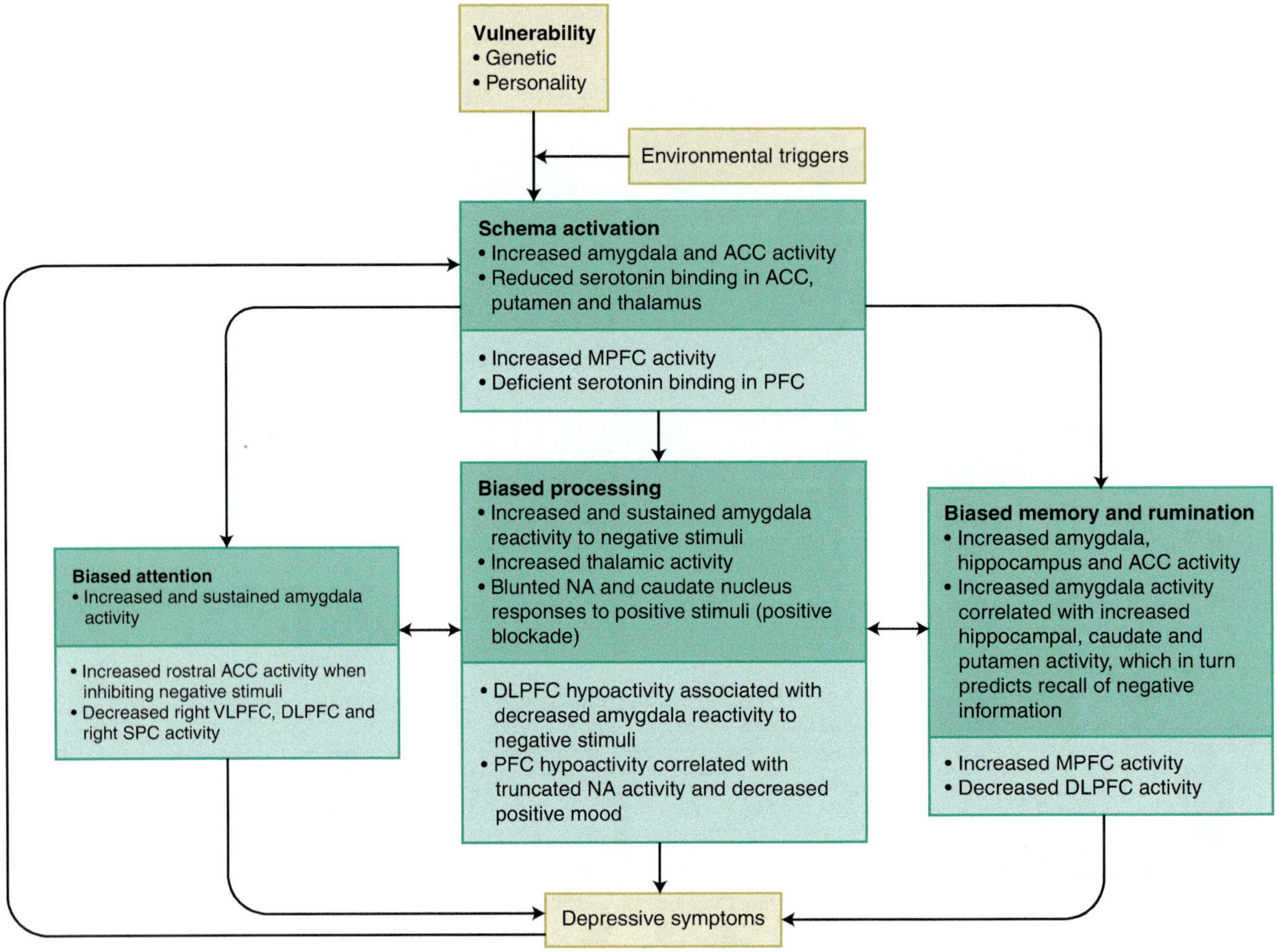

Fig. 25.23 Summary of an integrated cognitive neurobiological model of depression. This flowchart shows the sequence of events that is proposed to be involved in the development of depression, beginning with depression vulnerability factors and environmental stressors and resulting in depressive symptoms. The figure outlines the neurobiological events that are associated with each step of the cognitive model: schema activation, biased attention, biased processing, and biased memory and rumination. The brain regions in this flowchart are divided into two groups: regions associated with bottom-up, limbic system influences (shown by the blue boxes), and regions that maintain bottom-up influences through altered top-down, cognitive control (shown by the gray boxes). Note that all elements contribute directly to depressive symptoms and that depressive symptoms also feed back into the system, thus exacerbating schema activation. *ACC* anterior cingulate cortex; *DLPFC* dorsolateral prefrontal cortex; *MPFC* medial prefrontal cortex; *NA* nucleus accumbens; *PFC* prefrontal cortex; *SPC* superior parietal cortex. (From Disner et al. [27]; with permission)

Old and New Targets

The targets for drug action for psychopharmacological agents are highlighted below [29] (see Fig. 25.25) showing that there is still significant room for more agents.

Innovative Medication Combinations

Innovative medication combinations as the ones in the figure below [30] will need to be tested in comparative effectiveness studies (see Fig. 25.26).

Drug Repositioning for Psychiatric and Neurological Disorders

"Drug repositioning" is a novel approach that uses already approved medications for new purposes for psychiatric and neurological disorder (PNDs) and represents a promising alternative method of treatment. In this example [9], researchers used a powerful machine learning text-mining application to connect PNDs and genes or drugs from 50 years of published scientific literature revealing a several drugs that have not used for the identified PNDs before, paving the road for research trials (see Fig. 25.27).

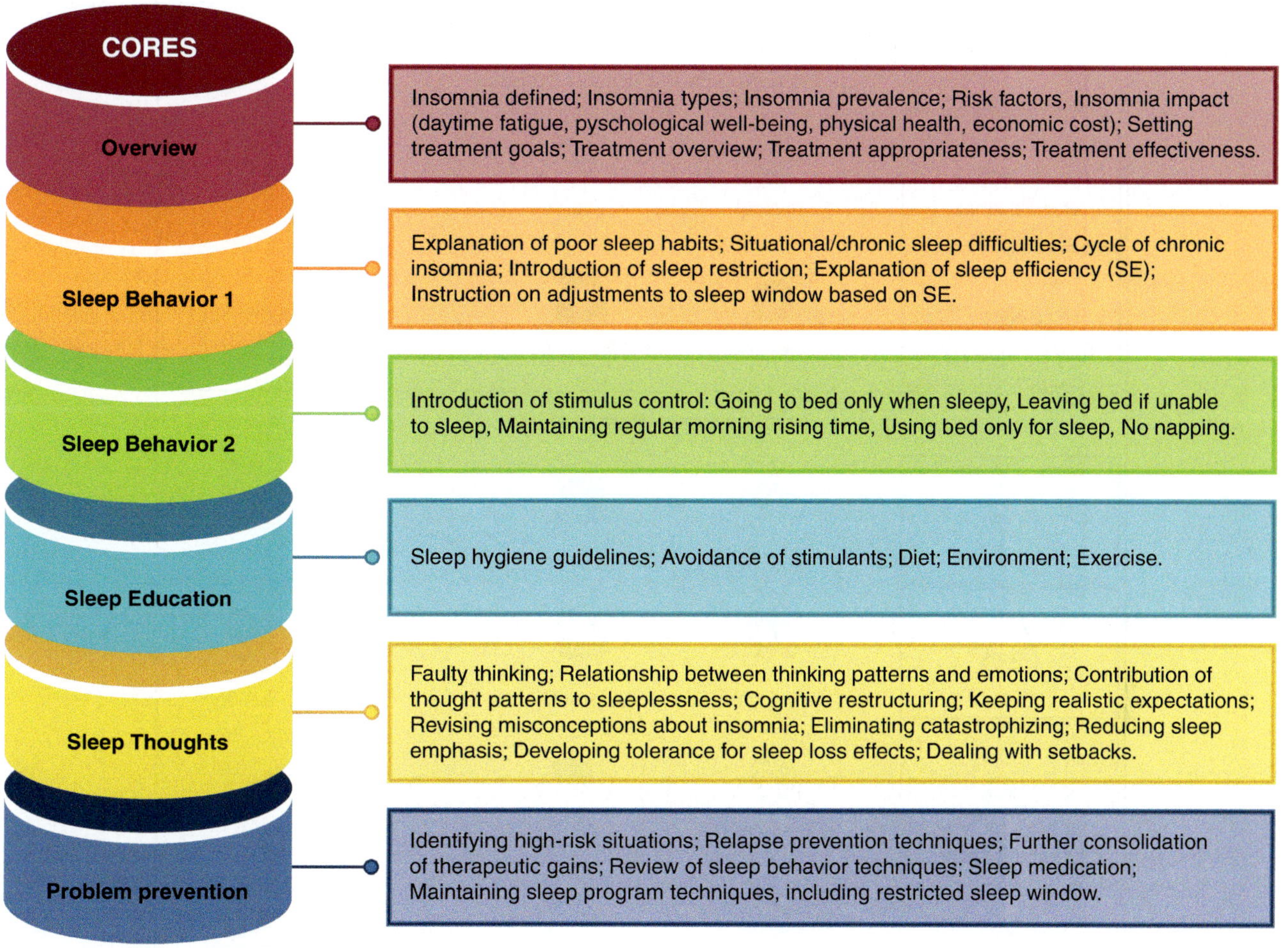

Fig. 25.24 Online CBT for insomnia exemplified by SHUTi Cores and core descriptions. Adapted from "Development and Perceived Utility and Impact of an Internet Intervention for Insomnia," by Thorndike et al., 2008 (Thorndike FP, Saylor DK, Bailey ET, Gonder-Frederick L, Morin CM, Ritterband LM. Development and perceived utility and impact of an Internet intervention for insomnia. E J Appl Psychol. 2008;4(2):32–42.) (From Brooks et al. [28]; Creative Commons CC BY)

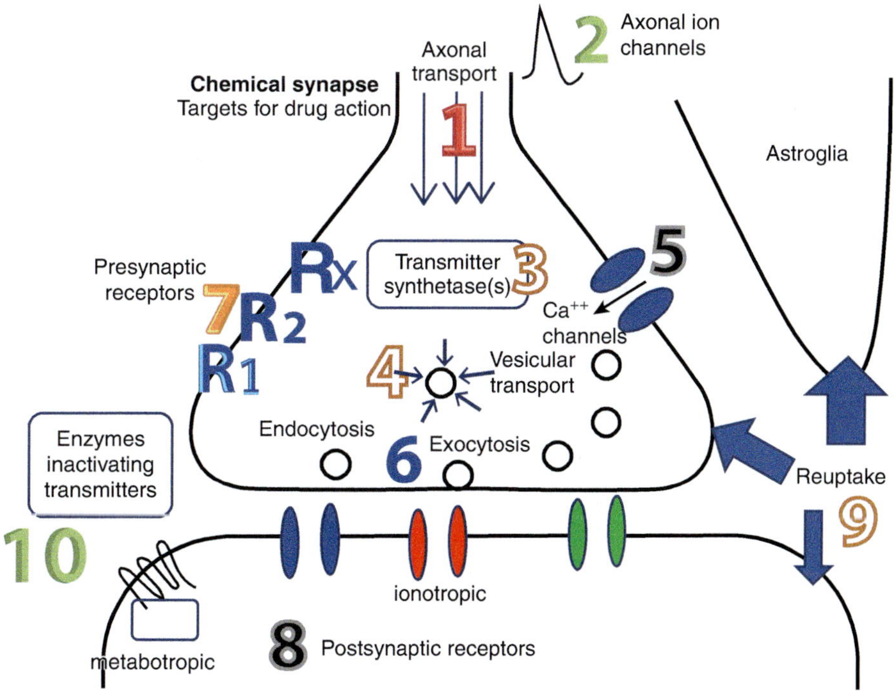

Fig. 25.25 Sites or mechanisms that can influence synaptic chemical transmission. (From Zeise [29]; with permission)

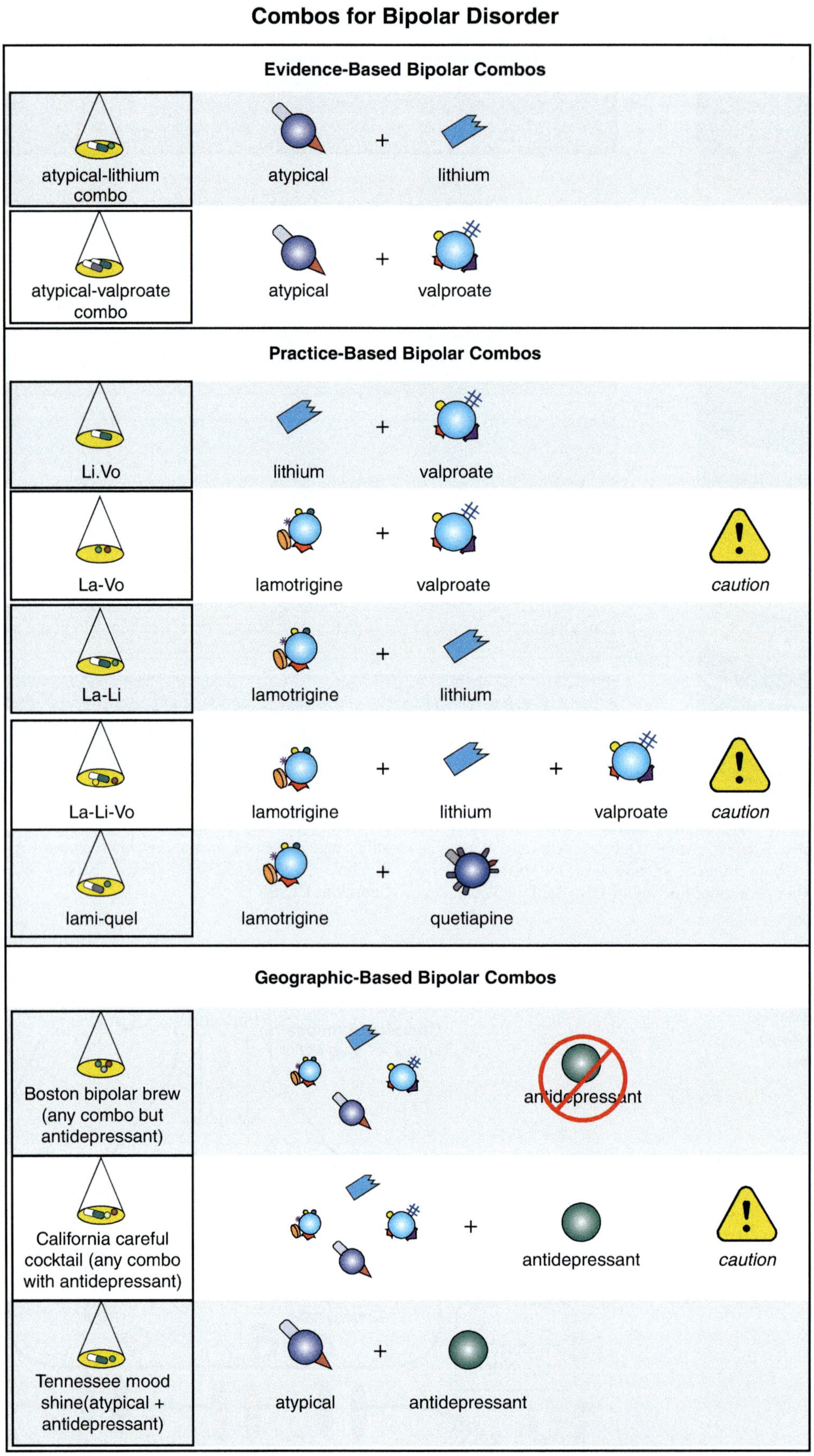

Fig. 25.26 Psychopharmacological combinations in bipolar disorder. (From Stahl [30]; with permission)

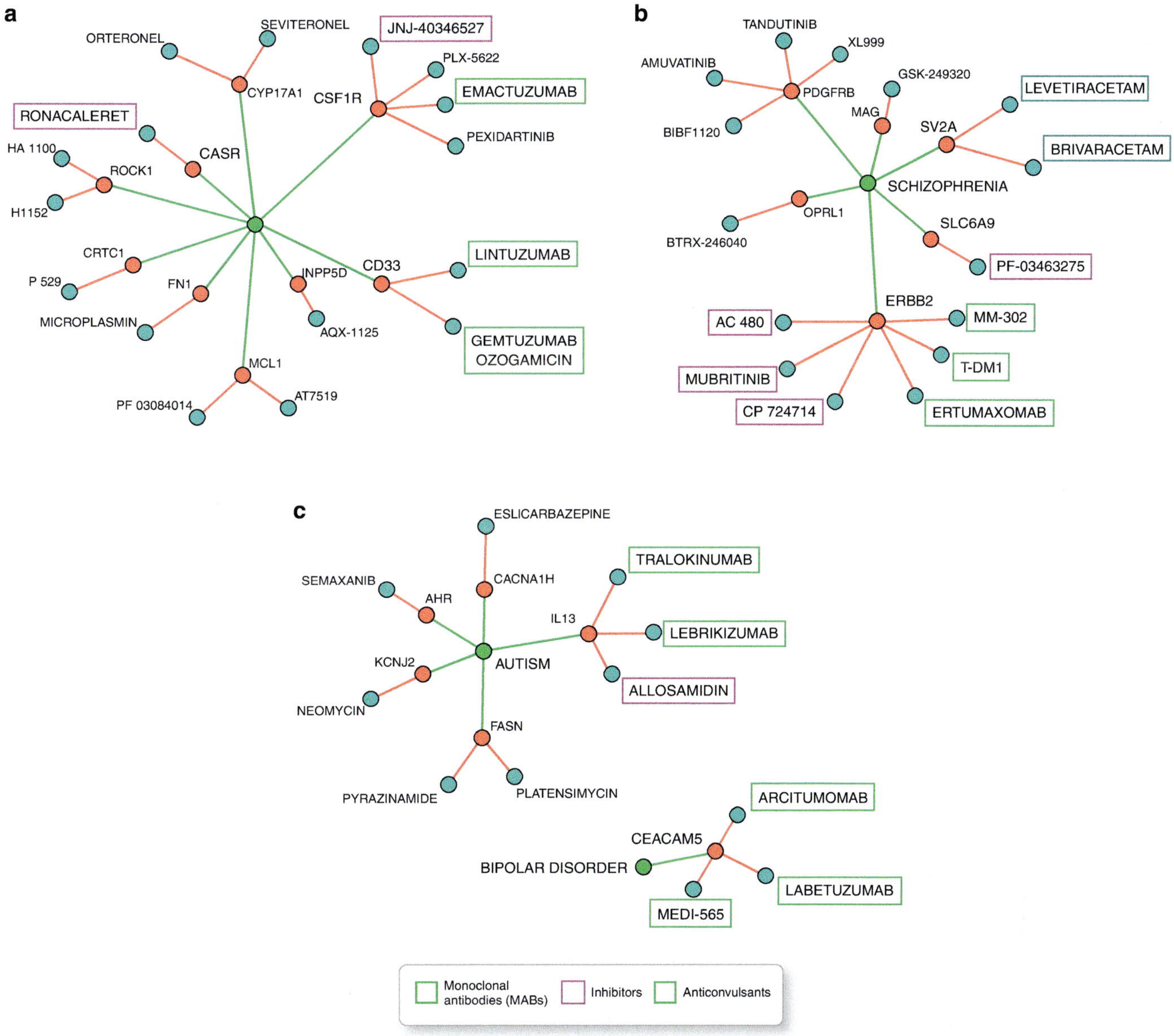

Fig. 25.27 Drugs with high repositioning potential for psychiatric and neurological disorders. (**a–c**) The most promising repositioning drug candidates (blue) that target the genes (red) unique to Alzheimer's disease (**a**), schizophrenia (**b**), and autism and bipolar disorder (**c**). The drugs discussed in the main text are highlighted here: monoclonal antibodies (green), inhibitors (magenta), and anticonvulsants (cyan). (From Lüscher Dias et al. [9]; Creative Commons CC BY)

New Uses of Available Drugs: The Psychedelics Example

Psychedelics such as psilocybin, lysergic acid diethylamide (LSD), and dimethyltryptamine (DMT) have been shown to improve depressive and anxiety symptoms. The number of active studies registered on ClinicalTrials.gov that are focused on psychedelics in psychiatry had surpassed 70 studies by the end of 2020 [31]. The mechanism of action of psychedelics is highlighted in the figure below [32] (see Fig. 25.28).

Psilocybin and other psychedelics such as ayahuasca with or without psychotherapy have been shown to be effective with long-term positive effects in mood disorders especially depression. The functional magnetic resonance imaging (fMRI) study below demonstrates that the effects of psilocybin with psychological support in patients with treatment-resistant depression by examining cerebral blood flow (CBF) and blood oxygen-level dependent (BOLD) resting-state functional connectivity (RSFC) were measured. The study revealed following treatment decreased CBF in the amyg-

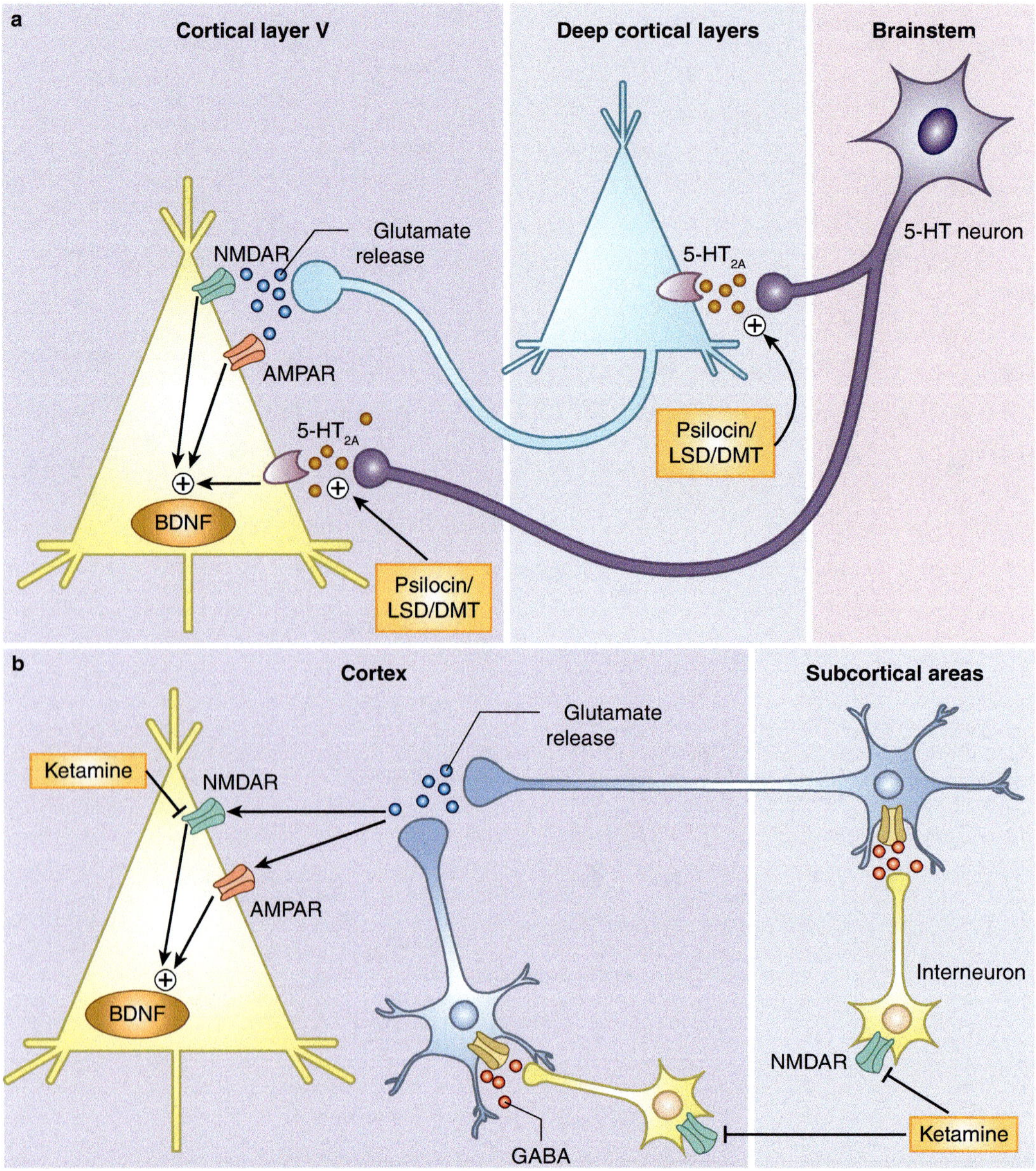

Fig. 25.28 Activation of the prefrontal network and glutamate release by psychedelics. (**a**) The figure shows a model in which hallucinogens, such as psilocin, lysergic acid diethylamide (LSD), and dimethyltryptamine (DMT), increase extracellular glutamate levels in the prefrontal cortex through stimulation of postsynaptic serotonin (5-hydroxytryptamine) 2A (5-HT_{2A}) receptors that are located on large glutamatergic pyramidal cells in deep cortical layers (V and VI) projecting to layer V pyramidal neurons. This glutamate release leads to an activation of AMPA (α-amino-3-hydroxy-5-methyl-4-isoxazole propionic acid) and NMDA (*N*-methyl-D-aspartate) receptors on cortical pyramidal neurons. In addition, hallucinogens directly activate 5-HT_{2A} receptors located on cortical pyramidal neurons. This activation is thought to ultimately lead to increased expression of brain-derived neurotrophic factor (BDNF). (**b**) This figure shows a model in which dissociative NMDA antagonists, such as ketamine, block inhibitory GABA (γ-aminobutyric acid)-ergic interneurons in cortical, and subcortical brain areas, leading to enhanced firing of glutamatergic projection neurons and increased extracellular glutamate levels in the prefrontal cortex. As ketamine also blocks NMDA receptors on cortical pyramidal neurons, the increased glutamate release in the cortex is thought to stimulate cortical AMPA more than NMDA receptors. The increased AMPA-receptor-mediated throughput relative to NMDA-receptor-mediated throughput is thought ultimately to lead to increased expression of BDNF. (From Vollenweider and Kometer [32]; with permission)

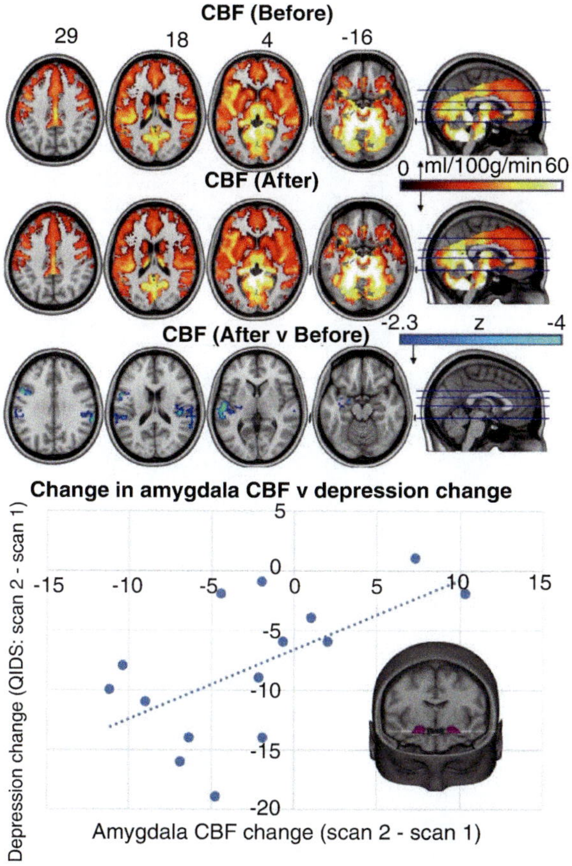

Fig. 25.29 Pre- and post-treatment whole-brain and amygdala CBF. Whole-brain cerebral blood flow maps for baseline versus one-day post-treatment, plus the difference map (cluster-corrected, $p < 0.05$, $n = 16$). Correlation chart shows post-treatment changes in bilateral amygdala CBF versus changes in depressive symptoms ($r = 0.59$, $p = 0.01$). One patient failed to complete the scan 2 QIDS-SR16 rating, reducing the sample size to $n = 15$ for the correlation analysis. In all of the images, the left of the brain is shown on the left. (From Carhart-Harris et al. [33]; Creative Commons CC BY)

dala correlating with decreased depressive symptom severity as well as increased RSFC within the default-mode network (DMN) as seen in Fig. 25.29 [33].

The same study revealed that the predictors of response to psilocybin included increased RSFC in the ventromedial prefrontal cortex, bilateral inferior lateral parietal cortex, and decreased RSFC in the parahippocampal (PH)-prefrontal cortex (PFC) as seen in Fig. 25.30 [33].

Ayahuasca (single dose) was found to exert a rapid antidepressant effect compared with placebo in treatment-resistant depression [34]. The pharmacokinetic and pharmacodynamic aspects of ayahuasca are shown below [35] (see Fig. 25.31).

New Drug Discovery

New drug discovery is extremely costly. Safety issues continue to be the primary driver for discarding new agents even after long development time periods. The model described below [36] integrates safety assessment early in drug discovery (see Fig. 25.32).

The pipeline of new psychiatric medications is increasingly active especially in the last decade. The future decades bring more medication options in terms of mechanism of action, mode of delivery, and promising impact (see Table 25.3) [37, 38].

Antidepressants acting on G protein-coupled receptors (GPCRs) have been detected to have faster onset and more efficacy. **Novel GPCR-based strategies in brain regions involved in major depression have been most recently detailed by** Mantas et al. in 2021 as seen in Fig. 25.33 [39].

Nanotechnology and Drug Delivery Across Barriers

Nanotechnology is a major development in the facilitation of CNS agents crossing over several barriers, the most important of which is the blood brain barrier (Fig. 25.34) [40].

Medication Dosing Personalization

Digital technology could be used to personalize medication dosing. This application described below [41] could be incorporated into hospital and clinic electronic health systems using machine learning for dose optimization (see Fig. 25.35).

Brain Modulation Treatments

Brain modulation treatments are also called brain stimulation therapies or neuromodulation. Neuromodulation is defined as "technology that acts directly upon nerves. It is the alteration—or modulation—of nerve activity by deliver-

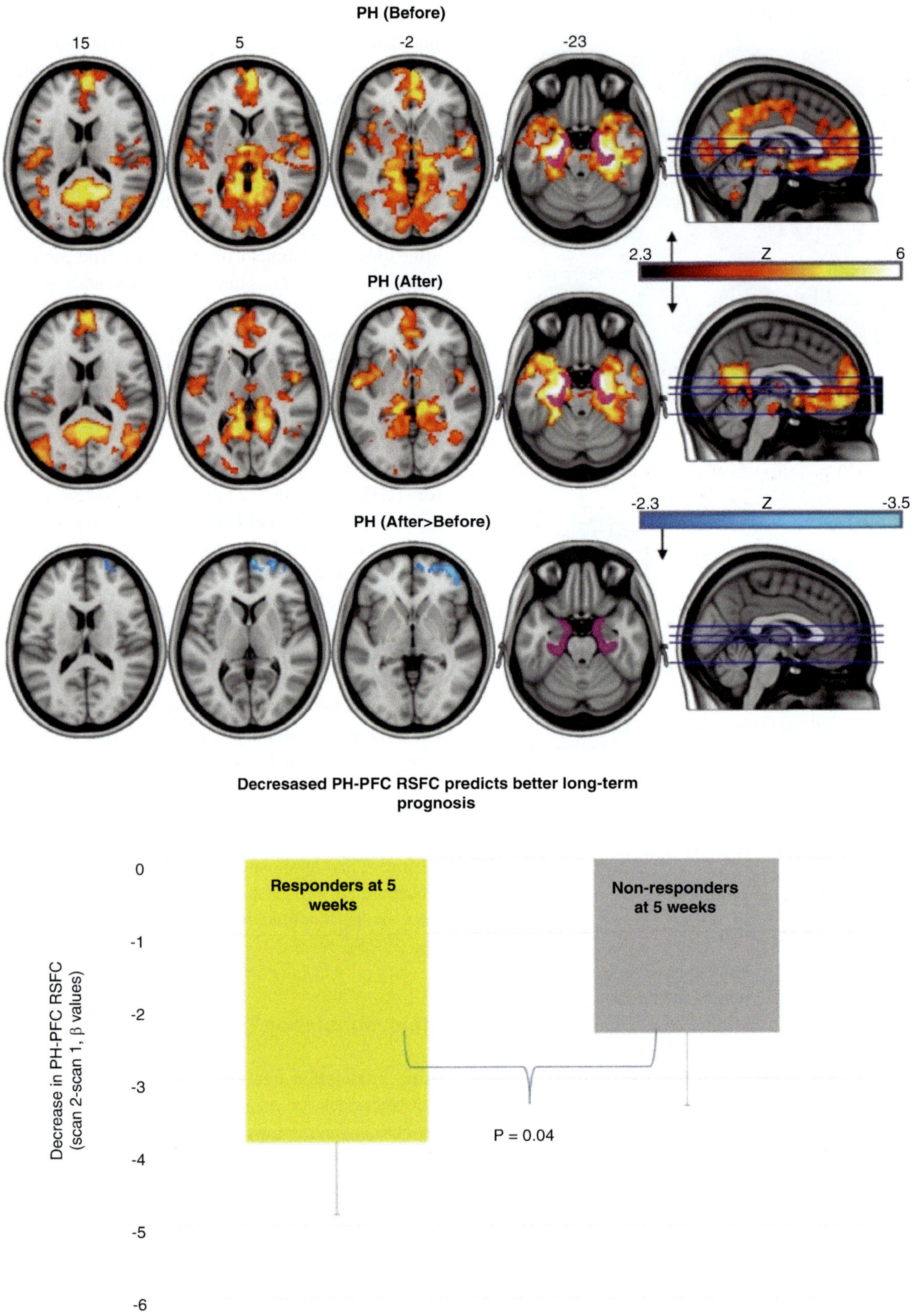

Fig. 25.30 Pre- and post-treatment parahippocampal (PH)-prefrontal cortex (PFC) RSFC. Top two rows = Bilateral PH (purple) RSFC before and after psilocybin treatment (hot colors = regions of significantly positive coupling). Bottom row reveals regions where there was a significant decrease in PH RSFC post-treatment (cold colors). All maps are cluster-corrected, $p < 0.05$, $Z > 2.3$. Decreased coupling between the PH and the displayed regions (bottom row) was predictive of clinical response at 5-week post-treatment ($t = -1.9$, $p = 0.04$). Chart shows mean values and negative standard errors. (From Carhart-Harris et al. [33]; Creative Commons CC BY)

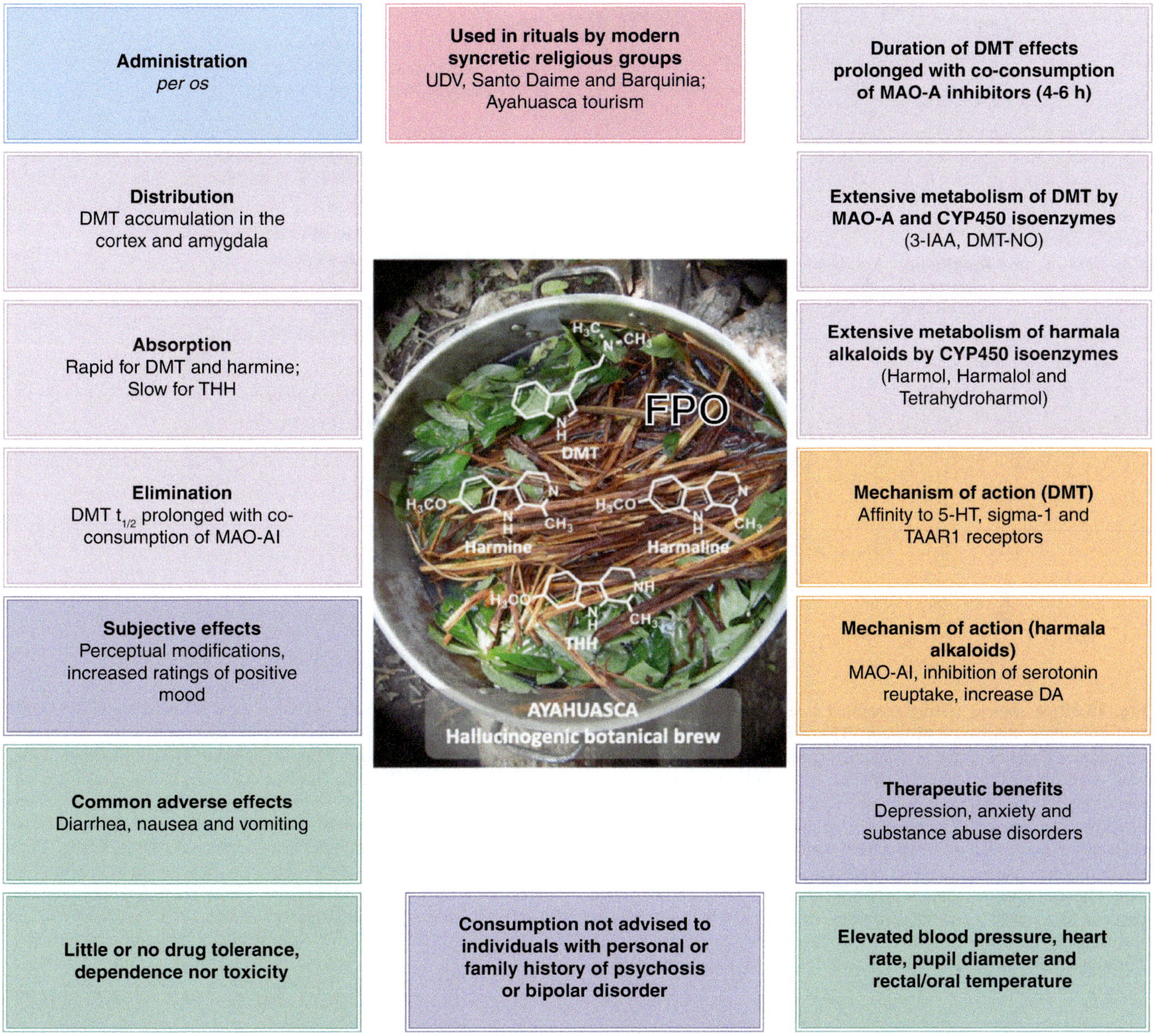

Fig. 25.31 Pharmacokinetic and pharmacodynamic aspects of ayahuasca. *3-IAA* 3-Indole-acetic acid; *5-HT* serotonin; *DA* dopamine; *DMT* N,N-dimethyltryptamine; *DMT-NO* DMT-N-oxide; *MAO* monoamine oxidase; *TAAR1* trace amine-associated receptor type 1; *THH* tetrahydroharmine, *UDV* União do Vegetal. (From Brito-da-Costa et al. [35]; Creative Commons CC BY)

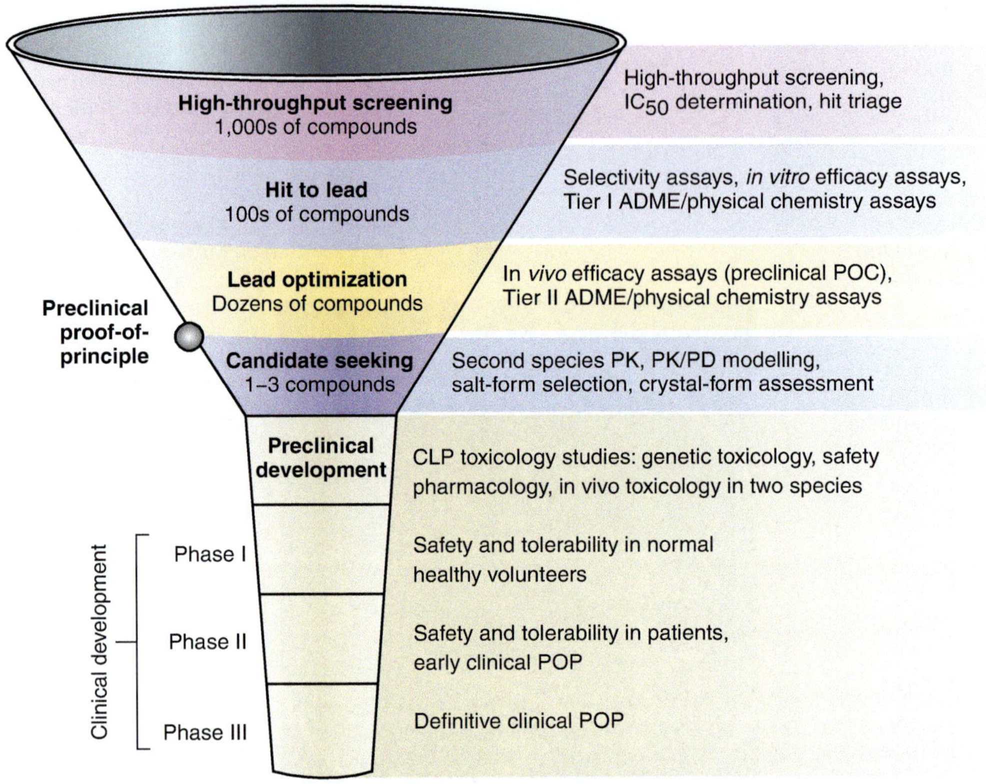

Fig. 25.32 A typical testing scheme for an orally delivered small-molecule drug discovery program. The primary goal of the high-throughput screening stage is to identify chemical hits from which lead series may be derived. Confirmed hits are then divided into broad chemical series, and each series is evaluated with respect to potency, physical and chemical properties, predicted ease of synthesis, cost of goods, scalability, target selectivity, structural alerts, freedom to operate, and the ability to create and protect intellectual property. The hit to lead stage represents an evaluation of those series that survived this triage process to identify potential liabilities associated with each series. Focused libraries may be generated to build a structure-activity relationship (SAR) in target binding and cell-based target modulation assays. Potent and selective leads are then evaluated in early ADME (absorption, distribution, metabolism, and excretion) assays to measure properties such as metabolic stability, plasma-protein binding, permeability, cLogP, and solubility. Upon selecting the most promising chemical series, efforts are made in the lead optimization stage to achieve proof-of-principle in a widely accepted preclinical model of disease, while optimizing drug properties with additional ADME assays. In the candidate-seeking stage, safety, ADME, and formulation liabilities are addressed to identify a candidate for formal preclinical development. *PK/PD* pharmacokinetic/pharmacodynamic; *POC* proof-of-concept; *POP* proof-of-principle. (From Kramer et al. [36]; with permission)

ing electrical or pharmaceutical agents directly to a target area" [42]. A couple of neuromodulation treatments are shown below (Fig. 25.36) [43].

Table 25.4 highlights the advantages of neuromodulation treatments in depression, including investigational treatments for the future [44].

Researchers highlighted invasive and noninvasive neuromodulation strategies for obsessive–compulsive disorder (OCD) [45] and depression [46] for the purpose of personalizing brain stimulation interventions as shown in Fig. 25.37 [47].

Advanced Treatments

Molecular Level

Studies of the molecular level in mood disorders such as depression reveal more disease mechanisms and opportunities for interventions at the molecular level as shown in Fig. 25.38 [48].

Cascade Level

In addition to the similar effects of lithium and valproic acid at the cascade level in bipolar disorder described by Chen

Table 25.3 New psychiatric medication pipeline

Disorder	Name	Mechanism	Mode/Phase/Reference
Depression	Psilocybin	Metabolized to psilocin, which stimulates serotonergic receptors: 5HT2A, 5HT2C, and 5HT1C	**Oral. Phase 3** Carhart-Harris R, Giribaldi B, Watts R, Baker-Jones M, Murphy-Beiner A, Murphy R, Martell J, Blemings A, Erritzoe D, Nutt DJ. Trial of Psilocybin versus Escitalopram for Depression. N Engl J Med. 2021 Apr 15;384(15):1402–1411. https://doi.org/10.1056/NEJMoa2032994
Depression	Hydroxy-nor-ketamine	NMDAR inhibitor through activation of AMPAR-mediated synaptic potentiation	**Intravenous. Phase 1** Highland JN, Zanos P, Riggs LM, Georgiou P, Clark SM, Morris PJ, Moaddel R, Thomas CJ, Zarate CA Jr., Pereira EFR, Gould TD. Hydroxynorketamines: Pharmacology and Potential Therapeutic Applications. Pharmacol Rev. 2021 Apr;73(2):763–791. https://doi.org/10.1124/pharmrev.120.000149
Depression	Dextromethorphan + Bupropion (AXS-05)	Dextromethorphan is an NMDA-glutamate antagonist; sigma-1 agonism; and nonselective serotonin reuptake inhibition. Bupropion is a selective norepinephrine/dopamine reuptake inhibitor	**Oral. Phase 3** O'Gorman C, Jones A, Iosifescu DV, Tabuteau H. Efficacy and safety of AXS-05, an oral NMDA receptor antagonist with multimodal activity, in major depressive disorder. Results from the GEMINI phase 3, double-blind, placebo-controlled trial. Poster presented at: American Society of Clinical Psychopharmacology, May 29–30, 2020; virtual. Oral Session/Poster. Accessed December 4, 2020. https://pmg.joynadmin.org/documents/1005/5ece89c7ef0d261a143a92ac.pdf
Depression, major and postpartum	Zuranolone	γ-Aminobutyric acid (GABA) type A receptor positive allosteric modulator	**Oral. Phase 3** Arnaud A, Suthoff E, Stenson K, Werneburg B, Hodgkins P, Bonthapally V, Jonas J, Meyer K, O'Day K. Number Needed to Treat and Number Needed to Harm analysis of the zuranolone phase 2 clinical trial results in major depressive disorder. J Affect Disord. 2021 Apr 15;285:112–119. https://doi.org/10.1016/j.jad.2021.02.027
Depression	NV-5138	Sestrin modulator leading to activation of mammalian target of rapamycin Complex 1 (mTORC1) similar to ketamine	**Oral. Phase 2** Hasegawa Y, Zhu X, Kamiya A. NV-5138 as a fast-acting antidepressant via direct activation of mTORC1 signaling. J Clin Invest. 2019 May 20;129(6):2207–2209. https://doi.org/10.1172/JCI129702
Bipolar depression and acute suicidal ideation	D-cycloserine + lurasidone (NRX-101)	D-cycloserine, is an N-methyl-D-aspartate (NMDA) receptor modulator, and lurasidone, is a D2/5-HT2a receptor antagonist	**Oral. Phase 3** Wilkinson ST, Sanacora G. A new generation of antidepressants: an update on the pharmaceutical pipeline for novel and rapid-acting therapeutics in mood disorders based on glutamate/GABA neurotransmitter systems. Drug Discov Today. 2019 Feb;24(2):606–615. https://doi.org/10.1016/j.drudis.2018.11.007.
Schizophrenia	Xanomeline + Trospium (Kar-XT)	Xanomeline is a muscarinic M1/M4 agonist. Trospium is a peripheral muscarinic antagonist	**Oral. Phase 3** Brannan SK, Sawchak S, Miller AC, Lieberman JA, Paul SM, Breier A. muscarinic cholinergic receptor agonist and peripheral antagonist for schizophrenia. The New England Journal of Medicine. 2021;384(8):717–726
Schizophrenia	SEP-856	Trace amine-associated receptor 1 (TAAR-1) agonist (indirectly decrease dopamine activity and 5HT1A agonist	**Oral. Phase 3** Begni V, Sanson A, Luoni A, Sensini F, Grayson B, Munni S, Neill JC, Riva MA. Towards Novel Treatments for Schizophrenia: Molecular and Behavioural Signatures of the Psychotropic Agent SEP-363856. Int J Mol Sci. 2021 Apr 16;22(8):4119. https://doi.org/10.3390/ijms22084119
Schizophrenia	Roluperidone (MIN-101)	5-HT2A antagonist and sigma-2 receptors antagonist	Oral. Phase 3 Strauss GP, Zamani Esfahlani F, Sayama H, Kirkpatrick B, Opler MG, Saoud JB, Davidson M, Luthringer R. Network Analysis Indicates That Avolition Is the Most Central Domain for the Successful Treatment of Negative Symptoms: Evidence From the Roluperidone Randomized Clinical Trial. Schizophr Bull. 2020 Jul 8;46(4):964–970. https://doi.org/10.1093/schbul/sbz141
Schizophrenia	Olanzapine+Samidorphan (ALKS 3831)	Samidorphan is a potent mu-opioid receptor antagonist, to reduce weight gain from olanzapine	**Oral. Phase 3** Sun L, McDonnell D, von Moltke L. Pharmacokinetics and Short-term Safety of ALKS 3831, a Fixed-dose Combination of Olanzapine and Samidorphan, in Adult Subjects with Schizophrenia. Clin Ther. 2018 Nov;40(11):1845–1854.e2. https://doi.org/10.1016/j.clinthera.2018.09.002

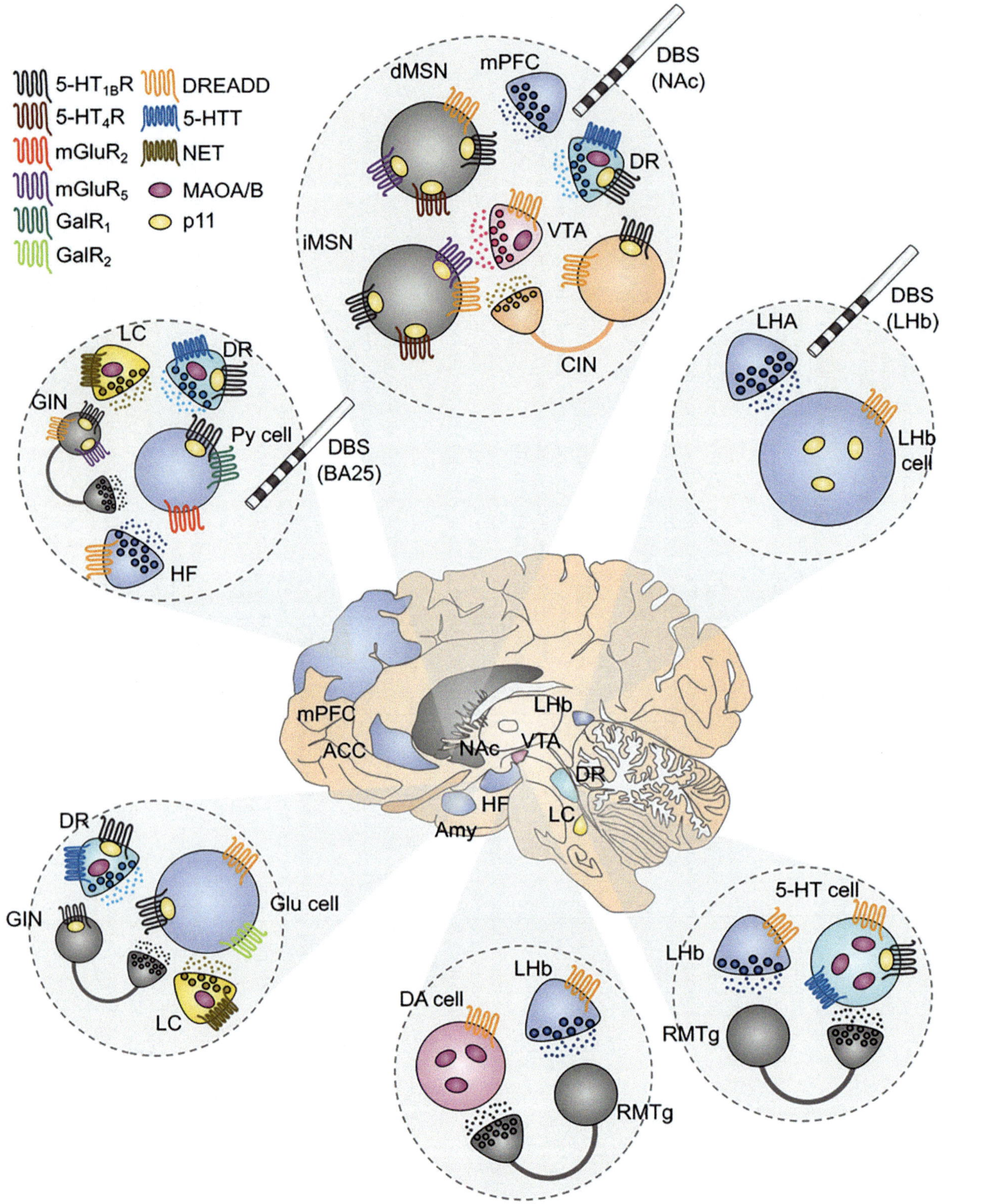

Fig. 25.33 Novel G protein-coupled receptor-based therapeutical strategies in brain regions involved in major depressive disorder. In the center, the human brain is depicted together with different brain areas that are involved in the symptomatology of MDD. Each circle panel shows the neuronal types that have been found to affect depressive-like behavior together with the receptors that they express. GABA neurons/terminals: gray, glutamate neurons/terminals: blue, DA neurons/terminals: pink, 5-HT neurons/terminals: cyan, NE neurons/terminals: yellow, cholinergic neurons/terminals: orange. *VTA* ventral tegmental area; *mPFC* medial prefrontal cortex; *LHA* lateral hypothalamic area; *NAc* nucleus accumbens; *DR* dorsal raphe; *LHb* lateral habenula; *RMTg* rostromedial tegmentum; *ACC* anterior cingulate cortex; *BA25* Brodmann area 25; *HF* hippocampal formation; *Amy* amygdala; *dMSN* direct medium spiny neuron; *iMSN* indirect medium spiny neuron; *CIN* cholinergic interneuron; *GIN* GABAergic interneuron; *Py* pyramidal; *Glu* glutamate; *DA* dopamine; *5-HT* serotonin; *5-HTT* serotonin transporter; *NET* norepinephrine transporter; *MAOA/B* monoamine oxidase A/B. DREADD designer receptors exclusively activated by designer drugs, DBS deep brain stimulation. (From Mantas et al. [39]; Creative Commons CC BY)

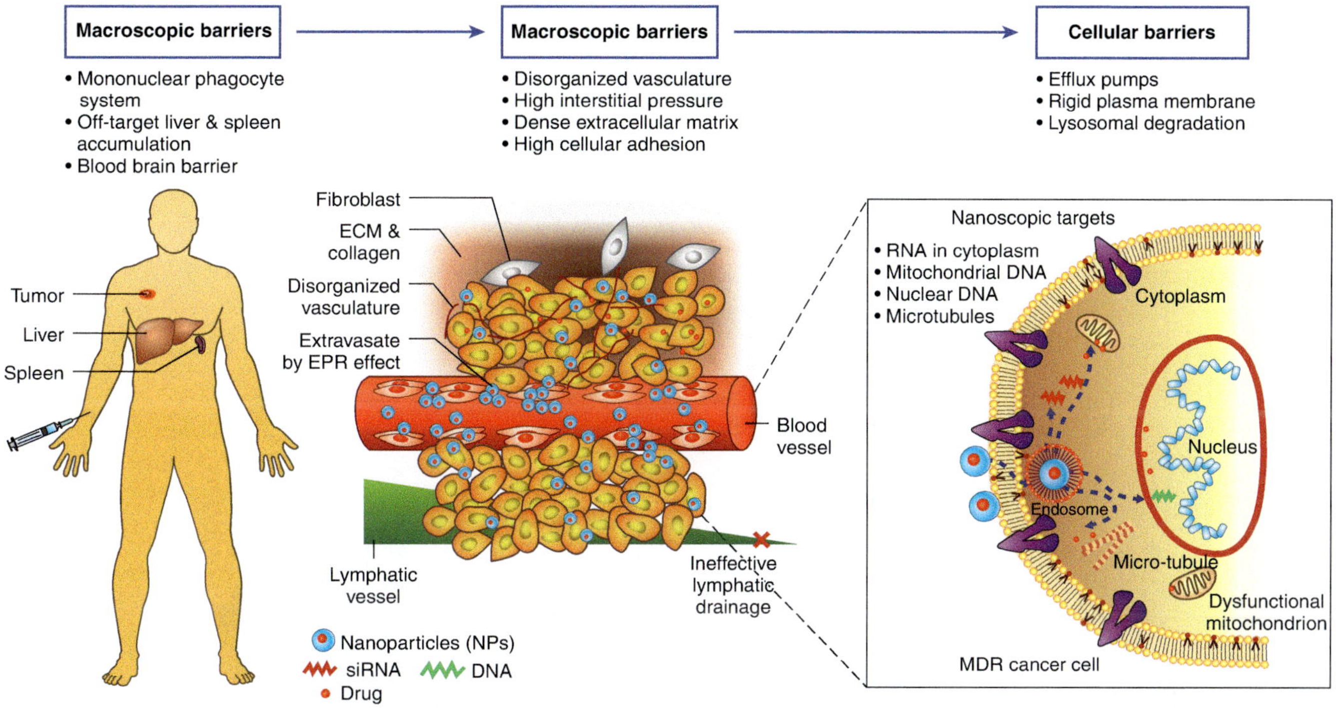

Fig. 25.34 Illustration of multiple biological barriers to nanoparticles (NPs) and its delivered drugs before reaching nanoscopic targets of diseased cells. Left panel: at the macroscopic level (non-cellular), iv administered NPs are sequestered, accumulated, and eventually eliminated by mononuclear phagocytic system (MPS) consisting mainly of the liver and spleen. In addition, the blood-brain barrier (BBB) is highly selective for many foreign substances, thus preventing the entry of drug containing NPs into the brain. Middle panel: at the microscopic level (non-cellular), the complex tumor microenvironment (TME), e.g., poor neo-vasculatures and dense extracellular matrix (ECM), limits the tumor permeation and retention of NPs, leading to low drug accumulation at the tumor necrotic region. Right panel: at the cellular level, the nucleus and mitochondrion are the primary organelles of genetic mutation responsible for complicated MDR phenotypes, such as overexpression of efflux transporters (e.g., P-gp), membrane rigidity, lysosomal sequestration, apoptosis evasion, drug detoxification, and altered drug target. All of the MDR mechanisms can occur simultaneously to confer drug resistance, leading to suboptimal therapies. (From Zhang et al. [40]; with permission)

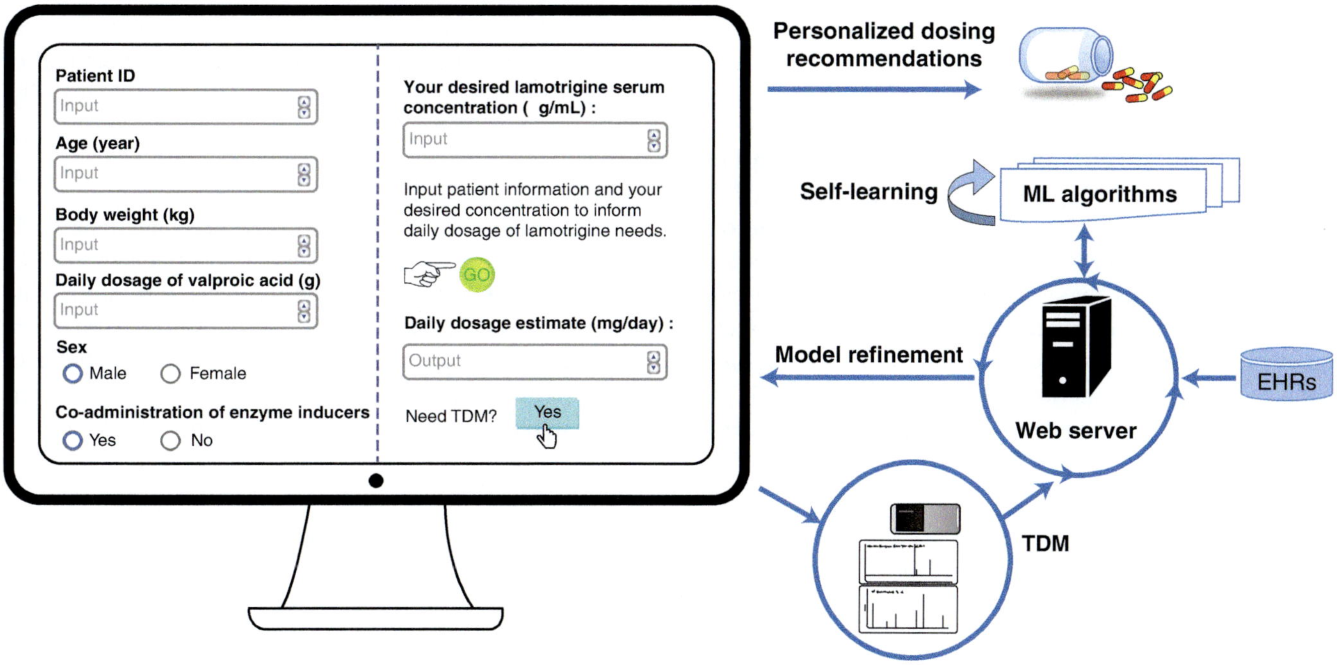

Fig. 25.35 Web application to personalize dosing adjustments of lamotrigine and the model's self-learning and refinement processes. *ML* machine learning; *TDM* therapeutic drug-monitoring; *EHRs* electronic health records. (From Zhu et al. [41]; Creative Commons CC BY)

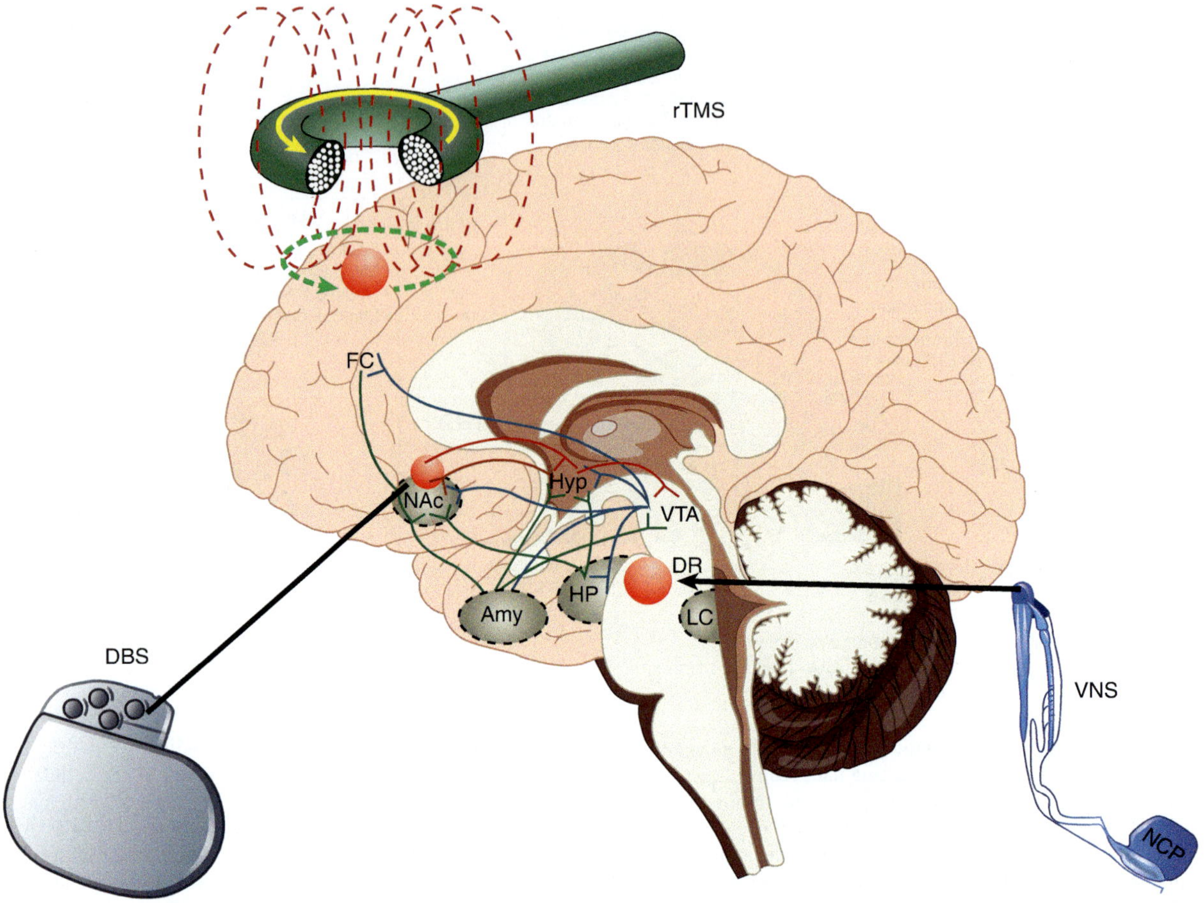

Fig. 25.36 Neuromodulation treatments: Repetitive transcranial magnetic stimulation (rTMS), vagus nerve stimulation (VNS) and deep brain stimulation (DBS). *FC* frontal cortex; *HYP* hypothalamus; *NAc* nucleus accumbens; *Amy* amygdala; *HP* hippocampus; *VTA* ventral tegmental area; *DR* dorsal raphe; and *LC* locus ceruleus. (From Yildiz et al. [43]; with permission)

and Manji in 2006 (see Fig. 25.39) [49], similar or different cascade level interventions are also being pursued for other psychiatric disorders [50].

Cellular Level

The discovery of neurogenesis in the adult human brain was a major breakthrough in 1998 [51]. Evidence for new neurons forming in subventricular zone of the anterolateral ventricle and the subgranular zone of the hippocampal dentate gyrus has generated significant research studies leading to exponential growth in our knowledge about brain repair mechanisms, migration, neural stems cells, neuroblasts, interneurons, and astrocytes [52], as well as the factors involved in neurogenesis as seen in Fig. 25.40.

Stem Cells

The introduction of stem cells in regenerative medicine was a major advancement in the field and has the potential of enhancing precision medicine, especially in psychiatric disorders (see Fig. 25.41) [53].

Embryonic Stem Cells

Recent knowledge of the role of GABAergic interneurons in psychiatric disorders has triggered basic science research (using mouse models) regarding the feasibility of creating human periventricular endothelial cells (PVECs) from human embryonic stem cells and potential transplantation of human stem cell-derived interneurons as a form of cell therapy for psychiatric disorders as shown in Fig. 25.42 [54].

Table 25.4 Neuromodulation treatments for major depression

Treatment	Primary advantages	Primary disadvantages	Comments
Food and Drug Administration–approved treatments			
Electroconvulsive therapy (ECT)	Excellent database in geriatric treatment-resistant depression (TRD), continuation, and maintenance treatment. ECT is the "gold standard" for the treatment of the most severely ill patients including patients with psychotic depression	Potential for cognitive and cardiac side effects; significant costs to providing an appropriate medical setting for ECT; the social stigma related to the treatment	ECT techniques continue to evolve. For example, ultra brief right unilateral ECT has been shown to limit the cognitive side effects of ECT while maintaining efficacy in depression
Transcranial magnetic stimulation (TMS)	No discernable cognitive or cardiac side effects; good data in the elderly to maintain efficacy with specific treatment modifications (e.g., increasing the intensity and number of pulses)	Six weeks of daily treatments may present practical problems; insurance coverage often limits modifications to the TMS protocol	TMS technique will need to be refined (increased intensity and/or pulses) to be effective in the most treatment-resistant geriatric patients
Vagus nerve stimulation (VNS)	Evidence that VNS is an effective long-term treatment for chronic depression with no apparent cognitive or cardiac side effects; evidence that VNS may be effective in patients who have failed a trial of ECT	Surgical procedure and efficacy may take months to become apparent; insurance coverage is difficult to obtain; limited data in the elderly	Centers for Medicare and Medicaid Services (CMS) will cover VNS when provided under the CMS-approved Coverage Evidenced Development plan
Investigational treatments			
Magnetic seizure therapy (MST)	More focal stimulation than ECT that may provide the efficacy of ECT with fewer cognitive side effects	Involves anesthesia and the medical setting for ECT; limited data particularly in the elderly	More focal brain stimulation may provide a therapeutic effect without significant cognitive side effects
Focal electrically administered seizure therapy (FEAST)	More focal stimulation and the potential to decrease cognitive side effects with similar efficacy to ECT	Involves anesthesia and medical setting for ECT; limited data in the elderly	This is a similar approach to MST
Transcutaneous vagal nerve stimulation (tVNS)	Noninvasive form of VNS, which has been shown to be safe and well-tolerated	Limited data in the elderly and TRD	This approach may have the advantages of VNS with a less-invasive procedure
Transcranial direct current stimulation (tDCS)	Preliminary data supports tDCS in the treatment of depression; safe, low cost, and easy accessibility	Limited data in the elderly and TRD	Has a number of potential advantages for the elderly if shown to be effective
Deep brain stimulation (DBS)	Published data shows that TRD patients, even patients who have not responded to ECT, respond to DBS	Invasive surgical procedure; may take months to show response	Data in Parkinson's disease may be useful in determining safety in geriatric TRD patients

From van Rooij et al. [44]; with permission

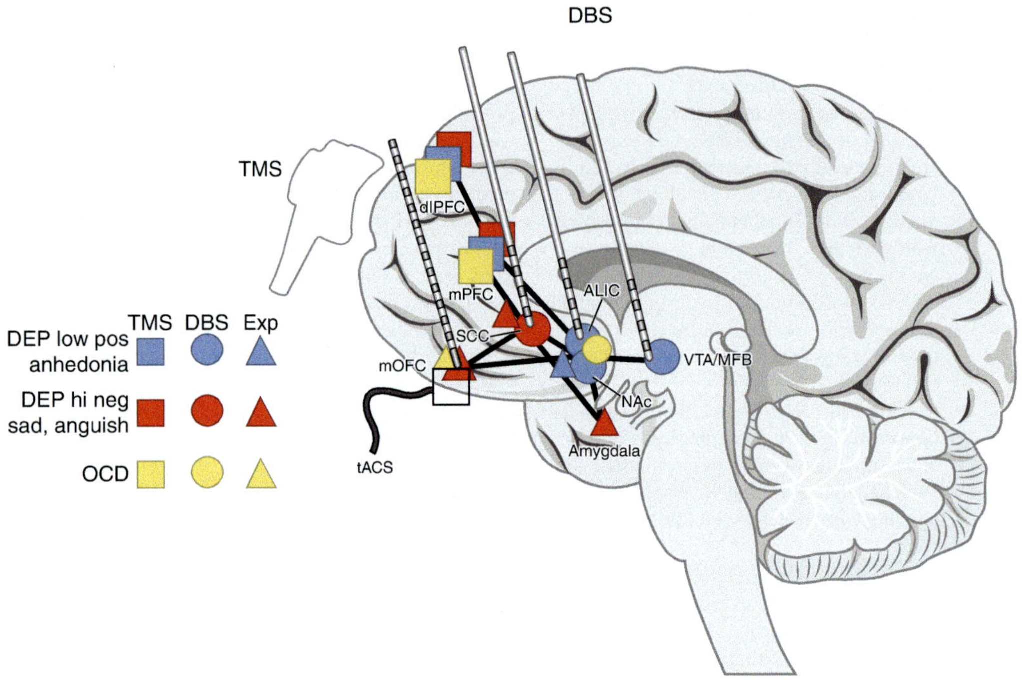

Fig. 25.37 Typical targets in the brain network for invasive and noninvasive neuromodulation in OCD and depression (DEP). These typical targets are the nucleus accumbens (NAc), anterior limb of internal capsule (ALIC), subcallosal cingulate (SCC), ventral tegmental area (VTA), medial forebrain bundle (MFB), dorsal lateral prefrontal cortex (dlPFC), and medial prefrontal cortex (mPFC). Triangles indicate targets that showed promise for personalized stimulation in the studies by Grover et al. and Scangos et al.; these uniquely included the mOFC. *TMS* transcranial magnetic stimulation; *low pos* low positive affect; *hi neg* high negative affect; *Exp* experimental; *tACS* transcranial alternating-current stimulation. (From Figee and Mayberg [47]; with permission)

Human-I nduced Pluripotent Stem Cells

The breakthrough of the development of human-induced pluripotent stem cells (hiPSCs) had triggered innovative research in disease modeling. Recent advances in hiPSC research led to the development of advanced techniques such as three-dimensional organoids, tissue engineering, microfluidic organ chips, and humanized animal systems as seen in Fig. 25.43 [55].

Recent developments led to the creation of the human-induced pluripotent stem cells model systems shown below [56] to study psychiatric disorders (see Fig. 25.44).

Recent developments in regenerative medicine in psychiatry show growing evidence for the utility of human-induced pluripotent stem cells (iPSCs) in examining the etiology and pathogenesis of psychiatric disorders such as schizophrenia, bipolar disorder, depressive disorders, anxiety disorders, and alcohol/substance use disorders [57]. iPSC research allows for describing cellular phenotypes and potentially producing or testing new therapies or diagnostic tests, as well as studying effects of antidepressant therapies, and predicting benefits or risks of medications (see Fig. 25.45) [58].

New research points to the potential of predicting of the response to antidepressants. Avior et al. examined patients from the STAR*D trial of major depressive disorder (MDD) and showed that patient-derived cortical neurons revealed potential biomarkers for antidepressant response to bupropion (see Fig. 25.46) [59].

In a prospective study, pharmacogenomics in bipolar disorder could be examined similarly to predict response to lithium in-vitro using hiPSC (see Fig. 25.47) [60].

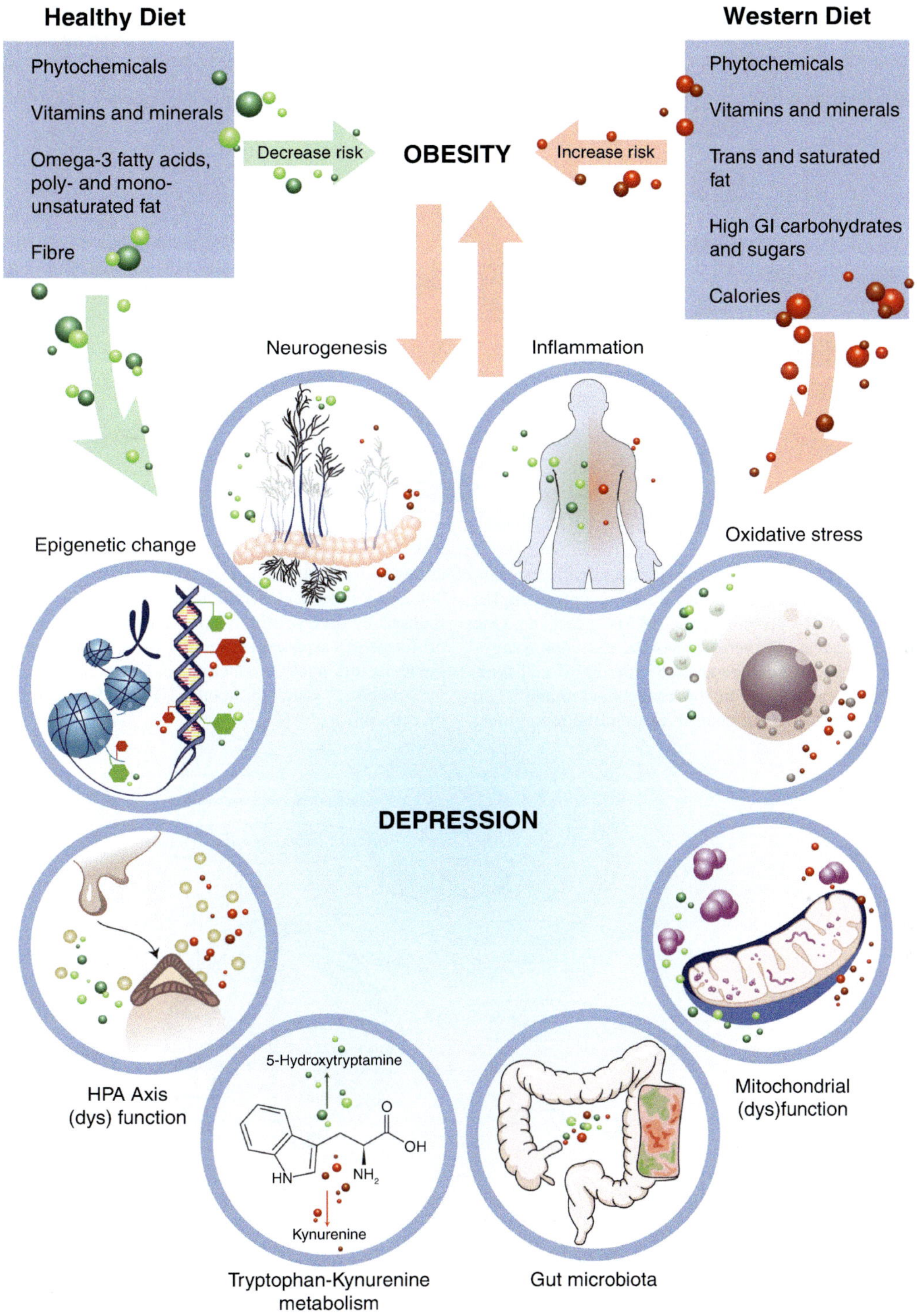

Fig. 25.38 Overview of the role of diet quality on implicated mechanisms of depression. This figure details the identified pathways implicated in depression that may be amenable to dietary manipulation. The black arrows represent increased or decreased consumption related to the opposing dietary patterns. Green arrows represent a posited beneficial modulation of the included pathways while red represent potentially detrimental modulation. (From Marx et al. [48]; with permission)

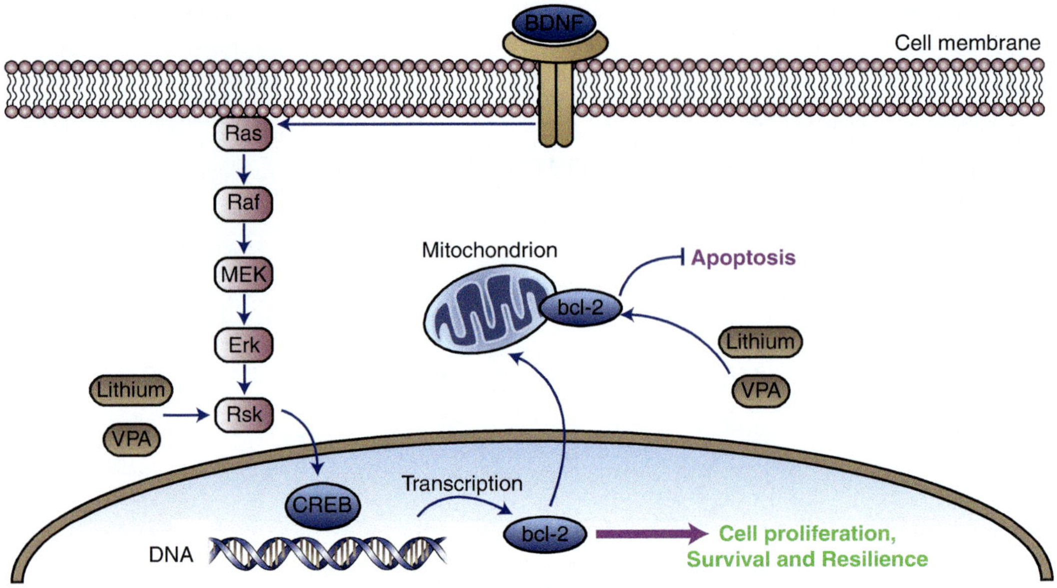

Fig. 25.39 Lithium and valproate (VPA), at therapeutically relevant concentrations, robustly activate the extracellular receptor-coupled kinase (ERK) mitogen-activated protein kinase (MAPK) cascade. One of the major downstream targets of the ERK MAPK cascades is arguably one of the most important neuroprotective proteins, B-cell lymphoma-2 (bcl-2). Bcl-2 is expressed in the rodent and mammalian nervous system and is localized to the outer mitochondrial membrane, endoplasmic reticulum, and nuclear membrane. It is now clear that bcl-2 is a protein that inhibits both apoptotic and necrotic cell death induced by diverse stimuli. Bcl-2 attenuates apoptosis by sequestering proforms of caspases, preventing the release of mitochondrial apoptogenic factors such as calcium and cytochrome c, and by enhancing mitochondrial calcium uptake. (From Schloesser et al. [50]; with permission)

Fig. 25.40 Factors involved in neurogenesis. (From Kucharska-Mazur et al. [52]; with permission)

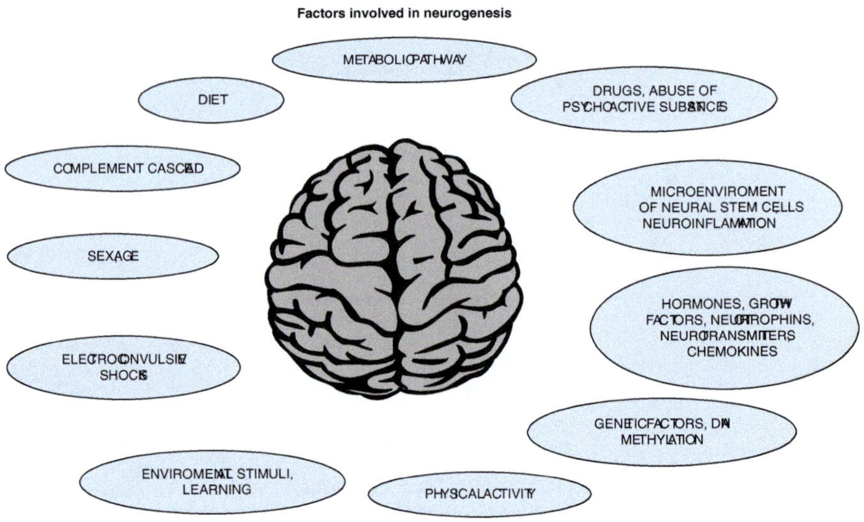

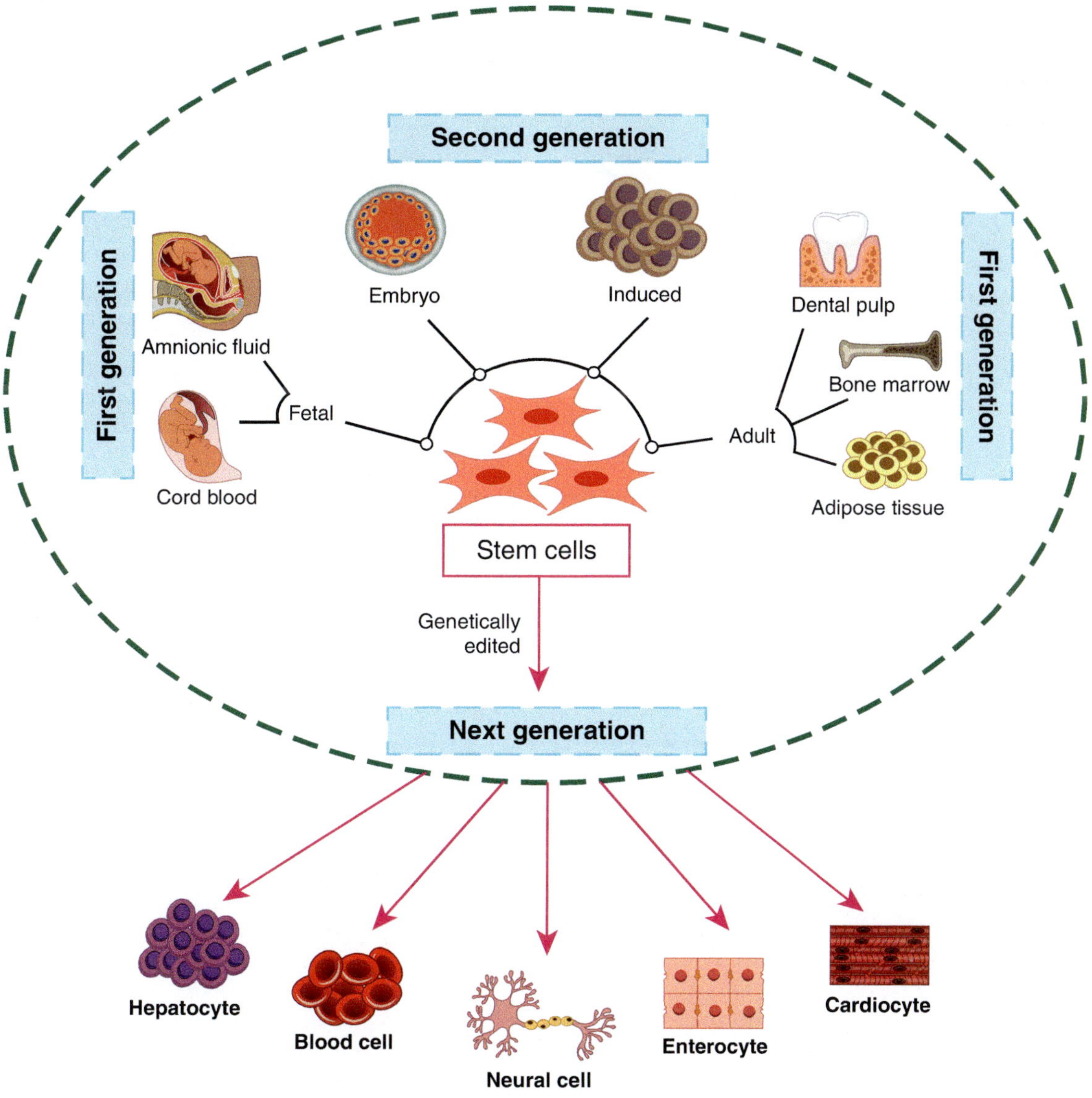

Fig. 25.41 Types of stem cells. First-generation stem cell types, including adult stem cells and fetal membrane-derived stem cells, demonstrated feasibility and safety; however, they were heterogeneous results and low efficiency in the clinical application. To resolve some limitations, second-generation stem cells suggest the advantage of pluripotent stem cells, including embryonic stem cells and induced pluripotent stem cells. Next generation of stem cells for the enhancement of stem cell therapy is directed toward cell engineering. (From Basiri et al. [53]; with permission)

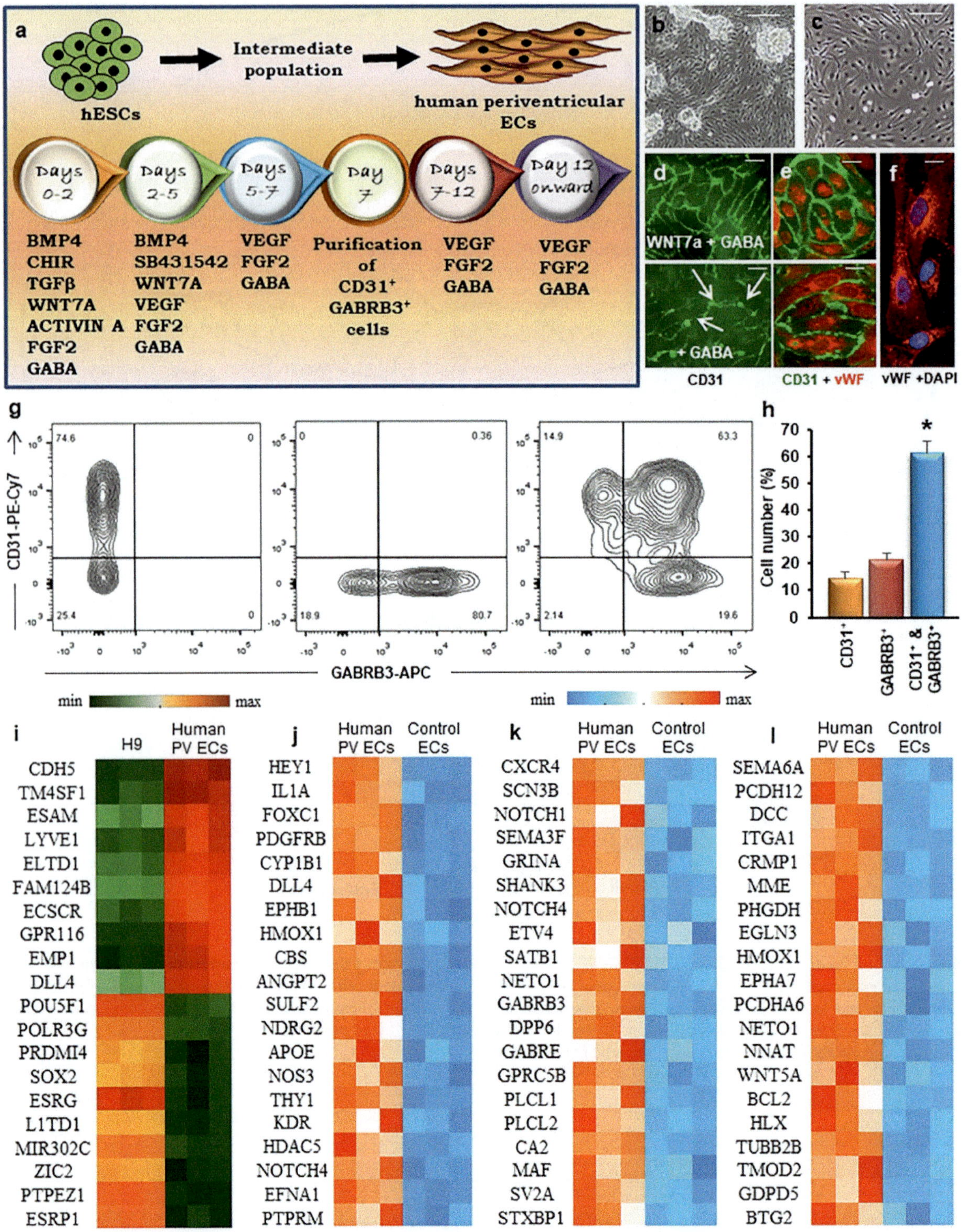

Fig. 25.42 Human forebrain endothelial cell therapy for psychiatric disorders. (**a**) Schematic of the human periventricular endothelial cell differentiation protocol. Phase contrast images of the day 6 cell population (**b**) and pure population of human periventricular endothelial cells at day 10 (**c**). (**d**) Periventricular endothelial cells showed robust CD31 expression upon addition of WNT7A and GABA from day 0–5 of differentiation, while addition of GABA alone, selectively increased CD31 expression on endothelial cell–cell junctions. (**e**) Co-labeling with endothelial cell markers, vWF (red) and CD31 (green) of human periventricular endothelial cells. (**f**) High-magnification image of vWF labeling of periventricular endothelial cells. (**g**) Flow cytometry analysis showing $CD31^{+}GABRB3^{-}$, $CD31^{-}GABRB3^{+}$, and double positive $CD31^{+}GABRB3^{+}$populations. (**h**) Frequencies of human periventricular endothelial cells are $CD31^{+}/GABRB3^{+}$. Data represent mean ± SD ($n = 6$, $^{*}P < 0.05$, student's t test). (**i**) Heatmap showing top 20 differentially expressed genes in H9 cells versus H9-derived periventricular endothelial cells (PV ECs), indicating efficient endothelial cell differentiation. Heatmaps showing top 20 upregulated genes in H9-derived periventricular endothelial cells versus control endothelial cells in three different categories: angiogenesis (**j**), GABA pathway (**k**), and neurogenesis (**l**) categories. Scale bars: (**b**) 100 µm (applies to **c**), (**d**) 50 µm (applies to **e**, **f**). (*From* Datta et al. [54]; Creative Commons CC BY)

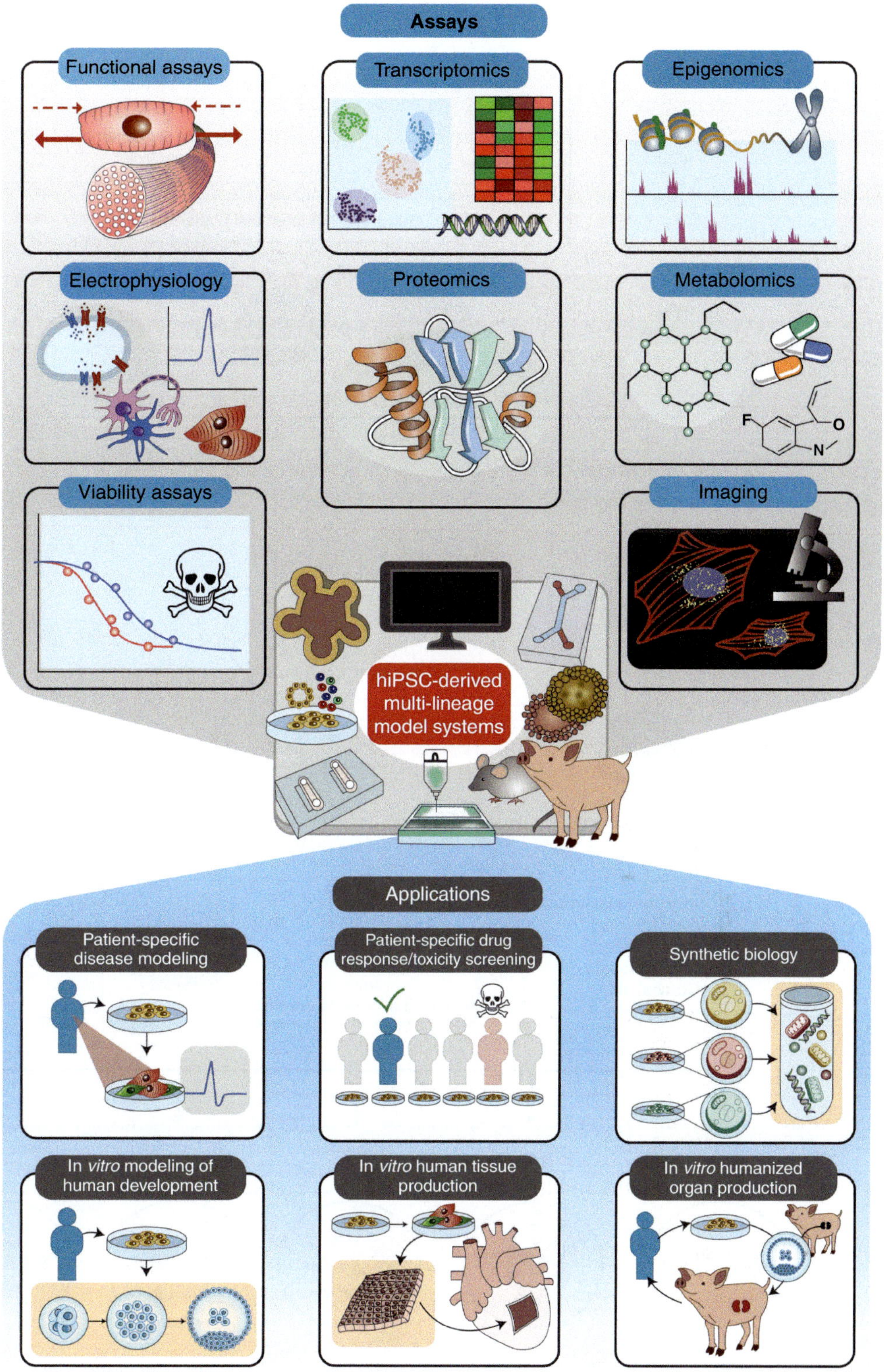

Fig. 25.43 Assays for interrogating cells within human-induced pluripotent stem cells (hiPSC)-derived multilineage model systems and potential downstream applications. A variety of technical readouts can be considered when evaluating the properties of multiple cell types within an hiPSC-derived multilineage model system. Analyses are widely applicable across multilineage model systems, in particular those analyses that examine functional, visual, electrophysiological, and omics level properties of cells. Ideal assays are able to interrogate multiple cell types simultaneously, such as in the case of single-cell transcriptomic, epigenomic, proteomic, and metabolomic analyses. Downstream applications for multilineage hiPSC-derived systems include patient-specific disease modeling, personalized drug response screening, and human tissue production. (From Sharma et al. [55]; with permission)

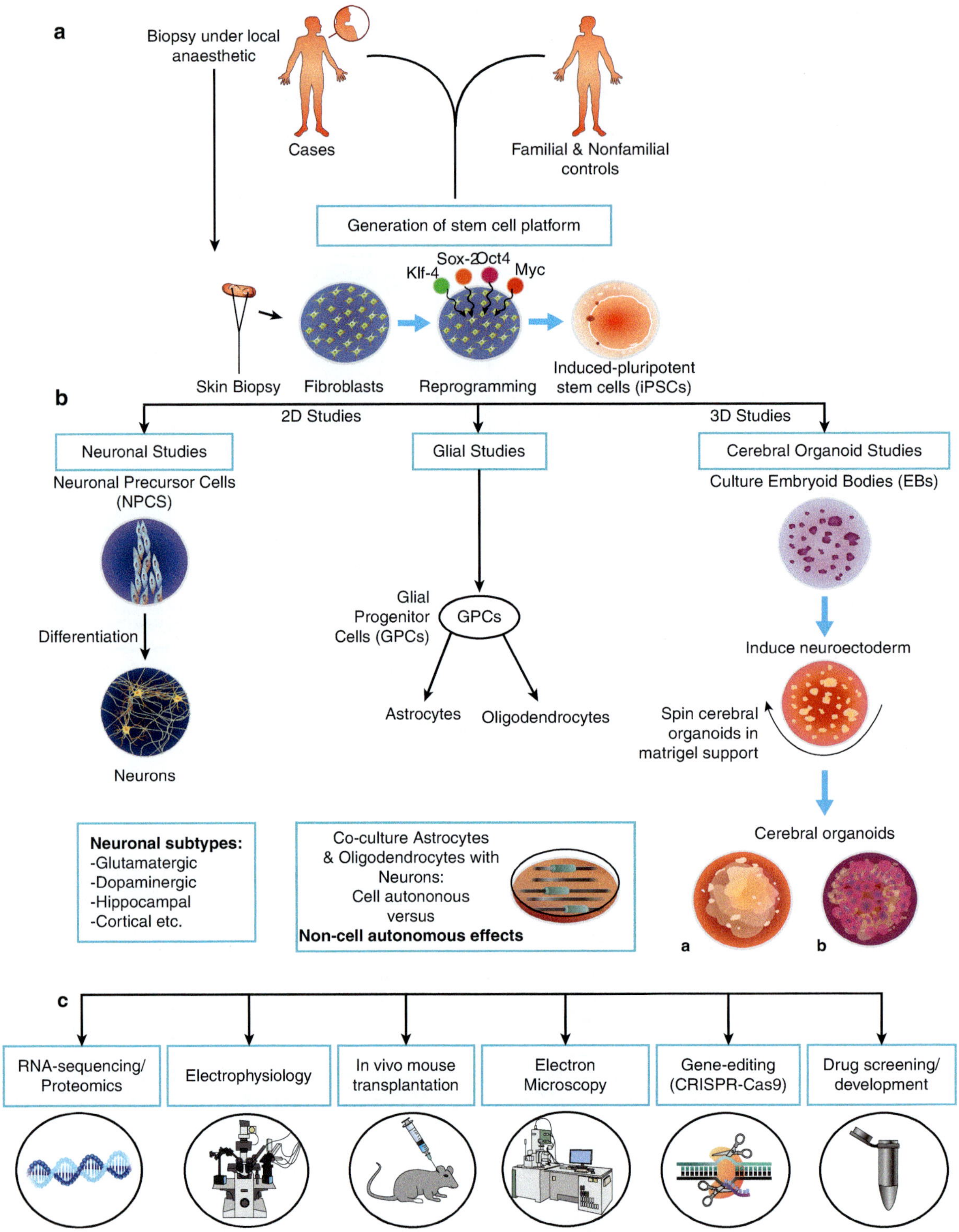

Fig. 25.44 Overview of human iPSC model systems to study psychiatric disorders. Human iPSC is generated by reprogramming fibroblasts from skin biopsies from volunteers with a variety of techniques, most commonly using standard Yamanaka factors, delivered in nonintegrative episomal vectors. Other starting cellular materials can be used such as keratinocytes from hair or from peripheral blood mononuclear cells. Once generated and extensively tested, the hiPSCs can be used to either make neuronal precursor cells or glial precursor cells (e.g., oligodendrocyte/astrocyte precursors) or grown and lifted to make 3-D organoids as shown in frame (**a**) phase-bright image of a cerebral organoid at 2 months of age, and frame (**b**) shows an organoid that has been sectioned and stained with antibodies to Pax6 and phospho-histone H3, clearly demonstrating a ventricular zone. (**c**) The cellular platforms generated can then be used for further downstream studies including electrophysiology, transcriptomic and proteomic studies, drug screening, and morphological studies and coculturing with other cell types. In addition, the hiPSCs can be gene edited using CRISR-Cas9 to attempt to rescue phenotypes observed. (From Johnstone et al. [56]; with permission)

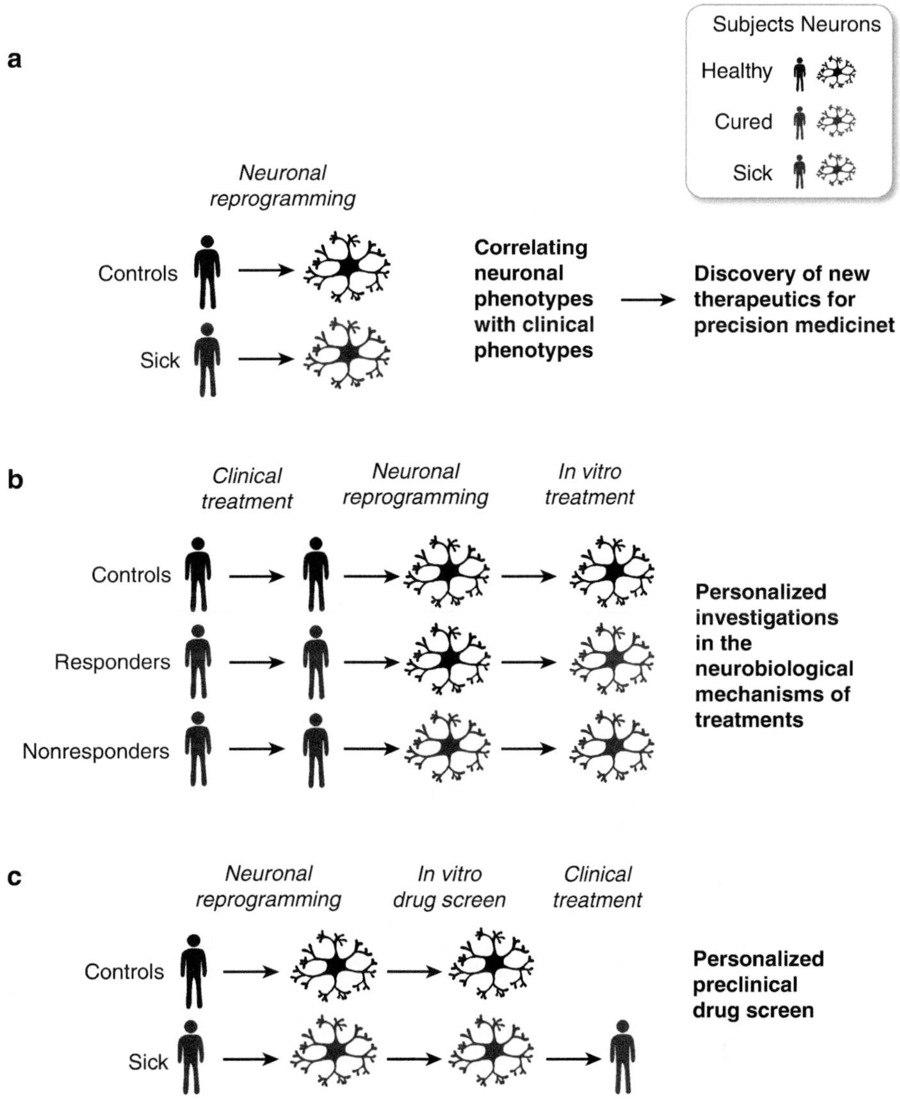

Fig. 25.45 Using patient-derived brain cells in-vitro for personalized medicine. (**a**) Correlating the clinical phenotypes of patients with their neuronal phenotypes to produce new therapeutics and diagnostics tools. (**b**) Reprogrammed neurons can be used to distinguish which patients will benefit from a specific drug (responders) to patients that show little or no benefit from treatment (nonresponders), ultimately improving efficacy of treatments. (**c**) High-throughput drug screening can be performed on patient vs healthy control-derived neurons, to provide evidence-based predictions of drug benefits, side-effects, and/or toxicity to patients. (From Bardy et al. [58]; with permission)

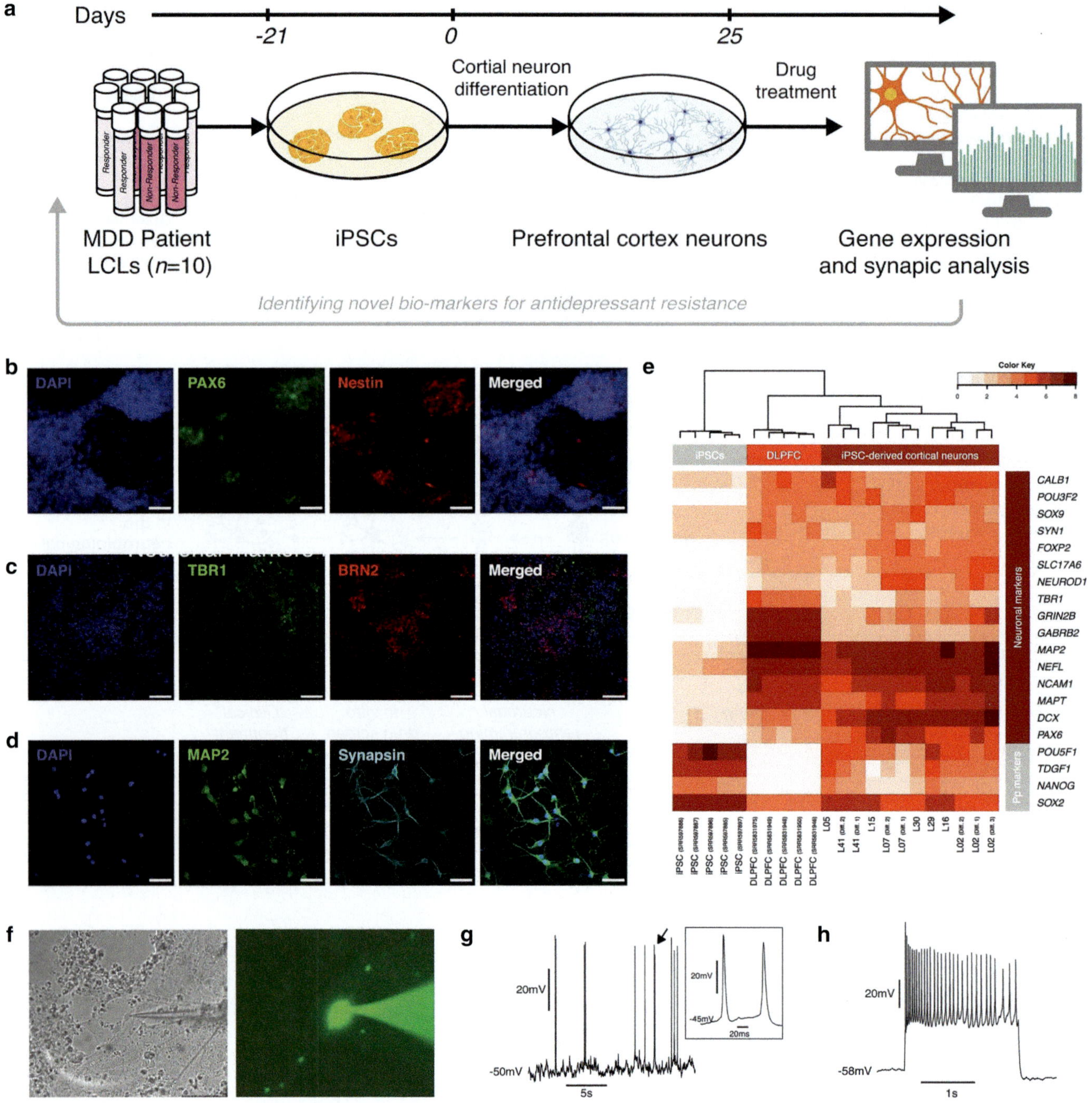

Fig. 25.46 Major depressive disorder (MDD patient lymphoblastoid cell lines reprogrammed to induced pluripotent stem cells and differentiated into functional cortical neurons. (**a**) Schematic illustration protocol and analysis. Major depression disorder (MDD) patient lymphoblastoid cell lines (LCLs) were reprogrammed into induced pluripotent stem cells (iPSCs) using Sendai viruses. iPSCs were then rapidly differentiated into cortical neurons, treated with an antidepressant and analyzed thereafter using immunofluorescent staining and RNA-sequencing. (**b**) Five days into the differentiation protocol, patient-derived cells were positive for the neural progenitor markers PAX6 and Nestin. Scale bars represent 260 μm. (**c**) After 25 days, neurons were positive for the cortical neural markers TBR1 and BRN2. Scale bars represent 100 μm. (**d**) Mature neurons were also positive for synapsin and MAP 2. Scale bars represent 50 μm. (**e**) Neural gene expression of iPSC-derived cortical neurons is similar to postmortem dorsolateral prefrontal cortex (DLPFC) tissues and different from undifferentiated iPSCs. (**f**) Differential interference contrast (DIC) (left) and fluorescent (right) representative microscopy images taken during electrophysiological recording. (**g**) Representative whole-cell intracellular recording of spontaneous activity. Inset: two individual action potentials marked by an arrow. (**h**) Representative firing pattern of a recorded neuron following a prolonged high amplitude depolarization current step. (From Avior et al. [59]; Creative Commons CC BY)

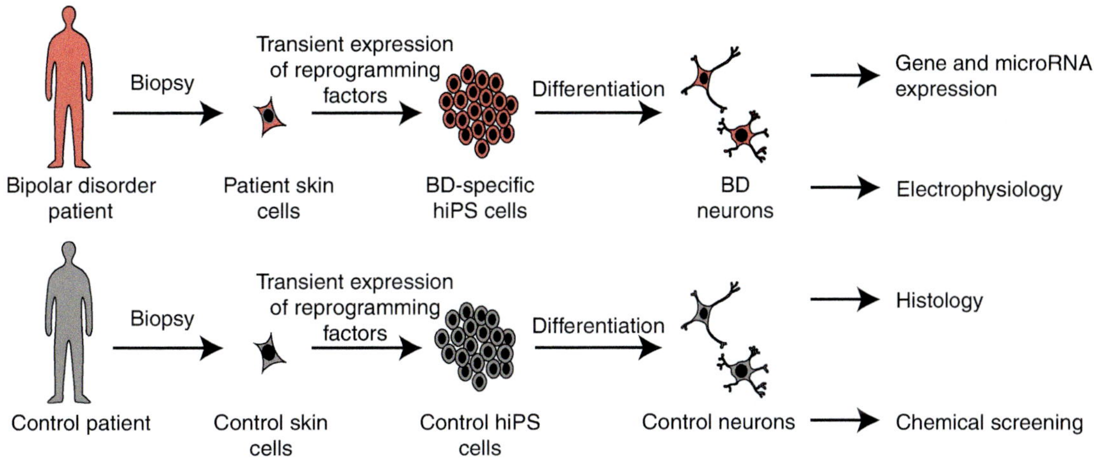

Fig. 25.47 iPSC-derived neurons as a cellular model of bipolar disorder and lithium response. Fibroblasts are grown from skin biopsies taken from participating subjects. These cells are treated with a combination of four transcription factors that reprogram the cells to stem cells. These iPSCs are then treated with a series of growth factors to differentiate them into a variety of neuronal types. In this way, neurons from patients can be compared with controls or lithium responders to nonresponders. (From Oedegaard et al. [60]; Creative Commons CC BY)

Network Level: Nuclei, Tract, and Pathway Level

Interventions at the network level could be tested on evolving hypotheses such as the one highlighted in Fig. 25.48 [61].

Person Level

Person level interventions include not only psychotherapy, psychopharmacology, brain modulation as the mainstays of treatment but also advanced and futuristic interventions such as digital therapeutics and monitoring, music therapy, psychosurgery, and from illness to wellness interventions.

Digital Therapeutics and Monitoring

The future of wearable technologies includes the devices shown below [62]. These technologies will become components of Internet of Health Things (IoHT) systems in order to understand people and patients (Fig. 25.49).

Mood and Behavioral Monitoring

The new field of edible electronics is focused on ingestion of safe, cost-effective, electronics that get digested or metabolized after performing their function (see Fig. 25.50) [63]. The FDA approved Abilify MyCite incorporating an ingestible sensor to track compliance (see Fig. 25.50d).

Advances in smartphone and sensor technology now allow the passive collection of useful data that could be helpful in monitoring mood, behavior, or even suicide risk (Fig. 25.51a, b) [64].

Similarly, large NIH studies have shown the feasibility of such continuous monitoring as shown below (see Fig. 25.51c) [65].

Digital therapeutic apps such as GET.ON PANICAPP aim at using digital technology to deliver evidence-based therapy for anxiety (see Fig. 25.52) [66]. More CBT-delivery apps have been cleared by the FDA such as Someryst for insomnia and Parallel for irritable bowel syndrome.

Randomized controlled trials of smart phone or web-based gaming apps designed to improve resilience and mood have shown initial evidence of efficacy with large effect sizes such as the Superbetter (SB) trial where SB participants had greater reductions in depression scores compared with waiting list participants at posttest (Cohen's $d = 0.67$) and at follow-up ($d = 1.05$) [67]. The use of "gamification" in mental health is depicted in Fig. 25.53 [68].

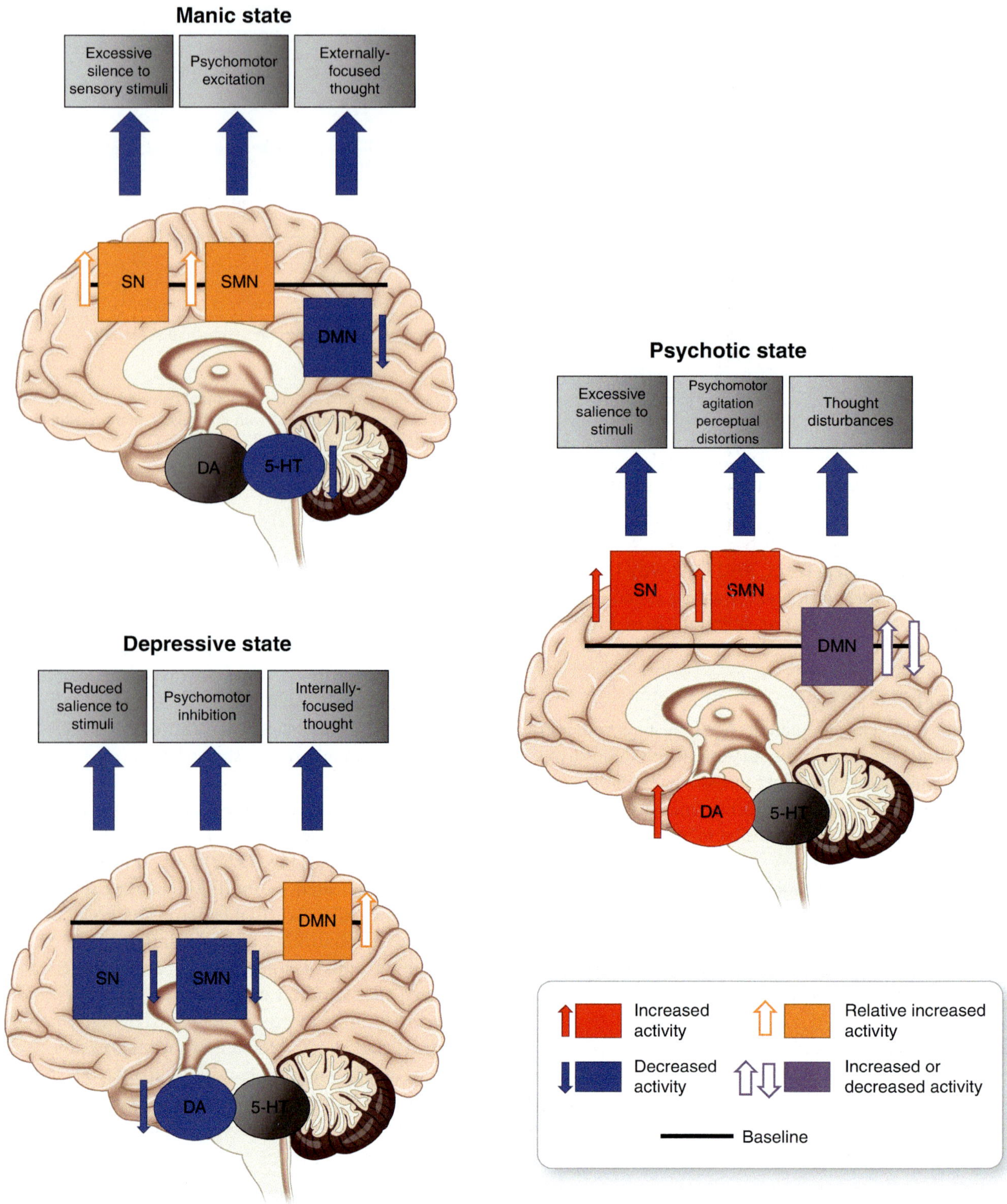

Fig. 25.48 Hypothesis on the functional reorganization and resting-state networks disbalancing mediated by alterations in neurotransmitters signaling in different psychopathological states. Neurotransmitters signaling affects the functional architecture and balances of resting-state networks. Thus, we hypothesize that: deficit in 5-HT signaling may result in DMN deficit with relative predominance of SMN-SN activity, manifesting in the manic state; deficit in DA signaling may result in SMN-SN deficit with relative predominance of DMN activity, manifesting in the depressive state; and hyperactive DA signaling may result in over-activity of SMN-SN, manifesting in a psychotic state. *SMN* sensorimotor network; *DMN* default-mode network; *SN* salience network; *DA* dopamine; *5-HT* serotonin. (From Conio et al. [61]; with permission)

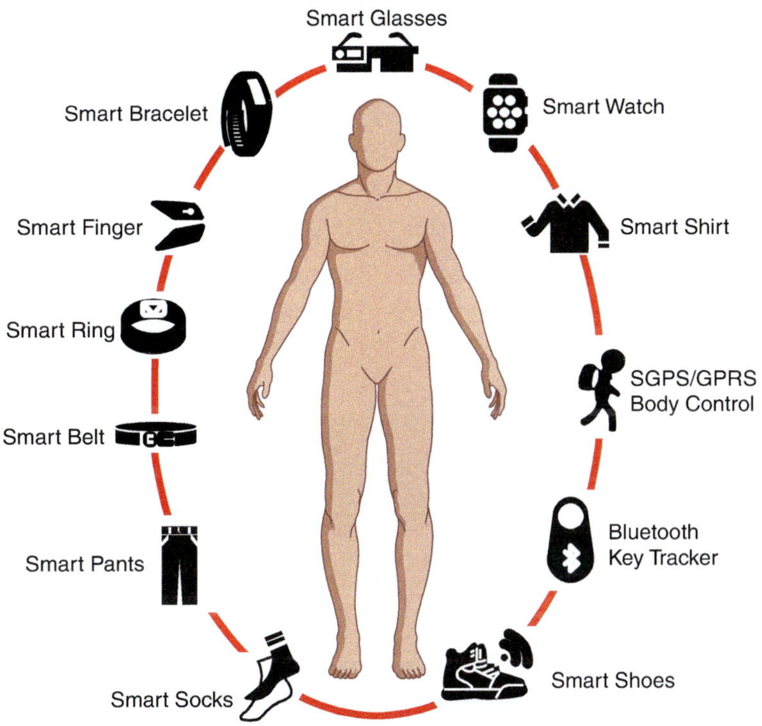

Fig. 25.49 Wearable technologies. (From Kose et al. [62]; with permission)

Wellness and mental health service delivery apps have also been developed for indigenous populations (e.g., ibobbly) with the components highlighted in Fig. 25.54. The same components are applicable for all-in-one apps and services for urban, suburban, and rural populations.

The future of Music Therapy

Music therapy is the clinical and evidence-based use of music interventions to accomplish individualized goals within a therapeutic relationship, which has gained much traction in the last several decades. There are many different types of music therapy, encompassing many forms of treatment from listening to performing. One of the most promising is improvisation, which gives participants the basic materials (instruments, microphones, etc.) to create melodies of their own. With increasing technology of digital music, future improvisational therapy may involve participants guiding a trained studio player in making a personalized tune. MacDonald and Wilson proposed a model that takes account of all routes by which musical improvisation between individuals may influence a given health condition in a given population as seen in Fig. 25.55 [69].

The Future of Psychosurgery

The history of neurosurgery for psychiatric disorders, i.e., psychosurgery, has been marred with ethical and medical complications. Despite the pharmacological, psychotherapeutic, and neuromodulatory advances, there is still a sector of treatment refractory patients, especially those with OCD and depression that might be candidates for surgical interventions given the advances in neuroscience and image-guided stereotactic techniques (Fig. 25.56) [70].

Nijensohn and Dagi pointed that "the future of psychosurgery likely includes sonogenetics, brain augmentation, neuromorphic chips, cyborgs, trans-humanity technologies, the field of brain-machine technologies (carbon nanotubes, nanowires, nanoscale coating), labs-on-a-chip, and other fusion technologies." [71]. Brain transplantation including controversial pursuits of human head transplantation continue to make headlines in the past decade [72, 73]. The integration of structural and functional connectivity is fundamental to the restoration of any CNS disorders (see Fig. 25.57) [74].

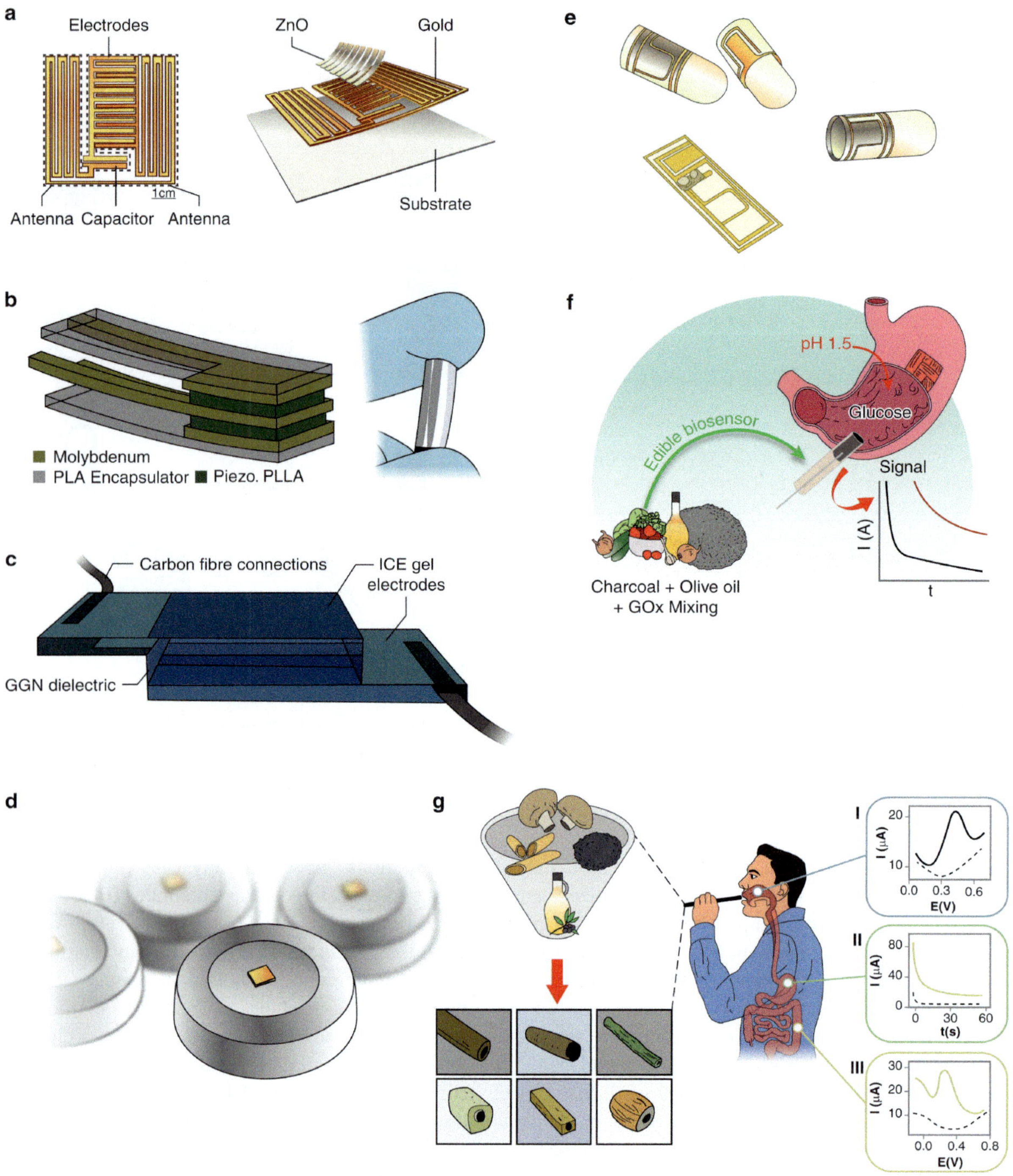

Fig. 25.50 Potentially edible sensors for in-body operation. (**a**) Photograph and illustration of an edible pH sensor on a sugar paste substrate. Sensor is made of Au–ZnO, connected to an Au antenna for wireless signals transmission and an edible capacitor made of thin gelatin sheets coated with edible Au. (**b**) Biodegradable piezoelectric PLLA pressure sensor. The sensor structure includes two layers of piezoelectric PLLA, sandwiched between Mo or Mg electrodes, and a PLA encapsulation (left); optical image of a fabricated biodegradable piezoelectric PLLA sensor (right); the device dimensions are 5 mm × 5 mm, with a thickness of 200 μm. (**c**) Schematic of a capacitive pressure sensor. The device consists of ionic-covalent entanglement (ICE) hydrogel electrodes based on gellan gum and gelatin, carbon additional connections, and dielectric prepared from 10% w/w genipin to gelatin hydrogel. (**d**) Photograph and schematic of ingestible Abilify MyCite sensor embedded in a tablet. (**e**) The gelatin ID-Capsule containing the ingestible sensor with an RF tag that activates in contact with gastric acids. The digital pill has the size of an 800 mg ibuprofen tablet. The ID-Tag is composed of an integrated circuit (Ag traces, Mg, and AgCl electrodes) on a flexible film. (**f**) Edible electrochemical biosensors for direct and controlled glucose sensing in gastrointestinal fluids of different pH ranges (gastric, pH 1.5 and intestinal, pH 6.5). The sensors are based on GOx enzyme protected from the harsh acid conditions by the matrix of activated charcoal conductor and olive oil binder. (**g**) Food-based electrochemical sensors. The electrodes are made of edible activated charcoal, edible food sleeves (penne, cookie, green bean, milk candy, cheese, and almond), and olive oil. Electrochemical data: detecting (i) salivary uric acid (0.5×10^{-3} m) in artificial saliva using penne electrode, (ii) ascorbic acid (0.2×10^{-3} m) in artificial gastric fluid using candy electrode, and (iii) dopamine (0.4×10^{-3} m) in artificial intestinal fluid using almond electrode. (From Sharova et al. [63]; Creative Commons CC BY)

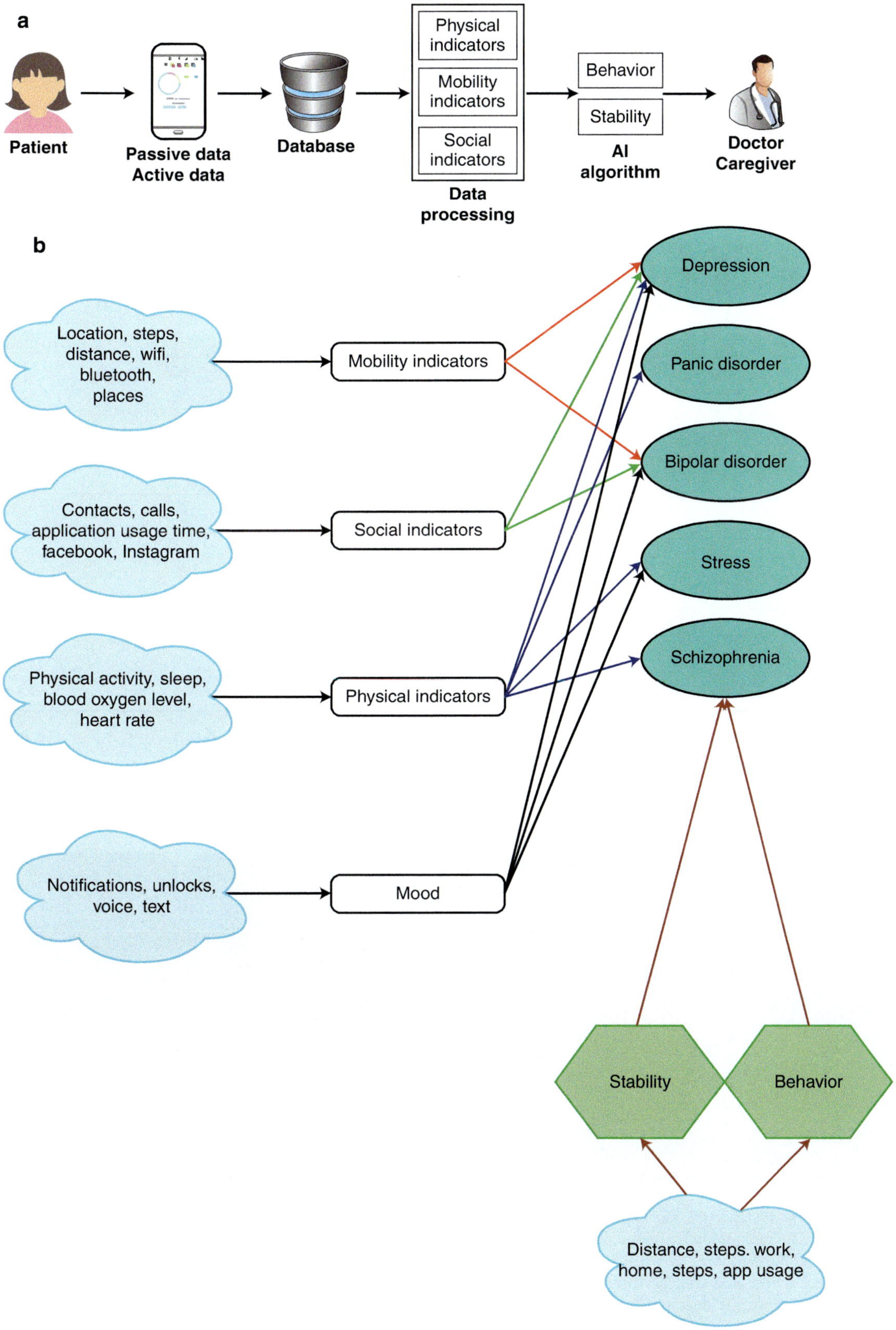

Fig. 25.51 (**a**) Continuous and objective monitoring of Mood and Activity: the Eb2 system. (**b**) Continuous and objective monitoring of mood and activity: Relation between data and indicators (From Carretero et al. [64]; with permission.) (**c**) The domains assessed in the NIMH Family Study through simultaneous objective and subjective ratings tracked in real time in bipolar disorder. Continuous objective measures of sleep and heart rate are derived from accelerometry with a wrist-worn device and analog ratings of mood, energy, anxiety, and a range of other emotions, contextual information, stressors, food intake, sleep timing and quality, exercise, and saliva samples are collected four times per day on a mobile phone application. (From Dunster et al. [65]; with permission)

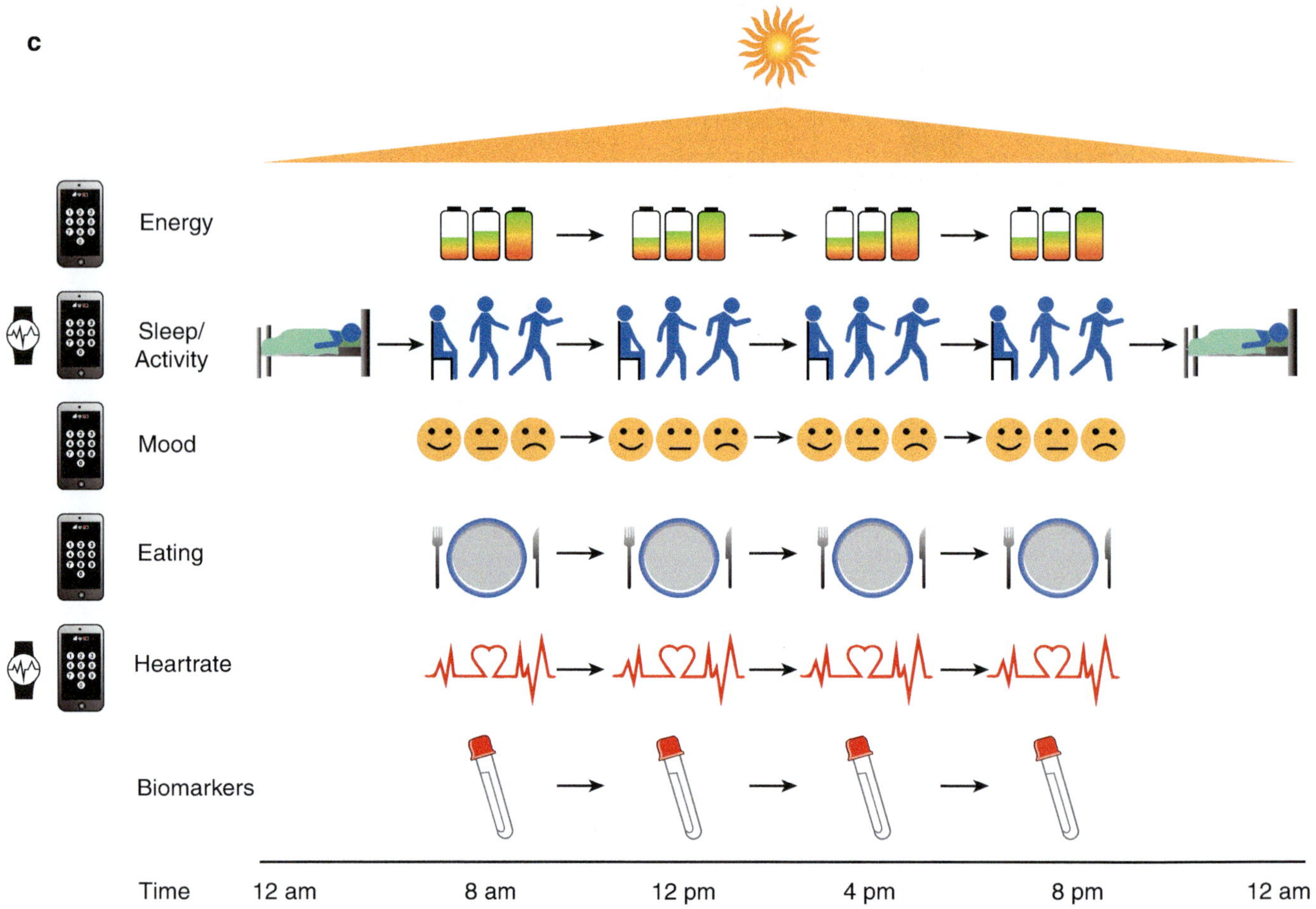

Fig. 25.51 (continued)

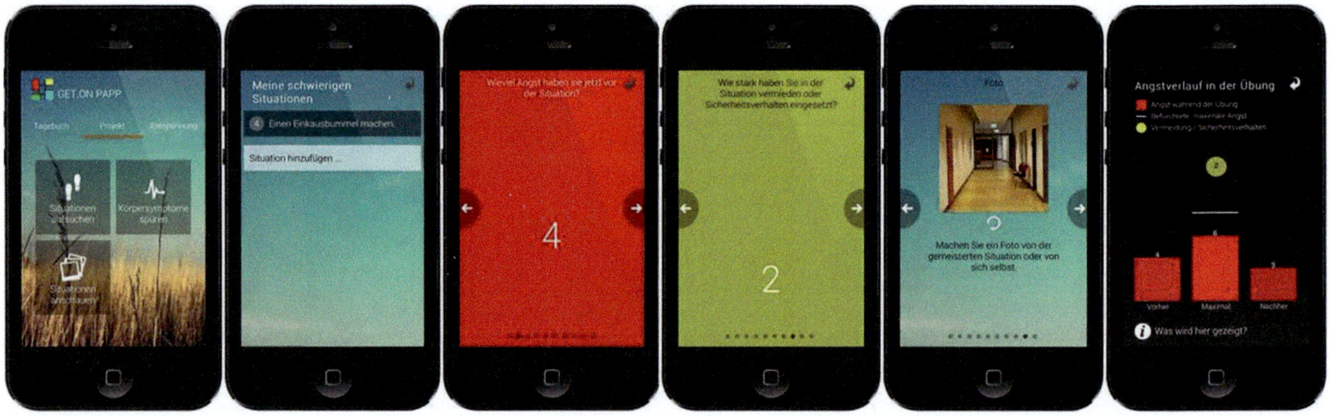

Fig. 25.52 App screenshots of GET.ON PANICAPP. The app supports in vivo exposures. Participants start with ranking their anxiety provoking situations in a hierarchical order. Furthermore, they are asked to answer questions about their anxiety before and after performing the exposure exercise (e.g., the level of anxiety, the degree of avoidance, and the severity of body symptoms). In addition, they have the ability to take a photo after an in vivo exposure exercise is completed. The bar chart in the end offers graphical feedback to the participants regarding the exposure performance. (From Ebenfeld et al. [66] Creative Commons CC BY 4.0; Sinha [68]; with permission)

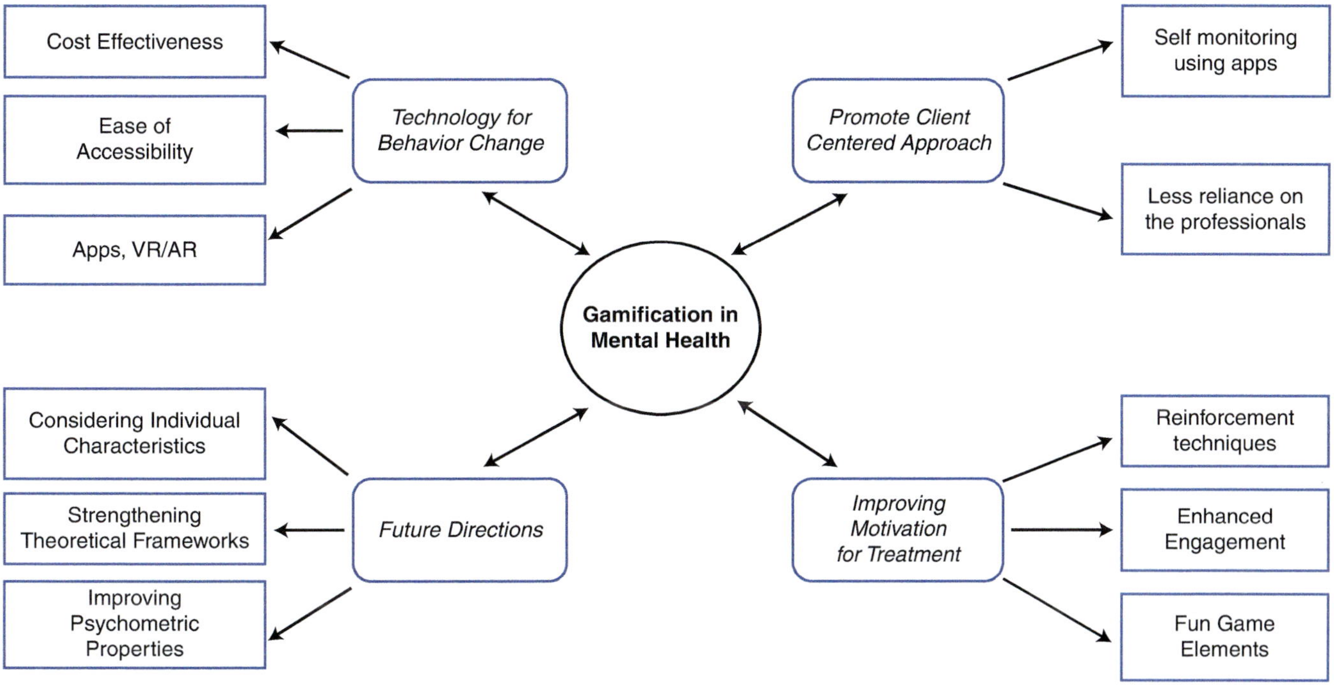

Fig. 25.53 Current description and future directions in gamification. (*From* Sinha [68]; *with permission*)

Fig. 25.54 Digital health solutions for Indigenous mental well-being depicted around the Indigenous Medicine Wheel with the individual located at the center. (From Hensel et al. [113]; Creative Commons CC BY)

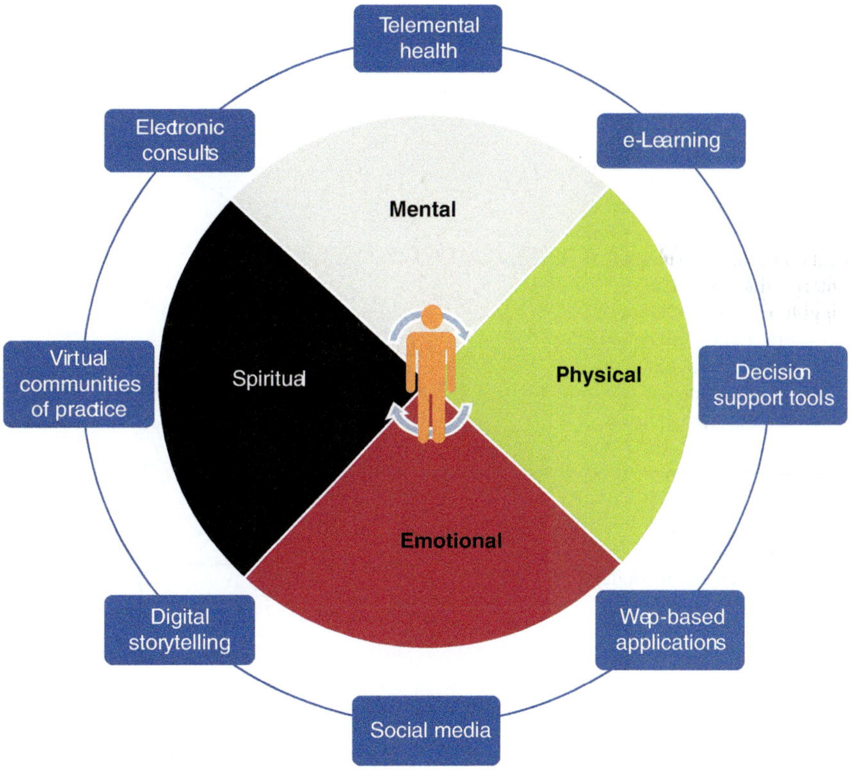

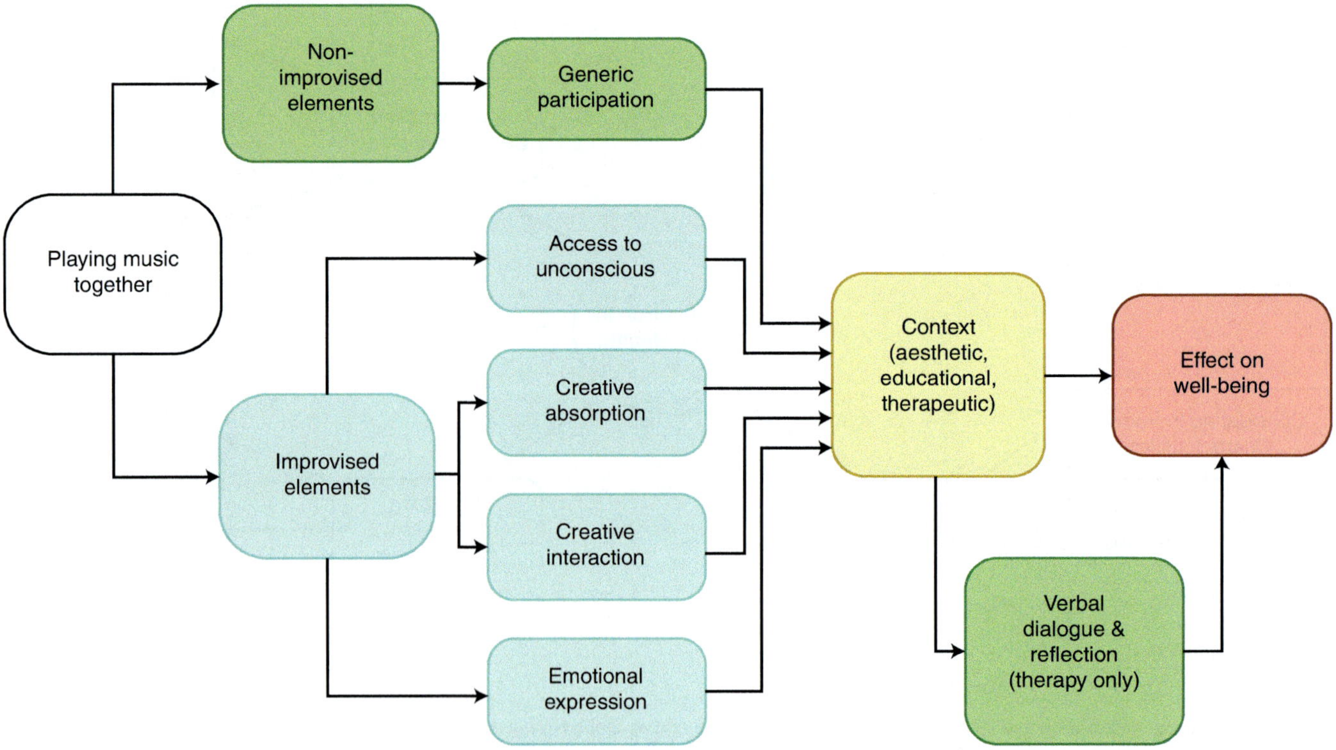

Fig. 25.55 Model for the effects of group music on well-being. Music therapy is rapidly changing from a social science (a general understanding that music promotes quality of life) to one that is heavily based on neuroscientific evidence on brain function and music perception. Thus, the future of music therapy may involve prescribing pieces of music that produce different neurological responses catered to certain illnesses. (From MacDonald and Wilson [69]; Creative Commons CC BY)

Fig. 25.56 Overview of brain structures and pathways targeted by stereotactic psychosurgical operations. *A* amygdala; *ALIC* anterior limb of the internal capsule; *AT* anterior thalamus; *CB* cingulum bundle; *CC* corpus callosum; *CG* cingulate gyrus; *DMT* dorsomedial thalamus; *F* fornix; *G* nucleus of Gudden; *HC* hippocampus; *HT* hypothalamus; *MB* mammillary bodies; *OFC* orbitofrontal cortex; *P* periaqueductal gray; *S* septum; *UF* unicate fasciculus. (From Neumaier et al. [70]; with permission)

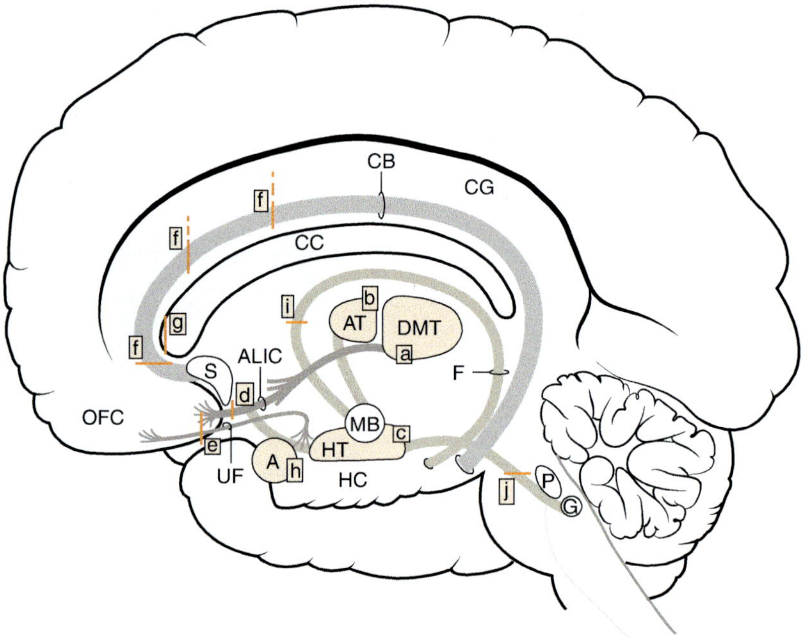

a Dorsomedial thalamotomy	f Cingulo(mo)tomy
b Anterior thalamotomy	g Mesoloviotomy
c Posteromedial hypothalamotomy	h Amygdalotomy
d Anterior capsulotomy	i Fornicotomy
e Subca udate tractotomy	j Mesencephalic reticulotomy

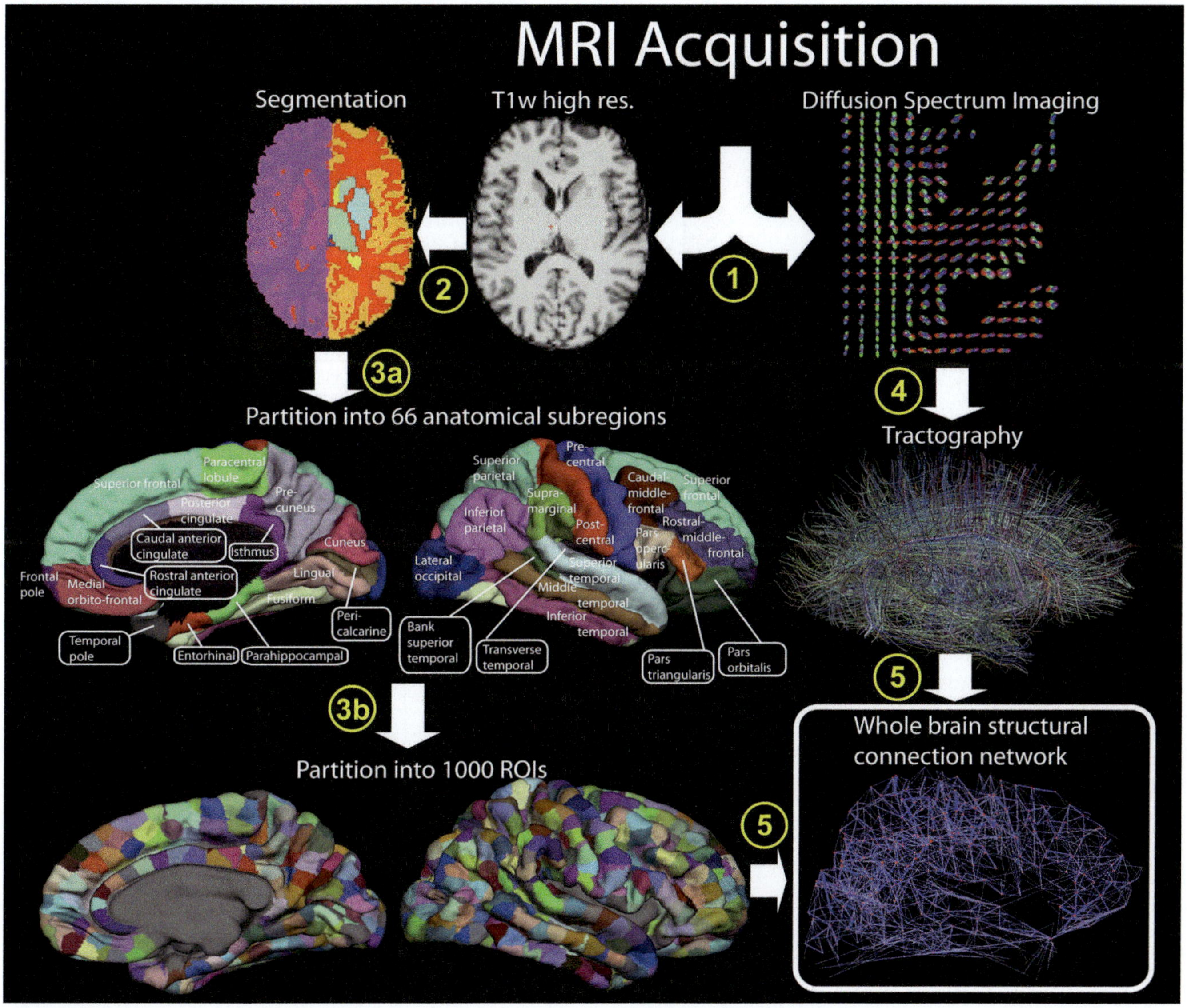

Fig. 25.57 Extraction of a whole brain structural connectivity network. (1) High-resolution T1-weighted and diffusion spectrum MRI (DSI) is acquired. DSI is represented with a zoom on the axial slice of the reconstructed diffusion map, showing an orientation distribution function at each position represented by a deformed sphere whose radius codes for diffusion intensity. Blue codes for the head-feet, red for left-right, and green for anterior-posterior orientations. (2) White and gray matter segmentation is performed from the T1-weighted image. (3a) Sixty-six cortical regions with clear anatomical landmarks are created and then (3b) individually subdivided into small regions of interest (ROIs) resulting in 998 ROIs. (4) Whole brain tractography is performed providing an estimate of axonal trajectories across the entire white matter. (5) ROIs identified in step (3b) are combined with result of step (4) in order to compute the connection weight between each pair of ROIs. The result is a weighted network of structural connectivity across the entire brain. (From Hagmann et al. [74]; Creative Commons)

From Illness to Wellness Interventions

Wellness has been pioneered by John Travis in 1972 who was influenced by Halbert L. Dunn's 1961 book, High-Level Wellness, when he first proposed and popularized the well-being concept seen in Fig. 25.58 [75].

Envisioning the Future Wellness Center and Wellness Medicine

A Wellness Center is where interventions are delivered in-person or online with the help of a wellness coach, who then helps each individual develop and maintain a personalized wellness plan. This plan incorporates wellness interventions along the eight WHO wellness dimensions shown below (Fig. 25.59) [76], along with medical involvement from an evolving the medical subspecialty of Wellness Medicine.

Population Level

The Internet of Healthcare Things (IoHT) and sensor technologies will play an integral role in healthcare and mental health and will be more involved in the future of pandemic control systems (see Fig. 25.60) [62].

Fig. 25.58 The illness-wellness continuum

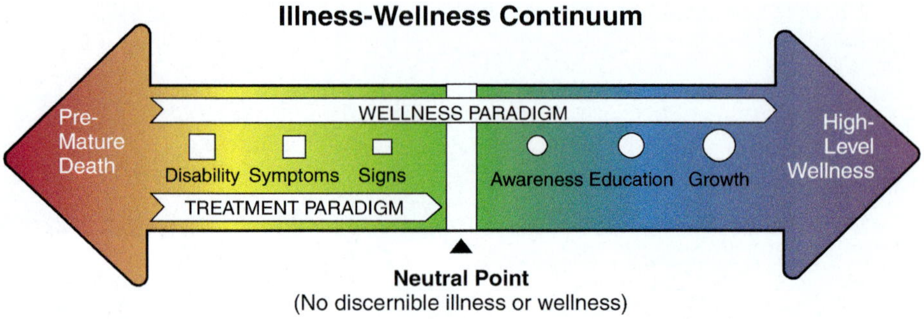

Fig. 25.59 Wellness interventions

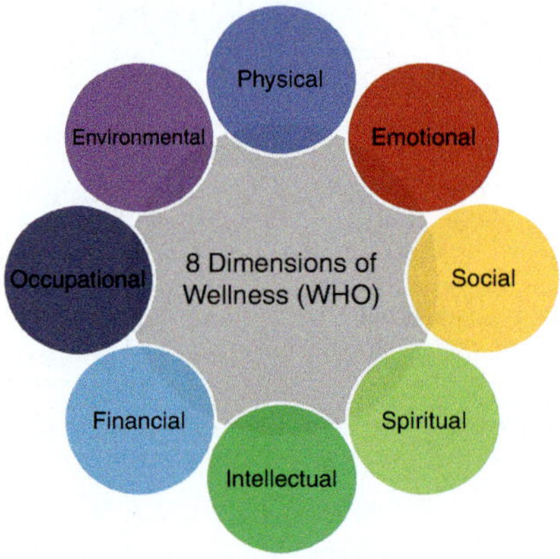

Nutrition
Nutraceuticals
Pharmaceuticals
Exercise, Dance, Tai Chi, Pilates
Sleep, Rest, and Relaxation
Sex and Intimacy
Mindfulness, Meditation, and Yoga
Gratitude, Forgiveness, and Spirituality
Positive Neuropsychology, Cognitive Rehabilitation, and Neuroenhancement
Acupuncture, Herbs, and Ayurvedic Medicine
Aesthetics
Massage, Humor, and Music
Nature and Pets
Circadian Rhythm
The Arts in Health Settings
Engaging the Five Senses: Taste, Scent, Sight, Hearing, and Touch
Emotional Intelligence
Psychotherapy and Positive Psychology
Resilience and Wellness
Developing Purpose, Meaning, and Achievements
Healing
Connection, Compassion, and Community

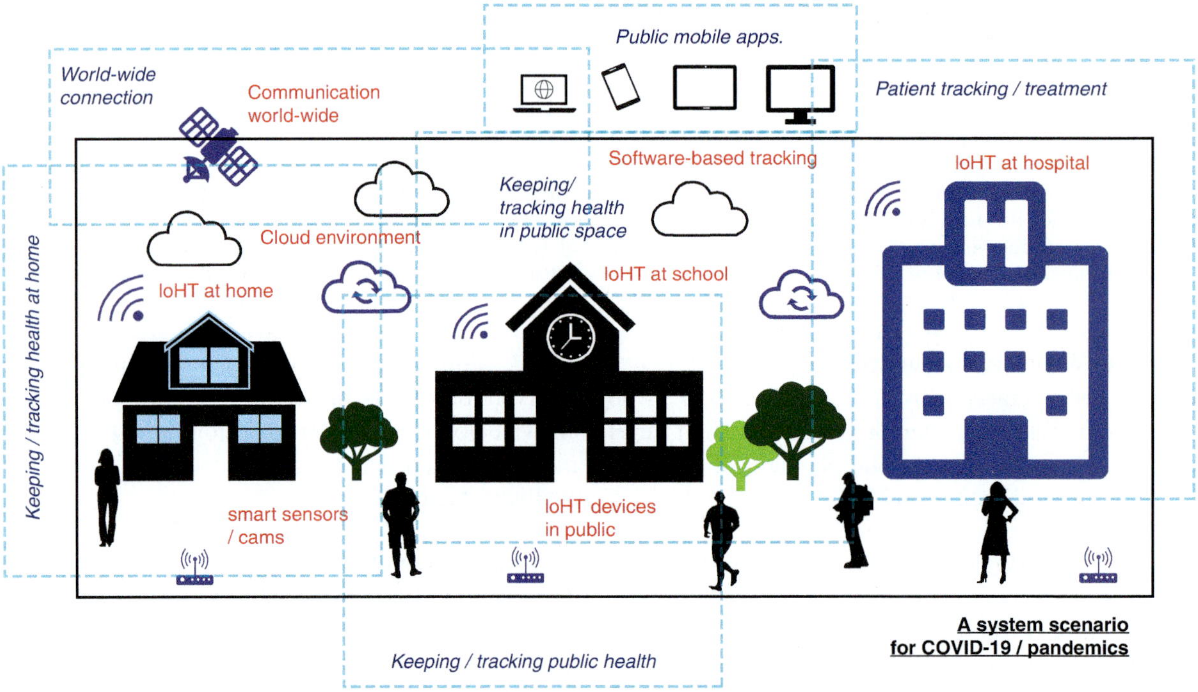

Fig. 25.60 A possible system scenario for COVID-19 and pandemics digital control. (From Kose et al. [62]; with permission)

The Future of Prediction and Prevention of Psychiatric Disorders

Rashid and Calhoun in 2020 reviewed 250 neuroimaging studies of different psychiatric disorders using multivariate brain network features and incorporating them into a predictive model and called this approach the "predictome" as detailed in the figure below (see Fig. 25.61) [77].

Colizzi, Lasalvia, and Ruggeri in 2020 highlighted the importance of prevention and early psychiatric interventions

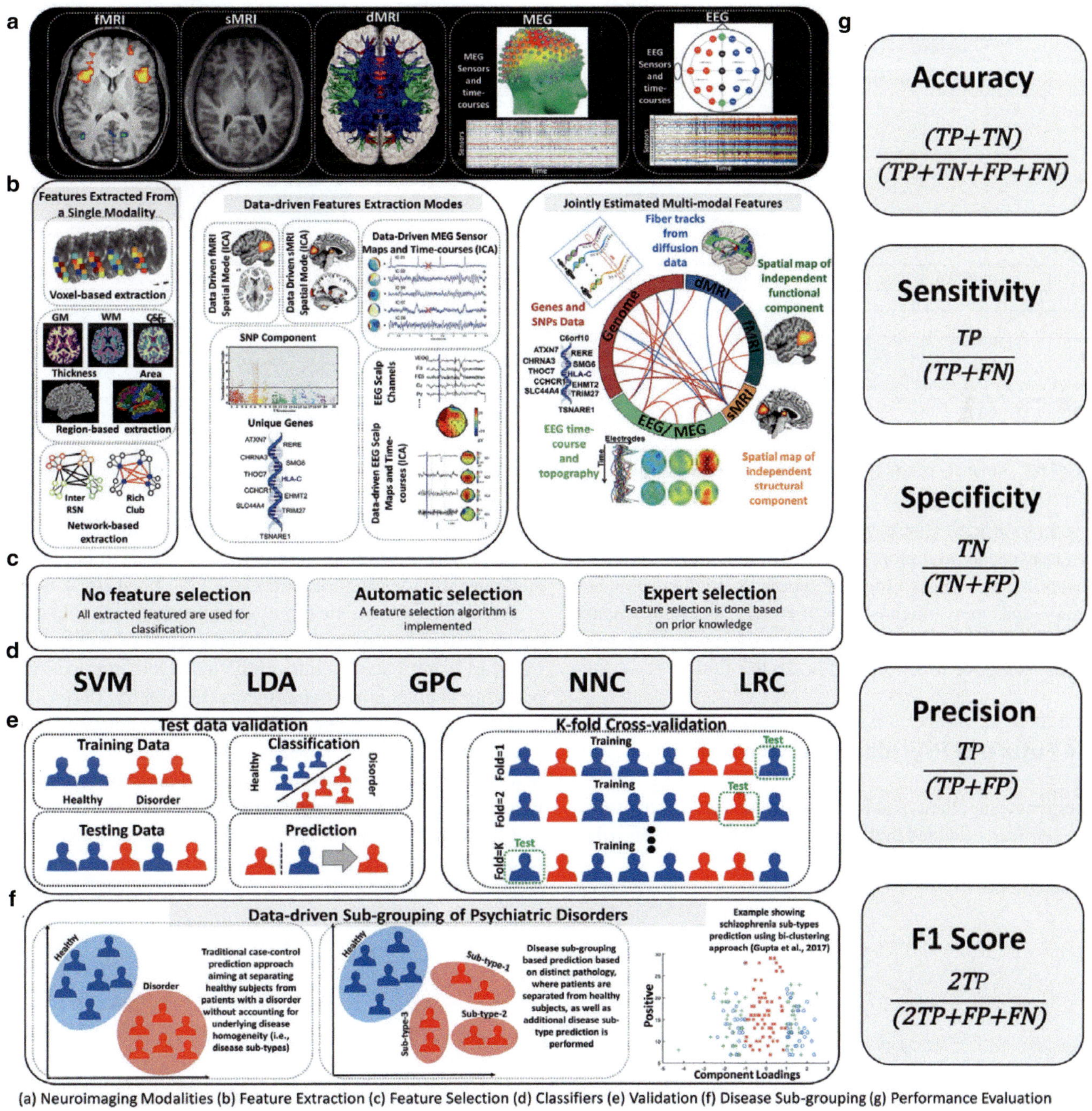

Fig. 25.61 Predictome pipeline. An overview of neuroimaging-based predictome pipeline. (**a**) Neuroimaging modalities typically used for mental illness prediction. (**b**) Current approaches for feature selection. Feature extraction can include (i) voxel-based, (ii) network-based, (iii) data-driven approaches (e.g., independent component analysis, ICA), or (iv) jointly estimated features from multiple modalities (e.g., fMRI and genomics). (**c**) Types of feature selections can include automatic or expert selection approaches. (**d**) Choice of classifiers may include support vector machine (SVM), linear discriminant analysis (LDA), Gaussian process classifier (GPC), neural network classifier (NNC), or logistic regression classifier (LRC). (**e**) Model validation can be performed using either a test-validation setup or using a k-fold cross-validation scheme. (**f**) Data-driven subtype identification can also be performed for homogeneous disorders. (**g**) Various measures for performance evaluation such as accuracy, sensitivity, specificity, precision and F1-score. *FN* false negative; *FP* false positive; *TN* true negative; *TP* true positive. (From Rashid et al. [77]; Creative Commons)

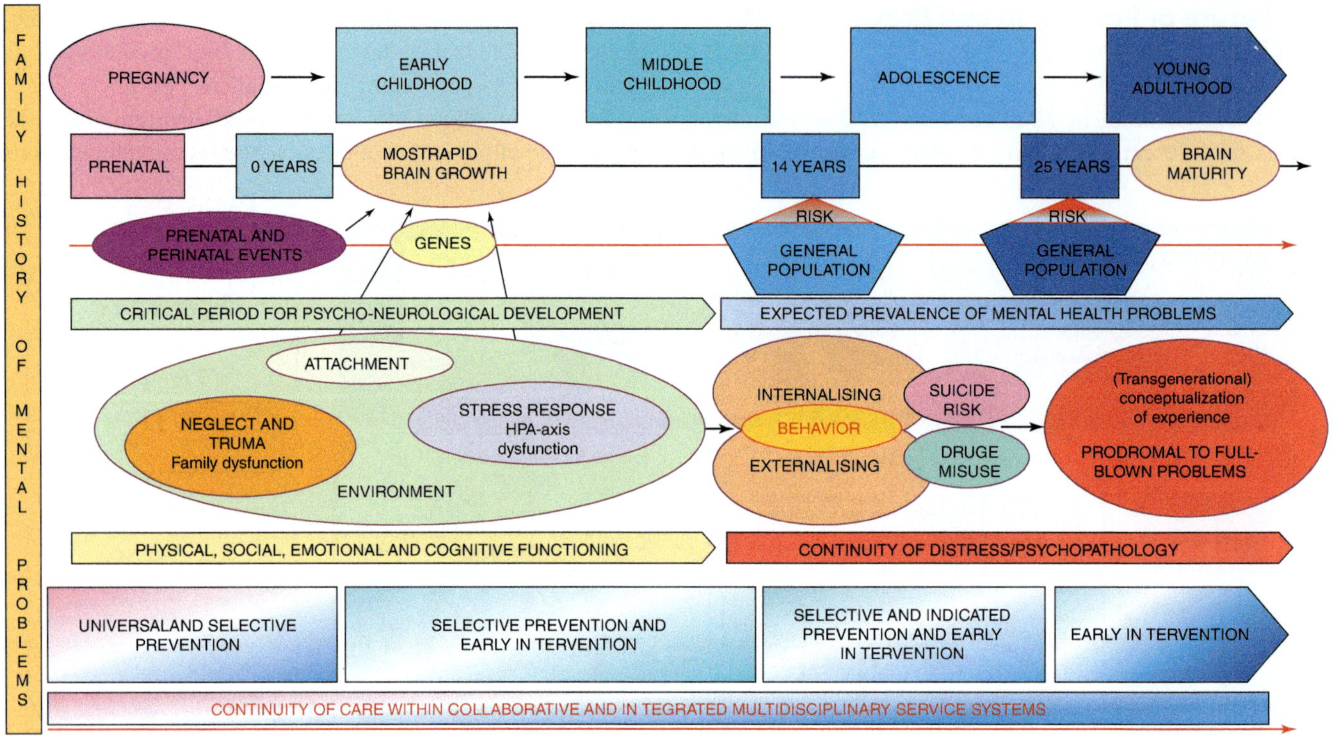

Fig. 25.62 Summary of risk factors and pluripotent pathological trajectory for mental disorders. (From Colizzi et al. [78]; with permission)

in youth, since 50% of psychiatric disorders start by age 14 with nonspecific symptoms that evolve into major disorders. Prevention will need to focus on youth using the multidisciplinary and trans-diagnostic framework, including mental health professionals, health professionals, researchers, institutions, and governments (see Fig. 25.62) [78].

The Future of Psychiatry Service Delivery

Emergency, inpatient, and intermediate levels of care psychiatric services provided in the continuum of care are described in Fig. 25.63 [79].

A decline in the number of community mental health centers and partial hospitalization/day was found to be associated with suicide mortality rates (see Fig. 25.64) [80].

It has also become clear that a similar decline in inpatient psychiatric beds, especially with the decline of public funding, has contributed significantly to psychiatric patients' boarding in emergency departments (Fig. 25.65) [81].

The American College of Emergency Physicians (ACEP) issued an information paper that highlighted a number of practical solutions due to the boarding of psychiatric patients in the emergency department (see Fig. 25.66) [82].

Psychiatric services delivery is in critical need for a reform that would include the interventions highlighted below in Fig. 25.67 [83].

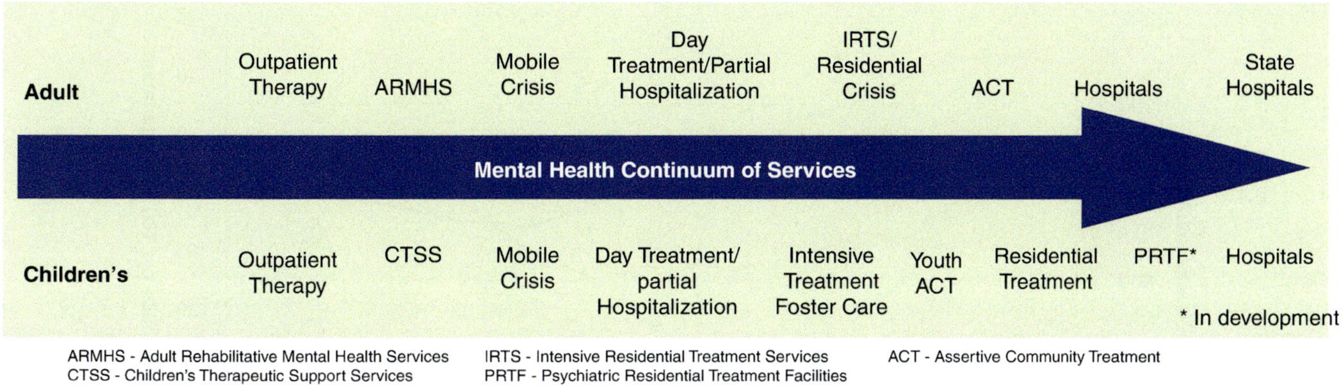

Fig. 25.63 Continuum of care for psychiatric services. (From Hector and Khey [79]; with permission)

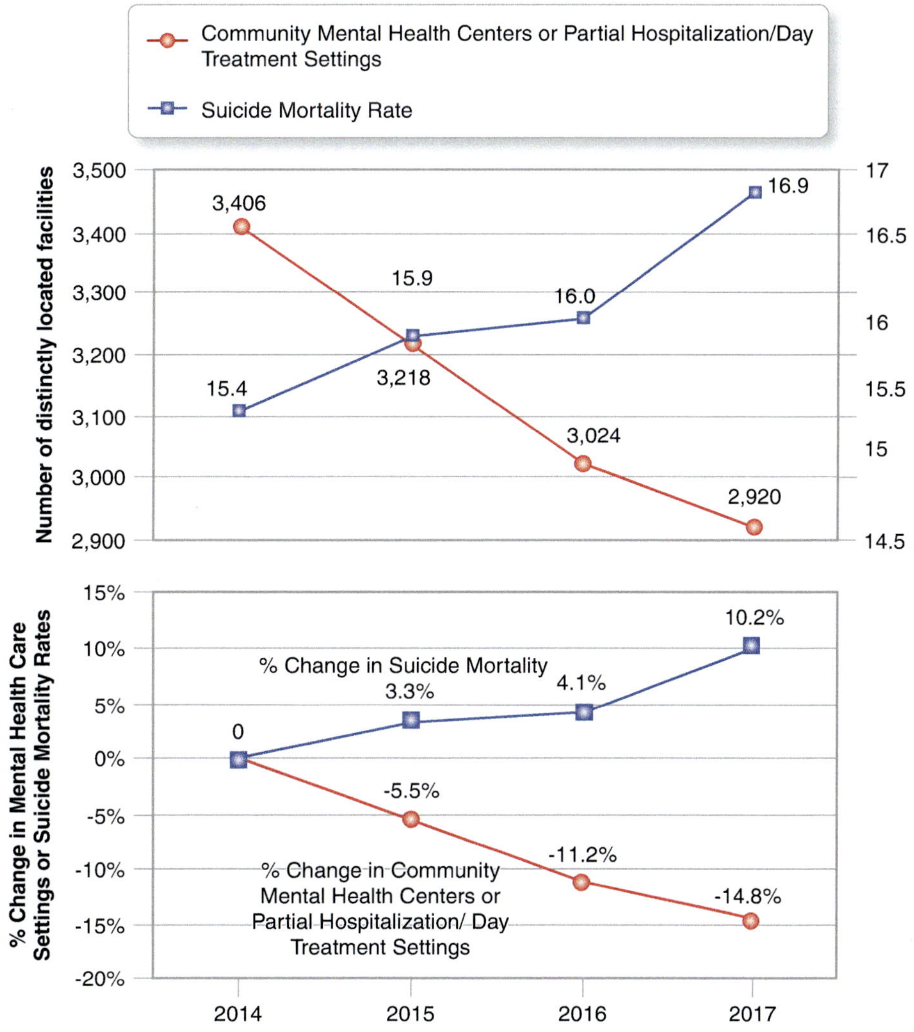

Fig. 25.64 Trend of Mental Health Facilities Supply and Suicide Mortality in the United States 2014–2017. Data were from 2014 to 2017 National Mental Health Services Survey (N-MHSS) to identify state-level community mental health center status during 2014–2017 and from Centers for Disease Control and Prevention (CDC) Wide-Ranging Online Data for Epidemiologic Research (WONDER) data for suicide rates, identified as intentional self-harm by ICD-10-CM diagnosis codes U03, X60-X71, X72-X74, X75-X84, Y87.0. A Community Mental Health Center was defined as a facility that provided any of the following services: (1) outpatient services, (2) 24-h emergency care services, (3) day treatment or other partial hospitalization services or psychosocial rehabilitation services, and (4) screening for inpatient services to state mental health facilities, and that met applicable licensing or certification requirements for community mental health centers in a state where it is located. Mental health care facilities self-identified as a partial hospitalization or day treatment facility were also categorized as a community mental health center. (From Hung et al. [80]; Creative Commons CC-BY)

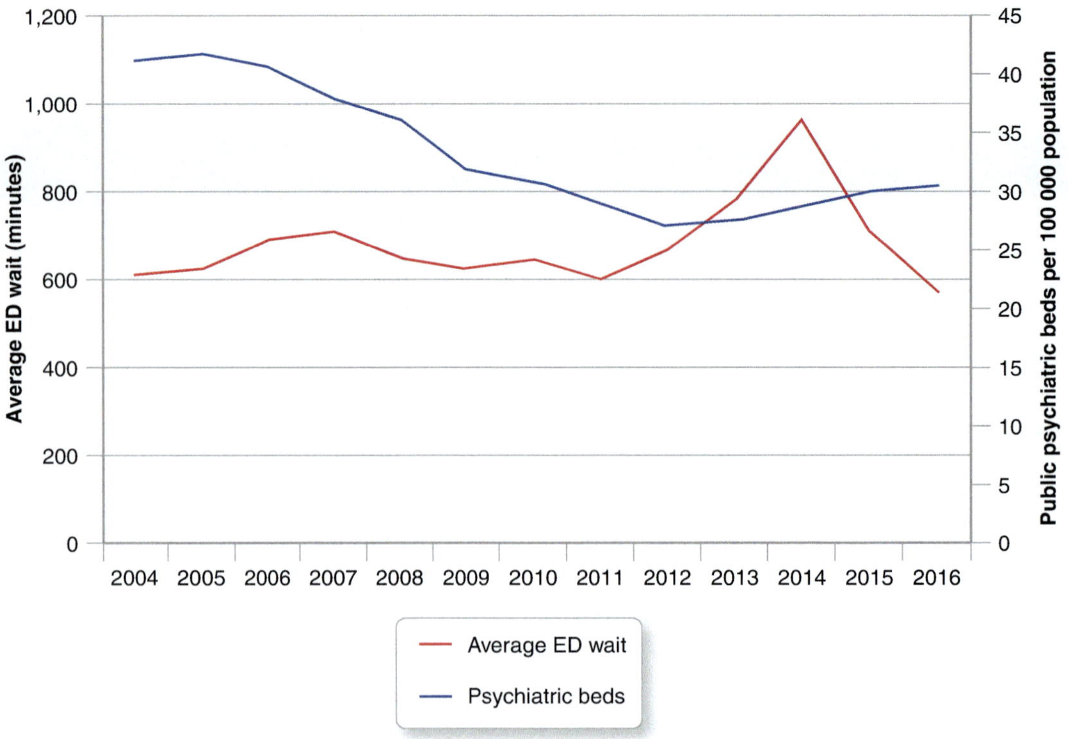

Fig. 25.65 Publicly funded psychiatric beds and Emergency Department (ED) average wait times for the general hospitals (from the Australian Institute of Health and Welfare, Australian Government). (From Allison et al. [81]; with permission)

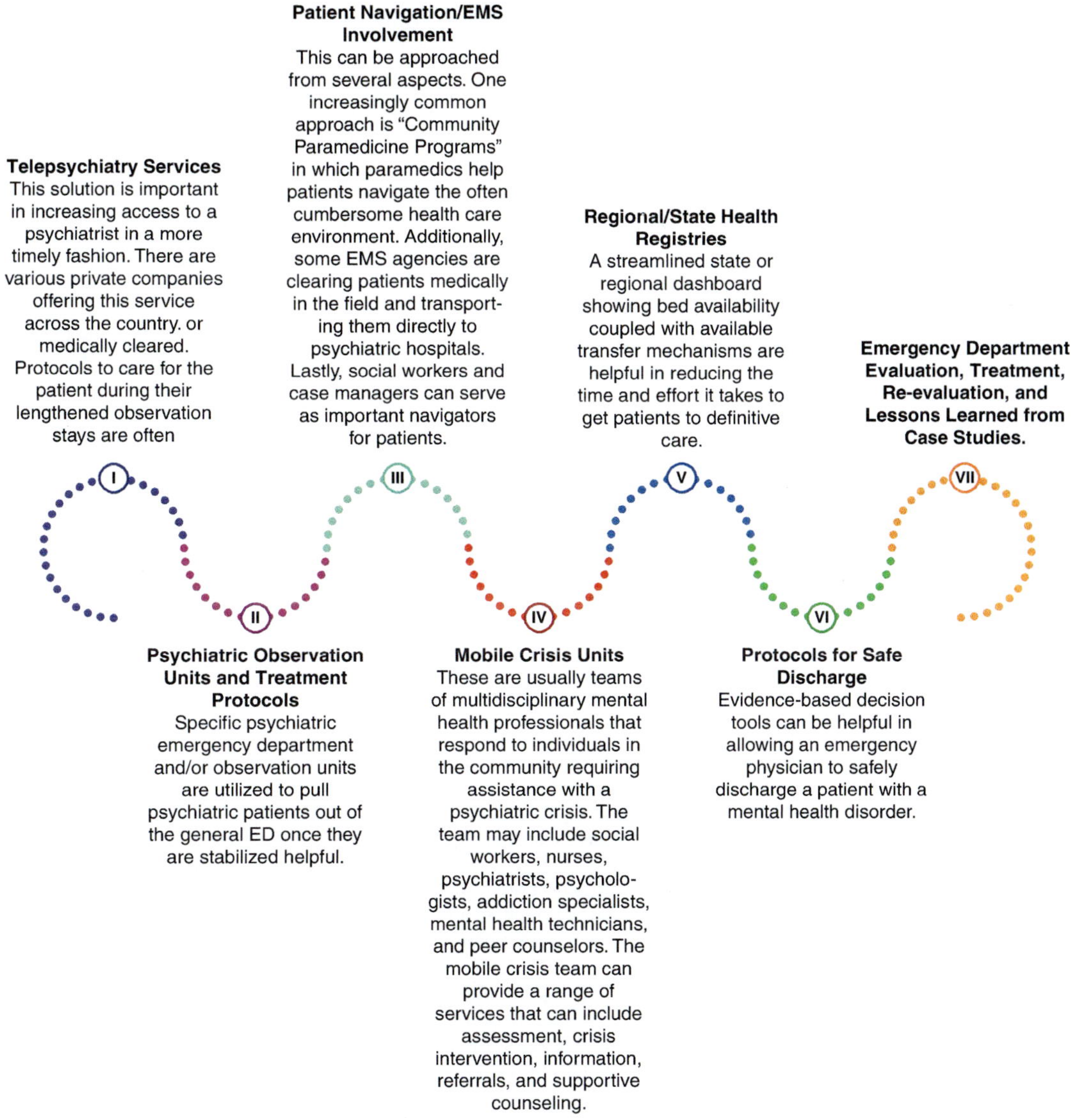

Fig. 25.66 Practical Solutions to Boarding of Psychiatric Patients in the Emergency Department

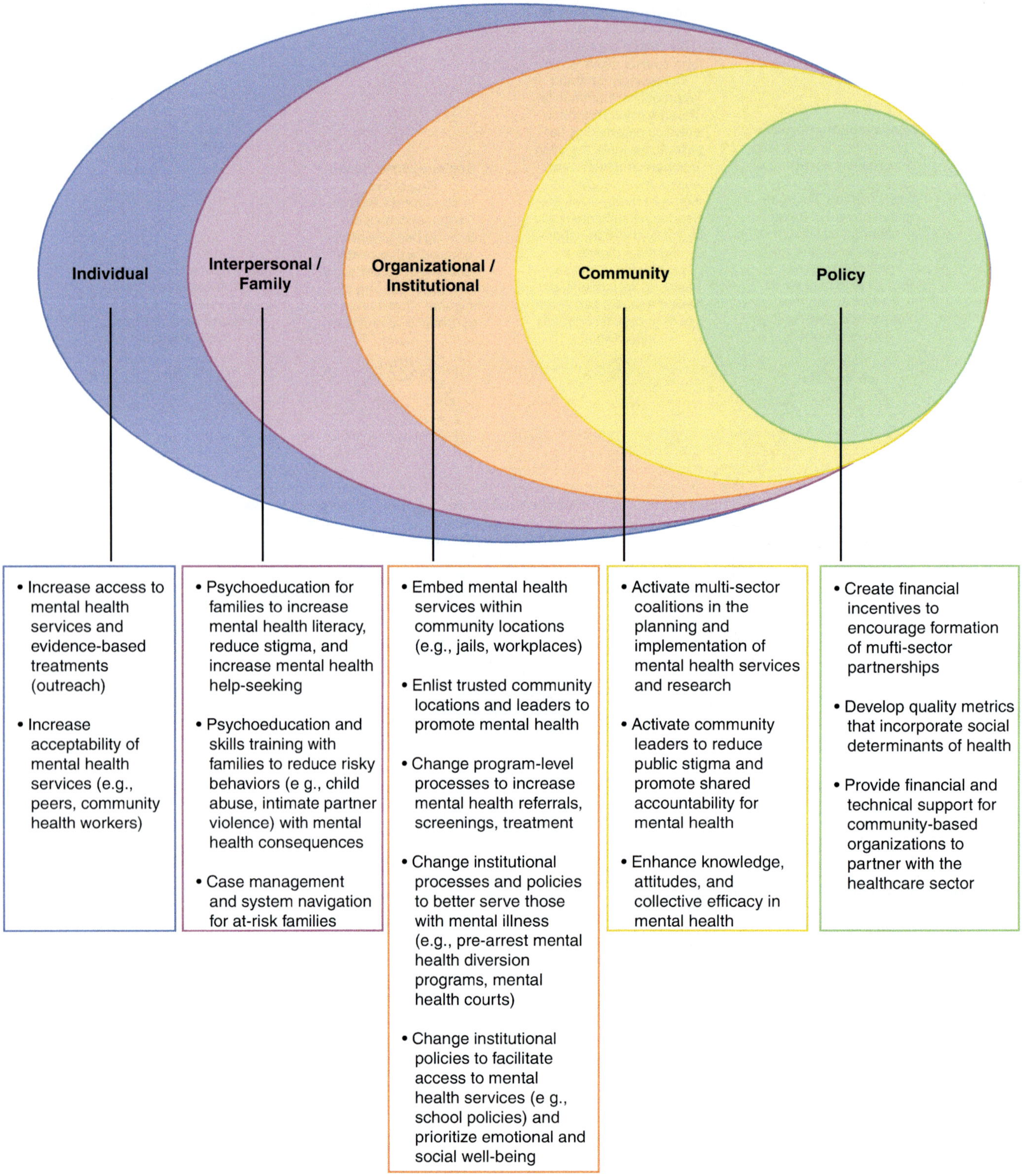

Fig. 25.67 Overview of community intervention processes by social-ecological level. (Adapted from McElroy, KR, Bibeau D, Steckler A, Glanz K. An ecological perspective on health promotion programs. Health Educ Q. 1988;15:351–377). (From Castillo et al. [83]; Creative Commons CC-BY)

Financing Psychiatric Services of the Future

Psychiatry has relied primarily on public funds for financing mental health care for decades; however, a new trend with private sector involvement has been detected in recent years. Shah and Berry reported that in 2019, venture capital firms invested $637 million in "mental health companies," almost 23 times that same figure in 2013 according to data obtained from Pitchbook [84]. The most recent data published by Pitchbook placed the funds invested in such companies at higher figures. By the end of the third quarter of 2020 (ending September 30, 2020), venture capital funding reached $1.37 billion in US mental health startups [85]. It was believed that this was driven by the rising demand in mental health services due to the COVID-19 pandemic's impact [85]. In May of 2021, Business Insider announced that mental health startups have raised a record $1.9 billion in 2021 [86]. This exponential growth in funding is shown in different graphs from a Google search from May 21, 2021, in Fig. 25.68 [87].

Mental health companies and startups have reached a total of 1403 in May 2021 according to AngelList, which is a platform for startups [88]. Many startups are focusing on creating apps on meditation, breathing, sleep, journaling, and education. Others are tackling Telepsychiatry, employee assistance services, tracking and measurement, peer advising, and digital therapeutics such as prescription apps delivering CBT or other modalities. The CBT for insomnia app called Someryst [89] and the CBT app for irritable bowel syndrome called Parallel [90] have been cleared by the FDA in 2020 after showing both short-term and long-term efficacy in randomized controlled trials.

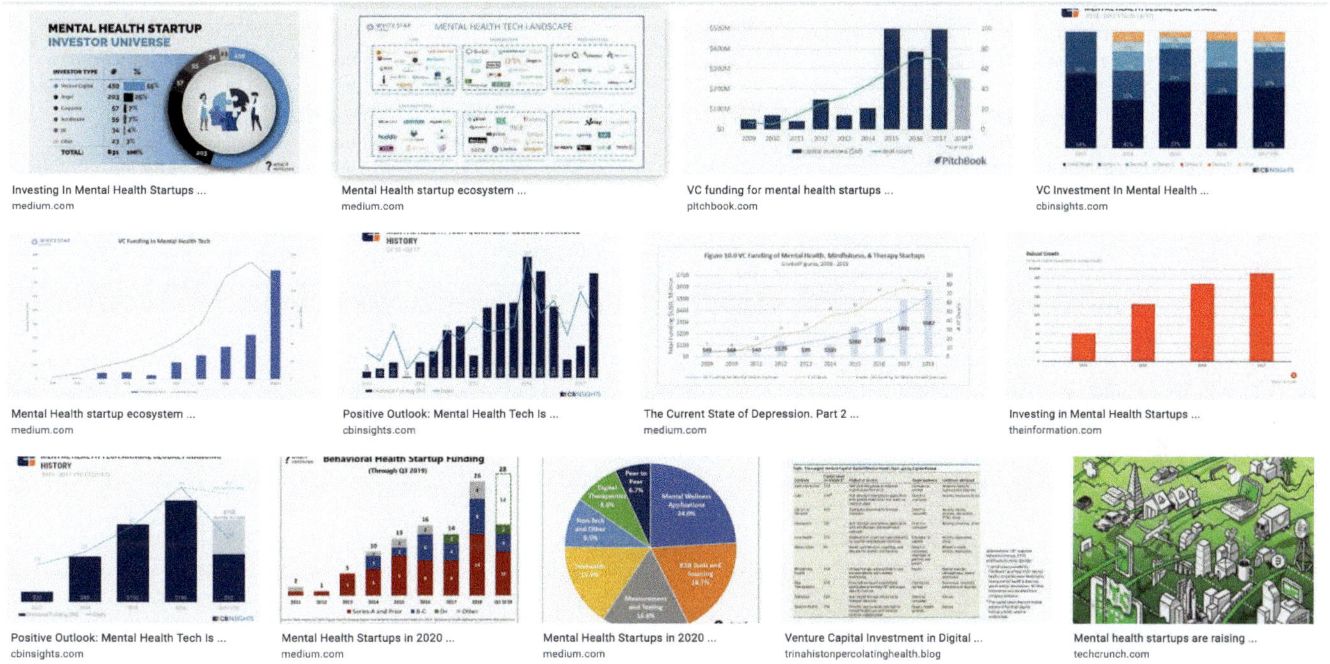

Fig. 25.68 The results of a Google search for keywords "venture capital" and "mental health" on May 21, 2021, showing different graphs demonstrating the exponential growth in funding of mental health startups

The Future of Psychiatry Laws

The reorganization of the DEA schedules is warranted based on new scientific evidence since their development more than 50 years. The reader is invited to examine how close or different the schedules are from current knowledge by reviewing them below (Table 25.5) [91].

The Future of the Psychiatry Training

Curriculum mapping of didactics during postgraduate residency training in psychiatry is an innovative approach that will enable a visual examination of training topics and will help create an advanced process of curricular improvement (see Fig. 25.69) [92]. A wordle based on the process above brings an additional level of clarity about what is being emphasized in the curriculum and the improvement opportunities (see Fig. 25.70) [92].

Table 25.5 Drug Enforcement Agency (DEA) drug schedules

Schedule	Description	Example drugs
Schedule I	No currently accepted medical use and a high potential for abuse	Heroin, lysergic acid diethylamide (LSD), psilocybin, marijuana (cannabis), 3,4-methylenedioxymethamphetamine (ecstasy), methaqualone, and peyote
Schedule II	High potential for abuse, with use potentially leading to severe psychological or physical dependence. These drugs are also considered dangerous	Combination products with less than 15 milligrams of hydrocodone per dosage unit (Vicodin), cocaine, methamphetamine, methadone, hydromorphone (Dilaudid), meperidine (Demerol), oxycodone (OxyContin), fentanyl, Dexedrine, Adderall, and Ritalin
Schedule III	Moderate to low potential for physical and psychological dependence. Schedule III drugs abuse potential is less than Schedule I and Schedule II drugs but more than Schedule IV	Products containing less than 90 milligrams of codeine per dosage unit (Tylenol with codeine), ketamine, anabolic steroids, and testosterone
Schedule IV	Low potential for abuse and low risk of dependence	Xanax, Soma, Darvon, Darvocet, Valium, Ativan, Talwin, Ambien, and Tramadol
Schedule V	Lower potential for abuse than Schedule IV and consist of preparations containing limited quantities of certain narcotics. Schedule V drugs are generally used for antidiarrheal, antitussive, and analgesic purposes	Cough preparations with less than 200 milligrams of codeine or per 100 milliliters (Robitussin AC), Lomotil, Motofen, Lyrica, and Parepectolin

For an alphabetical listing of all controlled substances and their DEA schedule designation, please check: https://www.deadiversion.usdoj.gov/schedules/orangebook/c_cs_alpha.pdf

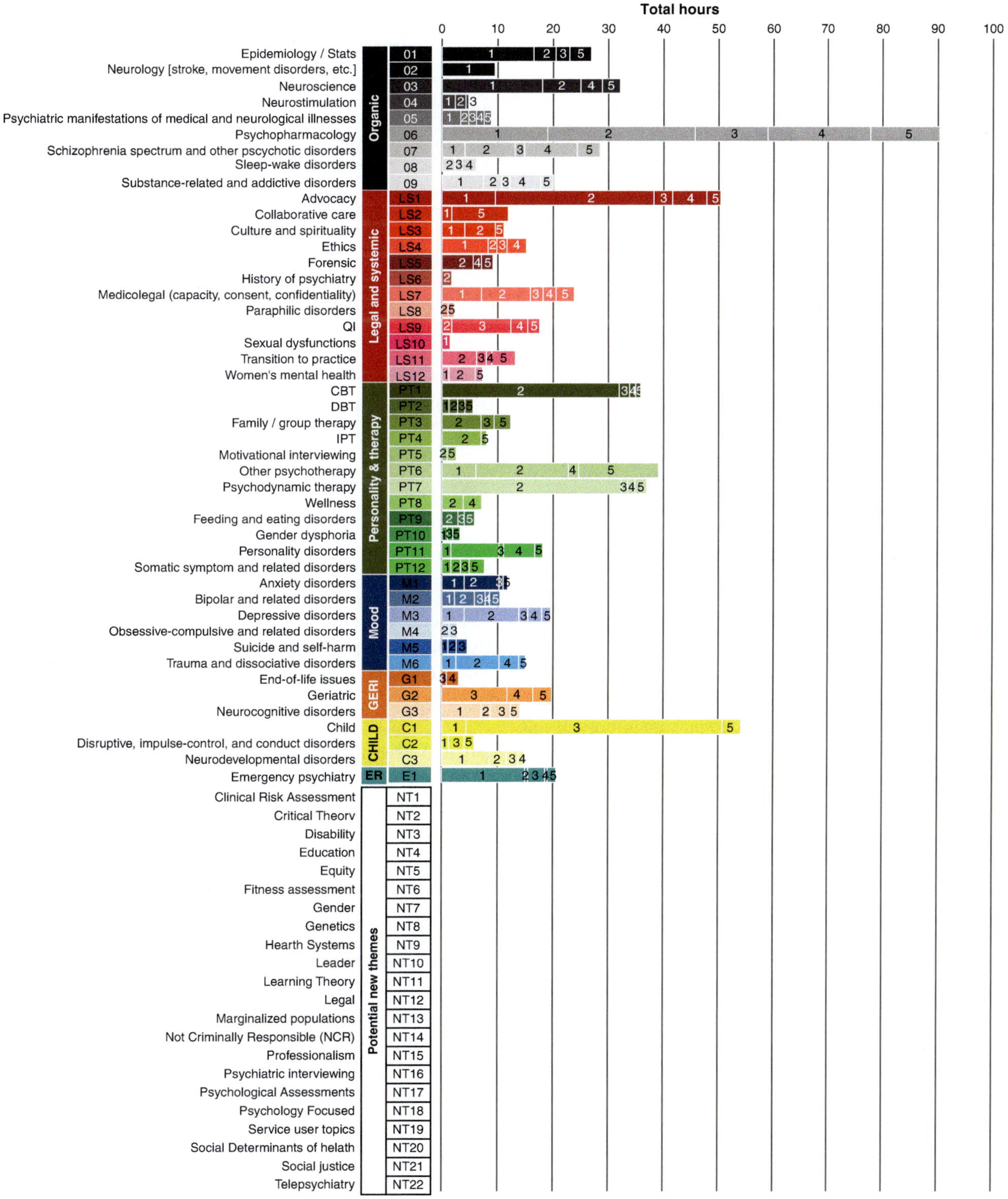

Fig. 25.69 Topics and duration spent in hours on content topic over 5 years of postgraduate psychiatry residency training (from the University of Toronto Postgraduate Psychiatry). (From Colman et al. [92]; with permission)

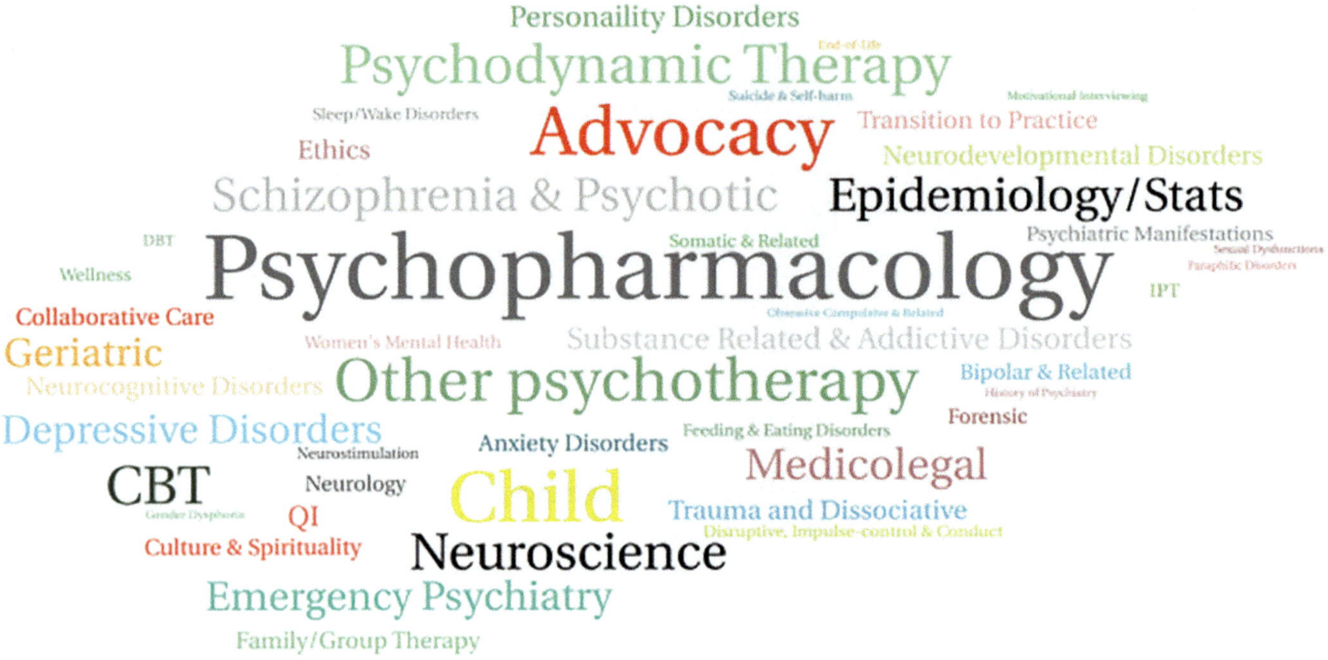

Fig. 25.70 Wordle displaying weighted content taught throughout residency. (From Colman et al. [92]; with permission)

The Future of the Psychiatry Research

Data Science and Big Data

Data science and big data are going to play an important role for the advancement of psychiatric research in diagnosis, treatment, and future prevention (see Fig. 25.71) [93].

Big data will be integrated in the future to link with focused hypothesis-driven studies in order to scale genomics and digital approaches to phenotyping of psychiatric disorders as shown below in bipolar disorder (see Fig. 25.72) [94].

Computational Psychiatry

Computational psychiatry combines data-driven approaches, such as machine-learning and theory-driven approaches, in order to improve the understanding of relationships between symptoms, classification of disorders, treatment selection, and outcome prediction. For example, data on patients with major depressive disorder were reanalyzed from the large STAR*D and the COMED trials showing that combining supervised dimensionality reduction and multivariate classifiers ended up by yielding a cross-validated prediction of remission (see Fig. 25.73) [95, 96].

Potential solutions from machine learning to the ongoing challenges for precision medicine in psychiatry are shown below (see Fig. 25.74) [97].

Digital Phenotyping

Future methods of psychiatry research include enhancement of digital phenotyping technology platforms hand in hand with improving collaboration between patients, healthcare professionals, and researchers (see Fig. 25.75) [98].

Real-World Data Collection

Psychiatric research relies heavily on real-world data collection. Future approaches include the use of Amazon's Mechanical Turk (mTurk https://www.mturk.com/mturk/welcome), which enables researchers to recruit large samples of research participants. These paid individuals enable businesses to perform repetitive tasks that still need human involvement. mTurk has been shown to be a valid and reliable research method (see Fig. 25.76) [99, 100].

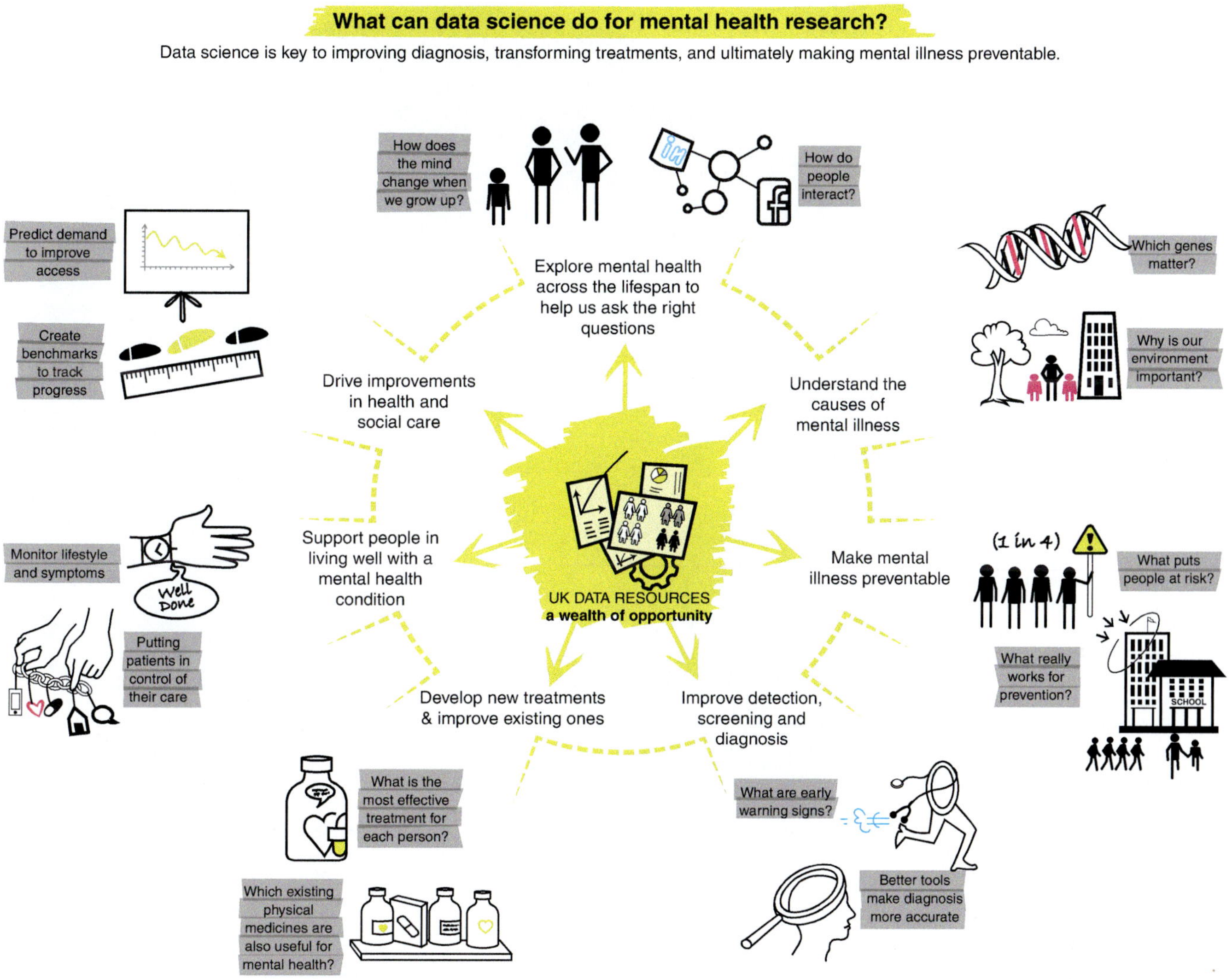

Fig. 25.71 Data science is key to improving diagnosis, transforming treatments, and ultimately making mental illness preventable. (From Russ et al.; MQ Data Science group [93]; with permission)

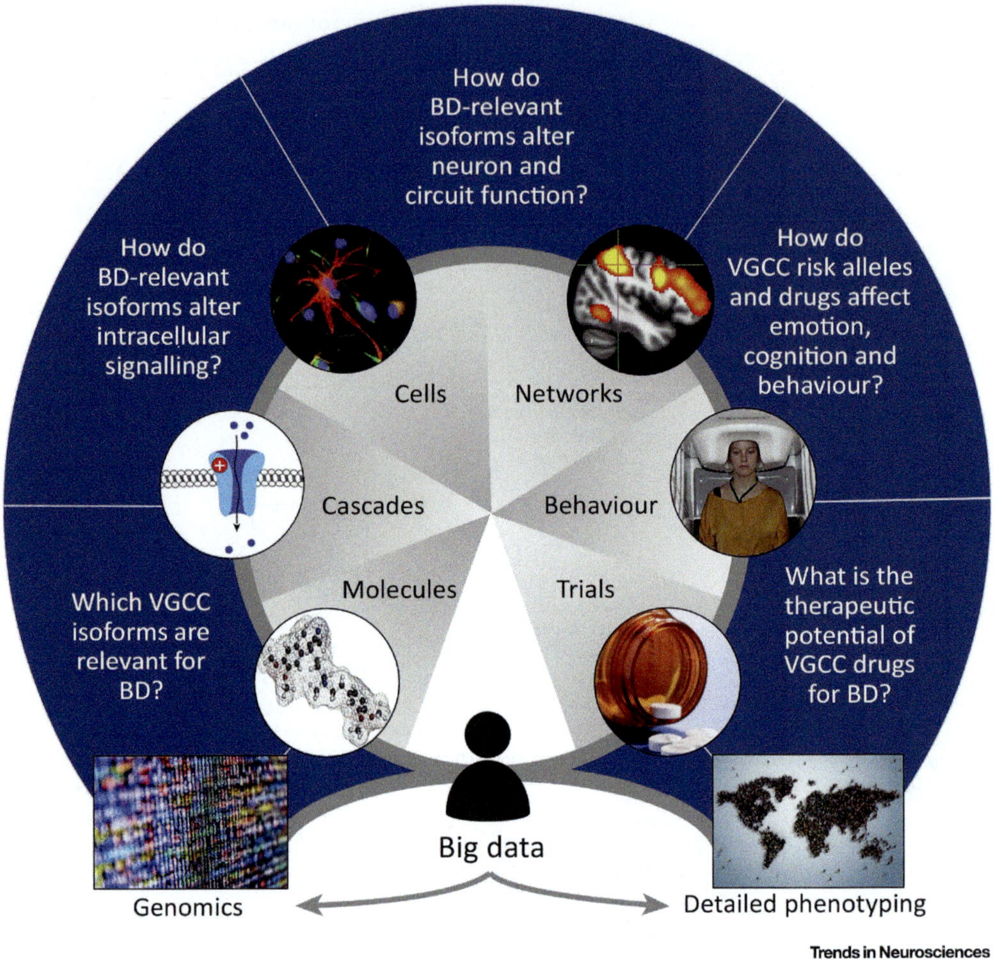

Fig. 25.72 Genomics, neuroscience, and treatment innovation in bipolar disorder (BD). The study of voltage-gated calcium channels (VGCCs) in BD exemplifies the potential and the challenges of translating genomic discoveries into pathophysiology and therapeutics. Although sometimes portrayed as a one-way, bottom-up, process from genes to treatments, the wheel-like figure emphasizes that it is iterative. Underpinning this approach is the increasing wealth of "big data," since it is the scale of both the genomics and the contemporary digital approaches to phenotyping that have driven the developments discussed in the review. Looking ahead, an integrative, collaborative approach will be essential to link the power of big data with the more-focused, hypothesis-driven studies that are required for most of the intervening segments. (*From* Harrison et al. [94]; Creative Commons CC-BY license)

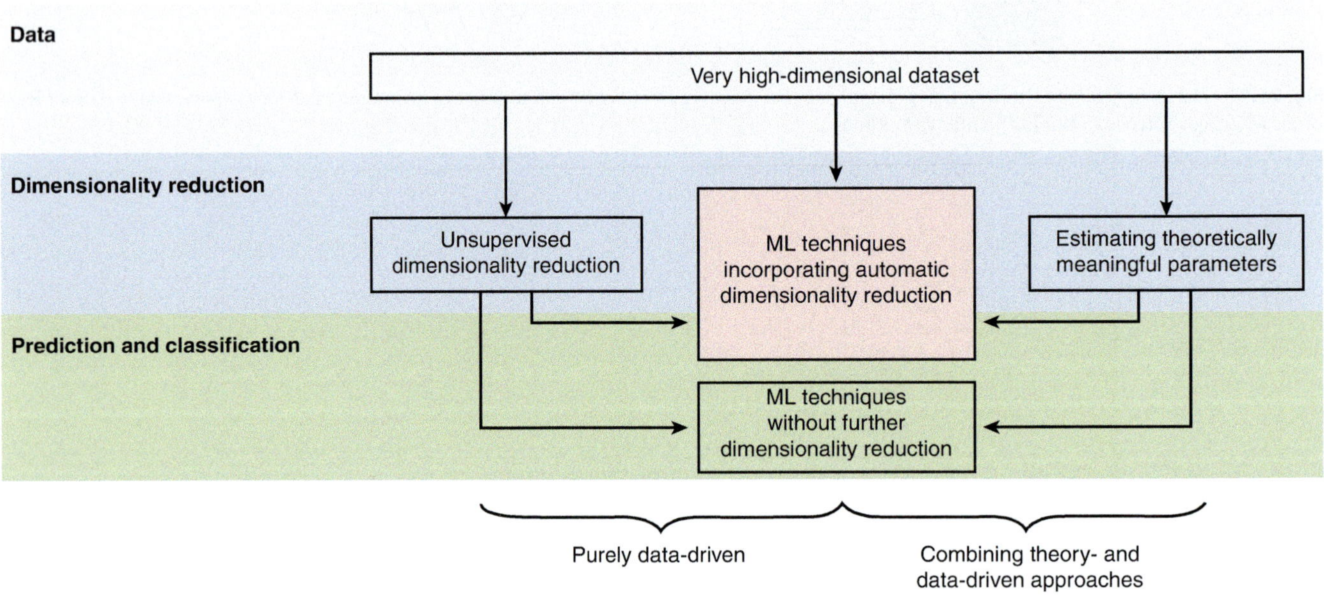

Fig. 25.73 Exploiting and coping with high dimensionality in psychiatric data sets. Purely data-driven approaches (left and middle branches) and combinations of theory- and data-driven approaches (right branch) can be used to analyze large data sets to arrive at clinically useful applications. Dimensionality reduction is a key step to avoid overfitting. It can be performed as a preprocessing step using unsupervised methods before application of other ML techniques with or without further dimensionality reduction (left branch; Box 1); using ML techniques that automatically limit the number of variables for prediction; using regularization or Bayesian model selection (middle branch; Box 1); or using theory-driven models that in essence project the original high-dimensional data into a low-dimensional space of theoretically meaningful parameters, which can then be fed into ML algorithms that may or not further reduce dimensionality (right branch). (*From* Huys et al. [96]; with permission)

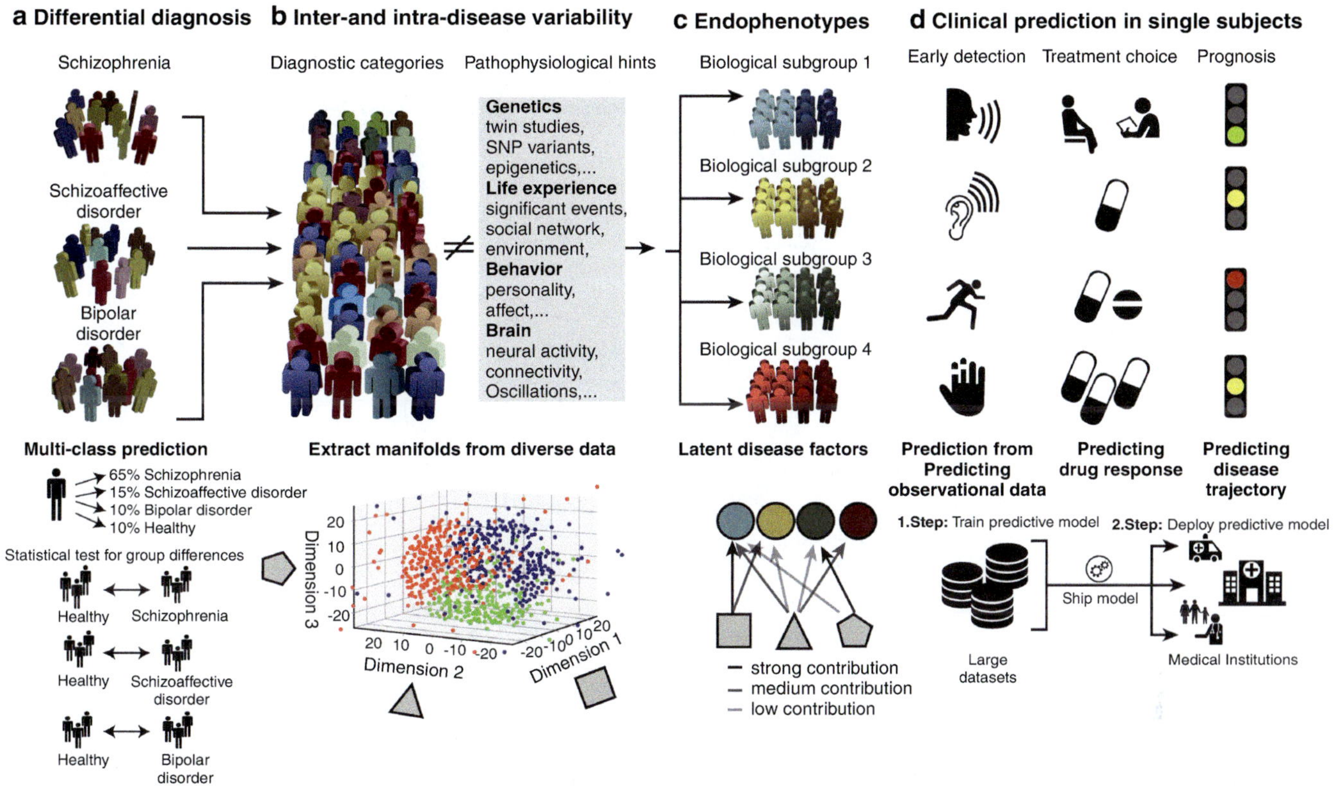

Fig. 25.74 Current challenges for precision medicine in psychiatry and possible solutions from machine learning. (**a**) Basic and clinical psychiatric research frequently investigates a given patient population by group comparison against the healthy population, possibly creating artificial dichotomies. Many machine learning approaches can be extended to compare observations from a number of groups in the same statistical estimation (i.e., multiclass prediction). (**b**) The diagnostic categories in the ICD and DSM manuals were primarily designed to reliably describe symptom phenomenology and are frequently incongruent with new behavioral, neural, and genetic research evidence. Machine learning methods can automatically extract currently unknown patterns of variation in individuals simultaneously from heterogeneous data that cut across traditional diagnoses (i.e., manifolds). (**c**) Assigning a patient to only one diagnostic category may ignore that different pathophysiological mechanisms (i.e., endophenotypes) can contribute to the same clinical picture. Instead of relying on categorical assignments, biologically defined subgroups can be described by continuous contributions of several disease processes in graded degrees (i.e., latent factor models). (**d**) Psychiatric care today often resorts to trial and error. Predictive models could improve patient care by earlier detection, treatment selection and adjustment, and inference of disease trajectory. After a machine learning algorithm has been trained in extensive data (i.e., in sample), the trained predictive model can be used for personalized prediction without database access (i.e., out of sample). *SNP* single nucleotide polymorphism. (*From* Bzdok et al. [97]; with permission)

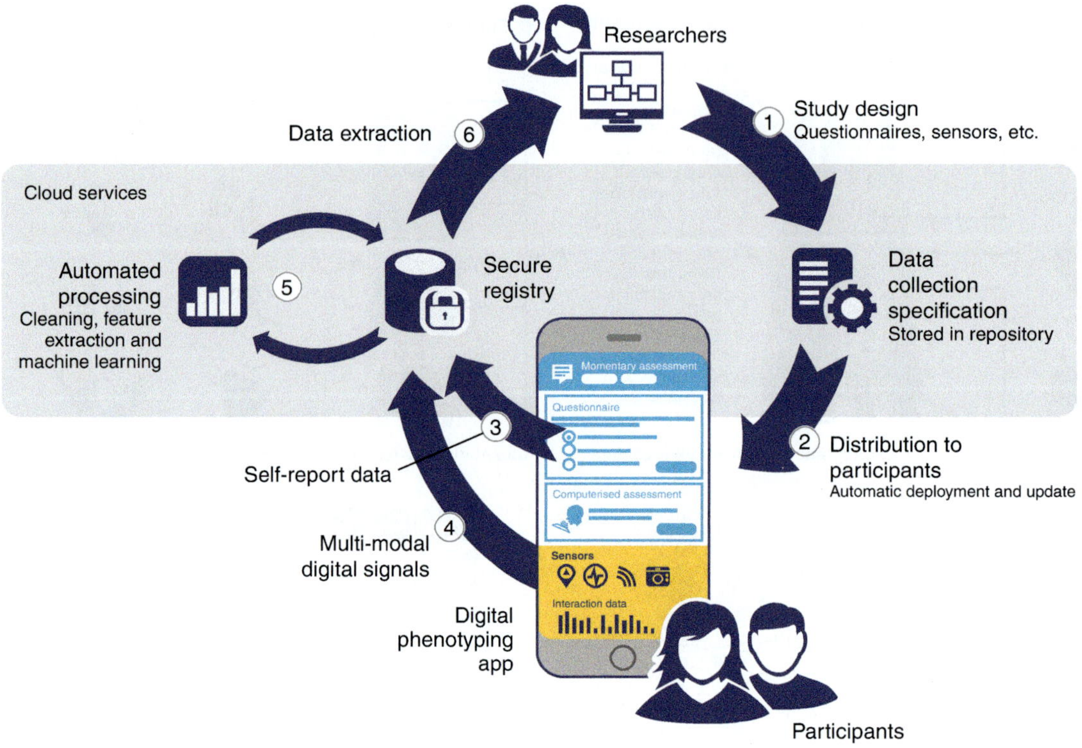

Fig. 25.75 Black Dog Institute/Deakin model for a scalable, integrated multi-user platform for digital phenotyping research. Figures and letters refer to those shown in the diagram. In this model, (1) researchers specify the study design and define which questionnaires and sensors are required to deliver a digital phenotyping study (and optionally how these are integrated with any intervention components, such as self-guided therapy.) This specification is then hosted alongside others in a secure online repository. When each study commences, the specification is automatically downloaded (2) to users' devices by a digital phenotyping app. This app can be a multi-study coordination tool that acts to coordinate data collection, a bespoke, study-specific data collection app, or a hybrid data collection intervention. Collected (3) self-report (e.g., questionnaires and momentary assessments) and (4) digital data (e.g., sensor measurements and device interaction data) is uploaded automatically to a secure online registry. Platform modules automatically manage potential barriers to data collection, such as user battery life and limited connectivity, through smart scheduling and caching. Automated processing pipeline (5) normalizes and converts raw data into standardized intermediate features and labeled outputs using machine learning. Researchers can start to extract registry data (6) as soon as it is received, accelerating analysis, permitting study designs that involve expert feedback, and allowing any data collection issues to be identified and addressed early in the research process. Rights management enables future researchers to request from users' access to previously collected data. (From Huckvale et al. [98]; Creative Commons CC-BY)

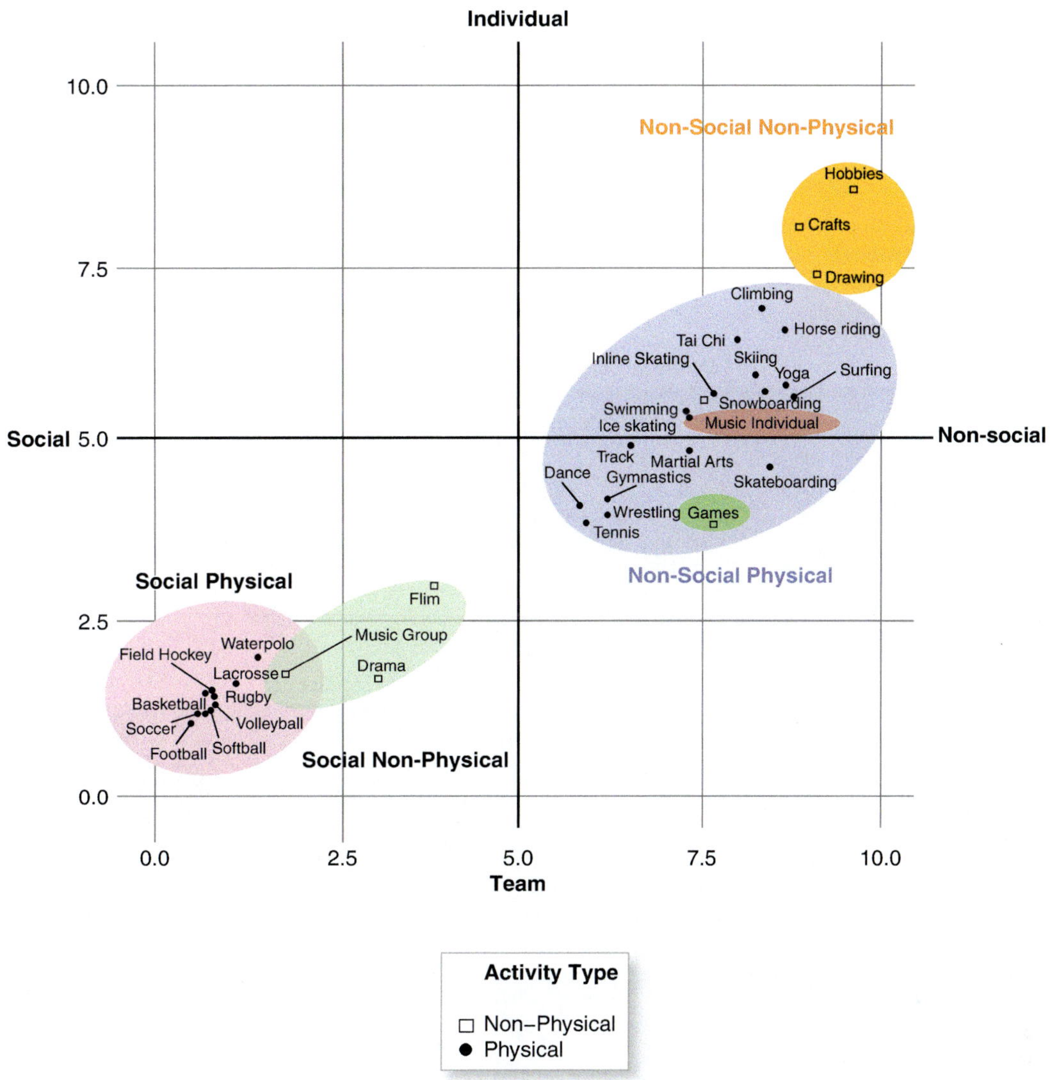

Fig. 25.76 MTurk youth activities categorization in depression research. This study was conducted using 500,500 observations collected from MTurk participants. Quadrant plot of MTurk Youth Activities Survey showing results of k-means clustering of Sports Activities Involvement Questionnaire (SAIQ) activities. Social–non-social and team–individual dimensions are visualized across the x- and y-axes, respectively, and the physical–non-physical dimension is visualized with shading and bullet shape. (From Conley et al. [100]; Creative Commons CC-BY)

The Future of Important Additional Roles of Psychiatry

Role of Psychiatry in Society Wellness and Happiness

Psychiatry has a role to play in promoting wellness and even happiness in society in the future.

The Neuroscience of Happiness

The brain's default network and eudaimonic-hedonic interactions are described in Fig. 25.77 [101].

The graph below focuses on the three primary factors that influence happiness. Lyubomirsky et al. postulated that 50% of the variance in well-being could be explained by genetic factors, 10% by life circumstances, and up to 40% by intentional activities (see Fig. 25.78) [102]. Psychiatry could play

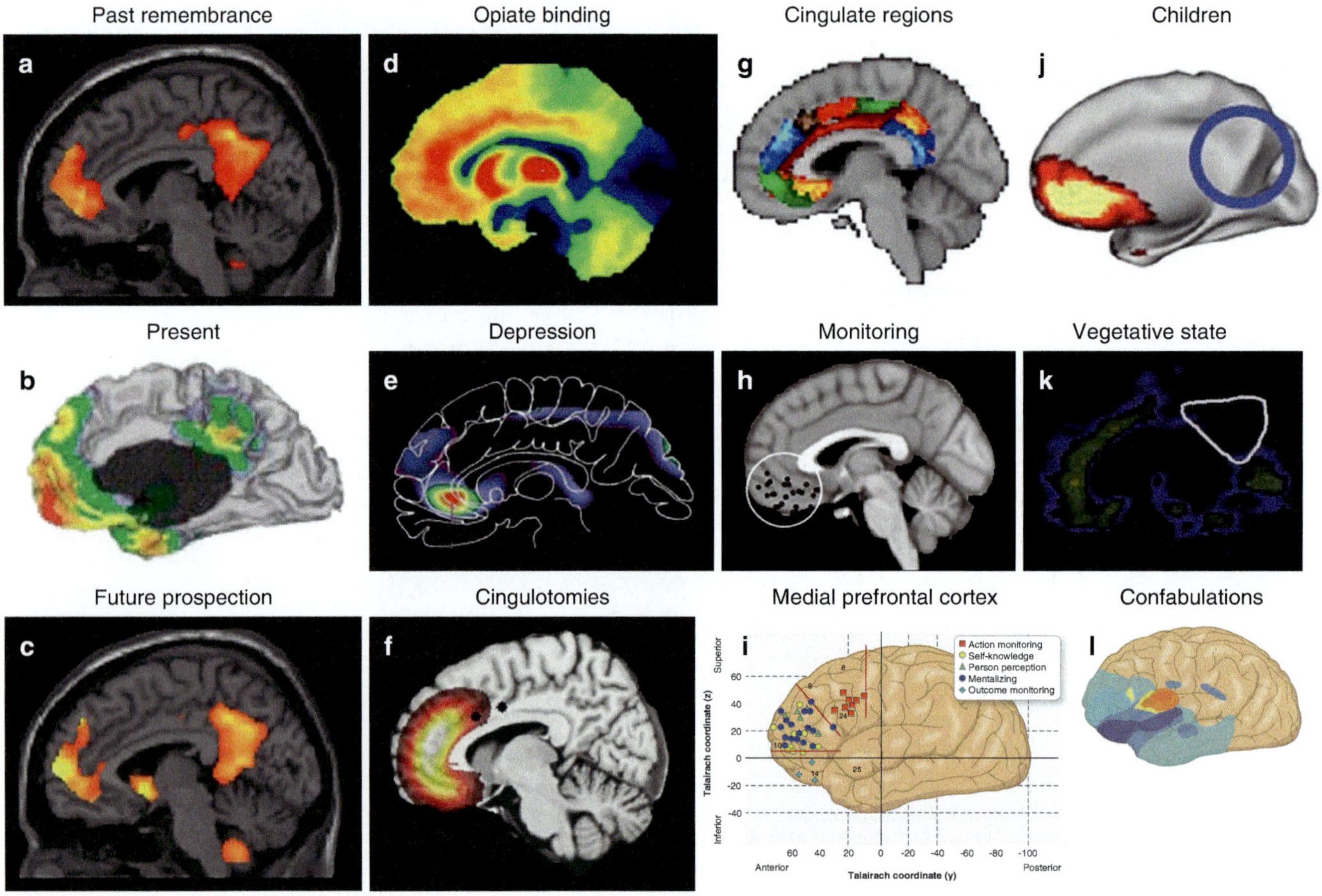

Fig. 25.77 The brain's default network and eudaimonic—hedonic interaction. (**a–c**) The brain's default network has been linked to self-awareness, remembering the past and prospecting the future. Some components overlap with pleasure networks, including midline structures such as the orbitofrontal, medial prefrontal, and cingulate cortices. We wonder whether happiness might include a role for the default network, or for related neural circuits that contribute to computing relations between self and others, in evaluating eudaimonic meaning and interacting with hedonic circuits of positive affect. Examples show key regions of the default network such as (**d**) the anterior cingulate and orbitofrontal cortices that have a high density of opiate receptors, (**e**) have been linked to depression, and (**f**) its surgical treatment, (**g**) have been implicated by connectivity analyses, (**h**) and are implicated in pleasure-related cognitive functions such as monitoring, learning and memory, (**i**) or in self-knowledge, person perception and other cognitive functions. (**j**) The default network may change over early life in infants and children, (**k**) in pathological states including depression and vegetative states, (**l**) and after cortical lesions that disrupt reality monitoring and create spontaneous confabulations. (From Berridge and Kringelbach [101]; Creative Commons CC-BY)

an important role in promoting these 40% volitional activities that could boost happiness, such as expressing gratitude, cultivating optimism, practicing acts of kindness to others, nurturing relationships, and promoting growth and purpose [103].

Future directions in the prevention and treatment of psychiatric disorders will incorporate all of the interventions described below, in terms of personalized activities that generate positive emotions, thoughts, and behaviors, which could contribute to the 40% intentional activity to boost happiness (see Fig. 25.79) [102].

Transdisciplinary approaches along with psychiatry could influence four domains of active living: recreation, transport, occupation, and household as seen below (see Fig. 25.80) [104].

The Role of Psychiatry in Promoting Wellness in the workplace

Workplaces and companies that utilize *ESG Principles* are gaining more traction in recent years. *ESG* stands for "Environmental, Social, and Governance." Such metrics judge how a company treats the natural environment, the general population, and its employees, respectively. JP Morgan's Asset Management division detailed in a recent report showcased the significance of investing in high ESG score companies, which have seen increased investment returns [105].

Burnout, satisfaction, and wellness are interrelated. A conceptual graph of their relationship between them is depicted below (see Fig. 25.81) [106].

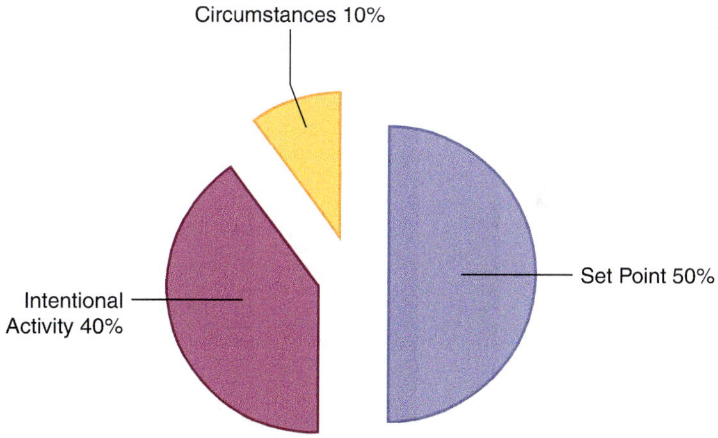

Fig. 25.78 The "happiness pie." (From Brown and Rohrer [103]; Creative Commons CC-BY)

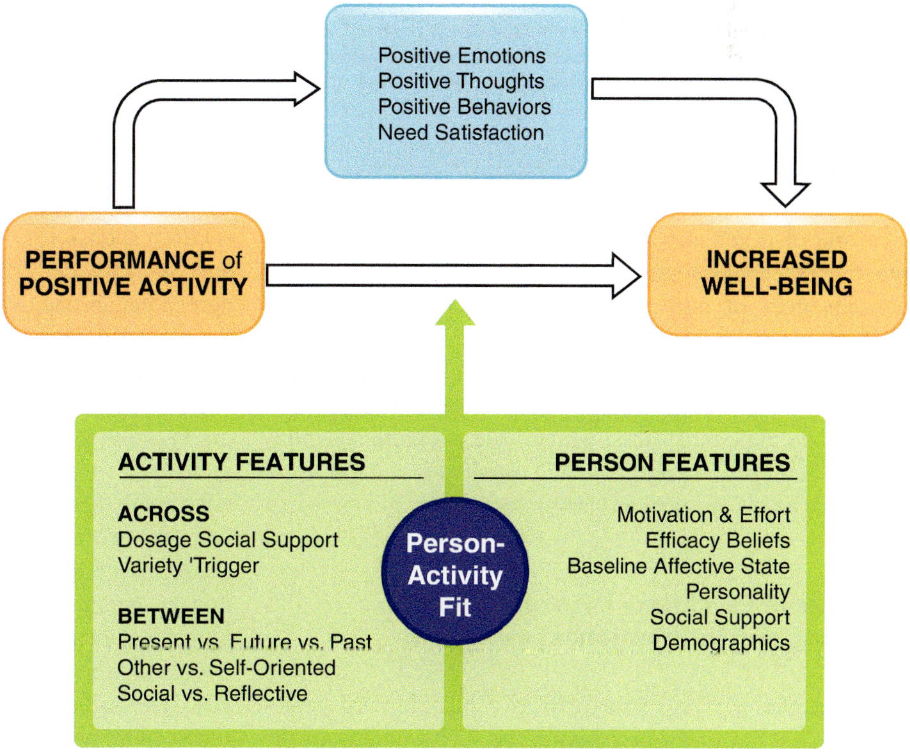

Fig. 25.79 The positive-activity model, which aims to explain how and why performing positive activities makes people happier. As illustrated at top, positive activities increase positive emotions, positive thoughts, positive behaviors, and need satisfaction, all of which in turn enhance well-being. Features of positive activities (e.g., dosage and variety) and of the person (e.g., motivation and effort) influence the degree to which the activities improve well-being. An optimal person-activity fit (i.e., the overlap between activity and person features) further predicts increases in well-being

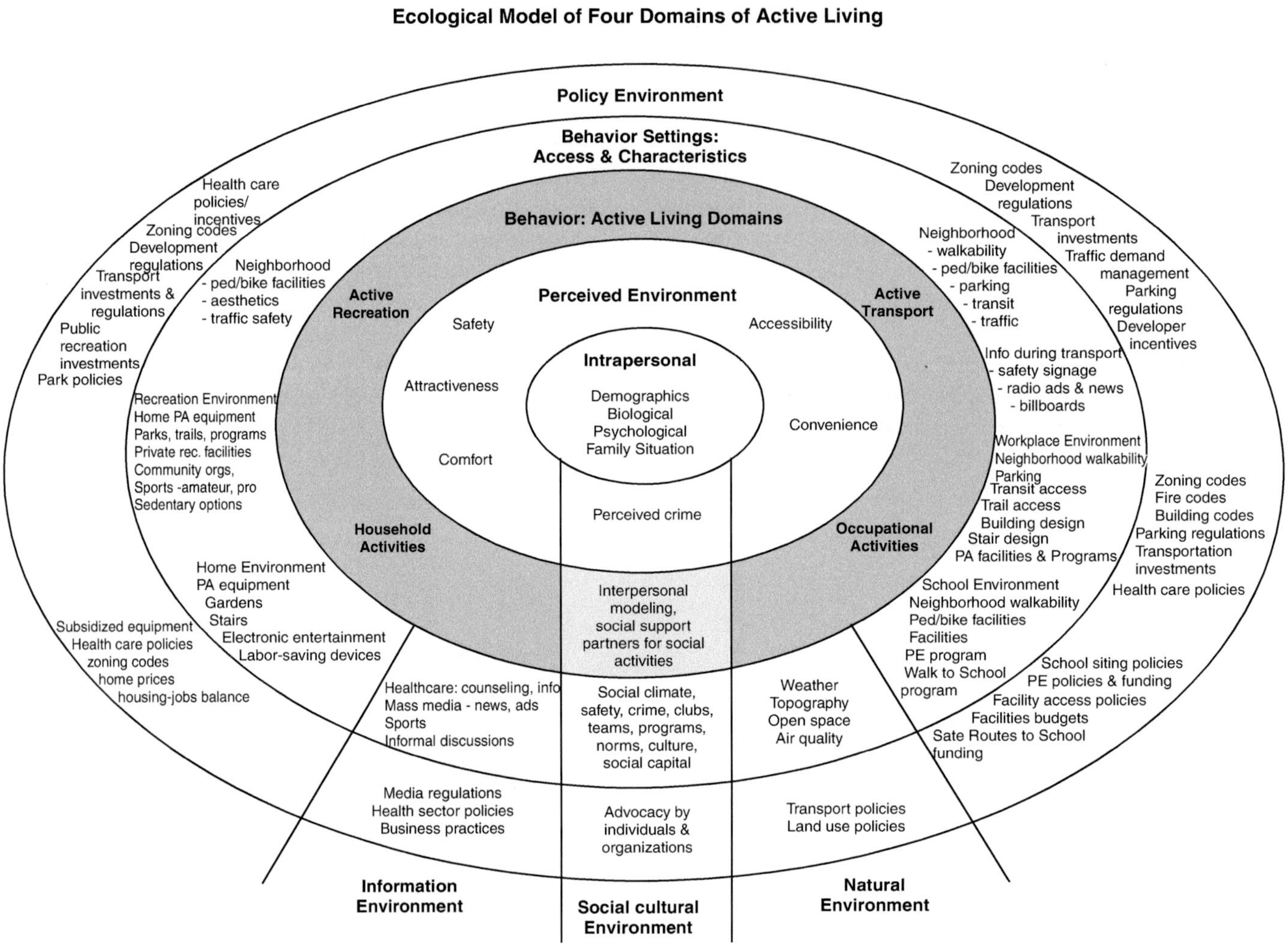

Fig. 25.80 Ecological model of four domains of active living with multiple levels of influences specific to each domain. A multilevel model was developed to illustrate the roles numerous disciplines can play in research on active living. This is an ecological model built around four domains of active living

The Role of Psychiatry in Physician Wellness

The role of psychiatry in the well-being of physicians and other healthcare professional cannot be understated given the consequences of burnout highlighted below (Fig. 25.82) [107].

In the future, psychiatry needs to play a leadership role in advocating and addressing the individual, work unit, organization, and national factors, which have a significant influence on burnout and engagement in physicians as depicted in the figure below (Fig. 25.83) [108].

The Role of Psychiatry in Local, Regional, National, and International Leadership

After the end of World War II, Brock Chisholm, a psychiatrist and first Executive Secretary of the WHO, addressed the American Psychiatric Association meeting in May 1947, stating that the future of psychiatry "lies in two directions-social responsibility at home through all possible channels and world-wide collaboration, compromise, and public agreement abroad. All the other psychiatric activities, care of the mentally ill, psychotherapy, psychiatric research, and so on should be merely the laboratories where the pathology and etiology of intra- inter-human relations are studied, in the interests of prevention of personal and social maladjustment, and in the hope of racial survival" [109]. Chisholm advocated that psychiatrists and psychologists should get involved in leadership both at home and abroad and viewed clinical work to be complementary to the mission of prevention of personal and social maladjustment. Leadership at home includes membership of governing or policy-making bodies in schools, places of worship, workplaces, city councils, state legislature, and federal houses. Leadership abroad included involvement in national and international organiza-

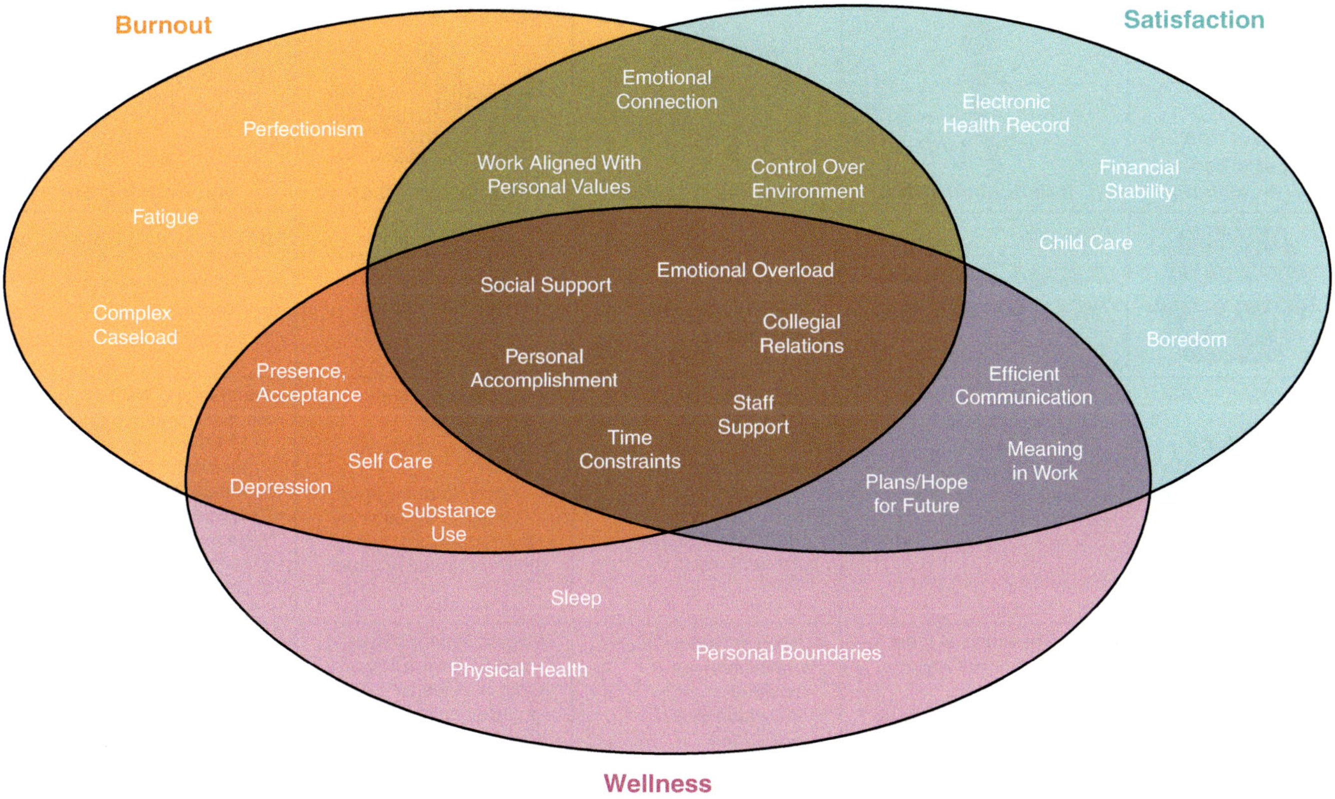

Fig. 25.81 Conceptual illustration of burnout, satisfaction, and wellness. These constructs share many common elements, but each also has unique aspects. For example, wellness includes an emphasis on physical health, whereas satisfaction includes more concepts related to practice logistics. All three constructs influence each other and are substantially correlated. (From Stan et al. [106]; Creative Commons CC-BY)

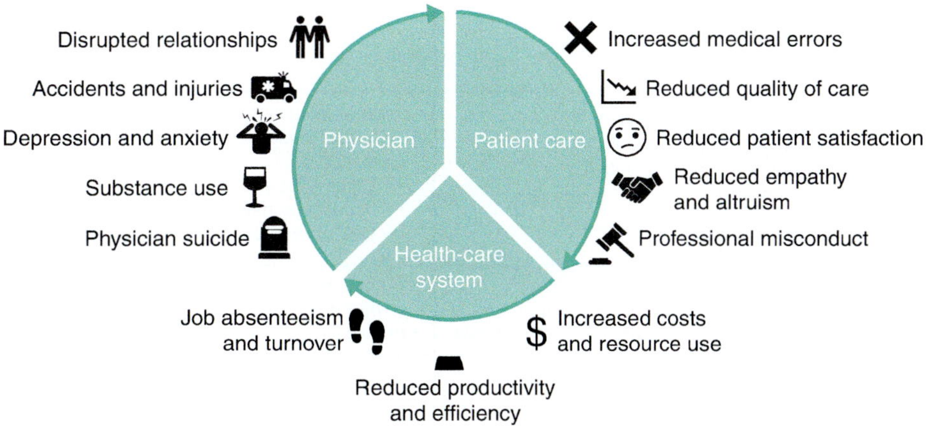

Fig. 25.82 Consequences of physician burnout

tions. As the WHO defined health in 1947 as "a state of complete physical, mental, and social well-being and not merely the absence of disease or infirmity," it became clearer that psychiatry has an important role in local, regional, national, and international leadership. Advanced leadership research over the years including the most recent work by Haslam et al. in 2021 (using COVID-19 pandemic management as an example) showed that effective leadership is grounded in the leader's "ability to represent and advance the shared interests of group members and to create and embed a sense of shared social identity among them (a sense of 'us-ness')" as depicted in Fig. 25.84 [110, 111].

Drivers of burnout and engagement in physicians	Individual factors	Work unit factors	Organization factors	National factors
Workload and job demands	• Specialty • Practice location • Decision to increase work to increase income	• Productivity expectations • Team structure • Efficiency • Use of allied health professionals	• Productivity targets • Method of compensation - Salary - Productivity based • Payer mix	• Structure reimbursement - Medicare/Medicaid - Bundled payments - Documentation requirements
Efficiency and resources	• Experience • Ability to prioritize • Personal efficiency • Organizational skills • willingness to delegate • Ability to say "no"	• Availability of support staff and their experience • Patient check-in efficiency/process • Use of scribes • Team huddles • Use of allied health professionals	• Integration of care • Use of patient • Institutional efficiency: - EHR - Appointment system - Ordering systems • How regulations interpreted and applied	• Integration of care • Requirements for: - Electronic prescribing - Medication reconciliation - Meaningful use of EHR • Certification agency facility regulations (JCAHO) • Precertifications for tests/treatment
Meaning in work	• Self-awareness of most personally meaningful aspect of work • Ability to shape career to focus on interests • Doctor–patient relationships • Personal recognition of positive events at work	• Match of work to talents and interests of individuals • Opportunities for involvement - Education - Research - Leadership	• Organizational culture • Practice environment • Opportunities for professional development	• Evolving supervisory role of physicians (potentially less direct patient contact) • Reduced funding - Research - Education • Regulations that increase clerical work
Culture and values	• Personal values • Professional values • Level of altruism • Moral compass/ethics • Commitment to organization	• Behavior of work unit leader • Work unit norms and expectations • Equity/faimess	• Organization's mission - Service/quality vs profit • Organization's values • Behavior of senior leaders • Communication/ messaging • Organizational norms and expectations • Just culture	• System of coverage for uninsured • Structure reimbursement - What is rewarded • Regulations
Control and flexibility	• Personality • Assertiveness • Intentionality	• Degree of flexibility: - Control of physician calendars - Clinic start/end times - Vacation scheduling - Call schedule	• Scheduling system • Policies • Affiliations that restrict referrals • Rigid application practice guidelines	• Precertifications for tests/ treatments • Insurance networks that restrict referrals • Practice guidelines
Social support and community at work	• Personality trails • Length of service • Relationship-building Skills	• Collegiality in practice environment • Physical configuration of work unit space • Social gatherings to promote community • Team structure	• Collegiality across the organization • Physician lounge • Strategies to build community • Social gatherings	• Support and community created by Medical/specialty societies
Work-life integration	• Priorities and values • Personal characteristics - Spouse/partner - Children/dependents - Health issues	• Call schedule • Structure night/weekend coverage • Cross-coverage for time away • Expectations/role models	• Vacation policies • Sick/medical leave • Policies - Part-time work - Flexible scheduling • Expectations/role models	• Requirements for - Maintenance certification - Licensing • Regulations that increase clerical work

Fig. 25.83 Drivers of burnout and engagement with examples of individual, work unit, organization, and national factors that influence each driver. *EHR* electronic health record; *JCAHO* Joint Commission on the Accreditation of Healthcare Organizations. (From Shanafelt and Noseworthy [108]; with permission)

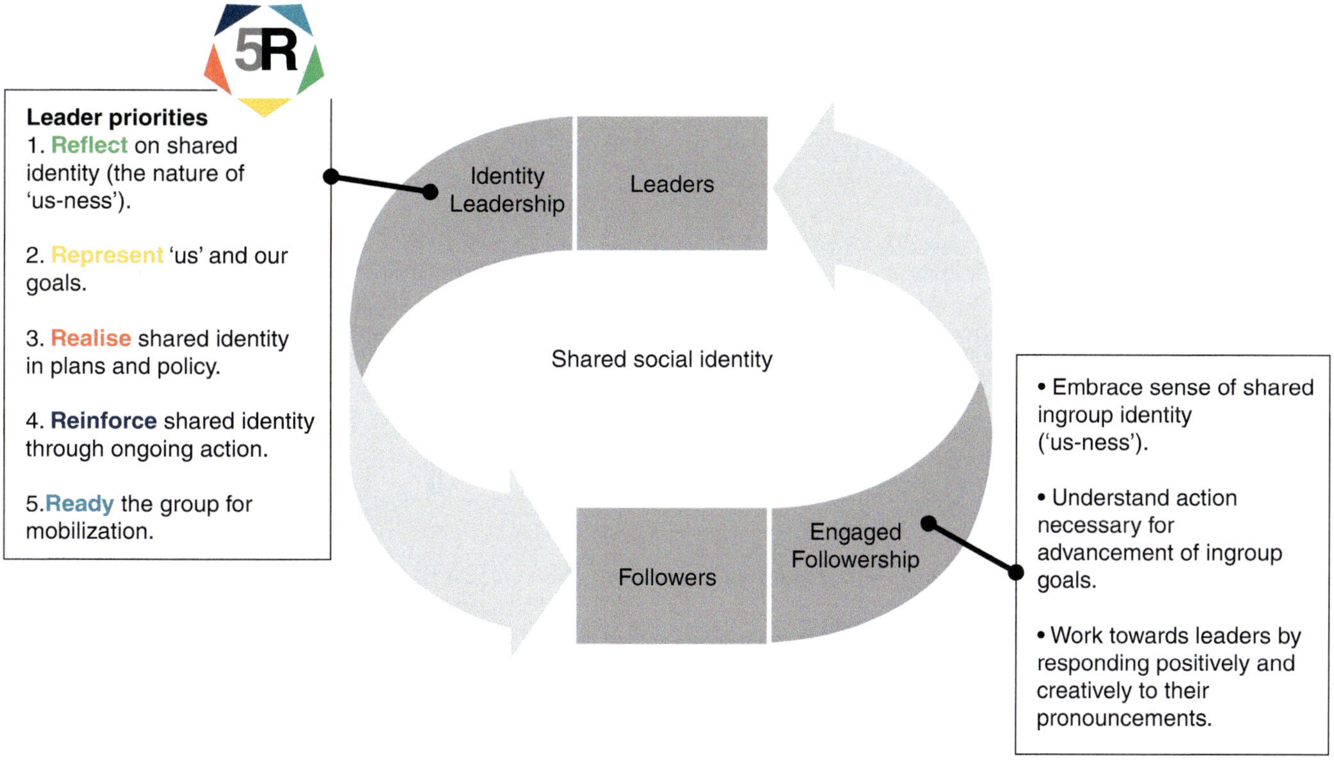

Fig. 25.84 Shared social identity as a focus for priorities of identity leadership (the 5Rs) and a platform for engaged followership. (From Haslam et al. [110]; with permission)

Conclusion

Psychiatry is a major contributor to mental health; yet the future will place it as a major contributor to mental wealth. The Foresight Project on Mental Capital and Wellbeing (UK) introduced this concept in their report Mental Wealth of Nations back in 2008, and much of the descriptions still hold true to this day. Psychiatry is envisioned to contribute to mental wealth at every step as shown in Fig. 25.85 [112].

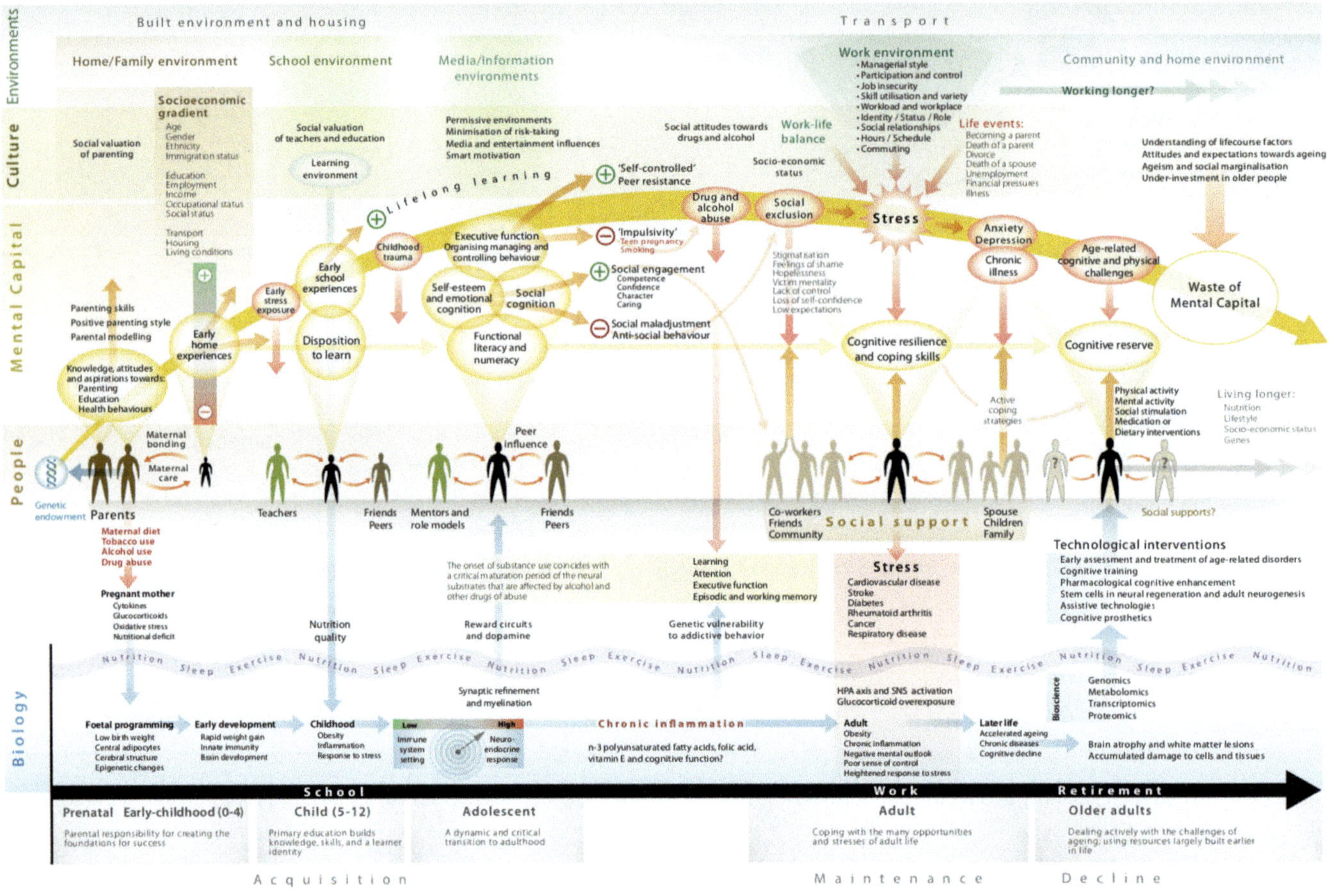

Fig. 25.85 How could psychiatry contribute to mental wealth. The Foresight Project on Mental Capital and Wellbeing (UK) states that: "Mental capital encompasses both cognitive and emotional resources. It includes people's cognitive ability; their flexibility and efficiency at learning; and their 'emotional intelligence', or social skills and resilience in the face of stress. The term therefore captures a key dimension of the elements that establish how well an individual is able to contribute to society and to experience a high quality of life. Mental wellbeing, on the other hand, is a dynamic state that refers to individuals' ability to develop their potential, work productively and creatively, build strong and positive relationships with others and contribute to their community." (From Beddington et al. [112]; with permission)

References

1. Bhugra D, Tasman A, Pathare S, Priebe S, Smith S, Torous J, et al. The WPA-Lancet Psychiatry Commission on the Future of Psychiatry. Lancet Psychiatry. 2017;4(10):775–818. https://doi.org/10.1016/S2215-0366(17)30333-4.
2. Swiaczny F. Demographic and health development in the long run. In: Glatzer W, Camfield L, Møller V, Rojas M, editors. Global handbook of quality of life. International handbooks of quality-of-life. Dordrecht: Springer; 2015. https://doi.org/10.1007/978-94-017-9178-6_2.
3. WHO. Improving health systems and services for mental health. WHO mental health policy and service guidance package. Geneva: World Health Organization; 2009. https://apps.who.int/iris/bitstream/handle/10665/44219/9789241598774_eng.pdf. Accessed 1 May 2021.
4. Ahrendt D, Dubois H, Mezger E. An overview of quality of life in Europe. In: Glatzer W, Camfield L, Møller V, Rojas M, editors. Global handbook of quality of life. International handbooks of quality-of-life. Dordrecht: Springer; 2015. https://doi.org/10.1007/978-94-017-9178-6_29.
5. United Nations. Convention on the Rights of Persons with Disabilities. https://www.ohchr.org/Documents/Issues/HRIndicators/MetadataRatificationStatus.pdf from Database of the United Nations Office of Legal Affairs (OLA) https://treaties.un.org. Accessed 1 May 2021.
6. HidalgoMazzei D, Murru A, Reinares M, Vieta E, Colom F. Big data in mental health: a challenging fragmented future. World Psychiatry. 2016;15:186–7.
7. Tolks D, Schäfer C, Raupach T, et al. An introduction to the inverted/flipped classroom model in education and advanced training in medicine and in the healthcare professions. GMS J Med Educ. 2016;33:Doc46.
8. Fountoulakis KN. Ethology, evolutionary psychology, sociobiology, and evolutionary psychiatry. In: Fountoulakis K, Nimatoudis I, editors. Psychobiology of behaviour. Cham: Springer; 2019. https://doi.org/10.1007/978-3-030-18323-3_12.
9. Lüscher Dias T, Schuch V, Beltrão-Braga PCB, et al. Drug repositioning for psychiatric and neurological disorders through a network medicine approach. Transl. Psychiatry. 2020;10:141. https://doi.org/10.1038/s41398-020-0827-5.
10. Hernandez LM, Kim M, Hoftman GD, Haney JR, de la Torre-Ubieta L, Pasaniuc B, Gandal MJ. Transcriptomic insight into the polygenic mechanisms underlying psychiatric disorders. Biol Psychiatry. 2021;89(1):54–64. https://doi.org/10.1016/j.biopsych.2020.06.005.

11. Courtet P, Gottesman I, Jollant F, et al. The neuroscience of suicidal behaviors: what can we expect from endophenotype strategies? Transl Psychiatry. 2011;1:e7. https://doi.org/10.1038/tp.2011.6.
12. Danese A, Lewis J, S. Psychoneuroimmunology of early-life stress: the hidden wounds of childhood trauma? Neuropsychopharmacology. 2017;42:99–114. https://doi.org/10.1038/npp.2016.198.
13. Kaur P, Sharma M. Diagnosis of human psychological disorders using supervised learning and nature-inspired computing techniques: a meta-analysis. J Med Syst. 2019;43:204. https://doi.org/10.1007/s10916-019-1341-2.
14. Brückl TM, Spoormaker VI, Sämann PG, et al. The biological classification of mental disorders (BeCOME) study: a protocol for an observational deep-phenotyping study for the identification of biological subtypes. BMC Psychiatry. 2020;20:213. https://doi.org/10.1186/s12888-020-02541-z.
15. Torrente-Rodríguez RM, Tu J, Yang Y, Min J, Wang M, Song Y, Yu Y, Xu C, Ye C, IsHak WW, Gao W. Investigation of cortisol dynamics in human sweat using a graphene-based wireless mHealth system. Matter. 2020;2(4):921–37. https://doi.org/10.1016/j.matt.2020.01.021.
16. Pratt JA, Morris B, Dawson N. Deconstructing schizophrenia: advances in preclinical models for biomarker identification. In: Pratt J, Hall J, editors. Biomarkers in psychiatry. Current topics in behavioral neurosciences, vol. 40. Cham: Springer; 2018. https://doi.org/10.1007/7854_2018_48.
17. Le-Niculescu H, Roseberry K, Gill SS, et al. Precision medicine for mood disorders: objective assessment, risk prediction, pharmacogenomics, and repurposed drugs. Mol Psychiatry. 2021. https://doi.org/10.1038/s41380-021-01061-w.
18. Herron JW, Nerurkar L, Cavanagh J. Neuroimmune biomarkers in mental illness. In: Pratt J, Hall J, editors. Biomarkers in psychiatry. Current topics in behavioral neurosciences, vol. 40. Cham: Springer; 2018. https://doi.org/10.1007/7854_2018_45.
19. Notter T. Immunological processes in schizophrenia pathology: potential biomarkers? In: Pratt J, Hall J, editors. Biomarkers in psychiatry. Current topics in behavioral neurosciences, vol. 40. Cham: Springer; 2018. https://doi.org/10.1007/7854_2018_43.
20. Kim S, Webster MJ. The Stanley Neuropathology Consortium Integrative Database (SNCID) for psychiatric disorders. Neurosci Bull. 2019;35:277–82. https://doi.org/10.1007/s12264-018-0314-7.
21. Downar J, Blumberger DM, Daskalakis ZJ. The neural crossroads of psychiatric illness: an emerging target for brain stimulation. Trends Cogn Sci. 2016;20(2):107–20. https://doi.org/10.1016/j.tics.2015.10.007.
22. Long M, Verbeke W, Ein-Dor T, Vrtička P. A functional neuro-anatomical model of human attachment (NAMA): insights from first- and second-person social neuroscience. Cortex. 2020;126:281–321. https://doi.org/10.1016/j.cortex.2020.01.010.
23. DeRubeis R, Siegle G, Hollon S. Cognitive therapy versus medication for depression: treatment outcomes and neural mechanisms. Nat Rev Neurosci. 2008;9:788–96. https://doi.org/10.1038/nrn2345.
24. Bolt T, Nomi JS, Arens R, et al. Ontological dimensions of cognitive-neural mappings. Neuroinformatics. 2020;18:451–63. https://doi.org/10.1007/s12021-020-09454-y.
25. National Research Council (US) Committee on A Framework for Developing a New Taxonomy of Disease. Toward precision medicine: building a knowledge network for biomedical research and a new taxonomy of disease. Washington, DC: National Academies Press (US); 2011. https://doi.org/10.17226/13284.
26. Fernandes BS, Williams LM, Steiner J, et al. The new field of 'precision psychiatry'. BMC Med. 2017;15:80. https://doi.org/10.1186/s12916-017-0849-x.
27. Disner S, Beevers C, Haigh E, et al. Neural mechanisms of the cognitive model of depression. Nat Rev Neurosci. 2011;12:467–77. https://doi.org/10.1038/nrn3027.
28. Brooks AT, Tuason RT, Chakravorty S, et al. Online cognitive behavioral therapy for insomnia (CBT-I) for the treatment of insomnia among individuals with alcohol use disorder: study protocol for a randomized controlled trial. Pilot Feasibility Stud. 2018;4:183. https://doi.org/10.1186/s40814-018-0376-3.
29. Zeise ML. Basics of neuropharmacology. In: Zeise ML, editor. Neuroscience for psychologists. Cham: Springer; 2021. https://doi.org/10.1007/978-3-030-47645-8_3.
30. Stahl SM. Stahl's essential psychopharmacology: neuroscientific basis and practical applications. Cambridge University Press. https://www.cambridge.org/us/academic/subjects/medicine/mental-health-psychiatry-and-clinical-psychology/stahls-essential-psychopharmacology-neuroscientific-basis-and-practical-applications-4th-edition?format=HB&isbn=9781107025981.
31. Siegel AN, Meshkat S, Benitah K, Lipsitz O, Gill H, Lui LMW, Teopiz KM, McIntyre RS, Rosenblat JD. Registered clinical studies investigating psychedelic drugs for psychiatric disorders. J Psychiatr Res. 2021;139:71–81. https://doi.org/10.1016/j.jpsychires.2021.05.019.
32. Vollenweider F, Kometer M. The neurobiology of psychedelic drugs: implications for the treatment of mood disorders. Nat Rev Neurosci. 2010;11:642–51. https://doi.org/10.1038/nrn2884.
33. Carhart-Harris RL, Roseman L, Bolstridge M, et al. Psilocybin for treatment-resistant depression: fMRI-measured brain mechanisms. Sci Rep. 2017;7:13187. https://doi.org/10.1038/s41598-017-13282-7.
34. Palhano-Fontes F, Barreto D, Onias H, et al. Rapid antidepressant effects of the psychedelic ayahuasca in treatment-resistant depression: a randomized placebo-controlled trial. Psychol Med. 2019;49(4):655–63. https://doi.org/10.1017/S0033291718001356.
35. Brito-da-Costa AM, Dias-da-Silva D, Gomes NGM, Dinis-Oliveira RJ, Madureira-Carvalho Á. Toxicokinetics and toxicodynamics of ayahuasca alkaloids N,N-dimethyltryptamine (DMT), harmine, harmaline and tetrahydroharmine: clinical and forensic impact. Pharmaceuticals. 2020;13(11):334. https://doi.org/10.3390/ph13110334.
36. Kramer J, Sagartz J, Morris D. The application of discovery toxicology and pathology towards the design of safer pharmaceutical lead candidates. Nat Rev Drug Discov. 2007;6:636–49. https://doi.org/10.1038/nrd2378.
37. Miller JJ. The psychiatric pipeline: 10 agents to watch. Psychiatric Times. 2021;38(1). https://www.psychiatrictimes.com/view/psychiatric-pipeline-10-agents-watch. Accessed 21 May 2021.
38. Wilkinson ST, Sanacora G. A new generation of antidepressants: an update on the pharmaceutical pipeline for novel and rapid-acting therapeutics in mood disorders based on glutamate/GABA neurotransmitter systems. Drug Discov Today. 2019;24(2):606–15. https://doi.org/10.1016/j.drudis.2018.11.007.
39. Mantas I, Saarinen M, Xu ZD, et al. Update on GPCR-based targets for the development of novel antidepressants. Mol Psychiatry. 2021. https://doi.org/10.1038/s41380-021-01040-1.
40. Zhang R, Li J, Zhang T, et al. Importance of integrating nanotechnology with pharmacology and physiology for innovative drug delivery and therapy—an illustration with firsthand examples. Acta Pharmacol Sin. 2018;39:825–44. https://doi.org/10.1038/aps.2018.33.

41. Zhu X, Huang W, Lu H, et al. A machine learning approach to personalized dose adjustment of lamotrigine using noninvasive clinical parameters. Sci Rep. 2021;11:5568. https://doi.org/10.1038/s41598-021-85157-x.
42. International Neuromodulation Society (INS). Neuromodulation defined. https://www.neuromodulation.com/about-neuromodulation. Accessed 1 May 2021.
43. Yildiz A, Ruiz P, Nemeroff CB. The Bipolar book. Oxford, UK: Oxford University Press; 2017. p. xxii-xxiii.
44. van Rooij SJH, Riva-Posse P, McDonald WM. The efficacy and safety of neuromodulation treatments in late-life depression. Curr Treat Options Psych. 2020;7:337–48. https://doi.org/10.1007/s40501-020-00216-w.
45. Grover S, Nguyen JA, Viswanathan V, Reinhart RMG. High-frequency neuromodulation improves obsessive-compulsive behavior. Nat Med. 2021;27(2):232–8. https://doi.org/10.1038/s41591-020-01173-w.
46. Scangos KW, Makhoul GS, Sugrue LP, Chang EF, Krystal AD. State-dependent responses to intracranial brain stimulation in a patient with depression. Nat Med. 2021;27(2):229–31. https://doi.org/10.1038/s41591-020-01175-8.
47. Figee M, Mayberg H. The future of personalized brain stimulation. Nat Med. 2021;27:196–7. https://doi.org/10.1038/s41591-021-01243-7.
48. Marx W, Lane M, Hockey M, et al. Diet and depression: exploring the biological mechanisms of action. Mol Psychiatry. 2021;26:134–50. https://doi.org/10.1038/s41380-020-00925-x.
49. Chen G, Manji HK. The extracellular signal-regulated kinase pathway: an emerging promising target for mood stabilizers. Curr Opin Psychiatry. 2006;19(3):313–23. https://doi.org/10.1097/01.yco.0000218604.63463.cd.
50. Schloesser R, Huang J, Klein P, et al. Cellular plasticity cascades in the pathophysiology and treatment of bipolar disorder. Neuropsychopharmacology. 2008;33:110–33. https://doi.org/10.1038/sj.npp.1301575.
51. Eriksson PS, Perfilieva E, Björk-Eriksson T, Alborn AM, Nordborg C, Peterson DA, Gage FH. Neurogenesis in the adult human hippocampus. Nat Med. 1998;4(11):1313–7.
52. Kucharska-Mazur J, Ratajczak MZ, Samochowiec J. Stem cells in psychiatry. In: Ratajczak M, editor. Stem cells. Advances in experimental medicine and biology, vol. 1201. Cham: Springer; 2019. https://doi.org/10.1007/978-3-030-31206-0_8.
53. Basiri A, Mansouri F, Azari A, et al. Stem cell therapy potency in personalizing severe COVID-19 treatment. Stem Cell Rev and Rep. 2021;17:193–213. https://doi.org/10.1007/s12015-020-10110-w.
54. Datta D, Subburaju S, Kaye S, et al. Human forebrain endothelial cell therapy for psychiatric disorders. Mol Psychiatry. 2020. https://doi.org/10.1038/s41380-020-0839-9.
55. Sharma A, Sances S, Workman MJ, Svendsen CN. Multi-lineage human iPSC-derived platforms for disease modeling and drug discovery. Cell Stem Cell. 2020;26(3):309–29. https://doi.org/10.1016/j.stem.2020.02.011.
56. Johnstone M, Hillary RF, St. Clair D. Stem cells to inform the neurobiology of mental illness. In: Pratt J, Hall J, editors. Biomarkers in psychiatry. Current topics in behavioral neurosciences, vol. 40. Cham: Springer; 2018. https://doi.org/10.1007/7854_2018_57.
57. McNeill RV, Ziegler GC, Radtke F, Nieberler M, Lesch KP, Kittel-Schneider S. Mental health dished up-the use of iPSC models in neuropsychiatric research. J Neural Transm (Vienna). 2020;127(11):1547–68. https://doi.org/10.1007/s00702-020-02197-9.
58. Bardy C, Greenberg Z, Perry SW, Licinio J. Personalized psychiatry with human iPSCs and neuronal reprogramming. In: Personalized psychiatry. Amsterdam, The Netherlands: Elsevier; 2020. p. 127–46. https://doi.org/10.1016/B978-0-12-813176-3.00012-2.
59. Avior Y, Ron S, Kroitorou D, et al. Depression patient-derived cortical neurons reveal potential biomarkers for antidepressant response. Transl Psychiatry. 2021;11:201. https://doi.org/10.1038/s41398-021-01319-5.
60. Oedegaard KJ, Alda M, Anand A, et al. The Pharmacogenomics of Bipolar Disorder study (PGBD): identification of genes for lithium response in a prospective sample. BMC Psychiatry. 2016;16:129. https://doi.org/10.1186/s12888-016-0732-x.
61. Conio B, Martino M, Magioncalda P, et al. Opposite effects of dopamine and serotonin on resting-state networks: review and implications for psychiatric disorders. Mol Psychiatry. 2020;25:82–93. https://doi.org/10.1038/s41380-019-0406-4.
62. Kose U, Deperlioglu O, Alzubi J, Patrut B. Future of medical decision support systems. In: Deep learning for medical decision support systems. Studies in computational intelligence, vol. 909. Singapore: Springer; 2021. https://doi.org/10.1007/978-981-15-6325-6_10.
63. Sharova AS, Melloni F, Lanzani G, Bettinger CJ, Caironi M. Edible electronics: the vision and the challenge. Adv Mater Technol. 2021;6(2):202000757. https://doi.org/10.1002/admt.202000757.
64. Carretero P, Campana-Montes JJ, Artes-Rodriguez A. Ecological momentary assessment for monitoring risk of suicide behavior. In: Baca-Garcia E, editor. Behavioral neurobiology of suicide and self harm. Current topics in behavioral neurosciences, vol. 46. Cham: Springer; 2020. https://doi.org/10.1007/7854_2020_170.
65. Dunster GP, Swendsen J, Merikangas KR. Real-time mobile monitoring of bipolar disorder: a review of evidence and future directions. Neuropsychopharmacology. 2021;46:197–208. https://doi.org/10.1038/s41386-020-00830-5.
66. Ebenfeld L, Kleine Stegemann S, Lehr D, Ebert DD, Jazaieri H, van Ballegooijen W, et al. Efficacy of a hybrid online training for panic symptoms and agoraphobia: study protocol for a randomized controlled trial. Trials. 2014;15(1):1–10.
67. Roepke AM, Jaffee SR, Riffle OM, et al. Randomized controlled trial of SuperBetter, a smartphone-based/internet-based self-help tool to reduce depressive symptoms. Games Health J. 2015;4:235–46.
68. Sinha N. Introducing gamification for advancing current mental healthcare and treatment practices. In: Marques G, Bhoi AK, Albuquerque VHC, K.S. H., editors. IoT in healthcare and ambient assisted living. Studies in computational intelligence, vol. 933. Singapore: Springer; 2021. https://doi.org/10.1007/978-981-15-9897-5_11.
69. MacDonald RA, Wilson GB. Musical improvisation and health: a review. Psych Well-Being. 2014;4:20. https://doi.org/10.1186/s13612-014-0020-9.
70. Neumaier F, Paterno M, Alpdogan S, Tevoufouet EE, Schneider T, Hescheler J, Albanna W. Surgical approaches in psychiatry: a survey of the world literature on psychosurgery. World Neurosurg. 2017;97:603–634.e8. https://doi.org/10.1016/j.wneu.2016.10.008.
71. Nijensohn DE, Dagi TF. Neurosurgical intervention for treatment-resistant psychiatric disorders. In: Kim YK, editor. Treatment resistance in psychiatry. Singapore: Springer; 2019. https://doi.org/10.1007/978-981-10-4358-1_25.
72. Tyson P, PBS. The Future of Brain Transplants. https://www.pbs.org/wgbh/nova/article/brain-transplants/. Accessed 1 May 2021.
73. Canavero S. Head transplantation: the future is now, TEDx Talk. https://www.technologynetworks.com/neuroscience/videos/head-transplantation-the-future-is-now-tedx-talk-by-drsergio-canavero-295184. Accessed 1 May 2021.
74. Hagmann P, Cammoun L, Gigandet X, Meuli R, Honey CJ, Wedeen VJ, Sporns O. Mapping the structural core of human cerebral cortex. PLoS Biol. 2008;6(7):e159. https://doi.org/10.1371/journal.pbio.0060159.

75. Travis J. Illness-Wellness Continuum. https://en.wikipedia.org/wiki/John_Travis_(physician)#/media/File:Illness-Wellness_Continuum.jpg. Accessed 21 May 2021.
76. IsHak WW. The handbook of wellness medicine. Cambridge, UK: Cambridge University Press; 2020.
77. Rashid B, Calhoun V. Towards a brain-based predictome of mental illness. Hum Brain Mapp. 2020;41(12):3468–535. https://doi.org/10.1002/hbm.25013.
78. Colizzi M, Lasalvia A, Ruggeri M. Prevention and early intervention in youth mental health: is it time for a multidisciplinary and trans-diagnostic model for care? Int J Ment Health Syst. 2020;14:23. https://doi.org/10.1186/s13033-020-00356-9.
79. Hector J, Khey D. Treatment: intersection with criminal justice. In: Criminal justice and mental health. Cham: Springer; 2018. https://doi.org/10.1007/978-3-319-76442-9_4.
80. Hung P, Busch S, Shih YW, et al. Changes in community mental health services availability and suicide mortality in the US: a retrospective study. BMC Psychiatry. 2020;20:188. https://doi.org/10.1186/s12888-020-02607-y.
81. Allison S, Bastiampillai T, Licinio J, et al. When should governments increase the supply of psychiatric beds? Mol Psychiatry. 2018;23:796–800. https://doi.org/10.1038/mp.2017.139.
82. American College of Emergency Physicians. Practical solutions to boarding of psychiatric Patients in the emergency department. https://https://www.macep.org/Files/Behavioral%20Health%20Boarding/Practical%20Solutions%20to%20Boarding%20of%20Psych%20Patients%20in%20EDs.pdf. Accessed 2 Dec 2022.
83. Castillo EG, Ijadi-Maghsoodi R, Shadravan S, et al. Community interventions to promote mental health and social equity. Curr Psychiatry Rep. 2019;21:35. https://doi.org/10.1007/s11920-019-1017-0.
84. Shah RN, Berry OO. The rise of venture capital investing in mental health. JAMA Psychiatry. 2020. https://doi.org/10.1001/jamapsychiatry.2020.2847.
85. Thorne J, Pitchbook. Driven by pandemic demand, mental health startups surpass 2019 funding. 2020. https://pitchbook.com/news/articles/mental-health-startups-venture-capital-outpace-2019. Accessed 1 May 2021.
86. Burrough C, Business Insider. Mental health startups have raised a record $1.9 billion in 2021 as COVID-19 pushes VC investors further into the space. 2021. https://www.businessinsider.com/mental-health-startups-hit-quarterly-funding-records-amid-vc-interest-2021-5. Accessed 21 May 2021.
87. Google. Search for "venture capital" and "mental health". https://www.google.com/search?q=venture+capital+mental+health&client=safari&hl=en&source=lnms&tbm=isch&sa=X&ved=2ahUKEwj48ZKn_eLwAhXOJzQIHa7tC7sQ_AUoAnoECAEQBA&biw=1440&bih=789. Accessed 21 May 2021.
88. Angelist. https://angel.co/mental-health-3. Accessed 21 May 2021.
89. Ritterband LM, Thorndike FP, Ingersoll KS, et al. Effect of a web-based cognitive behavior therapy for insomnia intervention with 1-year follow-up: a randomized clinical trial. JAMA Psychiat. 2017;74(1):68–75.
90. Everitt HA, Landau S, O'Reilly G, Sibelli A, Hughes S, Windgassen S, Holland R, Little P, McCrone P, Bishop FL, Goldsmith K, Coleman N, Logan R, Chalder T, Moss-Morris R. Cognitive behavioural therapy for irritable bowel syndrome: 24-month follow-up of participants in the ACTIB randomised trial. Lancet Gastroenterol Hepatol. 2019;4(11):863–72. https://doi.org/10.1016/S2468-1253(19)30243-2.
91. Sadock BJ, Ahmad S, Sadock VA. Kaplan & Sadock Pocket handbook of clinical psychiatry. London, UK: Wolters-Kuwer; 2018. https://shop.lww.com/Kaplan---Sadock-s-Pocket-Handbook-of-Clinical-Psychiatry/p/9781496386939.
92. Colman S, Wong L, Wong AHC, et al. Curriculum mapping: an innovative approach to mapping the didactic lecture series at the University of Toronto Postgraduate Psychiatry. Acad Psychiatry. 2020;44:335–9. https://doi.org/10.1007/s40596-020-01186-0.
93. Russ TC, Woelbert E, Davis KAS, Hafferty JD, Ibrahim Z, Inkster B, John A, Lee W, Maxwell M, McIntosh AM, Stewart R, MQ Data Science Group. How data science can advance mental health research. Nat Hum Behav. 2019;3(1):24–32. https://doi.org/10.1038/s41562-018-0470-9.
94. Harrison PJ, Geddes JR, Tunbridge EM. The emerging neurobiology of bipolar disorder. Trends Neurosci. 2018;41(1):18–30. https://doi.org/10.1016/j.tins.2017.10.006.
95. Chekroud AM, Zotti RJ, Shehzad Z, Gueorguieva R, Johnson MK, Trivedi MH, Cannon TD, Krystal JH, Corlett PR. Cross-trial prediction of treatment outcome in depression: a machine learning approach. Lancet Psychiatry. 2016;3(3):243–50. https://doi.org/10.1016/S2215-0366(15)00471-X.
96. Huys Q, Maia T, Frank M. Computational psychiatry as a bridge from neuroscience to clinical applications. Nat Neurosci. 2016;19:404–13. https://doi.org/10.1038/nn.4238.
97. Bzdok D, Meyer-Lindenberg A. Machine learning for precision psychiatry: opportunities and challenges. Biol Psychiatry Cogn Neurosci Neuroimaging. 2018;3(3):223–30. https://doi.org/10.1016/j.bpsc.2017.11.007.
98. Huckvale K, Venkatesh S, Christensen H. Toward clinical digital phenotyping: a timely opportunity to consider purpose, quality, and safety. NPJ Digit Med. 2019;2:88. https://doi.org/10.1038/s41746-019-0166-1.
99. Chandler J, Shapiro D. Conducting clinical research using crowdsourced convenience samples. Annu Rev Clin Psychol. 2016;12:53–81. https://doi.org/10.1146/annurev-clinpsy-021815-093623.
100. Conley MI, Hindley I, Baskin-Sommers A, et al. The importance of social factors in the association between physical activity and depression in children. Child Adolesc Psychiatry Ment Health. 2020;14:28. https://doi.org/10.1186/s13034-020-00335-5.
101. Berridge KC, Kringelbach ML. Building a neuroscience of pleasure and well-being. Psychol Well Being. 2011;1(1):1–3. https://doi.org/10.1186/2211-1522-1-3.
102. Lyubomirsky S, Layous K. How do simple positive activities increase well-being? Curr Dir Psychol Sci. 2013;22(1):57–62. https://doi.org/10.1177/0963721412469809.
103. Brown NJL, Rohrer JM. Easy as (happiness) pie? A critical evaluation of a popular model of the determinants of well-being. J Happiness Stud. 2020;21:1285–301. https://doi.org/10.1007/s10902-019-00128-4.
104. Sallis JF, Cervero RB, Ascher W, Henderson KA, Kraft MK, Kerr J. An ecological approach to creating active living communities. Annu Rev Public Health. 2006;27:297–322. https://doi.org/10.1146/annurev.publhealth.27.021405.102100.
105. Ward K, Wu J. How is ESG affecting the investment landscape? 2019. https://am.jpmorgan.com/no/en/asset-management/adv/insights/market-insights/on-the-minds-of-investors/how-esg-affects-investment-process/#. Accessed 1 May 2021.
106. Stan VA, Correa R, Deslauriers JR, et al. Support, technology and mental health: correlates of trainee workplace satisfaction. Perspect Med Educ. 2020;9:31–40. https://doi.org/10.1007/s40037-019-00555-2.
107. Riddell T, Hategan A. Physician Health and Wellness. McMaster Textbook of Internal Medicine. Kraków: Medycyna Praktyczna. https://empendium.com/mcmtextbook/chapter/B31.II.21.26. Accessed 24 Apr 2021.
108. Shanafelt TD, Noseworthy JH. Executive leadership and physician well-being: nine organizational strategies to promote engagement and reduce burnout. Mayo Clin Proc. 2017;92(1):129–46. https://doi.org/10.1016/j.mayocp.2016.10.004.

109. Chisholm B. The future of psychiatry. Am J Psychiatry. 1948;104(8):543–7. https://doi.org/10.1176/ajp.104.8.543.
110. Haslam SA, Reicher SD, Platow MJ. The new psychology of leadership: identity, influence, and power. 2nd ed. New York: Psychology Press; 2020.
111. Haslam SA, Steffens NK, Reicher SD, Bentley SV. Identity leadership in a crisis: a 5R framework for learning from responses to COVID-19. Soc Issues Policy Rev. 2021;15(1):35–83. https://doi.org/10.1111/sipr.12075.
112. Beddington J, Cooper C, Field J, et al. The mental wealth of nations. Nature. 2008;455:1057–60. https://doi.org/10.1038/4551057a.
113. Hensel JM, Ellard K, Koltek M, et al. Digital health solutions for indigenous mental well-being. Curr Psychiatry Rep. 2019;21:68. https://doi.org/10.1007/s11920-019-1056-6.

Index

W. W. IsHak (ed.), *Atlas of Psychiatry*, https://doi.org/10.1007/978-3-031-15401-0